FOCUS ON THE FAMILY RESOURCES

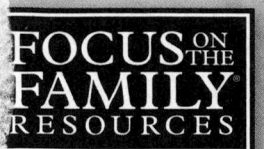

COMPLETE GUIDE TO

FAMILY HEALTH,

NUTRITION & FITNESS

PRIMARY AUTHOR PAUL C. REISSER, M.D.

THE OFFICIAL BOOK OF THE FOCUS ON THE FAMILY PHYSICIANS RESOU COUNCIL, U.S.A.

TYNDALE HOUSE PUBLISHERS, INC., CAROL STREAM, ILLINOIS

The information contained in this book provides a general overview of many health-related topics. It is not intended to substitute for advice that you might receive from your physician, whether by telephone or during a direct medical evaluation. Furthermore, health-care practices are continually updated as a result of medical research and advances in technology. You should therefore check with your doctor if there is any question about current recommendations for a specific problem. No book can substitute for a direct assessment by a qualified health-care professional.

Visit Tyndale's exciting Web site at www.tyndale.com

Complete Guide to Family Health, Nutrition, and Fitness

Designed by Dean H. Renninger and Zandrah Maguigad

Library of Congress Cataloging-in-Publication Data

Reisser, Paul C.
Complete guide to family health, nutrition, and fitness.
p. cm.
Includes bibliographical references and index.
ISBN-13: 978-0-8423-6181-1 (hc)
ISBN-10: 0-8423-6181-2 (hc)
1. Family—Health and hygiene. 2. Health. I. Title: Family health, nutrition, and fitness. II. Title.
RA777.7.R36 2006
613—dc22 2005028941

Printed in the United States of America

10 09 08 07 06
6 5 4 3 2 1

Table of Contents

Foreword by Dr. James Dobson

August 15, 1990, began much like any other day for me. I awoke early in the morning and headed to the gym for a game of basketball with a group of friends and colleagues—some of whom were as much as twenty or thirty years younger than I! Because I frequently hit the court with these "youngsters," and because I had reached middle age with the lanky build that allowed me to still move easily, I assumed that I was in the prime of physical health.

A sharp pain in my chest on that late summer morning told me otherwise. I excused myself from the game and drove alone to the hospital (something I do *not* recommend to anyone who suspects he or she is experiencing a serious medical problem!). Hoping and praying that I was merely battling fatigue, I knew deep down that there was something else terribly wrong. It didn't take the doctors long to confirm that, sure enough, this "healthy" basketball enthusiast had transformed, in the blink of an eye, into a heart attack victim.

As I lay in the hospital in the days following that ordeal, I realized that, early-morning basketball games notwithstanding, my predicament was directly related to my lifestyle choices and, in particular, the fatty foods I was allowing in my diet. I asked the Lord to give me another chance, resolving to use every resource at my disposal to safeguard my heart and my health through a combination of healthy diet and exercise. Despite some setbacks (I suffered a stroke in 1998 but recovered from it almost immediately), I have endeavored to keep that commitment, and today I am feeling better than ever.

Like so many Americans, prior to my heart attack, I was extremely busy—but not necessarily *active* in a way that would ensure optimal physical health. Indeed, statistics show that, despite our frantic pace of living and continued advances in the medical field, Americans suffer from an alarming number of health problems, many of which could be prevented or at least decreased by changing bad habits.

Research confirms just how serious the situation has become. The latest figures from the American Heart Association show that 13 million Americans have coronary heart disease; 5.4 million have suffered a stroke; and 65 million have been diagnosed with high blood pressure. Unfortunately, a large number of these cases are related, at least in part, to lifestyle choices. The AHA also reports that 48.5 million American adults (nearly 23 percent) are smokers. From 1995 to 1999, an average of 442,398 Americans died annually of smoking-related illnesses (32.2 percent of these deaths were cardiovascular related). The American Cancer Society estimates that 180,000 of the cancer deaths in 2004 could be attributed to smoking. Further, one-third of cancer deaths in 2004 were related to nutrition, physical inactivity, being overweight or obese, and other lifestyle issues. In other words, many of them were *preventable*!

As I suggested earlier, perhaps the biggest factors in maintaining proper physical health are diet and exercise. Unfortunately, a recent study revealed that a full 25 percent of Americans reported participating in *no* physical activity during their leisure time. Perhaps that is why more than 65 percent of adults in the United States are overweight, including 30 percent who are clinically obese. Between 1971 and 2000, the average daily caloric intake for men grew by about 7 percent, which translates into seventeen pounds of additional body fat per year. Obesity dramatically affects life span, as well. The life expectancy of a twenty-year-old white male who is clinically obese decreases by an estimated thirteen years, and for black males, an astonishing average of twenty years are lost due to obesity. One recent study revealed that the number of annual deaths attributable to obesity among adults in the United States is about 300,000. And perhaps most telling of all, airlines are telling us that they now have to carry additional fuel in order to transport more overweight customers.

This situation is sobering, but I am living proof that a dramatic change in eating habits, combined with a focused regimen of heart-strengthening exercise, can significantly improve one's overall health. I'll admit that the prospect of making such radical lifestyle changes can be daunting, but let me assure you that it is worth the investment. Choosing a healthy lifestyle *now*, while you still can, is infinitely preferable to being sidelined by a stroke, heart attack, cancer, or some other health crisis in the future.

This excellent resource is designed to answer many of the questions that may arise as you endeavor to put you and your loved ones on the road to a healthier life. You'll find detailed chapters on the three most common health problems—cardiovascular disease, cancer, and diabetes—as well as practical advice on those critical disciplines that I have mentioned several times already: *diet and exercise*.

And that's only the beginning. This guide has been designed to be a comprehensive reference for your entire family. It can help you find a pediatrician for your kids; identify medical tests that might prevent health problems before they occur; foster *emotional* and *spiritual* health in addition to physical fitness; discover answers to specific health-related questions for women and seniors; understand our country's often-confusing health-care system, and so much more. The information presented here is based on the most up-to-date medical research as well as the firsthand experiences of members of Focus on the Family's Physicians Resource Council. These experts will help you distinguish your triglycerides from your polyunsaturates and your cholesterol from your lipoproteins.

Perhaps you consider yourself generally healthy and are simply looking for a plan to help you stay that way. Or maybe you or someone you love is dangerously overweight or suffering from a serious health problem related to poor lifestyle choices in the past. Either way, the *Complete Guide to Family Health, Nutrition, and Fitness* will provide you with the tools you need—as a complement to the advice of your personal physician, of course—to live smarter and healthier. Change is never easy, but it *is* possible, and I pray that God will bless you as you endeavor to be a good steward of the body He has given you.

James C. Dobson, Ph.D.

Acknowledgments

This book is the product of four years of ongoing research, writing, review, discussion, revisions, and prayer, involving dozens of dedicated and talented individuals. Indeed, over such an extended time it literally developed a life of its own, and when its content was finally committed to print and paper, we experienced both relief (that it was finally done) and regret (that we couldn't add or update material, even as news continues to break in the world of health, fitness, and nutrition). We owe a debt of gratitude to many who contributed in various ways to this project, and we apologize for any oversights in this brief statement.

First of all, the following members of the Focus on the Family Physicians Resource Council served as primary reviewers for all or parts of this manuscript, and their input, suggestions, and insights have been of critical importance:

Byron Calhoun, M.D., F.A.C.O.G., F.A.C.S.
Maternal-Fetal Medicine—Rockford, Illinois

Douglas O. W. Eaton, M.D.
Internal Medicine—Loma Linda, California

Elaine Eng, M.D., F.A.P.A.
Psychiatry—Flushing, New York

J. Thomas Fitch, M.D., F.A.A.P.
Pediatrics—San Antonio, Texas

Donald Graber, M.D.
Psychiatry—Elkhart, Indiana

W. David Hager, M.D., F.A.C.O.G.
Gynecology—Lexington, Kentucky

Daniel R. Hinthorn, M.D., F.A.C.P.
Infectious Disease—Kansas City, Kansas

Gerard R. Hough, M.D., F.A.A.P.
Pediatrics—Brandon, Florida

Gaylen M. Kelton, M.D., F.A.A.F.P.
Family Medicine—Indianapolis, Indiana

John P. Livoni, M.D.
Radiology—Little Rock, Arkansas

Robert W. Mann, M.D., F.A.A.P.
Pediatrics—Mansfield, Texas

Marilyn A. Maxwell, M.D., F.A.A.P.
Internal Medicine/Pediatrics—St. Louis, Missouri

Paul Meier, M.D.
Psychiatry—Richardson, Texas

Gary Morsch, M.D., F.A.A.F.P.
Family Medicine—Olathe, Kansas

Mary Anne Nelson, M.D.
Family Medicine—Cedar Rapids, Iowa

Gregory Rutecki, M.D.
Internal Medicine—Columbus, Ohio

Roy C. Stringfellow, M.D., F.A.C.O.G.
Gynecology—Colorado Springs, Colorado

Margaret Cottle, M.D.
Palliative Care—Vancouver, British Columbia

Peter Nieman, M.D., F.A.A.P.
Pediatrics—Calgary, Alberta

We greatly appreciate the careful review and editing by Lisa Jackson, Kim Miller, and their team at Tyndale. Their diligence in double-checking and updating facts has served as a vital safety net for the contents of this book.

Finally, we cannot overlook the importance of supportive family and friends in a project of this magnitude.

From Paul C. Reisser, M.D.—I would like to offer special thanks to:

- My long-suffering co-laborers at Conejo Oaks Medical Group who have been hearing me talk about "the book" for four years and have provided extended practical support and encouragement. In particular I want to thank my teammate in medical school and family practice for more than thirty years, Frank Dawson, M.D., and my extraordinarily efficient and competent office nurse, Dorothy Dalenberg, R.N.
- Three good friends, prayer partners, and wise counselors (over countless Friday morning breakfasts and other occasions): Dan Collins, Dan Miller, and Dean Dods.
- My very patient and encouraging family—son, Chad, his wife, Erica, and their sweet daughter, Ella; daughter, Carrie; and most of all my wife and best friend of thirty years, Teri. Her wisdom and experience as a marriage and family therapist has impacted several chapters, especially those dealing with sexual, emotional, and spiritual health. Above all, however, for four years she served as a wellspring of encouragement and good cheer, and on a number of occasions provided well-timed exhortations when my energy was flagging. Without her I could not have stayed this course.

From David Davis—I extend heartfelt appreciation to:

- Linda Beck, Vicki Dihle, and Barbara Siebert at Focus on the Family, who have expertly assisted and supported Dr. Brad Beck and me as we labored on this book.
- My wonderful family. Thanks to my sons, Christopher and Matthew, and my daughter, Lauren, for their support and love. Special thanks to my wife, Kim, who has strengthened and encouraged me in ways she will never know and to whom I am most sweetly indebted.

From Brad Beck, M.D.:—I would like to offer my gratitude and thanks to:

- The best staff I have ever worked with here at Focus on the Family (as mentioned above, Barb, Linda, and Vicki) and Dave himself who has worked so diligently in the past few years on so much of this book. All of you do amazing work and I am privileged to get to work alongside each of you.
- My enduring and wonderful family, my daughter, Brianne, and son, Chris. I am so proud to be your dad. I am also grateful to my beautiful wife, Lisa, who has walked alongside me while I worked on this book, as well as supported me during so many "adventures" in our twenty years together. You are the best.

Editorial Staff

Paul C. Reisser, M.D., *Primary Author*
David Davis, *Managing Editor/Contributing Author*
Lisa Jackson, *Tyndale Editor*

Focus on the Family

Bradley G. Beck, M.D., *Medical Issues Advisor/Research Editor/Contributing Author*
Vicki Dihle, PA-C, *Medical Research Analyst/Contributing Author*
Barbara Siebert, *Manager, Medical Outreach*
Linda Beck, *Administrative Support*
Reginald Finger, M.D., *Medical Issues Analyst*
Kara Angelbeck, *Health and Wellness Coordinator*
Tom Neven, *Book Editor*

Tyndale House Publishers

Douglas R. Knox, *Publisher*

Richard L. Regenfuss, *Senior Director, Focus on the Family Alliance*
Pamela Cortez, *Product Development Manager*

Kimberly Miller, *Copy Editor*
Karin Buursma, *Editorial Support*
Elizabeth Gosnell, *Editorial Support*
Amanda Haring, *Editorial Support*
Kathy Olson, *Editorial Support*
Betty Free Swanberg, *Editorial Support*
Shawn Harrison, *Technical Support*
Anisa Baker, *Administrative Support*

Lisa Murphy, *Project Manager*
Dean Renninger, *Art Director*
Zandrah Maguigad, *Senior Designer*
Judy Stafford, *Typesetter*
Janine Bollhoefer, *Typesetter*
Mary Choate, *Print Buyer*

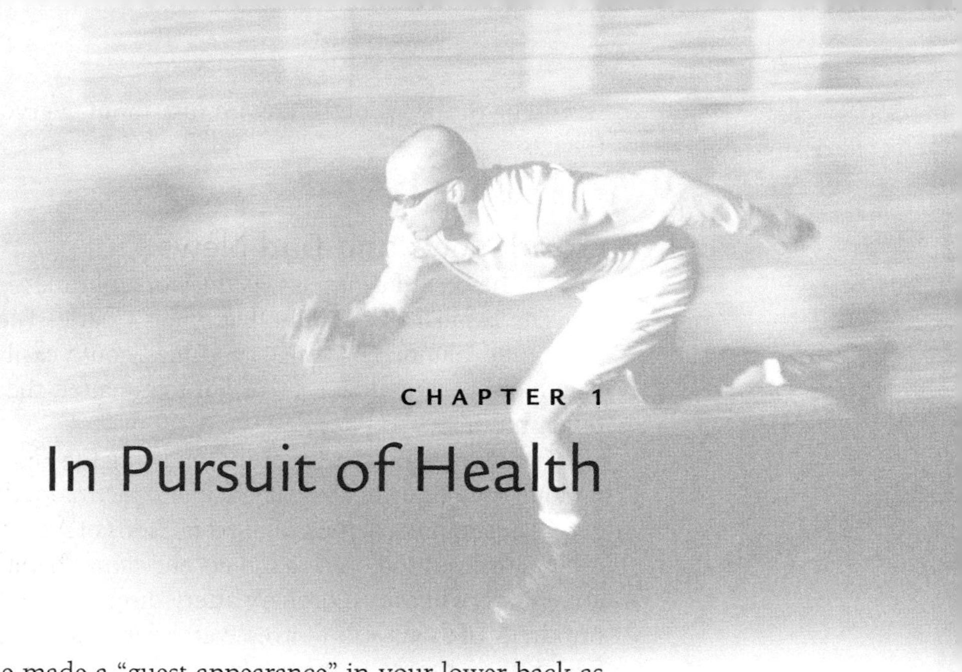

CHAPTER 1

In Pursuit of Health

Perhaps an unfamiliar ache made a "guest appearance" in your lower back as you got out of bed this morning . . .

. . . or your favorite belt just ran out of holes . . .

. . . or you heard about a new supplement that sounds as if it might replenish some of the energy you've been missing in your life lately . . .

. . . or you haven't had a checkup in several years, and you're a little concerned about what the doctor might find "under the hood" . . .

. . . or you *did* have that checkup and found out that your blood pressure, cholesterol, and blood sugar have risen to worrisome levels . . .

. . . or the kids just completed their health-ed class and are nagging you about having tobacco breath . . .

. . . or you just noticed that *they* have tobacco breath . . .

. . . or you're wondering whether any of the twenty-five surefire weight-loss plans on sale at your local bookstore might actually work for you . . .

. . . or a close friend your age (or younger) has been diagnosed with a serious medical problem . . .

. . . or you simply feel a conviction that it's time to start taking better care of yourself and your family.

Whatever the reason for your interest in improving your family's health or preventing problems in the future, you can be certain of one thing: You're not alone. Millions of people in the United States and around the world are pursuing better health—and spending billions of dollars every year doing so—through conventional or alternative health providers, in bookstores, on the Internet, in health-food stores, in gyms and spas, and even through personal trainers. Given the spectacular advances in medical science over the past several decades and the steady stream of health advisories we now receive on a daily basis, one might expect that good, or even great, health would be the order of the day for just about everyone. But, in fact, this is not the case.

Good News and Bad News

"It was the best of times, it was the worst of times."

The familiar declaration that opens Charles Dickens's classic novel of the French Revolution, *A Tale of Two Cities,* could easily be applied to the state of health of the United States—or, for that matter, the entire world—in the third millennium.

For more than a half century following the Second World War, developed nations have enjoyed a sustained abundance of food, both in quantity and variety, that is unprecedented. *And yet* millions of Americans, and millions more in other countries that have adopted our eating habits, are mired in diet-driven epidemics of obesity, coronary artery disease, and diabetes, all of which claim hundreds of thousands of lives every year. Tragically and ironically, more than 840 million people in the world, nearly 800 million of them from developing countries, are malnourished. Of these, more than 150 million are under the age of five, and 6 million of these children die every year from hunger.[1]

Many diseases and infections that terrified our ancestors just a few generations ago are no longer a concern for today's American doctors or their patients. Smallpox, which for centuries claimed millions of lives and even destroyed entire civilizations, was eradicated from our planet by the late 1970s. New cases of polio, a disease that can paralyze the limbs of great and small alike, have been drastically reduced through extensive worldwide vaccination efforts. *And yet* other ancient infectious foes—malaria, cholera, typhoid, to name a few—continue to make their deadly rounds throughout the world, claiming the lives of millions every year and making millions more who survive them miserable for a season or a lifetime. Even technologically advanced cultures are not immune to the threat of serious epidemics. In fact, in recent times many Western countries, especially the United States, have been confronted with the horrifying prospect that highly lethal organisms—anthrax, pneumonic plague, Ebola, and even smallpox—could be used as weapons by terrorists bent on causing death on a monumental scale.

Malaria alone causes 300 million acute illnesses and one million deaths every year. The World Health Organization estimates that a child in Africa dies of malaria *every thirty seconds*.[2]

Immunization campaigns in the United States have made once-familiar diseases such as measles, rubella (German measles), and mumps so uncommon that primary-care physicians rarely have to deal with them. Within one generation, the introduction of routine childhood vaccinations against the bacteria *Haemophilus influenzae* has made a serious dent in the number of cases of pneumonia and meningitis among American infants and toddlers. *And yet* every year tens of thousands of children in North America are not immunized because their families lack the health-care coverage or funds to obtain vaccinations, or because their parents are convinced that immunizations represent an unacceptable hazard. And millions of other children around the world are vulnerable to dangerous but preventable diseases primarily because they cannot get access to (let alone afford) the vaccines that would prevent them.

Modern biotechnology has created a host of antibiotics, which routinely vanquish infections that would have been lethal a few generations ago. *And yet* extensive and at times indiscriminate use of antibiotics by well-meaning physicians has led to the emergence of resistant strains of common bacteria (a few now sporting the nickname *superbugs*) that defy our medical armaments. And an alphabet soup of sexually transmitted infections and syndromes—HSV, HPV, PID, and the deadly HIV/AIDS, among others—continues to percolate through developed and developing nations alike, especially among the young.

F.Y.I.

HSV stands for herpes simplex virus, HPV for human papillomavirus, and PID for pelvic inflammatory disease. HIV stands for human immunodeficiency virus, the virus that causes AIDS (acquired immune deficiency syndrome). Some strains of HPV are implicated in nearly every case of cancer of the cervix (the opening of the uterus). HPV and cervical cancer are discussed in chapter 4 (see page 107).

In sub-Saharan Africa, AIDS has become a modern-day plague. The leading cause of death in that region, this illness is wreaking personal, social, and economic havoc and has left millions of children orphans.

America's health-care system is arguably the most sophisticated in the world, as anyone who has been treated in an emergency room or critical-care unit can testify. *And yet* health-care costs have soared over the past half century, now amounting to well over a trillion dollars every year.

F.Y.I.

Between 1960 and 2000, the United States' gross domestic product increased from approximately $526 billion to nearly $8 trillion, about fifteenfold. At the same time, health-care costs soared from $27 billion to $1.12 trillion—more than a fortyfold increase. (The percentage of GDP spent on health care increased from 5.1 percent to 14 percent over this period.)[3]

And partly as a reaction to skyrocketing costs, long waits, less-than-satisfactory interactions with harried practitioners, and a host of problems that conventional Western medicine has not been able to conquer, millions are turning to alternative therapies, some of which represent a radical departure from the most basic understandings of contemporary science.

A proliferation of books, magazines, videos, and Internet sites has given the average citizen unprecedented access to information about health and disease, wellness and illness, exercise and diet. *And yet* in many ways we seem to have an abundance of information and a shortage of discernment. Wheat mingles with chaff, fact and fancy compete for the limelight, and irrelevant details obscure what could be take-home lessons. So much of the current avalanche of facts and advice seems contradictory, especially in the realm of nutrition and weight loss. One day we hear that a particular food, drug, or supplement is the key to health or a research breakthrough. And then within a month comes the somber news that it may cause irreparable harm.

Americans and our counterparts in developed nations enjoy a standard of living unprecedented in human history. By all rights we should be the happiest, healthiest, and most productive people on earth. *And yet* depression, anxiety, addiction, violence, sexual anarchy, broken families, and boredom abound. Tobacco, alcohol, and drug abuse claim hundreds of thousands of lives and cost billions of dollars in health care, loss of productivity, injury, and crime each year. We spend billions more every year evaluating symptoms—chronic fatigue, headache, abdominal pains, sleeplessness, and a host of others—that all too often arise from our stressful and discontented lifestyles. Our forebears worried about storing enough provisions to survive the winter. Far too many of us store enough provision for ten winters in our own body fat. Our ancestors thanked God fervently for daily bread. We complain when the line is too long at a fast-food restaurant. Too many of us are doing better by almost any comparison with most of the world (and human history), yet feeling worse.

Our lives and times prove that health is much more than the absence of disease, as wonderful as that absence might be. They also demonstrate that the most sophisticated technical developments of modern civilization still cannot prevent a host of serious disorders that afflict millions every year. Nor can these advancements automatically cause us to behave in ways that would maintain our health at optimal levels.

That brings us to the first of several basic questions as we begin this book.

What Exactly Is Health?

We might be at a loss to find the exact words to define health, but most of us would probably be willing to say that we know it when we see it. On a more personal level, some of us would say that we know it when we feel it. Health encompasses a broad range of functions and experiences, and we cannot truly grasp what it means to be healthy without considering all of them.

Physical functions usually come to mind when the word *health* is mentioned. We typically think of **physical health** as a state in which "all (or most) systems are go," where a host of phenomenally complex organ systems function smoothly, if not at peak performance. These include:

The **nervous system:** the brain, spinal cord, sensory organs (for example, eyes and ears), and a network of nerves that send and receive information throughout the body. In a very real sense, all of the other systems exist to support this one, because through it we experience and express our very humanity—our thoughts and emotions, our prayers and our plans, and the actions that they generate.

The **circulatory system:** the heart and blood vessels, which deliver blood to every tissue and cell in the body. The Old Testament declared with complete accuracy that "the life of a creature is in the blood" (Leviticus 17:11). Blood carries oxygen, without which no tissue can survive. The brain is particularly dependent on a steady supply; only a few minutes of oxygen deprivation to any part of the brain can cause irreparable damage. If the entire brain loses its supply for more than three minutes, damage is likely; after eight minutes, coma and death are virtually inevitable.

The **respiratory system:** the lungs and airways that provide oxygen carried by red blood cells throughout the body. The respiratory system also removes carbon dioxide generated by the metabolism of our cells. A well-functioning heart pumping blood that lacks oxygen will be working in vain and will not pump for long.

The **gastrointestinal system:** the esophagus, stomach, and intestines that swallow, break down, and absorb the food we consume, as well as the liver that further processes materials sent to it from the intestine. This system supplies and refines the fuel used by the rest of the body.

The **renal/excretory system:** the kidneys that filter the blood and excrete waste products into the urine, which in turn is removed from the body. The kidneys are far more than generators of liquid waste. Their ability to regulate body-fluid levels, maintain blood pressure, and control the levels of a number of critical elements (called electrolytes) and several other chemical compounds is a marvel of engineering.

The **musculoskeletal system:** the bones, joints, muscles, tendons, and ligaments that allow us to express ourselves through physical action: standing, walking, reaching, and a host of other functions.

The **hemapoietic system:** the tissue (called marrow) safely hidden within bones throughout the body that continuously produces red blood cells (which carry oxygen, as previously noted), white blood cells (which serve a vital role in immunity), and platelets (which begin the clotting process whenever a blood vessel is damaged).

The **immune system:** a complex network of specialized cells and proteins (called antibodies) that defend us from bacteria, viruses, fungi, and other invaders.

The **endocrine system:** a diverse collection of organs and tissues that manufacture compounds (called hormones), which in turn regulate a vast number of bodily functions, including growth, metabolism, and reproduction.

The **reproductive system:** the structures, organs, and hormonal interactions that allow us to create new human beings and to enjoy pleasure, intimacy, and bonding with another.

In the best of all worlds, these systems would perform perfectly prior to birth, grow and develop without a hitch, and continue to work unhampered by disease, injury, or destructive habits throughout a lifetime extending to a ripe old age. Of course, we live in anything but the best of all worlds, and we would be hard-pressed to find anyone who, for eight or nine decades, has scaled such a pinnacle of physical perfection. Furthermore, as soon as we set forth a vision of what exceptional health might look like, we can begin to find any number of conspicuous exceptions.

For example, it is clearly possible for someone to live a productive, if not bountiful, life even though physically impaired in some significant way. Helen Keller lost her sight and hearing before the age of two but ultimately became a renowned and eloquent author and advocate for the blind. Joni Eareckson Tada suffered a devastating neck injury as a teenager, leaving her wheelchair-bound and dependent on others for the rest of her life. Yet she has flourished as an artist, speaker, musician, writer, and founder of a worldwide ministry serving the disabled. British theoretical physicist Stephen Hawking, author of the best-selling *A Brief History of Time,* has maintained a distinguished career despite being stricken with amyotrophic lateral sclerosis (or ALS, also known as Lou Gehrig's disease), which has severely impaired his ability to move and communicate.

We could use these and many other examples to illustrate another definition of health: making the most of the physical and intellectual resources available to us, regardless of how they have been shaped by our genetics, by events before and during our birth, by our upbringing, or by our experiences later in life. Just as a person with significant disabilities or other afflictions can still enjoy a fruitful life, it is also possible—indeed, all too common—for someone who is in good or even peak physical health to be sullen, lazy, hostile, or even dangerous to those around him. Clearly we cannot paint a picture of health using only the narrow brushstrokes of physical strength, attractiveness, a collection of normal organs, or an abundance of candles on a person's birthday cake. We need to consider other elements as well.

Emotional health, like physical health, may be easier to describe than to define precisely. We could propose a number of characteristics: stability and resilience; a positive but also realistic outlook on life; or a sense of humor, joy, contentment, and general calm in the face of difficulty, for example. Most of us could also suggest several indicators of problems with emotional health: persistent anxiety, depression, irritability, frequent outbursts of anger, overt hatred, pessimism, suspicion, and despair. Like physical health, our emotional well-being (or lack thereof) is a by-product of genetics, a certain degree of inborn temperament, childhood and adult experiences, personal habits, and everyday decisions.

Closely related to emotional health are a number of important arenas in life that we could evaluate for well-being or illness. We could speak, for example, of the health of one's relationships, including those with parents, friends, spouse, children, coworkers, and a community of faith. We could evaluate the quality of a person's work and career, not merely as a means of earning a living but as a source of fulfillment or frustration. We would be remiss if we did not also consider the state of a person's **spiritual health.** Not only does the "faith factor" impact physical and emotional well-being, but at some point we must also address an all-important and universal issue. To paraphrase Jesus' timeless question, what does it benefit a person to enjoy a long lifetime of superb health, wonderful relationships, and a stellar career—and lose his or her soul?

Why Invest Time and Effort Pursuing Better Health?

Presumably if you have bought (or merely picked up) this book, you already have one or more reasons. But how compelling are they? So often it seems as if health advisories are little more than "fun regulators," nudging us toward eating foods we don't like, spending endless hours in repetitive and boring exercise, subjecting us to medical pokings and proddings in areas we'd prefer be left alone, and generally disparaging anything that's remotely enjoyable. All the warnings about keeping track of cholesterol, blood pressure, and myriad other concerns seem oriented toward some vague and very distant problems that may or may not actually materialize. We wonder whether healthy habits really make a difference: *I really want that dish of ice cream sitting in front of me. It's calling my name, and I can taste it already. Will it really make that much of a difference in the long run? Will avoiding it really do anything for me, other than add a few minutes to my life when I'm eighty years old? By then I probably won't care or even notice, except perhaps to regret all of the pleasure I passed up!*

For many people, there are very obvious and immediate reasons to pay closer attention to health: a blood test showing elevated glucose (blood sugar), for example, or a bronchial infection aggravated by smoking. But even in the face of a clear and present danger, making meaningful changes can prove to be much easier said than done. No one begins his or her day with the specific objective of ruining body and mind, but it is often difficult to jettison long-established habits or simply make minor course corrections in lifestyle, even if the failure to do so may lead to an unpleasant payoff. But in the face of such obstacles, and many others we'll consider later on, there are some very important reasons to focus on maintaining and improving our health:

1. Life is a precious gift, and the meter is running. Our life and body are priceless and irreplaceable. In an eloquent passage in Psalms, King David praised both the intricacy of our earthly frame and the One who designed it.

> *For you created my inmost being;*
> *you knit me together in my mother's womb.*
> *I praise you because I am fearfully and wonderfully made;*
> *your works are wonderful,*
> *I know that full well.*
> (PSALM 139:13-14)

Furthermore, it is no secret that, no matter how indestructible we might feel (especially early in life), our days are numbered. David wrote in another psalm,

For [the Lord] knows how we are formed,
he remembers that we are dust.
As for man, his days are like grass,
he flourishes like a flower of the field;
the wind blows over it and it is gone,
and its place remembers it no more.
(PSALM 103:14-16)

Our bodies are indeed "fearfully and wonderfully made" and have fabulous powers of recuperation and regeneration. But those powers are limited in a number of ways. They do not work indefinitely. They cannot overcome years of bad choices (or in some cases, one bad choice). And, like it or not, maintaining them in optimal condition does not occur automatically but rather requires ongoing effort. Their proper maintenance is a lifetime project.

An example from a different realm might help to illustrate the implications of this reality. Imagine that the government decreed that every citizen capable of driving could receive, free of charge, a brand-new car of his or her choosing, loaded with every possible accessory. But this incredible, once-in-a-lifetime offer would come with a very important catch. If your fabulous free car should fall apart, suffer damage beyond repair, or simply wear out, you could never own another one. Furthermore, you could not borrow another person's car. In fact, you couldn't even ride in someone else's car or in any other type of transportation. You would have to remain wherever your car "breathed its last," whether in your own garage or by the side of the road.

If you were the proud owner admiring this vehicle on the day it was delivered, sleek and shiny, to your driveway, what sort of commitments would you make? Would you read the owner's manual carefully or stash it in the glove compartment? Would you follow the recommended maintenance schedule to the letter or take your car to the mechanic only when you noticed some new and strange noise emanating from the engine? Would you buy the finest fuel to fill its tank, or would you look for the cheapest, no-name brand you could find? Would you leave it outside to brave the elements or keep it safely in the garage when you weren't driving it? Would you let it sit for weeks or months at a time and then expect it to leap into traffic at a moment's notice? And when you were behind the wheel, would you drive like a maniac, play chicken with other drivers, and generally disobey all of the rules of the road?

The point of this simple analogy should be obvious: The body you have been given can be repaired (to a degree) but cannot be replaced. Once it has worn out, you can't use anyone else's. So will you treat it with respect, protect it, maintain it, and give it the best fuel possible?

2. Health increases our degree of freedom. A healthy person nearly always has the capacity to do more, see more, experience more, and most important, serve God in more ways than the person whose health is significantly impaired. Some of the more effective appeals to quit smoking or other unhealthy habits focus on what can be gained by giving up the life-threatening pursuit: more sunsets, walks on the beach, trips to the park with children or grandchildren, books to read, opportunities to reach out and change another person's life, and so forth. Poor health ultimately translates into limitations of all sorts, not merely physical impairments (such as difficulty moving, poor vision, shortness of breath, low energy, and chronic pain), but also a host of other tethers such as doctors' visits, drugs and their associated side effects, and expenses that can be astronomical, even for those with health insurance.

All of us have observed, and some of us have already experienced, the numerous effects of advanced age on body and mind. All too often these are a sad sight: gnarled limbs that carry the body with difficulty (if at all), vision and hearing problems, and, worst of all, loss of memory, comprehension, or even total communication with family and friends. While these changes aren't inevitable, they occur often enough to inspire heroic efforts by researchers to find causes and cures for aging and to support a booming industry of would-be cures. What generates far more sorrow, however, is to behold someone who has suffered a catastrophic health problem at a young age, especially when the loss easily could have been prevented.

A CAUTIONARY TALE: THE RAVE DRUG

Eighteen-year-old Rona (not her real name), once an honor student and a proficient athlete, now struggles to walk, talk, and carry out such simple functions as working a zipper or telling the time of day. She spends most of her waking hours in a rehabilitation unit, and it is yet uncertain whether she will ever live independently.

The cause of this disaster: the drug **ketamine**, an animal tranquilizer identified on the street as "Special K" or "cat Valium," among other colorful nicknames. Ketamine has become a popular item at all-night dance parties known as raves, where Rona first tried it.

But several months ago when she and her boyfriend snorted ketamine, she convulsed and stopped breathing for eight very long minutes. Lack of oxygen resulted in a two-week coma. When she finally awoke, the severity of damage to her brain became all too apparent.

One needless drug exposure on one ill-fated night severely and permanently damaged a young woman's capacity to communicate, learn, run, travel, marry, and have her own children. Ketamine has made her the prisoner of her own body, in which she will now serve a life sentence.[4] ■

3. We are accountable for the gift of life we have been given. We have just noted that good health allows greater personal freedom. But absolute autonomy—the freedom to do whatever we want, whenever we want—is a fantasy, one of many popular fairy tales for adults in which our culture remains heavily invested. The reality is that, whether we care to recognize it or not, we are accountable to a Higher Authority. The universe has a Boss, and we're not here as a result of a long series of random coincidences. We've been given life for a purpose, that of knowing and serving the God who designed us. All of our resources, including our life, belong to Him. They are not ours to squander.

The apostle Paul made this elemental fact abundantly clear when he wrote to those in the city of Corinth who claimed to be followers of Christ but were not behaving accordingly. A number of them were willing participants in the worship at the temple of Aphrodite, where "religious services" involved consorting with temple prostitutes. He first reminded them that they were directly involving Christ in their activities. "Do you not know that your bodies are members of Christ himself?" he asked them. "Shall I then take the members of Christ and unite them with a prostitute? Never!" (1 Corinthians 6:15). He then addressed the issue of ownership: "Do you not know that your body is a temple of the Holy Spirit, who is in you, whom you have received from God? You are not your own; you were bought at a price. Therefore honor God with your body" (1 Corinthians 6:19-20).

It is not unreasonable to extend this notion of God's ownership of our body—and our obligation to honor Him with it—into areas well beyond sexual behavior (although that one is of particular importance). We could easily apply it to the food we eat, the substances we ingest, the shape we allow our body to take over time, and our general presentability to the world around us. In another letter to the Corinthians, Paul described all who have entered into a relationship with Christ as His ambassadors, whom God is using to share His message. If that's the case, how are we maintaining our individual embassy? Is it thriving and well-preserved, or crumbling, overgrown with weeds, and in dire need of a fresh coat of paint? Even if our body is relatively well-kept and attractive, is it being put to good use? Is it teeming with activity that advances the cause of the One it claims to represent, or is it bogged down in wasteful, or even destructive, pursuits?

Pursuing Health—Oblivious or Obsessed?

We all have known people who have earned the label "health nut" because of their obsession with foods, supplements, and bodily functions—often to a degree that seems motivated more by endless anxiety than by a positive outlook on life. We've also known people who have acted as if they were determined to end their lives as quickly as possible, consuming tobacco, alcohol, drugs, and calories in extraordinary quantities (or by starving themselves with an eating disorder).

While a few who read this book may actually be drawn to one of these extremes, most of us fall into a broad group of people who don't spend a lot of time thinking about health unless something goes wrong. "If it ain't broke, don't fix it"—or more specifically, "If it ain't hurting, don't go looking for trouble"—probably expresses the way we usually feel, whether we admit it or not.

Unfortunately, there are many ways that "doing what comes naturally" can get us into trouble. All too often our own appetites or the common routines of our culture lead to some unpleasant but avoidable problems. And even if we have exceptionally healthy habits, some diseases, both common and unusual, can literally sneak up on us unless we subject ourselves to basic screening on a regular basis.

The pursuit of good health, like any worthwhile project, needs to be carried out with wisdom and balance. We need to avoid extremes—whether they take the form of destructive habits, ignorance, food or fitness obsessions, or the mere disregard for well-established, well-grounded health recommendations that might give us an ounce of prevention and help prevent a pound (or a ton) of cure.

What This Book Is—and Isn't—About

With this in mind, the Focus on the Family *Complete Guide to Family Health, Nutrition, and Fitness* has been written with some very specific objectives:

It focuses on the promotion of health and prevention of illness—and thus it will not be a medical encyclopedia. We fervently encourage healthy lifestyles, and we also provide basic information about common health problems (for example, coronary artery disease and cancer) in order to explain how they might be prevented and detected. But this book does not contain hundreds of pages detailing diseases and syndromes. Nor does it outline all of the possible causes of symptoms, such as headache or abdominal pain. Such information is readily available in reference books or on the Internet. Including hundreds of pages of

AN INSPIRATIONAL TALE: ALIVE AND WELL IN THREE CENTURIES

Born in 1899, Helen witnessed the grand panorama of the entire twentieth century, from the horse and buggy to the space shuttle. At 102 she was still living independently in a retirement community, alert, keenly interested in other people, and an avid reader of the Bible.

Trained as a nurse, she spent many years organizing public-health programs in northern California. For those who had the time to ask and listen, she provided a wealth of stories about the delivery of health care decades ago.

She attributed her longevity to "good genes," but her abstinence from tobacco, her prudent diet, her sense of humor, and her rock-solid faith no doubt made a significant contribution not only to her many birthdays but also to her continued ability to enjoy them. ■

medical details here would reinvent a very large (and not particularly interesting) wheel.

It is both biblically sound and scientifically accurate, to the best of our ability. There are many books on the market that are medically solid but presume that the physical world is all there is and that God does not enter the health equation in any way. Others seek to honor God and the Bible but unfortunately wander into the fringes of health care, often promoting questionable information or even irrational claims about the workings of our body and mind. A number of books—some of them best sellers—are literally out in left field both scientifically and spiritually. Some of these attempt to blend quasiscientific or even mythological ideas about health with spiritual teachings that are incompatible with, or vigorously hostile to, the teachings of the Old and New Testaments. While we cannot claim to have the last word on either medical research or biblical scholarship, we have attempted to be diligent in our pursuit of scientific accuracy, as well as to be workmen who correctly handle the word of truth (2 Timothy 2:15).

It focuses on the whole person—not only the physical body, but also emotions, relationships, and spiritual well-being as they impact health. An expanding body of research supports such an approach, not to mention timeless wisdom found in the Old and New Testaments, which lay the foundation for physical, emotional, and spiritual health.

It is practical. What good are health advisories that are so demanding that only the most enthusiastic or determined person can follow them? Most of us live with all sorts of demands on our time and energy, and spending hours every day doing vigorous exercise or in intricate preparation of "health-conscious" meals is simply not an option. This brings us to an important aspect of practicality.

It focuses on the process of change. A huge number of medical problems can be helped, or avoided altogether, by what medical journals politely call "lifestyle modification": changing the way we eat, exercise, relate to other people, and generally order our life. Most of us have areas of health that need a tune-up, and some need a major overhaul. One week after any New Year's Day, we can usually testify that making and sticking to changes is easier said than done. How do we rise above the ingrained habits, the inertia, the schedule, the false starts, the discomfort, the discouragement?

Each chapter will end with some questions and suggested action items to help you in the process of change.

It is meant to be used as a hands-on resource by your family. Most medical guides are written for the individual; this book was written with families in mind. We hope it will serve as an aid when your family seeks to adopt healthy lifestyle habits or wrestles with a health issue.

It will help you become a wiser and more discerning consumer of health products and resources. Many people who are well-educated and savvy about everyday decisions sometimes seem to throw caution to the wind when dealing with their health. Because it is impossible to include information about the validity of every approach to promoting health, we hope to assist you in separating the wheat from the chaff. How can you determine whether a claim for a product or therapy is realistic or bogus? Is taking vitamins and supplements worthwhile? Are alternative therapies worth exploring? What about the endless flow of health advice from the news media and the Internet? In addition, navigating the health-care system can be a daunting task. How can you get the most for your money (and time!) when visiting a doctor, clinic, or emergency room? How do you deal with the alphabet soup of health-care insurance plans (PPOs, HMOs, etc.), and what do you do if you can't obtain insurance at all? We will attempt to address these and many other concerns related to the complexities of obtaining appropriate health screening and medical care.

An Important Reminder before We Begin . . .

Medical research and information continues to proliferate at a dizzying pace. While we always seek to provide the most current information on any given topic, it is quite possible that what was hot off the press when this book was published may be old news in a matter of months. Needless to say, it is very important that you build and maintain a relationship with a primary-care physician who can advise you—not only about any new developments in health promotion and prevention, but also about medical decisions in light of your own individual status and needs. No book, no matter how thorough, can substitute for the one-on-one assessment of a caring professional.

That being said, let's begin our journey, a step at a time, toward making the most of the body and mind that God has given us.

QUESTIONS TO PONDER:

1. What are *your* reasons for wanting to improve your family's health?
2. Why do these reasons matter to you?

Action item: If you keep a personal journal, write in it the answers to these questions (and others that you'll find later in this book). If you don't keep a personal journal where you take note of your experiences, thoughts, and prayers, it's never too late to start. Years from now, what you have written will be an irreplaceable gift to yourself (not to mention any future generations you permit to read it).

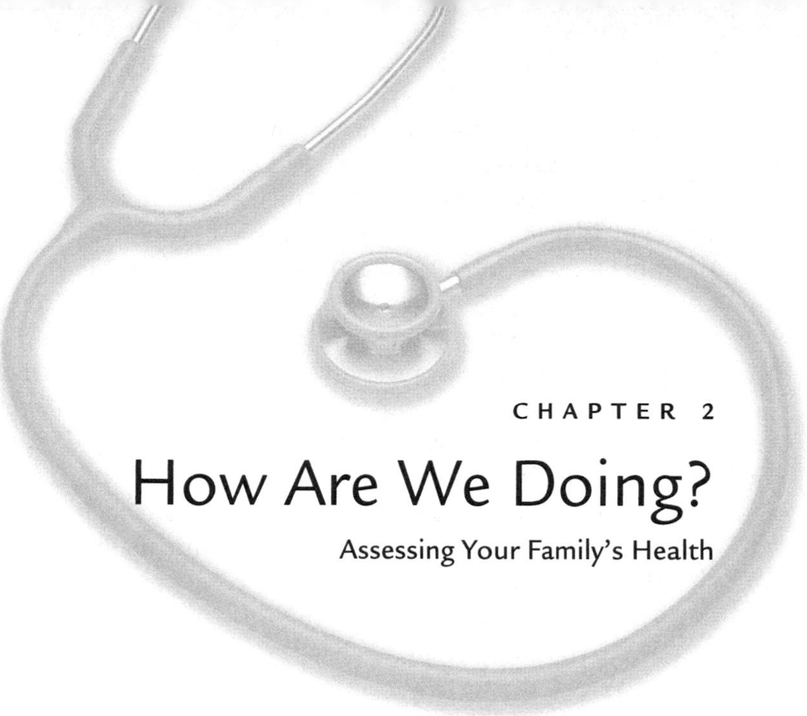

CHAPTER 2

How Are We Doing?

Assessing Your Family's Health

Whether you've just decided to begin a journey toward excellent (or at least improved) health or you feel that you're already well on your way, you need to address an important question: *Do you know where you are?* The paths you choose to follow will be determined not only by the places you want to go, but also by your current location.

If this were a book about your personal finances, the first order of business would be to answer a number of basic questions about money matters. What do you own, and how much is it worth? What do you owe? How much money are you taking in every month, and how much are you spending? Are you reducing your debt load each year, or are you digging the hole deeper? Then comes the pivotal question: *If you continue on your current course, where will you be in five, ten, or twenty years?* Are you likely to be satisfied and independent or frustrated with financial burdens and shortfalls? Of course, even with the best information and planning, life might throw you some curveballs that could drastically alter your future. You might receive a windfall, or lose your job, or land a big raise, or suffer a change in health that torpedoes your earning capacity.

Similarly, if you're going to improve or protect your health, you need to assess how you're doing right now. What are your assets and liabilities? How are you treating your body, mind, and spirit? What are you doing, whether on an occasional or regular basis, that enhances—or threatens—your health? As with finances, a pivotal question should be addressed: *If you continue on your current course, where are you likely to be in five, ten, or twenty years?* Unfortunately, predicting the course of a person's health is even more uncertain than making an economic forecast. Even worse, positive "windfalls" in health are uncommon (unless you count situations in which a frightening symptom turns out to be a false alarm). More often, unexpected events that impact our health prove to be the kind we would rather avoid. An exception to this is a dramatic improvement in a health problem, whether it occurs spontaneously or in response to prayer, that "beats the odds" or flies in the face of medical predictions.

This chapter will provide an overview of several steps you can take to assess your health, and your family's as well. For some of these, you will need the services of a physician and (depending on your age and other factors) additional resources. Many of the subjects mentioned here will be discussed in more detail in other chapters. If you have a particular interest in pursuing one of them, you can take a detour to visit that topic. But this chapter should serve as your road map to the information found in the rest of the book.

When assessing your health, you need to consider these five areas:

- Your family history
- Your own health history
- Your lifestyle
- Screening examinations by a physician
- Screening tests (lab, X rays, scans, scopes, etc.)

In the rest of this chapter, we will look at the first three, as well as overview the screening examinations (otherwise known as checkups) for all age groups. In chapter 3, we will take an important detour to examine three important health problems you and your family want to avoid: cardiovascular (heart and blood vessel) disease, cancer, and diabetes. This will set the stage for much of what follows in chapter 4: a guided tour of the world of health-screening tests for adults.

Your Family History: Handicap or Head Start?

Whether you realize it or not, you have inherited a lot more from your parents (and their ancestors) than the color of your eyes or the shape of your chin. Many other characteristics that can impact your health, most of which you can't see, are transmitted within the complex genetic code that was established when twenty-three chromosomes from each of your parents first combined to begin your life. Some diseases (for example, hemophilia) have very specific inheritance patterns. When a family member is found to have one of these problems, it's important to receive **genetic counseling** from a qualified professional in order to understand the potential risk for transmitting it to future offspring.

While exploring the length and breadth of specific genetic disorders is beyond the scope of this book, in the next two chapters we will look at a number of important and common medical conditions that can have roots in previous generations. If your mother, father, or siblings have had one or more of these problems, you or your children may be at higher risk as well. Understanding that risk may help you take measures to prevent similar problems or even lead you to undergo appropriate screening tests that might otherwise seem unnecessary.

Unlike genetic disorders with clear-cut inheritance patterns, it is usually not possible to give more than a rough estimate of your risk for the more common diseases with family ties. However, you can generally assume that the odds of your having a given problem will increase with

- the number of blood relatives, especially immediate family members, who have been affected by the same problem,
- how early in their lives it appeared, and
- how severe it was.

For example, if your parents and one or more of your siblings have very high cholesterol levels and have suffered damage to the heart because of clogged coronary arteries before their fiftieth birthday, you'd better pay close attention to your own risk factors for this common but dangerous problem. On the other hand, if both sides of your family tree are full of people who live well into their nineties, always have low blood pressure and cholesterol levels, and never have heart attacks or strokes, you can figure that you've been blessed with a favorable genetic outlook with respect to cardiovascular disease. (This does *not* mean, however, that you would be free to smoke, avoid exercise, or become careless about the quality and quantity of food you consume. As in many areas of life, you can squander a nice hereditary advantage by making a lot of small, unwise decisions—or a few big ones.)

What if you have no idea what kind of health problems your immediate blood relatives have faced? Perhaps you were adopted and have had little or no contact with your biological parents and siblings. If this is the case, you might see little need to read up on the role of heredity in common diseases, but keep in mind that *your* health status might reveal a genetic factor that could play a major role in your own children's health.

Your Health History: A Single Paragraph or *War and Peace*?

Depending on your age, genetics, habits, and surroundings, as well as the vicissitudes of your life, you may have a very short health history ("Nothing has happened to me and I feel great!") or enough medical events to fill several folders in your doctor's chart rack.

For the most part, your medical history impacts decisions you make with your doctor, who hopefully at some point has collected this information. But some health events can have consequences that affect everyday life for decades.

Vicissitudes is a wonderful, nonmedical word for "ups and downs," the sudden and often unexpected twists and turns that our life may take.

Even if you don't spend a lot of time ruminating on the state of your health, you would be wise to create a basic summary of the major events in your health history. In an emergency, or at your next physical, your doctor will appreciate having this information and may even admire your organization.

HOT TIP

If you have a computer with simple word processing, you can create a health-information document for each member of your family. You can easily update this whenever something new and interesting happens.

Key topics on this list should include:

Significant health problems in the past that aren't causing trouble now: For example, asthma during childhood that disappeared when you grew up; obesity during an earlier era of life; or depression after a baby was born.

Surgeries: When they occurred and for what problem.

Other hospitalizations: For example, a heart attack, pneumonia, or other problems that couldn't be handled at home.

Immunizations: Childhood, adult, travel, military.

Ongoing concerns: These could include specific health problems that already have been identified (such as high blood pressure or diabetes) or recurring symptoms that may or may not have a diagnosis (such as headaches or back pain).

Family history: Significant medical problems that have occurred among your parents, siblings, or even children—especially if any of these led to serious illness or death. Particularly important is knowing a family history of cardiovascular disease, especially heart attack and stroke, and its various risk factors, as well as cancer and diabetes.

Substance use/problems: Current or past use of tobacco, alcohol, or illegal drugs.

Current medications and supplements: This includes any tablet or tonic that you take regularly or once in a while, whether prescribed by a physician, purchased without a prescription, borrowed from a friend (not a good idea), or bought on the street (a really bad idea). Remember that vitamins, supplements, and herbal products may have unexpected effects or may interact with other medications, even if they are billed as "100 percent natural." St. John's wort, for example, can interact with some prescription drugs and alter their effectiveness, while ginkgo biloba can cause bleeding problems when taken with medications that affect clotting, such as aspirin or Coumadin. During a medical evaluation it is very important to list *everything* you are using, even if you don't think of it as a drug.

Known allergies: This includes allergic reactions to foods, insect stings, or environmental factors such as pollens or mold.

F.Y.I.

Even grapefruit juice, a 100 percent natural product if there ever was one, can change the metabolism of a number of medications. This may result in higher (or sometimes lower) blood levels of these medications, thus altering their effects. You should let your doctor know if you're a regular consumer of grapefruit juice, because this could impact decisions about drugs prescribed for you (or, if necessary, lead to a recommendation that you change your juice habits).

Past reactions or other problems with medications: Often the term *drug allergy* is used whenever something goes wrong after taking a medication. While that phrase may or may not be accurate in a specific case (see sidebar "Drug Reactions: Allergies, Adverse Reactions, Side Effects, or Coincidence?" on p. 20), you would be wise to keep a list of any problems you have had with medications. This not only can save time during a medical evaluation but also can prevent future suffering and expense.

HOT TIP

You might also list medications (especially prescriptions) that you have used in the past, even if they didn't cause any problems. For a physician, knowledge of what has worked for you (and what hasn't) for a given problem can be very useful.

Your Lifestyle: Health Booster—or Buster?

Like it or not, a number of your everyday decisions are like brushstrokes on an extensive canvas. Individually, they may not appear monumental. In fact, they may seem irrelevant to the total picture. But repeated over months and years, they can create a work of art—or an eyesore. While medical research and technology continue to make dramatic advances in diagnosing and treating disease, all too often they are deployed (at considerable expense) to clean up a preventable mess. Most primary-care physicians will tell you, for example, that their average workday would be dramatically altered if everyone in their practices maintained an appropriate weight, exercised regularly, and never used tobacco.

What follows is a list of questions that are meant to give you a heads-up about several areas of your daily life that could have a serious impact on your health. We will also direct your attention to related chapters in this book that could help you make some useful course corrections for you and your family.

1. What's the quality of your fuel?

Your body needs a steady supply of high-quality nutrients to build, maintain, and repair itself, and to provide energy for millions of critical metabolic reactions. We're designed with a powerful mechanism—hunger—that drives us to seek fuel, but not necessarily to choose the best quality when many options are available. Furthermore, despite an unprecedented abundance and variety of foods that are available to the average American shopper, some have raised concerns that the foods we buy at the local supermarket aren't as nutritious as they could or should be because of the way they have been grown, packaged, or prepared. As a result, we are exposed to an endless stream of advice (of variable credibility) about the type of food we should eat and the vitamins and supplements we apparently need. We will review this important topic in chapters 5

continued on page 22

DRUG REACTIONS: ALLERGIES, ADVERSE REACTIONS, SIDE EFFECTS, OR COINCIDENCE?

To risk stating the obvious, none of us would take a medication or supplement and expect it to do absolutely nothing. Based upon someone's professional judgment or our own understanding, we normally assume (correctly or not) that a substance we deliberately swallow, inhale, or rub on our skin will end an illness, relieve symptoms, or prevent a problem in the future. But any product that does something we like—no matter how natural, mild, or safe it may be—can also cause problems, at least for somebody.

When something goes wrong after taking a medication, most people assume they are allergic to it. But that might not always be the case. In fact, there are several possibilities.

An **allergic reaction** occurs when a drug provokes an inappropriate—or even extreme—response from the immune system. The most common manifestation of an allergic reaction is a rash, which may be a nonspecific-looking collection of spots on any or all parts of the body, or the irregular, raised itchy areas called **hives** that are constantly shifting in size and location. A more alarming (but less common) manifestation is swelling or puffiness, especially of the face or tongue, known as **angioedema**. The most serious type of allergic reaction is called **anaphylaxis**, which can be life-threatening. Symptoms can include wheezing, hoarseness, dizziness, nausea, diarrhea, and abdominal cramps. The most severe manifestation of anaphylaxis is a drastic drop in blood pressure known as **anaphylactic shock**.

One of the most common reactions to antibiotics is a rash provoked by ampicillin or amoxicillin, variations of penicillin that have been widely used for many years. This typically occurs when one of these drugs is given to a child during an acute illness—often one in which the physician was concerned about a **strep** throat (that is, a throat infection caused by a specific type of streptococcal bacteria). In some cases, this may not be a true allergic reaction, but rather an interaction between the drug and a specific virus. The person may not actually be allergic to penicillin, but until he or she knows for sure it would be prudent to avoid using penicillins of any type.

Mild symptoms caused by an allergic reaction are often treated with a nonprescription antihistamine such as **diphenhydramine** (Benadryl). More serious symptoms may require prescription medications (such as oral **cortisone**), or even emergency care to stop an anaphylactic reaction. A person who is having difficulty breathing should be seen immediately in an emergency room. If you are uncertain where the nearest facility is or cannot get there, call 911 for immediate assistance.

An allergic reaction to any substance requires at least one previous exposure, so you would not expect it to occur on the first dose. (However, it is possible to be exposed to a substance without remembering—for example, if it occurred during childhood or perhaps involved another drug that was similar and caused a sensitizing effect.) Once a true allergic response has taken place, the next exposure is likely to cause a more severe reaction. Two of the oldest families of antibiotics, the **penicillins** and the **sulfa drugs**, are well-known for provoking allergic reactions. Other types of drugs that more commonly cause allergic reactions include anti-inflammatory medications, barbiturates, local anesthetics such as **lidocaine** (Xylocaine), and X-ray contrast dyes that contain iodine.

An **adverse reaction** is one that is not allergic and may—or may not—be predictable from the drug's known properties. For example, the common anti-inflammatory pain relievers **ibuprofen** (Advil, Motrin, and others) and **naproxen** (Aleve and others) may irritate the stomach, but taking them with food can decrease the chance of this happening. In addition, when taken continuously for weeks or months, any of these medications occasionally cause abnormalities in kidney or liver function. All of these are potential by-products of the mechanisms by which anti-inflammatory drugs are known to work.

A different type of adverse reaction was observed after word got out that two mild appetite suppressants already on the market for many years—**phentermine** and **fenfluramine**—were very effective at promoting weight loss when taken together. As millions tried what became known as **fen-phen**, a small number eventually developed a heart-valve abnormality. The culprit, fenfluramine, was eventually taken off the market. But before the fen-phen craze, when this relatively obscure drug was suddenly being ingested by an enormous number of people, there had been little reason to suspect that it would have this effect.

With few exceptions, most medications on the market have a *generic* name (for example, ibuprofen) and one or more **trade** or **brand names** (such as Advil or Motrin). Needless to say, keeping all of them straight can be a challenge. Throughout this book we will usually refer to a drug by its generic name, but also note one or more common trade names, which often are more familiar.

A **side effect** is a predictable consequence of taking a drug that is usually (but not always) annoying or even hazardous. For example, the antihistamine diphenhydramine (Benadryl) is very effective not only at reducing the sneezing and itching of nasal allergy, but also at curbing allergic reactions in general. But it also causes drowsiness so often that many people cannot tolerate it during waking and working hours. That side effect, however, has given diphenhydramine another common role as a nonprescription sleep aid.

Coincidence and the **nocebo effect** may also be to blame for a bad response to a drug. When you don't feel well, it's a normal response to wonder what you did, where you went, or what you ate within the last day or two that might have caused the problem. If you just started a new medication, the likely culprit may seem obvious—but it may have been an innocent bystander. Before dumping that new prescription in the trash, check with the physician who prescribed it, because your symptoms may have been caused by something else. Also, if you weren't too keen on taking the medication in the first place, your negative expectations could actually play a role in how you feel. This phenomenon is called the nocebo effect, the evil twin of the **placebo effect**. A placebo is a substance with no biological effect—sometimes called a "sugar pill," although it need not contain any—that in bygone days was given by physicians to patients with an abundance of symptoms but no apparent illness. While deliberately doing this today would be considered deceptive, other actions that create a positive expectation of recovery—especially reassurance from someone who is perceived to be both knowledgeable and caring—can provide a noticeable benefit. Unfortunately, uneasiness or fear of any treatment, whether medication or something else, can definitely have the opposite effect. ■

The word *placebo* comes from the Latin for "I will please," which is what the doctor was supposedly trying to do. Now placebos are used primarily in research, where one group of people receiving a medication under investigation is compared to a similar group given an inert substance. The inactive substance is called the placebo, although it isn't intended to "please" anyone in particular.

continued from page 19

and 6 (which begin on page 119), as well as in appendix B (which begins on page 869), but for now think about the following "food for thought" questions:

- Do you know the approximate number of calories you need each day? Do you know how many you actually consume on a typical day?
- Do you look at the nutritional information printed on virtually every product in the supermarket? Do you understand most of it, or does it seem like a foreign language?
- What are the proportions of protein, fat, and carbohydrate in your daily food intake? Do you know how to estimate those proportions?
- How many servings of fruit and vegetables should you and your family eat every day? How many do you actually consume? (By the way, do you know what constitutes a "serving"?)
- How many times every week does your family eat at fast-food restaurants? Have you ever checked the nutritional content of some of your (or your kids') favorite fast foods?
- How often does your family eat together during the week? Is it really worth the effort to eat together as often as possible?
- Do you eat breakfast every day?

2. Are you carrying too much—or too little—fat storage?

By far the most common, and most serious, nutritional problem in America (and in other developed countries) is consuming too much food. A much smaller number of people struggle with a powerful compulsion to eat very little, or to deliberately throw up much of what they take in. We will look at eating disorders in chapter 8 (beginning on page 331) and examine the problem of excessive weight in chapter 6, but to whet your appetite, so to speak, see if you know the answers to the following questions:

- What is your body mass index (BMI)? Do you know whether it is a threat to your health?
- If you are carrying too much weight, have you tried one or more methods for losing it? Have any worked? Have you had trouble keeping it off?
- Which is more effective: a low-fat or a low-carbohydrate diet (or neither)?
- If you are overweight, do you believe the primary problem is a genetic or metabolic defect? bad habits? uncontrollable cravings? lack of exercise? emotional or spiritual conflict? a combination of these?
- If you exercise regularly, is your activity likely to help you lose weight? Do you know how many calories you burn each time you exercise?
- Is there any specific food, supplement, or medication that can help you lose weight and keep it off?

If you can't wait to find out, you can use the charts on page 924 to determine your BMI.

3. Do you exercise regularly?
Most of us do not earn our living by the "sweat of our brow," and too many of our children spend too many hours exercising only their thumbs on a video-game controller. As a result, obtaining even a reasonable level of physical conditioning often requires deliberate effort, planning, tweaking of our schedules, and overcoming a lot of inertia. Yet the rewards for doing so include not only better long-term health, but also heightened energy and alertness. We will walk you, so to speak, through these benefits in chapter 7, but for now think about the following:

- Do you deliberately do some type of exercise at least five days every week? If not, what are your biggest obstacles? (Hint: At least one of them probably involves your calendar.)
- Do your school-age (and older) children move their muscles at school or home on a regular basis? (Another hint: Their overall physical condition may be inversely proportional to the number of hours they spend staring at the TV or computer screens.)
- Do you know how much exercise—and what kind—will enhance your health and improve how you feel?
- Is it safe for you to exercise? If you're just getting started or planning to upgrade your exercise routine, can you do so without risking a heart attack or a pain in the whatchamacallit?
- Do you know what muscle-strengthening (or "bodybuilding") exercise might do for you beyond reducing embarrassment around the swimming pool?

4. Do you swallow, drink, smoke, or chew any substances that could wreck your health and shorten your life?

- Do you use tobacco in any form (smoked or chewed) on a regular basis?
- Do you use alcohol? How much and how often? Do you know how much (if any) is safe to consume on a day-to-day basis? Is anyone in your family concerned about your use of alcohol (even if you believe it's not a problem)?
- Are you taking any prescription medications in amounts that you, your family, or your physician feel are excessive?
- Do you use any illegal drugs?
- Is your use of *any* substance creating turbulence in your body, mind, spirit, family, workplace, or community?

If any substance has a choke hold on your life, you will probably need more help than any single book (including this one) can offer. Nevertheless, in chapter 10 we will do a "flyby" over the blighted realm of bad habits and addictions. It won't be a pretty sight, but if you or a family member is struggling with one or more habit-forming substances, we hope it will provide some motivation to take whatever steps are necessary to break the chains. We will also address a critical question for your family: How can you keep your kids away from tobacco, alcohol, and drugs—and what can you do if they become ensnared by them?

5. How is your emotional health?

The connection between your body and your mind is not speculative psychobabble, although all of its dimensions are far from understood. But any primary-care physician will tell you that the agenda for a substantial number—perhaps the majority—of any week's appointments involves diagnosing and managing physical symptoms that have roots in emotional turbulence, or specifically treating a mood problem. We will look at emotional health in chapter 8, but for now consider the following questions:

- Do you feel anxious or depressed much (or all) of the time?
- Do you struggle with fatigue, headaches, aches and pains, and other symptoms for which no one can find a cause?
- Are your relationships healthy or toxic? Can you identify characteristics that impact the health of your relationships (including those with your spouse and children)?
- What changes and stresses have you been dealing with recently?
- Do you have trouble relaxing?
- Do you feel that there is balance among important arenas of your life such as family, career, church, and leisure?
- Do you observe a day of rest every week for worship, restoration, and recharging your batteries?

6. How is your spiritual health?

A robust amount of research indicates that spiritual commitment plays a definite role in overall health. There are many sensible reasons why this should be the case, and we will review them in detail in chapter 9. For now, here are some questions to consider:

- Do you have a personal faith that affects your outlook on life (and death)? Does it have an impact on the choices you make on a day-to-day basis? Does it bring you comfort, joy, peace, or other emotional benefits?
- Do you sense any connection between your physical and emotional health and your understanding of—and relationship with—God? Does your faith affect any decisions you make about the way you treat your body?
- Do you pray or meditate on a regular basis? Do you feel that doing so has any impact on your health?
- When you become ill, do you see God as playing any part in your recovery? Do you ask others to pray for you?
- Are you involved with other people in a community of faith?

7. Do you play it safe or do you take chances with your life and health?
There are more ways to put yourself in jeopardy besides exposing yourself to harmful and addictive substances. Before we look at several safety issues in chapter 11, try this pop quiz:

- Are you and your children current with your immunizations? Do you know which are currently recommended? Are you avoiding immunizations for yourself or your children, and if so, what are your reasons?
- Before you start the ignition on your car, is everyone properly buckled up? If you have infants and small children, are they fastened into appropriate car seats on every trip, no matter how short?
- Do you know the keys to proper vehicle maintenance and focused driving that can reduce your odds of being involved in an automobile accident?
- Do your children wear helmets whenever they ride their bikes? Do they use appropriate safety gear for in-line skating and other pursuits involving speed and wheels? If you are a cyclist (motor or self-propelled), do you always wear a helmet?
- Do you have smoke detectors installed in one or more strategic places in your home? Are they in good working order? What about carbon monoxide detectors?
- Do you use sunscreen for yourself or your children whenever you are in the sunlight for any length of time (whether at the beach or in the backyard)? Do you visit tanning salons, and if so, do you consider them to be safer than tanning in the sun?
- If you travel abroad, do you know how to avoid common problems, such as traveler's diarrhea and potentially more serious infections such as malaria?
- If you have crawling infants, toddlers, or preschoolers, is the home "baby-proofed"? If you have a pool or spa, is it surrounded by barriers that will prevent young explorers from falling in?
- Do you know how to reduce the risk of accidental poisonings and how to respond if you suspect your child has ingested poison?
- Do you know the top causes of foodborne illnesses and the steps you can take to prevent them?

8. Is your sex life a source of great fulfillment or frustration? Is it truly safe, or is it more risky than you may realize?
Our culture is saturated with sexual messages, and most of them say or imply something like this: "Sex with any person [or persons] of either gender is okay as long as everyone consents, no one is too young [with that boundary becoming fuzzier every year], no one gets pregnant [unless she wants to], and no one gets a disease. Therefore everyone, starting in grade school, should be well-aware of reliable birth-control methods and the proper use of condoms." Even

in this age of sexual candor and general overexposure, myths and misconceptions about what kind of sex is "safe" and satisfying—and what isn't—are abundant. We will look at healthy sexuality in chapter 12, but for now consider the following:

- According to current research, who is more likely to enjoy the most sexual satisfaction: a married couple or singles who engage in sex without a formal commitment to (or even a relationship with) their partners?
- What enhances, or undermines, sexual satisfaction in a marriage? If this area of your marriage isn't doing as well as you'd like, where might you seek help?
- You have no doubt heard of AIDS and the human immunodeficiency virus (HIV) that causes it, as well as syphilis and gonorrhea. Are you also aware of some other sexually transmitted infections such as HPV (human papillomavirus), HSV (herpes simplex virus), and chlamydia, which are much more common?
- Despite their high profile in sex-education classes for the past two decades, condoms do not provide complete protection against sexually transmitted infections. Do you know which organisms are likely to be acquired from an infected partner even when condoms are used consistently and correctly?
- Is there any way to tell whether a potential partner has a sexually transmitted infection?
- Do you think of pornography as harmless entertainment or a potential threat to a person's sexual integrity?
- How can you help your children preserve the gift of sex for the right time and place (i.e., their wedding night)?

9. Are you getting enough refreshing, restorative sleep?

We spend roughly a third of our life sleeping, yet most of us don't know that much about it. We'll take a closer look at this crucial activity in chapter 15, but for now consider the following:

- Do you feel as though you get enough sleep most nights?
- Do you have trouble falling or staying asleep?
- Do you awaken feeling refreshed or groggy (or even more tired than when you went to bed)?
- Can you fall asleep at the drop of a hat during the day? Do you have trouble staying awake during a meeting or a class, or while behind the wheel?
- Do you know how many hours of sleep you or your children need every night?
- If you work a night shift, are you able to get enough sleep at other times of the day?

- Do you feel tired most (or all) of the time, even if you've had enough sleep?

Chronic fatigue generates millions of visits to health practitioners (both conventional and alternative) every year, not to mention billions of dollars in annual sales of vitamins, supplements, and other concoctions that promise more energy. This is usually a different problem from daytime drowsiness, although the two may be related. While ongoing fatigue usually *isn't* caused by a serious medical problem, it is important to have a medical evaluation to make sure this is the case before considering other possibilities. We will take a look at this common and frustrating problem in chapter 16.

10. How well do you navigate the health-care system?

In addition to all that you might do to enhance or undermine your health, your well-being (or even your life)—and your family's as well—may someday hinge on your ability to gain access to and utilize the health-care system. We will look at this challenging topic in chapter 17, but for now consider the following:

- Does each member of your family have a primary-care physician? In this era of medical specialization, it's possible to have a different doctor for every organ system in your body. But ideally one physician (or clinic) serves as home base for your health care and knows (or has a chart containing) the big picture—the history, current problems, medications, and so on—for you and your children.
- Do you have health insurance? For many families on a tight budget, health insurance may seem like a luxury or a complete impossibility. But without it, the fear of overwhelming medical bills may delay or prevent necessary care when there is a problem or when preventive measures should be taken.
- If you do have insurance, do you know what it covers? Does it include checkups or any screening tests? What about medications? Do you know how to get access to care? Does your coverage pay for some practitioners and not others? Do you have to see a "gatekeeper" physician before you can see a specialist?
- Do you know how to get the most out of a doctor's visit? Do you get your problems addressed and questions answered satisfactorily?
- Are you aware of the wide variety of alternative therapies that are available on the health-care market? How can you evaluate these approaches to determine whether they are effective and appropriate?

11. Are you sixty-five or older?

If you have reached this important milestone, congratulations! We hope that you will have many more birthday celebrations and that you will be thriving at each one. Unfortunately, however, for obvious reasons health problems are more likely to knock on your door now than when you were in your twenties.

Paying attention to the advisories in this book about food, exercise, and health-promoting habits is particularly important now. If you have spent many years overweight, out of shape, hooked on cigarettes, or overly fond of alcohol, for example, their unpleasant consequences are more likely to come home to roost during the next several years. If you've been angry and depressed much of your life, things may not spontaneously improve as you continue to grow older. *But it's never too late to make meaningful changes.* In addition, a few other health issues come to the surface more often at this time of life. We will review these in chapter 14, but for now think about these questions:

- Are you keeping physically and mentally active? The old adage "Use it or lose it" has particular relevance to life in the senior lane. Both muscles and mental alertness can be maintained with appropriate exercise and may dramatically decline without it.
- Are you getting appropriate checkups? The fact that you have "seniority" doesn't mean that you're off the hook for screening tests that could spare you some grief. (See chapter 4 for details.)
- Do you see your future as golden or ghastly? As you approach retirement, how can you fill the hours between nine and five with meaningful activities that will enrich your life while improving the lot of others? If you are already retired, are you planning for productivity or inactivity?
- How do your nutritional needs change as you age? Should you take a supplement, and if so, should you take one formulated specifically for seniors?
- How important is exercise in keeping you healthy? What special precautions should you take as you age?
- Are you at risk for a fall? Have you already been injured in one?
- Are you taking one or more prescriptions? If so, do you know the purpose, dose, precautions, and possible side effects for each one? Does everyone writing prescriptions for you know all that you are taking, including nonprescription drugs and supplements? Seniors have a tendency to accumulate multiple prescriptions as various medical problems develop. Sometimes the list can be daunting—and dangerous.
- Do you know which immunizations are strongly recommended for seniors? Why are they so important to maintaining health?
- Are you as conscious of your emotional and spiritual well-being as you are of your physical health? Many seniors suffer from anxiety and depression—often for the first time in their lives. Are you aware of the risk factors and symptoms? Do you know how to respond if you notice them in yourself or your loved one?
- To quote another old adage (but all-important question), "Are you ready to meet your Maker?" Even if you are in great condition, your body has probably notified you in a few ways that "it ain't what it

used to be" and that your time on this planet isn't indefinite. Have you thought about what will happen to you after the clock stops ticking? Just as it's never too late to make meaningful changes in your health habits, it's also never too late to become acquainted with your Creator. (See chapter 9 for further details.)

Do You or Your Family Members Need a Checkup?

Obviously, if you are having pain, difficulty breathing, or some other symptom that can't be ignored, you will (hopefully) seek appropriate medical care. But what if you and your kids have been feeling okay for years or your health problems have been minor annoyances, such as a sore throat or a cut finger, that didn't require a complete evaluation? How often do you need a complete checkup by a physician? What about labs, X rays, scans, or other tests? What about dental and eye checks?

Ideally, you have a primary-care physician who is advising you on this subject, especially if you have one or more significant medical problems. What follows are some basic recommendations that can help you gauge how your family is doing.

Infants and children

For babies and children through the teen years, the guidelines for checkups are well-established and followed by nearly all primary-care physicians (pediatricians and family physicians) who see children. These visits typically include several agenda items:

- Measuring height and weight (and, in infants, head circumference). In older children, the body mass index (BMI) may be calculated if there is any concern about their being under- or overweight.
- Reviewing developmental milestones and behavioral status.
- Checking the fuel intake: nursing (or formula) patterns in infants, quantity and variety of foods in toddlers and preschoolers, and the nutritional quality of food choices in older children and teenagers.
- Immunizations.
- Addressing specific parental concerns: Why does she cry so much at night? When will he stop wetting the bed? How can we improve school performance? What can we do about her acne?
- Safety, prevention, and "anticipatory guidance"—advice about what may be coming around the next bend.

HOT TIP

You can get a detailed look at all of these topics for newborns through teens in the* Complete Book of Baby & Child Care *(Colorado Springs: Focus on the Family, 1997), which you can find at your local bookstore or the Focus on the Family Web site: http://www.family.org.

Depending on what is going on in your child's life at a particular age, getting all of this accomplished during a single office visit may be a by-the-numbers snap or an impossibility. If there are more problems or items on your question list than can be fielded during the time allotted for the appointment, you can always make another one to deal with any unfinished business.

HOT TIP

Want to get the most bang for the buck out of your next doctor's appointment? See chapter 17 for some useful tips.

It is not uncommon for a parent to bring a child faithfully to the newborn and baby checks and then let visits during the school and teen years fall by the wayside. Often a cursory (or even assembly-line) camp or sports exam serves as a substitute for a more detailed visit with a primary-care doctor. This is not a wise idea. As we will see in a moment, regular checks are recommended through the high school years, even if your older child or teenager isn't having any obvious medical problems.

What follows is a timetable of visits from prebirth through the teen years, based upon recommendations from the American Academy of Pediatrics and the American Academy of Family Physicians. This includes immunizations that are commonly given at specific visits, but timing may vary depending on your child's health status and your (and the physician's) preferences.

F.Y.I.

Details about specific immunizations—the diseases they prevent, the way they are given, their benefits and risks—can be found in chapter 11. Also, recommendations for immunizations and how they are to be given change frequently, and new ones are introduced on a regular basis. Therefore *you should always check with your child's physician about the "current wisdom" in this important aspect of your child's health.*

Before birth. If your first baby is on the way, a prebirth visit with the doctor who will care for him or her is a wise idea. Ideally, this will accomplish more than "meeting and greeting" the physician. This is a good time for you to review any information about the pregnancy and other health matters that might have an impact on the baby at birth or later. And you can clarify expectations and procedures for care of your baby immediately after birth and during the months to follow. If you already have one or more children and know the physician, you generally won't need this appointment unless there is a problem with the pregnancy or a suspected abnormality with the baby that might require special care.

HOT TIP

Find out who's who on the office staff—especially the nurse(s) and appointment personnel—and treat them well. Your phone calls and other interactions will probably go much more smoothly as a result.

Newborn care. A new baby should be examined by a physician within the first twenty-four hours after birth. Normally the newborn is rechecked daily while in the hospital, including a reexamination at the time of discharge (usually at two or three days of age). If a baby is sent home less than forty-eight hours after birth, a recheck in the office is advisable a few days later. Another check may be done at the first week or two of age, especially if this is your first baby. (Typically the baby's first few days—and nights—at home generate a million questions for rookie parents; be sure to bring a list.) In addition to being looked over from stem to stern by a doctor, a new baby will usually have a few specific screening tests:

- **A hearing test.** Out of a thousand otherwise normal newborns, between one and three have significant hearing loss that can have a major effect on speech, language, and learning. Often this problem is not detected until after the first birthday, but the American Academy of Pediatrics recommends that care for hearing loss begin before six months of age. Tests that are both painless and relatively simple can now be done to check hearing, typically before the newborn leaves the hospital.
- **Tests for metabolic birth defects.** These are biochemical abnormalities that are usually not apparent at birth but can cause serious medical problems, retardation, and even death if not treated properly. Testing usually involves pricking the infant's heel to obtain a few drops of blood, which are then sent to a lab for analysis. This type of screening is mandated in every state, but the tests that are required vary from state to state. The most commonly screened conditions include:
    1. **Phenylketonuria (PKU),** which can cause mental retardation unless a special diet is followed.
    2. **Congenital hypothyroidism,** in which a deficiency of thyroid hormone interferes with growth and brain development. Thyroid hormone given orally corrects this problem.
    3. **Galactosemia,** which involves an inability of the baby to convert a form of sugar found in milk, called **galactose,** into glucose. The accumulation of galactose can cause retardation or death and can be prevented by removing milk and other products containing lactose or galactose from the infant's diet.
    4. **Sickle cell disease,** which involves a slight alteration of the protein hemoglobin that carries oxygen within red blood cells. This disease affects about one in 600 people of African-American descent. Early detection can help parents and physicians anticipate (and thus prevent) some of its complications.

PKU, congenital hypothyroidism, and galactosemia are the only three metabolic conditions for which screening is required in all fifty states.

F.Y.I.

The term *sickle cell* refers to a characteristic curved distortion of red cells that can occur in this disease. This change in shape (from their normal disclike configuration) causes "sludging" in the smaller blood vessels and capillaries, resulting in impaired blood flow to vital organs. This decreased blood flow leads to more rapid destruction of red cells, leading to anemia and other potentially dangerous consequences.

Examinations during the first year are typically carried out at one, two, four, six, nine, and twelve months of age. A number of immunizations—**diphtheria, tetanus, pertussis (DTaP), *Haemophilus influenzae* type B (Hib), polio, pneumococcus, and hepatitis B**—are typically given at or between the two-, four-, and six-month visits (see chapter 11). In addition, a **hemoglobin** or **hematocrit,** a simple test to check for anemia (a shortage of red blood cells), may be recommended at nine months of age or after. At that age, depending upon certain risk factors, screening tests may also be done to check blood lead levels and exposure to **tuberculosis.**

The American Dental Association recommends that a child's first dental checkup occur after the eruption of the first tooth but before the first birthday. The timetable for further checks can be discussed at that time, but you can assume that everyone in the family who has teeth should have a rendezvous with the dentist or dental hygienist every six months.

Examinations during the toddler and preschool years include an eighteen-month visit. After that checkups should occur annually. Toddlers normally receive the first **MMR (measles, mumps, rubella)** and **chickenpox (varicella) vaccinations** and the DTaP, polio, Hib, and pneumococcus boosters at twelve to eighteen months of age. At the beginning of influenza season in the fall, infants six to twenty-three months of age should receive the flu vaccine. Normally immunizations are not given at ages two, three, or four unless there is a need to catch up on any that were missed earlier in infancy. Because a number of vaccinations and tests are routinely done at age five before entering school (see below), some practitioners will carry out part of this assignment at age four. If the child's behavior raises any questions about vision or hearing, more formal testing may be done at this time. (Obviously this becomes easier to carry out as the child gets older and can cooperate.)

Examinations during the grade school years (ages five through ten) often "start off with a bang" at age five, when a number of immunizations and other tests must be completed before beginning kindergarten. Preschool booster doses of MMR, DTaP, and polio vaccines are given at this time. In addition, usually a tuberculosis (TB) skin test will be applied, the urine checked, and a finger poked for a drop of blood to look for anemia. Often the number of discomforts in this lineup, necessary though they may be, can be so unpleasant for the child (not to mention parents and nursing staff) that the physician may elect to do some of them at the four-year checkup. Routine exams are recommended at ages six, eight, and ten, including vision and hearing checks.

Examinations during the adolescent years (ages eleven through the teen years) are the most likely to be skipped or relegated to camp or sports physicals that may cover only some of the important bases. But because of the important developments—physical, emotional, and behavioral—that occur during this passage from childhood to adulthood, yearly checkups are definitely a wise idea. In addition to a general review and troubleshooting, frank discussion of teenage risk behaviors is strongly recommended at this time.

- **Immunizations need to be rechecked** at the adolescent visit at age eleven or twelve. At this time a DTaP (tetanus, diphtheria, and pertussis) booster and a dose of **meningococcal vaccine** are given, as well as any other "catch-up" immunizations that might be needed. (See chapter 11.)
- **Hearing and vision screening** every three years (for example, at ages twelve, fifteen, and eighteen).
- **A blood count** to check for anemia or any blood-cell abnormalities at least once during the adolescent years.
- **A urinalysis** at least once during these years.
- **A pelvic exam and Pap smear** for females who have had vaginal intercourse, regardless of age. Routine pelvic exams and Pap smears should be initiated between the ages of eighteen and twenty-one, even for those who have not been sexually active.
- **Discussions about risky behavior:** tobacco, alcohol and drug use, sexual activity, and unsafe use of things with wheels (bicycles, skateboards, scooters, motorcycles, and automobiles). Remember that your teenager's physician may—or may not—have the time or the inclination to delve into these subjects during a busy day in the office. Also, you may want to inquire about his or her views on these subjects, especially teen sexuality, to confirm that they are compatible with the values you embrace and teach to your children. And though a well-timed conversation with a wise and caring professional can have a real impact on an adolescent's life, your son or daughter spends far more waking hours in *your* company. The values you instill (and live out) at home every day are the primary barriers to risky behavior.

The reasons for pelvic exams and Pap smears are discussed in detail in chapter 4.

F.Y.I.

We will take a more detailed look at the subject of preventing a variety of risky behaviors among children and adolescents in chapters 10–12. The important task of passing the baton, transferring your values to the next generation, is also covered in detail in the Focus on the Family *Parents' Guide to Teen Health* (Colorado Springs, Colo: Focus on the Family, 1997).

Adult Checkups

Once you have reached adulthood, how often should you have a general physical exam, assuming nothing in particular is bothering you? Do you need an annual physical, or is some other interval more appropriate? You might be

continued on page 38

WHAT EXACTLY IS A BLOOD COUNT?

This common lab test may be done at your child's five-year checkup, at a routine visit sometime during the teen years, and at any number of times throughout life for screening or troubleshooting.

The term *blood count* may refer either to a simple hemoglobin or hematocrit, or to a more elaborate study called a complete blood count (or CBC) that includes these two measures and many others. A CBC looks at the status of **red blood cells** that carry life-sustaining oxygen, **white blood cells** that play a vital role in immunity, and **platelets**, smaller but complex cells that circulate in the blood and are "first on scene" to begin the clotting process when the lining of a blood vessel is damaged. A CBC can be carried out on blood drawn from a vein or gently squeezed from a prick on the fingertip. (In a newborn or young infant, the heel is usually pricked rather than the finger.)

Important measurements involving the red blood cells include:

- Hemoglobin, the vital protein within red cells that carries oxygen.
- Hematocrit (often called the "crit" by doctors when they're in a hurry) is the volume of blood that consists of red cells, expressed as a percentage of the total. A hematocrit of 45, for example—a robust number for an adult—indicates that 45 percent of a given amount of blood is red cells, and the rest is the watery liquid (the serum) in which they are suspended plus a small amount of other solid materials (primarily white cells and platelets).
- Other measurements of red cells, including their actual number (there are roughly 4 to 6 million in a cubic millimeter of blood), their size, and the average amount of hemoglobin each one contains.

A person who is short on red cells is said to be **anemic**, a condition that may develop relatively quickly (usually after a sudden loss of blood), or over weeks or even months. The various red cell measurements can provide helpful clues to the cause of anemia. For example, small red cells are seen in iron deficiency or in certain hereditary hemoglobin abnormalities. Certain types of anemia, in which the red cells are abnormally large, may be caused by a deficiency of vitamin B_{12} or folic acid.

With red cells it is also possible to have too much of a good thing. In a condition called **polycythemia** (which is far less common than anemia), there are too many red cells in circulation. If the hematocrit rises too high, circulation can be impaired as the blood flow becomes more sluggish (as when too many cars are jammed on the freeway).

Polycythemia is one of a very few medical conditions that may require periodic bloodletting to restore a normal blood count. In the eighteenth century, physicians mistakenly believed that this practice would help or cure a vast number of problems. Overzealous removal of blood almost certainly speeded the death of George Washington, who at the time was suffering from a severe sore throat. Had he lived two hundred years later, he would have been treated with antibiotics—and his red cells would have been left where they belonged.

A CBC also looks at the number of white blood cells in circulation, which typically number several thousand per cubic milliliter of blood (5,000 to 10,000 is a common result). The significance of a high or low white count depends on what else is going on. An elevated count (over 11,000) could indicate that a bacterial infection is under way, for example, but several other factors—acute arthritis, a burn, certain medications, even exertion or anxiety—could have the same effect. A much higher white cell count—30,000 to 50,000 or more—could represent an exaggerated white cell response to infection or inflammation, but it also raises more ominous concerns about overproduction of white cells, specifically **leukemia**, which can afflict both children and adults. A count in this range should prompt a thorough medical evaluation. A low white cell count (2,500 to 5,000) may be seen in many viral infections or may have other causes. (For some individuals, however, this may be their normal count throughout life, without any ill effect.) White cell counts below 2,000 may affect a person's ability to resist infections.

In addition to the number of white cells in circulation, the type of white cells roaming through the bloodstream at any given time may provide clues to a medical problem. A CBC includes a listing of several different types of white cells (usually five) and the percentage of each in circulation. This is called the **differential** (or the "diff" in medical shorthand), and it may be generated by the machine that runs the CBC or by a technologist looking at the white cells under a microscope. A significant departure from the expected range of percentages in one or more cell types can be an important clue in a medical evaluation.

Finally, the **platelet count** is included in most CBCs. Normally it ranges from 150,000 to 450,000 per cubic millimeter of blood. Lower numbers (called **thrombocytopenia**) may occur when the production of platelets declines, their destruction accelerates, or both. Levels below 50,000 may result in excessive bleeding from injury or surgery, and platelet counts below 20,000 can result in significant bleeding even without provocation. Less common is **thrombocytosis**, in which the platelet count is excessively high. When there are a million or more platelets per cubic millimeter of blood, abnormal clotting may occur. Abnormally low or high platelet counts can have many causes, and consultation with a **hematologist**—a physician who specializes in disorders of the blood—is usually needed for a diagnosis and list of appropriate treatment options. ■

A cubic millimeter is a tiny volume—the space occupied by a cube whose sides measure one millimeter, or about one-twenty-fifth of an inch. The fact that millions of red cells, thousands of white cells, and hundreds of thousands of platelets are present and functioning in every cubic millimeter of blood is truly astonishing.

Platelets are also called **thrombocytes**, from the Greek roots *thrombo* or "clot," and *cyte* or "cell." The suffix *penia* comes from the Greek word for poverty, so the fancy word *thrombocytopenia* boils down to mean "poor in clot cells." The suffix *-osis,* which shows up constantly in medical terminology, can mean "abnormal," "diseased," or "increased." The word *thrombocytosis* literally means "increased clot cells."

WHAT EXACTLY IS A URINALYSIS?

A urinalysis (or "UA" in doctor shorthand) is one of the more useful (and one of the least expensive) tests for basic screening and also for evaluation of a number of medical problems. Medical laboratories, hospitals, clinics, urgent-care centers, and most primary-care physician offices can carry out this procedure. It consists of three components.

First, the **color** and **general appearance** of the urine is noted. Obviously most of the time it will be clear and yellow, but the presence of blood, bilirubin (in someone who is jaundiced), or certain medications can change its color, usually to amber, orange, or red. Urine may also be cloudy for a variety of reasons (for example, because of debris present during an infection).

Second is the **chemistry** portion, which involves using a disposable plastic "dipstick" that is inserted into the freshly voided urine, then pulled out and observed over the next couple of minutes. Attached to it is a row of several small square chemical pads, which change color in response to various characteristics of the urine. These usually include:

- Concentration (called the **specific gravity**).
- Acidity (called the **pH**).
- The presence of **hemoglobin,** which usually (but not always) reflects the presence of at least some red blood cells in the urine.
- The presence of **protein,** which may be trivial or significant depending upon the amount and the clinical situation.
- The presence of **glucose** (blood sugar), which indicates that blood glucose levels were high enough above normal to "spill" into the urine.
- The presence of **ketones**, which may reflect a recent absence of food (or specifically carbohydrates). Ketones may also be present in the urine of a diabetic—and nearly always in the sample of someone with type 1 (also called insulin-dependent) diabetes whose blood glucose is significantly out of control.
- The presence of **bilirubin**, a by-product of the normal breakdown of hemoglobin that accumulates in the bloodstream when the liver is not functioning properly. (People with very high levels of bilirubin in the blood appear yellow or **jaundiced**.) If bilirubin is not being properly excreted by the liver into the intestinal tract, it may appear in the urine, giving it a darker, amber color.

Based on the degree of color change, the dipstick can provide a crude indication of the amount of these substances, but not a direct measurement. While abnormalities may require further evaluation, the significance of any of these findings must be put into perspective by the examining physician.

The third component of a urinalysis is called the **microscopic** evaluation of what is called the urine sediment. The **sediment** is the solid material that collects at the bottom of a test tube full of urine when it is spun in a centrifuge for a few minutes. Nearly all of the liquid is poured off, and then a drop containing the sediment is placed on a glass slide and checked under a microscope. The examiner makes note of any red and/or white blood cells, bacteria, casts (which are microscopic cylinders, composed of various substances that may be formed within the kidney), crystals, and cells from various parts of the urinary tract. A detailed account of the significance of these findings is beyond the scope of this book, and (as with the dipstick) the results must be assessed by a qualified practitioner in light of a person's history, symptoms, examination, and other tests.

One very important component of a meaningful urinalysis is obtaining a good specimen. Unfortunately, cells, bacteria, and other debris that are not actually in the urine can easily wind up in the collection cup, especially in infants and in females of all ages. For this reason you will typically be asked to obtain what is called a **clean-catch midstream urine specimen**. This involves first cleaning the area around the urethra (the narrow tube from which urine exits the body) to remove any local contaminants. The lab or office should have a supply of small moist individually wrapped towelettes available in the lavatory for this purpose.

Men and boys should clean the head of the penis. Women and girls should part the area between the labia (or lips) at the opening of the vagina and gently clean between them; ideally, the urine should be obtained while the labia are still being held apart. Then, as urine begins to flow, a small amount should be allowed to fall into the toilet before the collection cup is brought into the stream. After an ounce or two flows into the cup, it should be removed from the stream. This avoidance of urine from the beginning and the end of the stream helps reduce the amount of contaminating material in the specimen. Needless to say, young children will need a little help from a parent to complete this task. For an infant, a small plastic bag with an adhesive lining may be placed over the penis or the labia after a gentle cleansing. When urine appears in the bag, it can be transferred into a sterile container and taken as soon as possible to the office or lab.

There are some situations in which it is so important to obtain an uncontaminated specimen that these basic collection methods will not be adequate. Very often this involves the need to determine if an infection is present, and if so what bacteria is the culprit. In an adult (more often a woman), a physician or nurse may need to insert a thin sterile plastic catheter into the bladder via the urethra, obtain the urine, and then remove it. In an infant who is very ill, a small catheter may be used or a physician may obtain a urine specimen by briefly and very carefully inserting a thin needle directly into the bladder through the lower abdominal wall. This may sound like a drastic measure, but it is in fact a relatively straightforward procedure and can provide vital information, especially when a baby under three months of age is running a fever over 100.4°. At that young age, an infection may be more serious and symptoms may be vague, so accurate information about any possible bacterial infection is very important. ■

continued from page 33

surprised to learn that, unlike the widely accepted guidelines for children, there is no universally accepted set of recommendations for *general* screening exams in adults. Instead, as you will discover in the next two chapters, there are a host of guidelines for screening *specific* problems, many of which apply only to men or women. How do you cover all of these bases?

Women are more likely to have a regular physical in the context of routine pelvic exams and Pap smears, which are commonly done every year throughout adulthood by a gynecologist, family physician, or internist. Depending on the time allotted and the thoroughness of the physician, these may or may not cover other important areas such as cholesterol screening. Men have no counterpart to this exam, although some may make a regular visit to a urologist when a problem develops in the prostate gland. However, these visits are rarely comprehensive.

One recommendation for broad-based screening comes from the American Cancer Society, which suggests that adults regularly undergo a cancer-related checkup as part of a routine screening visit every three years between the ages of twenty and thirty-nine, and annually thereafter. The cancer-related checkup involves a look at possible trouble spots such as the mouth, thyroid, lymph nodes, skin, breasts, and ovaries in women, and the prostate in men fifty and over. It also includes a review of any risky behaviors (such as smoking) and any specific tests (such as a colonoscopy) that might be appropriate. Of course, other screening unrelated to cancer could be carried out at such a visit, when appropriate.

A reasonable approach would be to follow this basic game plan of a general review every three years until age forty and then annually thereafter, modifying it according to the recommendations of your own physician. (As already noted, most women younger than forty will be having Pap smears on a more frequent basis.) This schedule does not require that a full gamut of screening tests be done at each visit, but rather provides an opportunity to do a basic once-over and then decide what (if any) studies might be appropriate.

We will look at all of the tests currently recommended for screening specific cancers in chapter 4.

And what studies might those be? The next two chapters will tell you all about them.

QUESTIONS TO PONDER:

1. The section in this chapter entitled "Your Lifestyle: Health Booster—or Buster?" contains enough questions to keep you thinking for weeks. If you find them a bit overwhelming, look through that section again (beginning on page 19) and pick out three or four questions that you find particularly interesting (or worrisome). Then feel free to take a look at the chapters that deal with them in more detail.
2. When was the last time you had a general checkup? Based on the suggestions in the last section ("Adult Checkups"), do you need one? What about your other family members?
3. Do you have a primary-care physician—someone who looks after the whole person—for you and your children?

Action item: If you haven't done so already, begin compiling a basic summary of health history and current status for each member of your family. (See "Your Health History," beginning on page 17.) If you have a computer with basic word processing, you can easily update these.

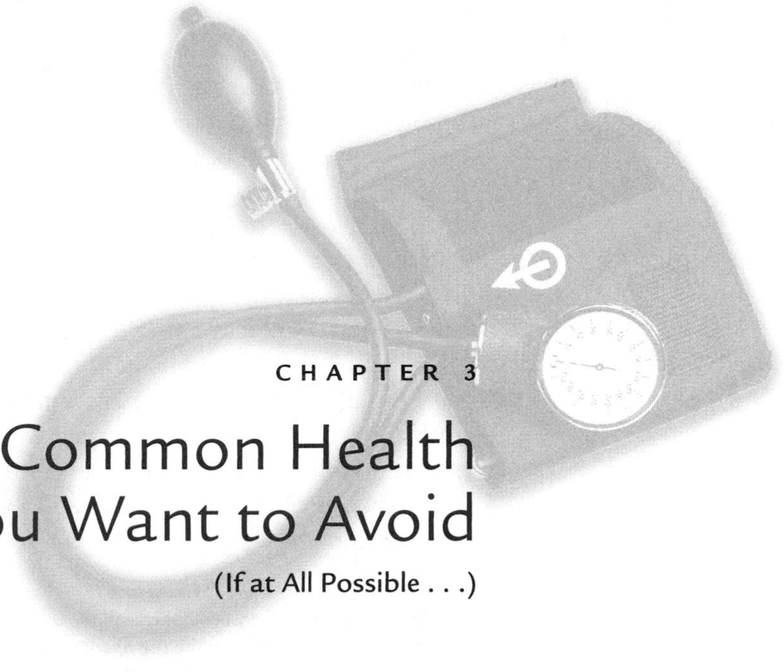

CHAPTER 3

Three Common Health Problems You Want to Avoid

(If at All Possible . . .)

While this book is not an encyclopedia of diseases, it *is* intended to help you avoid a number of major health robbers that are potentially preventable—especially when appropriate screening is done on a regular basis. In order to be informed and motivated to do what is necessary to avoid them, it's wise to know your enemy. Three health problems—cardiovascular disease, cancer, and diabetes—are very common and frequently serious, but with due diligence they often can be intercepted at an early stage or prevented altogether. Since we will be mentioning them on a regular basis throughout this book, some introductions are in order.

Arteries Behaving Badly: Cardiovascular Disease

Year after year, without fail, arteries that become obstructed (or, less commonly, that rupture) cause more deaths among adults in the United States and other developed countries than any other type of problem. **Arteries** are the blood vessels that carry blood from the heart to every organ and tissue in the body. The major arteries divide into smaller and smaller branches, eventually reaching a microscopic diameter (in what are called **capillaries**) through which red blood cells pass single file to deliver their life-sustaining oxygen before returning to the heart via the veins. Nothing in our body can function properly for any length of time without a steady supply of oxygen; if deprived long enough, a cell, tissue, organ—or person—will die. While we might think of arteries as passive tubes through which blood flows like water through a drainpipe, they are actually complex, active structures. Unfortunately, they can also become diseased.

Under the influence of our heredity and our habits, the tissue that forms the inner lining of arteries can be damaged, allowing deposits of fatty material called **plaque** to form. This nasty-looking stuff can accumulate locally or extensively throughout one or more arteries, until only a fraction of the normal blood flow can pass, much like a freeway littered by wreckage that slows normal traffic. If the demand for blood in some part of the body outstrips what a clogged artery can deliver to it, the affected area may begin to protest. For example, the muscles in our legs need a lot more blood when we are walking or running than when we are sitting still. If the arteries that supply them become obstructed, these muscles will sound off with pain after one walks a short distance, a phenomenon called **claudication**.

F.Y.I.

Over the past few centuries, medical practitioners have created a vast and intimidating vocabulary, which often involves the use of convoluted terms for everyday experiences. But behind nearly all of its ninety-eight-cent words are some basic Greek or Latin roots that translate "medicalese" into very simple concepts. Throughout this book we will include a number of margin notes that will explain the derivations (and thus the meaning) of many medical terms. The word *claudication* comes from the Latin word for limping, *claudicare,* which is what happens when this pain occurs.

Even more critical are the **coronary arteries** that supply the heart itself. When these become so narrow that they cannot supply enough blood to satisfy the immediate need of an area of heart muscle, a distress signal known as **angina pectoris** may arise. This is a discomfort felt as pain or pressure across the chest, sometimes described as squeezing or "like someone standing on me," lasting for a few minutes or longer and then subsiding. Usually this is felt on the left side but can also be felt in the center of the chest. The discomfort may also occur in the arm, neck, jaw, shoulder, or back, most commonly on the left side. Like many symptoms we might experience, angina doesn't always go by the book. It may skip the chest and show up merely as arm or jaw pain, or even as an unexpected shortness of breath from mild exertion such as climbing a flight of stairs. An adult who feels this type of discomfort for the first time needs urgent medical evaluation to determine whether or not the problem involves the heart and to take whatever action is appropriate.

If the blood and oxygen supply catches up with the demand relatively quickly (whether on its own or when medication such as nitroglycerin is given), the pain/pressure will fade away. But if any area of the heart is deprived of oxygen long enough, the muscle involved will be injured and eventually die, an incident commonly called a **heart attack**. This is a highly dangerous situation, because damaged heart cells have a tendency to become unstable, provoking rhythm patterns that can be erratic or sometimes even lethal.

The coronary arteries were so named because their distribution around the upper end of the heart vaguely resembles a crown.

The Latin phrase *angina pectoris* literally means "strangling of the chest," an apt description of this feeling.

The medical term for a heart attack is **myocardial infarction** (or **infarct** for short), usually abbreviated by the initials *MI. Myocardial* literally means "muscle of the heart." The word *infarct,* which refers to any tissue that has died from loss of its blood supply, comes from a Latin verb meaning to "cram" or "stuff." The word was undoubtedly picked because the artery supplying the dead tissue is typically "stuffed" with blood clot or plaque.

The most feared complication of a heart attack is called **ventricular fibrillation**. The ventricles are the larger, lower chambers of the heart that pump blood into the lungs (right ventricle) and the rest of the body (left ventricle). Fibrillation is rapid, chaotic, uncoordinated movement of heart muscle. In ventricular fibrillation, therefore, the life-sustaining lower chambers of the heart suddenly stop contracting and merely vibrate or quiver, effectively stopping the flow of blood to the rest of the body. If this is not quickly reversed, life will end within a matter of minutes. Those who survive a heart attack may have other problems if enough muscle was damaged to impair the heart's overall performance.

IS THAT PAIN IN MY CHEST COMING FROM MY HEART?

If you tell your doctor that you've been "having a little chest pain," don't be surprised if you receive a series of rapid-fire questions about its severity, duration, location, and relationship to activities such as walking, lifting, eating, or sex. The purpose of this interrogation is usually to determine whether coronary artery disease can be ruled out as a suspect. Characteristics that suggest that the discomfort does *not* come from the heart include:

- Pain that comes in sudden twinges lasting a few seconds or less. (Pain arising from the heart usually rises and falls more slowly, and typically lasts at least a few minutes.)
- Pain that is localized in a very small area of the chest (for example, the size of a fingertip). People experiencing discomfort from the heart usually use their entire palm or a fist to show where it hurts.
- Pain that changes with touch—in other words, local tenderness—or with body movement, position, or deep breaths.

All of these examples are typical of pain arising from the chest wall (ribs, muscles, and ligaments, and the nerves that supply them) or from the **pleura**, the thin but highly sensitive membrane that covers the lungs and lines the inside of the chest cavity. Unfortunately, many problems can mimic the pain or pressure of a heart deprived of oxygen. A wayward gallstone, a spasm of the esophagus (which carries food from mouth to stomach), a blood clot that has floated from a vein in a leg or the pelvis to the lung, or even intense anxiety are some of the events that can generate some alarming discomfort in the chest. Because an error in judgment and diagnosis could be disastrous, it is always wise to have any chest pain addressed immediately by a qualified health professional. Unless a competent physician advises otherwise on the phone, this will usually entail a visit to the nearest emergency room, where an appropriate evaluation can be carried out as quickly as possible. ■

Appropriately enough, the word *pleura* comes from the Greek word for "rib" or "side." When the pleura becomes irritated on one or both sides of the chest, the pain that results (called **pleurisy**) is usually very intense, but sharp and quick, like a sudden jab in the side.

There are two sobering realities of **coronary heart disease**, or **CHD**: One is the enormous number of lives it affects every year. According to the American Heart Association:

One out of every five deaths in the United States is the result of coronary heart disease.

- CHD causes or contributes to approximately 656,000 deaths every year in the United States—more than any other health problem.
- Although CHD commonly affects men at an earlier age than women, it is an equal opportunity killer: The number of deaths each year among women is nearly equal to the number among men.

F.Y.I. Many women tend to be more concerned about cancer—especially of the breast or cervix—than coronary heart disease. Appropriate screening for cancer is very important, as we will see in chapter 4. But every year more than five times as many women die from coronary disease than from breast cancer and cervical cancer combined. Needless to say, coronary heart disease isn't just a "guy thing."

- More than 13 million Americans are estimated to have CHD. Of these approximately 865,000 will have a heart attack this year, and about four out of ten will die as a result. This translates to an astonishing frequency of coronary events: one every twenty-six seconds and a death almost every minute.[1]

The second reality is more chilling. About 335,000 people die every year from CHD either in an emergency room or before reaching a hospital, typically the result of a heart attack suddenly provoking a lethal cardiac rhythm. This means that for a significant number of people with narrowed coronary arteries, the *first indication that something is wrong will be sudden death.* Because of this potential for instantaneous catastrophe and because cardiologists (physicians who specialize in caring for the heart) now can perform interventions that preserve heart muscle if action is taken quickly enough, it is imperative that a person having chest discomfort seek immediate medical attention.

The traditional medical term for a stroke is *cerebrovascular accident,* or *CVA* for short. (*Cerebrovascular* is a fancy word combining terms for brain and blood vessels.) The newer term **brain attack** also refers to a stroke.

The other place in which diseased arteries can wreak havoc is in the brain. Every year in the United States some 700,000 people suffer a **stroke,** and more than 162,000 die—the third most common cause of death among adults, after heart disease and cancer. If strokelike symptoms resolve within twenty-four hours, the incident is called a **transient ischemic attack,** or **TIA.** The original and still widely used term *stroke* was inspired by the sudden, lightning-like loss of function that occurs when the flow of blood to an area of the brain is interrupted. Virtually anything controlled by the brain can be affected by a stroke—speech, movement of an arm or leg (or both), balance, vision, consciousness, or life itself.

The term *ischemic* comes from two Greek words that mean "to keep back blood." It usually refers to a reduction in the blood supply to a part of the body that is significant enough to cause symptoms, but it may be reversible.

More than 60 percent of strokes involve the sudden closure of a diseased artery, while about one in four occurs when a clot floats into an artery in the brain from some other part of the body. The most dreaded form of stroke doesn't arise from the sudden obstruction of an artery but rather a leak or rupture that allows blood to flow freely into the brain (called a **cerebral hemor-**

rhage). Sudden severe headache, nausea and vomiting, and loss of consciousness are common symptoms of a cerebral hemorrhage, and more than a third of these result in death within thirty days.

F.Y.I.

A **clot** (or some other type of material) that drifts through the bloodstream from one part of the body to another and blocks an artery is called an **embolus,** from the Greek word for a stopper or plug. A clot (usually from a vein in the pelvis or leg) that floats into an artery in the lung is called a **pulmonary embolus,** and a stroke arising from a drifting clot is called an **embolic stroke.**

Stroke is the leading cause of long-term disability in the United States. Among 4.6 million stroke survivors, more than a million experience some form of long-term limitation in daily activities. While 50 to 70 percent of stroke victims are able to eventually regain their independence, 20 percent require care in a nursing home or similar facility three months after the initial episode.[2]

F.Y.I.

Many but not all strokes arise from an **aneurysm,** an abnormally dilated or bulging segment of one of the blood vessels within the brain. This may arise from a local defect present from birth or from factors such as high blood pressure, atherosclerosis, or trauma. An aneurysm may remain stable for decades and not cause any symptoms until it ruptures, or it may generate a variety of symptoms as it gradually enlarges.

What causes arteries to become diseased and obstructed? The most common culprit is a process called **atherosclerosis,** which refers to a mix of fatty material, cholesterol, calcium, fibrin (a protein ingredient of blood clots), and miscellaneous cellular debris that can form a dense plaque within the lining of a major artery. Damage to the inner lining of an artery allows this material to gain a toehold, which in turn stimulates the growth of new cells, accumulation of more fat and debris, and so on until the plaque begins to impair the flow of blood. This may by itself cause symptoms (such as chest pain with exertion) or remain silent for years, even when as much as 90 percent or more of the artery's diameter is obstructed.

The word *atherosclerosis* was invented in the early twentieth century by combining Greek words for "hard" and "porridge." Anyone who has actually seen this stomach-churning material can confirm that "hard porridge" is an apt description.

If an artery suddenly closes, the results are usually dramatic and often catastrophic—a stroke, a cool and painful leg, gripping chest pain, or sudden collapse with an abnormal heart rhythm—depending on the size and location of the particular artery involved. Occasionally, the closing of an artery causes milder symptoms or none at all. Usually this occurs when more than one artery supplies blood to the same tissue, or if the amount of tissue involved is very limited. Some people, for example, have "silent" heart attacks in which the symptoms are vague or nonexistent, and damaged heart muscle isn't detected until months or years later, if ever. (Usually, these involve the closing of a narrow, distant branch of one of the coronary arteries.)

Why does a particular artery suddenly close? Often a damaged segment attracts platelets, the microscopic structures (smaller than red or white cells) circulating in blood that begin the clotting process, which can suddenly block the artery. Sometimes blood will suddenly seep into a thick plaque lining an artery, causing the plaque to swell and obstruct blood flow. Unfortunately, either of these events can occur whether an artery is tightly or only partially narrowed by plaque. Indeed, a lot of current research effort is focused on understanding why some plaques remain stable while others suddenly swell or attract a clot.

Numerous risk factors can contribute to this scenario, and it is vitally important to identify any that could potentially threaten your health and shorten your life. Keep in mind that there are degrees of severity for many of these. Furthermore, the risk factors compound one another; in other words, the total risk may be worse than the sum of its various parts.

The risk factors for cardiovascular disease fall into two main groups: those you can't change and those you can. The first group includes:

Your age. The more birthday candles on your cake, the longer any other risk factors have to stir up trouble. Over 80 percent of those who die from coronary artery disease are sixty-five or older. The risk of a stroke doubles every decade past the age of fifty-five.

Your sex. While overall deaths from coronary artery disease are about equally divided between men and women, men are more likely to experience heart attacks and sudden death, and to have them earlier in life. Overall, women lag behind men by about twenty years in the timing of these events, but they make up for lost time after menopause. Each year about 40,000 more women than men have a stroke, and more than 60 percent of stroke deaths occur among women.

Your heredity—family history and race. Without question, all of the other risk factors play out against a background of a basic genetic vulnerability, or resistance, to developing diseased arteries. Some of us are blessed with a heritage in which long lives are common and heart attack or stroke is completely absent from the family tree. But if any immediate family members—one or both parents, one or more brothers and sisters—have had coronary artery disease or a stroke, you are at higher risk. The more family members affected and the earlier the trouble began, the more concerned you should be. In addition, African-Americans are more vulnerable to coronary disease and stroke than Caucasians. This is due in part to their tendency toward higher blood pressure, but other factors (including socioeconomic issues and access to health care) may play a role as well. Similarly, Latinos, Native Americans, and native Hawaiians are more prone to coronary artery disease, partly because of higher rates of obesity and diabetes in these groups.[3]

The second group of risk factors includes those we can modify by changing our habits or through a physician's intervention, or both. A number of these, especially those involving lifestyle, are so important that we will spend a good deal of time reviewing them later in this book.

Cigarette smoking leads the pack, so to speak, because it stimulates the formation of plaque, increases blood pressure, tightens arteries, promotes clot formation, and makes the heart more irritable. As a result, smokers not only have twice the risk of a heart attack compared to nonsmokers, but they are also much more likely to die suddenly as a result. A smoker's exhaust irritates nonsmoking bystanders who are unfortunate enough to inhale it, and it tampers with their arteries as well. Furthermore, smoking amplifies the effects of any other risk factors that may be present. For those who have racked up a few other risk factors for arterial disease, cigarettes are literal gas on the fire. The more smoke inhaled every day, the more likely an untimely trip to the hospital—or the mortuary—lies ahead.

We will take a detailed look at the entire gamut of problems caused by tobacco use (and some strategies to quit smoking) in chapter 10.

High blood pressure, also called **hypertension,** is the most important risk factor for stroke but also ranks highly as a cause for coronary artery disease, heart attack, heart failure, and kidney damage. Consistent readings of 140/90 or more (see sidebar "Blood Pressure Basics" on page 52) indicate an increased risk and a need for action, including lifestyle changes and, when appropriate, medication. (For some people with a significant collection of risk factors—for example, known diabetes and coronary artery disease—treatment may be started for pressures that are a little lower.) The higher the pressure, the larger the risk and the more urgent the need for intervention. There are a number of ways to help reduce blood pressure without using medication. But even the best efforts often fail to bring adequate results, and medications that lower blood pressure (called **antihypertensive drugs**) may be recommended. It is now possible to control a wayward blood pressure without having to endure any side effects, other than the inconvenience of purchasing and taking the medication every day. Many antihypertensive medications actually provide added benefits, such as protecting the lining of arteries or preventing migraine headaches.

HOT TIP

Most of the things you can do to lower your blood pressure without drugs involve lifestyle changes that are wise whether or not you have hypertension.

Elevated levels and unfavorable blends of cholesterol and triglycerides. A mountain of research has connected these circulating compounds, collectively known as **lipids,** with the risk of developing diseased, congested arteries. Like blood pressure, higher levels mean higher risk—but in this case the equation involves more than one number. Reducing cholesterol and triglycerides to safe levels is an extremely important project and may involve weight loss, improved eating habits, exercise, and sometimes medications.

How do you lower your cholesterol? Like high blood pressure, cholesterol can be lowered through lifestyle changes, medication, or both. The nondrug approaches include some advisories that may sound familiar by now:

- **Lose excess weight.** This can be amazingly effective at lowering cholesterol. Very often a modest loss—ten or fifteen pounds, for example—is enough to send cholesterol plummeting.

- **Increase physical activity.** Consistent exercise helps lower total cholesterol and tends to raise the HDL ("good") cholesterol.
- **Reduce saturated fats** to less than 7 percent of total daily calories and cholesterol to less than 200 mg per day. How do you do *that*? If you want the details, see pages 179–186 in chapter 5.
- **Consume 20 to 30 grams of fiber every day.** This nondigestible component of plant foods can bind cholesterol in the intestine and carry it out of the body.

We will review the basics of dietary fiber in chapter 5.

For some people with stubborn or very high cholesterol levels (which often run in families) or with a very high risk for coronary artery disease, medication may be not only appropriate, but also life preserving. Deciding whether to go this route, which medication to use, and how to follow your progress will require input from your physician. For years a high daily dose of niacin was widely used, but its acceptability was limited by an annoying tendency to cause skin flushing. It is, however, effective if taken in large enough doses (time-release formats are better tolerated), but these require lab follow-up to confirm that the dose is working and that the liver isn't being irritated.

Currently a group of drugs called **statins** rule the cholesterol roost, and for good reason. Not only are they highly effective at sinking the total and LDL cholesterols while preserving HDL, but by a separate mechanism they also appear to stabilize the linings of arteries, reducing the likelihood that plaques will form, expand, or generate clots. They are also very well-tolerated by most people, although some users have to change brands (or abandon them altogether) because of widespread muscle aching. Liver functions also are usually checked periodically while a person is taking a statin, although for the vast majority of users the liver shows no sign of distress.

The other statins currently on the market include, in alphabetical order, **atorvastatin (Lipitor), fluvastatin (Lescol), pravastatin (Pravachol), rosuvastatin (Crestor),** and **simvastatin (Zocor).**

Many people have heard about using red rice yeast extract as an alternative to prescription drugs to lower cholesterol. This substance is indeed effective, because it contains variable amounts of lovastatin, the compound used in the first prescription statin on the market (**Mevacor**) and the first available in a generic format. The bad news is that red rice yeast extract is unregulated, so you have little idea how much drug you may actually be taking. Those who choose this route will need medical monitoring (including liver function checks), just like those taking the prescription statins. Remember, a drug is a drug, whether it is extracted from a plant or manufactured by a pharmaceutical company.

Physical inactivity. It might come as a surprise to learn that a sedentary lifestyle—that is, one lacking in physical exercise—is as dangerous to your heart as smoking cigarettes. As we will describe in detail in chapter 7, this risk can usually be reduced by a relatively simple regime of moderate exercise, such as walking thirty minutes, five times per week.

WHAT ARE THE ODDS? — FOR MEN

How to calculate your chances of developing coronary heart disease

To get an idea of your risk of developing coronary heart disease over the next 10 years, use the Framingham Point Scores system below.[4]

1. Select your age. Circle your points.

AGE	POINTS
20–34	-9
35–39	-4
40–44	0
45–49	3
50–54	6
55–59	8
60–64	10
65–69	11
70–74	12
75–79	13

2. Select your HDL level. Circle your points.

HDL (mg/dl)	POINTS
≥60	-1
50–59	0
40–49	1
<40	2

3. Select your systolic level. Circle your points. Notice that you get more points (and thus have a higher risk) for a given blood pressure level that is *treated,* rather than untreated. That's because it is assumed that your pressure before treatment was higher, which carries some added residual risk.

SYSTOLIC BP (mmHg)	IF UNTREATED	IF TREATED
<120	0	0
120–129	0	1
130–139	1	2
140–159	1	2
≥160	2	3

4. Are you a smoker? Circle your points depending upon your answer and your age.

	POINTS (by age)				
	20–39	40–49	50–59	60–69	70–79
NONSMOKER	0	0	0	0	0
SMOKER	8	5	3	1	1

5. Select your cholesterol level. Circle your points depending upon your age.

	POINTS (by age)				
TOTAL CHOLESTEROL	20–39	40–49	50–59	60–69	70–79
<160	0	0	0	0	0
160–199	4	3	2	1	0
200–239	7	5	3	1	0
240–279	9	6	4	2	1
≥280	11	8	5	3	1

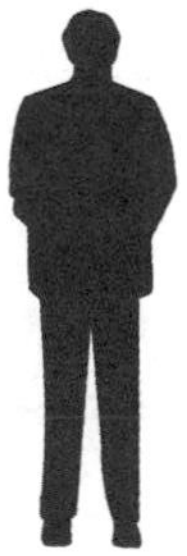

6. Circle your points. Determine your risk of getting coronary heart disease.

POINT TOTAL	10-YEAR RISK %	POINT TOTAL	10-YEAR RISK %	POINT TOTAL	10-YEAR RISK %
<0	<1	5	2	11	8
0	1	6	2	12	10
1	1	7	3	13	12
2	1	8	4	14	16
3	1	9	5	15	20
4	1	10	6	16	25
				≥17	≥30

If your 10-year risk for coronary disease is 20 percent or more, you should talk with your doctor about lowering your LDL cholesterol to 100 mg/dl or less—*the same goal recommended for those who have diabetes or who have already had a heart attack.* (See section "When do I need to think about lowering my cholesterol?" in the sidebar "Cholesterol Basics" on page 58.)

Source: The National Heart, Lung, and Blood Institute, a part of the National Institutes of Health and the U.S. Department of Health and Human Services.

Obesity. Carrying extra baggage, especially if a lot of it is concentrated around the waistline, increases your risk for developing diseased arteries. Much of obesity's role in this problem arises from its association with higher cholesterol, blood pressure, and glucose (blood sugar) levels.

Diabetes. This common disorder can exact a terrible toll on blood vessels and many other organ systems. We will look at diabetes a little later in this chapter.

All of the risk factors we have discussed so far have been well-established by current research. Some others have been proposed, although their impact on arteries is probably indirect. For example:

Stress. The impact of stress on arteries and the heart is unpredictable because it depends on two kinds of responses: how our bodies react and how we behave when life becomes unpleasant or threatening. For example, one person's antidote for a lousy day may be a pack of cigarettes or an entire box of cookies. Another's may be a good workout and a hot bath. One motorist responds to a colossal traffic jam with a shrug and thinks, *Hey, it gives me more time to think.* Another greets every red light with fists slamming the dashboard, a surge of adrenaline, and a soaring heart rate and blood pressure.

Excessive use of alcohol. More than two drinks per day for men and more than one for women can raise blood pressure. It can also elevate levels of triglycerides (which may contribute to clogged arteries), add enough calories to worsen obesity, increase the odds of having a stroke, and lead to heart failure.

The ebb and flow of hormones. The role of hormones in cardiovascular disease is a complex and controversial subject, whether the hormones are manufactured in our body or taken as supplements. We know that men are more likely to have heart attacks at an earlier age than women. We also know that after menopause the risk for coronary disease among women increases, and that this is particularly notable among women who have surgery to remove their ovaries before natural menopause. These observations led to a widespread assumption that if every woman took an estrogen supplement after menopause, the number of heart attacks in this age group could be significantly reduced. Unfortunately this idea has not been validated by controlled studies, and as a result, women are no longer being advised to take estrogen to protect their heart after natural menopause. The confusion is probably due to a mixed bag of effects: a modest improvement in cholesterol combined with a small (but not negligible) increase in the risk for forming blood clots, especially among women who smoke. The effects of progesterone, which has been routinely given to women along with estrogen if they have a uterus (to reduce the risk of cancer in its inner lining), have also muddied the water. The question of using (or avoiding) hormone supplements before or after menopause will no doubt continue to be a subject of research and controversy for many years to come.

continued on page 60

WHAT ARE THE ODDS? — FOR WOMEN

How to calculate your chances of developing coronary heart disease

To get an idea of your risk of developing coronary heart disease over the next 10 years, use the Framingham Point Scores system below.

1. Select your age. Circle your points.

AGE	POINTS
20–34	-7
35–39	-3
40–44	0
45–49	3
50–54	6
55–59	8
60–64	10
65–69	12
70–74	14
75–79	16

2. Select your HDL level. Circle your points.

HDL (mg/dl)	POINTS
≥60	-1
50–59	0
40–49	1
<40	2

3. Select your systolic level. Circle your points. Notice that you get more points (and thus have a higher risk) for a given blood pressure level that is *treated,* rather than untreated. That's because it is assumed that your pressure before treatment was higher, which carries some added residual risk.

SYSTOLIC BP (mmHg)	IF UNTREATED	IF TREATED
<120	0	0
120–129	1	3
130–139	2	4
140–159	3	5
≥160	4	6

4. Are you a smoker? Circle your points depending upon your answer and your age.

	POINTS (by age)				
	20–39	40–49	50–59	60–69	70–79
NONSMOKER	0	0	0	0	0
SMOKER	9	7	4	2	1

5. Select your cholesterol level. Circle your points depending upon your age.

	POINTS (by age)				
TOTAL CHOLESTEROL	20–39	40–49	50–59	60–69	70–79
<160	0	0	0	0	0
160–199	4	3	2	1	1
200–239	8	6	4	2	1
240–279	11	8	5	3	2
≥280	13	10	7	4	2

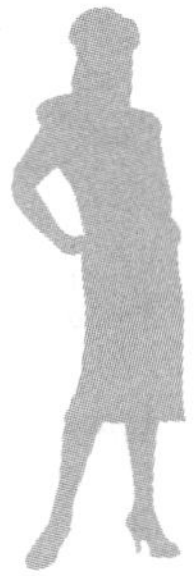

6. Circle your points. Determine your risk of getting coronary heart disease.

POINT TOTAL	10-YEAR RISK %	POINT TOTAL	10-YEAR RISK %	POINT TOTAL	10-YEAR RISK %
<9	<1	14	2	20	11
9	1	15	3	21	14
10	1	16	4	22	17
11	1	17	5	23	22
12	1	18	6	24	27
13	2	19	8	≥25	≥30

If your 10-year risk for coronary disease is 20 percent or more, you should talk with your doctor about lowering your LDL cholesterol to 100 mg/dl or less—*the same goal recommended for those who have diabetes or who have already had a heart attack.* (See section "When do I need to think about lowering my cholesterol?" in the sidebar "Cholesterol Basics" on page 58.)

Source: The National Heart, Lung, and Blood Institute, a part of the National Institutes of Health and the U.S. Department of Health and Human Services.

BLOOD PRESSURE BASICS

The term *hypertension* sounds like a psychological condition—the affliction of someone who is talking a mile a minute and seriously stressed. But the word actually has nothing to do with emotions. The *tension* in *hypertension* refers strictly to blood pressure, and *hyper* means literally "above" or "over," so the word indicates that blood is pulsing through the arteries at a pressure that is above normal. (Similarly, somebody whose blood pressure is too low is said to be **hypotensive**—*hypo* meaning "low"—and someone with normal pressure is **normotensive**.)

Blood doesn't flow through your arteries in a steady stream like water through a faucet, but rather in pulses produced by each contraction of the heart. As a result, a blood pressure measurement always includes two numbers, called the **systolic** and **diastolic** pressures, representing the high and low pressure of each beat. Blood pressure readings are expressed in the same units of measure used by weather forecasters when they talk about the barometer: millimeters of mercury or, more specifically, the pressure exerted by a column of mercury a given number of millimeters in height.

Blood pressure is typically measured using a **sphygmomanometer**—better known as a blood pressure cuff, an inflatable band connected by a flexible tube to a meter, digital display, or even an honest-to-goodness column of mercury that you can see rising and falling as the cuff wrapped around your upper arm is squeezed and released. The cuff is inflated to a level estimated to be higher than your systolic (peak) pressure. The momentary discomfort of this tight squeeze quickly fades as the cuff deflates, while the person checking the pressure uses a stethoscope or an electronic pickup to detect the sound of blood flowing through the main artery of the arm (called the **brachial artery**) as it passes the elbow joint. Nothing can be heard when the cuff is squeezing hard enough to stop the flow of blood altogether. As the cuff relaxes, a pulse can be heard as the blood begins to spurt past it, and then it will be silent again as blood flows without hindrance. (The sound is caused by turbulence, much like that made by water passing through a kink in a hose.)

The pressure at which the pulse is first heard is the peak or systolic level, and the point at which it disappears is the diastolic pressure. The two numbers are expressed as "systolic over diastolic," (for example, "120 over 80") and written as the two numbers separated by a line (120/80). Using the right-sized blood pressure cuff is important. If it is too small for a large arm, the pressure reading may be elevated above the true value because the cuff has to squeeze harder to compress the artery; less commonly, the reading may be low if the cuff is too large.

Blood pressure is a moving target, shifting constantly in response to all sorts of conditions in the body (and mind). Current research indicates that heart attack and stroke risk begins at pressures as low as 115/75 and doubles with each 20 mm rise in systolic pressure or 10 mm rise in diastolic pressure. As a result, blood pressures of 119/79 or less are considered normal while pressures in the range of 120–139/80–89 are classified as **prehypertension**, and pressures of 140/90 or more are considered to be elevated. Those with prehypertension should begin lifestyle modifications, and if other conditions such as diabetes or a history of heart attack are present, medical treatment may be recommended as well. A number of readings may need to be taken over time before a decision to treat blood pressure is made. (However, consistent readings of 180/110 or higher usually call for more immediate action.) With rare exceptions involving extremely high blood pressures (more than 220/120), hypertension by itself is usually completely unnoticeable. Very few people request medical care to relieve blood pressure symptoms. The problems hypertension ultimately causes, on the other hand, are anything *but* silent.

Many people buy a blood pressure cuff to check readings at home. This can be particularly useful if the pressure varies a lot from one reading to another (the medical term is **labile**). Indeed, more than a few of us are prone to "white-coat hypertension"—a blood pressure elevation that occurs at the doctor's office and not at home. While this may represent some sort of deep-seated response to dimly remembered but unpleasant experiences at doctors' offices during childhood—or simple anxiety over being the object of medical attention—it may also reveal how a person's blood pressure responds to stressful situations. Even if blood pressure isn't elevated all of the time, by the way, it still may need to be treated.

Most home blood pressure machines make use of electronic sensors and digital readouts to simplify the process. Devices that compress a finger or wrist to obtain a blood pressure may not be as reliable as those that squeeze the upper arm. If you purchase a home blood pressure unit, take it to the next visit with your physician to confirm that his or her cuff obtains readings similar to yours.

WHAT—BESIDES MEDICATION—CAN HELP LOWER BLOOD PRESSURE?

Weight reduction. Excessive weight is associated with an increased risk of high blood pressure and many other health problems as well. Losing as little as ten pounds can lower pressure to some degree in many overweight people, and will also enhance the effect of any medications that might be prescribed to treat hypertension. However, a significant number of people with high blood pressure are *not* overweight. Furthermore, because a number of diverse factors can drive up blood pressure, losing excessive weight doesn't always resolve this problem.

We will take a look at the common—and frustrating—problem of excessive weight in chapter 6.

BLOOD PRESSURE BASICS ***continued on page 54***

BLOOD PRESSURE BASICS *continued from page 53*

Limited—or no—alcohol. Most people assume that intoxicating beverages have a relaxing effect on the body, just as they do on inhibitions. But the regular use of alcohol above certain levels can actually have the opposite effect on blood pressure. As we will discuss in detail in chapter 10, there are a host of good reasons to abstain altogether. (Those of legal age who choose to drink should limit their daily intake as follows: for men, less than one ounce of pure alcohol per day—roughly the amount contained in 2 twelve-ounce beers, ten ounces of wine, or two ounces of distilled spirits—and for women, half that amount.)

Physical activity. Moderate physical exercise, such as a brisk thirty-minute walk five or more times per week, reduces the risk of a host of health problems, including hypertension and stroke. For those who already have high blood pressure, exercise may help lower it. Even if one or more medications are necessary to maintain satisfactory control, physical activity should definitely continue. While most people can begin and continue a walking program without medical clearance, those with hypertension and other risk factors for heart disease and stroke should review their exercise plans with their physician, especially if they have more vigorous activities in mind.

We will take a detailed look at the important topic of physical exercise in chapter 7.

Watch the salt. Sodium in our food, which we encounter every day as sodium chloride or table salt, has a tendency to raise blood pressure, especially in African-Americans, the elderly, and diabetics. The National High Blood Pressure Education Program (under the auspices of the National Institutes of Health) recommends keeping the sodium intake to less than 2.5 grams every day—a little more than is contained in a level teaspoonful of salt.[5]

Increase potassium intake. This approach to lowering hypertension has been studied by medical researchers since the 1920s. The effect of potassium on blood pressure is quite modest when compared with medications now available, but it may be helpful for those with high pressure and low levels of potassium in the diet. This is particularly true for African-Americans, whose sensitivity to salt may be reduced by adding potassium through diet or supplements. Potassium is found in a number of foods, especially fruits (and fruit juices) and vegetables. Bananas, orange and tomato juices, potatoes, and squash are particularly rich sources. In addition, salt alternatives such as Morton Lite Salt and Cardia substitute potassium for some of the sodium. You should speak with your physician if you're thinking about using a potassium supplement, because other health conditions and medications may also need to be considered.

What about calcium and magnesium? Some studies have suggested that inadequate amounts of calcium and magnesium in the diet are associated with high blood pressure. Surprisingly, the current evidence suggests that taking these minerals as supplements has minimal, if any, effect on hyper-

Interested in vitamin and mineral supplements? We take a detailed look at them in appendix B.

tension.[6] (There are, however, other good reasons to make sure that you take enough calcium and magnesium every day, both in food and, if needed, supplements.)

And how about caffeine? One would think that caffeine's stimulant effects would send blood pressures soaring among coffee and tea lovers. First-time users may in fact have a brief and mild increase in pressure, but this effect is only transient and does not continue with regular use. The weight of evidence does not implicate caffeine as a culprit in the cause of hypertension, stroke, or cardiovascular disease. (It can, however, cause other symptoms, such as an increased heart rate, jitteriness, and insomnia, which may make switching to decaf a good idea.)

What about stress management and relaxation techniques? There is no question that blood pressure rises when we are excited, angry, uncomfortable, or tense. This is but one of our body's many responses to stress, and it helps prepare us to take appropriate action, whatever that might be. However, the connection between such responses, or stress in general, and high blood pressure isn't always obvious. It is not uncommon in medical practice to see individuals with dramatic hypertension who aren't particularly stressed, and also to see people who are in the midst of grievous trials and tribulations, or who are extremely anxious, with normal blood pressure. On the other hand, some people are physiological "hot reactors" whose blood pressure takes off like a rocket when they have a fight with their boss or get stuck at a red light. Currently claims abound for biofeedback, meditation, relaxation, and various stress-management techniques as effective treatments for blood pressure. While short-term studies suggest some benefit from these, the National High Blood Pressure Education Program has not been impressed with the evidence (in the form of controlled studies) supporting their routine use for treating hypertension.[7] (This no doubt reflects the great variety of factors that can raise blood pressure.)

We will examine the question of stress and its effects on health in chapter 8.

Religious activity. A 1998 Duke University study of nearly four thousand adults sixty-five and over found that those who attended weekly services and prayed or studied the Bible daily were likely to have blood pressures consistently lower than those who did so less often or not at all.[8] The researchers noted that nine out of eleven prior studies of blood pressure and religious involvement had yielded similar results. This is but one of many studies that have suggested a positive impact of religious commitment on overall health, a fascinating subject we will explore in more detail in chapter 9. ■

CHOLESTEROL BASICS

For all of the negative press it receives, one might imagine that cholesterol is rat poison under an assumed name. In fact, it is an important and necessary compound—but one for which there can definitely be too much of a good thing.

What is cholesterol? Cholesterol is a member of a class of compounds called **sterols**, which also includes vitamin D and the sex hormones (such as estrogen and testosterone)—vital molecules that are themselves derived from cholesterol. Cholesterol is necessary for the formation and maintenance of the complex membranes that surround every cell in our body. It is also a component of **bile**, the liquid formed by the liver that helps disperse fat molecules in the intestine so that they can be absorbed. When they are going about their appointed errands, cholesterol molecules are our lifelong allies. But when floating through the bloodstream in excessive numbers, they can get us into trouble.

About 85 percent of the cholesterol in our body—in fact, all that you can possibly use—is generated internally, mostly by the liver, in quantities affected dramatically both by our genetics and our weight. The rest comes from animal sources in our diet: meats (especially the so-called "organ meats," such as liver and kidney), eggs, fish, and dairy products. The fact that so much of your cholesterol comes from within, rather than from food, helps explain why some people who are relentless carnivores and couch potatoes can still have ridiculously low levels of cholesterol, while some well-conditioned, fastidious vegetarians may be stuck with high levels. (These are, of course, exceptions rather than the rule. Dietary habits do play an important role.)

What do the terms "good" and "bad" cholesterol mean? Cholesterol belongs to the family of nutrients called lipids—we usually refer to them as fats—which are, among other things, generally not soluble in water. As it turns out, this chemical detail has some major implications for our health. Think of what happens when you pour a little vegetable oil into a pan of water: The oil clumps into droplets and dollops of various sizes, and floats to the surface. Blood is essentially a water-based liquid. If cholesterol molecules were released directly into the bloodstream, they would likewise form clumps and would not disperse to all of the cells that need them. Instead, cholesterol molecules, as well as other lipid molecules such as the triglycerides, are escorted through the bloodstream by carrier proteins (called **apoproteins**) that *are* water/blood soluble. Apoproteins and various combinations of lipid molecules are packaged together to form **lipoproteins**, which researchers have

Technically fats are only one member of the lipid family, but they comprise about 95 percent of the lipids in our diet. The other members are the sterols, which include cholesterol, and phospholipids, such as lecithin.

sorted into categories based on their density. Two of these—the **low-density lipoproteins** (or **LDL**) and the **high-density lipoproteins** (or **HDL**)—are particularly important to our health.

LDL packages are larger, lighter, and loaded with more cholesterol. They also have an unfortunate tendency to deposit cholesterol in the walls of arteries, contributing to the buildup of blood-blocking plaque. HDL packages, on the other hand, are smaller and heavier, and carry more protein and less cholesterol than LDL. More important, they help "clean up the mess" left by LDL, removing some of the excess cholesterol and other lipids from tissues and bringing them back to the liver. An abundance of research has shown that the more cholesterol you have associated with LDL, the more likely you are to have atherosclerotic disease congesting your arteries. The more you have riding on HDL, the more you will be protected from this problem. It's not uncommon to hear about "bad" cholesterol, referring to that which is attached to LDL, and "good" cholesterol that rides with HDL. In fact, cholesterol is cholesterol, but what makes it "good" or "bad" depends a lot on how much you have in circulation and the company it keeps.

What should I have checked, and how often? When you have your cholesterol checked, it isn't enough to know the total that is circulating in the bloodstream. You also need to know how much is attached to HDL and LDL carriers. Most physicians or clinics typically order what is called a **lipid profile** or **coronary risk panel**, which includes not only these numbers but also the level of triglycerides. Triglycerides are the predominant form of fat in the body. As we will describe later in chapter 5, they consist of three chainlike molecules called fatty acids attached to a short molecular "backbone" called **glycerol**. High triglyceride levels in the blood increase the risk for developing diseased arteries and other problems. (The common blood panels don't include a lipoprotein breakdown for triglycerides, by the way, because most of it is carried by what is called **very low-density lipoprotein**, or **VLDL**.)

A number of professional and governmental organizations have weighed in on the question of screening lipids, and a common recommendation is that a fasting profile (no food for nine to twelve hours before the blood is drawn) be done periodically—every five years is reasonable—on men thirty-five and older and women forty-five and older. Younger adults should be considered for screening starting at age twenty if they have other risk factors, such as smoking, diabetes, or a family history of problems with lipids or heart disease.[9] In the United States, the most widely followed guidelines for assessing and treating cholesterol are those issued by the National Cholesterol Education Program (or NCEP) of the National Heart, Lung, and Blood Institute. In its 2001 update, the NCEP took a stronger position on screening, recommending

CHOLESTEROL BASICS ***continued on page 58***

CHOLESTEROL BASICS *continued from page 57*

that a fasting lipid profile be obtained once every five years (and more often if needed) for every adult twenty and over.

What levels of cholesterol are desirable? Not too many decades ago, a "normal" cholesterol level was considered to be one below 300 mg/dl. Today we know that there can be a big gap between what is common or normal in a population and what is desirable. In its 2001 update, the NCEP summarized desirable (and undesirable) levels of various lipids as follows:

TOTAL CHOLESTEROL

Less than 200 .... Desirable
200 to 239 .... Borderline high
240 or greater .... High

LDL CHOLESTEROL

Less than 100 .... Optimal
100 to 129 .... Near optimal
130 to 159 .... Borderline high
160 to 189 .... High
190 or greater .... Very high

HDL CHOLESTEROL

Less than 40 .... Low
60 or greater .... High (desirable)

TRIGLYCERIDES

Less than 150 .... Optimal

When do I need to think about lowering my cholesterol? While some people now obtain total cholesterol readings and lipid profiles on their own, you would be wise to review any numbers you obtain with a health professional—typically a primary-care physician such as a family practitioner or internist, or if appropriate, a specialist such as a cardiologist. The type of action you might take, and how vigorously you pursue it, depends not only upon the results of the test but also on your overall health status.

Based on current research, the LDL ("bad") cholesterol has become the primary marker for determining whether action is needed and what kind. The latest NCEP guidelines identify three LDL target levels, based on other risk factors for having diseased arteries. Basically, the more risk factors you have, the lower your LDL should be:

The National Heart, Lung, and Blood Institute is one of twenty-seven institutes and centers within the National Institutes of Health (NIH), which is the primary federal agency conducting and promoting health research.

Like many common blood tests, the levels of cholesterol and its various components are most commonly expressed in mg/dl, or milligrams per deciliter of serum. A deciliter is a tenth of a liter, or 100 milliliters—a little over three ounces. Serum is the liquid that is left when the red cells are removed from blood. Fortunately, only a small amount of blood—a lot less than three ounces—is needed to test for cholesterol.

RISK CATEGORY	LDL GOAL (in mg/dl)
Zero to one risk factor	160
Two or more risk factors	130
Coronary heart disease or equivalent risk	100

What are the factors that determine your risk category?

- Cigarette smoking
- Age—for men, forty-five and older; for women, fifty-five and older
- High blood pressure (140/90 or greater) or blood pressure that is normal as the result of medical treatment
- HDL ("good") cholesterol less than 40
- History of coronary heart disease in a parent, brother, or sister at an early age: fifty-five years old or younger in a male; sixty-five or younger in a female

Those who need the lowest LDL cholesterol levels are people who have had a heart attack or other clear evidence of blocked coronary arteries. In addition, a few other situations create a risk level that is just as high—what the NCEP calls "equivalent risk":

- Significantly diseased arteries in other areas, such as the neck, abdomen, or leg. If arteries in one part of the body are clogged, the same process is likely to be going on elsewhere.
- Diabetics are at significant risk of developing coronary artery disease within ten years of being diagnosed. Furthermore, diabetics who suffer a heart attack have an unusually high death rate, both immediately and in subsequent years.
- A combination of risk factors severe enough to create more than a 20 percent chance of developing coronary artery disease within ten years. The NCEP guidelines include a relatively simple point system for estimating your ten-year risk for coronary artery disease, which is included in the sidebar "What Are the Odds? How to Calculate Your Chances for Developing Coronary Heart Disease" (pages 49 and 51). ■

More recent research suggests that individuals at very high risk for coronary heart disease are likely to benefit from lowering their LDL cholesterol to levels below 70mg/dl. For most people, this requires the use of one or more lipid-lowering medications.

continued from page 50

Cells Behaving Badly: Cancer

This much-feared foe that takes the lives of more than 500,000 Americans every year, second only to cardiovascular disease, is really a collection of disorders that can affect virtually any tissue in the body. The common denominator for all of them is a loss of self-control: cells multiplying in numbers that interfere with surrounding tissues or with organs far removed from them. Many cells in our body, such as our red and white blood cells or those that line the intestine, undergo constant turnover. Others, such as nerve and brain cells, usually assume their assigned function and are never replaced. The mechanisms that cause cells to remain at their appointed tasks without increasing in number beyond what is needed (or preordained) are complex. Understanding them, let alone gaining control of them when they malfunction, remains a frontier of biological research.

A mass of cells that shows up where it doesn't belong is called a **tumor,** which in turn can be designated as **benign** or **malignant.** A benign tumor is so named because it does not invade its surroundings or spread to other parts of the body. A common example is the everyday wart (caused by a virus) or a **lipoma**, a nodule of fatty tissue that may develop on the arms, legs, or trunk. The fact that a tumor is benign doesn't mean that it can't cause trouble; ask anyone who has had to deal with a collection of warts on the hands or feet. Some benign tumors can become quite large—certain types that arise in the ovary may become gigantic—but in nearly all circumstances they can still be removed completely.

The term *cancer* always refers to a malignant tumor (also called a **malignancy**). Cancer cells tend to be disorderly both in appearance and behavior. Indeed, they can be so misshapen and primitive in appearance that it may be impossible to determine from what tissue they originated. Certain organs are more prone to generate cancers than others, and what's common (and what isn't) will also vary with gender and age. The ten most common cancers among adults are listed in the table on page 61. The types of cancers that affect children under fifteen are very different from those seen in adults. (See sidebar "Cancer in Children" on page 62.)

F.Y.I.

The word *cancer* comes from Latin and Greek words for "crab," and its use to describe a tumor has been attributed to Hippocrates, the ancient Greek physician whom historians have generally considered to be the father of Western medicine. It is thought that the appearance of a spreading tumor at the skin surface (as can occur, for example, when breast cancer grows without restraint and extends through the skin) suggested the claws of a crab.

Altogether there are roughly two hundred varieties of cancer. Cancers begin as microscopic nests of cells, which, depending upon where they are located and how fast they multiply, may not be noticeable for months or even years. As they increase in number, they may compress normal tissues adjacent to them, or actually invade them like an advancing army. Unfortunately, many

THE MOST COMMON CANCERS IN ADULTS

ESTIMATED NEW CASES* MALE	FEMALE	ESTIMATED DEATHS MALE	FEMALE
Prostate 232,090 (33%)	**Breast** 211,240 (32%)	**Lung & bronchus** 90,490 (31%)	**Lung & bronchus** 73,020 (26%)
Lung & bronchus 93,010 (13%)	**Lung & bronchus** 79,560 (12%)	**Prostate** 30,350 (10%)	**Breast** 40,410 (15%)
Colon & rectum 71,820 (10%)	**Colon & rectum** 73,470 (11%)	**Colon & rectum** 28,540 (10%)	**Colon & rectum** 27,750 (10%)
Urinary bladder 47,010 (6%)	**Uterine corpus** 40,880 (6%)	**Pancreas** 15,820 (5%)	**Ovary** 16,210 (6%)
Melanoma of the skin 33,580 (5%)	**Non-Hodgkin's lymphoma** 27,320 (4%)	**Leukemia** 12,540 (4%)	**Pancreas** 15,980 (6%)
Non-Hodgkin's lymphoma 29,070 (4%)	**Melanoma of the skin** 26,000 (4%)	**Esophagus** 10,530 (4%)	**Leukemia** 10,030 (4%)
Kidney 22,490 (3%)	**Ovary** 22,220 (3%)	**Liver** 10,330 (3%)	**Non-Hodgkin's lymphoma** 9,050 (3%)
Leukemia 19,640 (3%)	**Thyroid** 19,190 (3%)	**Non-Hodgkin's lymphoma** 10,150 (3%)	**Uterine corpus** 7,310 (3%)
Oral cavity 19,100 (3%)	**Urinary bladder** 16,200 (2%)	**Urinary bladder** 8,970 (3%)	**Multiple myeloma** 5,640 (2%)
Pancreas 16,100 (2%)	**Pancreas** 16,080 (2%)	**Kidney** 8,020 (3%)	**Brain** 5,480 (2%)
All sites 710,040 (100%)	**All sites** 662,870 (100%)	**All sites** 295,280 (100%)	**All sites** 275,000 (100%)

*Excludes basal and squamous cell skin cancers and in situ carcinoma except urinary bladder. Percentages do not total 100% because not all cancers are listed in this table. Source: American Cancer Society's Cancer Facts and Figures—2005. www.cancer.org. Reprinted with permission.

We will look in more detail at a number of the most common cancers—lung, breast, prostate, colon, and several others—in chapter 4, beginning on page 86.

cancers are not content to stay in one general location but spread through the most readily available distribution systems: the lymph channels and the bloodstream.

When blood reaches the smallest vessels, the capillaries, some of the liquid portion (called **plasma**) oozes into the surrounding tissue. This clear fluid, known as **lymph** (from the Latin word for water), eventually returns to the bloodstream via an intricate network of nearly invisible vessels known as **lymph channels** that drain every cubic inch of the body. Lymph routinely contains white blood cells and some red cells. In addition, bacteria and viruses that have invaded local tissue may float into local lymph channels, as can any tumor cells that have broken away from a growing mass. Strategically placed throughout the lymphatic system are battle stations called **lymph nodes** (or, less correctly, *lymph glands*) packed with white cells called **lymphocytes**, **monocytes**,

Technically, a **gland** is a structure that generates a substance and then secretes it to be used elsewhere or eliminated. (Sweat glands are a good example.) Lymph nodes may resemble glands, but they are filters rather than secretors.

CANCER IN CHILDREN

More than 9,000 children under fifteen are diagnosed with cancer every year in the United States, and about 1,500 die from this disease, making it the second most common cause of death among children (after accidents). In general, the types of tumors most commonly seen among children are very different from those in adults:

- **Leukemia**, in which white cells multiply uncontrollably, is the most common cancer in children, accounting for about 30 percent of cancer cases through age fourteen. Leukemia involving a particular type of white cell called the lymphocyte is the most common.
- **Central nervous system tumors** (involving the brain and spinal cord) are the second most common type of cancer in this age group.
- **Neuroblastoma** originates in the sympathetic nervous system (one of the divisions of the autonomic nervous system that regulates those body functions not under conscious control). Neuroblastomas can occur anywhere, but most arise within the abdomen.
- **Wilms' tumor** arises from the kidney.
- **Hodgkin's disease and non-Hodgkin's lymphoma** arise from lymph tissue and may cause enlargement of lymph nodes in the neck, under the arm, or in the groin.
- **Rhabdomyosarcoma** is a cancer arising from muscle.
- **Retinoblastoma** arises in the eye, most commonly before the age of four.
- **Osteosarcoma** is a cancer originating in bone. (In adults, cancer in bone is nearly always metastatic—that is, spread from some distant site.)
- **Ewing's sarcoma** is another type of cancer originating in bone.

There are a number of recommendations for cancer-screening tests among adults, and we will look at these in some detail in chapter 4. But there are no routine screening recommendations for cancer in children (other than getting routine checkups by a pediatrician or family physician), not only because cancer in the young is so uncommon, but also because the signs and symptoms are not very specific. Nevertheless, parents should be aware of complaints or problems that *might* indicate trouble. These include:

- An unusual lump or swelling anywhere in the body
- Persistent fever, fatigue, and/or weight loss
- Unusual bruising
- Frequent or persistent headaches, especially with nausea or vomiting
- Ongoing pain in a specific part of the body

Remember that when symptoms such as these are checked out, they nearly always turn out to be caused by something *other* than cancer. Nevertheless, it is important not to ignore any of them, but rather to have your child's pediatrician or family physician carry out an appropriate evaluation. ■

and **plasma cells.** Lymph nodes are clustered in certain areas of the body, such as the neck, groin, and armpit, and provide an important line of defense against any incoming microscopic threats. Normally they are quite small, but in response to a local infection they may swell dramatically. (The familiar bumps in the neck that often show up with a sore throat are a common example.)

Tumor cells that arrive in lymph nodes may be contained, but they may also stage a hostile takeover and send more of their destructive emissaries into lymph channels upstream, where they eventually enter the blood. In a worst-case scenario, cancer cells spread throughout the body, establishing beachheads in areas far removed from their origin. Liver, lung, bone, and brain are common sites for these invasions, which are called **metastases.** (A tumor that has broken loose from its origin is said to be **metastatic**.) Some cancers arise in more than one location. **Leukemia** involves excessive production of white blood cells throughout the **marrow**, the tissue packed within the core of our bones. **Lymphomas** may develop in multiple lymph nodes and other sites where lymphocytes are concentrated. The unchecked spread of cancer cells eventually saps the body of vital nutrients, causing weight loss and weakness. As they relentlessly replace, displace, obstruct, or otherwise interfere with normal tissues, important body functions—and eventually life itself—come to an end.

The specter of a pitiless "enemy within," often remaining silent until it's too late to overcome and then laying waste to health and life itself, is certainly intimidating. Whether the diagnosis of cancer is a sure thing or merely one of many possibilities when one isn't feeling well, some may be tempted to raise the mental white flag when they receive the bad news. But it is important to understand that cancer is by no means the automatic victor whenever it establishes a base of operations somewhere in the body. Some tumors arrive late in life and then don't seem to be in any hurry to grow, so that their hosts eventually pass away from some other problem. (Autopsies of elderly men, for example, frequently reveal cancer within the prostate gland that was a cause neither of death nor of any symptoms.) Many cancers respond to a combination of medical treatments and lifestyle changes that either eliminates them or stifles their growth.

It is well beyond our purposes here to review all of the therapeutic possibilities for dealing with cancer, for two reasons. First and foremost, the options will depend upon the contenders in the conflict: the tumor and the person who has it. For the tumor, its origin (if known), the appearance of its cells, how far (and fast) it has spread, and the treatments that are known to affect it are important variables. For the individual, sex, health status, access to medical care, and willingness to undergo whatever treatments are appropriate are all crucial elements in the decision-making process. Second, the treatment options are evolving as research continues to uncover the mechanisms of tumor growth and the most effective ways to slow or stop it. As a result, a person with cancer needs input from a professional (usually a physician specializing in **oncology,** the study and treatment of tumors) who can apply the best current information to his or her own unique situation. This may take place within a local medical community or at a major center for cancer research and treatment.

What causes cells to behave so badly, and why would the body allow a gang of unruly, often primitive cells to continue to multiply? The ultimate answers lie in the intricate biochemical mechanisms that regulate the production and maturation of new cells, as well as the ability of the immune system to recognize and destroy those that are malfunctioning. There doesn't appear to be a single underlying cause that applies to all tumors, but rather a variety of risk

WHERE DO I GET RELIABLE INFORMATION ABOUT CANCER?

Because cancer is such a complex problem, and because conventional treatment can be a challenging, expensive—and frankly scary—undertaking, there is no shortage of people and organizations weighing in on this subject. Needless to say, the quality of information and opinions in the public square ranges from the reasonable to the ridiculous. The Internet is ripe with Web sites dealing with this topic from every conceivable angle. Generally speaking, when hunting through the bookstore or the Internet, you would be wise to stick with researchers and institutions that have resources, scientific credentials, and most of all accountability to the health-care community at large. Remember: When it comes to difficult medical issues, there are no Lone Rangers who come up with the answer that everyone else has missed. Talk is cheap, but good research isn't.

The following are some excellent resources for information about cancer in general, as well as specific types of tumors:

- The **American Cancer Society** is a national community-based health organization, with more than thirty-four hundred local units and some 2 million volunteers. It provides research grants, promotes prevention through a variety of programs, provides patient support and education services, and works to impact public policy on behalf of cancer patients and their families. Phone: (800) ACS-2345; Web site: http://www.cancer.org.
- The **National Cancer Institute** (NCI), a component of the National Institutes of Health, is the federal government's principal agency in the field of cancer research and training. With a 2005 budget of almost $5 billion, NCI coordinates the National Cancer Program and its extensive activities related to research, education, and patient care. Phone: (800) 4CANCER; Web site: http://www.cancer.gov.

factors that may increase the likelihood that a malignant process may be set in motion. These include:

Heredity. Some types of tumors (or more precisely, the vulnerability to certain cancers) run in families. This is particularly important for cancer of the breast, ovary, colon, and prostate. A history of one of these in a parent or sibling may affect what type of screening a person should have.

Age. More birthdays mean more time for cells to misbehave, and as a result cancer tends to show up later in life—most of the time. Some types of cancer, including certain leukemias, lymphomas, kidney, and bone tumors affect children, and most testicular tumors occur among men in their twenties and thirties. Overall, however, it is more common for cancer to rear its ugly head after the age of fifty.

- For those with Internet access, **MedlinePlus** is an excellent resource for information about cancer and virtually any other health topic. This commercial-free Web site (http://www.medlineplus.gov), a service of the National Library of Medicine, provides access to information compiled by the National Library of Medicine and the National Institutes of Health, as well as an illustrated medical encyclopedia, drug information, interactive health tutorials, and news. In addition, the site provides links to hundreds of other Web sites that have been selected using several criteria for overall quality and accuracy.
- Many professional organizations have useful information available at their Web site or upon request. For example: The Mayo Clinic has a Web site (http://www.mayoclinic.com) that provides reliable information about a variety of subjects, including cancer. Major cancer centers such as Memorial Sloan-Kettering Cancer Center in New York (http://www.mskcc.org or 212-639-2000), M. D. Anderson Cancer Center at the University of Texas (http://www.mdanderson.org or 800-392-1611), and City of Hope near Los Angeles (http://www.cityofhope.org or 626-256-HOPE) not only provide diagnostic and treatment services for cancer but also information about current developments and research. Medical specialty organizations such as the American Academy of Family Physicians (http://www.aafp.org or 800-274-2237), the American Lung Association (http://www.lungusa.org or 800-LUNG-USA), the American Academy of Dermatology (http://www.aad.org or 888-462-DERM), and the American College of Obstetricians and Gynecologists (http://www.acog.org) can provide educational material about cancer in general or in relation to their specific fields. Medem, a communications network founded by seven professional organizations including the American Medical Association and the American Academy of Pediatrics, provides an online medical library (http://www.medem.com) and a number of other services. ■

Tobacco use. Tobacco is literally the world's biggest "smoking gun." Not only does cigarette use aggravate disease of the heart and blood vessels, as we have already discussed, but tobacco in all of its forms—smoked, chewed, or exhaled for someone else to endure—is implicated in one-third of all cancer deaths in the United States. Smoking is of course notorious for its role in lung cancer. Some 87 percent of deaths from this cancer, the number-one cancer killer every year, are smoke related, and the pack-a-day cigarette user is ten times more likely than a nonsmoker to be afflicted with it. Unfortunately, cigarette users are also more likely to develop malignancies in a number of other locations, including the mouth, vocal cords, esophagus, pancreas, kidney, bladder, and cervix (the opening of the uterus). Cigar and pipe smokers, as well as tobacco chewers, all share an increased risk for cancer of the oral cavity—the lip, mouth, tongue, and throat—a particularly unpleasant place to deal with a tumor. Cigar smokers, depending upon how many they puff per day and how deeply they inhale, are also at greater risk for cancer of the lung and esophagus.

Alcohol. Roughly 75 percent of cases of cancer of the esophagus, which kills more than thirteen thousand Americans every year, and half of the malignant tumors of the mouth, throat, and vocal cords (altogether more than ten thousand annual deaths) are related to chronic, heavy alcohol use. This risk increases dramatically when excessive alcohol use is combined with smoking. Alcohol also may play an indirect role in the development of breast cancer.

Diet. Announcements that certain foods may cause or prevent cancer are now about as common as stock tips and are often equally unreliable. Nevertheless there is evidence to suggest that a high-fat diet increases the risk for cancers of the colon, prostate, and uterus. Furthermore, obesity is linked to breast cancer (probably because of higher estrogen levels generated by body fat), as well as cancer of the colon, pancreas, prostate, ovary, and uterus.

Ionizing radiation. Radiation is basically energy traveling in the form of particles and waves that crosses our path in a variety of ways. Visible light, microwaves, and radio waves are examples of **nonionizing radiation** that has enough energy to cause atoms to move or vibrate, but not enough to change them chemically. **Ionizing radiation**, on the other hand, has both a higher frequency and more energy—enough to remove electrons from atoms, creating positively and negatively charged particles (known as **ions**). We are exposed to variable but small amounts of ionizing radiation every day from the sun and from radioactive material in the soil, such as radon and uranium. Larger amounts may enter our body during X-ray procedures or through contact with radioactive substances. Very large exposures may increase the risk for developing cancer later in life, as occurred among many survivors of the Hiroshima and Nagasaki atomic bombs in 1945.

Before 1950, X rays were used for purposes now considered inappropriate, such as treating enlarged tonsils and even acne. Some individuals who were exposed to such procedures have been found to be at higher risk for developing thyroid cancer. Improvements in technology over the past few decades have reduced the amount of radiation exposure during standard X-ray procedures, although more exposure occurs during CT scans. X rays (including CT scans) taken for appropriate medical diagnostic purposes appear to pose minimal if any risk, and no formal limit has been placed on the number of procedures that a person may have if they are considered medically necessary. However, limiting one's X-ray exposure is one consideration for avoiding screening "total body" CT scans, which at this time are not recommended by any professional organization. (We will discuss this topic in chapter 4, beginning on page 114.) Furthermore, a woman of childbearing age should notify her doctor *before* any X ray or CT scan if there is a possibility that she might be pregnant.

MRI scans and ultrasounds do not involve ionizing radiation.

Ultraviolet (UV) radiation. Along with the life-giving heat and light that we receive every day, the sun also sends us a steady stream of this radiation with a wavelength shorter than that of blue or violet light. Most of it is filtered by the ozone layer in our atmosphere, but enough penetrates to be a potential threat to our skin—especially at higher altitudes; lower latitudes (that is, nearer the equator); during the late morning and early afternoon; and in areas where sand, water, or snow can reflect it onto any nearby exposed skin. We are all familiar with sunburn, UV's most well-known calling card, as well as the aging and wrinkling effect of chronic sun exposure. But the damage the UV exposure can cause in skin also increases the risk for skin cancer (especially among those with lighter complexions), the nonmelanoma form of which is the most common malignancy (but fortunately not the most lethal) in the United States, affecting about a million people every year.

We will look at skin cancer and its prevention in more detail in chapter 4.

Chemical exposure. A number of substances used in the workplace have been found to be **carcinogenic** (that is, cancer inducing). Among the most notorious are asbestos, nickel, cadmium, arsenic, vinyl chloride, and benzene. The list of potential offenders is lengthy—more than forty are listed at the American Cancer Society Web site (http://www.cancer.org) in a section under "Health Information Seekers: Prevention and Early Detection" called "Environmental and Occupational Cancer Risks"—and a number of industrial processes such as aluminum production, nickel refining, and rubber manufacturing are known to be associated with an increased cancer risk. In order to reduce, or even eliminate entirely, their risk for developing cancer, it is critically important for those who work with these materials to follow guidelines set both by industry and government agencies such as the Occupational Safety and Health Administration (OSHA).

Infections. Infection with certain viruses is associated with an increased risk for developing cancer. For example, a relatively small percentage of people infected with hepatitis B and a larger percentage infected with hepatitis C develop chronic inflammation of the liver that can lead to cirrhosis and cancer. Human immunodeficiency virus (HIV), the virus that causes AIDS, is linked to a number of cancers, including a form of lymphoma, an aggressive type of cancer of the cervix in women, and Kaposi's sarcoma, a cancer involving soft tissue beneath the skin that affects a significant percentage of homosexual men with

A FEW IMPORTANT CAUTIONS ABOUT RISK FACTORS FOR CANCER

Having one or more risk factors does not guarantee that you will get cancer. It does mean that your odds are increased compared with people who don't have that particular risk—but by how much? Consider this illustration: A woman wants to take hormone therapy but wants to use estrogen only. Her doctor is reluctant to write this prescription because she still has a uterus. Unless she uses progesterone at the same time, her risk of developing **cancer of the endometrium**—the lining of the uterus—would increase by 800 percent. While the physician's concern is appropriate, it is worth noting that a woman who never takes estrogen therapy has about a 1 in 1,000 chance of developing cancer of the uterus. The patient who wants estrogen alone would therefore increase that risk to 8 in 1,000—or, looking at it another way, 125 to 1 against her developing cancer of the uterus. An important take-home lesson is that, with rare exception, the majority of people with one or more risk factors for developing a certain type of cancer won't get it.

Having no risk factors doesn't guarantee that you won't get cancer. As a matter of fact, most people diagnosed with cancer have no known risk factors. This may sound paradoxical and not exactly fair, but it brings into focus an important truth about health and medicine: More often than not, doctors are much better at determining what is wrong than *why* it happened. Your physician may be able to attach a name to your symptoms and offer a description of your illness—be it lung cancer, pneumonia, or asthma—but rarely can he or she say why *you* became ill instead of your spouse or coworker, or why it occurred *now* instead of last week or next year, or even what (if anything) you might have done to prevent it. This is not to say that there isn't an explanation, but rather that our current understanding and technologies are not capable of uncovering it with absolute certainty.

AIDS. Sexually transmitted infection with certain strains of the human papillomavirus (or HPV) has been identified as the cause of nearly all cases of cancer of the cervix, which kills more than 3,700 women in the United States every year.

Hormone therapy. Long-term use of estrogen during and after menopause may be associated with an increased risk of developing cancer of the breast, uterus, and ovary. This has generated a lot of concern and controversy about the risks and benefits of this common treatment for symptoms such as hot flashes and vaginal atrophy, as well as long-term problems such as osteoporosis. Needless to say, there is no one-size-fits-all approach to hormone therapy.

Chapter 13 reviews the pros and cons of hormone therapy in depth, beginning on page 666.

Put the "risk factor of the week" into perspective. Hardly a week passes without a breathless news report about a new study showing a link between _____ (a particular food, herb, drug, or activity) and _____ (a certain cancer or some other disease), usually including an incredibly alarming statistic. Consider this example involving a fictitious organ: As you wipe the sleep from your eyes one sunny morning, you make the mistake of flipping on the morning news. The glamorous anchorwoman furrows her brow and gravely announces, "A new study just published this week in the *New Zealand Journal of Phrenology* reveals that people who sleep facing southeast are 50 percent more likely to develop cancer of the left corpsuckle, compared with those who sleep in other directions."

You immediately snap to attention, because *you* sleep facing southeast. "What did she say? I have a 50 percent chance of developing cancer in my left corpsuckle? I better call the doctor!" Your alarm (not the one on your nightstand) would be premature.

Upon hearing that you might have a 50 percent increased risk of developing cancer of the left corpsuckle, you must immediately ask "*How* often does this cancer occur?" If the answer is two cases for every 100,000 people, then a 50 percent increase would change the odds to 3 in 100,000—not 1 in 2. Furthermore, another news flash may arrive in a couple of months announcing a newer study showing that people who sleep facing southeast are less likely to develop impacted molars. Now what? Are you more worried about your teeth or your left corpsuckle? At this point, you may need to ask your doctor or proceed to a reputable Web site to seek some informed guidance. Bottom line: You should beware of making significant changes in your life based on the results of one news report, especially if it contradicts a lot of previous research. (Please note, however, that the risk factors for cancer listed in this chapter, and those for other major diseases described elsewhere in this book, represent a consensus of mainstream medical opinion, unless stated otherwise.) ■

Metabolism Behaving Badly: Diabetes

Some 18 million people in the United States are diabetic, more than 6 percent of the population. Of these, more than 5 million have no idea that they have this problem. Most people are aware that diabetes has something to do with blood sugar and insulin, but few have an understanding of how much damage it can cause or in how many places. The word **diabetes** (from a Greek term for "pass over" or "pass through") refers to a profuse output of urine, a symptom that actually does not appear until the underlying process has gotten way out of hand. The vast majority of people with diabetes are diagnosed before they ever begin making frequent trips to the bathroom, but unfortunately many of them will deal with setbacks that are far more serious.

F.Y.I.

When speaking of diabetes in this section and throughout this book, we are referring to **diabetes mellitus,** sometimes called "sugar diabetes," in which blood sugar levels are abnormally high. (Before physicians could measure blood sugar, they noted that the urine of diabetics was sweet, a result of the presence of glucose in the urine.) The relatively rare condition **diabetes insipidus** is an entirely different disorder in which the kidneys cannot maintain a normal fluid balance, leading to a large output of extremely dilute urine.

To understand what goes wrong in diabetes, you need to know a little about how the human body manages a crucial fuel supply. The simple molecule **glucose** (often called blood sugar) serves as a primary energy source for cells throughout the body and is the exclusive fuel for the brain and central nervous system, which cannot function without a steady supply. As a result, we are designed with several mechanisms that maintain blood glucose at an adequate level, and only one hormone—**insulin**—that lowers it. Insulin is created by special cells (called **beta cells**) scattered throughout the **pancreas,** a large organ tucked behind the stomach in the upper abdomen. (In addition to manufacturing insulin, the pancreas also secretes large amounts of digestive enzymes into the intestine to disassemble complex food molecules before they are absorbed.)

The word *insulin* comes from the Latin word for island. It was given this name because the beta cells where insulin is produced are located in numerous clusters that resemble small islands in the pancreas.

Glucose molecules do not simply float through the blood and then ooze into the nearest cell. They must be escorted inside by insulin, which serves somewhat like a key that opens the door to the cell, allowing glucose to enter. Normally after a meal the level of glucose in the blood rises, and the pancreas responds by sending enough insulin "keys" into the bloodstream to open the cellular "locks." As glucose enters cells throughout the body, the blood glucose level goes down again. Diabetes occurs when there aren't enough keys, or when the locks don't work properly.

Type 1 diabetes, previously called **juvenile-onset** or **insulin-dependent** diabetes, affects only 5 percent to 10 percent of diabetics, usually children and young adults. In type 1 diabetes, the insulin-producing beta cells in the pancreas are destroyed by what is called an **autoimmune** process. This is a friendly-fire scenario in which the immune system mistakenly attacks normal tissue. What sets off this self-destruction is unclear, although many researchers suspect that genetic vulnerability interacting with some type of environmental event (such as a viral infection) is to blame. While it may take a while (perhaps years in some cases) to deplete the beta cells, once symptoms appear they are usually dramatic. As blood glucose levels soar and cells are starved of the fuel they need, a number of metabolic consequences kick into high gear.

Normally the kidneys prevent glucose in the blood from appearing in the urine. When blood levels reach a critical level, however, glucose begins to spill into the urine, drawing extra water with it. This leads to the classic symptom of excessive urine flow, and with it an intense thirst. Because so much fuel is literally going to waste, weight loss is common, despite (at first) an increase in appetite. Unless the correct diagnosis is made and treatment started, the hapless individual—all too often a child—eventually develops a dangerous mix of severe dehydration, increased acidity of the blood, and other serious abnormalities that together are known as **diabetic ketoacidosis.** If this metabolic runaway train is not stopped, coma and death are inevitable.

Before the early 1920s, the diagnosis of diabetes in a young person was nearly always a death sentence. But in 1922, Toronto researchers Frederick Grant Banting and Charles Best successfully treated a dying fourteen-year-old diabetic with animal pancreatic extracts containing insulin. The discovery of insulin won the Nobel Prize in 1923, and soon thereafter, this compound became available to patients all over the world. Because it is broken down in the digestive tract, insulin must be injected under the skin (or, in an emergency, into a vein). Various short- and long-acting forms are available, and many type 1 diabetics now use a sophisticated electronic pump that gradually releases insulin throughout the day.

Type 2 diabetes, previously called **adult-onset** or **non-insulin-dependent diabetes,** represents 90 percent to 95 percent of cases of this disorder. As its prior names suggest, type 2 diabetes usually occurs later in life—usually after age forty, and most commonly after age fifty-five—and does not arise from a shortage of insulin. Instead, there are plenty of keys (insulin) available to open the biochemical locks at the surface of the cells, but the locks don't work properly, a problem called **insulin resistance**. Glucose thus has greater difficulty entering the cells that need it, and higher levels gradually appear in the bloodstream. At first, the pancreas responds by sending out more keys, but eventually it can "burn out" and production of insulin may fall, aggravating the problem. Unlike type 1 diabetics, those with type 2 do not need insulin to survive, although in some cases it may be prescribed when other efforts are unsuccessful.

An alarming development in recent years has been the increasing number of cases of type 2 diabetes among younger adults and even children. This has been linked to the increasing presence of obesity among young people.

Researchers now believe that by the time blood sugars are first noted to be above normal levels, the metabolic processes—and consequences—associated with type 2 diabetes have been present for ten to twelve years. Very often, insulin resistance or overt diabetes is accompanied by obesity, high blood pressure, and abnormalities of lipid (cholesterol and triglyceride) levels in the blood. The

continued on page 74

HEALTH PROBLEMS FOR DIABETICS

Heart and blood vessel disease. All of the processes that clog arteries throughout the body are aggravated by diabetes. As a result, diabetics are two to four times more likely than nondiabetics to have a heart attack or stroke. The fact that type 2 diabetics frequently have other risk factors for these calamities—high blood pressure, elevated cholesterol and triglyceride levels, and obesity—increases their likelihood even more. Furthermore, diabetics are vulnerable to clogging of both large and small arteries in the legs. Without adequate blood flow, small wounds on the legs and feet may not heal, and infections may fester and spread despite proper medical care. For this reason more than eighty thousand diabetics lose a foot or leg every year in the United States. Because cigarette smoking dramatically accelerates disease in all arteries, anyone with diabetes must avoid smoking at all costs.

Six out of ten amputations done for reasons other than trauma occur in diabetics.

Kidney disease. Diabetes is not kind to the kidneys, and a specific disease known as **diabetic nephropathy** is the leading cause of end-stage kidney disease that requires dialysis or transplant.

The word *nephropathy* is a fancy term for kidney disease created by combining the roots *nephro,* meaning kidney, and *path,* meaning disease. A **nephrologist** is a physician who specializes in disorders of kidney function.

Eye disease. In diabetics a number of changes within the retina (including the abnormal proliferation of small blood vessels) can lead to serious visual loss. Diabetes is the leading cause of new cases of blindness among adults over twenty. In order to take early preventive action if needed, anyone with diabetes should see an ophthalmologist (a physician trained to diagnose and treat eye disease) every year.

Nervous system disease. Diabetes can cause a variety of troubling nerve malfunctions. Altered sensations—especially burning, tingling, or numbness of the hands or feet—can be particularly irritating. If sensation is decreased or lost altogether, a diabetic may not feel pain that would normally serve as a warning that something is wrong. This may allow an injury or infection (especially in the feet) to progress before it is discovered.

Periodontal (gum) disease is more common among diabetics, and as many as one in three may have significant problems in this tissue.

Complications of pregnancy. Between 3 and 5 percent of pregnant women develop **gestational diabetes**, an elevation in glucose provoked by the hormonal changes of pregnancy. Their babies are more likely to be above average in size and weight (which may cause deliveries to be more difficult), and up to half of these mothers will develop type 2 diabetes later in life. Women with poorly controlled diabetes at the time of conception and during early pregnancy carry a 15 to 20 percent chance of suffering a miscarriage and a 5 to 10 percent chance of having a baby with a significant birth defect.[10] ■

TOP 10 GOALS FOR PEOPLE WITH DIABETES

Attain and maintain a body mass index (BMI) of 25 or less. We'll explain body mass index in chapter 6.

Begin and maintain moderate exercise at least five days per week, if not daily. We'll discuss exercise (and what is "moderate") in detail in chapter 7.

Avoid tobacco—your worst enemy. We review the damage wrought by tobacco in all of its forms, and how to free yourself from its grip, in chapter 10.

Maintain blood pressure of 120/80 or under. (Discussed earlier in this chapter.)

Keep LDL cholesterol at 100 or less. (Also reviewed earlier in this chapter.)

Get your blood glucose under control. For many people with type 2 diabetes (and nearly everyone with metabolic syndrome), this can be accomplished by achieving a healthy weight and exercising regularly. For people with type 1 diabetes and many with type 2, this will be a joint venture with a physician, involving blood glucose monitoring and, when appropriate, prescription medications. (Type 1 diabetics will need to become experts on the use of insulin.) You should become familiar with the blood test called the **glycohemoglobin** (also called **hemoglobin A1C**), which gives diabetics and their physicians feedback about overall glucose control over the previous three months.

Have your urine screened for a type of protein called microalbumin. This is an important marker for early kidney disease that can be slowed or stopped with appropriate medication.

Have your eyes checked by an ophthalmologist every year. Early changes in the retina that can lead to significant loss of vision can be detected and treated if the eyes are screened regularly.

Take good care of your feet. Diabetics are at risk for losing sensation, blood supply, or both in their feet. As a result, a minor injury can go unnoticed and eventually evolve into an ulcer (or a more severe infection) that will not heal. Your doctor or podiatrist can provide you with information about diabetic foot care. (Or check online—for example, the National Diabetes Education Program has an excellent summary called "Take Care of Your Feet for a Lifetime" at http://ndep.nih.gov/materials/pubs/feet/brochure/index.htm.)

Become a lifelong learner. There is a constant flow of new developments and helpful ideas for people with diabetes. Get on the mailing list or—if you are connected to the Internet —become a "frequent flyer" at one or more of the Web sites listed in the margin. ■

AMERICAN DIABETES ASSOCIATION
www.diabetes.org
(800) DIABETES

CENTERS FOR DISEASE CONTROL AND PREVENTION
Diabetes Public Health Resource
www.cdc.gov/diabetes
(877) 232-3422

NATIONAL DIABETES EDUCATION PROGRAM
www.ndep.nih.gov
(800) 438-5383

AMERICAN PODIATRIC MEDICAL ASSOCIATION
(for information about foot care)
www.apma.org
(800) FOOTCARE

continued from page 71

combination of these problems is now called the **metabolic syndrome,** a silent but hazardous convergence that significantly increases the risk of cardiovascular disease.

If the only problems caused by diabetes were thirst and frequent trips to the bathroom when glucose levels reached very high levels, this disease would now be more of a medical curiosity than a major national health problem. People with type 1 would merely take just enough insulin to keep out of trouble, and some with type 2 might eventually need to do the same, though for most the elevated glucose would represent little more than a high number on a lab report. Unfortunately, however, this disease can cause trouble from one end of the body to the other, and poor control of glucose aggravates all of its complications. For those with type 2 diabetes, all kinds of damaging events can be set in motion long before any symptoms appear. As a result, diabetes contributes to more than 200,000 deaths and more than $90 billion in direct health-care costs every year in the United States.

In spite of all of the terrible health problems that may be associated with diabetes, this problem and its complications can be contained—and an excellent quality and length of life enjoyed—with proper self-care and good medical management. While exploring the entire gamut of treatment options for diabetes is beyond the scope of this book, people with diabetes would do well to pursue several important goals. (See sidebar on page 73 "Top 10 Goals for People with Diabetes.") In addition, there are two very important "bottom-line" points that we want to emphasize here.

First, diabetes and two silent conditions, high blood pressure and elevated lipid levels, can be easily screened. Furthermore, these can also be dramatically improved through a combination of lifestyle changes and, when appropriate, medical treatment.

Second, and even more crucial, is the fact that we have seen a dramatic rise in the number of people with type 2 diabetes and its associated disturbances over the past few decades. While some of this can be accounted for by an increasing number of people over fifty, another major factor is that more of us are overweight and not exercising. We will take a long look at these issues later in this book, but we can say without hesitation—and we will say many more times—that *prudent dietary habits and a reasonable level of fitness can prevent a huge amount of expense, suffering, and death.*

Now that you have taken a look at these three common and important health problems, how do you find out whether or not any of them are already present, looming on the horizon, or potential troublemakers in your future? The next chapter will give you a guided tour of some important screening options. (We'll try to keep the discussion interesting.) These medical examinations and tests may not be the most enjoyable activities you'll ever encounter, but they may enhance, extend, or even save your life.

According to the Food and Drug Administration (FDA), about 1.6 million Americans had diabetes in 1958, compared with more than ten times that number today. Even allowing for differences in the measurement and reporting of diabetes over this forty-plus year period, this is a startling increase.[11]

QUESTIONS TO PONDER:

1. Do you or your family members have any of the basic risk factors for cardiovascular disease, cancer, or diabetes that were mentioned in this chapter?
2. If you are aware that you're at risk for one of these diseases, does that by itself provide enough motivation to make some changes (such as losing excessive weight or quitting smoking)? If not, what other types of motivation might work for you? (Look again at the section in chapter 1 entitled "Why Invest Time and Effort Pursuing Better Health?")

Action item: Read the next chapter to determine whether you or a family member should undergo any health screenings.

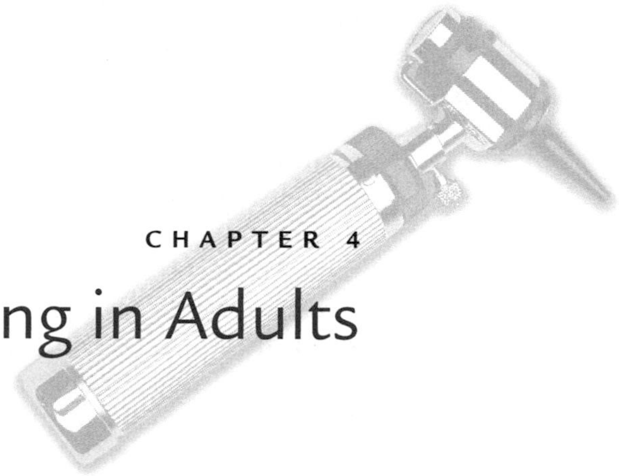

CHAPTER 4

Health Screening in Adults

Let's face it: Medical examinations and tests are no one's idea of a good time. They typically involve poking and probing into areas we would rather have left alone, not to mention bloodletting, X rays, and other procedures we would prefer be done only when absolutely necessary, especially when we may have to pay hundreds or even thousands of dollars for the privilege. This is particularly true when all of this is being done for screening purposes (and thus we don't have any symptoms) and when the results might spell B-a-d N-e-w-s. To make matters worse, well-informed physicians, government agencies, and major medical organizations often disagree regarding the necessity and frequency of commonly recommended screening tests. Adding to the confusion are entrepreneurs who promote medical screening tests directly to the public—but with questionable benefits, especially given the costs involved.

Despite all of these potential drawbacks, health screening can be worthwhile for a number of conditions. The goal, of course, is summarized by the old proverb "A stitch in time saves nine." We want to detect problems early, ideally before they're causing symptoms and definitely before they become big problems. But deciding what problems to screen for, how often, and what test(s) to use can be challenging. In order to make well-informed choices, you need to understand first what makes a screening test useful—or a waste of time and money.

1. The problem being screened should be relatively common in the general population, at a particular age, or in an identifiable group of people. Screening large numbers of people for a rare condition is like playing a state lottery; for every "winner"—the unfortunate person found to have the problem—there are many thousands who take the particular test with normal results. For example, not too many years ago it was common practice to order a chest X ray as part of a routine checkup in adults. Eventually it became apparent that a chest X ray rarely revealed a treatable problem when no symptoms were present.

2. An exception to the idea of screening for relatively common problems is a situation in which it is imperative that certain rare conditions be detected. For example, all blood donors must be screened for HIV (the virus that causes AIDS), as well as hepatitis B and C, even when there may be no reason to suspect that a given donor might carry one of these viruses. Why? Because it would be disastrous to give blood containing any of these viruses to an unsuspecting patient. Another exception would be a problem that isn't particularly common but that fits the other criteria described below. For example, newborn infants are routinely screened for a number of congenital syndromes, such as PKU, for which the tests are relatively inexpensive and the impact profound if the disease is not detected and treated. (See page 31 for more details on newborn screening tests.)

3. The problem being screened must have the potential to make a significant impact on future health if undetected and left alone. Obvious examples would include high blood pressure, which increases the odds of having a stroke or a heart attack and most (but not all) cancers.

4. The screening test must be able to detect the problem early enough to allow for action that will improve the quality and length of life. A corollary to this idea is that there should be an advantage to detecting the problem while it is silent, rather than waiting until symptoms have developed. One reason that chest X rays have not been considered useful in screening for lung cancer is the discouraging fact that in most cases a tumor large enough to be visible is also too far advanced for treatment to make a meaningful difference. By contrast, a colonoscopy can detect tumors or polyps in the large intestine at a stage when treatment can interrupt growth and prevent both local and distant spread.

5. The test should be reasonably sensitive and specific for the condition being screened. If a test isn't sensitive enough, it won't detect the presence of the problem you're concerned about, and you might get what is called a *false negative* result. Here the test results give a false sense of security, suggesting that nothing is wrong when in fact the condition is present. If a test isn't specific enough, a worrisome positive test result might actually be a false alarm (or what is called a *false positive* result), caused by some other condition. Not only can this create considerable anxiety, but additional tests that could be much more expensive and unpleasant may be needed to settle the question.

6. The test should be safe. This may seem like stating the obvious, but not every screening test is completely without risk.

7. The test should be reasonably comfortable. Fear of pain or other discomfort keeps many people away from tests that might prove to be life preserving. For some tests (for example, colonoscopy), special measures must be taken to ensure a reasonable level of comfort, if not a totally pain-free experience.

8. The test should be affordable or covered by insurance. Unfortunately, the opposite is true for many screening tests.

9. The test should be cost-effective. This concept is not necessarily related to affordability. Rather, it has to do with how many people must be tested for a given condition—and at what total price tag—to make a difference in the life and health of one person. Like it or not, decisions about the value and availability of screening tests often boil down to what sounds like cold economics: "If we decide to cover this test, we will have to spend X million dollars to save one life, and so it isn't cost-effective." Obviously, if you're the one whose life is on the line, cost-effectiveness may involve completely different calculations.

Considering all of these factors, it should come as no surprise that health professionals don't always agree on who should be screened, for which problems, at what age, and how often. There is even less harmony among insurance providers and government health-care programs (such as Medicare and Medicaid)—collectively known as the "payers"—on the subject of who should pick up the tab for all of this. While you might assume that payers would be interested in covering screening tests that could save them money in the long run, the economics of performing exams and tests on large numbers of people often dictate otherwise. But the fact that checkups and screening tests aren't covered by insurance doesn't mean that they are a waste of time and money. However, some activities definitely give you more bang for the buck than others, and throughout this section we will highlight those that are particularly worthwhile.

In chapter 2 we described how screening typically takes place for infants and children during age-related checkups carried out by a pediatrician or family physician. For adults, on the other hand, screening may or may not take place in the setting of a comprehensive examination. Therefore, our tour of screening tests for adults will be organized around several specific conditions. As you might expect if you have read chapter 3 ("Three Common Health Problems You Want to Avoid"), a major portion of current screening recommendations for adults is focused on preventing and detecting cardiovascular disease, cancer, and diabetes.

Screening for Cardiovascular Disease

Why is this important? As we discussed in detail in chapter 3, more adults die from this problem than any other, including all forms of cancer combined. Diseased arteries can obstruct the flow of blood to vital organs, especially your heart and brain, both of which you want to protect at all cost. Unfortunately, the first sign that anything is wrong may be sudden death or a devastating stroke, without any prior symptoms to warn you that major trouble is brewing.

How do I determine my risk factors? You do not need any medical tests for several of these: your age, your sex, your weight, a history of coronary artery disease (or certain risk factors for it) among your parents or siblings, your use of cigarettes, and whether or not you exercise on a regular basis. To determine the others, you need to answer the following questions:

What is my blood pressure?

Detailed information about high blood pressure (also called *hypertension*) may be found in chapter 3 beginning on page 52.

How do I find out? Blood pressure is measured using an arm cuff (sphygmomanometer) in a health-care setting, a machine in a pharmacy or supermarket, or a device at home. (Of these, the reading at the drugstore or market is likely to be the least accurate.) At home, a machine that uses an arm cuff (as opposed to a wrist or finger) is preferable, although for someone with a very large upper arm, a wrist cuff may be more practical to use. (Readings from a finger cuff may not be as reliable as those from an arm.)

During virtually any type of medical encounter, it is customary to record your **vital signs:** blood pressure, temperature, pulse, and respiratory rate (that is, how many times per minute you take a breath).

How often should I have this done? Regardless of your age, your blood pressure should be checked every time you see a doctor for any reason. Many dentists routinely check blood pressure, and other venues such as senior centers and health fairs typically offer free blood pressure screening. Even if you rarely need medical care, you should have your blood pressure checked every two or three years if you are younger than forty, and every year thereafter. If your pressure is borderline (120–139/80–89, now called **prehypertension**) or elevated (140/90 and over), you should be evaluated and followed more closely by a physician.

What is my cholesterol?

Detailed information about cholesterol and its impact on your health may be found in chapter 3 on page 56.

How do I find out? You will need to have a fasting blood specimen drawn at a laboratory or physician's office. Typically your physician orders this test, although it may also be requested as part of screening for life insurance. Health fairs usually offer this type of screening, as do some drugstores. You can even buy your own blood cholesterol testing kit, although this usually tests only the total cholesterol. In order to obtain a complete assessment of your risk, you should obtain a **lipid profile**, which includes not only total cholesterol but also the HDL and LDL components, as well as the triglycerides.

How often should I have this done? This test should be done every five years, beginning at age twenty.[1] Some experts do not recommend routine screening of adults older than seventy-five,[2] although this decision is affected by a person's health history and other risk factors for coronary artery disease. If your lipid profile represents a risk to your future health, or if you are being treated for abnormal lipids, you will need to be checked more often.

Fasting means that you haven't had any food or liquid containing calories for twelve to fourteen hours before the blood is drawn. Water, coffee, or tea without any creamer or sugar won't change the results of the test.

What is my blood sugar?

Elevated glucose (blood sugar) is an important diagnosis in and of itself, but it is particularly important as a risk factor for cardiovascular disease.

How do I find out? As with cholesterol, a fasting blood test is necessary and may be obtained in the same places as blood pressure readings (e.g., laboratories, physicians' offices, health fairs). If this is borderline or slightly elevated, additional blood sugar readings may be recommended, including tests taken one and two hours after a predetermined amount of glucose (usually a solution containing 75 grams) is taken by mouth. Blood glucose meters can also be purchased at any drugstore, although they are normally used by diabetics to follow their progress rather than for screening.

In a nonfasting test, only the total and HDL cholesterol results will be usable. If the total is more than 200 mg/dl or the HDL less than 40 mg/dl, a complete fasting lipid profile should be done. Are you a little fuzzy on what HDL, LDL, and triglycerides are? Check out pages 56–59.

F.Y.I.

Blood sugar measured at one or more specific intervals after a certain amount of glucose is swallowed is commonly called a glucose tolerance test (or GTT). Years ago this involved an ordeal of multiple blood draws over five or six hours. Nowadays, GTTs typically involve only a fasting glucose level and then repeating readings one and two hours after the glucose is swallowed.

At the present time, the diagnosis of diabetes may be based on any of the following findings:

- A fasting glucose level of 126 mg/dl or greater
- A nonfasting glucose of 200 mg/dl or greater when symptoms of diabetes (such as increased urine output, thirst, and unexplained weight loss) are present
- A glucose level of 200 mg/dl or more two hours after drinking the glucose solution during a glucose tolerance test

In order to confirm the diagnosis, a second abnormal result should be obtained on a different day.

A detailed look at the significance of elevated blood sugar and diabetes may be found in chapter 3, beginning on page 70.

How often should I have it done? The American Diabetes Association (ADA) recommends a fasting glucose test every three years to screen for type 2 diabetes in all individuals over forty-five years of age, regardless of their risk factors. Testing should be considered at a younger age, or should be carried out more frequently, in individuals with one or more risk factors for type 2 diabetes. These include

- A history of type 2 diabetes in a brother, sister, or parent.
- Excessive weight.

The definition of overweight used by the ADA is a body mass index (BMI) of 25 or greater. (A table to determine your BMI can be found on page 924.)

- A habitual lack of physical activity.
- Race/ethnicity—specifically Native American, Latino, African-American, Asian-American, and Pacific Islanders.
- An elevated fasting glucose or abnormal glucose tolerance test in the past.
- Hypertension (blood pressure of 140/90 or higher).
- HDL cholesterol less than or equal to 35 mg/dl and/or a triglyceride level greater than or equal to 250 mg/dl. (These lipid abnormalities are commonly found in people with type 2 diabetes.)
- For women, a history of diabetes during pregnancy (called gestational diabetes) or delivery of a baby weighing nine pounds or more. A disorder known as **polycystic ovary syndrome** is also associated with a risk of developing type 2 diabetes.[3]

Other Screening Tests for Cardiovascular Disease

A number of other tests to screen for cardiovascular disease are available, none of which are recommended on a routine basis for every adult. However, depending on your risk factors, symptoms, and other considerations, your doctor or a cardiologist may recommend any of the following:

C-reactive protein (CRP)

What is it? Many researchers now believe that chronic inflammation within the walls of arteries plays an important role in the process that leads to heart attacks and strokes. **CRP**, a protein manufactured in the liver and released into the bloodstream, has served for years as a marker for inflammatory diseases such as rheumatoid arthritis. A number of studies have suggested that CRP levels may also predict an increased risk for heart attack and stroke, even if cholesterol levels are normal. One theory holds that cholesterol levels reflect how much plaque is developing within the arteries, while CRP indicates the likelihood that the plaque may rupture. Interestingly, CRP also rises with—guess what—smoking and excessive weight, and decreases when cigarettes and extra pounds disappear.

How do I find out? Your doctor will need to order a blood test called a **high-sensitivity CRP** (or **hs-CRP**), which is different from the standard CRP test used to detect other diseases. This distinction is important, because variations in CRP that predict your risk for heart attack and stroke occur at relatively low levels, low enough to be considered normal on the standard CRP test.

See page 48 for more information about statins, which are widely used to treat high cholesterol levels.

What do I do with the results? If your hs-CRP is high, it is critically important that you quit smoking and achieve a desirable weight (if these are problem areas for you). In addition, your doctor may recommend taking a low-dose (81 mg) aspirin and a type of lipid-lowering drug called a statin that may reduce not only cholesterol but also inflammation (and thus CRP levels as well).

Homocysteine

What is it? The compound **homocysteine** is created during the metabolism of methionine, an essential amino acid that is one of the building blocks of proteins. Decades ago researchers noted that children with a rare genetic disorder called **homocystinuria**, which is marked by (among other things) very high homocysteine levels in the blood, had diffuse atherosclerosis—the diseased, thickened linings of blood vessels associated with heart attack and stroke. More recent studies have suggested that in the general population the risk of atherosclerotic disease rises with homocysteine levels in the blood. When present in abnormally high levels, this compound may injure arterial walls, provoke inflammation, and enhance the clotting process, which could lead to a sudden obstruction.

For some basic information about proteins, check pages 155–158 in chapter 5.

As we described in chapter 3, *atherosclerosis,* a word that literally means "hard porridge," is the medical term for the buildup of plaque that obstructs the flow of blood through arteries.

How do I find out? Your homocysteine level is determined by a blood test. While organizations such as the American Heart Association do not recommend screening everyone for this, your doctor may recommend it if you are at high risk for atherosclerotic disease, if you have already experienced a heart attack or stroke before the age of sixty, or if you have had this problem without other known risk factors.

What do I do with the results? If homocysteine levels are elevated, your doctor may recommend that you take **folic acid,** a safe and inexpensive supplement that lowers homocysteine levels. (Vitamins B_{12} and B_6 are also helpful.) How much you might be advised to take will depend upon the blood level—the higher the level, the higher the dose. Follow-up blood tests will be needed to gauge how the homocysteine level is responding. It is important to note that research has yet to determine whether lowering homocysteine levels actually reduces the likelihood of having a heart attack and stroke. Also, remember that one good reason to eat five or more servings of leafy green vegetables, fruits, and legumes every day is that they contain folic acid, B_6, and B_{12}.[4]

F.Y.I.

CAUSE AND EFFECT ALERT: If elevated homocysteine levels are associated with more heart attacks and strokes, wouldn't it make sense that lowering them would reduce this risk? That conclusion seems obvious, but in the realm of health, cause and effect are easy to assume and often hard to prove. The fact that elevated homocysteine levels are associated with more heart attacks and strokes does not mean that one causes the other, although it is reasonable to suspect that this could be the case. Furthermore, it is possible that lowering the level may not change an underlying process that is causing the problem. Only well-designed research will settle this question.

An electrocardiogram (ECG)

What is it? An **ECG** takes a snapshot of the heart's electrical activity over a period of several seconds. A number of electrically conducting patches connected by wires (called **leads**) to an ECG machine or a computer equipped with appropriate software are attached (using a gentle adhesive) to the chest, arms, and legs. These record the electrical impulse that travels through the heart with each beat, producing a tracing that looks like a series of blips and spikes on a continuous strip or (more commonly) on a single 8 ½-by-11-inch sheet of paper. Each of the leads looks at that impulse from a different "angle" of sorts, and the typical ECG contains twelve different views of the heart's electrical activity. The apparent hieroglyphics of an ECG reveal not only the heart's rate and rhythm pattern, but also specific changes that suggest that part of the heart isn't functioning (usually from a prior heart attack), or that some area isn't receiving enough blood at the moment—in essence, a distress signal. It also reveals abnormalities in the path taken by the electrical impulse as it travels through the heart.

Most people (including doctors) refer to this test as an "EKG," a throwback to the original German spelling of the word: electrokardiogram.

Should I have one done? The ECG is an important tool in the emergency department or any setting in which people are experiencing chest discomfort, pounding or fluttering sensations, faintness, or other symptoms that might indicate a problem with the heart. But if you have no symptoms, this test offers surprisingly little help in assessing your risk for coronary artery disease; it may, for example, appear completely normal in a person who is on the brink of a massive heart attack. Even if your ECG suggests that part of your heart has been damaged by a blocked coronary artery in the past, it does not provide the final answer, and further testing is necessary to determine the significance of that finding. For these reasons, an ECG may not necessarily be on the agenda for your routine physical. For someone over forty, however, one of these can be very useful as a baseline for future reference and comparison, if and when needed.

A stress exercise (treadmill) test

What is it? A **stress test** monitors the heart while exercising to see how it performs when subjected to an increased workload. The exercise usually involves walking on a treadmill at gradually increasing rates of speed, with the machine periodically tilting so that you are moving not only faster but also uphill at an ever increasing angle. The speeds and angles are predetermined according to a protocol that is designed to cause the heart to reach a maximal rate within nine to twelve minutes. For those who cannot walk (for example, because of bone and joint problems), the heart can also be put through its paces using medication that increases its rate in a predictable way.

Using harmless (and painless) high-frequency sound waves, an echocardiogram allows a physician to analyze the shapes and movement of the four chambers of the heart, as well as the thickness of the muscle that forms their walls. It also provides a look at the heart valves and the **pericardium,** the fibrous sac that surrounds the heart.

Blood pressure, pulse, and an ECG tracing are monitored and recorded during the test. Abnormalities of the blood pressure and pulse, and especially of the ECG tracing, during exercise may indicate problems. More elaborate monitoring can be done if the ECG tracing is difficult to interpret or mildly abnormal, in which case more information may be needed. One option is to do an **echocardiogram,** an image of the heart created using ultrasound equipment, at rest and then again just after the peak level of exercise is achieved. Heart muscle that's short on blood during exercise won't contract normally, which the echocardiogram will often detect. Another option is to inject a small amount of a specific radioactive isotope just before the exercise and then again afterward. A scan of the heart detects the distribution of the isotope and then creates an image reflecting the supply of blood to various areas.

Should I have this done? Exercise stress tests are not recommended as a routine screening for every adult at any given age. Instead, they are normally done in order to answer one of the following questions:

- *Do you have one or more symptoms that suggest coronary artery disease?* These would include chest pain or pressure that cannot be clearly written off as stemming from something other than the heart, an unexplained fainting episode, especially in someone over sixty, or unusual shortness of breath with minimal exertion.
- *Do you have so many risk factors that a date with the coronary-care unit is likely in the near future?* If you are an overweight, sedentary, hypertensive, hyperlipidemic, diabetic, chain-smoking, fifty-plus man whose parents and brothers all had heart attacks before the age of sixty, your doctor has probably already suggested (among other things) some type of stress test. You probably don't have *all* of these risk factors, but if you have enough of them to elicit this recommendation from your physician, give it some serious thought. The results may be revealing, motivating, and lifesaving.
- *Is it safe for you to exercise?* This is where the concept of the treadmill as a test drive can be particularly important, but whether you need one will depend on several factors, including the opinion of your doctor. Professional organizations have proposed various criteria for ordering a stress test. For someone planning to do moderate exercise—usually defined as a level of exertion at roughly 50 percent of one's maximal capacity and easily sustained for thirty to sixty minutes, such as a brisk walk—a treadmill would be appropriate if there is known cardiovascular disease, multiple risk factors, or symptoms as described above. For anyone over forty who is planning vigorous exercise—usually defined as jogging, running, cross-country skiing, mountain biking, or any activity that results in fatigue within twenty minutes or less—a treadmill test is usually recommended. (Obviously, *anyone* with multiple risk factors should have one before trying vigorous exercise.)

F.Y.I.

Why *not* do a stress test on everyone at a certain age? Wouldn't that uncover a lot of unsuspected disease and save thousands of lives? It would undoubtedly save some, but many (if not most) of those could have been predicted by a careful review of risk factors and symptoms. Unfortunately, if we were to screen every adult, there would be more than a few false positive results. These abnormal studies then require follow-up tests—which, by the way, are much more expensive—to determine more clearly whether the heart is actually in danger. The cost (and worry) generated by this "exercise" would be enormous.

Electron beam computerized tomography (EBCT)

What is it? EBCT is a high-speed computerized tomography (CT) scan of the coronary arteries (those that supply the heart) that specifically detects and measures the amount of calcium deposited in the walls of these blood vessels. Researchers have known for decades that calcium deposits are found in diseased (atherosclerotic) arteries, but not in normal ones. The development of plaque takes many years, and calcium deposits in the arteries increase both with age and the amount of plaque present. The scan provides what is called a calcium score, which generally, but not perfectly, correlates with the severity of coronary artery disease.

Should I have this done? The EBCT is not yet recommended by any professional organization as a screening tool for the general public. Current research suggests that while EBCT may be able to predict a heart attack in the future, it has not yet conclusively proven that ability. (Large-scale studies to address that question are now underway.) While the EBCT definitely is successful at finding plaque, arteries containing a lot of calcium may not necessarily be tightly narrowed or (more importantly) unstable. And coronary arteries may also become obstructed by "soft plaque," which contains little if any calcium but may still be unstable, especially among people younger than fifty. Like many of the tests just described in this section, EBCT may be a useful tool to help guide decisions about treatment when there is some uncertainty about the best course of action.

F.Y.I.

Later in this chapter we describe the pros and cons of "total body" CT scans that are now offered to the public as a screening test without a doctor's prescription. (This segment, starting on page 114, also includes some basic information about CT scans.) A total body scan may or may not include a high-speed scan of the coronary arteries; often this test is done separately.

Screening for Cancer

We would all love to have a simple, painless, reliable, and inexpensive test that would warn us early about a cancer that is just starting to grow (or better yet, one that is about to develop) somewhere in our body. Unfortunately, we don't have any wondrous *Star Trek* technology that fits this description. Instead we must rely on a patchwork of tests and procedures with great variability in cost, complexity, and comfort. Some tests to detect cancer (or precancerous conditions) are widely accepted as appropriate for nearly everyone; some are recommended specifically for people who may be at higher risk for a particular cancer; and some are controversial. The following is a field guide of sorts, a brief tour of a number of screening options that you should know about.

Remember that by definition, a screening test is one that is done for someone without symptoms. A person with symptoms—a persistent cough, pain, unexplained weight loss, or blood in the stool, to name a few—will need to be evaluated to find out what is wrong. Some of the tests that might be ordered will be similar or identical to those done for screening, but the strategy will be quite different. In this book, we will not attempt to outline what should be done about various symptoms because to do so appropriately requires a proper medical evaluation. As always, decisions tailored to your concerns, risks, coverage, and budget are best made in consultation with your own physician. Unless otherwise noted, the screening recommendations described here generally reflect those of the American Cancer Society.

Lung cancer

Lung cancer kills more people in the United States—about 160,000 every year—than any other type of tumor. More than 170,000 new cases are diagnosed each year.

Who is at risk? In a word, smokers. The more years and the more packs per day, the higher the risk. Unfortunately, those exposed passively to other people's cigarette exhaust (so-called "secondhand" smoking) and those who have inhaled smoke (of all kinds) at the workplace are also at higher risk.

What screening tests are available?

- One would think that a **chest X ray** would be useful for the smoker worried about his or her lungs. Unfortunately, in most cases by the time a tumor is visible on a chest X ray, treatment is not likely to be successful in curing it or even prolonging life. As a result, no professional organization recommends routine screening of smokers, or anyone else, for lung cancer. However, one large-scale study now underway is reevaluating the use of screening chest X rays in high-risk individuals, and future recommendations may change depending upon its outcome.
- **Sputum cytology** is a fancy term for a microscopic evaluation of cells brought up in phlegm from the chest. For a while it was thought that looking for abnormal cells in this material might prove useful in screening for lung cancer, just as the Pap smear has served well as a way to detect early changes in a woman's cervix (the opening of the uterus). But like the chest X ray, this approach has not proven to save or extend life, and no professional organization recommends it for routine screening. In the future, however, sputum may be evaluated for other biochemical markers that could indicate an increased risk for (or the actual presence of) cancer.
- **Spiral (helical) CT of the chest** is a rapid form of computerized tomography (CT) scanning that provides a detailed cross-sectional view of the chest with a relatively low dose of radiation. It is definitely more sensitive than a chest X ray in picking up abnormalities at an early stage. Therein is its greatest benefit and one major liability. The scan

can detect small nodules that may—or may not—be cancerous, and figuring out which is which can be difficult. One concern about doing this study on tens of thousands of people as a screening test is that this may result in thousands of elaborate evaluations, at an enormous cost, for abnormal (but ultimately benign) scans. At the present time no professional organization recommends screening chest CT scans, even for those who are definitely at risk for lung cancer. However, the technique has shown enough promise that large-scale studies are underway to determine whether it should be used widely for this purpose.

Technically the most common type of cancer for both men and women are skin cancers called basal cell and squamous cell carcinomas, which outnumber all other types of cancer combined. However, they cause far fewer deaths. Unless otherwise noted, when we mention that a certain type of cancer is the most common, second most common, etc., we are referring specifically to tumors not arising from the skin.

The bottom line: Lung cancer is common, lethal, and tough to screen. Low-dose spiral CT scanning may prove to be the most useful screening test for people at risk (i.e., smokers), but its routine use is controversial, it costs several hundred dollars, and in most cases it will not be covered by insurance.

Any way to prevent it? You know the answer: If you are a smoker, it's never too late to quit, and the sooner the better. Also, you should do whatever it takes to keep your kids from becoming tobacco users.

Breast cancer

Breast cancer is the most common nonskin cancer in women (more than 210,000 new cases every year) and the second most common cause of death from cancer (more than 40,000 deaths) in the United States.

Breast cancer is not a problem exclusive to women. About 1,700 cases and over 400 deaths from breast cancer occur in men every year in the United States.

Who is at risk? The following factors increase a woman's risk for developing breast cancer:

- Age: Most breast cancer occurs in women over fifty.
- A history of breast cancer in one's mother or in one or more sisters.
- Menstrual periods beginning early (before the age of twelve) and/or ending later in life (after fifty-five).
- Never having a baby or having one's first child after the age of thirty. Having a baby at a younger age reduces breast-cancer risk, as does bearing more than one child.
- Prolonged use (more than five years) of hormone therapy—specifically estrogen with progesterone—after menopause.

F.Y.I.

What about oral contraceptives? Most studies suggest either no risk—or at most a slight increase—among women who have used birth control pills. The risk may be associated with prolonged use, an early start, or use before one's first pregnancy. Note, however, that oral contraceptive use decreases the risk of ovarian cancer.[5]

- Exposure of the breast to radiation (other than diagnostic procedures such as mammography or chest X rays), especially at a young age.
- Inheriting an altered BRCA1 or BRCA2 gene. (See sidebar "Should I Be Tested for an Altered BRCA Gene?")

SHOULD I BE TESTED FOR AN ALTERED BRCA GENE?

About 5 to 10 percent of all cases of breast cancer, and 25 percent of cases in women under the age of thirty (which are, needless to say, very unusual), may be linked to an alteration of genes that control the growth of cells in breast tissue. These have been dubbed **BRCA 1** and **BRCA 2**, short for **br**east **ca**ncer **1** and **br**east **ca**ncer **2**, and a mutated form of one of these may be involved when there are multiple cases of breast cancer, or breast and ovarian cancer, in the same family. This genetic link may also be present when a person develops two completely different types of cancer. It is more common in members of certain Eastern European (Ashkenazi) Jewish families. Women born with the altered form of one of these genes have a three- to sevenfold higher risk for developing breast cancer than women without the alteration. (Their risk of developing ovarian cancer is also much higher—as much as ten- to thirtyfold.)

Checking for BRCA alterations involves taking a blood sample that is sent to a qualified laboratory. As simple as this sounds, the test is definitely *not* a routine screening exercise for every woman. There should be some selection based on family history or other specific reasons for concern. (If multiple family members have breast cancer, testing one who actually has this disease may help other family members decide whether to be screened as well.) The test is expensive—from several hundred to more than two thousand dollars—and may not be covered by insurance. In fact, many choose *not* to involve their health insurance out of concern that a positive result might adversely affect current or future coverage. Furthermore, a normal gene does not guarantee a life free of breast cancer, nor does an abnormal result mean that one is destined to have cancer.

Perhaps most thorny is the problem of deciding what to do about the finding of an altered BRCA gene. Certainly careful surveillance of breasts and ovaries is in order, but what about more aggressive measures? While removal of normal breast tissue and/or ovaries might seem a rather drastic approach to cancer prevention, certain women at very high risk may need to weigh this option. Medications such as tamoxifen (see page 93) that can reduce the risk of breast cancer are under evaluation for their usefulness in women with altered BRCA genes.

Needless to say, testing one's BRCA status should be done in concert with a physician who is well versed in the appropriate use, interpretation, and follow-up of this test. ■

- Obesity, excessive alcohol use, and possibly the consumption of a high-fat diet.
- Interruption of pregnancy by therapeutic abortion—a possible but hotly debated risk factor. (See appendix A on page 865.)

What screening tests are available? The American Cancer Society recommends the following for routine screening. (Remember that these advisories may be altered for a woman at higher-than-average risk or one who has had one or more abnormalities, biopsies, or surgeries needing closer follow-up.)

- **Breast self-exam (BSE)** every month for women over the age of twenty. This of course cannot diagnose breast cancer, and some have questioned whether self-examination is worthwhile because a tumor large enough to feel is likely to have been present for many months or even a few years. Furthermore, a woman with **fibrocystic breast changes,** which can create an ever-changing landscape of lumps and bumps from one month to the next (or even one part of the month to another), may feel that monthly self-checking is an exercise in futility. Nevertheless, more than a few women have found a cancerous lump before the doctor or a mammogram made the discovery.
- **Clinical breast exam (CBE)** every three years for women aged twenty to thirty-nine and annually for women forty and older. CBE is a fancy term for an exam by a physician (or an appropriately trained nurse practitioner or physician's assistant), typically carried out at the same time as a Pap smear.

F.Y.I.

The results of one recent large-scale study suggested that monthly breast self-examinations do not lower a woman's risk of dying from breast cancer and may lead to unnecessary biopsies. Based upon this and other research, some have suggested that teaching women to do this is counterproductive. While there is no question that breast self-examination *in the absence of regular mammograms* does not appear to save lives, it does enhance a woman's sense of what is normal (and what isn't) and thus may alert her to a change that should be evaluated.[6]

- **Mammography** every year starting at age forty. Why subject yourself to this procedure so often? Because breast cancer typically has a phase in which the tumor is large enough to be detected by mammography but too small to be felt by you or your doctor. This phase tends to be shorter before menopause (less than two years) than after menopause (more than three years). If at all possible, it's better to have a mammogram *after* the CBE (physician's exam), because any abnormality found on the exam can be brought to the attention of the radiologist interpreting the mammogram, who may recommend special views or even additional tests, such as an ultrasound study, to clarify the situation. If something is found during a breast exam done shortly after a normal mammogram, there may be a temptation to

For many years mammography was recommended every other year starting at forty and every year starting at fifty. More recent research has supported more frequent screening for women in their forties. Women at a higher risk for developing cancer based on family history may be advised to begin earlier.

BREAST SELF-EXAMINATION

First and foremost, remember the purpose of this exercise: to become familiar enough with the landscape of your breasts so that you will notice any changes that might need to be evaluated.

Because the consistency of your breasts may change during the course of your menstrual cycle, it is wise to self-examine at roughly the same time of each cycle. For most women the best time is during the week after a menstrual period ends, when the breasts are less likely to be lumpy or tender. Women with very irregular cycles may need to pick a more arbitrary date, such as the beginning of each calendar month. It's also a good idea to self-examine on a morning of the week when you're not pressed for time.

You'll get more accomplished if you examine yourself in two positions: lying down (typically, before you get up in the morning) and standing up (either in the shower or in front of a mirror). In each case, feel each breast using the pads of the three middle fingers of the opposite hand. When lying down, put a pillow under the shoulder of the side being examined, and place the hand on that side under your head. You'll want to press firmly enough to feel the texture (and any lumps) well below the skin surface, but without jabbing yourself or causing pain. You will probably notice a firm ridge along the lower curve of each breast; this is normal.

Move your hand around the breast in a circular motion or up and down, being sure to cover not only the entire surface of the breast but also the "tail," the upper, outer segment of breast tissue that extends to the armpit. *Roughly half of all breast cancers are found in this area,* which is felt most easily while you are standing up, so don't overlook it. If you examine your breasts the same way every month, you'll be more likely to pick up changes. Also, check in the mirror for any suspicious changes at the surface: inflammation of the skin, dimpling, crusting, or discharge from the nipple.

If you detect something that doesn't seem normal to you, be sure to have your physician check it. You should do this *even if you have had a normal mammogram within the previous year.* ■

ignore it. But the examiner may pick up something that a routine mammogram missed, and so his or her findings should not be brushed aside, even after a normal mammogram.

The bottom line: The best strategy for early breast-cancer detection is to undergo *all three types of examinations on a regular basis,* starting at the appropriate age. Ignoring any of them because you have done one or two of the others is a bad idea. It is particularly unwise to skip the mammogram—certainly a temptation because of the cost and discomfort involved—even if

MAMMOGRAM QUESTIONS AND ANSWERS

What's the difference between a screening and a diagnostic mammogram? A *screening* mammogram is carried out to detect changes in the breasts when there are no symptoms or abnormalities. A *diagnostic* mammogram, on the other hand, is done to investigate a suspicious area in one or both breasts.

I really don't like the part during a mammogram when they squeeze my breast. Why is that necessary? Flattening the breast allows for more detail to be seen with less radiation. Fortunately this portion of the exam takes a relatively short amount of time—usually a minute or so. This discomfort can be minimized if the mammogram is done shortly after a menstrual period (if they are still occurring), when the breasts are least likely to be tender.

Speaking of radiation, is it safe to have a mammogram every year? The radiation exposure during a mammogram is extremely low, and there is no evidence that an annual mammogram, even when done for decades, increases the risk for any cancer (including breast).

Once I have had the mammogram, "no news is good news," right? Probably, but you should always receive some type of communication—either a phone call or a letter—from the facility that performed the study or from your own doctor. If the radiologist—the physician who "reads" the mammogram—is available, you may get feedback on the spot. If not, it may take a few days for the interpretation to be completed and for you to hear about it. Sometimes additional views or even a different type of study (such as an ultrasound) may be recommended in order to clarify what is going on in a certain area.

If the radiologist recommends further tests, is that bad? Not necessarily.

Should I have them done? Absolutely. Roughly one in ten of these women who have a mammogram is advised to have additional testing. Of these, about one in ten evaluations leads to a biopsy, and of these only about one in ten of these women will actually have cancer. All in all, this means that only about one in one thousand mammograms reveals a tumor. This is good news—but it would be foolhardy to ignore the advice of the radiologist or your physician when additional tests have been recommended. ■

you have had consistently normal exams by yourself and your physician.

Any way to prevent breast cancer? Obesity and lack of exercise increase your risk for developing breast cancer, so it only makes sense that maintaining physical fitness and an appropriate weight will pay off. Because breast cancer is more common in populations that consume a high-fat diet, shifting the menu away from fatty foods may be prudent, although there is no conclusive evidence that doing so will reduce your risk. Avoiding excessive alcohol use is a wise idea as well. A woman contemplating an abortion should be aware of its potential contribution to her chances of developing breast cancer—especially if she has other risk factors. Prolonged use of estrogen and progesterone after menopause is associated with an increased risk of breast cancer, and you should thus weigh carefully the pros and cons of taking this supplement for more than five years. (The data are inconclusive about whether estrogen-only hormone therapy is a risk factor.) In addition, women at increased risk (especially those with a history of breast cancer in a close family member) may be candidates for medications called selective estrogen receptor modulators (or SERMs).

How much alcohol is too much? See chapter 10 for some input on this important topic.

"SERMs" AND BREAST CANCER

A group of medications called **selective estrogen receptor modulators**, or **SERMs**, might be considered "estrogen imposters." They attach to cells and tissues in the body that are normally stimulated by estrogen, but then affect them in different ways. On the plus side, they block the stimulation of breast-cancer cells (if any are present) by estrogen. They also imitate estrogen's bone-strengthening effects. **Tamoxifen** (Nolvadex) has been used for years as a treatment for breast cancer, and more recently has been used to lower the likelihood of breast cancer in properly selected women who are at increased risk. **Raloxifene** (Evista), which is prescribed as a treatment for osteoporosis (thinning of bone), may reduce breast-cancer risk as well, although research data has not been released as of the date of publication of this book.

So why not put every woman on a SERM after menopause? Because these drugs also have a minus side: They imitate estrogen's tendency to increase the risk of blood clots but block its benefits in the genital area. They can also generate hot flashes or bring them back for an encore in women who have already endured this particular rite of passage. Tamoxifen, like estrogen, can also stimulate some worrisome changes in the lining of the uterus.

SERMs can be health-preserving (even life-preserving) tools for some women, but they are not without risks and drawbacks. Optimal use requires appropriate selection by a gynecologist or family physician and a careful discussion of benefits and risks. ■

Prostate cancer

For men, **prostate cancer** is the most common nonskin cancer (over 230,000 new cases each year) and the second most common cause of cancer death (about 30,000 per year). As these numbers suggest, a man is much more likely to develop prostate cancer than to die from it. If he lives well into his eighties or beyond, he is even more likely to harbor cancer cells in his prostate without knowing it.

The prostate is a walnut-sized gland in the male reproductive system, located just in front of the rectum and below the bladder. In fact, it surrounds the urethra—the tube that carries urine and semen through the penis—where it exits the bladder. The prostate manufactures most of the fluid (but not the sperm cells) in semen.

F.Y.I.

Vocabulary lesson: The sound-alike words **ureter, urethra,** and **uterus** can be a source of confusion in the doctor's office or hospital. The *ureters* are a pair of narrow tubes that conduct urine from each kidney to the bladder. If obstructed by a stone, a ureter can generate severe pain. The *urethra* is the tube that transports urine from the bladder to the outside world. The male urethra is much longer, because it passes through the penis. The *uterus*—otherwise known as the womb—actually is not part of the urinary tract, but rather the pear-shaped muscular organ in which a baby grows during a woman's pregnancy.

Who is at risk? Men, obviously, but more specifically:

- Older men. Prostate cancer is primarily (but not exclusively) a disease of men over fifty. More than 70 percent of cases are diagnosed in men sixty-five years and older, and in the United States, the average age at the time of diagnosis is seventy-two. It is estimated that by the age of eighty, half of all men have cancer cells in the prostate, though the vast majority will die of something else.
- African-American men have the highest rates of acquiring and dying from prostate cancer. Asian-American and Pacific Island men have the lowest rates of disease and death.
- Family history. A man whose father or brother(s) have had prostate cancer has a higher risk.
- A diet high in fat may increase a man's risk for developing prostate cancer.

F.Y.I.

Several years ago, one study suggested that a *vasectomy*—the procedure for male sterilization in which the tubes (*vas deferens*) that carry sperm away from the testes are cut—might increase a man's risk for prostate cancer. Subsequent studies have not shown any connection between vasectomy and this or any other disease.

What screening tests are available?

- The **digital rectal exam** (or **DRE**) is a time-honored, quick, low-tech and—for those both on the giving and receiving end—not terribly popular method of checking the prostate. Since one side of the prostate is directly adjacent to the rectum, a physician can insert a gloved, lubricated finger through the anal canal and check the size, shape, and consistency of the prostate. A definite **nodule** would need to be investigated in more detail. Unfortunately, this method will rarely pick up an early tumor, because a growth must be relatively large and protruding from the gland before it can be felt. Nevertheless, a small percentage of prostate cancers are discovered this way, even when the more sensitive PSA test (see below) is normal.

- **Prostate-specific antigen (PSA)** is a protein that is produced by the normal prostate gland. It is present in semen, but more importantly also measurable in blood. The PSA level in blood is found in tiny amounts: the norm is less than 4 *nanograms* per milliliter (expressed as 4 ng/ml) of blood. A PSA level can be obtained from a small blood sample, which may be drawn at a doctor's office, clinic, lab, or hospital. Many men have their PSA level checked at health fairs or prostate-screening clinics sponsored by their employer. While a PSA level can be elevated for a variety of reasons (see sidebar "Does an Elevated PSA Level Mean I Have Cancer?"), the higher it goes, the more likely a prostate cancer is present. A man with a PSA between 4 and 10 has roughly a one in four chance of having prostate cancer; at a PSA of 10 or more, the chances increase to more than two out of three. Note also that the medication **finasteride** (known as **Proscar** when it is prescribed for reducing the size of the prostate gland and as **Propecia** when it is used to grow hair) can lower the PSA level.

A nanogram is a *billionth* of a gram, and a gram weighs about one-thirtieth of an ounce. A milliliter, also known as a cubic centimeter (or cc), is one-thousandth of a liter. (A liter is a volume roughly equal to a quart.) Obviously, we're dealing with very small quantities here.

The bottom line: With the availability of a relatively inexpensive, sensitive test such as the PSA test, one would think that screening for prostate cancer would be a slam-dunk process. Surprisingly, most of the major professional organizations do *not* recommend any specific routine screening for prostate cancer. Why? Because (more surprisingly) it has yet to be shown conclusively that screening large numbers of men will lower the overall death rate. Critics of screening have pointed out that chasing down borderline PSA results that prove to be false alarms can involve costly and uncomfortable procedures. Furthermore, even when an early cancer is detected in the prostate, it is impossible to know whether the tumor is destined to grow and spread aggressively, or whether it will sit quietly within the gland and never cause problems. The American Cancer Society and the American Urological Association, on the other hand, have expressed the opinion that this screening *does* save lives, although their recommendation is merely that physicians offer a digital rectal exam and a blood test to check the PSA level to men fifty and over and that they discuss carefully the pros and cons of pursuing abnormal results.

The popular herb **saw palmetto**, which improves urine flow in men with prostate enlargement, does not appear to affect PSA measurements. However, some experts recommend checking a baseline PSA prior to using this herb and then rechecking a few months later, because herbal preparations are not always pure and may contain other compounds that could affect the PSA level.

It is certainly important to evaluate and debate the overall costs and benefits of screening large populations for any type of cancer. For an individual

DOES AN ELEVATED PSA LEVEL MEAN I HAVE CANCER?

Before you lose a lot of sleep over the news that your PSA is elevated, remember that the test is measuring prostate-*specific* antigen, not prostate-*cancer* antigen. Yes, the level goes up when cancer is present. But it also goes up:

- **With age.** There is a gradual increase in the normal range for PSA with each passing decade, and so a level that might cause alarm in a fifty-year-old would not be as worrisome in an eighty-year-old.
- **With enlargement of the gland that is not cancerous.** As men age, the prostate tends to enlarge and may interfere with the flow of urine from the bladder, even when no cancer cells are present. This condition is called **benign prostatic hypertrophy**, one of the most common problems for which men seek help from urologists.
- **With inflammation.** An infection in the prostate (called **prostatitis**) will send the PSA soaring. Any screening for cancer must be done well after any such infection has resolved.
- **After ejaculation.** The PSA level goes up after semen is released. Abstaining for two days prior to the test will avoid a false elevation.

What other tests might reveal the cause of an elevated PSA?

- **Repeating the test at a later date.** This may be appropriate if there is any doubt about the validity of the result, or if the physician wants to see if a borderline level is increasing over time.
- **Checking the percent of free PSA.** Most PSA circulates through the bloodstream attached to a carrier protein, while some travels on its own. These are called **bound** and **free PSA**, and the more free the better. If your PSA is mildly elevated—between 4 and 10 ng/ml—you have a 50 percent chance of having prostate cancer if your free PSA is less than 10 percent of the total. On the other hand, if your free PSA is more than 25 percent, your odds of having cancer are definitely lower (but not zero).
- **Calculating the PSA velocity.** This "speed test" actually involves checking successive PSA levels over at least eighteen months and then calculating how rapidly it is rising. A biopsy may be appropriate if the PSA increases at a rate of more than 0.75 ng/ml per year.
- **Transrectal ultrasound and biopsy.** These tests are carried out by a urologist when all of the risk factors, exam, PSA, and other variables indicate that more information is needed. The transrectal ultrasound creates sound-wave images of the prostate using a small probe that is inserted into the rectum. This helps locate suspicious-appearing areas that can be biopsied using a fine, hollow needle to remove a very small sample of tissue. If no suspicious areas are seen, the urologist may take a few samples (typically six) from different areas of the prostate. These tissue specimens are evaluated by a pathologist. ■

A **urologist** is a physician trained in surgery who deals with diseases involving the urinary tract in which something needs repair, revision, or removal. He or she also deals with male reproductive problems. A **nephrologist**, on the other hand, is an internal-medicine specialist who has special training in and experience treating nonsurgical kidney disease; for example, nephrologists perform **dialysis** as a treatment for acute or chronic kidney failure.

man over fifty, however, it is difficult to decline a prostate exam and a blood test for PSA based on national cost-effectiveness statistics. The only alternative would be to look the other way and hope for the best, waiting for the cancer to announce its presence after it has become advanced or widespread. Granted, it can be difficult to decide what to do about a mildly elevated PSA—or even how best to treat an early prostate cancer. This requires a careful review of the options with a urologist (perhaps a second opinion as well). But the prostate exam and PSA test provide at least *some* information rather than leaving a man completely in the dark about the condition of his prostate.

At the very least, we recommend that men fifty and over discuss a digital rectal exam and PSA screening with their physician and certainly consider having these done. Those at higher risk, such as African-American men or those with a father or brother who has had prostate cancer, should begin this process at age forty-five. (An exception would be a man whose life expectancy is less than ten years.)

Any way to prevent prostate cancer? Unlike many other types of cancer, the possibilities for preventing prostate cancer are currently a list of "maybe's." Steering clear of fats and including lots of fruits, vegetables, and grains in your diet—a common thread in cancer prevention—may help prevent prostate cancer. Compounds called **lycopenes** that are found in tomatoes, tomato products, grapefruit, and watermelon may have antioxidant properties that reduce prostate cancer risk. Vitamin E (at 400 units per day) and the trace mineral selenium have been proposed as possibly protecting against prostate cancer, but the results of a major study designed to address that question will not be available until 2013.

The drugs finasteride (Proscar) and dutasteride (Avodart) reduce the size of the prostate by blocking the effect of testosterone on it. Recent research suggests that prolonged use of this drug may reduce the likelihood of developing prostate cancer—but if cancer does occur in men using this drug, it is more likely to be of a higher **grade**, which is bad news. (Pathologists evaluate prostate-cancer cells using what is called the **Gleason system,** which assigns a grade from one to five based on how closely the cells resemble normal tissue. Higher grade cells are more abnormal in appearance and are considered more likely to grow and spread more rapidly.) Future research will no doubt clarify this situation, but for now men and their physicians will have to sort through the pros and cons of using this drug.

The popular herb saw palmetto, which can relieve symptoms caused by benign prostate enlargement, is not known to treat or protect against prostate cancer.

Colon cancer

Colon cancer (also called **colorectal cancer** to include the very end of the colon, called the rectum) is, for both men and women, the third most common type of cancer (nearly 145,000 new cases every year in the United States) and also the second most common cause of cancer death (more than 56,000 every year). Cases and deaths are about equally divided between men and women, with women affected slightly more frequently than men. Like breast cancer, colon cancer often develops slowly enough to be intercepted at an early stage, when a cure is possible if appropriate steps are taken. In fact, it typically begins as a **polyp,** a fleshy growth on a stalk that can be snared and removed during a sigmoidoscopy or colonoscopy. During its early growth, *colorectal cancer is usually completely silent.* By the time a tumor in the colon or rectum becomes large enough to cause symptoms, it may be advanced and much more difficult to treat. Therefore, screening is very important and may be lifesaving.

A terminology note: The **colon** (also called the **large intestine**) is the final segment of bowel through which undigested food and other waste products pass before being eliminated. It serves primarily to absorb water and thus convert the liquid outflow from the **small intestine** (which is actually much longer) into solid stool. It forms a shape roughly resembling an inverted U. The first segment, which begins in the right lower abdomen, is called the **cecum.** Stool moves "uphill," through what is called the **ascending** (or simply **right**) colon, then crosses the upper abdomen in the **transverse** colon, and finally flows downward again through the **descending** (or **left**) colon. Before leaving the body, stool passes through the **sigmoid** colon into the **rectum,** where it is held before receiving the signal (voluntary or otherwise) to be pushed out via the anus during a bowel movement.

THE COLON

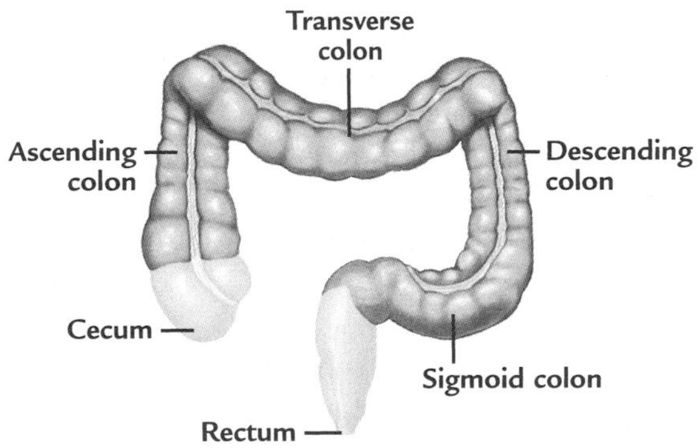

The term *sigmoid* means "like the letter S," suggested by the curving shape of this part of the colon, while the word *rectum* comes from the Latin for *straight* (as in *rectify* or *rectitude*), reflecting its direct path between sigmoid and anus.

Who is at risk? The risk for this type of tumor increases with:

- Age. Most cases occur in people over sixty-five years of age, but screening for most people should begin at fifty.
- Family history of colorectal cancer in a parent or sibling that appeared before the age of sixty, or in two immediate family members at any age. About 65 percent to 85 percent of colon cancers are called **sporadic**, because no one in the family is known to have this problem. About 10 percent to 30 percent of colon cancers are called **familial**, which means that more than one family member is affected, but without a known genetic abnormality. Finally, about 5 percent of colon cancers involve a specific, identified inherited gene mutation, which results in a markedly higher risk among

members of the affected family. (See sidebar "Hereditary Colon Cancer Syndromes.")

- A history of **inflammatory bowel disease**, specifically **ulcerative colitis** or **Crohn's disease**, for an extended period of time. Cancer risk significantly increases after eight years of widespread involvement of the colon, or twelve to fifteen years of involvement of the left colon.
- A history of colon cancer or polyps. If you had a colon cancer in the past, you have an increased risk for developing cancer somewhere else in the colon, even if the first tumor was completely removed. Likewise, if you have had polyps diagnosed (and hopefully removed) in the past, you also have an increased risk of developing colon cancer, especially if they were large or plentiful. Because all polyps are not created equal—that is, some types are more worrisome than others—your physician should guide you regarding fol-

HEREDITARY COLON CANCER SYNDROMES

About one percent of all colon cancers are caused by **familial adenomatous polyposis**, in which large numbers of polyps (often numbering in the thousands) develop throughout the colon, beginning during the teen years. Cancer inevitably develops in one or more of these polyps between the ages of thirty and fifty, and without identification and treatment the development of colon cancer by the age of forty-five is nearly a certainty. Because it is impossible to deal with hundreds or thousands of polyps on a long-term basis, complete removal of the colon is commonly recommended as a preventive measure. This might seem to be a drastic measure, but it is nearly always preferable to enduring treatment for (or dying from) colon cancer. Members of families affected by this syndrome should begin having colonoscopies on a regular basis beginning at age ten.

Three to 4 percent of colon cancers occur in people with **nonpolyposis colorectal cancer** (or **Lynch's syndrome**), which results from an abnormality in one or more of five specific genes. Lynch's syndrome should be suspected if

- Three or more members of the same family have colon cancer, and at least one person is a **first-degree relative**—that is, the parent, son, daughter, or sibling—of one of the other two.
- Colon cancer has occurred in at least two generations.
- At least one individual developed cancer before the age of fifty.
- Familial adenomatous polyposis is not involved.

Because people with Lynch's syndrome have about a 70 percent chance of developing colon cancer (more often on the right side), colonoscopy should begin at age twenty and continue every one to three years if this problem is suspected or known to exist within the family. ■

low-up, which usually involves having a colonoscopy at regular intervals.

- Bad habits. Smoking, heavy alcohol use, and lack of physical exercise are all associated with a higher risk of developing colon cancer.
- Obesity.
- Diabetes. People with this problem have a 40 percent greater chance of developing colon cancer.
- A diet high in fat from animal sources.

What screening tests are available? Since the colon is hidden from any direct view, screening for cancer involves "looking" for it in three possible ways: directly with colonoscopy or sigmoidoscopy, indirectly with X-ray imaging, and *very* indirectly by detecting blood in the stool.

- **Fecal occult blood testing (FOBT)** is the very indirect approach, but it is a simple, low-tech, and inexpensive way to get a heads-up that something might be wrong. Tumors and polyps are more fragile than normal tissue and may lose small amounts of blood as stool passes by them. But they usually bleed slowly and intermittently; so slowly, in fact, that the blood may not be visible at all. The term *fecal occult blood* thus refers to blood that is "occult" in the sense of "hidden" within the feces. It can, however, be detected using a simple chemical test (known as a **guaiac test**) that involves applying small samples of stool onto a card specifically designed for this purpose. When a chemical "developer" is placed on the specimen, a blue color heralds the presence of blood. (When a doctor or nurse says that a sample of stool is "guaiac positive," he or she is saying that it contains blood you can't see.) That does not, of course, automatically mean that cancer is present. The blood could have come from a hemorrhoid or a small crack (called a **fissure**) at the anal opening. Even some undercooked meat eaten during the previous day or two might give a positive result. A properly executed FOBT every year starting at age fifty is one of five possible options recommended by the American Cancer Society for colorectal-cancer screening. Note that a single specimen collected by the doctor during a rectal exam is not by itself an adequate test. Your odds of picking up blood that is oozing sporadically from a polyp or tumor increase if you get samples from three bowel movements. (See sidebar "Dealing with the Dreaded Stool Card.") The newer **fecal immunochemical test** is essentially performed the same way as an FOBT, but it is more precise and results in fewer false positives. It detects a specific portion of a human blood protein. Like the conventional FOBT, it will not detect a tumor that is not bleeding.
- **Sigmoidoscopy** provides a direct look into the colon using a flexible, narrow (finger-width) hollow tube containing special fibers that send light to the tip and an image back to an eyepiece or video moni-

DEALING WITH THE DREADED STOOL CARD

If you are fifty or over, at any routine checkup your doctor may hand you an envelope containing a little card and some short wooden sticks before giving you a daunting assignment: "You'll need to collect some samples from three bowel movements on this card. . . ." You have just been invited to enter the wonderful world of fecal occult blood testing.

I need to do what?? you ask yourself. Nobody looks forward to collecting a stool specimen for any reason, but *three* of them? No way! Very often this card ends up gathering dust in a dresser drawer. But since the lowly card could save your life, it is worth treating respectfully, even if not with total enthusiasm. To get the most bang for your screening buck, you should observe the following:

- Don't cheat yourself. The odds of finding something improve dramatically if you collect two samples from each of three different stools (thus a total of six in all). The three stools don't have to be consecutive, although you'll get this over more quickly if they are.
- For each of the three stools, there should be two little "windows" on the card into which you will dab your samples. These should be from different parts of the stool. (For example, you could take one from the toilet paper, and the other out of the bowl, but you should let any water drip off before applying the specimen to the card.) You don't need a large amount—a modest smear will do.
- Watch what you ingest—including medications—for two days prior to starting your collection and for however long it takes to finish it. Red meats, vitamin C (more than 250 mg daily), iron supplements, aspirin, or anti-inflammatory drugs such as ibuprofen (Advil, Motrin, and others) or naproxen (Aleve and others) may set off a false alarm. If you are taking low-dose aspirin to prevent a heart attack or stroke, however, you should continue your usual dose.
- Once you have done your duty, return the card promptly to the doctor, clinic, or lab to have it processed. *Don't mail it* unless you were given a special reinforced envelope in which to send it. (The postal service does not want to have any direct contact with your sample.)
- Be sure to put your name on the sample card before you return it.
- Even if you did not adhere perfectly to the dietary recommendations during the collection period, *return the card*. The worst thing that could happen would be a more thorough evaluation (specifically, a colonoscopy) that will give you a clear understanding of your colon's status. This is far better than not returning the card at all. ■

tor. This procedure is typically performed by a specialist called a **gastroenterologist**, although many family physicians and general internists do flexible sigmoidoscopies as well. (It is less common for physicians who are not gastroenterologists to do colonoscopies.) A sigmoidoscopy allows the examiner to peer into the last fifty to sixty centimeters (about twenty to twenty-four inches) of the colon, which includes the rectum and the sigmoid. The test can be done in a physician's office, requires only a modest preparation (typically a couple of enemas taken two hours apart), and is relatively inexpensive (under two hundred dollars). Unfortunately, a sigmoidoscopy leaves a large segment of the colon unseen and thus will detect only about half of all tumors of the colon. (This is like having a mammogram of one breast but not the other—definitely better than nothing, but not exactly a complete screening.) If any polyps are seen during a sigmoidoscopy, however, the patient will need a full colonoscopy at a later date.

F.Y.I. Years ago, sigmoidoscopies were done using a rigid metal scope which could only be inserted about twenty to twenty-five centimeters (about eight to ten inches). Needless to say, these were rather uncomfortable and very limited in what they could visualize. The curving sigmoid is not particularly interested in conforming to the shape of a straight object.

- **Colonoscopy** involves passing a longer flexible scope through the entire colon. Currently the gold standard for cancer screening, this procedure allows a complete inspection of the colon (provided that it is properly cleared of stool that would obstruct the view) and has the ability to remove any polyps or take samples from areas that appear abnormal. With few exceptions, colonoscopy is performed using sedation that effectively allows the person to doze through the entire procedure, usually with very little or no memory of it. This involves an intravenous line (to give medication directly into the vein) and monitoring of heart rate and oxygen levels. For this reason, colonoscopy can be done only in a properly equipped office or clinic, or in a hospital. This pushes its potential cost to several hundred dollars, if not into the thousand-plus range. Medicare will now pay for a screening colonoscopy every ten years for those sixty-five and older, but most insurance plans will cover this procedure only when specific problems are being addressed: rectal bleeding or a stool card that tests positive, unexplained anemia (low red blood cell count), a history of colon cancer in a parent or sibling, or abdominal discomfort for which this is an appropriate test. In an adult over forty, colonoscopy is usually one of the first tests to be considered when a low red blood cell count is found and there is no obvious underlying cause.

For more information about health insurance in general, and Medicare in particular, see chapter 17.

F.Y.I.

Those who have had both sigmoidoscopy and colonoscopy will typically declare their preference for snoozing through the more complex procedure over being wide-awake during the simpler one. However, while a colonoscopy takes only about thirty minutes, it's common to feel groggy or at least tired for several hours afterward. When you include the time involved to "prep" (clean out) the colon with one or more laxative materials, the entire process involves the better part of a day.

- **Imaging tests for the colon** include both old and new technologies. The old is the **double-contrast barium enema (BE)**, which was the primary test to view the contents of the colon before the advent of fiber-optic technology. A BE involves a laxative prep to clear out as much stool as possible and then the insertion of a chalky liquid and some air via the rectum. Several X rays are taken of the colon as its owner is moved in several positions, providing a black-and-white image of its inner contours. All of this is about as much fun as it sounds—no sedation is involved, and a sensitive colon may cramp in protest. Many people have become intrigued by the newer technology popularly called **virtual colonoscopy** (sometimes called **virtual colonography**), which utilizes helical CT scanning technology to create an image similar to that seen by a physician performing a colonoscopy. The amount of X-ray exposure is likely to be less than that from a barium enema, but the procedure is no less uncomfortable. The preparation utilized to cleanse the colon of stool needs to be at least as vigorous as that for a barium enema, if not more so, and the colon must be inflated with air (via a thin tube in the rectum) prior to the scan, as it is during a BE. No sedation is needed, however, and so either procedure takes much less time than a colonoscopy. Barium enema and virtual colonoscopy are likely to be less expensive than a colonoscopy (although the virtual colonoscopy is likely to be the more expensive X-ray procedure), and both can detect polyps larger than one centimeter (about a half-inch) in diameter, though not smaller ones. (However, growths smaller than one centimeter are extremely unlikely to be cancerous.) There may even be situations where virtual colonoscopy may have the advantage of being able to "see" segments of colon that are out of reach of conventional colonoscopy or a barium enema (for example, because of spasm or partial obstruction). Neither barium enema nor virtual colonoscopy can show the color or subtle changes of the lining of the colon, which can be important if problems other than tumors or polyps, such as inflammation of the colon, are present. Virtual colonoscopy may mistake a small bit of leftover stool for a polyp, which will lead to a colonoscopy, although newer technologies may make that problem less common. And, most important, neither procedure can obtain a specimen for biopsy. If something looks sus-

What's a helical CT scan? Check the sidebar "Should I Have a 'Total Body' CT scan?" beginning on page 114.

picious, a full colonoscopy will need to be done. At present, medical insurance plans do not cover either procedure for screening purposes, and no professional organization has endorsed virtual colonoscopy as a screening procedure.

The bottom line: Colon cancer is common but definitely detectable—and often curable if detected early. American Cancer Society guidelines recommend one of the following screening strategies for everyone who has an average risk for colon cancer, beginning at age fifty:

- Fecal occult blood testing every year, or
- Sigmoidoscopy every five years, or
- Fecal occult blood testing every year *plus* sigmoidoscopy every five years, or
- Double-contrast barium enema every five years, or
- Colonoscopy every ten years.

These options, however, are not of equal value: the third option (combining fecal occult blood testing and sigmoidoscopy) is better than the first two (the individual tests), and colonoscopy is preferable to a barium enema or virtual colonoscopy. But any is better than none.

If you have a higher risk for colon cancer, you may need to begin screening before age fifty and have procedures such as colonoscopy more often. If one or more family members have had colon cancer, you should begin having a colonoscopy at age forty or ten years before the earliest age at which cancer was diagnosed, whichever is sooner. Anyone in a family beset with one of the hereditary colon cancer syndromes (Lynch's syndrome or familial adenomatous polyposis) should have a first colonoscopy at a much earlier age, and regularly thereafter. (See page 99.) Needless to say, you should review these options with your physician to determine which is most appropriate for you.

Any way to prevent colon cancer? Current research links obesity, physical inactivity, and smoking with a higher risk for developing colorectal cancer. Therefore, as with so many other health problems, losing excessive weight (see chapter 6), exercising regularly (see chapter 7), and quitting smoking (see chapter 10) will help reduce your risk. In addition, an abundance of vegetables (especially the highly regarded leafy greens) and fruit in the diet reduces the risk for this cancer. For many years it was assumed that the fiber content of fruits and vegetables accounted for this benefit, but more recent research has not supported this idea. Instead, it may be years of consistent intake of folic acid (or folate), which is abundant in these foods, that helps provide this protection. A daily dose of aspirin may reduce colon-cancer risk, but you should check with your doctor before taking this approach, since aspirin can cause stomach ulcers, bleeding, and other problems.[7]

Ovarian cancer

Ovarian cancer is a source of both fear and frustration among women, especially those over fifty, because it is common enough to hit close to home—more than 22,000 new cases and over 16,000 deaths every year in the United States—but at the same time, difficult to detect at an early stage. Furthermore, even when it is advanced enough to cause symptoms, they are typically vague: nonspecific pain in the abdomen or pelvis, fullness, bloating, nausea, diarrhea, constipation, or fatigue.

The **ovaries** are relatively small organs, one on each side of the pelvis near the uterus, which are responsible for producing one or more microscopic eggs each month during a woman's menstrual cycle.

Who is at risk? Roughly one out of seventy women will develop ovarian cancer, and several factors can increase—or decrease—these odds. The risk is *increased* with:

- Age. Most cases occur after menopause, and half after age sixty-three.
- Family history. Your risk is higher if your mother or sister (or daughter) has had ovarian cancer.
- Early onset of menstrual cycles (before twelve), late onset of menopause, no pregnancies, or first pregnancy after age thirty. It appears that ovarian-cancer risk is affected by the number of uninterrupted menstrual cycles in a woman's lifetime.
- Use of fertility drugs, and in particular long-term use of the drug **clomiphene** (Clomid), especially if pregnancy is not achieved. This appears to be an added risk beyond that related to infertility itself.
- Use of estrogen therapy after menopause. While a connection between ovarian cancer and taking hormones after menopause has been debated for many years, more recent observational studies have suggested that prolonged use—more than ten years—of estrogen nearly doubles a woman's risk of developing ovarian cancer.[8] (Keep in mind, however, that without added risk factors, a woman's lifetime likelihood of developing ovarian cancer is relatively low, less than 2 percent.) The risk similarly appears to be increased for women using the combination of estrogen and progesterone.
- A history of breast cancer. This is particularly significant for a woman who has been found to have an altered BRCA1 or BRCA2 gene, which is associated with a markedly higher risk of developing ovarian cancer. (For more information see the sidebar "Should I Be Tested for an Altered BRCA Gene?" earlier in this chapter on page 89.)

The risk for developing ovarian cancer is *decreased* with:

- Childbearing and breast-feeding, presumably because these interrupt menstrual cycles for extended periods of time.
- Oral contraceptives, which also override the normal menstrual cycle, are known to decrease the risk of developing ovarian cancer later in life. This effect increases with the duration of their use.
- Hysterectomy (surgical removal of the uterus) or tubal ligation (cutting the fallopian tubes that transport a woman's egg to her uterus

every month) also appears to reduce the risk of ovarian cancer, for reasons that are unclear. (It is possible that this association is artificial—not the result of removing the uterus or cutting the tubes but because the ovaries are inspected during surgery. Only ovaries that appear normal, and are thus less likely to become cancerous, are left behind.)

What screening tests are available?

- A pelvic exam done at the time of a Pap smear (see "What screening tests are available?" on page 108) may detect an ovarian tumor—but only after it has grown large enough to be felt by the examiner. Unfortunately, this rarely occurs at an early stage.
- **CA-125** is a protein that can be measured in the blood. It is present in high levels in about 80 percent of women with advanced ovarian cancer and about half of women with early disease. It may also be elevated in women who do not have ovarian cancer. As a result, this test is used primarily to follow the progress of women who are already known to have this tumor rather than to screen women without symptoms.
- A pelvic ultrasound, which creates an image using sound waves, can detect an abnormality in one or both ovaries much earlier than a pelvic exam, but it isn't cost-effective for routine screening. However, this study is extremely helpful in evaluating pelvic pain or an unusual finding from a pelvic exam. Additional evaluation may be needed to determine whether an abnormal ultrasound finding is worrisome or not.

The bottom line: Ovarian cancer is tough to detect early, with no test that's considered ideal for screening. However, women who are at high risk, especially those with one or more close relatives who have had ovarian cancer, should discuss pelvic ultrasound and CA-125 testing with their physician.

Any way to prevent it? You may have noted that the factors that increase and decrease the risk for ovarian cancer offer few immediate action items. No one should become pregnant or have a hysterectomy strictly for the purpose of preventing ovarian cancer, although some women with an altered BRCA1 or BRCA2 gene who are at extremely high risk for this disease may be advised to consider surgical removal of the ovaries after childbearing has been completed. Even this drastic procedure does not completely eliminate the risk, however, because a tumor that behaves exactly like ovarian cancer can still develop in the abdominal wall lining (called the **peritoneum**) that once covered the ovaries. The presence of other risk factors might also impact a woman's decision about timing of childbearing (i.e., sooner—before age thirty—better than later), breast-feeding (i.e., longer better than shorter), or the use of oral contraceptives. Taking birth control pills for six years or more may decrease a woman's risk of ovarian cancer by as much as 60 percent, and that use does not need to be continuous to be effective.

A detailed look at the pros and cons of using oral contraceptives may be found in chapter 13.

Some research suggests that taking aspirin three or more times per week for at least six months may decrease the risk of ovarian cancer. And—guess what—a diet low in fat may also reduce the risk, as it appears to do for other cancers.[9]

Cervical cancer

Cancer of the cervix (also called cervical cancer) involves cells at the narrow "neck" of the uterus, where it enters the upper end of the vagina. It's actually less common, and causes fewer deaths, than cancer that develops elsewhere in the uterus. But cervical cancer is notable for two reasons: It can be detected at a very early stage through routine screening and it is largely preventable.

F.Y.I.

More than 10,000 cases of cervical cancer are diagnosed each year in the United States, and about 3,700 women die of this disease. Cancer occurring in the rest of the uterus, which is also called "cancer of the uterine body" or "corpus," nearly always arises from the inner lining or **endometrium.** More than 40,000 new cases are diagnosed and about 7,300 women die from this cancer every year in the United States.

Who is at risk? The predisposing factors for cancer of the cervix are well-established—and nearly always avoidable:

- Infection with human papillomavirus (HPV) is the most important risk factor for this cancer. There are some 100 types of HPV, of which thirty can be transmitted sexually. In fact, HPV is now recognized to be the most common sexually transmitted infection (or STI). More than 95 percent of sexually transmitted HPV infections do not cause any noticeable symptoms. Some, however, result in the growth of so-called **genital warts** (also called condylomata), which can occur anywhere on or around the genitals or anus. These can develop weeks, months, or even years after the contact that transmitted them, and may vary enormously in size. Only a small percentage of HPV infections lead to cervical cancer—but virtually all cases of cervical cancer are linked to one of several high-risk HPV types. Interestingly, the high-risk HPVs tend to cause growths that are flat and nearly invisible, while the larger, fleshy genital warts are usually caused by low-risk HPVs. Unfortunately, it is possible to become infected with more than one kind of HPV, including both low- and high-risk types. A woman with one or more visible warts, which are likely to be of the low-risk type, can have a less visible but higher-risk HPV infection as well.
- Other sexually transmitted infections appear to increase the likelihood that a high-risk HPV infection will lead to cancer. Some research links **chlamydia**, a very common (and often silent) bacterial infection, with increased odds of developing cervical cancer. Human immunodeficiency virus (HIV) infection also increases this risk,

Other types of HPV are responsible for the everyday warts that grow on the hands and feet.

Sexually transmitted HPV infection is also linked to cancers of the vagina, vulva (the woman's external genitals), penis, and anus, as well as certain areas of the mouth, including the tonsils, soft palate, and base of the tongue.

probably by impairing the immune system's response to HPV. Among women infected with HIV, precancerous abnormalities in the cells of the cervix may progress to full-blown cancer more rapidly.

- Smoking damages more than the lungs. Tobacco by-products have been detected in the secretions of the cervix in female smokers, who are twice as likely as their nonsmoking counterparts to develop cervical cancer.
- **Diethylstilbestrol (DES)**, a hormone used between 1940 and 1970 to prevent miscarriage, has been linked to unusual forms of vaginal and cervical cancers among women whose mothers took this medication.
- Oral-contraceptive use has been associated with an increase in cervical cancer, but this is probably not a direct effect of this medication on the cervix. The common thread may instead be an increased likelihood that women who are taking birth control pills—especially adolescents—may be having early sexual experiences and multiple partners.
- A family history of cervical cancer in a woman's mother or sister(s) may predict an increased risk, but not in the absence of HPV. Rather, it may reflect a greater genetic vulnerability to a high-risk HPV infection, should one be acquired.

What screening tests are available? The Pap smear is the cornerstone of screening for cervical cancer. This painless test, which normally is done as part of a woman's routine pelvic examination, collects cells from her cervix to check for abnormalities that might indicate that cancer is present or may develop in the future. A duck-bill-shaped instrument called a **speculum** is gently inserted into the vagina and then carefully opened to allow the examiner to see the cervix. Using a wooden or plastic spatula, the outer surface is scraped, and then a swab or thin brush is used to collect material from the opening of the cervix. These specimens may be spread on microscope slides or placed in a liquid preparation before being placed on a slide. The latter approach is newer and somewhat more expensive, but also more likely to remove extraneous debris from the specimen and spread the cells more evenly. The slide, however it is prepared, is read by a specially trained technologist and/or a **pathologist** (a physician who, among other things, is an expert at identifying abnormalities in cells). The specimen will be interpreted as normal, abnormal to some degree but not appearing to be cancerous, or highly likely to be cancer. The action taken in response to an abnormal Pap smear will depend on several factors, including the severity of the changes that are observed. If they are mild, the physician may recommend that the Pap smear simply be rechecked in four to six months. More worrisome findings will often lead to a procedure called a **colposcopy**, during which a physician closely examines the cervix using an optical in-

Some laboratories use computerized equipment to scan Pap smears for abnormal cells. This approach may be used as a backup check on smears read as normal by a technologist, or even as the primary check, with humans evaluating any specimens identified as abnormal.

With thin-prep Pap smears, it is also possible to identify HPV types and even to diagnose two other sexually transmitted infections: gonorrhea and chlamydia.

strument similar to binoculars. Small amounts of tissue may then be taken from suspicious areas, using one of several techniques, in order to make a formal diagnosis.

F.Y.I. The Pap smear was named for Greek-born physician George Papanicolaou (1883–1962) who, in the 1920s, began to identify cancer cells in human vaginal and cervical smears. Formally validated as a screening technique in the 1940s, the Pap smear has been credited with saving thousands of lives by detecting cervical cancer at an earlier, treatable stage.

The bottom line: The American Cancer Society recommends that a woman should have her first Pap smear within three years of her first vaginal intercourse and no later than age twenty-one. Assuming that the results are normal, the test should be repeated annually. If the newer, liquid-based tests are used, testing every other year may be considered. In addition, a woman over thirty who has had three consecutive normal tests and is not at increased risk for cervical cancer may consider having a Pap smear every two or three years. However, less frequent testing should *not* be considered unless a woman has had no new sexual partners—and her partner has not had any new partners—since the last Pap smear. Similarly, a woman over seventy who has had at least three normal Pap smears and no abnormal results over the previous ten years may elect not to continue having this test done. While the Pap smear has become the centerpiece of routine screening for women, there are other items on the health agenda (such as blood pressure and breast checks) that should be carried out whether or not a Pap is done. *The fact that a Pap may not be considered necessary every year does not mean that other appropriate screening should be neglected.* Above all, it is important to review the plans for decisions about health screening with your own physician.

F.Y.I. Many physicians believe it is wise for a woman to be screened as soon as possible after her first intercourse and then yearly (or more often if needed) thereafter. Not only does this uncover any early changes in the cervix, it also enables her physician to check for any other sexually transmitted infections, which often do not cause any symptoms.

Any way to prevent it? Absolutely. Before the connection between cervical cancer and HPV was understood, it was well-known that cervical cancer is much more common among women with a history of multiple sexual partners, especially if those experiences began at a young age. Unfortunately, condoms offer little if any protection against HPV, probably because the virus can be transmitted by skin-to-skin contact anywhere in the genital area. Furthermore, the HPV subtypes that are most commonly associated with cervical cancer generate warts that are essentially invisible—and the virus can be passed even when warts are absent.

For a woman who has abstained from nonmarital sex and has maintained an exclusive sexual relationship with a husband who has done likewise, cervical cancer is extremely unlikely. For one who has not practiced that level of sexual exclusivity, the risk of developing cervical cancer can be markedly reduced by obtaining regular Pap smears and carefully following up on any abnormalities. Research is also in progress to develop a vaccine against one or more strains of HPV that are most commonly associated with cervical cancer.

Finally, quitting smoking—or better yet, never starting—may also decrease a woman's risk for developing cervical cancer.

Testicular cancer

Testicular cancers are not particularly common—about 8,000 cases and nearly 400 deaths every year in the United States—but they are worth noting because they are responsive to treatment and often can be detected through a simple self-examination.

Who is at risk?

- Younger men. Unlike many tumors, the risk of testicular cancer does not increase with age. Instead, it is most common between the ages of fifteen and forty, although it may occur at any age.
- Those who have had an undescended testicle (**cryptorchidism**). Normally the testes develop within the abdomen and then migrate into the scrotum before birth. In about 3 percent of male infants, however, one or both testes fail to make the trip, either remaining within the abdomen or hung up in the groin. In most infants the undescended testicle assumes its rightful position before the first birthday, but occasionally surgery is needed to correct this abnormality. In nearly 15 percent of men with testicular cancer, there is a history of an undescended testicle. Interestingly, as many as one in four of these tumors may develop in the testicle that descended properly, suggesting that some underlying factor, rather than the lack of descent itself, increases the risk for tumor.
- Race. Testicular cancer is five times more common among white males than in African-American men, and it is twice as common among whites as in Asian-American men.
- Occupational exposure. For reasons that are unclear, men who work in certain industries are more likely to develop a specific testicular cancer (called a **nonseminoma germ cell tumor**). These include miners, those involved in oil and gas production, leather workers, and janitors, among others.
- Family history. A man whose brother has had testicular cancer is more likely to develop it.

What screening tests are available? A simple check for swelling or a nodule on either testicle can be done by a physician during a routine exam. Some also recommend that men—especially those younger than forty and especially those with a history of an undescended testicle—briefly check their own testicles every month. This can be done after a shower or bath, when the scrotum is relaxed, by gently rolling each testicle between a thumb and the other fingers of one hand. Check for any obvious difference between the two sides, and especially for swelling or any lump or nodule that seems unusual. (Remember, however, that it is normal for one testicle to be a little larger than the other.) If you feel anything that seems abnormal or different, have it checked by your physician or by a urologist. *Don't put off being checked merely because you don't have pain.* While a heaviness or dull pain in the scrotum or abdomen might be a sign of a testicular tumor, in the vast majority of cases no discomfort is present.

The bottom line: Testicular cancer is not very common but also not hard to detect. Because most testicular tumors are very responsive to treatment, an early diagnosis provides a definite advantage.

Skin cancer

Skin cancer is the most common type of cancer in the United States, with more than one million cases every year, nearly as many as all other types of cancer combined. Because only a very small percentage of these spread to other parts of the body, fewer than one in one hundred cases lead to death. The vast majority of skin cancers arise from the outer layer of skin known as the **epidermis**, which contains three types of cells that can cause trouble:

A person who lives to be sixty-five has about a 50 percent chance of developing one of the three main types of skin cancer.

The flat, scalelike superficial **squamous** cells at the surface can develop **squamous cell carcinoma**. About 250,000 of these occur every year in the United States, and a small percentage spread to other parts of the body, leading to 2,500 deaths.

The round **basal** cells lie deeper in the epidermis. Some 800,000 cases of **basal cell carcinoma** occur every year in the United States, but these rarely cause death because they grow very slowly and nearly always remain where they started. They can, however, cause extensive local damage if they are allowed to grow for many years without treatment.

About 75 percent of all skin cancer deaths are caused by **malignant melanoma**, a tumor that arises from the pigment-producing **melanocytes** deep in the epidermis that give our skin its color. Unlike basal and squamous cell cancers, melanomas are much more likely to spread to distant areas of the body. Nearly 60,000 cases of melanoma, and over 7,700 deaths, occur every year in the United States.

Who is at risk?

- People who are fair-skinned, blond or red-haired, freckled, easily sunburned
- People who have had a lot of exposure to ultraviolet (UV) light, whether from the sun or in a tanning salon
- People who have had two or more blistering sunburns during childhood or adolescence

- People who have had a skin cancer or have a family history of skin cancer

What screening tests are available? In a nutshell, the best screening is something you can do yourself: inspect your own skin and have worrisome areas checked by your doctor or a dermatologist. Individuals who have had a skin cancer already or who have had moles removed that were not entirely normal should consider having regular inspections by a dermatologist.

The bottom line: When in doubt, check it out. If you see a suspicious area of skin (see sidebar "Inspecting the Skin"), have your personal physician or a dermatologist take a look at it. He or she may be able to tell you immediately that you have nothing to worry about or may recommend further action. Often this involves taking a small sample of skin (known as a **biopsy**) and sending it to a pathologist to be analyzed. This procedure normally includes the injection of a small amount of local anesthetic just under the skin, so that the biopsy won't hurt.

Any way to prevent it? Fair skin and UV exposure are a worrisome combination. Since you can't change the skin into which you were born, limiting your exposure to sunlight and tanning salons is the key to prevention.

Other cancers

What about screening for other types of cancer? We have looked at many types of cancer that are either very common, good potential candidates for screening, or both. But what about cancer of the pancreas (the fourth most common cause of cancer death), bladder, kidney, brain, lymph tissue, liver, esophagus, and so on? What about leukemia? All of these are important, but none have a test available that meets the solid criteria for sensitive, specific, reliable, cost-effective screening for people with no symptoms. Some may be picked up during testing that is done for some other reason. For example, a simple urinalysis done prior to a surgery might detect red blood cells that cannot be seen with the naked eye but which could be the first indication that a tumor is present in the bladder or kidney.

F.Y.I.

The medical term for blood in the urine is **hematuria**, a word concocted by combining two roots that mean "blood" (*heme*) and "urine" (*uria*). Blood that is directly visible is called **gross hematuria.** Blood detected in the urine by lab tests or inspection under the microscope is called **microscopic hematuria.** However it is detected, blood in the urine *always* demands an explanation—even if it is seen only one time—because one possible reason could be the presence of a tumor.

Many tumors are discovered during a physician's examination, during a routine checkup, or while tracking down the cause of a specific symptom. The American Cancer Society recommends that adults without any particular symptoms have a cancer-related checkup on a regular basis—every three years between the ages of twenty and thirty-nine and annually after age forty. This

continued on page 116

INSPECTING THE SKIN

Unless you have regular checks by a dermatologist, you should consider doing a brief but systematic survey of your skin on a regular basis. Your goal is not only to identify suspicious areas, but also to become familiar enough with your own surface "landmarks" to be able to detect changes that might signal trouble. Here are some basic pointers for this project, which normally is best carried out after a bath or shower in front of a full-length mirror, with good lighting and a hand mirror available to check nooks and crannies:

- Check the front and then, with arms raised, the sides of your body.
- Take a specific look at your arms—especially the back of the forearms and hands, which are often the site of sun damage—legs, and feet, including the soles and between the toes.
- Take a closer look at your face, ears, and neck, which are common sites of skin cancers.
- You may need help with your backside. If you can't see your back well with mirrors, you may want to ask your spouse or a trusted friend to take a closer look.
- While your children are young, check all of these areas during bath time. As they approach the adolescent years and modesty overrides your checking their skin, talk about self-checking and remind them to show you any areas that have changed or look unusual.

What exactly are you looking for during your "mole patrol"? Basically, any lump, bump, sore, scaly area, freckle, or other local abnormality that appears to be new or active in some way over time (more than two weeks). Changes you might observe include crusting, bleeding, scaling, spreading, or thickening—but rarely pain.

In addition to these signs of trouble, dermatologists also describe the following specific "ABCDE's" of melanoma as signs that a mole might need additional attention:

- A = Asymmetry. One side of the mole is not the mirror image of the other.
- B = Border irregularity. The edge of the mole isn't smooth and doesn't make a clean transition to normal skin. Instead, it is irregular, ragged, or even blurry.
- C = Color. Instead of a uniform color, the mole contains various shades of black, brown, tan, and even white.
- D = Diameter. A mole is of greater concern when it is more than six millimeters in diameter (about a quarter of an inch, or roughly the size of a pencil eraser).
- E = Elevation. The surface of the mole is raised above the skin.

While these signs do not automatically mean that a skin cancer is present, one or more of them should trigger a check by a physician to determine whether a biopsy is needed. ■

SHOULD I HAVE A "TOTAL BODY" CT SCAN?

CT stands for **computerized tomography**, sometimes referred to as a **CAT scan** (for **computerized axial tomography**, unrelated to felines). *Tomography* literally means "imaging of a section," and a CT scan does indeed provide a cross-sectional look at the body. A regular (or plain) **X ray** involves passing a single dose of x-radiation through a part of the body onto a sensitive film. Depending on their density, tissues in the same area will absorb different amounts of the X ray. The variations in the intensity of X rays arriving at the film create an image with recognizable patterns.

CT uses the same principle, except that the X-ray beam electronically rotates around a patient who lies on a table moving slowly through the scanner. A detector records the variations in X-ray penetration, and sophisticated computer software crunches this information to generate a series of images. Depending on the area being evaluated, the patient may be given contrast material by mouth, through a vein, or both, in order to help the radiologist see various structures more clearly. When introduced during the early 1970s CT scanning was a dramatic breakthrough providing a cross-sectional view of the body with unprecedented detail.

As computers have become more powerful, scans performed using newer techniques (such as the spiral CT) can be performed very rapidly—often in a minute or less. CT scanning remains a staple for diagnosing tumors, fractures in complex structures (such as the skull and spine), certain types of infections, and other problems in which disease has caused changes in the shape and size of internal structures. Until a few years ago a CT could be obtained only through the order of a physician, who would request that a specific area (such as the head or chest) be scanned to evaluate a particular problem or symptom. More recently, however, medical entrepreneurs began offering "total body" or "whole body" CT scans to the public for health screening. These typically include the chest, abdomen, and pelvis—but not the head—and do not use contrast material. Very often a scan of the coronary arteries is included as well. This experience can cost anywhere from six hundred to one thousand dollars—some facilities even offer group rates (such as half price for a second family member)—but it is never covered by insurance. Total body CTs have a certain high-tech appeal: If you can afford it, why not scan your body and detect cancer or coronary artery disease before it causes a major problem?

At the present time, three types of CT scans are being evaluated for their potential usefulness as screening procedures, and each has already been discussed in this chapter:

- Electron beam CT (EBCT) of the coronary arteries to detect calcium deposits that could predict the risk for a heart attack (page 86)
- CT scans of the chest in smokers (page 87)
- Virtual colonoscopy, in which the CT scanner creates an image of the inside of the colon without the insertion of a flexible scope (page 103)

A radiologist is a physician who has specialized in performing and interpreting a variety of tests that collectively are known as **diagnostic imaging**. These include conventional X rays, ultrasound, CT scans, MRI (magnetic resonance imaging), and nuclear scans. (Nuclear scans utilize extremely small amounts of radioactive material that are injected into the patient and concentrate in certain tissues, allowing them to be detected and visualized.) Radiologists also perform certain procedures that require special imaging; for example, a radiologist may collect tissue through a syringe (a procedure called a **needle biopsy**) from an area that can be seen only on a CT scan.

The term *spiral* (also called *helical*) *CT* refers to the path traced by the X-ray beam through the patient. In this technique, the X-ray tube rotates continuously as the table (on which the patient lies) moves through it. Spiral CTs are not only faster, but they also produce a better image with less radiation exposure. This is particularly important for patients who are very young, very old, or very ill. When CT scans were first introduced, a baby or toddler who needed this procedure would have to undergo a general anesthetic so he or she wouldn't wiggle during the long exposure times.

Aside from these three applications, no professional organization recommends this type of exam, and the Food and Drug Administration (FDA) has never approved CT scanning for screening purposes. The American College of Radiology stated in 2000 that it "does not believe there is sufficient scientific evidence to justify recommending total body computed tomographic (CT) scanning for patients with no symptoms or a family history suggesting disease."[10]

Why not recommend a CT scan? Consider the possible outcomes:

- **Your scan is normal.** You feel relief, but you also have received a radiation dose that may be equivalent to that of several hundred chest X rays.[11] While this doesn't pose any immediate danger to you, most authorities recommend exposing yourself to radiation only when there is a specific need to do so.
- **Your scan is normal and there is actually a significant problem that the study failed to detect (a false negative result).** This, of course, is the last thing you want: a false sense of security, time and money wasted, and a disease in progress that will cause you grief in the not-too-distant future.
- **Your scan is abnormal, but the problem isn't significant (a false positive result).** This is not uncommon with total body CTs, especially if the radiologist interpreting the study is very concerned about missing something that could cause trouble for the patient (and a possible lawsuit) in the future. If a tiny nodule is found in an internal organ, for example, it may be impossible to evaluate its significance except by waiting for a few months and then repeating the CT. Or a larger abnormality may be spotted but prove to be benign when a more detailed study (such as another CT scan with appropriate contrast material) is carried out.
- **Your scan is abnormal and the problem is in fact important, even though you had no symptoms.** This is why you did the scan in the first place, but will it make a difference? The problem may actually be too advanced for treatment or you may obtain treatment that appears at first to be effective, but in the long run doesn't actually add to the quantity or quality of life. (This outcome, of course, can occur even with the most widely accepted screening procedure.) However, if the problem was in fact significant, wasn't causing any symptoms, was picked up by the CT scan, and appropriate treatment was rendered that prevented a great deal of grief (or even death), then the procedure was a rousing success.

The very last of the above scenarios is, of course, the big payoff for a total body scan—and unfortunately one that isn't very common. The FDA, in its advice to the public on this subject, notes: "The surprising fact about a CT interpretation of abnormality when there is nothing significant wrong is that it is *far more likely* to happen to you than the finding of any actual life-threatening disease, since the likelihood that you actually have any deadly disease is so small to begin with"[12] (emphasis in original text). ■

continued from page 112

would encompass not only the various assessments and tests that have already been discussed in this section, but also a brief check for other signs that something is wrong. These might include:

- A look into the nose, mouth, and throat
- Checking the thyroid for any nodules
- Feeling the neck, armpit, and groin areas for any enlarged lymph nodes
- Feeling the abdomen for any masses or enlargement of organs such as liver or spleen
- Checking the testicles for any nodules or swelling

Even this type of targeted exam, however, cannot uncover tumors within the brain or deep inside the abdomen. Some medical entrepreneurs have proposed that adults should periodically have a computerized X-ray (CT) scan of the lungs, abdomen, and pelvis rather than waiting for symptoms to develop, and they have offered this service (for several hundred dollars) without a physician's prescription. While theoretically appealing, this idea has not been endorsed by any professional organization. (See sidebar "Should I Have a 'Total Body' CT Scan?") Unfortunately, until other effective screening tests become available, we must rely on symptoms and warning signs of other tumors to trigger an evaluation that leads to the diagnosis. Some of these include:

- Unexplained, unintentional weight loss
- Coughing or hoarseness that continues longer than two or three weeks, especially if it did not begin as a cold
- Blood in urine or stool
- Vaginal bleeding after menopause
- Difficulty swallowing, or food "hanging up" somewhere in the esophagus before it reaches the stomach
- A lump or nodule that appears in any part of the body
- A change in bowel habits: more difficulty passing stool or loose stools
- A change in bladder function: difficulty passing or controlling urine
- A new and persistent headache, especially one that is relentless, worsening, and interfering with sleep
- Changes in moles or a skin sore that does not heal

The presence of one or more of these symptoms does not automatically mean that someone has cancer. In fact, in most cases they are found not to be caused by a tumor. But they should not be ignored or left to smolder for weeks or months out of fear, wishful thinking that they will disappear, or under the mistaken belief that "if it doesn't hurt, it probably isn't cancer." Letting a physician review the problem will usually relieve some anxiety, and more often than not, the symptoms as well. Furthermore, if a tumor is present, it is always better to know sooner rather than later.

Screening for Other Problems

Diabetes carries with it a host of potential complications, including its contribution to disease in blood vessels throughout the body. We covered the basics on diabetes in chapter 3, and screening strategies for it earlier in this chapter (pages 81–82).

The **thyroid gland** lies at the base of the neck just below the Adam's apple. The hormone it releases into the bloodstream, known simply as thyroid hormone, plays a vital role in setting the overall metabolic rate of the body, somewhat like the idle speed of your car. If the gland is making too much (a condition called **hyperthyroidism**), a person's metabolic "engine" is literally revved up, producing symptoms such as a rapid heart rate (or even irregular rhythm), tremors, sweating (and feeling hot most of the time), hair loss, weight loss, fatigue, and menstrual periods that are less frequent, with less flow. If the gland is underproductive (a condition known as **hypothyroidism**), the opposite occurs: The body seems to slow down, with a slower heart rate, weight gain, heavy menstrual flow, poor memory and concentration, and a general sense of being cold, sluggish, and drowsy.

Many people look at a list of symptoms for hyper- and hypothyroidism and exclaim, "That sounds just like me!" A number of these complaints (especially fatigue) are indeed very common, but more often than not they arise from other

HOW TO CHECK THYROID FUNCTION

In bygone years the state of one's thyroid was assessed by symptoms and physical findings—which often aren't apparent until the hormone abnormality is relatively severe—or by a cumbersome (and now extinct) test called the basal metabolic rate. Now a straightforward combination of blood tests can determine whether the gland is producing too much or too little.

Measurement of the thyroid hormone known as **T4**, along with another hormone called **TSH**, can tell the tale in the majority of cases. T4 (or **thyroxine**) is the main product of the thyroid gland, although a derivative called **T3** does most of the work in the body. In some situations, a physician may want to measure T3 as well. (The "4" and "3" in T4 and T3 refer to the number of iodine atoms bound to each molecule.) TSH stands for **thyroid stimulating hormone**, an important product of the **pituitary gland**, which resembles a tiny punching bag extending from the base of the brain. The pituitary, long known as the "master gland," secretes a number of hormones that give orders to other organs. TSH is no exception. If the thyroid gland's output is low, TSH levels rise, as if to say "Get busy and make more of your hormone!" If the thyroid is churning out too much, on the other hand, TSH levels are driven very low. For screening alone, many physicians order only the TSH level. Note that these tests only determine whether too much, too little, or the right amount of hormone is being produced; they do not tell *why* there is an abnormality, which may require further investigation. ■

F.Y.I. Because high thyroid-hormone levels can cause weight loss, some weight-loss clinics have attempted to "help things along" by giving this hormone in relatively high doses to clients who are not actually hypothyroid. This is definitely a bad idea, because at levels high enough to cause weight loss, other symptoms and side effects abound.

conditions—especially anxiety and depression—rather than a misbehaving thyroid gland. It's usually not difficult to determine whether the thyroid is responsible for any of these symptoms, and therefore thyroid hormone levels are usually checked as part of an evaluation for a specific concern. There isn't a clear consensus, however, about routine screening of thyroid function when there are no symptoms. One organization, the American Thyroid Association, recommends that adults thirty-five and over have hormone screening every five years in order to detect cases of hypothyroidism that may be causing minimal or no symptoms. In addition, people with type 1 diabetes may be screened more frequently for thyroid abnormalities (especially hypothyroidism), because autoimmune processes (that is, the immune system damaging a person's own tissue) may underlie both types of problems.

Osteoporosis, or thinning of the bones, affects some 8 million women and 2 million men in the United States, causing some 1.5 million fractures every year. Risk factors, screening options, and preventive measures for this important problem are reviewed in detail in chapter 13, beginning on page 661.

QUESTIONS TO PONDER

1. If your family has health insurance, do you know whether your policy covers routine health screenings, and if so, which ones? If you have no coverage for such screenings, do you think it is worth paying a few hundred dollars to have them done? (Hint: How much do you spend on routine maintenance for your car?)
2. Do you know what your blood pressure, cholesterol, and blood glucose levels are (or were within the last couple of years)? If not, now would be a good time to find out.

Action items: Look again at the "Who is at risk?" sections for the various types of cancer. If you or a family member seems to have multiple risk factors for one or more of these, make an appointment with your physician to outline a game plan for appropriate screening.

If you have read through the previous two chapters and feel that, based on your family history and lifestyle, you or a family member is not at any particular risk for cardiovascular disease, cancer, or diabetes, keep up the good work. However, you should still consider checking in with your physician every three years if you are under forty and yearly thereafter. (Most women younger than forty will be having Pap smears on a more frequent basis.) If this sounds too frequent, check with your own physician for his or her recommendations.

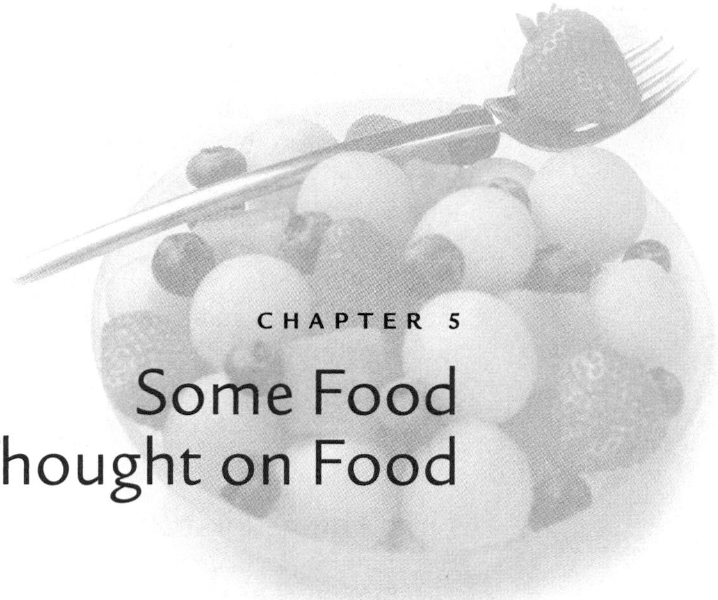

CHAPTER 5

Some Food for Thought on Food

Have you ever asked yourself any of the following questions?

For years I've been hearing that fats are bad and that I should gravitate toward foods that say "low fat" or "nonfat" on the label. Now I'm hearing that carbohydrates are bad and that I should avoid eating them. What gives?

I hardly eat anything, but I keep gaining weight. Is there something wrong with me?

Do I get enough vitamins and minerals out of my foods or should I take a supplement? What about my kids—do they need to take something?

Every weekend on my local radio station, I hear infomercials for nutritional products that sound too good to be true. Are they?

Sure, I'd like my family to eat healthier foods, but what exactly does that mean, and how do we break some of our bad habits?

It seems like every other month someone comes out with a new surefire way to lose weight. I've tried most of them, and nothing seems to work for long. What am I doing wrong?

I feel tired and irritable most of the time. Should I change something in my diet?

The capacity to eat and enjoy food is one of God's wonderful gifts to our physical body, as are sleep, sex, and the ability to exercise. Furthermore, we live in a nation blessed with a richer bounty and variety of foods for the average citizen than at any other time or place in history. One would think that deciding what to eat would be a straightforward task, or even a pleasant diversion from the normal routines of life. But too many of us don't feel well, or aren't as healthy as we would like, or are overweight. And so we are bombarded every day with advice (half of which seems to contradict the other half) about what we should or shouldn't eat, drink, and take as supplements, accompanied by promises of boundless energy and the Body Beautiful if we will only follow it.

This chapter and the one that follows will not set forth imaginative theories of how the body works, magic formulas for losing weight, lists of miracle supplements for you to buy, or recommendations that you eat exotic foods that you may have a hard time swallowing (let alone finding). They will, however, attempt to give you a reality-based orientation to this subject and a handle on a lot of words and catchphrases that you've probably heard but perhaps never entirely understood. (*What exactly is a saturated fat? What in the world is a trans fatty acid?*) Hopefully this will help you make better-informed decisions about the foods you buy and prepare for yourself and your family. We also hope that it will give you a clear-eyed (and, when needed, skeptical) vantage point to evaluate advertising slogans used by the food industry and extravagant claims that are often made for diets or supplements.

First Things First: Giving Credit Where It's Due

Hopefully your mealtime routine, whether a quick bite on the way to work or Thanksgiving dinner with family and friends, includes at least a moment to thank the true "Father of the feast." We're so accustomed to a steady bounty of food, usually available at one of several supermarkets within a short drive of home, that it's all too easy to forget what must happen before the food we enjoy ever reaches our plate.

We of course appreciate those who have prepared our food. But we should never take for granted the productivity of our farmers year after year and the stable and efficient methods of distribution that set our national table with a spread that most of the world would consider a vision of paradise. We should also offer thanks every day to the Creator of the natural resources of our land, for seed and sun and rain that must converge at the right time and in the necessary amounts to produce huge amounts and varieties of crops.

Before we consider the basics of nutrition, we also need to stop, marvel, and give thanks for an incredibly complex phenomenon that is even more fundamental than the planting, harvesting, and distributing of food. In order for any of God's creatures to obtain any nourishment, energy must be captured from one source: the sun. Trees, plants, grasses, algae, and some bacteria do this every day on a monumental scale, in a process called **photosynthesis**. The biochemistry involved is well beyond the scope of this book, but we want to call attention to a crucial bottom line: Plants take the energy in sunlight and apply it to carbon dioxide and water to generate **glucose**, the basic carbohydrate fuel of both plants and animals. In exchange they return oxygen into the atmosphere. Humans and animals cannot survive without oxygen that the plant kingdom continually replenishes, and our metabolic engines in turn generate carbon dioxide that plants need for photosynthesis. All of the food consumed by animals and people—including meat—contains energy that was originally captured from the sun and stored by plants.

The complexity of this interdependent system is truly remarkable, and it becomes even more breathtaking when we consider the other factors, both colossal and intricate, that must interact perfectly for us to take our next breath. These include the size of our planet, its distance from and orbit around the sun, the size and stability of that nearby star, the presence and composition of the earth's oceans, and so on. "The heavens declare the glory of God; the skies proclaim the work of his hands," wrote King David (Psalm 19:1). The marvelous processes that allow our body to function every day do likewise, and so should we who inhabit them.

First Things Second: The Benefits of Breaking Bread Together

Before we look at the ABC's of nutrients, we also need a reminder about the importance of the *context* of our nourishment. We are not animals that graze in a field or gather at a trough; we do not inhale our food and then wander away. We are meant to be nourished at the table in more ways than merely transporting food from plate to stomach. Meals are a time for socializing, conversation, sharing, and celebration. Family meals can be particularly powerful events in the lives of both children and adults. They can and should be the occasion to share the day's events, decompress, commiserate and encourage one another, laugh, learn how to speak and listen politely, instill values, establish one's identity as a member of a family, welcome guests, and acknowledge God's provision on a day-to-day basis.

"If more of us valued food and cheer and song above hoarded gold, it would be a merrier world."
—J. R. R. TOLKIEN

In a classic case of scientific research bearing witness to common sense, a study of more than five hundred adolescents reported in 1997 by the American Psychological Association found that those who ate dinner more often (five times per week) with their families at home were less likely to be depressed or involved in drug use, more likely to have better relationships with friends, and better motivated at school, compared with teenagers who ate with their families less often (three times per week).[1]

Family dinners are, unfortunately, an endangered species, threatened by overcommitment, crowded calendars, and electronic distractions such as TVs and phones. If you take away nothing else from this chapter, make a decision that shared family meals will become a priority in your home. As part of that process, consider the following:

- Set aside three, if not more, nights per week (perhaps including a "cook's day off" meal after church on Sunday) that are designated for family meals. The expectation is that "all hands will be on deck," even young children, unless prior notice is given.
- After considering the ages and abilities in your family, establish routines that will spread the work around. The tasks involved in

planning the menu, preparing the various components of the meal, and cleaning up can be rotated among the able-bodied family members who are living at home. Younger children can learn to set the table, and everybody should help clear it.

- Table manners (including such niceties as pulling out chairs for the ladies and not starting to eat until everyone is seated and grace has been said) can and should be encouraged.
- Televisions should be turned off and phones unanswered, taken off the hook, or (in the case of cell phones) turned off. This is a time to talk to one another, unhindered by the yammering of the tube or the demands of whomever decides to dial your number.
- Speaking of talking, without being too restrictive on the topics of conversation, it is wise to address hot issues in the family at some other time. If mealtimes are a constant hotbed of bickering and animosity, no one is going to want to show up. Ideally, the family table should be a place of warmth, respect, safety, genuine interest in what everyone has to say, and mutual support. If the kids are having a little trouble with this, some role modeling of respectful conversation from Mom and Dad will speak volumes. And, if no one seems to have much to say, ask a few open-ended questions such as, "What was the highlight of your day?" or "What didn't go well today?"
- While you're at it, mealtimes can also provide opportunities to talk with your children about the foods they (and you) eat and why some are definitely better than others. Obviously, learning by example at the table—sampling the foods you're discussing—also speaks volumes and helps set patterns that will continue long after children have left home to live on their own.

"Better a meal of vegetables where there is love than a fattened calf with hatred." Proverbs 15:17

Ladies and Gentlemen, This Is a Nutrient

Now that we've offered these important public-service messages, it's time for some basic training about the components of the foods we enjoy every day. Vince Lombardi, the legendary coach of the Green Bay Packers, started every training season by announcing, "Gentlemen, this is a football." In that tradition, we will not gloss over the fundamentals. No prior knowledge of this subject will be assumed.

If you stop and think about it, the utilization of food by our body is an incredible accomplishment and a marvelous feat of engineering. An enormous number and variety of substances that we chew and swallow (usually with some pleasure) are broken down into basic components that serve three general purposes:

1. Provide a steady supply of fuel for thousands of mechanical, electrical, and chemical processes that go on twenty-four hours a day

2. Build, maintain, and repair structures of incredibly diverse shapes, sizes, and constituents

3. Provide some protection against certain destructive processes

We may buy the best fuel and additives for our car, but they can only power the engine and perhaps reduce wear and tear. A vehicle that could take gasoline and other raw materials and then repair itself exists only in the realm of fantasy. The fact that our body does all of this and more without our awareness, supervision, or understanding is mind-boggling.

There are six types of nutrients: carbohydrates, fats, proteins, vitamins, minerals, and water. The first three are called **macronutrients** because we use them in substantial quantities. They are also known as **energy-yielding nutrients** because they provide the fuel for our bodily functions. Vitamins and minerals are called **micronutrients** because of the tiny amounts that we use. They do not provide any energy but play a number of important roles in releasing and regulating it. Macronutrients and vitamins are called **organic** compounds. This word has acquired all sorts of meanings over the years (such as "natural" or "unadulterated") but the word *organic* simply means that the substance contains **carbon**, the element found in every living thing. Minerals and water are **inorganic**, though no less important (or natural).

The Macronutrients

Carbohydrates: More than sugar and starch

We hear a lot about "carbs" today, and based on what you have heard, you may think of carbohydrates as the staff of life or the root of all illness. Neither viewpoint is particularly accurate, and in this chapter we'll try to explain what some of the fuss is about.

F.Y.I.

The word *carbohydrate* comes from joining the roots *carbo* for "carbon" and *hydr* for "water" (as in the words *hydrant* or *dehydrated*). This reflects not only the usual presence of one oxygen and two hydrogen atoms for each carbon atom in these molecules, but also the by-products that remain when glucose is oxidized (burned) to release energy: water and carbon dioxide.

First, a little terminology

Carbohydrates fall into two basic categories: **simple** (commonly called **sugars**) and **complex**.

Three of the most important simple carbohydrates are glucose, fructose, and galactose, which are also called **monosaccharides** because each consists of a single ring of carbon molecules. These are the building blocks of other carbohydrates.

- **Glucose** (which in the bloodstream is also called **blood sugar**) is the primary energy source for almost every cell in the body, and the body's biochemical machinery is programmed to break down more complex carbohydrates into glucose or to convert the other simple sugars into it. The central nervous system has no fuel storage capability and requires a continuous flow of glucose. If blood

A FEW ABC'S OF MEASUREMENT

You can't read or understand a food label without having some familiarity with a number of measurements that are used in general science, medicine, and nutrition—terms that we'll mention many times in this book as well. Unfortunately, in the United States and many other countries we use two "languages" of measurement, often in the same breath: the **metric system** (officially called the **International System of Units** since 1960), which is the universal standard for all scientific endeavors throughout the world, and the quirky but more familiar (for us) **English system**. To complicate matters, nutritional materials add a third and often confusing type of measurement for quantities of food: "portions" and "servings."

In the early 1600s English settlers in North America brought with them the "inch-foot-yard-mile" measurements of distance, the "ounce-pound" measures of weight, and the "ounce-pint-quart-gallon" measures of volume. We've all been brought up with this system—twelve inches to the foot, three feet to the yard, sixteen ounces to the pound, thirty-two liquid ounces to the quart, and so forth—but it doesn't make any particular sense.

The metric system originated in France in the late eighteenth century as an attempt to standardize the world's weights and measures based on a single measurement from nature: the **meter**, which was defined as one ten-millionth of the distance from the North Pole to the equator. (The length of a meter established at that time was based on the best available estimate of that colossal distance, and today the standard keepers use far more sophisticated methods to define it.) Other measures were then built around the meter, using powers of ten:

- 1000 meters = one **kilometer** (a little over six-tenths of a mile)
- 1/100 of a meter = one **centimeter** (about four-tenths of an inch)
- 1/1000 of a meter = one **millimeter**, etc.

Volume measurements were based on the cubic centimeters (or "cc")—the volume of a cube whose sides are one centimeter in length. A cube whose sides are ten centimeters in length contains one thousand cubic centimeters, which is

glucose falls drastically (a condition called **hypoglycemia**), consciousness rapidly becomes cloudy. If blood glucose levels are not restored quickly, brain damage can result.

- **Fructose** (also called **fruit sugar**) is the sweetest of the sugars. It is abundant in fruits and honey and readily converted to glucose.
- **Galactose** is a component of **lactose** (see next page) and appears only when lactose is digested.

The other important simple sugars are the **disaccharides**, which consist of two monosaccharides joined together.

called a **liter** (so a cubic centimeter is also called a **milliliter**). Weight measurements were originally based on the weight of water occupying a certain volume at sea level at a temperature of 4 degrees Celsius, the temperature at which water is most dense. The **gram** was defined as the weight of a cubic centimeter of water and the **kilogram** as the weight of one thousand cubic centimeters (one liter) of water. **Celsius** (also called **centigrade**, and abbreviated C) is the metric system's scale of temperature measurement, with **0°C** set at the freezing point of water and **100°C** the boiling point.

Why wade through these definitions? Because when we talk about nutrition, we talk a lot about **calories**, a measure of energy in the metric system defined as the amount of energy needed to raise a cubic centimeter of water by one degree Celsius. A **kilocalorie** (or **kcal**) is one thousand calories: the amount of energy needed to raise the temperature of a thousand cubic centimeters (or a kilogram) of water one degree Celsius. One somewhat confusing tradition in nutritional literature (and reflected on every food label) is the use of the word *calories* to refer to kilocalories. In other words, if we say that a slice of bread provides 130 calories, technically we mean 130 kcal—or 130,000 actual calories. For our purposes, it will be simpler to follow tradition and use the word *calorie* instead of *kilocalorie*.

Like it or not, you can't avoid dealing with the metric system. To help you get a handle on some common quantities, note the following:

- A pound weighs a little less than half a kilogram (0.454 kg, to be exact), so a kilogram weighs 2.2 pounds.
- An ounce weighs a little more than 28 grams, so a gram doesn't weigh much—only 0.035 ounces.
- A fluid ounce is just under 30 ml.
- A tablespoon is about 15 ml, and a teaspoon about 5 ml.
- A cup is 8 fluid ounces, or a little less than 240 ml.
- A pint is 2 cups, 16 fluid ounces, or a little less than 480 ml.
- A quart is 2 pints, 32 fluid ounces, or a little less than a liter.

If you're not used to using some of these measures, don't panic. We'll provide reminders of some of these equivalents as we go. ■

- **Sucrose** (also called table sugar) consists of one glucose and one fructose molecule joined together.
- **Lactose** (also called milk sugar) consists of one glucose and one galactose molecule joined together.
- **Maltose** (also called malt sugar) consists of two glucose molecules joined together.

F.Y.I. **The words *monosaccharide* and *disaccharide* come from the roots *mono* meaning "one," *di* meaning "two," and *sacchar* meaning "sweet." From the latter we derive the words *saccharin,* the artificial sweetener, and *saccharine,* meaning perhaps a little *too* sweet (as in "he wasn't taken in by her saccharine smile").**

The complex carbohydrates (also called **polysaccharides**) include two important types of structures that are wonderfully designed to store energy in plants and animals. While the sugars consist of various combinations of glucose, fructose, and galactose, the complex carbohydrates are built almost entirely of huge numbers of glucose molecules chained together. Starch is the general term for a long chain of hundreds or even thousands of glucose molecules linked together and packed into certain parts of plants. Glycogen (which is made only by animals) also consists of chains of glucose molecules, though with many more branches. Found in muscle and the liver, it serves as a short-term fuel supply when food isn't available.

The chemical bonds that link the glucose molecules together in starch and glycogen can be readily broken down to provide glucose. In the third important type of complex carbohydrate, **fibers**, the chemical bonds linking the sugar molecules together cannot be broken during human digestion. Fibers are components of the cell walls of plants and include **cellulose**, **hemicellulose**, **pectins**, **gums**, **mucilages**, and **lignins**.

Lignins are not like the other fibers in that they are not polysaccharides. Instead, they are composed of chains of a type of organic alcohol called a phenol.

More on sugar (and perhaps less of it)

Apparently we like sugar, since as a nation we consume a lot of it. A widely quoted report released in 2000 by the United States Department of Agriculture (USDA) raised national eyebrows when it reported that annual sugar consumption in America had reached 158 pounds per person—a whopping fifty teaspoons per day—in 1999, up 30 percent from 1983.

The United States is the largest consumer of sweeteners and among the four largest sugar producers in the world.[2]

Actually these numbers were based on the amount of sugar available in the wholesale market. Estimates based on surveys of people's eating habits (also conducted by the USDA) revealed somewhat lower (but still impressive) numbers: 109 pounds per year for a typical teenage boy and sixty-four pounds for the average American citizen.[3]

Why so much? Obviously, we all like one or more sweet foods, and for some of us many of them seem to be addicting. But in addition, many foods we buy—including some, such as ketchup, that are not particularly sweet—include significant amounts of one or more types of **added sugars** under a variety of

continued on page 130

SUGAR BLUES AND CRAVINGS

Many books and articles have painted a vivid picture of the ways sugar can provoke mood and behavior disorders, including anxiety, depression, irritability, fatigue, and even violent or psychotic (delusional) episodes. A variation on this theme describes cravings or even outright addiction to sugar as a major cause of personal and social ills. For example, William Duffy's popular book *Sugar Blues,* published in 1975, is a particularly colorful if extreme treatment of this subject, proclaiming sucrose to be not only as dangerous and addictive as morphine or cocaine, but also the root of mental illness, war, plague, pestilence, and every other scourge of civilization for the past five hundred years. (Duffy also accused both conventional medicine and the Christian church of numerous crimes against humanity, and waxed eloquent in his praise for any "sorceress"—his term for a natural healer—who bucked these two institutions.)

Is it possible to be addicted to sugar or carbohydrates? The answer is yes in the general sense that a person's desire for sweets or carbohydrate-rich foods (primarily starches) can range from pleasant enjoyment to craving to compulsive consumption of large amounts in the face of obvious consequences (such as obesity). The nature of craving and compulsion, however, is complex. *Sugar Blues* and similar books have argued that sugar's effects and potency are similar to those of narcotics. This is a gross overstatement. That being said, however, what drives excessive consumption?

- The same factors that lead to other compulsions involving alcohol, addictive drugs, sex, gambling, or spending money: physical and emotional pleasure. There is pleasure in the taste and feel of food, the relief of hunger, the time-out from a difficult day, camaraderie with family and friends, and associations with comforting memories from the past.
- Swings in blood glucose after eating sweets and refined carbohydrate foods may provoke a rebound hunger, which in turn leads to more eating.
- Changes in brain neurochemistry are associated not only with increased (or decreased) appetite, but also with desires for certain foods. Carbohydrate cravings are often seen among people with certain types of **endogenous depression**—that is, depression related to alterations of chemical messengers or neurotransmitters in the brain, such as serotonin, norepinephrine, and dopamine. Some researchers have proposed that these cravings are an attempt by the brain to provide raw materials to create more of these compounds.

Can sugar contribute to a person's mood problem? It's not likely to be the underlying cause or the main contributor, but there's a simple way to find out. For details read the sidebar "Do I Have Hypoglycemia?" on page 128. ■

For a closer look at the subject of depression and its various causes, see chapter 8.

DO I HAVE HYPOGLYCEMIA?

True hypoglycemia or low blood sugar (glucose) is not a common event because, barring unusual circumstances, our body is designed to maintain adequate blood glucose levels at all cost. Remember that the brain and central nervous system cannot function without a steady flow of this fuel and that they have no way to store it. As we described in chapter 3 in our look at diabetes (page 70), when glucose enters the bloodstream after a meal, insulin is released by special cells located in the pancreas. Insulin serves as a "key" that opens the biochemical "door" of the cells, allowing glucose to enter and be utilized as fuel. In so doing, insulin prevents blood glucose from rising to potentially harmful levels—but it is the only hormone in the body that does so. The normal range for blood glucose in humans is between 60 and 150 mg/dl. (Reminder: *dl* stands for deciliter, or one-tenth of a liter, which equals one hundred milliliters of blood.)

The symptoms of true hypoglycemia typically appear when blood glucose drifts below 50 mg/dl. Fatigue, clouded thinking, light-headedness, anxiety, irritability, and restlessness arise from the brain, which is being deprived of its fuel. If hypoglycemia isn't rapidly corrected, confusion, seizures, loss of consciousness, and coma will follow.

The most common cause of true hypoglycemia is a problem with one or more medications used to treat diabetes. People with type 1 diabetes, who must give themselves injections of insulin on a regular basis, can overshoot the mark or not eat enough to compensate for a dose they gave themselves earlier in the day.

A severe drop in glucose following an injection of insulin is called **insulin shock**, a dangerous and potentially fatal event. Those who use insulin must have a glucose source (such as juice or another drink containing sugar) available at all times. This should be swallowed as soon as symptoms of hypoglycemia appear, and additional food should be eaten to maintain the glucose level, especially if symptoms do not improve over the next several minutes. Some diabetics carry a kit containing the hormone **glucagon** that can be injected if the low glucose persists.

Many people with type 2 diabetes (the more common form that occurs later in life, often associated with being overweight) take one or more medications that occasionally can cause hypoglycemia. (Some type 2 diabetics also take insulin, though usually as a last resort when other treatment options have failed.)

A variety of other medical conditions, such as severe liver or kidney disease, alcoholism, and anorexia nervosa, can occasionally be associated with low or borderline glucose levels. Very uncommonly, abnormal amounts of insulin may be secreted by a tumor arising from the pancreas, or an insulin-like hormone may be created by a tumor elsewhere.

During the 1970s and 1980s, fueled in part by *Sugar Blues* and dozens of other books about hypoglycemia, this condition also became a common self-diagnosis for chronic fatigue, headaches, aches and pains, dizziness, mood disturbances, and a host of other common symptoms. Most doctors find this idea difficult to swallow, because those who claim to have this problem rarely if ever are found to have low blood sugar, even if tested when they feel their worst.

A *very* small number of people have true **reactive hypoglycemia**, in which glucose rises and then plummets to dangerously low levels after they eat a meal loaded with carbohydrates. Many more, however, experience a drop that is not as severe, but enough to bring on a sense of fatigue, hunger, tremulousness, or other symptoms. An improvement in symptoms following a small snack is a clue that this might be occurring. If there is any question that shifting blood glucose levels might be causing symptoms, there are three relatively simple ways to find out. One is to have a physician check your blood glucose when you are fasting, after a meal, when you feel poorly, or perhaps as part of a more formal glucose tolerance test, which measures blood sugar one and two hours after you drink a standardized load of glucose. If there is still some doubt, a glucose meter can be purchased at a pharmacy or discount store. (These are used routinely by type 1 diabetics to monitor their responses to food and insulin and by some type 2 diabetics to track their progress.) Your glucose levels can be checked as frequently as needed to clarify their connection (if any) to symptoms.

A second, very practical approach is to make a straightforward (and for that matter healthy) change in eating habits: Take a time-out from foods that are likely to cause trouble. If you think that fluctuating blood glucose could be bringing you grief, try to eliminate the foods that are most likely to provoke rising and falling levels. These include foods in which added sugars are listed as one of the first two ingredients, as well as a number of foods (most of which are refined and processed members of the starch category) that have a high glycemic index, a concept we will introduce in the next section.

Third, fluctuations in blood sugar can be avoided by eating smaller amounts of food more frequently. The common convention of eating breakfast at 6 or 7 A.M., lunch at noon or one P.M., and dinner at 6 or 7 P.M. is based on the preferences of a majority of people—but not all of them. Many people feel hungry halfway between breakfast and lunch, or between lunch and dinner, no matter how much they have eaten at the previous meal. In fact, very often large meals lead to lethargy (or overt drowsiness), poor concentration, and hunger within a few hours, not to mention heartburn. This very practical approach of eating smaller meals more often ensures that a steady flow of nutrients enters your digestive tract—and thus your bloodstream—throughout the day. ■

continued from page 126

aliases. You might notice some of the following listed among the ingredients of the foods on your shelves.

- Sucrose, also known as white sugar, table sugar, refined sugar, granulated sugar, cane sugar, and beet sugar, consists of one glucose and one fructose molecule linked together. A teaspoon of sugar contains about sixteen calories.
- Powdered sugar, also known as confectioners' sugar, is basically white sugar pulverized to a fine consistency, with a little cornstarch added to prevent lumps from forming.
- Raw sugar, or partially refined sugar, is brown and coarser than white sugar. True raw sugar is banned in the United States because it may contain unsavory ingredients such as bacteria and insect parts, but the products sold here (such as Sugar In The Raw or "turbinado") have had impurities removed.
- Brown sugar is white sugar to which molasses has been added.
- Molasses is the thick, brown syrup produced during the extraction and refining of sugar from cane.
- Dextrose is another name for glucose.
- Levulose is another name for fructose.
- Invert sugar, a mix of glucose and fructose, occurs naturally (as in honey) or by chemical action on cane sugar.
- Corn syrup is a liquid (containing mostly glucose) derived from cornstarch.
- High-fructose corn syrup, a form of corn syrup that was introduced in the mid-1960s, contains glucose and fructose, but with a higher proportion (up to 55 percent) of fructose. This product is sweeter than corn syrup, cheaper than sugar obtained from sugar cane (but equally sweet), and not prone to crystallize, making it a popular sweetener that has been added to an enormous number of products. Between 1966 and 2001, high-fructose corn syrup consumption in the United States rose from zero to over sixty pounds per person annually.[4]

Honey contains primarily glucose and fructose, but typically with a higher percentage of fructose, making most forms sweeter than white sugar. It also contains a small percentage of sucrose and other simple sugars. Almost 200 million pounds (including more than three hundred unique flavors) of honey are produced every year in the United States by more than 2.5 million colonies of honeybees. Each pound of honey represents about 2 million visits to flowers by bees and about fifty thousand flight miles. A tablespoon of honey contains about sixty-four calories (compared to about forty-eight calories in a tablespoon of sugar).

If all the various forms of sugar are so pleasing to the taste buds, how might they cause us trouble? Some feel that sugar is literally the root of all evil, the cause not only of misbehavior in children and depression in adults, but also of worldwide plague and pestilence. As with many health issues, there is a fair distance between such allegations and reality. Nevertheless, some noteworthy concerns have been raised about our love affair with sugar.

Sugar and obesity: The number of Americans, young and old, who are overweight or obese has increased dramatically over the past two decades, as has our national consumption of added sugars. Currently Americans on average consume 16 percent of their calories from added sugars. Among children ages six to eleven, the number is 18 percent, while teenagers derive 20 percent of their calories from added sugars. Among the young, soft drinks—what some critics call "liquid candy"—are a major source of these calories. A typical twelve-ounce canned soft drink contains the equivalent of about ten teaspoons of sugar, yielding 140 calories. This by itself represents the maximum daily intake of added sugars recommended by the USDA. But fast-food restaurants, convenience stores, and movie theaters sell soft drinks in colossal serving sizes ranging from thirty-two to fifty-two ounces, often with free refills. A forty-two-ounce fast-food "supersize" nondiet soft drink packs more than four hundred calories.

Sugar and obesity (part 2): The contribution of sweets to obesity may involve more than calorie counts. In many people the metabolic response to surges of blood glucose from products containing a lot of simple sugars appears to promote fat storage. Unfortunately, the same may be happening with starches and other mainstays of the low-fat approach to eating that has been encouraged by government and health professionals for the past three decades. We will look at this question in the next section.

Empty calories: One of the strongest arguments against the wholesale consumption of sugar is that it is basically a raw energy source without any additional nutritive value. No vitamins, minerals, fiber, or other useful compounds are present in a typical can of soda. Enjoy a medium-sized orange and you get a total of eighty calories, of which about fifty-six come from sugars. But the orange also contains 7 grams of fiber, a gram of protein, a generous dose of vitamin C, and some vitamin A, iron, and calcium. Polish off a mere five ounces of a typical orange soda—less than half of a twelve-ounce can—and you get the same number of calories, all from sugar in one form or another, plus a little caffeine to jangle your nerves and—that's all, folks! Drink the entire can, and you'll consume twice as many calories as the orange contains. Of course, using artificial sweeteners is one way to indulge your sweet tooth without consuming empty calories, but some have questioned their safety. See the sidebar "Artificial Sweeteners: Help or Hazard?" on page 134.

Sugar vs. the teeth: Actually, this isn't just a shortcoming of sugar. Carbohydrates in any form serve as a food supply for bacteria within the mouth that produce enamel-eroding acid. What makes a carbohydrate bad for the teeth isn't necessarily how sweet it is—the bacteria can be as happy with

continued on page 136

DAIRY DIFFICULTIES: LACTOSE INTOLERANCE AND MILK ALLERGY

Years ago a dairy-industry advertising campaign proclaimed, "Milk is good for every body." This was a bold claim, given the fact that most adults in the world cannot tolerate milk. (The ads have long been replaced by the more playful milk-mustache photos and "Got milk?" commercials.)

All newborn mammals are designed to be nourished with mother's milk, which contains lactose as its primary carbohydrate. Appropriately called milk sugar, lactose is a disaccharide (two-sugar) molecule consisting of one glucose and one galactose molecule linked together. In this form it cannot be absorbed. An enzyme called **lactase**, produced in the lining of the intestine, breaks lactose into these two monosaccharide (single-sugar) molecules, which can then be absorbed and utilized. After weaning, all land mammals dramatically decrease the production of lactase. Thus, if lactose shows up in the small intestine, some or most of it will not be broken down and absorbed. This may actually draw fluid into the bowel. Then, when lactose arrives in the colon (large intestine), an army of bacteria cheerfully ferments it, yielding both increased gas and the component sugars glucose and galactose. These cannot be absorbed by the lining of the colon, but instead draw ever more fluid into it. Bloating, cramps, gas, and diarrhea may result.

We use the term **lactose intolerance** as if it were a disease, a malady that causes the afflicted person to experience a host of unpleasant symptoms after enjoying a perfectly harmless glass of milk. In fact, the ability to drink milk throughout life is the exception in the human race, rather than the rule. A small percentage (less than 15 to 20 percent) of northern and central European, as well as American, whites lose enough lactase to become lactose intolerant. But 50 to 80 percent of African-Americans and Ashkenazi Jews, 60 to 80 percent of Hispanics, and nearly 100 percent of Asians and Native Americans eventually become lactose intolerant. Only 20 to 30 percent of those living in northern India are lactose intolerant, but 60 to 70 percent in southern India are affected. (In general, most of those who tolerate lactose into adulthood come from populations that raise cows and use dairy products. But whether ongoing exposure to lactose maintains the lactase or whether more of those who were endowed with long-term supplies of lactase survived in locales where dairy products became a food source, no one knows for certain.)

Lactose intolerance can develop early or late in life. It may also follow on the heels of any gastrointestinal illness that damages the lining of the small bowel or causes food to move through it more rapidly. The severity of symptoms depends on the person's age and ethnic background, as well as the amount of lactose. Typically, the amount present in eight to twelve ounces of milk will provoke symptoms about two hours after it is swallowed. Usually lactose intolerance can be confirmed by an improvement in bowel symptoms (gas, cramps, rumbling, diarrhea) after a time-out from dairy products for several days, although specific medical tests for it are also available. (A discussion with one's physician is a good idea, however. A number of other medical problems can cause similar symptoms.)

People with lactose intolerance can eliminate dairy products altogether or adjust their intake to include whatever amounts and forms they can handle without symptoms. Milk that has been pretreated with lactase is available along with regular milk in the dairy case at the store, as are various forms of lactase (such as Lactaid or Lactrase) that can be added to milk or taken before drinking or eating dairy products. Often products such as ice cream or aged cheese will not provoke symptoms, and yogurts with live cultures are usually tolerated because the bacteria present generate lactase. Those who reduce or eliminate dairy products—especially if they are women over thirty-five—should make an effort to take adequate amounts of calcium from other dietary sources or supplements.

Milk allergy is an entirely different problem from lactose intolerance. It involves an overzealous response of the immune system to protein in milk, most often seen among infants drinking formula derived from cow's milk. As many as 7 percent of babies are allergic to cow's milk protein and manifest this problem in one of two ways. The less common is a sudden allergic response, with wheezing, swelling, hives, or even vomiting. Much more common (and often difficult to identify) is a slower reaction, which may include a variety of symptoms: failure to gain weight, irritability, and loose stools (occasionally containing blood). If the infant's doctor suspects that cow's milk allergy is the problem, a soy-based formula may be tried, although about 15 percent of infants with the sudden type of reaction, and about half with the slower reaction, may react to soy-based formula as well. Should that occur, the doctor might recommend a **hypoallergenic** formula, although these may be up to three times as expensive as regular formulas. Needless to say, this type of allergy to milk does not occur when an infant is breast-fed. ■

ARTIFICIAL SWEETENERS: HELP OR HAZARD?

Over the past hundred-plus years, a number of substances have been discovered—nearly all of them by accident, by the way—that provide sweetness without calories. But are they safe? And do they really do any good in the long run? Here is a look at the three most widely used sweeteners: saccharin, aspartame, and sucralose.

Saccharin was discovered in 1879, and by 1907 it was used as a substitute for sugar in the diets of diabetics. With no calories, no metabolic by-products, and sweetness about five hundred times that of sucrose, saccharin was the only nonnutritive sweetener available in the United States through the 1970s. It is still added to a wide variety of products (including cosmetics and medications) and is the sweetener found in Sweet'N Low.

Saccharin generated controversy during the 1970s when it was reported that high doses were associated with an increased risk for bladder cancer in rats. The Food and Drug Administration (FDA) proposed that saccharin be taken off the market, but in response to public protest Congress put the ban on hold in 1977. Subsequent research failed to demonstrate a risk of bladder (or any other) cancer among human users. Furthermore, the rats had been given huge daily doses of sodium saccharin—on a dose-per-weight basis, an adult human would have to drink hundreds of cans of diet soft drinks every day to consume an equivalent amount. Additional evidence suggested that the sodium rather than the saccharin in sodium saccharin was responsible for the tumors. Congress repeatedly extended the moratorium on the FDA's proposed saccharin ban, until the FDA withdrew its request in 1991.

While available evidence indicates that saccharin is safe when consumed in limited amounts, the FDA has set an **acceptable daily intake (ADI)** for this sweetener at 5 mg per kg of body weight per day. For a 150-pound adult, this is about 350 mg of saccharin—roughly the amount in ten packets of Sweet'N Low.

Aspartame was discovered (also accidentally) in 1965 and introduced in 1981 after extensive human and animal studies. (Some two hundred have been conducted to date.) Approved for use in one hundred countries, it is found in more than six thousand products and is the sweetener in Equal and NutraSweet. Aspartame consists of two amino acids, phenylalanine and aspartic acid, in a form which, when digested, yields these two molecules plus methanol. The amino acids are building blocks of naturally occurring protein, and methanol is found in foods in amounts larger than those generated by typical doses of aspartame.

People with the metabolic disorder **phenylketonuria** (or **PKU**), which occurs in about one in ten thousand individuals, do not metabolize phenylalanine normally. They must limit their intake of phenylalanine in order to avoid an accumulation in the body that could cause mental impairment or permanent brain damage. Products containing aspartame carry a warning for people with PKU, who should limit their use or avoid them entirely. The acceptable daily intake (ADI) of aspartame for a person without PKU is 50 mg per kg of body weight (or ten times that of saccharin). For a 150-pound person this is about 3,500 mg, the amount in about one hundred packets of Equal. (A twelve-ounce diet soft drink contains about 225 mg of aspartame.)

Aspartame has been the object of a vigorous campaign (much of which has been waged on the Internet) blaming it for a variety of symptoms and diseases. These include, among many others, headaches, visual disturbances, dizziness, confusion, fatigue, seizures, fibromyalgia, Alzheimer's disease, Parkinson's disease, multiple sclerosis, and brain tumors. However, no professional organization (including the American Academy of Family Physicians, the American Academy of Pediatrics, the Alzheimer's Association, the National Parkinson Foundation, the National Multiple Sclerosis Society, and many others) or government agency (not only in the United States, but also in England, France, and Canada) has found these claims credible. Both physiology and research findings argue strongly against the breadth and severity of these hazards.

The accusations against aspartame are not unlike those that have been raised about other products over the past few decades. We will take a closer look at the important question of evaluating the validity of health claims (both positive and negative) in chapter 17.

Sucralose is the only artificial sweetener derived directly from sucrose (table sugar). It is created by substituting chlorine molecules for three of the hydrogen-oxygen groups on the sugar molecule, resulting in a compound that is six hundred times as sweet as sugar but is not digested or absorbed by the intestine. Furthermore, it remains stable at high temperatures, so that it can be used in products that are cooked or baked. Sold as the sweetener Splenda, it has been approved for use in a wide variety of foods. Sucralose thus far has not earned any warning labels from the FDA or from health-regulatory organizations in thirty countries, based on more than one hundred studies over a twenty-year period. As with the other sweeteners, dire warnings about sucralose may be found on the Internet, though not from reputable sources.

One important question to ponder: Is there a long-term advantage to using products containing artificial sweeteners or to adding them to coffee or tea in place of sugar? The two major reasons would be to reduce the intake of calories for someone trying to lose weight and to limit sugar intake in diabetics. Both of these are worthy goals, but they may be undermined by other choices at the kitchen table. A number of studies have suggested that some dieters may rob Peter to pay Paul by reducing calories at one meal (or in one food) but adding many more elsewhere. Also, diabetics who are trying to prevent elevations in blood glucose by avoiding sugar need to remember that other unsweetened nutrients can also have a serious impact on blood glucose, as we will see shortly. Furthermore, the fact that a sweet food or drink is sugar free doesn't guarantee that its other ingredients are good for you.

The bottom line: Artificial sweeteners appear to be safe when used in moderation, despite Internet alarms that are usually undermined by doubtful credibility and shrill rhetoric. Nevertheless, whether sweeteners offer long-term benefit to dieters and diabetics is questionable, and no one can be completely certain of their effects when used over a lifetime. ■

continued from page 131

raisins as with candy—but how long it hangs around inside the mouth. Sticky, sugary foods are thus likely to be troublemakers, especially for those who don't brush after every meal. In general, the greater the percentage of one's daily calories that comes in the form of sugars, the greater the risk of dental caries (tooth decay).

Sugar and hyperactivity: The popular notion that hyperactivity or aggressive behavior in children is provoked by eating sugar has persisted for decades, despite a lack of any consistent support from scientific research. Numerous studies evaluating behavior and learning among children given variable amounts of sugar and artificial sweeteners have shown minimal, if any, objective impact. If Johnny seems "amped up" after a few rounds of soft drinks, cake, and ice cream at a friend's birthday party, the sugar he gobbled up might seem like a prime suspect. But the general excitement, games, presents, and perhaps the caffeine lurking in the sodas are more likely to blame. Nevertheless, if parents notice that a child's behavior seems to take a turn for the worse whenever sugary foods cross his lips, it certainly wouldn't hurt him to stay away from them.

Starches: "They fatten me, they fatten me not"

Starches have had a wild ride in the public consciousness over the past fifty years. A few decades ago they were considered to be the "eat it today, wear it tomorrow" foods, guaranteed to travel directly from the stomach to some unattractive location on the abdomen or hips. Then during the late 1970s starches began to earn big points for being nonfat, slow-release foods that would curb a national epidemic of heart attacks and strokes. From 1992 until 2005, they were given a prominent position at the base of the Food Guide Pyramid, the diagram from the U.S. Department of Agriculture and the U.S. Department of Health and Human Services that illustrated which foods should be the cornerstone of our diet and which should rarely, if ever, cross our lips. That esteemed position within the pyramid signified that, depending upon one's energy needs, three to ten ounces of starches in the form of grains (especially whole grains) should be eaten every day.

But starches came under unflattering scrutiny from some researchers who argued that they played a major role in an alarming national epidemic of obesity over the past two decades. Indeed, the conflict over whether starches are good or bad, and whether they should be promoted or discouraged, has become something of a nutritional "cold war," with advocates on both sides fervently defending their position. We will have more to say about this often heated discussion, and about the 2005 Food Guide Pyramid, later in this chapter. For now, we need to set forth a few more facts about these important forms of carbohydrate.

The word *starch* comes from an old English word for "stiffen," inspired by the usefulness of some forms of starch in adding a little of that quality to clothing.

As we noted earlier, starches consist of long chains of glucose molecules linked together and packed into certain parts of a variety of foods:

- **Grains** are the small, dry, one-seed fruit of cereal grasses—wheat, rice, corn, oats, and barley. We think of cereal, of course, as what we pour out of a box for breakfast, but a wondrous variety of foods derived from cereal grasses have fed the human race for millennia.

F.Y.I. The word *cereal* comes from the name Ceres, the ancient Roman goddess of agriculture. While we think of cereals primarily as sources of carbohydrate, cereal grains provide more than 85 percent of the total amount of protein consumed around the world.[5]

- **Legumes** are the fruits or seeds of the bean and pea family, which also includes lentils and peanuts.
- **Tubers** (also called **root vegetables**) possess a swollen segment of stem (usually underground) or root that plays a role in both reproduction and energy storage. Our most familiar tubers are potatoes and yams.

F.Y.I. The word *tuber* comes from a Latin word for "lump," which is what potatoes and yams look like. The word *tuberculosis* literally means "the condition of having small lumps," arising from the fact that an untreated tuberculosis infection can produce large numbers of tubercles (small lumps) in the lungs and other organs.

These foods have been the staple of cultivation around the world because they are both generous and generally inexpensive sources of carbohydrate fuel that can be prepared and consumed in a variety of ways. Their lack of fat content has given them a particularly esteemed status in the United States over the past thirty years, as dietary recommendations from government and professional groups stressed the importance of eating low-fat or nonfat foods. So why would a host of weight-loss programs such as the Atkins diet, Protein Power and Sugar Busters! conclude that starch is the root of most of our dietary ills, including excessive weight?

To address that question, we need to take a closer look at what happens when we consume these foods. Traditionally, complex carbohydrate foods (including all of the various forms of starches) have been considered time-release sources of fuel. Eat a candy bar or drink a soda, and one can reasonably assume that the sugars it contains will gain rapid access to the bloodstream. (Indeed, they usually do.) Have a piece of bread or a baked potato, on the other hand, and it will take awhile to disassemble all of those complex molecules and release their glucose into circulation—or will it? Depending upon what happened between their harvest and their arrival at the table, the constituents of many complex carbohydrate foods may be capable of releasing large amounts of glucose into the bloodstream very rapidly—even more rapidly, in fact, than sugar itself.

How do we know that this is happening? A measurement called the

glycemic index (or **GI**) has been utilized in recent years (though more widely among dietary professionals in Canada, Europe, and Australia than in the United States) as an estimate of the tendency of a food to raise blood glucose. Healthy volunteers are given a specific amount of pure glucose to swallow, after which their blood glucose levels are measured several times over the next few hours. Then they consume other foods in amounts containing the same quantity of carbohydrate as the original glucose sample, and blood glucose levels are measured at the same time intervals. The responses of blood glucose to the food and to the pure glucose are compared using a computer program. The tests are repeated a number of times with different volunteers to smooth out the effects of individual differences in digestion and metabolism.

Glucose, the reference food, is given a GI of 100. For other foods, a GI of 70 or more is considered high; one less than 55 is considered low; and one between 55 and 70 is intermediate. Researchers in various parts of the world have generated tables of GIs for a gamut of foods, and the results are often surprising.

F.Y.I.

Some researchers assign a GI of 100 to a slice of white bread and calculate those of other foods accordingly. With this as the reference, the GI for glucose ranges from 130 to 140. Since

What kinds of carbohydrate foods have the highest glycemic index? One would expect candy and soft drinks to lead the pack. They are, in fact, on the higher end of the list (especially jelly beans). But all of the following foods have a higher GI than white sugar: white, whole wheat, and rye bread; bagels; waffles; mashed, baked, or french fried potatoes; cornflakes; instant rice; corn chips and pretzels. What foods tend to have a lower glycemic index? With few exceptions, vegetables, fruits (except dried dates), and legumes (peas and beans); pumpernickel and heavy, mixed-grain breads; milk and low-fat yogurt; and (surprise) most pastas, especially when lightly cooked (the so-called al dente style).

What is it about certain foods that raises their glycemic index? Obviously, an abundance of simple sugars has an impact. But the preparation of many starch-laden foods (for example, baking or mashing potatoes) alters their physical characteristics in a way that allows them to be converted into glucose very rapidly. Unfortunately, one of the most common alterations of food over the past century—the processing and refining of grains, especially wheat and rice—significantly raises the GI of these everyday staples. For example, the outer bran and inner germ layers are removed from wheat in order to increase efficiency and stability in creating white flour, which may in turn be finely ground. These characteristics all lead to more rapid digestion and conversion into glucose, and thus more dramatic changes in blood sugar after these foods are eaten.

In the real world of real people eating real food (as opposed to a controlled laboratory setting), many factors impact how rapidly blood glucose changes after a meal. These include:

- **How much of a food is eaten.** Carrots have a moderately high glycemic index, but one would have to eat a huge number to provoke a dramatic effect on blood glucose.
- **What else is eaten with the food.** We rarely eat just one food at a time for a meal. If a high-glycemic-index carbohydrate is eaten with some protein and fat, absorption of the entire mix tends to be slower.
- **Individual characteristics** of the eater (such as age) may alter the rate at which food is digested and absorbed.
- **The presence of fiber.** Foods that are rich in fiber, such as vegetables and most fruits, are the true time-release sources of fuel. (Note that riper fruits tend to have a higher sugar content and thus a higher glycemic index.) Whole-grain breads, which are more abundant in fiber than their refined counterparts, may have a similar glycemic index if the flour has been finely ground. However, the benefits of their nutrients and fiber counterbalance the impact of their glycemic index.

If a food has a high glycemic index, does that make it bad? While some advocates of low-carbohydrate diets seem to imply that high-glycemic foods are literal poison, the picture isn't quite that black-and-white. Carrots, beets, bananas, cantaloupe, papayas, and pineapples, for example, have a moderately high GI, but that hardly qualifies them as foods to be avoided at all cost. Indeed, another factor that must be considered along with the glycemic index is the *amount* of carbohydrate in a given serving of food. The term **glycemic load** is obtained by dividing the glycemic index of a food by 100 and then multiplying it by the number of grams of carbohydrate in that portion. (A glycemic load for an entire meal can be calculated by repeating this process for every carbohydrate source on the plate—a rather laborious process.) Dietitians note that the glycemic load is equally if not more important than the glycemic index. For example, even though a medium-sized carrot has a relatively high glycemic index of 92, it contains only about 4 grams of carbohydrate, and so its glycemic load is 3.7. Mashed potato has a similar glycemic index of 97, but a typical serving contains about 23 grams of carbohydrate, for which the glycemic load is 22—six times greater than that of the carrot.

That being said, a diet heavy on high-glycemic foods—especially those that are calorie dense and have little additional nutritional value—could cause problems for many people because of the physiological response that they are likely to provoke. As we mentioned earlier in our look at sugars, eating foods that provoke a rapid rise in blood glucose causes the pancreas to release a surge of insulin so that the glucose can be escorted into all of the cells that need it.

But there are some downsides to this response: First, a relatively rapid rise and fall of glucose may provoke hunger, which leads to—that's right—more eating. In fact, the hunger may last well after the blood glucose has risen again. If the desire for more food leads to another round of high-glycemic-index treats, the cycle may repeat itself. Second, insulin not only moves glucose into cells. It also promotes storage of any excess calories as fat and slows the use of fat as a source of energy.

Perhaps the most worrisome issue related to foods with a high-glycemic index is their potential effect on people who have a genetic tendency toward what is called **insulin resistance**. If we think of insulin as the biochemical key that opens the lock on the surface of cells so that glucose can enter, we would consider people with insulin resistance to have sticky locks. Insulin is present and accounted for, but glucose levels remain elevated so the pancreas secretes more insulin in an effort to solve this problem. But as we have just noted, the increased insulin serves to promote storage of extra calories as fat and to inhibit the utilization (or "burning") of fat to provide energy.

Insulin resistance is a component of a hazardous and increasingly common phenomenon in developed countries, which we introduced in chapter 3 as **metabolic syndrome**. Previously known as Syndrome X and sometimes called insulin resistance syndrome, metabolic syndrome is characterized by the following:

- **Obesity**
- **Increased abdominal girth**—specifically, excessive fat in the abdomen, reflected in the waistline: forty inches or more for men, and thirty-five inches or more for women
- **Hypertension** (elevated blood pressure)—130/85 or greater
- **Abnormalities in lipids**—specifically, a tendency toward high levels of triglycerides (more than 150 mg/dl) and low levels of HDL (or "good") cholesterol (less than 40 mg/dl for men or 50 mg/dl for women)
- **Insulin resistance**, which is often reflected in mild elevations of fasting blood glucose, or more significant increases during a glucose tolerance test

For a refresher on the various types of lipids and their significance, see chapter 3 beginning on page 56.

A person with metabolic syndrome has a lot going against him (or her). For one thing, all of these features are specific risk factors for cardiovascular disease. *Unless the problem is addressed through a combination of lifestyle efforts (diet and exercise) and medical treatment, heart attack, stroke, and all of the other woes brought about by progressively congested arteries are likely to loom in the future.* In addition, this condition could also be considered "prediabetes." If allowed to continue, eventually blood glucose levels are likely to rise until diabetes arrives with all of its potentially devastating complications.

Cardiovascular disease and diabetes are reviewed in detail in chapter 3.

F.Y.I. Insulin resistance has also been implicated as the physiological problem underlying **polycystic ovary syndrome** (or **PCO**), an increasingly common condition in women characterized by obesity, infrequent menstrual cycles, and infertility. Along with weight loss, medications that reduce insulin resistance can help correct this problem.

What brings on metabolic syndrome and why it has become so common are important and provocative questions. One theory proposes that it arises from genetic programming that increases the odds for survival when food is scarce—a situation that humans have endured through most of history and still do in many parts of the world today. Indeed, we are so obsessed with losing weight in our culture—and are so upset when the pounds don't just melt off when we eat less or do a little exercise—that we fail to appreciate the magnificent design of our body that allows us to function with a highly unpredictable fuel supply. If little food is available most of the time or if life is a literal "feast or famine," we're built to make the most of any calories we find. This includes not only using them efficiently, but also storing any extra for a "rainy day" (or a lot of them).

This storage occurs in two forms: **glycogen** and **fat**. Glycogen is a complex carbohydrate (we might think of it as "animal starch") that is readily available as a source of fuel, like cash in a biochemical automated teller machine. Glycogen is stored in limited amounts in muscle and liver and can supply about two days' worth of calories for quiet activities if little or no food is available. When glycogen stores are full, we're designed not to allow any extra calories go to waste but rather to store them as fat. And, as we well know, our capacity for fat storage is enormous.

Some researchers have suggested that the metabolic syndrome may represent the downside of a "thrifty gene" that causes a rapid response to any carbo-

WATER WEIGHT AND "HITTING THE WALL"

TWO INTERESTING FEATURES OF GLYCOGEN

We store about a pound of **glycogen**, our quick-release fuel, in our muscles and the liver. When food—especially carbohydrate—is absent or in short supply, this is the first energy source to be tapped. Glycogen is also hydrophilic (literally "water loving"), meaning it binds as much as three times its weight in water. A person starting a weight-loss program—especially one that includes very little carbohydrate—will use up glycogen stores within the first couple of days, and as these stores disappear the water associated with them will disappear as well, in the form of a temporary diuresis (that is, increased output of urine). This accounts for the rapid initial weight loss of a few pounds that is so common (and so encouraging) for new dieters. Of course, those who fall off the wagon before they have mobilized a substantial amount of fat can expect to welcome back their glycogen and its associated water very quickly.

While our stored glycogen can serve as a fuel supply for a couple of days, long-distance running and other forms of endurance exercise burn through it much more rapidly. When it's gone, the body must shift gears to mobilize fuel from protein or fat. This transition causes what marathon runners call "hitting the wall," a point in the race when the bottom suddenly seems to fall out of one's energy supply. In order to delay it, before the event many partake in what is called "carbohydrate loading," a feast of starchy foods consumed for the purpose of topping off glycogen stores. ■

hydrates, efficient storage of extra carbohydrates as fat once glycogen stores are full, and resistance to letting any fat disappear. When food is scarce, people with the thrifty gene would have a distinct advantage: They would rapidly convert available food into energy for muscles and the brain to use and wouldn't squander any extra fuel, thus improving their odds of survival. But in modern-day America and other developed countries, the opposite is true—especially when an enormous number of calories arrive in the form of sugars and refined/processed starches. Now with a perpetual feast in progress, glucose and insulin levels soar, fat is both readily stored and resistant to being mobilized, and all of the woes of cardiovascular disease and diabetes multiply.

Whether insulin resistance is caused primarily by a person's genetic makeup, diet, or a combination of factors is unknown. Some postulate that a diet loaded with high-glycemic-index foods might actually induce metabolic syndrome and type 2 diabetes. Others argue that metabolic syndrome and type 2 diabetes are the natural consequences of exposing genetically susceptible individuals or ethnic groups to a diet that is poorly suited to their metabolism. Whatever the mechanism, the emergence of metabolic syndrome, type 2 diabetes, and obesity as modern-day epidemics has set off a lot of alarms in the public-health arena, along with much speculating and hand-wringing over their causes. One obvious equation—more calories plus less exercise equal weight gain—is addressed in chapter 6. But one well-intentioned public-health effort over the past thirty years may have made a major contribution to this problem.

In the 1970s the understanding that high levels of cholesterol in the blood is a risk factor for coronary artery disease led to what seemed like a logical conclusion: *If we could get the entire country to eat less fat and more carbohydrates, we'd see a drop in cholesterol, heart attacks, and obesity.* After all, carbohydrates contain only four calories per gram, whereas fat contains nine calories per gram, and saturated fat is definitely not good for the arteries, as we shall see a little later. The idea caught on and has been promoted by health professionals, the government, and the food industry for three decades. As we have already mentioned, grains were installed as a fundamental part of the USDA's Food Guide Pyramid, largely because of their lack of fat. In addition, some fifteen thousand products, both new and old, proudly announce on their labels that they are low fat or (better) nonfat. For example, one prominent brand of chocolate syrup—not exactly the most nutritious treat on the shelf—defends its guilty-pleasure status with the reassuring words "a fat-free food" on the label.

Statistics monitoring the eating habits of Americans suggest that we indeed reduced our consumption of fat as a percentage of total daily calories over the past few decades. That was not a bad thing to do, but it didn't prevent a massive national weight gain. Some proponents of low- or controlled-carbohydrate diets argue that the push to reduce dietary fat actually contributed to the obesity epidemic, because our low-fat replacements were often high-glycemic-index products. The explanation isn't that one-dimensional, and many nutritionists are not convinced that the glycemic index is the final authority on the quality of a food. Nevertheless, as we'll see later in this chapter, it's one of several factors to weigh when considering which carbohydrates are the best choices to fill your pantry and refrigerator.

Fiber: The regulators

Dietary fiber, the other major type of complex carbohydrate, plays a supportive but very important role in nutritional health. Remember that fiber is the component of plant foods that we cannot digest. (We do not obtain any fiber from animal or dairy products.) **Soluble** fiber partially dissolves in water, while **insoluble** does not. Sources of soluble fiber (such as gums and pectins) include many fruits (apples, pears, and strawberries), legumes (peas, beans, and lentils), oatmeal, and oat bran. Sources of insoluble fiber include many vegetables (carrots, celery, tomatoes, zucchini), whole-grain breads and cereals (especially whole wheat), wheat bran, brown rice, and couscous. Soluble or not, since we can't use it for energy or building materials, what good is it?

Fiber contributes to the time release of energy from carbohydrates by slowing both the release of food from the stomach and the absorption of digestible carbohydrate that accompanies it. This tends to prevent the spikes in blood glucose and insulin that we just described as undesirable features of high-glycemic-index foods (at least for people with metabolic syndrome and type 2 diabetes). Foods with a healthy component of fiber tend to have a lower glycemic index. A diet high in fiber may reduce the risk of developing type 2 diabetes.

Fiber can help reduce overeating and weight gain. Slowing the speed with which you consume a meal is a basic strategy in controlling the size of your food portions, and those higher in fiber content generally take longer to eat. Their larger bulk, increased even more by water they absorb, creates a feeling of fullness. Furthermore, they slow not only the stomach's rate of emptying food but also the passage of food through the small intestine, thus prolonging the sense of being full or even "stuffed" (called **satiety**, from the Latin word for "enough").

Fiber (especially the insoluble form) tends to soften and increase the bulk of stool and helps to move it through the colon more rapidly. It thus can prevent or relieve constipation, the most common intestinal complaint in the United States (especially among the elderly). Wheat and oat bran appear to be particularly effective at this, as is **psyllium seed**, derived from a Mediterranean plant, which swells and becomes gelatinous when moist. Psyllium seed is used in many bulk laxatives such as Metamucil.

Fiber (again, especially the insoluble type) helps prevent diverticulosis, a common condition in which small pouches called **diverticula** form in the wall of the colon. Diverticula can bleed, become infected (a condition called **diverticulitis**), or even perforate, resulting in a serious infection within the abdomen.

continued on page 146

The word *diverticula* literally means "little diversions." In North America, roughly one in three adults over forty-five, and two out of three over eighty-five, have diverticula.

HOW CAN I INCREASE MY DAILY DOSE OF FIBER?

The richest sources of dietary fiber are legumes (beans and peas), vegetables and fruits, and whole-grain products. You'll find less of it in refined grain products (white bread and cereals that aren't whole grain), and none in dairy or meat products. Here are a few ways to increase your family's daily dose of fiber:

1. **Buy bread that lists whole grain (wheat or otherwise) as the first ingredient on the label,** with at least 3 grams of fiber per slice. These tend to be heavier, darker, and more flavorful. If you bake your own bread, use whole-grain flour for a fourth to a half (or more) of the amount of flour in your recipe. (You will need more yeast or baking powder—about a teaspoon more baking powder for every three cups of whole-grain flour.)

2. **Look for breakfast cereals with 5 grams or more of fiber per serving.** Often they include the words *bran* or *fiber* in the name or display it on the packaging, but *check the Nutrition Facts label* to see how much fiber is actually present. (Remember also that fiber content may not be the only virtue a cereal offers.) If these cereals don't suit your taste, try adding some unprocessed wheat bran to the cereals you like. Some cereals that rank highest for fiber on the USDA's National Nutrient Database include the following (but note the varying serving sizes):
   - Kellogg's All-Bran: 9.6 grams of fiber in a half cup
   - Wheatena, cooked in water: 6.6 grams in one cup
   - Post Shredded Wheat: 5.3 grams in two biscuits
   - Kellogg's Complete Wheat Bran Flakes: 5.1 grams in three-quarters of a cup
   - Kellogg's Frosted Mini-Wheats: 5.5 grams in one cup (bite-size) and 5.1 grams in one cup (original)
   - General Mills Raisin Nut Bran: 5.1 grams in one cup
   - General Mills Total Raisin Bran: 5 grams in one cup

   Some cereals whose fiber content is in the medium range include:
   - Quaker 100% Natural Cereal (with oats, honey, and raisins): 4.2 grams in a half cup
   - Oatmeal, cooked: 4 grams in one cup
   - Quaker Honey Nut Heaven: 3.7 grams in one cup
   - General Mills Wheat Chex: 3.3 grams in one cup
   - General Mills Basic 4: 3.2 grams in one cup
   - General Mills Wheaties: 3 grams in one cup
   - General Mills Cheerios: 3 grams in one cup
   - General Mills Whole Grain Total: 2.4 grams in three-quarters cup

   The low end of the USDA fiber rank includes a number of popular brands:
   - Cream of Wheat and Malt-O-Meal: one gram in one cup
   - Kellogg's Corn Flakes, Frosted Flakes, Product 19, Apple Jacks, Cocoa Krispies, Smacks: one gram in one cup
   - Farina hot wheat cereal: less than one gram in one cup

- Kellogg's Special K: 0.7 gram in one cup
- General Mills Cocoa Puffs, Corn Chex, Golden Grahams, Kix, Total Corn Flakes, Trix: between 0.6 and 0.9 gram in one cup
- General Mills Rice Chex and Honey Nut Chex: 0.3 gram in one cup
- Kellogg's Crispix and Rice Krispies: 0.1 gram in one cup
- Last and least: General Mills Reese's Puffs and Kaboom: 0 grams

3. **Try some whole-grain variations on common products,** such as brown rice (rather than white) and whole wheat spaghetti, which contains more than twice the fiber found in regular spaghetti.

4. **Add more peas, beans, and lentils,** which are among the richest sources of dietary fiber, to your daily routine:
   - Baked, kidney, black, white, and pinto beans all contain from 12 to 17 grams of fiber per cup.
   - Lima beans, soybeans (mature), and chickpeas average 10 to 12 grams per cup.
   - A cup of cooked split peas contains over 16 grams of fiber, and an equal amount of frozen green peas contains nearly 9 grams.
   - A cup of cooked mature lentils contains more than 16 grams of fiber.

5. **Last, but certainly not least, eat a lot of fruits (at least three to four servings) and vegetables (four to five servings) every day.** (For children two to six, at least two fruit and three vegetable servings per day.) Some of the highest suppliers of fiber among fruits include:
   - Raspberries: 11 grams of fiber per cup (frozen, red) or 8 grams per cup (raw)
   - Pears: 5.1 grams in a raw pear (or about 4 grams per cup of canned pears)
   - Stewed prunes (dried plums): 7.7 grams per cup
   - Blackberries: 7.6 grams per cup (raw)
   - Pumpkin: 7.1 grams per cup (canned)
   - Papaya: 5.5 grams (raw)
   - Blueberries: 5.1 grams per cup (frozen)

   Other good sources of fiber among fruits include raisins, strawberries, peaches, oranges, apricots, bananas, strawberries, and apples.

   Good vegetable sources of fiber include:
   - Frozen mixed vegetables: 8 grams per cup
   - Spinach: 7 grams per cup (frozen, then cooked), or about 4 grams per cup cooked fresh
   - Artichoke: 6.6 grams (medium size)
   - Brussels sprouts: 6.4 grams per cup (frozen, then cooked), or about 4 grams per cup cooked fresh
   - Squash, winter: 5.6 grams per cup (cooked)
   - Broccoli: about 5 grams per cup (cooked, whether frozen or fresh)

   Other vegetable fiber sources include carrots and corn, as well as the tubers: potatoes and sweet potatoes. ■

continued from page 143

The soft, bulky stools produced by fiber in the diet are also less likely to form small, hard pellets that can lodge in the opening of the appendix, the first step in the development of **appendicitis**.

Some studies have shown lower rates of colon cancer in populations that consume large amounts of fiber, compared with those on a low-fiber diet. A reasonable explanation for this is that any potential carcinogenic (cancer-inducing) agents arriving in the intestine would be diluted and swept along by soft, bulky stools, and thus not allowed to have prolonged contact with the cells lining the colon. However, other research (including a Harvard study that followed eighty thousand women over sixteen years[6]) has not supported this particular benefit from eating dietary fiber.

Finally, dietary fiber—especially soluble fiber found in oats (including oatmeal and oat bran) and apples—can lower blood cholesterol to a modest degree. This occurs when cholesterol floating through the digestive tract binds to the fiber and is carried out of the body in stool, rather than being absorbed. While the impact of dietary fiber on blood cholesterol levels is usually not as dramatic as may be seen with weight loss or medications, it has been demonstrated to reduce the risk for coronary artery disease.

So how much fiber should we eat every day? The Institute of Medicine of the National Academies recommends the following daily amounts:

- For adults fifty and younger: 38 grams for men and 25 grams for women.
- For adults fifty-one and older: 30 grams for men and 21 grams for women.[7]

In addition, for children two and older, the current recommendation for fiber intake is an amount in grams equal to their age plus five.[8]

Unfortunately, Americans on average consume about half this amount of fiber or less on a day-to-day basis. If you are interested in tracking your fiber intake, one way to begin is by paying attention to the Nutrition Facts label found on every packaged food. As we will see later in this chapter, this label includes all sorts of useful tidbits, including grams of fiber per serving. (Of course, you have to note what the label identifies as a serving, and how many servings you are consuming at a given meal.)

A number of the best sources of fiber are vegetables and fruits that don't have nutrition labels slapped on them. We have included several foods and their fiber content in the sidebar "How Can I Increase My Daily Dose of Fiber?" on page 144. If you have access to the Internet, you can look up the nutritional content of foods at the U.S. Department of Agriculture's National Nutrient Database Web site at http://www.nal.usda.gov/fnic/foodcomp/search. The database allows you to view all of the nutritional characteristics of a specific food. And for each nutrient you can get a listing of its content in hundreds of foods, arranged either alphabetically or by the amount of the nutrient, from most to least.

If you don't feel like poring over labels, tables, and Web sites, refer to the sidebar we mentioned on pages 144–145, which offers several ways to ensure that your family's eating habits include a reasonable amount of fiber. As it turns out, these involve choices that enhance your health in many other ways as well, and it won't be the last time you see them in this chapter. If your eating habits up to this point have not included much fiber, you will want to make these changes gradually. A sudden increase in your daily fiber intake may provoke a few unpleasant responses from your intestinal tract, including cramping, bloating, and gas. If you find yourself getting constipated, drink more fluids, since fiber must absorb water to become soft and bulky.

Fats: More Than Excess Baggage

Just as it is dangerous to cast carbohydrates—a major class of nutrients—in the role of villain, the same is true of fats. We have been told for decades that we should eat as little fat as possible and that doing so will keep us thin, but that approach hasn't always worked. And now we hear other voices saying that eating fat is okay, and that doing so with gusto is apparently the way to lose weight. To complicate matters, the fat in so many of our favorite foods gives them the texture and flavor that we enjoy.

As it turns out, we need a certain amount of fat in both our diet and our body to live well. We noted in chapter 3 that fat is actually a member of a family of compounds called **lipids**, although we commonly use the word *fats* to refer to the entire group. The other members are **sterols**, which include cholesterol, and **phospholipids**, such as lecithin. All of these play a variety of important roles, including:

More than half of our ongoing energy needs at rest are supplied by fat stores. The percentage increases both when we're exercising and when we're deprived of food.

Energy storage. We've already described how we are designed to thrive when food is plentiful and survive when it isn't. One ingenious safeguard is the storage of extra calories as glycogen (see page 141) and in **adipose tissue**, which literally covers our body beneath the skin and is also found within the abdomen. Adipose tissue consists of unique cells (called, simply enough, adipose or fat cells) that can store almost unlimited amounts of fuel in the form of fat for immediate and future use. While other types of cells (such as liver or muscle cells) can store only a limited amount of fat, adipose cells can dramatically enlarge to accommodate whatever fat is available to them. One unfortunate result is that a human being can accumulate hundreds of pounds of adipose, to his or her peril.

A typical adult has the following energy reserves: about 650 calories as carbohydrate, 25,000 calories as protein, and 100,000 calories as fat.

Protection and appearance. The layer of fat that covers our body from one end to the other has several important functions beyond storing calories for the winter. It serves as a shock absorber for any part of the body that strikes, or is struck by, a blunt object. A wad of fat under the kidneys helps cushion those critical organs from injury when we jump or are jarred.

Adipose tissue serves as insulation against external heat and cold. And a certain amount of fat is necessary to give our body an appealing shape.

Structural and functional roles. Cholesterol and phospholipids are a vital component of cell membranes, the critical biochemical boundary that surrounds every cell. Far from being an inert "wall" between adjacent cells, these membranes regulate the passage of chemical elements and compounds in and out of cells. Lipids also play important roles in the nervous system. Among other things, they serve as a component of **myelin**, the sheath that functions as insulation around nerve fibers and allows for rapid transmission of nerve impulses. Lipids such as vitamin D, which is necessary for proper formation of bones, and the sex hormones estrogen, progesterone, and testosterone carry out important and far-reaching biochemical functions.

F.Y.I.

Multiple sclerosis is perhaps the most well-known **demyelinating disease**, in which damage to myelin sheaths can result in a disordered nerve function in various parts of the body, including numbness, weakness, lack of coordination, and visual disturbances.

Some basic fat vocabulary

You've probably heard that saturated fats and trans fats aren't good for you, and perhaps you're aware that omega-3 fatty acids and fish oils possess some sort of health benefit. If you look at food labels, you may see terms such as "polyunsaturated" and "partially hydrogenated" applied to a variety of products such as vegetable oils. Many of these ninety-nine-cent words have become part of our vocabulary, but what exactly do they mean? And what difference do they make?

In order to understand these terms and their importance, we're going to need to wade into some basic biochemistry and go a little deeper than we did with carbohydrates. But fear not: this isn't a textbook. If you find yourself losing track of some unfamiliar words and phrases, don't be afraid to back up a little, take a deep breath, and try again. This may take a little effort, but the payoff is that you can walk away from this book with more than a list of nutritional dos and don'ts.

While there are a variety of compounds in the lipid family, two are of particular importance in the world of nutrition. One is **cholesterol**, which we discussed in some detail in chapter 3 (starting on page 56). The other is a class of molecules known as **triglycerides**, which are the main constituents of fat in our food and in our body. Triglycerides consist of a short spine called **glycerol** containing three carbon atoms linked together; each of these carbon atoms is attached to a longer chain of carbon molecules, called a **fatty acid**. (Imagine three thin banners attached to the top, bottom, and middle of a short pole.) The length of the fatty acids and the chemical bonds they contain determine a number of important characteristics of various types of fats.

Now comes a simple but important foundation of fat biochemistry: Think of every carbon atom as having four chemical "outstretched hands" that can attach or **bond** to a maximum of four other atoms. In a fatty acid, each carbon atom (except for the one at the end of the chain) is bonded to two other carbon atoms, one on either side of it in the chain. When these bonds are broken, chemical energy is released. What about the other two bonds? Either both are attached to hydrogen atoms or one of them forms what is called a **double bond** with an adjacent carbon atom. Think of two adjacent carbon atoms holding on to each other with two hands instead of one. Among other things, this means that each of the carbon atoms in a double bond is holding on to one less hydrogen atom.

The energy storage in fat is quite efficient on a weight basis, yielding nine calories per gram. By comparison, carbohydrate or protein yields four calories per gram.

If every carbon atom in the chain (except those at the ends) is bonded to two hydrogen atoms, the fatty acid is said to be **saturated**. (In other words, the chain is saturated, or completely filled, with hydrogen atoms.) If there are one or more double bonds in the chain, the fatty acid is said to be **unsaturated**. If there is only one double bond in the chain, the fatty acid is **monounsaturated** (the prefix *mono* meaning "one"). If more than one carbon atom has formed a double bond in the chain, the fatty acid is said to be **polyunsaturated**. The particular combinations of saturated and unsaturated fatty acids that are attached to glycerol molecules to form triglycerides will vary from fat to fat and food to food.

A certain type of fat will be called saturated or unsaturated based on the type of fatty acid that is most abundant within it. **Saturated fats (SFAs)** are the form that the body prefers to store for future energy needs, and so not surprisingly they are abundant in animal fat. Solid or waxy at room temperature, they have been generally considered the "bad guys" in the world of fats, although they are present in some of America's favorite foods—red meats, butter, cheese, whole milk, and ice cream—as well as coconut, palm, and other tropical oils. The primary concern about eating a lot of saturated fats, other than their rich supply of calories, is that they increase cholesterol levels—in particular, the LDL or "bad" cholesterol—and are associated with a higher risk of developing congested arteries that can lead to heart attack or stroke. The American Heart Association and other organizations recommend that 10 percent or less of our daily calories come from saturated fat.

Monounsaturated fatty acids are abbreviated MUFAs and polyunsaturated fatty acids are abbreviated PUFAs.

F.Y.I.

Need a refresher on what HDL and LDL refer to? Chapter 3 contains a detailed look at cardiovascular disease, heart attack, and stroke, as well as HDL and LDL cholesterol.

Now here's where the rubber begins to meet the road for our health. One double bond, the difference between a saturated and a monounsaturated fatty acid (MUFA), turns a "bad fat" into a "good fat" (or at least a "better fat"). MUFAs are found in abundance in olive oil, canola oil, and peanut oil, as well as avocados and most nuts. They are liquid at room temperature but may solidify if refrigerated. They can be used by our body as fuel nearly as efficiently as saturated fats (SFAs), but unlike SFAs they appear to *reduce* cholesterol, and LDL cholesterol in particular. In fact, some research indicates that a diet in which MUFAs are abundant not only reduces LDL cholesterol but also tends to raise HDL ("good") cholesterol and lower triglycerides. MUFAs may also affect clotting in a beneficial way (that is, reduce the tendency to form unwanted blood clots in arteries).

F.Y.I. A low-fat, high-carbohydrate diet—the type that has been most commonly recommended for lowering cholesterol—can indeed lower LDL cholesterol, but it also tends to lower HDL and raise triglycerides, which is definitely not an ideal result.

Polyunsaturated fats (PUFAs) are liquid both at room temperature and in the refrigerator and, like monounsaturated fats, tend to lower cholesterol when substituted for saturated fatty acids. Indeed, a few decades ago this selling point led to a widespread shift from butter to various forms of margarine derived from polyunsaturated oils, on the assumption that these would be healthier for the heart. (There is, however, more to that story.) PUFAs also are important components of cell membranes and are used by our body in the synthesis of important hormones. Food sources that are rich in PUFAs include vegetable oils made from corn, safflower, cottonseed, flaxseed, soybean, sunflower, and others, as well as fish oils.

One definite liability of polyunsaturated fats is that their multiple double-bond sites make them susceptible to a process called **oxidation**, a chemical reaction that causes them to deteriorate and become rancid. Exposure to light, air, and heat speeds this process. If you leave butter, olive oil, and your favorite polyunsaturated oil sitting in an open dish, the butter will be the last to go rancid because its fat is saturated—that is, there are no double bonds in its fatty acids, so the oxidation proceeds much more slowly. Olive oil, which contains more monounsaturated fatty acids (MUFAs)—and thus fewer double bonds to react with oxygen—will be the second of the three to develop that nasty, rancid aroma. The polyunsaturated oil will be the fastest of the three to go bad, especially if the surroundings are warm. This tendency toward oxidation and rancidity can cause foods full of polyunsaturated fats to become unappetizing. It may also make them hazardous, because the oxidation process generates **free radicals**, highly reactive compounds that can damage cells in a variety of ways.

Food manufacturers realized that this particular drawback of polyunsaturated fatty acids could be countered if they could make them less "PUFA-like"—in other words, if they could reduce the number of double bonds in these fatty acids, which would make them behave more like saturated fats. By heating polyunsaturated oils under pressure in the presence of hydrogen gas, hydrogen atoms are added to the fatty acids, a process called **hydrogenation**. Actually, the reaction does not continue to completion, because this would turn the PUFAs into completely saturated fats—the ones we're supposed to limit in our diet. Instead, the hydrogenation process is stopped at a predetermined point, yielding fats that are called **partially hydrogenated**—a term that you will see on many food labels. This not only stabilizes PUFAs so that they won't go rancid, but it also converts liquid oils into more solid, spreadable, and generally more appealing products. Sounds good so far, but unfortunately research now suggests that the law of unintended consequences may be at work, canceling whatever benefits partially hydrogenated polyunsaturated fats might otherwise offer. In fact, it appears that we would be better off avoiding them. To understand the reason, we need to understand a little more basic fat biochemistry.

The carbon atoms chained together in a saturated fatty acid have a zigzag configuration that extends essentially in one direction. In an unsaturated fatty acid, however, every double bond bends the chain, and the shape of the bend will depend on the position of the single hydrogen atom attached to each carbon atom on either side of the double bond. (Remember that in the more common single bond, each carbon atom is attached to two hydrogen atoms.) If these hydrogen atoms are on the same side of the carbon chain, it is called a **cis fatty acid**. If they are on the opposite side, it is called a **trans fatty acid**. Polyunsaturated fatty acids that occur naturally in food are in the cis form. But both the process of extracting polyunsaturated oils from plants or seeds and the process of creating partially hydrogenated products from them generate a significant proportion of trans fatty acids.

F.Y.I. The prefix *cis* comes from a Latin word meaning "on this side." The more familiar prefix *trans,* as in "transcontinental" or "transfer," comes from the Latin for "across" or "on the other side."

So what's wrong with trans fatty acids? It turns out that they raise LDL ("bad") cholesterol nearly as efficiently as saturated fats, but at least the saturated fats also raise the HDL ("good") cholesterol. Trans fatty acids do not. Furthermore, they may also raise triglyceride levels, so that some researchers consider them at least as much of a threat to health—if not more so—than saturated fats. How much trans fatty acid is too much? No one knows, and thus far no professional organization or government agency has suggested a specific daily limit. While completely eliminating trans fatty acids from your diet is neither practical nor necessary, limiting them is definitely a good idea. (See the heading "Watch out for the trans fats" starting on page 183.) Indeed, in July 2003 the Food and Drug Administration (FDA) mandated that the amount of trans fatty acids in foods must be displayed on nutrition information labels by January 2006. (The FDA estimates that by 2009, reduced consumption of trans fatty acids resulting from food labeling, as well as voluntary efforts by manufacturers to reduce the amounts of these compounds in foods, will prevent 600 to 1,200 heart attacks and save 250 to 500 lives every year.)

The prefix *lin* in the word *linoleic* and *linolenic* comes from the Greek word *linon* which means "flax"—an excellent source of both of these.

Introducing some "good" fats—the essential fatty acids

There's one other important issue about the types of unsaturated fats that we eat, and to understand it we need to introduce just a little more biochemistry. (We promise this is the last you'll need to digest, so to speak—until the next section.) Our body is able to manufacture all of the fatty acids we need from other materials in our diet—carbohydrates, fats, and proteins—except for two, which have similar (and somewhat confusing) names: **linoleic acid** (abbreviated **LA**) and **linolenic acid** (abbreviated **LNA**). Because they must be taken directly from food sources, these are called **essential fatty acids**. From these two compounds, we make a number of other substances that play vital roles in immunity, the inflammatory response, clot formation, and the structure of cell membranes.

When chemists describe fatty acids, they use the Greek letter omega (Ω) to indicate the location of the last double bond in the fatty acid chain. The carbon atoms are numbered 1-2-3-4, etc., starting at the end of the chain. If a fatty acid has its last double bond located six carbon atoms from the end, it is called an **omega-6 fatty acid**. If the last double bond is three carbons from the end of the chain, it is called an **omega-3 fatty acid**.

As it turns out, plants are able to insert double bonds in fatty acids near the end of the carbon chain. Animals cannot accomplish this biochemical feat, which is why they must acquire omega-6 and omega-3 fatty acids from plant sources. Carnivorous animals get their omega-6 and omega-3 supply from other plant-eating animals that they eat. Linoleic acid is an omega-6 fatty acid and is relatively abundant in our food supply, occurring in seeds and any polyunsaturated oils made from them, corn and peanut oils, and animal fat (including poultry). Linolenic acid is an omega-3 fatty acid and, unlike linoleic acid, is far less plentiful in our diet. It is found in flaxseed, walnuts, soybeans, canola, and their oils. It is also present in dark leafy green vegetables, though in lesser amounts.

Two omega-3 fatty acids with tongue-twisting names—**eicosapentaenoic** and **docosahexaenoic acids**, better known by their initials **EPA** and **DHA**—have been identified as particularly important to the well-being of the heart, blood vessels, and nervous system. In particular, they appear to reduce triglyceride levels, lower blood pressure, decrease the growth rate of plaque that blocks arteries, and lower the risk for abnormal heart rhythms that can be lethal during a heart attack. DHA is also an important component of cell membranes in the brain, and both EPA and DHA are considered crucial to its development (as well as that of the eye) before birth and during infancy. DHA is transferred to the baby before birth via the placenta and is present in breast milk. (In fact, it is now being added to infant formula.) Some researchers have also been exploring the possibility that inadequate amounts of DHA play a role in the development of depression, schizophrenia, bipolar disorder, and other behavioral and neurological disturbances.

WHAT ABOUT THE MERCURY IN ALL OF THAT FISH I'M SUPPOSED TO EAT?

Fish is the only food that is considered spoiled once it smells like what it is.
P. J. O'ROURKE

The above quip notwithstanding, seafood is hardly a second-rate alternative to other types of meat. In addition to containing variable amounts of beneficial omega-3 fatty acids, fish is an excellent source of protein, with smaller amounts of saturated fats than many other types of meat.

A pregnant or nursing mother would appear to be a particularly good candidate to eat fish regularly, in order to obtain adequate supplies of DHA and EPA for the developing brain and eyes of her growing baby. But some fish contain a worrisome amount of **methylmercury**, a form of mercury that can harm a baby's central nervous system if he or she is exposed to it regularly. As an old commercial used to ask, "What's a mother to do?"

Mercury circulates in the atmosphere as a result of natural events and the release of industrial pollutants. Some of this settles and accumulates in rivers, streams, and larger bodies of water, where bacteria convert it to methylmercury. Fish in turn absorb this compound during their feeding, and as a result most contain tiny amounts of it that are not harmful to humans. But fish that are closer to the top of the food chain—especially the oldest and largest types that eat fish that have eaten other fish—are likely to have accumulated a fair amount of methylmercury before being pulled aboard the fishing boat. The most likely candidates to carry unwholesome quantities are shark, swordfish, king mackerel, and tilefish (sometimes called golden bass or golden snapper), and the FDA thus recommends that pregnant and nursing mothers, as well as young children, avoid eating them. They should also consider limiting their consumption of tuna to less than six ounces per week, based on recent concerns that have been raised about the presence of mercury in this popular fish. (The amount may vary depending on the type of tuna—tuna steaks and canned albacore tuna typically contain more mercury than canned light tuna, for example.)

What about other fish? Women who are pregnant (or may become so) and young children can enjoy up to twelve ounces of other types of fish per week without risk. (A typical serving is about three to six ounces.) Eating more than this amount in a given week isn't a big danger, but cutting back during the following week(s) to keep the overall average at twelve ounces is advisable.

Older children and women who are not pregnant need not adhere to a specific limit, although eating a variety of fish (and sampling shark, swordfish, king mackerel, or tilefish less frequently) will help minimize the risk of methylmercury exposure.

For updated advisories regarding mercury in fish, check the FDA Web site (http://www.fda.gov): In the "A to Z Index," go to "M," and then click on "Mercury in Fish." ■

Our body can make EPA and DHA from linolenic acid in our diet—but there's a catch. First, many of us don't consume significant quantities of flaxseed, canola, walnuts, and soybeans on a daily basis—they're not exactly staples at the drive-through. But in addition, our ability to generate EPA and DHA from linolenic acid depends on the relative quantities of omega-3 and omega-6 fatty acids that are available as raw materials. Basically, the more omega-6 fatty acids in the diet, the less efficient is our production of the beneficial EPA and DHA from omega-3 fatty acids. In fact, some have raised concerns about the ratio of omega-6 to omega-3 fatty acids in the modern Western diet, proposing that an ideal diet would contain no more than four times as much omega-6 as omega-3.

A widely recommended response to the research supporting the benefits of omega-3 fatty acids is to add some to our diet in the form of fatty, cold-water fish—salmon, mackerel, lake trout, albacore tuna, herring, and sardines. These contain the beneficial fatty acids EPA and DHA already formed and in more generous amounts than in their leaner counterparts, such as cod, orange roughy, sole, and flounder. While an ideal daily amount of omega-3 fatty acids has not been established, the American Heart Association recommends that the average adult have at least two servings of these fish every week, with some cautions for pregnant women. (See sidebar "What about the Mercury in All of That Fish I'm Supposed to Eat?" on page 153.)

People who are at high risk for coronary artery disease, or who already have

FLAXSEED: NOT JUST FOR VEGETARIANS

As we mentioned earlier in this section, an excellent source of omega-3 fatty acids and an alternative to fish sources is flaxseed. Those who want to insure an adequate intake of omega-3 fatty acids and are vegetarian—or those who simply don't care that much for fish—should become acquainted with this small, nutty-flavored seed widely used in Europe for baking. Flaxseed contains not only the beneficial linolenic acid, but also soluble and insoluble fiber and **lignans**. Lignans—not to be confused with lignin, a form of fiber we mentioned earlier in this chapter—are phytoestrogens (literally "plant estrogens") that mimic to a modest degree the effects of estrogens and may help prevent cancers of the breast and endometrium (the lining of the uterus).[9] Because the seeds have a tough, outer covering, crushing or grinding them can enhance their nutritional benefits. In this form they can be sprinkled on salads, soups, casseroles, or even cereals. Whole or ground flaxseed can also replace some of the flour used in baking anything from bread to cookies. Since its oil is heat sensitive, it's best to add it to hot foods after they've been prepared (except, of course, when baking) and to store unused seeds or oil in the refrigerator. ■

it, should try to consume enough omega-3 fatty acids to include about a gram per day of EPA and DHA. This can usually be obtained from a three- to four-ounce serving of any of the cold-water fish just mentioned, but not everyone may be ready to eat fish every day. However, EPA and DHA can also be obtained in supplements that are usually derived from fish oils. Higher doses—2 to 3 grams per day—may be appropriate for people with elevated triglycerides, but doses beyond 3 grams may lead to bleeding in some individuals and should be used only under medical supervision.

Proteins: Building Materials

If we think of carbohydrates primarily as a source of fuel for our body and fats as our long-term energy storage, proteins take the prize for the mind-boggling number of structures and functions in which they play a pivotal role. Altogether our body contains somewhere between ten thousand and fifty thousand different proteins. Of these, the functions of only about one thousand have been identified.

- **Proteins** are critical ingredients of nearly every **structure** in the body: skin, bones, muscles, ligaments, internal organs on the "macro" scale, and all of the varieties of cells and their internal components on the "micro" scale.
- **Enzymes** are incredible molecules that serve as **catalysts** for chemical reactions within the body. The overwhelming majority of these enzymes are proteins. A vast number of vital reactions would take place far too slowly at body temperature, and enzymes allow the various components of a reaction to interact at phenomenal speed. A single enzyme can facilitate several hundred reactions every second. These may involve the breaking down of nutrients into simpler compounds (the function of digestive enzymes secreted into the intestinal tract by the pancreas), assembling complex structures (including other proteins) out of simpler components, releasing energy, and hundreds of other functions. Life would not be possible without them.
- All of the **antibodies** that help defend us from invading organisms are protein molecules, and lack of resistance to infection is thus one of many problems facing those who are malnourished.
- Many **hormones**, chemical messengers that are created in one part of the body and have actions elsewhere, are proteins.
- Proteins serve as **carriers** for a host of other substances, transporting them through the bloodstream. In chapter 3, for example, we described how the carrier proteins called high-density lipoprotein (HDL) and low-density lipoprotein (LDL) play very important roles in transporting cholesterol throughout the body and in increasing or decreasing the risk for coronary artery disease and heart attack.

DO I NEED AN ENZYME SUPPLEMENT?

Many Web sites and nutritional advisers (of questionable credentials) claim that we need to take various enzyme supplements to aid digestion, give our "stressed" and "strained" pancreas a break, and provide any number of health services that our body apparently cannot do for itself. A variation on this theme is that enzymes found in plants are necessary for us to digest them; since cooking changes or alters these enzymes, we should eat only raw (also called "living") fruits and vegetables.

In fact, creating the enzymes we (or any other living thing) need is a specialized biochemical process, orchestrated by amazingly complex genetic blueprints for very specific purposes. Enzymes in our food are unceremoniously dismantled like any other protein, so that the amino acids they contain can be reassembled into other proteins that we need. They are not absorbed intact into the bloodstream. (This is why diabetics who require insulin must inject it. If taken by mouth, insulin would not be absorbed "as is" into the bloodstream to control glucose. Instead it would be disassembled into its component amino acids, which would then be absorbed to make other proteins.) Even our own digestive enzymes are themselves digested, and their amino acids recycled. Furthermore, the enzymes present in a fruit or vegetable are (or were) certainly important for the plant's well-being but weren't generated for our benefit, and they play no role in our ability to extract whatever we can use from it. (Remember also that there are structural elements of fruits and vegetables that we are not designed to digest. These provide fiber, which has numerous benefits that we have reviewed earlier in this chapter.)

With a few uncommon exceptions, the pancreas is quite capable of producing enough enzymes to digest our food without assistance from an expensive supplement. However, people who truly cannot produce or release enough enzymes because of significant damage to the pancreas or a condition such as cystic fibrosis (which can clog the ducts in the pancreas with sticky mucus, preventing enzymes from reaching the intestine) may in fact need supplemental enzymes. These are obtained from animal sources and typically utilize tiny pellets with an **enteric coating** that keep them intact in the stomach, allowing release in the small intestine.

One other potentially useful enzyme is **lactase**, which can be taken in various forms by people with lactose intolerance, a condition we discussed earlier in this chapter. (See page 132.) ■

- Proteins circulating in the blood play a vital role in maintaining the proper **balance of fluids** within blood vessels, in tissues, and within cells. They also are important in the regulation of the levels of **acids and bases** within body fluids. The acid-base balance must be maintained within very narrow limits for the body to function and survive.
- Finally, while we normally think of carbohydrates and fats as our primary energy sources, the building blocks of protein called amino acids (see below), also serve as an **energy source** if calories from carbohydrate and fat are in short supply. However, although we can store carbohydrate as glycogen and we have a virtually unlimited potential to store fat, we cannot store protein. If food is scarce and amino acids are needed as an energy source, protein from muscle and other body structures will be broken down to obtain them.

Proteins consist of compounds called **amino acids** assembled into long chains that can assume an enormous variety of shapes and sizes. Altogether twenty specific amino acids form the protein "alphabet," and typically one hundred to three hundred will be linked together to create a protein.

F.Y.I.

The term *amino* refers to the combination of one nitrogen and two hydrogen molecules (represented in chemical shorthand as NH_2), which is derived from ammonia. The presence of nitrogen in protein not only means that we must get enough of it from our food but also that we must deal with nitrogen waste products. The latter can become a particular problem for people with kidney or liver failure.

The chemical characteristics of the amino acids assembled in a particular sequence will cause the chain to fold, coil, or elongate into a shape uniquely suited for its function or structural role. The number of possible combinations is limitless, and the fact that thousands of different proteins can function day and night with such precision represents a mind-boggling marvel of engineering. Even more astonishing is the mechanism by which proteins are manufactured from DNA blueprints in the chromosomes that reside in the nucleus of every cell. Outlining that fascinating process is beyond the scope of this book, but among the many wonders of life on this earth it stands as one of the most eloquent testaments to the existence of a Designer.

Of the twenty amino acids, our body can make eleven. The other nine are called **essential amino acids**, because they must be supplied in our food. The ones we can make are called **nonessential**, which is no reflection on their importance. In order to make the proteins a cell needs, all twenty amino acids must be present and accounted for within that cell. This means that there must be enough nitrogen and energy available to manufacture the nonessential amino acids and enough of all nine essential amino acids as well. A protein source that fits this description is called a **complete protein**. Protein from animal sources—meat, fish, poultry, eggs, and milk—is usually complete, while protein from plant sources often is not. This does not mean that animal protein

In some situations, a person is unable to make enough of a particular nonessential amino acid, which is then called a conditionally essential amino acid.

is superior—indeed, it may have a fair amount of saturated fat or other undesirable compounds along for the ride.

Vegetarians can obtain all of the amino acids they need by eating foods in combination that provide **complementary proteins**, supplying adequate amounts of all of the essential amino acids. Legumes (beans and peas), for example, tend to be short on two amino acids (methionine and tryptophan) that are abundant in grains. Grains may fall short on two other amino acids (lysine and isoleucine) that legumes readily supply. But combinations of foods from these families, such as rice and beans or peanut butter and whole-grain bread, will supply adequate amounts of the essential amino acids. (These complementary sources do not have to be eaten at the same time, by the way, but can be spread throughout the day.)

How Shall We Eat? Some Summary Recommendations

Now that we have looked at the three basic categories of macronutrients, we need to step back, take a deep breath, and remind ourselves that we eat *food,* not isolated biochemical compounds. Furthermore, the length and breadth of cuisines, preparation techniques, cultural variations, cost factors, and individual tastes are so enormous that no single book, let alone one chapter, can possibly address all of the choices we have to make in setting our daily table. And, as we will see, not everyone is in complete agreement as to what constitutes the optimal diet for human health.

Nevertheless, we must start somewhere, and so as a point of reference we will begin with some basic recommendations known as **dietary reference intakes (DRIs)** from the **Institute of Medicine (IOM)**, one of the **National Academies**. These may not exactly make for fascinating bedtime reading, but bear with us, because we will then look at some of their practical implications and some variations on these recommendations.

How much fuel? The total number of calories you need every day depends on several factors: your age, gender, height, weight, activity level, and to some degree genetics (which affects the efficiency of your individual metabolic engine). You can see the genetic factor at work when someone consistently eats large amounts of food without gaining weight, while another person with a similar age, build, and activity level has to eat far less to prevent weight gain. Speaking of weight, calorie requirements must also be adjusted when a person is attempting to lose excess weight, as we will see in the next chapter.

The Institute of Medicine has estimated calorie needs for men and women at various ages, related to height, weight, and four levels of physical activity. These are not targets for people who are trying to lose excessive weight, by the way, but rather for maintenance of a stable weight. Some approximate daily calorie goals:

- For children between two and six, some older adults, and many women: 1,600 calories.
- For the "average adult": 2,000 calories. On nutrition labels you will typically see 2,000 listed as the total number of daily calories.
- For older children, teenage girls, and active women: 2,200 calories.
- For teenage boys and active men: 2,800 calories.

How much carbohydrate? The IOM recommends that 45 to 65 percent of total daily calories come from carbohydrates, or at least 130 grams for an adult, with no more than 25 percent of total daily calories from added sugars. Within those percentages there is a lot of room for good and not-so-good choices. As we have already pointed out, it is naive to think of one category of a nutrient as "good" or "bad." (For one thing, foods consist of combinations of nutrients, as should meals.) Instead, we need to pay attention to the type and quality of the sources of these nutrients.

How much dietary fiber? To recap, the IOM recommends these amounts:

- For adults fifty and younger: 38 grams for men and 25 grams for women
- For adults fifty-one and older: 30 grams for men and 21 grams for women

The current recommendation for children two and older is that they should eat an amount in grams equal to their age plus five.

How much fat? The IOM recommends that 20 to 35 percent of total daily calories come from fat. For children, the percentage of total fat may be a little higher because of the need for fat in the developing central nervous system. Among children four to eighteen years of age, 25 to 35 percent of daily calories may come from fat; for one- to three-year-olds, 30 to 40 percent. Remember the essential fatty acids, linoleic and linolenic acid, discussed on page 152? The IOM has recommended that adult men obtain 17 grams and women 12 grams daily of linoleic acid, and 1.6 grams (men) and 1.1 grams (women) of linolenic acid daily. These are considered adequate intake (AI) levels, because recommended daily allowances (RDAs) have yet to be determined. The IOM has not established specific guidelines regarding any other types of fats, but rather recommends simply that saturated fats, trans fats, and cholesterol be kept to a minimum.

How much protein? The IOM states its recommendation for daily protein intake as a range of 10 to 35 percent of total calories for adults, 10 to 30 percent for children ages four to eighteen, and 5 to 20 percent for children one to three years of age. An estimate based on a person's body weight is 0.8 grams of protein per kilogram (2.2 pounds) for adults, or 8 grams per 22 pounds of weight. For example, a woman weighing 150 pounds would need 56 grams of protein, which could be obtained by drinking two

8-ounce glasses of milk, having a slice of ham and cheese in a sandwich, and eating a three-ounce portion of meat for dinner. Unlike many impoverished areas of the world, most Americans get plenty of protein. An average-sized hamburger contains about 25 grams of protein, as does a cup of cottage cheese or a three-ounce portion of most types of meat (chicken, turkey, beef, lamb, or fish). An eight- or twelve-ounce steak can supply an entire day's protein for a large adult.

How do all of these recommendations relate to actual foods?

If you managed to read through the last several paragraphs without becoming glassy-eyed, congratulations. By now (if not earlier) you may have asked a very important question: How do I translate all of these recommendations

WHERE DO THE DIETARY REFERENCE INTAKES COME FROM?

The most widely quoted source of advice on what we should or shouldn't eat is the Institute of Medicine, a component of the National Academies. The National Academies is a private, nonprofit organization chartered by Congress in 1863 (originally as the National Academy of Sciences) with a mandate to advise the federal government on scientific matters and to promote the use of science and technology for the public welfare. Unlike the National Institutes of Health (NIH) and its various components, it is not an agency of the government. There are more than 4,000 members of the combined National Academies, as well as at least 500 foreign associates, among whom are more than 180 Nobel Prize winners. Election to membership is considered a high honor.

The Institute of Medicine (IOM), chartered in 1970, is one of four components of the National Academies. (The others are the National Academy of Engineering, the National Research Council, and the National Academy of Sciences, which is no longer the umbrella organization but is now a member organization of the National Academies.) The IOM is a private, nonprofit, nongovernmental organization whose mission is to provide information and advice to citizens, professionals, corporations, and government regarding health and science policy. All of its work is done in committees composed of experts who volunteer their time. Their reports and recommendations are **evidence based**—that is, built upon the best available research or on expert opinion when the published research is not conclusive—and **peer reviewed**, meaning they are formally reviewed by other experts who are independent of the committee. The IOM is organized into nine **oversight boards**, one of which is the **Food and Nutrition Board**, which was originally created in 1940 as a component of the National Academy of Sciences.

For more than half a century, nutritional guidelines in the United States were based on standards from the Food and Nutrition Board called the **recommended daily allowances** (or **RDAs**), which were focused on a somewhat

into actual decisions about the kinds of foods that I buy, prepare, order at a restaurant, and ultimately eat? How many of us actually calculate, or even have a rough idea, what percentage of our daily calories come from carbohydrates, fats, and proteins? And do these percentages tell the whole story of our nutritional health?

We could, of course, shrug our shoulders and proceed with business as usual: eat what and however much we like, guided by family traditions, taste buds, emotions, advertising, and convenience. In the United States, however, that approach has led to an epidemic of obesity and contributed to an increase in cardiovascular disease and diabetes. (Some cancers and a number of other chronic diseases may also be the by-product of this approach.) If we want to take some positive, proactive steps toward improving our personal and family

narrow but important goal: preventing nutritional deficiencies caused by inadequate amounts of specific essential nutrients. (The Canadian version of the RDA was the **recommended nutrient intakes**, or **RNIs**.) More recently, however, new research and a broader vision of the role of nutrition in health have led to major revisions of these standards, which are now called the dietary reference intakes (or DRIs). These guidelines are intended not only for the prevention of specific nutritional deficiencies, but also for reducing the frequency and impact of important chronic health problems such as cardiovascular disease, cancer, and osteoporosis. Furthermore, they have been geared to apply to individuals, whereas the older RDAs were focused on population groups. The DRIs for a variety of nutrient groups have been released in a series of reports beginning in 1997.

Recommended daily allowances (RDAs) were originally formulated for eight nutrients in 1941 at the request of the War Department (now the Department of Defense), which was concerned about the nutritional status of new recruits, soldiers in the field, and malnourished people who would be liberated by Allied troops. By 1989, the list of RDAs had expanded to twenty-seven nutrients.

The DRIs actually encompass four different guidelines:

- The familiar-sounding but revised **recommended daily allowance (RDA)**, which specifically refers to the amount of a nutrient necessary to meet the nutritional needs of 97 to 98 percent of healthy people of a certain age and gender (including pregnant and nursing mothers). You will see RDAs listed on the nutrition labels of packaged foods.
- The **adequate intake (AI)**, which is basically an educated guess of the necessary amount of a specific nutrient based on observations and scientific findings when the available evidence is not conclusive enough to arrive at an RDA.
- The **estimated average requirement (EAR)**, which is defined as the amount of a nutrient that will be adequate for half of the healthy members of a specific population. These EARs are used primarily as guidelines for groups and populations, rather than individuals. (You won't find EARs on nutrition labels.)
- The **tolerable upper intake level (UL)** applies to certain nutrients for which there can be "too much of a good thing." The UL is the highest daily intake of a nutrient that is not likely to have an adverse effect on the vast majority of individuals. ■

Why determine the levels of nutrients that would be adequate for *half* of the population? One way EARs are used is to determine the presence of certain nutritional problems in groups of people who might be at risk (for example, vitamin B_{12} deficiency among elderly patients in nursing homes).

fuel, how might we proceed? There are three basic approaches. All three have merit, and you may find it worthwhile to pick and choose certain elements from each approach that work for you and your family.

To get the most out of the next several paragraphs, you should look at the example below or grab a package of one of your favorite foods and look at its label.

1. **Get a notebook and calculator, and study those food labels.** In the United States, the Food and Drug Administration (FDA) requires that packaged foods bear a **Nutrition Facts label** that includes pertinent information about what's inside. Even if you don't keep a running tally of your daily nutrient intake, you should pay attention to at least some of the information on the label.

   Highlights include:

   - **Serving size.** This number is important, since all of the facts on the label are based on a serving size that the label assumes you will eat. The serving size may be obvious (such as the entire can of soda) or less so. For example, the serving size for dry cereal is typically listed as one cup, which may be a bit less than you pour into the bowl every morning. The label on a container of crackers or chips will list a certain number of these as a serving—but do we ever keep count when we're enjoying one of these snacks? Serving sizes for salad dressings are usually two tablespoons, but you may be surprised how that compares to your typical dollop on that bowl of greens. Measuring the amount of the serving size—and the amount you actually use—for a number of your favorite foods can be an eye-opening experience.
   - **Calories per serving.** All of the numbers on the label must be adjusted if you use more or less than the stated serving size.
   - **Calories from fat.** Divide this number by the calories per serving and multiply by 100. You'll get the percentage of calories derived from fat, which may or may not be useful, depending on the type of food. The fact that this number is included on the label is a reflection of the "fat is bad" doctrine that we have heard for decades. But the percentage of a food's calories derived from fat does not necessarily reflect its quality. Extra virgin olive oil is 100 percent fat, but it contains monounsaturated fatty acids that are beneficial to health.
   - **Total fat, cholesterol, and quantities of saturated, monounsaturated, and polyunsaturated fats, which are more useful numbers.** (Remember that trans fats are going to show up on labels as well.) These are listed in grams, and—for total fat, saturated fat, and cholesterol—as a **percent daily value**. The percent daily value (or **%DV**) is *not* the percent of calories in the serving, or the percent of total calories for the day, for fat or saturated fat in the serving. Instead, it is the percent of the maximum

Nutrition Facts

Serving Size 1 Cup (228g)
Serving Per Container 2

Amount Per Serving	
Calories 100	Calories from Fat 10
	% **Daily Value***
Total Fat 3g*	**5%**
Saturated Fat 1g	**5%**
Trans Fat 1.5g	
Cholesterol 0mg	**0%**
Sodium 188mg	**5%**
Total Carbohydrate 45g	**15%**
Dietary Fiber 4g	**16%**
Soluble Fiber 1g	
Sugars 20g	
Other Carbohydrates 21g	
Protein 5g	
Vitamin A	20%
Vitamin C	8%
Calcium	4%
Iron	15%
Vitamin D	20%
Vitamin E	25%
Thiamin	25%
Riboflavin	25%
Niacin	25%
Vitamin B6	100%
Folate	100%

WHAT DO THOSE PHRASES ON THE FOOD LABEL MEAN?

When the label on a food package says "low fat" or "good source of dietary fiber" or even "light," is that just an advertising gimmick to get your attention or does it actually mean something? As it turns out, the Food and Drug Administration (FDA) has spelled out specific guidelines for the various terms that you see when you browse the shelves at the supermarket. Here are some that may sound familiar:

No calories: Fewer than 5 calories per serving.

Low calorie, light or lite in calories: Fewer than 40 calories per serving. For a meal or main dish, fewer than 120 calories per 100 grams (about three and a half ounces).

Fat-free or nonfat: Less than 0.5 gram of fat per serving.

Low fat, light or lite in fat: Fewer than 3 grams of fat per serving. For a meal or main dish, fewer than 3 grams of fat per 100 grams, or less than 30 percent fat.

Saturated fat–free: Less than 0.5 gram of saturated fat per serving.

Low in saturated fat: Less than one gram of saturated fat and less than 15 percent of total calories from saturated fat per serving. For a meal or main dish, less than one gram of saturated fat per 100 grams or less than 10 percent saturated fat.

Cholesterol-free: Fewer than 2 milligrams of cholesterol and 2 grams or less of saturated fat per serving.

Low in cholesterol: Fewer than 20 milligrams of cholesterol per serving and 2 grams or less of saturated fat per serving.

Sugar-free: Less than 0.5 gram of sugar per serving.

No added sugar: No sugar or sugar-containing ingredient added during processing. (Not necessarily sugar-free, however, if the product naturally contains sugars.)

Reduced (less) calorie, fat, saturated fat, cholesterol, or sugar: At least 25 percent less of the particular substance than the same portion of a comparable product.

High fiber: Provides 5 grams or more of fiber per serving.

Good source of . . . : Provides 10 to 19 percent of the daily value of the specific nutrient per serving.

High in . . . : Provides 20 percent or more of the daily value of the specific nutrient per serving.

Lean (for meat and poultry products): Contains fewer than 10 grams of fat, 4.5 grams of saturated fat, and 95 milligrams of cholesterol per serving.

Extra lean: Contains fewer than 5 grams of fat, 2 grams of saturated fat, and 95 milligrams of cholesterol per serving. ■

recommended amount of these substances for a person eating two thousand calories per day. This number is intended to help you get a handle on how much of a contribution the particular food is making to what should be your daily maximum. At the bottom of the Nutrition Facts label is a listing of these recommendations, under a statement that begins "Percent Daily Values are based on a 2,000-calorie diet." Most labels include not only the recommendations for 2,000 calories but for 2,500 as well. If your calorie target is much more or less than 2,000, the %DV for the particular food will be less or more than the amount on the label. The %DV listings are based on the assumption that we should keep our fat calories below a maximum of 25 percent and our saturated fats below 10 percent of the total number of calories we consume every day. For cholesterol, the assumption is that we should eat foods containing a total of 300 mg or less per day. Note that you will not find any %DV listings for mono- or polyunsaturated fats. This means that the FDA hasn't provided recommended daily intakes for these nutrients.

F.Y.I.

Other organizations have suggested different percentages for the amounts of fat in our daily diet. The Institute of Medicine, as we noted earlier, suggests that fat calories can range from 20 to 35 percent of the total. Furthermore, other groups have recommended various daily percentages of calories from monounsaturated and polyunsaturated fats. A reasonable breakdown, assuming 35 percent of calories come from fat, is 10 percent of calories from saturated fat, 10 percent from polyunsaturated fat, and 15 percent from monounsaturated fat.

- **Total carbohydrate, dietary fiber, and sugars.** Of these, the most useful are the grams of fiber and sugars, since you want to get enough of the first and limit your intake of the second.
- **Protein.** The Nutrition Facts label includes grams of protein per serving, but without an estimate of the percent daily value, because the recommended amount for an individual is based on his or her weight.
- **Other nutrients.** The amounts of vitamins and minerals contained in a serving of the food are listed under the main nutrients. We will be looking at them in appendix B, which begins on page 869.

Few people are going to work through the laborious process of calculating the daily percentages of their various nutrients, a task that can be even more challenging if you are actually *cooking*—combining various ingredients to create a masterpiece in the kitchen—as opposed to eating prepackaged food. Nevertheless, you should know your way around the Nutrition Facts label, because several of its statistics can help you make informed choices.

2. **Follow the USDA Food Guide Pyramid—or perhaps another one.** For nearly a century the United States Department of Agriculture (USDA) has published a series of guides that combine foods into various groups and then recommend that we eat a certain number of servings from each group each day. For example, the first set of guidelines released in 1916 listed five food groups: milk and meat, cereals, fruits and vegetables, fats and fat foods, and sugars and sugary foods. Over the years the number of groups has expanded and contracted dramatically: Twelve food groups were identified in 1933, a Basic Seven in 1942, a Basic Four in 1956, and then back to five in 1979.

In 1980 the USDA and the U.S. Department of Health and Human Services (HHS) jointly published the first installment of the *Dietary Guidelines for Americans,* which have been updated every five years. The *Guidelines* represent what is called "federal nutrition policy," affecting nutrition-assistance programs and education messages for the general public. In 1992 the USDA and HHS introduced the Food Guide Pyramid as a learning tool to help us both visualize the recommended number of daily servings for five food groups and make better food choices. The underpinnings for the pyramid included the recommended daily allowances published by the National Academy of Sciences (which we discussed earlier in this chapter), the *Dietary Guidelines for Americans,* and USDA food consumption surveys that documented how Americans were actually eating. The dietary pattern represented by the pyramid was intended to meet the nutritional needs of healthy people over two years of age while limiting fat, cholesterol, sugar, and sodium.

For more than a decade the pyramid illustrated how we should eat more servings of some food groups and fewer of others. The base was occupied by the bread, cereal, rice, and pasta group because the USDA recommended six to eleven servings of foods from it every day. Vegetables, with three to five servings per day, shared the next level with fruits (two to four servings). The next level was shared by the milk and the meat groups, each with two to three daily servings. At the apex of the pyramid sat fats, oils, and sweets—not really food groups, but rather the foods we were advised to "use sparingly."

With the publication of the 2005 edition of the *Dietary Guidelines for Americans,* the Food Guide Pyramid got a major overhaul. The "layers" on the front of the new pyramid, representing five basic food groups—grains, vegetables, fruits, milk, and meat and beans—have been flipped to a vertical orientation, and they only vaguely suggest that some groups might be emphasized over others. Indeed, the pyramid offers virtually no nutritional information, but rather serves mainly as a symbol for the revised contents of the Dietary Guidelines and the new interactive Web site, http://www.mypyramid.gov, that supports it. Significantly, the left side of the

"Meat and beans" includes meats, poultry, fish, eggs, nuts, and seeds, as well as dry beans and peas.

pyramid is drawn as a stairway that a stick-figure human appears to be climbing rapidly—a visual message about the importance of exercise.

Those who enter the Web site may explore several informative options.

- "My Pyramid Plan" invites you to enter your age, gender, and an estimate of daily physical activity. The site then provides a semi-individualized outline of the recommended daily intake of foods from the five basic categories, along with oils and an allowance for extra fats and sugar.
- "Inside the Pyramid" not only lists the foods in each of the five basic food groups but also offers photo illustrations. For each group, you can learn about recommended quantities, health benefits, and specific tips to maximize enjoyment and nutritional value.
- "My Pyramid Tracker" is a more ambitious option for those who want a more detailed assessment of their eating and exercise habits. Users can enter detailed information about their daily food choices and receive feedback about the quality of their diet. They can also track their intake of specific food groups or nutrients over the course of a year. In addition, physical activity can be assessed and tracked for up to a year.

Unlike the original Food Guide Pyramid, the new version promotes exercise, emphasizes the benefits of whole grains, and makes an appropriate distinction between the healthier monounsaturated and polyunsaturated fats and the less healthy saturated and trans fats. Overall, the interactive Web site is a definite improvement over the old pyramid, provided one has access to a computer and the Internet. Those without these electronic tools can obtain a copy of the *2005 Dietary Guidelines for Americans* by calling the U.S. Government Printing Office toll-free at (866) 512-1800.

You should be aware that some other nutritional pyramids have generated interest among both health professionals and the public. Of these the most widely known is the **Mediterranean pyramid** (see sidebar "A Closer Look at the Mediterranean Diet" on page 170), but there are also **Asian**, **Latin American**, and **vegetarian pyramids**. These have been disseminated largely by the Oldways Preservation and Exchange Trust, a nonprofit "food issues think tank" that has gained respect in many professional circles for its efforts to integrate cutting-edge research with the culinary traditions of many cultures. You can learn about these alternative pyramids at http://www.oldwayspt.org.

3. **Orient (or reorient) your eating habits around some basic principles.** With some basic information about macronutrients, we can now look at several practical conclusions that are supported by a rising tide of research—

THE ORIGINAL FOOD GUIDE PYRAMID (1992–2004)

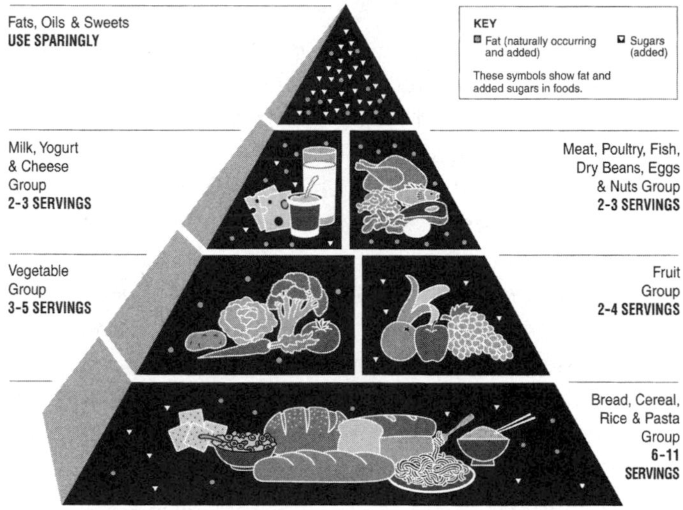

THE NEW FOOD GUIDE PYRAMID (AS OF 2005)

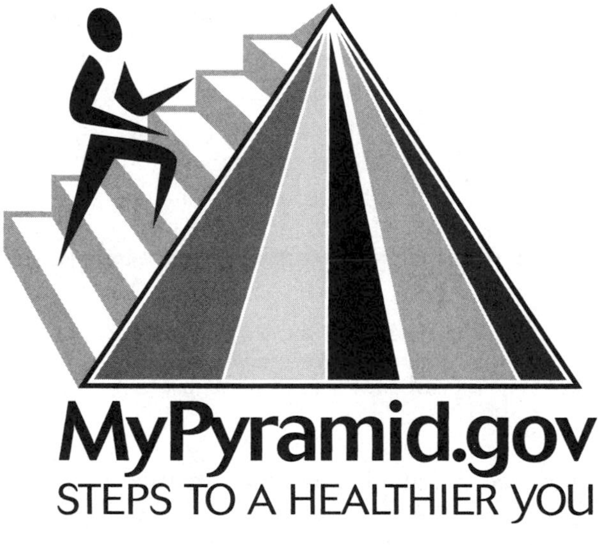

The 2005 Food Pyramid is designed to be an interactive tool that provides nutrition guidelines based on a person's age, gender, and level of physical activity. (To generate your own guidelines, visit **http://www.mypyramid.gov**.) The vertical shaded portions (from left to right) in the pyramid represent grains, vegetables, fruits, milk, and meat and beans.

Source: The U.S. Department of Agriculture and the U.S. Department of Health and Human Services.

HOT TIP

A simple trick to reduce portion sizes at home is to serve your meals on smaller plates. Not only is there less room for oversized servings, but this also creates a minor optical illusion suggesting to the brain that "less is more."

and some common sense. For most people, it is more helpful to think along these lines than to spend hours calculating percentages of calories from different nutrients. As with our tour of nutrients, we will start with a couple of those "this is a football" statements.

Don't eat too much. Talk about stating the obvious. We will be looking at the problem of obesity and the challenge of losing excess weight in the next chapter. But it bears noting that the freshest, most perfectly balanced, most exquisitely prepared food can still get you into trouble *if you eat too much of it.* If you are overweight, it is extremely unlikely that you will lose unwanted pounds without at some point addressing the portions of food that you are accustomed to eating. The most dramatic illustration of the wisdom of not eating too much is the so-called French paradox. The French enjoy a traditional cuisine that is known for its rich, calorie-dense sauces, cheeses, pastries, and other delights. Yet only 7 percent of the French are obese, compared to 30 percent of Americans. One reason appears to be *portion size*. A group of researchers actually weighed servings of foods at similar types of restaurants in Paris and Philadelphia, including fast-food outlets and ice-cream parlors. They found that the average portion size in Paris was 25 percent smaller than its counterpart in the United States. Even foods sold in American markets came in larger quantities than did those in France. And recipes in the classic book the *Joy of Cooking* yielded larger portions than those for similar dishes in a popular French cookbook *Je Sais Cuisiner (I Can Cook)*. The researchers also found that the French patrons at a Parisian McDonald's spent an average of twenty-two minutes enjoying their *hamburger, frites,* and *boisson,* compared to fourteen minutes for Americans consuming their burger, fries, and soft drink.

"Never eat more than you can lift."
—MISS PIGGY

HOT TIP

When dining out, you can conserve both cash and calories by splitting your meal with your companion (assuming that you can agree on the same one). If you're eating alone, plan on taking half of that huge entrée home. You won't offend your server, and you can enjoy it in a day or two.

One additional observation: At a truly upscale restaurant, French or otherwise, the portions are usually quite small. With fine dining, it is assumed that you will take your time, savor every morsel (especially when it's costing you a bundle), and walk out feeling pleasantly satisfied rather than stuffed. At less expensive restaurants that we're likely to visit more frequently, the portions are often colossal, and nearly every fast-food franchise has an option to buy "supersize" portions for a very modest bump in price. Avoid the temptation to get more for your money, because what you'll *really* get is more calories, saturated and trans fat, and sugar. Another way of looking at this principle: *Take your time and savor your food.* Put your fork down between bites and enjoy the taste and texture of what you're eating. By doing so you can have a longer, more enjoyable experience while consuming fewer calories.

Exercise on a regular basis—daily if possible. Yes, this is a chapter on nutrition, but moving your muscles on a regular basis is extremely important to your overall health and will help prevent accumulation of any extra calories as fat. We'll look at this critical topic in chapter 7.

Go easy on the added sugars. Contrary to the opinions found in a number of popular books over the past few decades, sugars aren't the cause of all disease, the root of all evil, or an imminent threat to world peace. But they are definitely a poor quality of fuel for our body, and the dramatic increase in their consumption in the United States and other developed countries has been a major step in the wrong direction. To put it bluntly, most of us could stand to cut back, and some of us need a major overhaul of our taste buds.

The upper limit for added sugars suggested by the Institute of Medicine—25 percent of total calories—is rather generous. The 2005 Food Pyramid does not include a specific recommendation for added sugar. Rather, it allows for a small number of "discretionary calories" that can be consumed after the recommended amount of nutrients has been met. These discretionary calories can come from either solid fats or added sugar. Remember that *these recommended amounts don't apply to the sugars that occur naturally in foods such as fruit and milk.* You can tally the number of grams of sugar in any packaged product at the store by checking the Nutrition Facts label. Unfortunately, this does *not* distinguish between naturally occurring and added sugars. Often the nature of the product leaves little doubt: In a soft drink, you can be certain that *all* 40 or so grams of the sugar were added, while in an orange all of the 12 or more grams of sugar were there to start with. On the other hand, a cup of raw blueberries contains 14 grams of natural sugar, while a cup of frozen sweetened blueberries contains 45 grams of sugar. The Nutrition Facts label wouldn't tell you that 31 grams were added.

Gravitate toward whole-grain foods, rather than those made from refined or processed grains. We have already described the potential for certain starches, and in particular foods derived from processed and refined grain products, to affect blood sugar in unfavorable ways. This isn't the only reason why whole grains are better for you than those that have been refined—an ironic term for this process:

- Fiber, vitamins, and minerals are lost during refining and processing (though some are replaced). Whole-grain products contain a variety of useful compounds, including antioxidants, phytochemicals (see page 177), folic acid, B vitamins, iron, and vitamin E.
- A number of studies have shown a link between eating whole grains and a lower risk of developing cardiovascular disease, diabetes, and cancer.[10]
- We have already described the many benefits of dietary fiber, and whole-grain foods generally have a more generous supply.

How do you get more whole-grain foods into your daily food routine?

- Buy whole-grain bread or other baked products, including crackers. Check the ingredient list for **whole wheat**, **whole oats**, **whole rye**, **whole barley**, **whole cornmeal**, etc., or a combina-

A CLOSER LOOK AT THE MEDITERRANEAN DIET

The Mediterranean diet has received considerable attention from the scientific community over the past several years, and for good reason. Between 1958 and 1970, nutrition researcher Ancel Keys surveyed the eating patterns of people living in eighteen areas of seven countries. Keys, who founded the Laboratory of Physiological Hygiene at the University of Minnesota in 1948, pioneered the investigation of the relationship between diet and chronic ailments such as heart disease and cancer.

Ancel Keys also developed the field rations used by American soldiers during World War II, which were dubbed K rations in his honor.

His landmark **Seven Countries Study** found, among other things, that people living on the island of Crete and in other areas of Greece and southern Italy had notably lower rates of heart disease and some cancers.[11] Keys became convinced that the traditional dietary patterns among these populations contributed to their longevity and relative freedom from the coronary artery disease that was becoming rampant in Western nations. In addition to developing a series of scientific articles related to the Seven Countries Study, he and his wife, Margaret, also published *How to Eat Well, Stay Well the Mediterranean Way* (now out of print) in 1975 to promote this diet to a larger audience. Its key characteristics include:

- An abundance of plant-based foods: fruits, vegetables, legumes and nuts, whole-grain cereals, and breads
- Olive oil as the primary source of fat
- Low intake of saturated fat
- Low to moderate amounts of dairy products, primarily in the form of cheese and yogurt
- Fish, poultry, and eggs a few times per week
- Red meat only a few times per month
- A moderate amount of wine with (at least some) meals

tion of these in a multigrain product. The term **cracked wheat** also is a good sign, referring to whole-wheat grains that have been cut or crushed, and **graham flour** refers to flour made from the entire wheat grain (also called the **wheat berry**). The term *wheat flour*, on the other hand, doesn't tell you whether it's whole wheat or a refined version. (Remember that the presence of whole-grain ingredients isn't the only item on your mental checklist. A whole-grain cracker, for example, may also contain trans fats that would be good to avoid.)

- Similarly, buy cereals made from whole grains. As with baked products, check the ingredient list and look for one or more of the whole grains as the first ingredient. Note that oatmeal is a whole grain, but "old-fashioned" or "steel-cut" oats are less processed than instant versions.

Some reviewers of Keys's work asked whether other factors besides diet might play a role in the favorable rates of heart disease. What about the effects of genetic (inherited) traits, exercise, or even portion sizes? As it turns out, some convincing research has suggested that Keys was on the right track. An important study from France, the **Lyon Diet Heart Study**, enrolled more than six hundred men and women who had survived their first heart attack and divided them into two groups. Half followed a low-fat diet widely recommended by the American Heart Association for people with coronary artery disease, while the other utilized a Mediterranean-type diet with characteristics similar to those listed above. (In place of olive oil, the researchers used a specially prepared margarine containing monounsaturated fats in amounts similar to those found in olive oil.) The study was interrupted less than halfway through its five-year course because the people following the Mediterranean diet were doing so much better than those in the other group, with 73 percent fewer coronary events and 70 percent fewer deaths from all causes.[12] A more recent study carefully evaluated the dietary habits of more than twenty-two thousand adults in Greece. It found that those who adhered more closely to a traditional Mediterranean diet were less likely to die not only from heart disease and cancer, but also from *all* causes.[13]

There are actually nearly twenty countries that border the Mediterranean Sea (not to mention the island nations of Cyprus and Malta), with widely varying dietary patterns. Furthermore, eating habits among many who live in Greece and other Mediterranean countries have changed since the 1960s (not necessarily for the better) with the introduction of Westernized foods high in saturated fat and refined carbohydrates. Nevertheless, a number of features of the traditional Mediterranean diet can be translated into some basic take-home principles. ■

- Eat brown rather than white rice.
- When baking, try substituting whole wheat flour for a quarter to a half of the flour needed in the recipe.
- Look for pasta made from whole wheat or from half-whole and half-refined wheat.

Eat lots of vegetables and fruits. You've heard this from your mother, your health education teacher, the American Dietetic Association, the government, and hopefully your doctor. Fruits and vegetables are supposed to be good for us (and they are), but

CONTROLLING THE SUGAR FLOW

If your family includes one or more members who are big fans of sweets, declaring a sudden moratorium in the name of good health may lead to a minor revolt. All of the following approaches are helpful, but they may be more successful if phased in over time.

1. On packaged foods, check the ingredient list for added sugar, whether named directly or under one of its many aliases—brown sugar, sucrose, fructose, dextrose, corn syrup, high-fructose corn syrup, molasses, or honey. Try to avoid foods in which some form of added sugar is the first or second ingredient on the list.
2. Some major sources of sugar (and calories) are those perennial favorites: cakes, pies, cookies, pastries, and candies. They won't kill anyone if eaten once in a while, but daily dosing should be avoided. Fruit is a better option for dessert.
3. Watch the sugar content of breakfast cereals, and choose brands that contain less than 8 grams per serving. (The Nutrition Facts label comes in handy here.)
4. You have a much easier time shaping the taste preferences of a baby who is just beginning to explore the world of foods beyond milk, compared with a ten-year-old who is already a confirmed lover of candy and soft drinks. Steer the growing toddler and preschooler toward fruit as a dessert, rather than cake and ice cream, and toward unsweetened cereal rather than Chocolate Frosted Sugar Wads.
5. A soft drink may be hard to resist at a ball game or the movies, but otherwise you should limit the number of soft drinks you—and especially your kids—consume every week. Of particular concern among children and teenagers is the replacement of other nutrients with the empty calories in soft drinks. Among teenagers, carbonated soft drinks supply 9 percent of daily calories among boys and 8 percent in girls' diets. One study of the eating habits of children found that those who drank the most soft drinks also ate the least amount of fruits and vegetables. For children, milk is a better option (unless they are lactose intolerant).

they're nearly always the side dish rather than the main event at a meal. (How many times have you picked up the menu at a typical restaurant and found a list of fruit and vegetable entrees?) Since 1991, the "5 a Day for Better Health" program, a joint project of several large federal agencies and private organizations, has been promoting the idea that we should eat five to nine servings of fruit and vegetables every day. But according to the Centers for Disease Control and Prevention's Behavior Risk Factor Surveillance System telephone survey (the world's largest telephone survey), as of 2000 fewer than one in four Americans

Appropriately enough, the word *fruit* comes from a Latin root meaning "enjoyment," while *vegetable* comes from a Latin word meaning "to enliven or invigorate."

6. While various fruit-flavored beverages may seem like a healthier alternative to soft drinks, most of these contain a small percentage of actual fruit juice (if any) and a lot of sugar. (Think soft drinks without the fizz.) If you're not sure, check the label for the amount of juice—and the amount of sugar.

7. Surprisingly, even pure fruit juice usually provides little more than the sugars found in the fruit, some vitamin C, and perhaps a little calcium if it's fortified. In babies and young children, fruit juice is not an appropriate substitute for breast milk, formula, or (after the first birthday) cow's milk. Those who come to favor juice over better sources of nutrition can develop diarrhea and gas, and may become malnourished. The following guidelines will allow children to enjoy fruit juice without becoming "juiceaholics" or damaging their teeth:
   - Infants younger than six months of age should not be given fruit juices at all. Indeed, you would be wise to avoid feeding juice to any infant or toddler from a bottle; wait until he can take it from a cup.
   - Limit juice intake to four to six ounces per day for children six and younger. Starting at age seven, you can set the limit at eight to twelve ounces per day. If he wants more than the daily limit, dilute juice with an equal amount of water.
   - Don't allow an infant or child to go to sleep sucking on a bottle containing juice, milk, or any other liquid that contains sugar. This not only promotes tooth decay but can also increase the risk for developing an ear infection.
   - Encourage children to eat whole fruit, which contains fewer calories and more fiber per serving than juice.
   - Since citrus fruits may provoke allergic responses during the first year, consider withholding orange juice until after the first birthday. (Check with your baby's doctor.)

8. Some of the most spectacular doses of sugar arrive in milk shakes and other frozen concoctions. A 24-ounce milk shake can clear 1,000 calories, more than 100 grams of sugar (about half of which is added) and—by the way—30 grams of saturated fat (roughly the amount in an entire pound of ground beef). ■

was actually following this advice, and one in three was consuming only one or two servings every day.

Why eat this many servings? Because Mom was right: An impressive and growing body of research supports her opinion that fruit and vegetables are good for you. Specifically, they can help reduce your risk of some of those "common health problems you want to avoid"—the ones we talked about in chapter 3:

- **Cancer.** More than two hundred studies conducted in various corners of the world support a fundamental conclusion: A diet plentiful

SOME BASICS ABOUT WHEAT AND BREAD

How can a nation be great if its bread tastes like Kleenex?
—JULIA CHILD

The smell of good bread baking, like the sound of lightly flowing water, is indescribable in its evocation of innocence and delight.
—M. F. K. FISHER, *THE ART OF EATING*[14]

The wheat grain (also called the kernel or the wheat berry) that we use for food is basically the reproductive structure of wheat grass and consists of three components:

- **Bran**, also called the **seed coat**, is the outer coating that makes up about 15 percent of the total kernel. It is a source of dietary fiber.
- **Wheat germ** is the embryo of the grain, the part that grows into a new plant if sown into the ground. While comprising only 3 percent of the kernel, wheat germ is rich in vitamins and also contains unsaturated fats.
- The **endosperm** is the starchy, soft white component that makes up the lion's share—nearly 85 percent—of the kernel.

Wheat was one of the first plants to be sown and harvested for food and is mentioned throughout the Old and New Testaments, from Genesis to Revelation. Wheat covers a larger surface of the earth than any other food crop, with some 600 million tons of wheat grown every year. More than a third of the world's population depends on it as a primary food source. Its popularity in baking arises from a protein it contains called **gluten** (from the Latin word for "glue"), which gives dough an elastic quality, allowing it to rise when yeast is present.

Gluten is also found in barley, rye, and possibly oats. For people with a disorder called **celiac disease** (also called **celiac sprue**), gluten provokes an abnormal immune response that damages the intestine, leading to an impaired absorption of nutrients and a host of symptoms. Once diagnosed, celiac disease is treated by avoiding foods containing gluten.

Flour is made by grinding wheat kernels into a fine powder. Whole wheat flour contains all of the components of the grain, while white flour consists only of finely ground endosperm, which includes the gluten and most of the starch but lacks the vitamins, minerals, and fiber. In order to make up for some of this deficit, manufacturers of white flour in the United States, Canada, and other countries add B vitamins and iron, yielding what is called **enriched flour**.

Since whole wheat flour is in fact much more enriched, why did white

in fruits and vegetables tends to protect you from at least some forms of cancer. This is not a universal effect. Not every food derived from plants is protective, and those that appear to offer some protection do not do so against every cancer. Nevertheless, reasonable evidence suggests that regular intake of certain fruits and vegetables may reduce the risk for developing cancer of the mouth, throat, esophagus, lung, colon, and prostate.[15]

- **Heart disease and stroke.** A growing body of evidence supports the idea that a diet rich in a variety of fruits and vegetables may

flour become so popular? It was perceived as purer and produced baked products that were lighter and fluffier—a victory of image and texture over nutritional value. A more practical reason is that whole wheat flour contains oils from the wheat germ and thus can become rancid over time. White flour will keep for six months at 70°F and two years at 40°F, while whole wheat flour should be refrigerated or frozen to prevent spoiling.

How do you sort through all of the offerings in your market's bread aisle? A few tips:

- **White bread** is the prototype of the refined/processed starchy carbohydrate. Even if made from enriched fiber, it lacks the nutritious contribution of the wheat.
- **Wheat bread** is a term that has been printed on packages of brown-colored bread for decades. Guess what? It is usually little more than refined/processed white-flour bread with some caramel or other ingredient added to color it brown. Check the ingredient list so that you won't confuse this for whole-grain bread.
- **Multigrain** breads may include a variety of grains and seeds—but often they are added to the basic refined wheat flour, which is the main ingredient, for flavor and texture. (Fiber content may not be impressive.)
- Many **rye breads** contain twice as much white flour as rye flour, which is also refined. As a result they may offer little fiber per slice and convert rapidly to glucose when eaten. If you enjoy rye bread, try one of the darker variations that contain more whole-grain rye flour. (Check the deli section.)
- White **sourdough** bread tends to be converted more slowly to glucose than regular white bread. Sourdough made from whole-grain flour is an even better choice.
- **Light bread** contains fewer calories per slice (thirty-five to fifty) than regular bread (typically sixty-five to ninety), though not by reducing fat content, which is minimal in bread. Instead, the slices are smaller and fluffier and their contents bolstered by some finely ground fiber that adds texture with fewer calories. However, this type of fiber may not be as nutritious as the unprocessed variety in regular bread. ■

Unbleached flour has been whitened by oxidation over several weeks. **Bleached flour** has been oxidized rapidly by exposure to a chemical agent such as chlorine gas, changing its structural properties in ways that make it more useful in cake and cookie production. The bleaching process is not known to change the nutritional quality of the flour or the finished baked product.

protect against these common and devastating conditions. One major study conducted by the Harvard School of Public Health, for example, found that eating five servings of fruits and vegetables per day was associated with a 30 percent reduction in the risk of stroke in healthy men and women.[16] Another Harvard study found that adults who took eight or more servings of fruit and vegetables every day were 30 percent less likely to have a heart attack than those who ate less than one and a half servings per day. Furthermore, the study suggested that for each serving added every day, the risk dropped by 4 percent.[17]

- **Cataract and macular degeneration.** A number of studies suggest that regularly eating dark, leafy green vegetables (such as spinach and kale) may reduce the risk of developing these com-

SHOULD I PICK CEREALS THAT ARE WHOLE GRAIN, HIGH IN FIBER, OR FULL OF VITAMINS?

Earlier in this chapter we listed cereals and their dietary fiber content (see pages 144–145) and recommended that you check the Nutrition Facts label to look for cereals with 5 or more grams of fiber per serving. If you spend some time looking at the Nutrition Facts label on the side of your favorite cereal box, you may notice that a whole-grain cereal may not be particularly high in fiber. Cheerios, for example, contains 3 grams per serving (one cup), and Wheaties also weighs in with 3 grams—respectable, but not on the high-fiber list. On the other hand, Kellogg's All-Bran cereal, the fiber champion at 9.6 grams per serving, isn't a whole-grain cereal. Since the bran (which contains the fiber) is only a small part of the grain, a whole-grain cereal will generally have less fiber than one that consists primarily of bran.

And what about those added vitamins? Cereal manufacturers have proclaimed the nutritional value of products to which they have added various combinations of vitamins to whatever is present in (or absent from) the actual cereal. But Whole Grain Total, bearing a 100 percent RDA package for several vitamins, contains 2.4 grams of fiber per serving. Kellogg's Product 19, which also contains a 100 percent RDA complement of several vitamins, offers but one gram of fiber per serving from ingredients that fall more into the refined than whole-grain category.

So which of these attributes are most important?

Whole-grain status and fiber content should definitely be your first two considerations, with vitamin content ranking a distant third. Kellogg's Complete Wheat Bran Flakes, for example, are not only made from whole wheat, but also contain 5 grams of fiber in a three-quarters-cup serving. Keep in mind that your cereal choices are not an all-or-nothing decision. You and your family probably

mon eye conditions. While cataracts—clouded lenses within the eye—can be removed and replaced with clear ones, there is no effective treatment for most cases of macular degeneration, the leading cause of blindness among those over sixty-five.

Fruits and vegetables don't walk and talk (except in cartoons), but that doesn't mean they are not amazingly complex. Nutritional science has identified a number of substances found in plants that do more than provide basic nutrients (carbohydrate, protein, and fat) for fuel and building materials. Some of these, such as vitamins C and E, are familiar to us. Others, with tongue-twisting names such as carotenoids and isothiocyanates, belong to a diverse group of compounds called **phytochemicals**. These are not necessary for life or health (as are the vitamins), but many of them appear to have a protective effect against

We take a closer look at cataracts and macular degeneration in chapter 14, beginning on page 710.

won't eat just one type of cereal every day of the year, and you should feel free to mix things up with a variety of options that will inevitably contain different amounts of fiber. And, by the way, you should enjoy whatever you eat. Few ideas are more oppressive than the notion that you have to repeatedly gag down some food you can't stand because it's "good for you."

Why are the vitamins a distant third? Because they're merely an added ingredient, and they don't improve the overall nutritional quality of the cereal itself. (You could add vitamins to a candy bar, but that doesn't make the contents of the candy any better for you.) As we'll discuss in appendix B (see page 869), you can take a multivitamin if you're concerned about getting an adequate supply every day.

One additional thought: Keep your eye on the sugar content. A serving of Cheerios contains only one gram of sugar with its 2.7 grams of fiber. Kellogg's Complete Wheat Bran Flakes contain more of each: 5 grams of sugar and 5 grams of fiber per serving. Popular raisin-bran cereals generally contain a generous amount of fiber—but at first glance also bear a major load of sugar. Kellogg's Raisin Bran contains 7 grams of fiber and 19 grams of sugar per serving; Post's contains 8 grams of fiber and 19 grams of sugar; and General Mill's Total Raisin Bran contains a mere 5 grams of fiber with its 19 grams of sugar. This is as much sugar as you'll consume in half of a twelve-ounce soft drink, and more than you'll find in a serving of a typical presweetened cereal. But here's the catch—a good chunk of that sugar comes from the raisins. (Half an ounce of seedless raisins contains more than 8 grams of sugar.) Raisin-bran cereals also contain added sugars, but unfortunately the Nutrition Facts label doesn't tell you how much of the sugar in each serving is added and how much occurs naturally in the food itself. This doesn't necessarily mean that everyone should shun raisin bran, but those (especially diabetics) who need to watch sugar intake may want to consider another source of fiber. ■

cancer and heart disease. Needless to say, researchers have only scratched the surface of this biological treasure trove. Furthermore, because of complicated interactions between various substances in fruits and vegetables, the most diligent human effort to reproduce or extract some useful "essence" of a plant for a surefire supplement usually doesn't come close to delivering the goods that are readily available by eating the real thing. We will look at vitamins, phytochemicals, and supplements in more detail in appendix B.

How can we incorporate more of these foods into our diet? Here are some practical suggestions:

- Try to eat a variety of colors every day. It appears that phytochemicals associated with different colors of fruits and vegetables provide a variety of health benefits. If you limit yourself to products bearing only one or two colors, you'll miss out.

WHAT'S A FRUIT? WHAT'S A VEGETABLE?

We tend to think of vegetables as the green stuff that sits between the meat and potatoes, and fruit as one of the sweet foods we might pick from a tree on a summer day or add to a bowl of cereal. On a regular basis most of us sample no more than a dozen of the common products from the garden or orchard, but there are many more choices for those who are willing to be a little adventurous.

By definition a fruit is the part of any plant that carries its seeds. A vegetable can come from anything else: the leaves (lettuce and spinach, for example), stems (asparagus), flower buds (broccoli and cauliflower), seeds (peas and corn), bulbs (onions and garlic), tubers (potatoes), or roots (carrots and beets). A few foods that we group with the vegetables are technically fruits: cut into tomatoes, avocados, eggplants, or squashes, for example, and you'll find seeds. And, for that matter, nuts and wheat grains also qualify as fruits. To keep us from losing sleep over these apparent contradictions, horticulturists have decided that in order to call a seed-bearing structure a fruit it must have fleshy tissue (which rules out nuts) and come from a perennial—a plant that lives at least two years without needing to be replanted. Thus an apple or orange tree can yield multiple crops, but you have to plant tomatoes every year. (We make an exception for watermelon, which we consider a fruit, but whose vines must be planted annually.) Some agricultural experimentation is focused on converting annuals into perennials.

Potatoes are vegetables, but because they consist almost entirely of starch they are, from a nutritional standpoint, far more similar to grains and the foods derived from them. (And, indeed, they don't offer a number of the nutritional benefits that you obtain from eating other vegetables.) For that reason, when we speak of eating five to nine servings of fruits and vegetables per day, we're *not* counting potatoes. ■

(See sidebar "What's in the Fruit and Vegetable Rainbow?" on pages 180–181.)

- Add some mixed frozen vegetables to your favorite soup as you heat it.
- Spice up your salads with some pieces of fruit.
- While most of us are used to the typical meat/starch/vegetable combination for a meal, try a second vegetable instead of the potato/rice/pasta.
- If you order a pizza for take-out or delivery to your home, order a salad with it or make one before it arrives. While you're at it, add a fruit or vegetable to balance out the meal.
- If the prospect of putting a salad together from scratch provokes you to reach for something simpler (like a box of macaroni), think about buying some precut salad mixes at the store. They're not as economical as using the original ingredients—you're paying for the convenience, after all—but they may be worth it if they increase your family's consumption of greens.
- Encourage your family (and yourself) to munch on carrot and/or celery sticks instead of chips for appetizers or snacks.
- Keep some fresh fruit in a bowl in the kitchen or family room for a healthy snack.
- Add slices of fruit to your favorite cereal. Be adventurous with the types that you try.
- Serve fruit with dessert . . . or as dessert.
- For a treat on a hot day, think about fixing or buying a fruit smoothie rather than a milk shake.

Limit the saturated fat to 10 percent or less of your total daily calories. We have already noted that the Institute of Medicine of the National Academies recommends that fat calories supply no more than 20 to 35 percent of daily calories. Other prominent health research and advisory groups such as the American Heart Association and the American Dietetic Association are in the same ballpark, recommending that we limit our daily fat intake to 30 percent of our total calories. But what about the different types of fat? The current guidelines from these organizations typically recommend limiting saturated fats to 10 percent or less of total calories per day. For someone on a 2,000-calorie diet, this means that 600 calories would come from all fats combined (or about 65 grams of fat), and 200 calories (about 22 grams) from saturated fat.

This is one situation in which the Nutrition Facts label displayed on many foods can be very helpful, since it lists not only the amount of saturated fat in the food, but also the percentage of the daily value (%DV)—that is, the percentage of the total day's allotment, assuming that you're trying to take no more than 10 percent of your total daily calories from saturated fat. (Remember that most Nutrition Facts labels also assume that your total daily intake is either 2,000 or 2,500 calories.)

The most abundant sources of saturated fats are red meats, dairy products, butter, and ice cream, as well as tropical (palm and coconut) oils. A mere tablespoon of butter, for example, contains 7 grams of saturated fat—about a third of the recommended daily amount for someone eating 2,000 calories per day. Coconut oil is 92 percent saturated fat, while 50 percent of palm oil is saturated fat. Some practical ways to keep the saturated fats at a reasonable level include:

WHAT'S IN THE FRUIT AND VEGETABLE RAINBOW?

The beautiful colors found in fruits and vegetables are not merely decorative touches.

Green: Remember the Harvard study mentioned on page 176? It suggested that each additional serving of fruits and vegetables reduced the risk of coronary artery disease by 4 percent. But each additional serving of green leafy vegetables was associated with a 23 percent reduction in risk. Why is that so? One reason could be that green leafy vegetables are a good source of **folic acid** (also called **folate**), which also is found in eggs and orange juice. As we discussed in chapter 4, folic acid helps reduce the level of **homocysteine** in the blood. This amino acid is associated with injury to the linings of arteries and the formation of blood clots in the wrong places, two factors that play a role in heart attack. Another compound found in green vegetables such as spinach, celery, and avocados is **lutein**, which may be protective against eye disorders, especially cataracts and macular degeneration. Green vegetables include some very familiar foods (especially at the salad bar)—lettuce, green peas and beans, broccoli, spinach, green peppers, asparagus, and zucchini—as well as a few that are not found as frequently in American refrigerators. The latter include the so-called "leafy greens"—collard and mustard greens, kale and Swiss chard—as well as okra, cabbage, and the ever popular brussels sprouts. While we think of "greens" as vegetables, there are several green fruits as well, including avocados, limes, honeydew melon, green apples, grapes, and pears.

Yellow/orange: Many fruits and vegetables of this color carry **antioxidants** such as vitamin C and **carotenoids**, which may protect against cancer and other diseases. (We will look at the importance of antioxidants in appendix B.) Familiar yellow/orange fruits include cantaloupe, grapefruit, lemons, nectarines, oranges, peaches, pineapples, tangerines, apricots, mangoes, and papayas. Carrots and corn are among the most commonly served yellow/orange vegetables, but don't forget sweet potatoes, squash (summer, winter, and butternut), pumpkin, and

- Limit your meat intake to about six ounces per day. Better yet, consider going "Mediterranean style" and eating red meat only a few times per month, and poultry and eggs only a few times per week.
- Choose leaner forms of beef. Avoid the marbled (fat-laden) cuts. Look for ground round containing lower percentages of fat—10 percent or less, if possible.
- Roasting, baking, grilling, broiling, and stir-frying meat are preferable to frying it.
- Trim the fat from your beef and pork, and remove the skin from your chicken.

yellow peppers. (Actually squash, pumpkin, and peppers, while commonly grouped with the vegetables, are actually fruits because they carry seeds.)

Red: Tomatoes and all of their various products (juice, soup, and sauce, among others) are technically fruits but usually grouped with vegetables. Whatever their category, they have gained favor for their abundant supply of **lycopene**, a member of the carotenoid family that is a powerful antioxidant and may protect against cancer (especially cancer of the prostate).

Red fruits and vegetables also contain varying amounts of **anthocyanins**, compounds that are members of the **flavinoid** class of phytochemicals. Anthocyanins are regarded as powerful antioxidants that may protect the integrity of blood vessels, among many other benefits. Familiar red fruits include apples, cherries, cranberries, raspberries, strawberries, pink grapefruit, red grapes, watermelon, and pomegranates. Red vegetables include beets, radishes, kidney beans, red peppers, red onions, red cabbage, and red beans.

Blue/purple: Familiar fruits (and less familiar vegetables) of this color also may contain anthocyanins, as well as **phenolics** (also called **polyphenols**), which are known to have antioxidant properties and may assist in the excretion of carcinogenic (cancer-causing) compounds. Blue/purple fruits include blueberries, blackberries, elderberries, purple grapes, plums, raisins, purple figs, and black currants. Aside from eggplant, most blue/purple vegetables are exotic-colored versions of more familiar relatives–purple asparagus, carrots, cabbage, and peppers, for example.

White/tan/brown: Perhaps the least colorful of fruits and vegetables, these are no less healthful. For example, the compound **allicin**, found in foods of the garlic and onion family, may lower cholesterol levels and reduce the risk of some types of cancer. Onions also contain **quercetin**, an antioxidant that may also inhibit the growth of cancer cells. Other vegetables in this color palette include cauliflower, turnips, and mushrooms, while fruits include bananas, dates, and pears. ■

Garden humor: What do you get if you divide the circumference of a pumpkin by its diameter? Pumpkin pi.

Lycopene is not absorbed well from raw tomatoes. Cooked tomato products, on the other hand, are a fine source of lycopene, especially when a little fat is present in the digestive tract to enhance their absorption.

WHAT CONSTITUTES A SERVING OF FRUIT OR VEGETABLE?

Many people struggle to eat enough fruits and vegetables each day. The old Food Guide Pyramid recommended five to nine daily servings, which is a good number to try to reach. Although the new Food Guide Pyramid guidelines make recommendations in terms of specific amounts (for example, cups or ounces), many people still think of fruits and vegetables in terms of servings. But what constitutes a serving?

- Six ounces (three-quarters of a cup) of fruit or vegetable juice.
- One medium-sized whole fruit (such as an orange, apple, or banana).
- One-quarter cup of dried fruit.
- One-half cup of raw, frozen, or cooked vegetables or fruit (sliced or chopped).
- One cup of raw leafy vegetables. Note that a large salad may contain three cups of greens and thus count as three servings.

These amounts reflect the most typical portion sizes determined by surveys of food consumption carried out by the USDA. (In other words, these are amounts that people typically eat.) You may find it interesting to get a measuring cup and see how much you actually serve or eat, compared with these amounts. You may notice that a helping of your favorite vegetable looks more like two servings rather than one. This can help you gauge your daily intake in light of these recommendations.

Some foods are easier to measure than others. Foods that you prepare in small pieces will fit into your measuring cup, but large broccoli spears won't. Here's what constitutes a serving for a few odd-sized items:

- Asparagus: six medium spears
- Broccoli: two spears
- Brussels sprouts: four sprouts
- Carrots: one medium-sized or eight baby-sized carrots
- Celery: two medium stalks
- Dates (dried): five dates
- Grapefruit: half of a medium grapefruit
- Strawberries: seven medium berries

Note: For smaller children, portion sizes will of course be smaller. Two- and three-year-olds, for example, will consume about half of the serving size that would be appropriate for adults. Remember to be cautious about excessive fruit-juice consumption in kids. (See point 7 on page 173 in the sidebar "Controlling the Sugar Flow.") For that matter, remember that fruit juice, nutritious as it may be, contains more sugar and calories than the fruit itself (and little if any fiber). ■

- When you buy tuna or other meats in a can, you're better off choosing those that are packed in water. If you get oil-packed meats, rinse them in warm water to remove the fat.
- If you're drinking whole milk, try switching to milk containing 2 percent fat. If you're used to 2 percent, try some one percent. If the watery texture isn't a turnoff, see how you do with nonfat. All of these forms are clearly marked in the dairy case.
- You can also try low-fat or nonfat versions of cheese, yogurt, sour cream, and ice cream.
- Try low-fat or nonfat versions of your favorite salad dressings. Remember, the regular forms can deliver more than 150 calories in two tablespoons.
- Before using butter (in whatever capacity), ask yourself whether olive oil would work just as well. It's a lot better for you.

Watch out for the trans fats. Foods that contain trans fatty acids (we'll call them "trans fats" for short) are pretty hard to avoid without subjecting your family to a rather spartan diet. But some that contain unhealthy portions of these compounds deserve to be reduced from your family's table, or eliminated altogether. The FDA estimates that the typical American adult consumes nearly 6 grams of trans fats every day. Some of this occurs naturally in animal products such as milk, cheese, butter, and red meats—the same foods that are rich in saturated fats. The vast majority, however, occur in products containing naturally occurring fats that have been processed in some way, usually involving partial hydrogenation. These include:

- **Stick margarine.** This spread contains nearly 3 grams of trans fat per tablespoon (and 2 grams of saturated fat). By contrast, butter contains a mere 0.3 grams of trans fat, but more than 7 grams of saturated fat per tablespoon. Some who have heard about the trans fat problem have dumped margarine and gone back to butter, but take note that tub margarine usually has much less of both trans and saturated fat. If you buy margarine, *read the labels* to find brands that have little or no trans fat.
- **Baked goods.** Perennial pleasures such as cakes, doughnuts, and cookies, aside from their sugar (and very often processed flour) content, are also likely to contain generous doses of trans fats. (A doughnut, for example, can pack 5 grams each of trans and saturated fat.) Ditto for packaged cake and baking mixes.
- **Chips and crackers.** A small bag of chips contains about 3 grams of trans fat. If it's fried or buttery in texture, you can assume trans fats are present.
- **Frozen treats.** Pizzas, pies, pot pies, waffles, and breaded fish and chicken also contain trans fat.

- **Fast foods.** The primary offenders are fried chicken and french fries. Their last moments prior to entering your digestive tract are spent in boiling hydrogenated or partially hydrogenated oil. While in recent years many fast-food restaurants have cut back on their use of trans fat, a medium serving of fries can still contain a sizeable 4 or 5 grams of trans fat.

HOT TIP

If you find partially hydrogenated oil of any type in the ingredient list of a food you're buying, trans fats are along for the ride. (You can learn how much from the Nutrition Facts label. That information is required as of January 1, 2006.)

Keep an eye on the cholesterol content of foods. The USDA recommends that adults limit their daily intake of cholesterol to 300 mg or less. The American Heart Association repeats this recommendation for healthy adults and sets 200 mg, less than the amount in a single egg yolk, as the upper limit for individuals with cardiovascular disease or its risk factors. In chapter 3 we noted that the vast majority of the cholesterol

THE FRESHER, THE BETTER

City and suburb dwellers often limit their fruit and vegetable intake to whatever they find in the produce section or the frozen-food aisle at the local supermarket. While frequent trips to these areas of the store are definitely a good idea, you may be missing out on some wonderful experiences if you haven't sampled truly fresh produce. Some suggestions:

- **Grow your own.** Even a very modest-sized yard can accommodate a variety of fruits and vegetables. Planning, preparing, planting, and tending to a garden (or even a fruit tree or two) can be a wonderful family project. Aside from the payoff of enjoying truly fresh food, these activities can also provide some education, conversation, physical activity, time away from vegetating in front of TV/video/computer screens, and (best of all) memory-making and bonding. Check with your local home improvement/garden store to find out what grows best in your climate. (Be sure everyone working outside wears sunscreen, by the way.)
- **Pay regular visits to nearby fruit and vegetable stands or (better yet) farmer's markets.** The produce you find will most likely be fresher than that shipped from afar, and the displays may tempt you to try some products that are new to you.
- **Raw is good, but . . .** If you enjoy your fruits and vegetables uncooked (properly washed, of course), eating them this way can give you an edge on benefiting from phytochemicals that may be altered by cook-

in our blood is generated by the liver, in amounts profoundly influenced by genetics and weight. Our daily intake of saturated and trans fats can also significantly affect blood cholesterol levels. The impact of the cholesterol that comes from our food, however, can be quite variable. For many people, eliminating or adding cholesterol in the diet has little impact on the amount circulating in the blood. For others, the effect is somewhat more significant. If you are trying to lower your cholesterol through dietary efforts, cutting back on saturated and trans fats will usually accomplish more than trying to limit cholesterol intake alone. Of course, a number of foods (such as red meats and cheese) contain generous amounts of both saturated fats and cholesterol, and so limiting foods with saturated fats often will reduce the cholesterol as well.

Eggs, on the other hand, pose a nutritional dilemma. Each contains more than 200 mg of cholesterol (all of it in the yolk), but also some polyunsaturated fat, very little saturated fat (about 1.5 grams), and about 7 grams of high-quality protein. Thus far no research has shown a clear relationship between eating eggs on a regular basis and

ing. (Don't forget one important exception: The availability of lycopene from tomatoes is enhanced when they've been cooked.) Otherwise, it's better to prepare them in ways that result in pleasant flavors and textures, rather than curbing everyone's interest in these foods by insisting that they all be eaten raw. (We will look at raw-food diets in the next chapter.)

- **When you cook, preserve the good stuff.** When you heat fresh or frozen vegetables in a pan of water, guess where some important nutrients go? Down the drain when you pour off the excess water. Lightly steaming, microwaving, or stir-frying your vegetables—keeping them on the crisp rather than the mushy side—will preserve more nutrients, not to mention taste and texture. If you can't resist cooking your vegetables in water, think about using the liquid that's left behind in a soup or sauce.
- **What about frozen or canned vegetables and fruits?** Frozen usually runs a close second to fresh produce in the nutrient and flavor department, although frozen foods may have an advantage over their would-be fresh counterparts that have been stored in such a way as to prevent ripening. Generally, canned products rank a distant third to fresh or frozen. Not only is flavor and texture affected by the canning process, but also a fair amount of salt and sugar may have been added. (Canned fruit, for example, often floats in syrup.) However, don't miss an important bottom line: Ultimately the best forms of fruits and vegetables are those *that you and your family will actually eat.* ■

developing coronary artery disease, and one could argue that an egg cooked using a little vegetable oil represents a more nutritious breakfast option than a doughnut full of trans fats or a few slices of white toast. Of course, eating the egg white without the yolk will eliminate the cholesterol, as will using a no-cholesterol egg substitute.

Get enough of the "good" fats. Earlier in this chapter we explained why monounsaturated fatty acids, especially omega-6 and omega-3 fatty acids, are beneficial to life and health. We also mentioned some good sources for these beneficial fats, and we'll recap them here:

- **Become a regular user of olive oil,** which contains more than 70 percent monounsaturated fatty acids. Buy the extra virgin oil, which comes from the first pressing of the fruit. Among other things, you can dip bread in it (rather than using butter) and use it when you stir-fry or sauté vegetables or meat. When not in use, keep it in a dark cupboard.
- **If you don't care for olive oil, try other vegetable oils that contain high percentages of monounsaturated fatty acids, including canola, peanut, and soybean oils.** You may find canola oil more to your liking for baking than olive oil.
- **Eat at least two servings of fish per week.** (See page 154.)
- **Try adding flaxseed to a variety of foods or as an ingredient in baking.** (See page 154.)

F.Y.I. A number of research studies have suggested that people who eat nuts on a regular basis are less likely to have heart attacks or heart disease than those who rarely eat them.

- **Add nuts and seeds to your diet,** especially as a substitute for less healthy snacks such as chips, or even as a source of protein. An ounce of nuts, for example, contains 8 grams of protein, roughly the same amount as in a glass of milk. Watch out, however, because these are calorie-dense foods—an ounce of walnuts contains 160 calories—and it's easy to down a bowlful without realizing that you've just swallowed several hundred calories. Depending upon their preparation, they also may have a fair amount of salt or sugar. Think *handfuls:* A serving size is an ounce; for example, roughly fifteen to twenty cashews.
- **Try avocado slices instead of cheese on your sandwiches.**

A Final Thought

We have covered a lot of ground, but we still haven't tackled two of the questions that opened this chapter: *Should I take vitamin, mineral, or other supplements?* and *How do I get rid of excess weight?*

To learn about vitamins and minerals, see appendix B. Excess weight is the subject of the next chapter. Here's a sneak preview: Don't expect a series of snappy, one-size-fits-all answers. After all, a number of these questions have kept diligent researchers occupied for decades. But we'll at least give you a basis for understanding the underlying issues and (when appropriate) a variety of viewpoints as well. Stay tuned.

QUESTIONS TO PONDER:

1. To what degree are the choices of foods you and your family eat every day driven by time pressure? How many times every week do you visit fast-food restaurants or order pizza because, as the old commercial went, "You're too tired to cook but you just gotta eat"? Are you into "instant everything" or do you actually have time to plan at least some meals? Consider whether improving the quality of your family's diet might require changes in schedules (specifically, simplifying them).
2. How often does your family eat a meal together . . . at the table . . . with the TV off? How could you make this happen more often?

Action Items: Buy (or dig out of that lower cupboard) a measuring cup—preferably one whose numbers haven't worn off and are easy to read. For a week or two, measure the amounts of foods and beverages that you and your family typically consume. Do you pour one cup (the typical serving size on the label) of your favorite cereal or a fair amount more? Is that glass of milk six, eight, or more ounces?

Spend some time looking at the Nutrition Facts labels for the foods you and your family most commonly enjoy. Pay particular attention to calories, cholesterol, sugar, saturated fats, and trans fats. (And be sure to check how the serving size compares to the amount you actually eat.) Are there some alternatives on the grocery shelves that have better numbers?

Work on implementing the basic principles in the last third of this chapter (beginning on page 158).

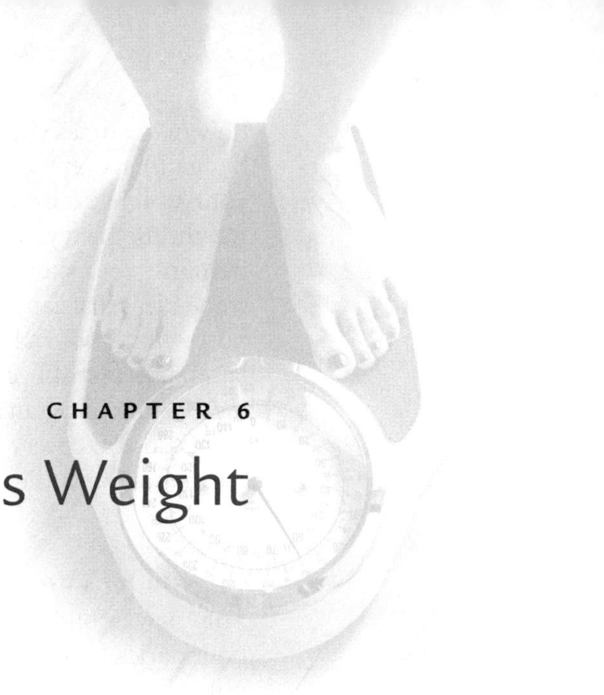

CHAPTER 6

Dealing with Excess Weight

I hate what I see in the mirror.

I can't fit into any clothes. Normal-sized seats on an airplane or at a theater are uncomfortable or just too small for me. My love life is nonexistent. People don't treat me with respect, or if they do, they're just acting. I've done every diet program on the planet, and I always gain back whatever I lose, with some extra pounds for good measure.

I'm such an utter failure.

For every person whose life is seriously affected by weight (and whose prevailing thoughts and feelings are as dark as these), there are many more who are annoyed and frustrated by a dozen or two extra pounds that they can't ever seem to shed. There are also a significant number who are overweight but not particularly concerned about it—at least until the doctor, or an episode of chest pain, sounds the alarm.

Speaking of alarms, the impact of excessive weight extends far beyond personal image or social acceptance, as important as those issues are. According to the American Obesity Association, it has been estimated that, as a nation, the United States is more than 2.5 billion pounds overweight. As we will see shortly, the health fallout is staggering: Overweight and obesity may soon overtake smoking as the leading cause of excess death in this country. America's mushrooming weight problem has morphed from a nagging concern into a four-alarm fire among health professionals and federal policy makers alike. This is all well and good, and we will no doubt benefit in a number of ways from attending to this problem as a nation. But for now many of us have some important work to do as individuals.

Whether you are squaring off against a weight problem for the first time, or feel like an old pro with a line of notches in your belt for all of the programs that you've tried without success, what you'll find in this chapter is some hope: No matter what your scale says, no matter how long you've struggled, no matter how many times you've lost weight only to see it come back again (or even rise higher than ever), it's *never* too late to make changes that will have an impact on your weight, your health, and your sense of well-being. If you don't have a weight problem yourself, you no doubt know many others who do—including, perhaps, your spouse or one or more of your children. This chapter will offer some ideas that can help you offer them both encouragement and practical support—along with a little basic training and a fair number of reality checks. The latter aren't terribly common in many best-selling, surefire, fat-melting miracle diet books, programs, and supplements that swallow billions of our hard-earned dollars every year. If any of these are actually working for you, by all means stay with them. For the other 95 percent of you, read on.

How Do We Define *Overweight* and *Obese*?

This may sound like a simple question, but in fact, for decades setting the boundaries between normal and excessive weight has been a thorny issue for nutrition experts and the general public alike.

What criteria might we use to determine whether our weight today is okay? There are several possibilities to consider, and over the past century all of these (and others as well) have been utilized by health-care professionals, researchers, government agencies, individuals, and entire cultures.

- **What does everyone else weigh?** By gathering data on what thousands of men and women at a given height actually weigh, we can develop averages and norms for a group of people or a whole nation. This can be somewhat helpful as a point of reference, but it can also be misleading if the people in question are in the midst of a famine or a rising tide of obesity. As with many areas of life, what everyone else is doing isn't necessarily the smartest, healthiest, or most virtuous path to follow.
- **What do other people (especially those of the opposite sex) find attractive?** This is a tricky question, with an answer that involves a variable blend of biological wiring, the shifting sands of cultural tastes, and personal preferences. It is also a treacherous question, because it can cause untold emotional pain for those (especially among the young) who are seeking to match whatever impossibly sleek and glamorous examples of physical beauty are currently appearing in magazines, music, movies, and television.
- **Do I like what I see when I look in the mirror or see my image in a picture?** This question is even more treacherous than the last one because too many people *never* like what they see. Indeed, for those with an eating disorder, the image in the mirror always appears to be too heavy, even when the person is "skin and bones" and dangerously malnourished.

- **What impact will my current weight have on my life expectancy?** This question was the basis of the widely disseminated "desirable weight" tables of the Metropolitan Life Insurance Company. On a personal basis, it can be very motivating—at least for a while.
- **How is my current weight affecting my health and overall quality of life?** This is by far the most useful and important question to address. If categorizing a person's weight as normal or excessive is strictly a matter of arbitrary personal or cultural preference, our most important priorities should be self-acceptance and promoting respect for others, regardless of their weight. And these *are* important priorities. But if the amount of fat we are storing (and the places we are storing it) is setting us up for a heart attack, cancer, painful joints, diabetes, and a host of other avoidable problems, we had better give it some thoughtful attention.

Some relatively new definitions of *overweight* and *obese* are not only widely used but also useful. You'll need to know something about them in order to get the most out of this chapter.

Body fat percentage. We need to remember that our concern about weight is rarely focused on the bone, muscle, internal organs, and other miscellaneous tissue that are all part of our weight, but rather on excess fat.

In some individuals, fluid retention can account for a significant number of extra pounds. While fluid retention often decreases as part of a general weight-loss effort, a substantial accumulation of fluid in the legs (or, less often, in other parts of the body) is called **edema** and represents a medical problem that needs diagnosis and treatment.

How much fat is too much? One basic approach to this question is to consider your **body fat percentage**. How much of your total body weight consists of fat tissue? As a rule of thumb, a healthy adult male carries 12 to 20 percent body fat, and a healthy female 20 to 30 percent. (The difference between genders is a by-product of changes during sexual maturation, as women acquire fat in breasts and hips under the influence of estrogen, while men more readily gain muscle mass in response to testosterone.) For a highly conditioned athlete, these numbers may be cut in half. At the other end of the spectrum, health problems are associated with:

- More than 22 percent body fat in younger men
- More than 25 percent in men over forty
- More than 32 percent in younger women
- More than 35 percent in women over forty

Contrary to popular wisdom, it *is* possible to be too thin. A woman of childbearing age whose fat stores reach a critically low level will stop her normal menstrual cycle. Not only will she be unable to become pregnant, but if this situation persists she may suffer osteoporosis, the loss of bone density that results in an increased risk for fractures.

A time-honored, low-tech method of estimating body fat involves taking **skinfold measurements**. A fold of skin in any of several locations—most commonly the triceps, or underside of the upper arm—is pulled away from underlying muscle and its width measured using a calibrated device called a **calipers**. The measurements are plugged into a formula to obtain the body fat estimate. The accuracy of this approach may be compromised by variations in technique, quality of calipers used, extremes in body fat, and even the basic assumption that fat under the skin in various locations accurately reflects total body fat.

There are a number of more sophisticated technical approaches to measuring body fat percentage, but many of these tests are expensive to perform and not available to the average individual. However, one measurement that estimates the percentage of body fat, known as **bioelectrical impedance**, can be done using devices available in some health clubs and doctors' offices, although it is less accurate in severely obese individuals. These instruments measure the resistance to the flow of a harmless (and painless) electrical signal between two points in the body. Based on the fact that current flows more readily through some tissues than others (fat in particular does not conduct well), the devices calculate an estimate of body fat percentage. (Note: Bioelectrical impedance varies with a person's level of hydration and will overestimate body fat content if a person is dehydrated. When tracking progress over time, the most reliable results are obtained if measurements are carried out under similar conditions—at roughly the same time of day, for example, and with proper hydration.)

Knowing your body fat percentage can be motivating (especially if you have a lot of weight to lose), but it isn't that useful for week-to-week monitoring. For that job we rely on the scale. Not surprisingly, there has been considerable research on the relationship between height, weight, body fat, and health.

One scenario in which tracking body fat percentage *can* be useful is when a person who is burning fat is also adding muscle through diligent exercise. He or she may feel thinner but may be discouraged because the scale isn't moving. In this case, seeing a decrease in body fat percentage can be useful and reassuring.

The Metropolitan Life Tables. If you visited a doctor as an adult one or two decades ago, you may have been confronted with "desirable weight" (originally called "ideal weight") charts, which were often posted in an accusing location on the wall next to the scale. Separate charts for men and women listed weight ranges for small-, medium-, and large-frame individuals, and unless you were rather trim, you would likely be discouraged when you compared your weight with the "desirable weight" range for your height. *I must be a person with a "large frame,"* you may have thought, because the weights under that column gave you a little more slack. More likely than not, you were looking at a set of numbers prepared by the Metropolitan Life Insurance Company, based on years of collecting data on life expectancy—a very important subject for an organization that is obliged to pay large sums of money when people die. First published in 1942 and then revised in 1959 and 1983, the tables reflected one basic concept: The weight ranges of the people who bought that company's life insurance policies and then took the longest time to die (delicately referred to as the lowest mortality rates) were identified as being ideal or desirable.

Though widely used in the United States for many years, the Metropolitan Life tables were somewhat limited in their usefulness for health assessment and research. For example, they reflected only one indicator of health—whether one was breathing or not—without any reference to other important aspects of wellness or illness. They did not reflect the population at large, but rather were derived from a single height and weight measurement of adults between the ages of twenty-five and fifty-nine who bought life insurance. People with known cancer, heart disease, or diabetes were excluded, and what happened to the policyholders' weight *after* they bought their insurance was unknown. Furthermore, as many as 20 percent of the heights and weights that comprised the data for the 1959 tables, and 10 percent of those for the 1983 edition, were self-reported by the customers based on their own bathroom scales—no doubt including a fair amount of "optimistic" fudging.[1]

Few people who stared at these numbers in their doctor's office decades later realized that the tables assumed you were wearing three pounds of clothing and one-inch heels when you were measured. Also, what determined whether you had a small, medium, or large frame was not what your great-aunt said about you when you were twelve years old, but rather the width of your elbow. Metropolitan published a handy table of elbow widths to help with this assignment, but measuring this distance was easier said than done and thus usually ignored by the busy physician. So while these tables gave an overview, they were generally skewed too low. They are rarely, if ever, used today as a reference for healthy weight ranges.

Body mass index (BMI). In recent years the Metropolitan Life tables have been displaced by an entirely different concept, the **body mass index** or **BMI**. Your BMI, which is based on your current height and weight, is calculated using the following formula:

$$\text{BMI} = \frac{\text{weight in kilograms}}{(\text{height in meters})^2}$$

Since few people in the United States know their weight in kilograms or height in meters, the formula can be adapted for the more familiar pounds and inches system used in the United States:

$$\text{BMI} = \frac{\text{weight in pounds}}{(\text{height in inches})^2} \times 703$$

For those who don't want to do the math, we have included a BMI table (see appendix C on page 924) for various heights and weights. Find your height in the vertical column on the left, and then look across the row until you find the column that is closest to your weight. The number in the table where your height and weight intersect is your BMI.

If you have Internet access, you can find BMI calculators on several Web sites. Two of these are http://nhlbisupport.com/bmi/bmicalc.htm (courtesy of the National Heart, Lung and Blood Institute) and http://www.cdc.gov/nccdphp/dnpa/bmi/calc-bmi.htm (Centers for Disease Control and Prevention, or CDC). Type in your height and weight, hit the button that says "calculate" or "compute," and you'll get the answer.

Note for detail people: Depending on the book you read or the Web site you visit, you may notice that the multiplier used to determine BMI using pounds and inches may range from 700 to 704.5. These variations do not make a significant difference in the result.

So what does the body mass index tell us? It correlates with body fat—not perfectly, but well enough to serve as a general indicator of the health risk associated with our weight. In 1998 the National Institutes of Health established the following categories for weight based on BMI among adults twenty years and older. These are now widely utilized among health professionals and researchers:

BMI	WEIGHT STATUS
Below 18.5	Underweight
18.5 to 24.9	Normal
25.0 to 29.9	Overweight
30.0 to 39.9	Obese
Over 40.0	Extremely obese

The BMI is an important and useful number—and you should know yours—but there are some important things to keep in mind. The BMI calculation for an adult is based solely on height and weight, without reference to age or sex. This makes it easier to use—no need for separate calculations and tables for men and women, for example—but the relationship between BMI and "fatness" is not absolute. Women tend to have a higher percent of body fat than men with the same BMI, and older adults are likely to have more body fat than their younger counterparts with the same BMI. A young male bodybuilder might have a BMI of 27, which is classed as overweight, but he may actually have a lot of lean body mass (i.e., bulging muscles) so that he would not be considered to have an excess of body fat.

Also keep in mind that the various categories of BMI—normal, overweight, and so on—are not absolute boundaries. Experts have argued back and forth about where to draw these lines, and there is not a sudden transformation in health status when a few pounds of weight loss bring a person from a BMI of 30 to 29.9, or from 25 to 24.9. Health risks generally rise with increasing BMI, and do so more dramatically as the BMI climbs past 25. In medical literature, a person with a BMI of 40 or more is said to have **morbid obesity**, reflecting the significant number of health problems associated with this level of excessive weight.

The popular use of the word *morbid* suggests horrific or ghastly, as in "Spare me the morbid details." In medical terminology it simply means "related to disease."

Finally, note that these BMI categories do not apply to children and teenagers. Between the ages of two and twenty, a different set of risk categories is used based not only on BMI but also on age and gender. (See "The Overweight Child and Teenager" beginning on page 260.)

Apples and pears. Weight-loss experts characterize overweight people as apple- or pear-shaped based on their fat distribution. Those with a prominent abdomen—shaped somewhat like apples—are thought to be at higher risk for health problems than those shaped like pears, with more fat deposited in the hips and thighs.

Two simple measurements related to apple and pear shapes tell us something about a person's health risk:

- **The waist circumference**, measured as the distance around the smallest area above the umbilicus (belly button) and below the rib cage. A measurement of more than forty inches in men and thirty-five inches in women is a cause for concern, because it suggests the presence of excessive fat within and around the abdomen. Fat stored here (a pattern more common in men) should be considered more dangerous to health than fat stored in the hips and thighs (a pattern more common in women). Note that waist circumference is a less meaningful measurement in adults five feet or under or with a BMI of 35 or more.
- **Waist-to-hip ratio** is another way to look at health risk from fat by comparing the amount of fat stored in the abdomen with the amount gravitating toward the hips and thighs. The waist circumference is measured as above, while the hip circumference is measured around the widest portion of the buttocks. Dividing waist by hip circumference gives the ratio, which ideally should be 0.90 or less in men and 0.80 or less in women. As you might expect from knowing that abdominal fat is more troublesome, a ratio of 1.0 or more (reflecting an apple- rather than a pear-shaped individual) suggests a greater health risk.

There are actually three components of abdominal fat: (1) fat deposited directly under the skin (called **subcutaneous fat**); (2) fat deposited around the internal organs (called **visceral fat**); and (3) fat deposited *deep* in the abdomen—in the space behind the internal organs and the tissue, called the peritoneum, that lines the entire abdominal cavity (**retroperitoneal fat**).

It is not certain how these three components stack up, so to speak, as far as their contribution to overall risk. Several studies suggest that excess visceral fat (surrounding the internal organs) is the most important contributor to health risk, but some research also correlates subcutaneous abdominal fat (the "padding" under the skin) with insulin resistance, the mechanism that leads to diabetes.

Several studies have suggested that an increased waist-to-hip ratio is associated with an increased risk for diabetes, high blood pressure, and coronary artery disease. However, compared to the waist-to-hip ratio, the waist circumference appears to be both a better indicator of abdominal fat content and a better predictor of future health problems. Indeed, waist circumference gives you an independent picture of your health risk above and beyond that of your BMI. For example, you should be concerned if your waist circumference is in the higher risk range (over forty inches for men, over thirty-five inches for women), even if your BMI is in the normal or modestly overweight range. However, if your BMI is over 35, measuring waist circumference offers little benefit, other than helping you decide what clothes are likely to fit.[2]

How Bad Is the Problem?

Excess weight is more than a number on one particular bathroom scale. Despite a national preoccupation with body image, despite a booming business in books and programs telling us how to lose weight, despite thousands of products advertised as light, reduced calorie, nonfat, or low carb, Americans are literally floundering in body fat. Obesity is now considered a national epidemic, one that adds billions of dollars to our country's annual medical bills, contributes to loss of health and life for hundreds of thousands every year, and wreaks daily emotional and spiritual havoc for millions more.

You may already have heard alarming statistics about our national weight problem, but they bear repeating. The most widely quoted figures come from the National Health and Nutrition Examination Survey (or NHANES), which has been carried out every few years by the National Center for Health Statistics (NCHS) of the Centers for Disease Control and Prevention (CDC). In the 2001–2002 survey, nearly two out of three American adults (65.7 percent) were overweight (defined as having a BMI of 25 or more), and nearly half of these (or 30.6 percent of all adults) were obese, with a BMI of 30 or more. Nearly one in twenty American adults (5.1 percent) was extremely obese, with a BMI of 40 or more.

While there was no significant change between this and the prior (1999–2000) study, all of these figures are higher than the 1988–1994 NHANES survey, which found that 55.9 percent were overweight, 22.9 percent obese, and 2.9 percent extremely obese.[3] Even more dramatic is the change since 1960, when the prevalence of obesity (BMI over 30) was 13.3 percent—less than half of the current rate—and extreme obesity (BMI over 40) was only 0.8 percent, compared with 5.1 percent now.

The problem is more pronounced among racial and ethnic minorities, especially women. The combined 1999–2002 NHANES survey data found the following percentages of people with a BMI over 25:

- Non-Hispanic black women: 77.2 percent
- Mexican American women: 71.7 percent
- Non-Hispanic white women: 57.2 percent
- Non-Hispanic black men: 62.9 percent
- Mexican American men: 73.1 percent
- Non-Hispanic white men: 69.4 percent[4]

The percentage of children and adolescents who are overweight has been rising dramatically as well over the past twenty years, as we will discuss later.

While we will focus on the impact of excessive weight in the United States, the epidemic of obesity is now a global issue for which a new term has been coined: *globesity*. According to the World Health Organization, more than a billion people in the world are overweight, and 300 million of these are obese (that is, with a BMI of 30 or more). Since 1980 dramatic increases in the

THE SPREAD OF OBESITY FROM SEA TO SHINING SEA

One of the most illuminating—and alarming—depictions of America's spreading weight problem is a map showing state-by-state percentages of adults with a BMI of 30 or more (the level that classifies a person as obese). A series of such maps compiled by the Centers for Disease Control (CDC) shows a startling rise between 1991 and 2003 in the number of states with higher percentages of obese adults. The first map (1991) shows only four states with 15 to 19 percent of adults having a BMI of 30 or more, and no states with more than 20 percent. The latest map (2003) shows *every* state having at least 15 percent of adults with a BMI of 30 or more:

- In fifteen states 15 to 19 percent of adults are obese
- In thirty-one states 20 to 24 percent of adults are obese
- In four states 25 percent or more of adults are obese

Want to see something *really* scary?

If you have Internet access you can download a dramatic PowerPoint presentation called "U.S. Obesity Trends 1985–2003" from the CDC Web site at http://www.cdc.gov/nccdphp/dnpa/obesity/trend/maps/index.htm. As you toggle through this "slide show" year by year, you will see U.S. maps with states marked in different colors representing the various percentages of obese adults. The maps are superimposed, and so the rising rates of obesity look like a plague that appears to rise from the Southeast and spread relentlessly across the country.

Watch this a few times and you'll think twice about that extra helping of pie. ■

OBESITY TRENDS AMONG U.S. ADULTS

BMI ≥ 30 (or about 30 lbs. overweight for a 5'4" person)

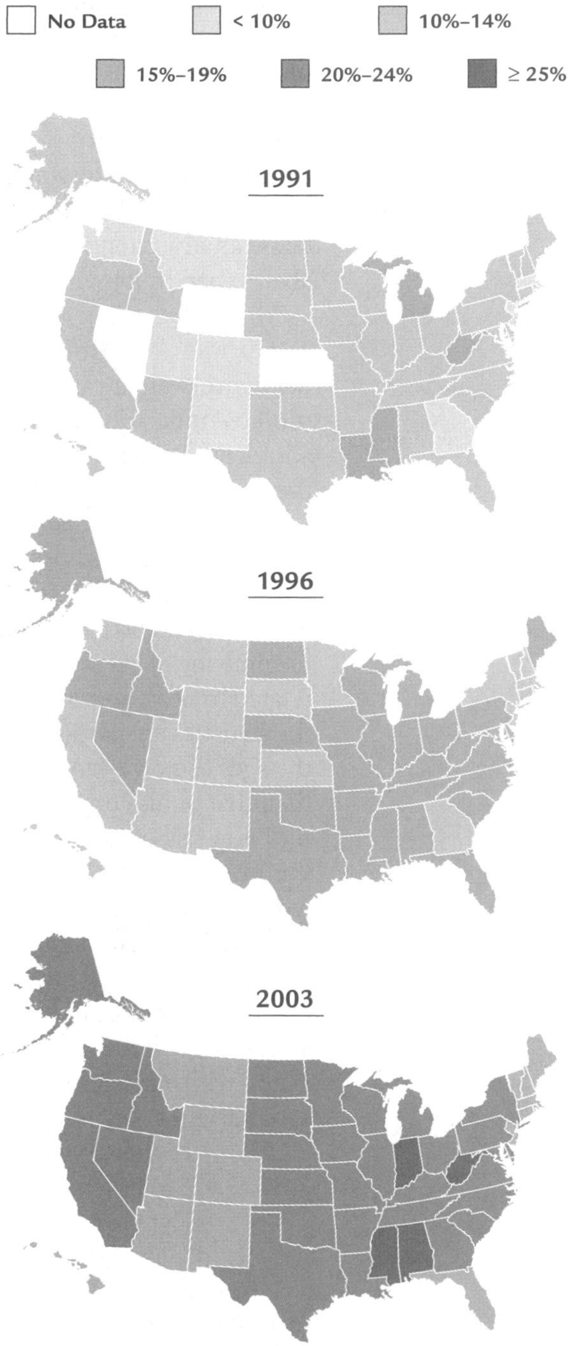

Source: Centers for Disease Control and Prevention

percentage of people who are overweight have been seen not only in North America, but also in the United Kingdom, Eastern Europe, the Middle East, the Pacific Islands, Australia, and Asia. Many of the same trends that have impacted the waistlines of Americans are at work in other parts of the world: modernization, urbanization, proliferation of cars and labor-saving devices, and perhaps most importantly, the increased availability of calorie-dense foods containing abundant fat, sugar, and processed carbohydrates. Ironically, in some developing countries where significant numbers of people remain undernourished, obesity rates are growing as fast as they are in industrialized nations. Furthermore, people who have been undernourished as children and then become obese as adults tend to have more severe manifestations of heart disease and diabetes than those who grew up with adequate amounts of food.[5]

What is our national weight problem costing us?

Being overweight can have such a profound impact on health that obesity may soon overtake tobacco use as the most significant cause of preventable disease and death in the United States. Excess weight and obesity take a toll, both on the nation's health and economy, in several ways:

Death from all causes. A 2001 Surgeon General's report estimated that as many as 300,000 adult deaths every year in the United States may be attributable to unhealthy eating habits and lack of physical activity. If your BMI is over 30 you have a 50 to 100 percent higher risk of dying from all causes compared to someone of your age and gender whose BMI is 20 to 25. (Most of the risk is related to heart and blood vessel disease.) For those with a BMI greater than 45, the statistics are particularly grim. The life expectancy for a white male between the ages of twenty and thirty with a BMI of 45 or more is thirteen years shorter than that of his counterpart with normal weight. The black male with a similar BMI is at risk of losing twenty years of his life. (For women with a BMI over 45, the numbers are somewhat less dramatic: up to eight fewer years for white women and up to five for black women.)

Cardiovascular disease. We just noted that most of the increased risk of death among the overweight and obese is related to cardiovascular disease—obstructed arteries in the heart and elsewhere that can lead to heart attack and stroke. This should come as no great surprise, because excessive weight is associated with a greater likelihood of having several important risk factors for diseased arteries:

- Higher levels of triglycerides, total and LDL ("bad") cholesterol
- Lower levels of HDL ("good") cholesterol
- Hypertension (high blood pressure)
- Type 2 diabetes

To make matters worse, body fat—especially that stored within the abdomen—may generate inflammatory substances that damage the lining of blood vessels and may participate in the formation of plaque that obstructs them.

Type 2 diabetes. There is a strong link between excessive weight and insulin resistance, the problem that eventually leads to type 2 (adult-onset) diabetes. More than 80 percent of people with type 2 diabetes are overweight, and for them losing weight is a crucial (if often challenging) component of treatment.

Cancer. Along with their other risks and burdens, the heaviest among us—those with a BMI of 40 or more—also suffer higher death rates for all forms of cancer: 52 percent more for men and 62 percent for women, compared to those with normal weight. In addition, in both sexes an elevated BMI is associated with higher death rates from cancers originating in several locations, including esophagus, colon and rectum, liver, gallbladder, pancreas, and kidney. Obese men have an increased risk of dying from cancer of the stomach or prostate, and obese women have a higher incidence of cancer of the breast, uterus, cervix, or ovaries than women with a normal BMI. The American Cancer Society estimates that as many as ninety thousand cancer deaths could be prevented every year in the United States if everyone maintained a BMI of 25 or less throughout life.[6]

For a review of cardiovascular disease and its risk factors, as well as diabetes and its consequences, see chapter 3.

Bone and joint disease. It should come as little surprise that the burden of supporting excessive weight increases the wear and tear in weight-bearing joints, leading to the ongoing discomfort and destruction of **osteoarthritis**. In addition, the searing pain of **gout**, in which uric acid crystals provoke intense arthritis in certain joints (especially the big toe), is more likely to occur among the overweight. It should be noted that one of the few advantages of excessive weight is a *reduced* likelihood of osteoporosis, the thinning of bone that is particularly troublesome for women after menopause.

Sleep apnea. As many as 18 million Americans have this disorder, in which the flow of air into the upper airway is repeatedly obstructed during the night, interrupting normal cycles of sleep and often causing fatigue and drowsiness during the day. Most people with sleep apnea are overweight, with the risk higher among men with a neck circumference greater than seventeen inches (for women, greater than sixteen inches).

A detailed discussion of sleep apnea may be found in chapter 15, beginning on page 755.

Reproductive problems. Irregular menstrual cycles, abnormal menstrual bleeding (including bleeding that is either excessive or unusually light), infertility, and several complications of pregnancy are more common in overweight women.

Other assorted health problems. Gallstones and a potentially dangerous condition called **fatty liver disease** are associated with excessive weight. The latter is specifically related to elevated blood sugar levels (which are in turn related to weight) and may provoke a form of inflammation and scarring similar to that seen among those who abuse alcohol.

Economic costs of medical care. Costs directly related to excessive weight are estimated to be more than $92 billion (or more than 9 percent of U.S. health-care expenditures), with indirect costs—lost wages from illness and the value of earnings cut short by premature death—estimated to be more than $55 billion.[7] But the flow of funds isn't limited to doctors' offices, hospitals, disability payments, and general losses. Millions of people live in various levels of desperation to find *something* that will help them lose weight, and there is no shortage of advisers, books, supplements, and programs promising to come to the rescue. According to the American Obesity Association, in the United States:

- About 40 percent of women and 25 percent of men are attempting to lose weight at any given time.
- About 45 million adults try some type of diet in a given year.
- An estimated $30 billion is spent every year in an effort to lose weight (or prevent gaining), including various forms of "diet" foods, appetite suppressants and other weight-loss supplements, books, videos, weight programs (both commercial and physician supervised), and health-club memberships.

Judging by the trends in weight among Americans over the past few decades, it would appear there has not been a good return on the hard-earned dollars invested in these various products and promotions.

Personal and emotional costs. While many who try to lose weight are motivated by health concerns, more commonly the driving force is very personal and very uncomfortable. For the mildly and severely overweight alike, a discouraging inner dialogue about how bad they look and feel is an ever-present runaway train of thought. Even for those who are actively seeking to silence the noisy critic residing in the brain, reminders from the environment are all too common.

Overweight people are confronted regularly with a harsh reality: Their weight is immediately apparent to others (except in the confines of the Internet chat room or in a sight-unseen exchange of letters) and thus is likely to have some impact on virtually every social interaction. Our culture sends powerful messages—especially to girls and women—that being slim is a prerequisite for desirability, sexiness, and a bright future. While there are a few exceptions, being overweight is widely perceived as a sign of poor self-control or even moral or spiritual failure, psychological or emotional disturbance, and decreased overall competence. A number of studies have documented negative attitudes toward the obese among both adults and children, among overweight people themselves (no big surprise), and also among health-care providers, who should know better. Other research has shown how these attitudes can affect employment, career opportunities, academic advancement, and marital prospects for those who are overweight. Obesity, or merely the accumulation of a few extra pounds, may become a divisive issue within a marriage if one partner is turned off by the other's weight. Again not surprisingly, studies of individuals seeking help in weight-loss programs have shown that a significant percentage are dealing with emotional distress, usually mild to moderate depression.[8] This ongoing emotional pain can in turn undermine efforts to deal with the weight, either through self-defeating inner dialogues (*I'm never going to overcome this, so why bother trying anymore?*) or through turning to food as a comfort after yet another lousy day.

Not everyone with an elevated BMI is convinced that weight loss is the key to life, liberty, and the pursuit of happiness. Some have come to accept their weight as a given, a fact of their life, feeling that if other people don't like it, that's their problem. A nonprofit advocacy organization called the National Association to Advance Fat Acceptance (or NAAFA) has squared off against negative cultural attitudes, seeking to "eliminate discrimination based on body size and provide fat people with the tools for self-empowerment through public education, advocacy, and member support."[9] Arguing that "just being fat does not signify poor health," NAAFA proposes that focusing on personal fitness rather than thinness per se is a more realistic approach to improving the health of those who are overweight.

While the health risks associated with obesity are in fact indisputable, there is no benefit whatsoever to a mind-set that concludes, *I won't have any basic worth until I'm no longer overweight.* There are valid and important reasons to strive for a healthy weight, but deriving one's identity from a number on the scale shouldn't be one of them. The person with a weight problem is no less precious to God than anyone else. Furthermore, Scripture makes it abundantly clear that He takes a dim view of bias, discrimination, harassment, or other expressions of judgment and contempt for a person based on appearance (see 1 Samuel 16:7, for example.)

How Does a Weight Problem Develop?

The simple and obvious answer is that *we gain weight when we consume more calories than we use over an extended period of time.* The simple and obvious conclusion we can draw from this answer is that *we lose weight when we consume fewer calories than we use over an extended period of time.*

In one way or another every bit of advice you will ever hear about managing weight boils down to these two pearls of wisdom. But if you struggle with the scale and the mirror and the clothes that don't fit, year after frustrating year, these words offer little comfort. And hidden beneath those statements are questions of surprising complexity: What controls feelings of hunger and of being filled? Why do some people seem to store every ounce of food they swallow, while others apparently can eat whatever they want without gaining any weight? What determines just how many calories are stored when we eat a sundae or how many are burned when we walk a mile?

Before we look at the variables that influence how you gain or lose weight, it's important to get a critical fact front and center in your thinking: *If you are overweight, with rare exception this has happened because your body has been doing exactly what it was designed to do.* Here's another way of looking at it: *We are better designed for life in the twenty-first century* B.C. *than for life today in the twenty-first century.* For most of human history, and for too many people on our planet today, a steady, reliable source of food has been the exception rather than the rule. In times of plenty, when more calories are available than we need, the capacity to store fuel for the "rainy day"—or the famine—is truly a gift from God, and He has provided you with 30 to 40 billion fat cells assigned to that duty. One could also argue that the pleasure most of us derive from sweets and fatty foods is programmed into our brain to steer us toward sources of calories that will provide quick energy and maximum long-term fuel storage on a bite-for-bite basis. If food supplies are erratic or scarce, guess who has a better chance of survival? The person who possesses the "thrifty gene" that allows him to store the extra calories most efficiently and burn through the stored calories most slowly.

We introduced the concept of the thrifty gene and its possible connection to excessive weight and type 2 diabetes on page 141 in chapter 5.

But what would promote our survival during famine is now the bane of our existence in a land flowing with milk, honey, burgers, and fries. We have more food at our disposal than at any other time in history. Much of that food is dense in calories and frequently processed in ways that promote rapid conversion to glucose and efficient storage as fat. At the same time, few of us are involved in "sweat of our brow" exertion from dawn until dusk. We enjoy the services of labor-saving devices and easily gravitate toward physically inactive lifestyles. We envy the person who seems to be able to eat anything and never gain weight or who seems capable of dropping ten pounds merely by skipping dessert for a couple of weeks. *That* person should regularly give thanks for an abundant supply of food, because at most other places or times in history he or she would be, well, history. We fret about the accumulation of extra pounds as the years pass. In fact, all things considered, we shouldn't be the least surprised that gaining weight is so easy and that obesity is currently an epidemic.

Another important reality check is an understanding of the basic components of energy expenditure—the different ways your body burns fuel. There are three basic ways in which this happens: basal metabolism, physical activity, and the thermic effect of food.

Basal metabolism (also called the **resting energy expenditure**) encompasses all the maintenance activities of the body going on behind the scenes to keep us alive and functioning: our 80,000 to 120,000 heartbeats and 17,000 to 23,000 breaths (give or take several thousand) every day, the contractions of muscles throughout the intestinal tract that move food from one end to the other, the biochemical processes within the liver, the filtering of blood by the kidney, the electrical activity within the brain and the rest of the nervous system, and so on. Roughly two out of three calories you burn every day are consumed by these activities, and the rate at which you use these maintenance calories—known as the **basal metabolic rate**—is affected by a number of factors:

- **Age.** Once you reach young adulthood, your basal metabolic rate slows by about 2 percent every decade.[10] Growing children and pregnant women have the highest basal metabolic rates.

- **Weight.** The greater your weight, the more energy you need for basal metabolic functions because you have a larger amount of tissue carrying out those functions. However, because lean body tissues (especially muscle) burn calories faster than fat, in an overweight person the *rate* of energy use per pound—that is, the total amount of energy burned divided by the number of pounds—may be less.
- **Height.** Metabolic rates tend to be higher in tall people because they have a greater surface area of skin through which heat is lost. Tall people may thus burn more calories simply to maintain body temperature.
- **Body composition.** How much of a person is fat and how much is lean tissue (especially muscle)? In general, women have a higher percentage of fat tissue than men, so men tend to have a faster metabolic rate.
- **Fasting, malnutrition, or starvation.** All of these conditions provoke a slowing of the metabolic rate, which should come as no great surprise. As we mentioned earlier, our body is designed to survive when food supplies are scarce.
- **External environment.** Adapting to both hot and cold environments raises the basal metabolic rate.
- **Internal environment.** Fever, stress, and certain diseases raise the basal metabolic rate.
- **Thyroid hormone.** Changes in this simple hormone, secreted by the thyroid gland located at the base of the neck, can raise or lower the metabolic rate as much as 50 percent. Some weight-loss clinics provide a prescription for extra thyroid hormone in a misguided effort to rev up metabolism in people who are not actually deficient. If they succeed in creating an artificial state of hyperthyroidism—too much thyroid hormone in circulation—a person's weight will indeed drop, but he or she usually also will experience sweating, shakiness, a pounding heart, and a dramatic loss of well-being. Even if it isn't enough to provoke these symptoms, a modest excess of thyroid hormone can also accelerate osteoporosis (thinning of bone).
- **Habits—smoking, caffeine, sleeping.** Yes, it's true—smoking increases metabolic rate, and smokers who quit without making an adjustment in eating habits may gain several pounds. But the *last* thing you need to compensate for a weight problem is a tobacco habit. If you are overweight *and* smoke, beware: Smoking aggravates all of the health risks that come with excess pounds. Caffeine increases your metabolic rate, but not enough to count on a pot of coffee to be your

primary weight-loss tool. And no great surprise, metabolic rate slows down during sleep. This doesn't mean that you'll automatically lose weight if you stay awake half the night. A good night's sleep is important for many reasons, not the least of which is feeling refreshed and ready for activity during the new day.

For a sobering survey of the risks of tobacco use, see chapter 10 (starting on page 433). We learn all about sleep in chapter 15.

Physical activity encompasses all of the muscle motion that we carry out every day, including simple activities such as standing, walking, and reaching, as well as more vigorous physical exercise. As you might imagine, this component of our daily energy expenditure can vary dramatically depending on our lifestyle.

The **thermic effect of food** is the total amount of energy used in food processing: moving food through the intestine, digesting, absorbing, and metabolizing it. This varies somewhat with the amount of food we consume, but generally accounts for only about 10 percent of our daily energy use.

When you consider all the factors that influence metabolic rate and the vast number of calories we consume over the course of a year—anywhere from 500,000 to a million for an adult, depending on age, gender, and activity—it is mind-boggling that the body maintains a stable weight year after year.

Now, back to the original question: *How does a person gain that extra weight, and why won't it go away?* As you might have guessed, there are several factors that affect how a person gains or loses weight, including a few that are affected by the rate of basal metabolism. As you read through this list, keep in mind an important fact: *The impact of each of these varies considerably from person to person.* For some, genetics is a driving force—these people gravitate toward being thin or overweight, no matter what they eat. Others are affected more by family traditions, the culture, or behaviors such as eating to calm the emotions. Most overweight people are impacted by a combination of these.

1. **Heredity.** Your genetic code affects your shape, size, hormone patterns, metabolic rate, regulation of hunger and fat storage, and numerous other biochemical characteristics, including many that have yet to be discovered. It is well-known that adopted children tend to follow the weight patterns of their biological rather than their adoptive parents and that identical twins are more likely to weigh the same than fraternal twins, even if they are reared in different families. Genes determine how susceptible you are to becoming overweight if you eat and behave in a certain way, but they don't cause it. Observations of certain isolated populations have demonstrated that a change from the group's traditional cuisine (typically involving little fat, lots of fiber, and limited quantities of food) to modern Western fare can lead to dramatic increases in the rates of obesity and diabetes, well beyond even those seen in America today. The fact that you may have been born with a tendency to gain and retain weight may seem unfair, but, as we mentioned earlier, that same tendency has been life preserving through most of human history.

2. **Age.** In general, we become more fuel efficient with age, and the quantities of food that meet our calorie needs as teenagers are enough to pack on the pounds a few decades later. Furthermore, as we age we tend to replace lean muscle mass with fat, although this may be affected by use—or more commonly disuse—of muscle because of changing activity patterns. As a result, unless one takes deliberate action to prevent it, between the ages of twenty-five and fifty-five an adult is likely to gain an average of half a pound per year.

3. **Gender.** Hormonal differences between genders can affect the storage or mobilization of fat. For example, women tend toward a higher percentage of fat and a lower percentage of muscle than men. Because a given amount of muscle burns more calories than an equal amount of fat (by weight), calorie needs tend to be greater (by about 10 to 20 percent) in men than in women on a per-pound basis.[11] Other hormonal influences may make women more resistant to weight loss, partly as a survival mechanism for the human race. When a woman of reproductive age reaches a critically low level of body fat, her menstrual cycles stop and she cannot become pregnant. (Indeed, this is a survival mechanism for her as well—a woman who is severely malnourished will have a difficult time maintaining her own and her baby's health during a pregnancy.)

DO I HAVE "FAT GENES"?

If you've struggled for years to lose weight, you may suspect that you're genetically destined (or doomed) to be heavy. Believe it or not, your weight isn't set in concrete. However, there are some clues that genetics may be playing a strong role in an ongoing weight problem:

- Obesity has been a persistent problem and began early in life.
- Obesity runs in your family. If this is the case, your risk is increased by 25 to 30 percent. (However, keep in mind that the impact of the family includes not only genetics, but also eating and activity patterns.)[12]
- Weight loss has been extremely difficult, even with persistent, supervised effort; calorie restriction; and consistent exercise.

Even if you are fighting a genetic uphill battle, you must never give up hope or decide that your ongoing efforts are a waste of time. More importantly, you must resist the temptation to begin or continue your membership in the Diet/Supplement-of-the-Month Club in a desperate search for "the Answer." You should instead find responsible, knowledgeable sources for ongoing help with nutrition, exercise, and counseling, and that's just for starters. Medication may provide limited assistance, and for some even bariatric (weight-loss) surgery may be appropriate. We will look at these options later in the chapter. ■

Fewer than 2 percent of people who are overweight have a specific medical disorder as a direct, primary cause of their weight problem.[13]

4. **Medical problems.** When a person is overweight, a medical evaluation is very important for a number of reasons, as we will see momentarily. One important agenda item will be to determine whether a medical condition or even a medication is contributing to weight gain and/or making losing weight more difficult. (See sidebars on pages 206–209.)

5. **Lifestyle.** This is the part of the equation we have the most control over and the one we usually least want to address. (Remember: Even if you have a genetic tendency to gain weight or are one of the small percentage of overweight people with a medical diagnosis underlying this problem, with rare exception addressing it will involve changing what you eat and increasing your activity level.) Several components of lifestyle play a role in weight gain (or loss):
   - **Activity.** How much do you move during the day, and how often do

MEDICAL CONDITIONS THAT MAY CONTRIBUTE TO WEIGHT GAIN

Polycystic ovary syndrome, metabolic syndrome, and type 2 diabetes are all variations on the theme of insulin resistance—the situation in which insulin becomes less effective at escorting glucose into all of the cells that use it. All of these conditions seem to involve a vicious circle: They are aggravated in the overweight and obese, but they also cause weight gain to be more likely (indeed, almost inevitable) when there is an abundance of food. To add insult to injury, they make weight loss much more difficult. (See pages 71–74 for more information about these common conditions.) Women with polycystic ovary syndrome are not only prone to obesity but also have an excessive supply of male hormones (called androgens) that can cause excessive hair growth, acne, fluid retention and—to make the weight problem more difficult—increased appetite.

Hypothyroidism. The thyroid gland, located at the base of the neck, regulates the body's metabolic rate, and a reduction in the hormones it secretes (which we identify simply as thyroid hormone) is not uncommon, especially in women over forty. Usually the change is very gradual, often discovered at an early stage when symptoms are minimal or absent. More severe hypothyroidism may slowly bring on a host of symptoms, including fatigue, depression, intolerance to cold, constipation, a gravelly voice, puffiness of the face, and unexplained weight gain. However, even severe hypothyroidism rarely accounts for more than about ten to twenty pounds of extra weight, much of which is fluid. Correcting the problem is important, straightforward, and gratifying—but by itself will not melt away

you exercise? How much time do you spend sitting in front of TV and computer screens? Many experts state that lack of exercise among both adults and children plays a major role in our current obesity epidemic. We'll take a detailed look at the why and how of exercise in chapter 7.

- **Family traditions.** You not only inherit genetic tendencies from your family, but also patterns of eating, including favorite foods, recipes and portion sizes. For some families, any get-together is an occasion for lots of food to appear, and not partaking enthusiastically is considered impolite (or a sign of illness).
- **Culture.** Most of us are presented with opportunities to eat throughout much of the day at home or work, and even when we're not eating we're bombarded by enticing advertisements for foods.

dozens of pounds of extra fat. (However, the improvement in energy may increase activity levels, which definitely helps.)

Cushing's syndrome results from an ongoing excess of cortisol in the body, either from an internal source (most often the adrenal gland) or from medications called **glucocorticoids** (such as prednisone) used to treat disorders such as asthma, serious arthritic disease (such as rheumatoid arthritis or lupus), and certain other conditions. A person with Cushing's syndrome has upper-body obesity, a round (or "moon") face, thin arms and legs, and a host of other disturbances. If your weight problem is primarily related to excess cortisol, there is a good chance that your doctor will recognize it from across the room. (Physicians use the term *Cushingoid* as shorthand for the classic appearance of this syndrome.) If not caused by medication, the primary goal will be to determine why it is occurring.

Cushing's syndrome was named for Dr. Harvey Cushing (1869–1939), a pioneering neurosurgeon—some say the greatest of the twentieth century—who first identified the pituitary disorder that can cause it.

Fluid retention is an entirely different problem from excessive fat storage, although some people tend to retain more fluid as a by-product of weight gain. Fluid accumulating in the legs, abdomen, and even hands can have a variety of causes, including congestive heart failure, chronic liver disease, hypothyroidism, kidney failure, or the use of certain medications. Some who are desperate to lose weight may seek **diuretics**, medications that increase the output of urine and mobilize excess fluid. These drugs may in fact be helpful (or even critical) for treating the underlying condition, and several pounds of fluid may disappear under their influence, but they won't move an ounce of fat. Needless to say, diagnosing and managing fluid retention are not tasks to attempt on your own, but should be addressed with your physician. ■

Furthermore, unless we've been brought up in rather strict isolation from our culture, the kinds of foods that have been the most popular, tasty, inexpensive, convenient, and heavily promoted for the past several decades are generally high in calories and low in nutrients. (An ample supply of these is readily available at your favorite fast-food franchise.) The abundance of products laden with fat (saturated and otherwise), added sugars of all types, and refined (i.e., processed) grains has been identified by a number of experts as creating a "toxic food environment."

- **Portion sizes.** Americans have long been exposed to supersize portions, especially in fast-food restaurants and convenience stores, and many restaurants serve entrées in quantities large enough to satisfy two people with some left over for the doggie bag. In chapter 5 we described the French paradox, which is that a country known for its rich cuisine is not known for its obesity rates, largely because

MEDICATIONS THAT MAY CONTRIBUTE TO WEIGHT GAIN

The medications on this list *may* contribute to weight gain in *some* people who are taking them. If you have a significant weight problem it is *unlikely* that a medication is the primary problem, and it's even more unlikely that stopping the medication will suddenly and dramatically turn the tide. *Don't stop what you're taking without discussing the problem with your physician.* There may be other options to consider, or it may be in your best interest to stay with what you're taking, even if you have to work to manage your weight.

The following medications may contribute to weight gain:

- **Certain blood pressure medications** in the families known as alpha-blockers and beta-blockers, as well as an older and rarely used agent called methyldopa. Some medications in the family called calcium channel blockers, especially amlodipine (Norvasc), may cause fluid retention, which can be annoying even though it doesn't involve added fat.
- **Antidepressants**, especially many of the older and less widely used tricyclics such as amitriptyline and doxepin. Variable weight gain can also occur with some of the more widely used selective serotonin reuptake inhibitors such as fluoxetine (Prozac) and paroxetine (Paxil).
- **A variety of medications that treat psychiatric conditions** such as bipolar disorder and psychosis, including lithium, olanzapine (Zyprexa), haloperidol (Haldol), and phenothiazines (a class of older drugs used to treat schizophrenia).
- **Valproic acid** (Depakene, Depakote), which prevents seizures and also is useful for preventing migraine headaches in some people.

portion sizes are typically smaller. To compound the problem, for a number of reasons (including the misguided clean-plate club we were told to join during childhood) we may feel compelled to polish off whatever shows up on our plate. This makes buffet lines, where quantities are essentially unlimited, particularly hazardous for the overweight.

- **Emotions.** Sharing a meal is a wonderful way to interact with family, friends, and strangers—indeed, it involves a certain intimacy unique in human experience. Food also soothes basic physical and emotional discomforts from the moment we leave the womb. Thus for most of us, eating isn't just a way to relieve hunger. It is an accompaniment to celebration and sorrow, socializing and solitude, excitement and boredom, working and relaxing, studying and goofing off, and especially to watching anything—TV, a movie, a sports event, you name it. For many, certain items—known famously as comfort

- **Hormonal preparations.** Long-term use of corticosteroids such as prednisone can also induce a specific type of obesity, as we noted in the sidebar "Medical Conditions That May Contribute to Weight Gain," which begins on page 206. For many years it was believed that oral contraceptives commonly cause weight gain, but controlled studies have not shown consistent or significant differences between users and nonusers.[14] Weight gain, if it occurs, will vary with the individual and medication, and may in fact involve fluid retention rather than increased fat storage. Similarly, many women gain weight just before, during, and after menopause, but the use of hormone therapy (HT) has not been shown to aggravate this effect. (Some research in fact suggests that HT may actually decrease menopausal weight gain, although this would not be an appropriate reason to take supplemental estrogen or progesterone.)[15]
- **Certain drugs used to treat type 2 diabetes.** These include some older medications called sulfonylureas (glipizide and glyburide are the most common), as well as the newer drugs pioglitazone (Actos) and rosiglitazone (Avandia). This potential effect on weight can be frustrating when one of the primary objectives with type 2 diabetes is losing excess weight. On the other hand, the commonly used medication metformin (Glucophage and other brands) normally does not contribute to weight gain. Needless to say, it is important to understand the benefits, risks, and proper use of the particular drugs a physician may recommend for this important problem, and to follow blood glucose and weight trends carefully after they are started. ■

foods—become a necessity for coping with anything, whether it be a bad day, the normal bumps in life's road, or a major crisis. Spiritual hunger that remains unfulfilled can lead to all kinds of cravings, including food, that serve as poor substitutes for intimacy with God.

Alas, the foods and the quantities that we elect to this role have a way of being highly caloric and rarely nutritious—how many people relax after a hard day by eating a bushel of carrots? In emotion-driven marathons known as binge eating, it's easy to finish off entire boxes of cookies, half gallons of ice cream, and other spectacular amounts in one sitting.

Then Jesus declared, "I am the bread of life. He who comes to me will never go hungry, and he who believes in me will never be thirsty."—John 6:35

- **Overcommitment and the frantic lifestyle.** These are perhaps *the* most important contributors to our national and personal weight problems. When there are too many irons in the fire and entries on the calendar, when we're rushed and racing and running around all day, there's no time to think about carefully shopping for and preparing nutritious meals. Who's got the time? Instead, it's instant whatever for breakfast (assuming we eat anything before dashing out the door), fast food for lunch, and "nuke and serve" for dinner—often involving concoctions that are highly processed, highly caloric, and admittedly highly satisfying to taste buds and stomachs. To make matters worse, dealing effectively with excess weight requires *time*. It should come as no surprise that so many Americans whose weight is a by-product of a frenzied lifestyle remain stuck because they want a quick solution—which, by the way, doesn't exist.

So What Can I Do to Lose Weight?

Whether your weight is a relatively new problem or you've tried everything without any long-term success, it's never too late to do something about it. If you're determined to do something about your weight, good for you! But you have an important decision to make at the outset, *especially* if you have struggled with weight for years and already feel utterly frustrated. Whatever else you do, get rid of the expectation that there is some supplement, medication, combination of foods, machine, or fifteen-minute exercise that will magically solve this problem for you. In other words, *stop looking for the quick fix.* The fact that there are so many different books, programs, and supplements all claiming to have the answer, and at the same time there are so many overweight people desperately looking for something that *really works,* tells you that (at least for now) there is no universal quick and easy cure for this problem.

Achieving and maintaining a healthy weight requires a steady, livable, step-by-step, day-by-day effort. It usually involves work on multiple fronts, including food choices and quantities, exercise, environment, habits, and emotions.

With rare exception it also requires more of our time than we would really like to give, which means that it may be necessary to make some fundamental changes in schedules, activities, and (above all) expectations. But the long-term benefits are definitely worth the effort. And, of equal importance, *anyone* can make these changes. A person doesn't need to be a nutritionist, a marathon runner, or a psychologist to bring them about. You do not need a will of steel, nor must you endure endless (or even short-term) hunger, to lose weight. Remember an important word in the first sentence of this paragraph: *livable.* What ultimately works are the adjustments that a person can live with indefinitely.

Here are some important steps that *everyone* who is overweight needs to address:

Meet with your doctor.

During your medical evaluation, it's important to ask your doctor if you have any health problems that are related to your weight. If you ask *that* question, your doctor will think that you are very astute and hopefully will investigate several factors:

- your actual height, weight, and body mass index (BMI), as well as their trend over the last several years (if your doctor has records extending back that far)
- your blood pressure
- your lipids: cholesterol (total, HDL, and LDL) and triglycerides
- your fasting blood glucose (blood sugar) level, which, if elevated, may lead your doctor to recommend a glucose tolerance test
- any symptoms that might suggest a medical problem aggravated by weight, including chest pain or pressure, shortness of breath, daytime drowsiness, fluid retention, irregular menses, or sore joints (especially knees and hips)
- an electrocardiogram, stress test, or other heart-related studies if you have worrisome chest symptoms or are contemplating vigorous exercise
- any medical problems that might be contributing to your weight problem, such as hypothyroidism or polycystic ovary syndrome

Identify* your *reasons for losing excess weight.

We say *your* reasons, because too many people try to lose weight in order to please someone else or to get another person (especially a spouse, a relative, or even a physician) off their back. This may provide motivation for a while, but it rarely sustains a long-term effort because resentment and resistance nearly always enter the picture. Sooner or later you need to identify, write down, and repeatedly review what it is about losing the weight that will keep you going when the going gets tough.

Big important hint to spouses and parents: If you don't like your wife's, husband's, or child's current weight, the best way to make matters *worse* is to provide a steady stream of criticism and sarcastic comments about his or her appearance. Believe it or not, he or she is well aware of this problem, and the last thing needed is another critic to chime in with the one already sounding off day and night in his or her mind. If you want to help, you need to become the individual's most steadfast source of love, support, reassurance, and safety. From that position you may then exercise the option (or in the case of a minor child, the responsibility) to express your heartfelt concern and your willingness to help in any way possible. Your message cannot be, *I can't love you at this weight,* but rather, *I love you too much to see you hurt—or your life threatened—by this problem.*

Adjust, amend, or eliminate any counterproductive expectations and beliefs. This is the most important part of the process. Here are some key things to keep in mind—and keep on keeping in mind:

- **Learn to appreciate slow and steady progress.** Fad diets and supplements always promise rapid and spectacular weight loss, and many career dieters cycle in and out of programs in a futile effort to lose twenty pounds by summer or to fit into a special outfit for a big occasion. Repeated cycles of weight loss and gain, often called yo-yo dieting, may actually cause your body to become more resistant to losing weight the next time you try. ***Reality check:*** The most reliable weight loss occurs *gradually*. A pound or two every week is very good progress. More than two pounds a week on an ongoing basis is uncommon and more likely to be hazardous. (Many people lose a few pounds of fluid during the first several days of calorie restriction, for reasons we explained in chapter 5 on page 141.) But once the water has passed, slower, steady weight loss should be the rule.
- **Adopt realistic expectations.** If you're nearing fifty and want to weigh what you did in college, think again. If you're looking at the models in the department-store ads or the muscular hulks in the typical men's-health magazine and want to be like them, good luck. Beyond whatever physical gifts God provided them, most of them spend a lot of time developing that look (and get a bit of help from photo enhancement techniques), which is likely to be beyond the reach of most mortals. ***Reality check:*** Your primary goal should be to arrive at a weight that improves your health and sense of overall well-being. For most adults the primary target will be a weight that gives you a BMI of 25. You can check the BMI table on page 924 as a point of reference, but you should also determine with your doctor or a registered dietitian whether that weight is in fact optimal for you. Remember also that if you are significantly overweight (that is, a BMI over 30), even a modest loss of 5 or 10 percent can make a major dif-

ference in some important risk factors, including cholesterol, triglycerides, blood sugar, and blood pressure.

- **Embrace your life in the present.** If you are perpetually discontented and think that losing weight will change everything, think again. Yes, there are personal and social benefits associated with being at a healthy weight, but if you're never satisfied with your life at your current weight, it's unlikely that your life minus several pounds will be much better. There are plenty of beautiful, thin, miserable people who can attest to this fact. ***Reality check:*** True happiness and contentment are "inside jobs," which unfortunately elude too many who seek them in all the wrong places. Remember, for starters, that God loves you unconditionally in the body you inhabit *now*. For more on this subject, see chapters 8 and 9, which deal with emotional and spiritual health.
- **Take personal responsibility.** If you continually blame your genes, your parents, fast-food restaurants, the sugar industry, or anyone else for your weight problem, you're wasting some perfectly good energy. ***Reality check:*** The bad news: No one can lose weight for you. The good news: No one can stop you from losing weight.
- **Realize that losing weight is not a prison sentence.** We often approach the day before we launch another weight-loss plan with dread and a self-defeating last grasp at food freedom: "Eat, drink, and be merry, for tomorrow we die(t)." Some consume impressive amounts of their favorite guilty pleasures, assuming that the next stretch of life is going to be a dry, dusty trail of deprivation. Indeed, the phrase "I'm going on a diet" carries a lot of emotional baggage: "I'm going to serve a sentence for my wrongdoing. When I'm done being punished, though, I'll be free again to do what I like." ***Reality check:*** Weight management requires an established pattern you can live with for the rest of your life. For some, this may feel like facing life in prison, but such a perspective needs to be tossed aside immediately, because only the most iron-willed individual can adhere to a program that involves perpetual hunger or a list of foods that make you gag. Believe it or not, a healthy diet can be one that allows you to lose weight, nourish your body, avoid hunger, and provide some eating pleasure as well. What you may not be able to find, however, is an approach that does all of these while soothing every emotional discomfort in your life. One of the biggest accomplishments of squaring off against excessive weight is figuring out ways to manage the stresses of life without reaching for food. More on that topic later.
- **Learn and grow from your mistakes.** Nearly everyone with long-term weight problems has felt as if an endless refrain of the pop song

"Oops! . . . I Did It Again" is playing. Whether you're attempting a well-reasoned eating plan or the latest fad diet, after a few days or weeks there's an inevitable slip—typically at the end of a hectic, stressed-out, exhausting day. The old comfort food beckons and there's no resisting it. The next day brings a barrage of mental accusations: *I blew it so badly last night. I just erased all of my efforts from the last three weeks, so there's no point in continuing this.* ***Reality check:*** If you think unbroken perfection is the only path to success with weight loss, take a moment to consider anything else you've ever accomplished or attempted: walking as a toddler (okay, you don't remember, but you've seen the pictures), reading, spelling, throwing a ball, driving a car, becoming a husband or wife, raising a child, gaining spiritual maturity. If you haven't experienced frustration, failures, and setbacks, you haven't accomplished anything. Furthermore, in the realm of weight loss and gain, what happens at one meal or in one day has far less impact on your weight than the ongoing pattern of food choices.

- **Be encouraged. You can succeed!** You may be frustrated, but "I'll never be able to lose weight" is a blues refrain you can't afford to be singing. ***Reality check:*** No matter how many times your weight seems to have defeated your efforts, you can make changes that will move this problem in the right direction.

Begin making smarter food choices.

This is perhaps the most confusing part of a weight-loss project, because there are so many contradictory views on what constitutes the "right" foods both for weight loss and for general nutrition. Should you go with a low-fat, low-carb, or high-protein diet, or none of the above? Do you have to eliminate certain foods to lose weight? We will take a brief tour of some current popular diet plans later in this segment. But even more important: If you haven't done so already, read (or perhaps reread) chapter 5, which reviews the basics of nutrition. Pay particular attention to the final segment, "How Shall We Eat?" beginning on page 158. Applying that basic advice to weight loss provides some commonsense, bottom-line advice:

- **Phase out the sugary foods.** Soft drinks (the nondiet variety), cookies, cakes, candies, pastries, and other sugary foods are the classic empty calories that need to be eaten sparingly, or phased out of your life entirely. This is one idea that both low-fat and low-carb advocates agree upon.
- **Gravitate toward whole-grain foods rather than those made from refined or processed grains.** For many people, especially those with type 2 diabetes or metabolic syndrome, limiting those foods (as well as sugars) that are rapidly converted into glucose may lead to

more effective weight loss. Whole-grain foods also contain more valuable nutrients, vitamins, and fiber.

- **Eat five to nine servings of fruits and vegetables (not counting potatoes) every day.** You need to think beyond the lettuce in your salad, by the way, and sample the rainbow of fruit and vegetable colors—green, yellow, red, orange, white, and even blue. Spend more time in the produce section or at a local farmer's market and less in the meat section.
- **Eat lean meats in modest portions**—three to four ounces, about the size of a deck of cards—and think baked, broiled, or grilled rather than deep fried.
- **Keep an eye on the cholesterol content of foods.** Cholesterol itself doesn't contribute to excess weight, but it tends to come along for the ride in many calorie-dense foods that do. (Important reminder: If you are overweight and a blood test shows that you have a high level of cholesterol, losing excess weight will lower the cholesterol level much more efficiently than simply limiting the amount of cholesterol you eat.)
- **Gravitate to the "good" fats.** These are the monounsaturated fats contained in olive and canola oils, as well as in cold-water-dwelling fish. When you can, substitute olive oil for butter or margarine in your food preparation. See page 186.

These are all generalities, of course, but if you read chapter 5 we hope you have picked up a number of specific, practical recommendations that you can begin using *today,* if you haven't already. Here's an important take-home message: *No single approach, formula, or plan for weight loss can work for every person.* You must learn basic, sound nutritional concepts and then adapt them to your (and your family's) unique circumstances, lifestyle, likes, and dislikes. This may sound like we're stating the obvious, but in the search for surefire formulas it's easy to miss the obvious: *If your approach to losing weight doesn't work for you, it isn't going to work at all.*

Eat less (and eat more slowly).

This obvious point is so often overlooked in the frantic search for the secret to losing weight. Whether you gravitate toward a plan that is low-fat, low-carb, both, or neither, you will need to deal with this part of the equation. If you're overweight and staying overweight (or getting more overweight with each passing year), guess what? Over the long haul, whatever you're eating contains more calories than your body needs. Keep in mind some basic arithmetic: A pound of stored fat represents an extra 3,500 calories of energy. That means an excess of only 100 calories per day—what you'll find in about eight ounces of your favorite nondiet soft drink—will add ten pounds to your body in a year.

The good news is that consistent small-scale reductions will also pay off if you give them enough time.

Obviously downsizing the amount of food we eat is easier said than done when so much is available everywhere we turn. Bariatric surgery, which is specifically intended to limit the amount of food eaten and absorbed, can accomplish this goal for people with serious, highly resistant weight problems, but it is anything but an easy, quick fix (see section starting on page 255).

Like it or not, even if you're choosing better quality food, it is very difficult to lose weight without addressing the amount of food you consume every day. So here's a top-ten list to help you adjust the amount of food you eat.

1. **Eat when you're hungry—and stop when you're not.** This is a profoundly simple idea, but we're so used to eating for every possible reason that this may prove harder than it sounds. Before you start eating, or before the next bite, get in the habit of asking yourself, *Am I (still) hungry?* You may be surprised at how often the answer is, *Not really,* at which point you need to ask, *So why am I reaching for something to put in my mouth?* If the answer is that you're upset, bored, or trying to relax, then ask yourself if there are other ways to solve that problem. If the answer is, *I'm enjoying this, and I don't feel like stopping,* then at least slow down (see number 3). Many people dread embarking on a weight-loss effort because they anticipate being hungry and miserable day and night. Here's a news flash—*you do not need to go hungry in order to lose weight.* In fact, you're more likely to yield to the worst food temptations if you're famished. If you're actually feeling hungry, you should eat something—but of course *what* and *how much* will be the critical issues.

   By the way, most of us eat so often that we don't know the difference between real hunger and every other vague uneasiness that seems to respond to food. If you have any doubt, try skipping one or two meals and note how you feel. (This can actually serve as an opportunity for some spiritual growth, as we'll discuss in chapter 9.) Then as an experiment, see how little food it takes to end that sensation.

2. **Stop eating when you're satisfied, but before you're really full.** We all enjoy eating a traditional Thanksgiving dinner, but how often have you left the table feeling more stuffed than the turkey? That bloated, heavy, drowsy sensation really isn't very pleasant, nor are the heartburn and gas that may join the party a little later. Unfortunately, eating a complete dinner at many restaurants—or perhaps at your dining-room table—will bring on the same sensation. In many cultures children are taught to stop eating before they feel full, and we should learn to do likewise. (Hunger will be gone long before you've eaten half of the amount that brings fullness.)

3. **Eat slowly.** If you've ever been interrupted for several minutes after the first

few bites of a meal, you may have noticed that you weren't particularly hungry when you sat down again. This is a very important validation of the fact that *whether we eat quickly or slowly, hunger goes away in about the same amount of time.* Think of it another way. After you begin eating, it takes about fifteen to twenty minutes for signals from the stomach and changes in blood glucose to signal that you're no longer hungry. If you are inhaling your food during that time, you can put away hundreds of calories—and yet be no more satisfied than if you took a fraction of that amount.

If you really enjoy food, eating slowly is the only way to go:

- Put down your utensils between bites.
- After cutting a piece of meat, put the knife down and pick up the fork with the hand that held the knife—then eat the piece of meat.
- Take smaller bites.
- Thoroughly chew, and savor the taste and texture of each mouthful.
- Pause between bites. If you're with others, enjoy the conversation. If everyone is too busy eating to talk, start a conversation so that *they'll* slow down. (If a TV is the yammering "guest" at your meal, turn it off.) A shared meal at which no one is talking is a wasted opportunity. When eating alone, stop and give thanks for every bite.

4. **Think differently about portions (part 1).** Here's the simplest, cheapest, most surefire weight-loss program, and it involves only three basic steps:
   - Put whatever you're used to eating at a given meal on your plate.
   - Take half of it away.
   - Eat what remains slowly enough to last as long as your regular portions.

Okay, so this advice was a little tongue-in-cheek, but not entirely. Assuming that you don't need a complete overhaul of your food choices (again, see chapter 5), if you're overweight and not making any progress, then whatever you're eating is sustaining (or building) your current weight. Removing half of your usual portions would be a pretty drastic change, but it would certainly work. Taking away a quarter or a third of your typical portions will almost certainly work over time, assuming you stick with it.

5. **Think differently about portions (part 2).** Here's another cheap and simple weight-loss program, also a little tongue-in-cheek:
   - Find a thin person your age and gender who appears to enjoy life and good health.
   - Observe carefully what and how much that person eats.
   - Go and do likewise.

There will of course be differences between you in genetics and activity level, but don't be surprised if you also find some important differences between the sizes of the portions you consume. Forget about sixteen-ounce steaks and baked potatoes the size of a football. Think instead about adopting some of the following portion sizes—none of which require you to use a food scale—for foods that are often sources of runaway calories:

- a piece of lean meat the size of a deck of cards
- a potato the size of a small lightbulb
- a serving of cheese the size of one or two pairs of dice
- a serving of butter the size of one of those dice
- a serving of pasta the size of your computer mouse
- a one-cup serving of cereal (one of the good kinds, without all of the added sugar), which is also the amount in one of those individual-sized boxes
- one slice of bread, half a bagel, half an English muffin, or half a bun

Notice we didn't list serving sizes for foods like broccoli, apples, and celery sticks. Most vegetables and fruits are part of the solution rather than part of the problem, unless they're swimming in rich sauces or syrups.

6. **Think differently about portions (part 3).** Here's our third and final cheap and simple weight-loss plan:
   - Instead of the typical dinner plate, use a salad plate to hold your usual fare. (You can have another salad plate for the salad.)
   - Don't eat any more than you can fit on that plate—no stacking allowed—and no going back for seconds.
   - Take your sweet time eating your meal.

   Remember the good old days when you would receive an actual hot meal on a long airline flight? Remember the tiny salad and the little rectangular container that held the main course? There wasn't much there, but because it filled the dish completely it always seemed like enough food. If you're trying to reduce portions and place some smaller servings on your old dinner plate, all of that open space may look alarming. *Is that all I get??* Put it on a smaller plate, however, and your brain will adjust its perception and your emotions.

7. **Avoid random or nonpurposeful eating.** We often eat not because we're hungry or even to comfort ourselves, but just because the food happens to appear before us. A lot of people have trouble with this at the workplace: Someone has a birthday or a coworker brings leftovers from a party at home, and suddenly there's an array of our favorite snack foods on the counter as we pass by. If it's something we like, it's all too easy to reach for it without thinking, an automatic reflex between brain, arm, and mouth. It takes some effort, but it's critical to ask yourself the all-important questions: (1) *Am I actually hungry?* (2) *If I am actually hungry, is this plateful of cake/cookies/chips the best way to relieve my hunger?*

   If you're an autopilot eater, you must create an environment at home that reduces the likelihood of this behavior. It's very simple: When you're done eating, put *all* of the food away. You can consider making an exception for a bowl of fruit, especially if you're trying to reprogram your household to enjoy more nutritious snacks. Some important variations on this theme:

- **The big one: eating in front of the TV.** This spells trouble in three ways. First, while engrossed in a program or a movie you can easily lose track of what you're eating and consume a tremendous quantity of food—especially those snacks that you don't actually put on a plate but rather pull out of a bag or box one after another. Second, TV watching is a sedentary (i.e., sitting or lying down) rather than active pastime. More hours in front of the tube mean fewer hours moving muscle. *This is especially important for children and adolescents,* for whom TV watching is frequently associated with excessive weight. Third, you're likely to see enticing ads for all kinds of food.

  Taming the TV and snacking monster may be a challenge, especially if this habit is entrenched in your (and your family's) life. It's all about taking charge: *You* decide how much and what you're going to watch, rather than simply turning the set on and mindlessly surfing through 150 channels. If there's going to be food in the TV room, *you* decide ahead of time what and how much. Don't just bring boxes, bags, and bowls of stuff to graze on. Another interesting option is to propose that anyone watching TV, including you, does some sort of exercise—aerobic, strength training, or stretching—at the same time. This not only solves the snacking problem but also improves everyone's physical condition and tends to cut the number of hours spent in front of the tube.
- **Eating at sporting events and movies.** Nowadays when you go out to the old ball game and other spectator sports you can buy a lot more than some peanuts and Cracker Jack. Giant hot dogs, pizza, ice cream, and king-size soft drinks are merely the basics, and for many fans a nonstop flow of food is as much a part of the show as rooting for the home team. The same can happen, of course, during a busy weekend of games on TV. Today's movie multiplexes likewise serve colossal buckets of popcorn dripping with butter and soft drinks the size of tankards, and then there's the candy and ice cream.

  Once again a little planning can save you hundreds of excess calories, not to mention a wad of cash. For one thing, don't come to the game or movie hungry. If the venue allows it, bring some healthier snacks of your own, such as fruit or sticks of carrots or celery. If not, look for smaller sizes or split larger quantities among two or more people. Consider getting ice water instead of a soft drink, and hold the butter on the popcorn. And as always, ask the important question: *Am I still hungry?*
- **Eating during other activities.** Many weight-loss programs advise

The typical box of movie popcorn in the 1950s held three cups and weighed in at about 170 calories. Today's large bucket can hold seven times that amount and, with butter added, deliver 1,700 calories.

that when at home you should eat only from one (modest-sized) plate, in one room, doing absolutely nothing else. If you want a snack, fine—just measure out a reasonable portion on your special plate, and then eat it at your kitchen or dining-room table without watching TV, reading, studying, or doing anything else. (Obviously, having a conversation with another person is okay—otherwise, eating becomes like sharing a trough in the barn.) In general this is a good idea for limiting random, unconscious eating, but with one exception. If you're eating an actual meal (as opposed to a snack) by yourself, reading may help you *take your time* with it, as long as you keep track of your hunger/fullness status.

8. **Get comfortable leaving food behind.** Many of us are driven by the insane notion that we are obliged to finish whatever food appears on our plate. This may arise from exhortations during childhood to "Join the clean-plate club" or "Remember that people are starving in Africa," or messages from Mom or Grandma that preparing food is a gesture of love and eating it is a way of saying thank you. How many times have we kept eating (especially in a restaurant and often long after being full) because we didn't want food to go to waste? If the only two destinations for that food are the trash bin or the bulging fat stores in our body, which is the better place for it to go? "I paid good money for that food," you might protest. But what is the excess fat costing you? And if you're in a restaurant, your server will gladly give you a box or bag to take home the extra for another day.

   Very important parenting tip: Don't encourage or exhort kids to eat when they're not hungry, and don't threaten to punish them for not cleaning their plates. There are much healthier ways to influence what they eat, which we'll cover later in this chapter.

9. **Be very careful when you eat out.** Enjoying restaurant meals can be both a treat and a trap. Yes, it's nice for special occasions, but all too often we opt for the drive-through, the pizza delivery, or even a complete sit-down meal because we're too rushed or hassled or tired to prepare food ourselves. About 25 percent of American meals are not home cooked, and that's not counting "nuke and serve" foods from the freezer. Not only can this be a drain on the pocketbook, but many restaurants serve up very large portions, whether or not they're designated as supersized. Here are some suggestions to help draw the line between dining out and pigging out:
   - Try to avoid bringing a ravenous appetite to the restaurant. You'll be tempted to order more items than you really need.
   - Take your time. The fact that families often go to restaurants because there isn't time to *prepare* a meal doesn't mean that "eating out" has to mean "eat and run." The best restaurant experiences are those in

which the meal is an occasion to share good conversation, not to rush through the food. The more expensive fine-dining establishments have this figured out: They tend to serve smaller portions (often exquisitely prepared) at a leisurely pace, leaving you satisfied but not bloated.

- Split entrees. If you and your companion can find something you both like, this will save both money and calories.
- As we just said, you don't have to clean your plate. Stop when you're pleasantly satisfied, and take home what remains.
- Skip dessert or order one for the whole table to share.
- Stay out of fast-food restaurants. Many overweight people can date some of their most dramatic weight gain to a period of time when the pressures of life led to frequent stops at fast-food franchises. The products they serve are carefully engineered to be highly satisfying—indeed, some would argue that they are addictive, especially to young palates whose business they aggressively court. In response to rising criticism about dispensing nutritional junk, the fast-food industry has started to offer some alternatives to the usual burgers and fries, including salads, broiled chicken entrées, and fruit. But their staple items remain highly processed, calorie dense, and loaded with saturated fat, salt, and sugar.
- If you can't stay out of fast-food restaurants, skip the fries and look for a salad. Avoid supersizing, the marketing ploy that seems like such a bargain but packs huge amounts of extra calories. The only items that get supersized are fries and soft drinks, which you should avoid anyway. Get the kids—and yourselves—milk or water instead of a soft drink.
- Avoid buffets, or at least don't come with a huge appetite. For the person with a weight problem, a buffet line represents a major challenge. Who can resist all of those appealing items, especially when it's all to be had for one price? Even small portions of a dozen different items can result in a calorie pileup. When faced with a buffet meal, follow some of the other guidelines in this section: Put your choices on a smaller plate (usually the salad plate), eat slowly, quit before you're full, and don't feel obliged to finish what's on your plate, even though you put it there yourself.

10. **Keep your eyes open for other ideas like these, and for recipes that utilize healthier foods and portions.** No single source of advice, including this book, will address *every* issue you might have related to weight or portions. While you don't want to obsess about what you eat or make food the center of your emotional universe, this is such an important topic that you would be wise to become a lifelong learner.

Get moving.

Regular exercise is a cornerstone of healthy living and weight loss for a number of reasons:

- Exercise builds (or at least maintains) muscle, which utilizes more fuel in its daily operations than fat does.
- When you are burning more calories than you are eating, your body may begin mobilizing protein in muscle as fuel, rather than tapping into fat stores. Exercise builds muscle mass and in so doing helps to limit this unwanted effect.
- Exercise reduces the risk of developing coronary artery disease, cancer, and diabetes, all of which are hazards of being overweight or obese. Exercise is also crucial to controlling type 2 diabetes.
- Exercise increases alertness, energy, and general well-being, all of which can improve one's ability to resist making poor food choices or eating to relieve stress or boredom. (*I just walked two miles this morning—I don't want to blow my progress by eating this doughnut.*)

As part of your weight-management program, you should set a goal to do some moderate aerobic exercise (such as walking, cycling, or swimming) for thirty minutes at least five days per week and do a simple strength-training routine two or three times per week. These important activities, their benefits, and some strategies to make them part of your weekly routine are discussed in detail in chapter 7.

Here's an important reality check: There is no question that exercise makes a vital contribution to your overall well-being and the efficiency of your weight-loss efforts. However, it is very unlikely that thirty to sixty minutes of exercise every day *by itself* will make a rapid dent in your weight. A brisk walk, for example, burns only about one hundred calories per mile. But your body fat, a terrifically efficient form of fuel storage, stores roughly 3,500 calories per pound. A little arithmetic indicates that if you decide to lose weight by walking without changing your eating habits, you need to cover thirty-five miles for every pound of fat you want to shed. If what you're eating is maintaining a stable weight and you begin walking two miles five to seven days every week, you'll lose between one and two pounds every month. Over time this adds up (so by all means keep it up), and ten to twenty pounds lost over the course of a year can offer some important benefits to your health—but it may not be as fast a rate of loss as you'd like.

Identify and address your triggers.

Spend some time thinking about the times and circumstances where you become vulnerable to overeating. For example: *At the end of the day, I'm exhausted and my resistance is definitely low. If the kids [or boss or customers] have been pushing me all day, I just need something that will relax me, and nothing works like a quart of ice cream.*

What else could you do at that moment that would distract you until the impulse passes? These alternatives to food need to be realistic, readily available, and capable of bringing you some satisfaction. Your options might include:

- going for a brisk walk
- taking a hot, relaxing bath
- doing some stretches (see chapter 7)
- praying or contemplating (see chapter 9)
- cleaning something
- getting rid of some clutter
- venting to a family member or friend
- watching a half hour of an upbeat, cheerful, or otherwise diverting program

My day is wall-to-wall with commitments: work, appointments, errands, church activities, chauffeuring kids, you name it. I don't even have time to nuke something out of the freezer, let alone prepare gourmet meals for myself or anyone else. When I'm hungry I need to grab and go, and fast food is my best friend. If you're a frequent flyer at the drive-through, or you stop at gas-station minimarts to fill your tank more often than the car's, or the take-out crew at the local pizza parlor knows your order and your address as soon as you say your name, you may be blowing too much cash for too many calories. Unfortunately, solving this requires some time and planning. Sometime when you're not going ninety miles per hour, sit down for a few minutes and think about preparing some healthier (and less expensive) food. Pace your intake throughout the day, so you don't become ravenous and head for the nearest vending machine or fast-food emporium. For what you'd save by bypassing the burgers and fries, you could buy an insulated food carrier for work or your car.

Every time the family [or congregation or work group] gathers for some socializing, all we do is eat. I don't want to be a snob or a party pooper, and I don't want to just sit there while everyone else enjoys the feast. Again, a little planning is in order, whether you're going to a birthday party, a church supper, or a corporate banquet:

- Avoid coming with a serious appetite. You'll be less tempted to overindulge.
- If the setting is informal, use the salad-plate approach (page 218) to downsize your meal, especially at a potluck.
- As mentioned earlier, take your time between bites. You can enjoy the meal and make it last as long as everyone else's, without the calories and bloating.
- Focus more on the conversation than the food.

You get the idea. Sometime when you're not rushed, think through your last—and your next—typical week. Recall when the eating got out of control and what prompted it. Then consider how you might avoid the same conclusion next time.

Another instructive approach is to keep a **food diary** for two weeks. Without adjusting what you normally do to make the diary look respectable, write down *everything* you eat, including snacks, using a format similar to that in the table below.

FOOD DIARY for 3/1/06

Time	Place	What food?	How much?	Was I hungry?	How was I feeling at the time?
Noon	Cafeteria	Small salad Tuna sandwich 2% milk	All of it Half 8 oz	Yes	A little rushed
4 P.M.	Desk	Bagel/ cream cheese	Half Thick layer	Not really	Tired/stressed

For the quantity, don't get hung up on the exact amount. An estimate based on size ("a steak the size of both hands") will do. More important is to identify the emotion that accompanied the food (happy, sad, bored, frustrated, celebrative, etc.). Getting a grip on how much and how often you eat, and what triggers your desire for food, can be very informative. Many people find that they begin to modify their eating habits just as a result of keeping these notes and becoming more aware of their patterns. In addition, if you seek help from a dietitian, bringing a two-week food diary will make his or her job much easier.

Modify your environment. (In other words, flee temptation.)

If you're trying to quit smoking or drinking alcohol, guess what you shouldn't have lying around your house? Cigarettes or alcohol. Similarly, if certain foods are your downfall, then by all means *get them out of sight and out of reach.* If your cupboards are full of cookies and chips and your fridge is bulging with ice cream and soft drinks, your job will be much harder. If these foods are beckoning you from open bowls or boxes, you can count on your weight-loss efforts failing. But if these temptations aren't readily available, you've created a line of defense against impulse eating.

But the kids and my spouse will complain if I don't bring this stuff home. The short answer is *too bad.* The longer answers are:

- Junk food isn't doing them any good. If your kitchen is full of healthier and more nutritious options, everybody wins.
- Are you buying these goodies for them . . . or for you?
- If anyone else in the family is struggling with weight—especially one or more children or teenagers—it's important to make their environment as temptation free as possible.

- Whether only one person in the family is too heavy or everyone could stand to shape up, the family needs to work as a team to support (or at least not undermine) the weight-loss effort.

Caution: Your efforts to purge the home of unhealthy, high-calorie snacks would be best done without becoming a dietary Darth Vader or a food fascist. Talk with your family about the changes you (and they) need to make and get their input. (Mom and Dad should already be on the same page before this conversation. If not, any disgruntled children will quickly divide and conquer to disrupt your efforts.) You may discover that they're not as attached to these foods as you thought. Your family may also prefer to phase in this process over time. For example, if you've been buying megabags of chips, try an assortment of individual servings instead. They're not as economical, but the calorie savings may well be worth it. The same goes for buying individual, smaller containers of soda or juice drinks rather than liter- or larger-sized bottles. Consider low-fat, reduced-sugar frozen yogurt rather than ice cream, or some fresh fruit instead of either of these for dessert.

Here are some other areas you need to be thinking about:

- Do you allow (or sneak) food all over the house?
- Do you do a lot of eating in the car?
- Does your workplace seem like an open vending machine?
- Does your route to and from work or your most common errands take you through "franchise row," from which all of your favorite foods call your name?
- Do you buy groceries from a list, or do you wander the aisles picking up whatever looks appealing?

All of these, and no doubt many others as well, are situations that cue you to eat, or at least to think about food, usually when you're not particularly hungry. Smokers who are trying to quit have to deal with this all day long, because so many events—a cup of coffee, a phone call, a ride in the car, and many more—become linked to lighting a cigarette. You can spend a lot of energy trying to uncouple the stimulus (that is, the sight, smell, or even thought of food) from the response (eating). But doing this involves exercising our willpower, which for most of us can fluctuate through the course of the day.

Some tips regarding trips to the store: (1) always go with a list; (2) don't shop for groceries when you're hungry; and (3) become a frequent visitor to the produce section.

Why make the battle harder than it already is? It's a lot easier and more practical to reduce the number of opportunities for the unwanted behavior. Someone who is trying to stay sober should stay out of cocktail lounges. A man who has problems with Internet pornography should avoid being alone with an online computer. A compulsive shopper shouldn't walk into a mall with a wallet full of credit cards. If you have a weight problem, it only makes sense to take some control of your environment in order to reduce the opportunities for snacking, impulsive eating, or even binging.

Address the emotional and spiritual issues related to eating.

This is extremely important, because for so many who are overweight or obese *food is the drug of choice to relieve emotional or even spiritual discomfort.* This is particularly critical if food binges (episodes in which hundreds or even thousands of calories are consumed) are part of your weight problem. Indeed, compulsive behaviors—whether involving eating, smoking, abuse of alcohol or other drugs, shopping, pornography, sex, gambling, you name it—all serve some emotional purpose, most often an immediate reduction of discomfort. These behaviors inevitably have serious, or even lethal, long-term consequences. Yet the most severe pain and suffering may not be enough to override whatever pleasure or relief the substance or behavior provides at the moment.

Wait a minute . . . I'm not like one of those drug addicts on the street. I'm behaving responsibly at home, work, and church, and getting quite a bit accomplished as well.

So noted, and much appreciated. But you can be a good person and do all of those good things, and still have a serious weight problem because eating is a form of release that happens to be legal, easily obtainable, quickly satisfying in public or in secret, and rarely singled out in church as a moral issue. Whether a full-blown compulsion or a quiet release, eating can be a response to any number of emotional aches and pains:

- the stresses of life, whether minor or monumental
- anxiety, whether short-term or chronic
- frustration over today's events—or all of life
- anger and its chronic cousin, bitterness
- fatigue
- boredom
- loneliness
- depression
- a defense against intimacy or attention from the opposite sex

The last item on this list might seem surprising—doesn't the overweight person long for a sexually attractive body? Certainly many do, but some women who have been sexually abused in the past may unconsciously seek protection from further exposure to this trauma by wrapping themselves in enough fat to ward off male attention.

People who are depressed can have an increased or decreased appetite. Also, as mentioned earlier in this chapter, some antidepressant medications can contribute to weight gain.

Acquiring and maintaining emotional health is a lifelong, multidimensional process, one that we will explore in more depth in chapter 8. It is also directly connected with spiritual health, because experiencing an intimate, nurturing experience with God plays a foundational role in the way you look at yourself, your life, and the people around you. (We'll examine this all-important topic in chapter 9.)

If you have a long-standing and seemingly unmanageable weight problem, it is unlikely that you will solve it merely by adjusting the types and amounts of food you eat. Even if you feel that any emotional issues are the result rather than the cause of the weight, it is essential that you begin to deal with them—and to do some exploring of underlying currents as well. This may involve individual counseling, a small group within your church in which you feel safe dealing with difficult and personal subjects, or a support group specifically focused on weight issues, such as Overeaters Anonymous.

Gather your support team.

If you are ten pounds over your target weight, you probably don't need to do this. But if you have a long way to go, and especially if you've had a long way to go for a long time, you shouldn't be traveling alone. Later in this book we will look at tobacco, alcohol, and drug addiction, and describe how breaking loose from these substances nearly always requires the support of others. In some ways a major weight problem is an even tougher challenge, because there is no way to be abstinent from food. You must interact with it and deal with the physiological and emotional impact of food in your life for months while you are losing weight and for the rest of your life thereafter.

You already know that this is an uphill battle. You want to make healthy eating choices, but your impulses, emotions, and most of the culture push you in the opposite direction. Though you might hope otherwise, you have probably figured out that there isn't a quick fix available now or in the foreseeable future. (Even surgery, for those who are candidates, is such a significant event that counseling and ongoing support, both before and afterward, are very important.) You need teammates and supporters for accountability, encouragement, and even inspiration. This is not a job for a Lone Ranger.

While each person's circumstances will differ, there are several basic sources of support that you should be thinking about:

- **God.** Acknowledging our dependence on Him for every heartbeat, let alone for success in a chronic struggle such as this, is the beginning of wisdom. Furthermore, if your eating patterns involve compulsive behaviors such as binges or addictions to certain foods, you will need to address the spiritual implications of this type of slavery sooner or later. One of these is acknowledging that a material object (in this case, food) may be displacing God, satisfying needs and forging emotional bonds that rightly should belong to Him alone. Another has long been known to those in Alcoholics Anonymous and other twelve-step programs, as we will discuss in chapter 10: realizing that we are powerless to manage the addiction (whatever it is), and that we must turn the reins of our lives over to God *daily* in order to do so.
- **A teammate.** One of the best resources you can find for this project will be someone who will cheer you on, hold you accountable in a spirit of love and respect, or (better yet) walk the journey with you. If this person happens to be your spouse and the support is genuine,

your likelihood of success will be greatly enhanced. If your spouse isn't interested in volunteering for this role, don't let that deter you, but rather look for another family member or a friend who will walk with you—in more ways than one. (As we'll discuss in chapter 7, you can benefit from an exercise partner as well.) Caution: If you are making significant changes in your eating habits, you may also have to deal with people, including one or more in your own family, whose words and deeds undermine your efforts. (See sidebar: "Dealing with Detractors" on page 232.)

- **A class or commercial weight-loss program.** In most communities you can find classes or other group programs in a variety of settings: hospitals, churches, community colleges, physicians' offices, a local mall. You should exercise some care before joining one of these, however, in order to avoid exchanging a chunk of your time and money for a lot of frustration. (See "Getting the Most from a Nutrition Program or a Weight-Loss Consultant" on page 246.)
- **A dietitian.** *I've been eating less and exercising more for three months, and the scale hasn't budged. What am I doing wrong?* If you're truly stuck in the process of losing weight, one or more troubleshooting visits with a dietitian can be time very well spent. Of course, you don't have to be at an impasse to seek this type of consultation. If you have a challenging medical or physical problem—you've just had a heart attack or you're newly diagnosed with diabetes or your kidneys aren't functioning properly, for example—you would be wise to have ongoing input from a dietitian. Some or all of your visits may be covered by medical insurance (especially if they are recommended by your physician). Like a private lesson or consultation in any field from skiing to financial planning, you pay extra for personal attention. And like any of those fields, how much you benefit will depend both on the skill of the consultant and your readiness for his or her input.
- **A support group.** Here the emphasis is on interacting with others who are dealing with the same struggle, rather than on hearing instruction from an expert. This may occur informally among friends; within the setting of a church, clinic, or hospital; or under the auspices of groups such as Take Off Pounds Sensibly (TOPS) or Overeaters Anonymous (OA). This is especially important if you need help with compulsive, out-of-control eating patterns. Many churches are now involved in ministries such as Celebrate Recovery that deal not only with alcohol and drugs, but with all forms of compulsions and addictions. (See chapter 10, page 483.)
- **A counselor.** Whether you have been waging a long-term battle with significant obesity or have been struggling to maintain your weight,

PROFILE: OVEREATERS ANONYMOUS

Do you struggle with uncontrolled eating binges in which you down an entire box of cookies or a half gallon of ice cream in one sitting? Is food your primary form of comfort when you're upset or stressed? Do you enjoy eating alone—or in secret? Has your compulsion to eat soundly defeated every New Year's resolution, diet program, and weight-loss commitment you've made to yourself and others? If so, you may want to look into Overeaters Anonymous (OA), which applies the principles of Alcoholics Anonymous, the oldest and best-known recovery group, to compulsive eating.

OA groups teach and practice the twelve steps of recovery that were originally set forth in Alcoholics Anonymous's *Big Book* in 1939 and have been adapted for groups dealing with various forms of addiction. These are often described as self-help groups, but in fact the central theme of the steps is the utter powerlessness of the individual to overcome the compulsive behavior and the need to turn the reins of one's life over to God. We describe the Twelve Steps in some detail in chapter 10 (see page 480), but in essence they embody strong themes of repentance, submission to God, confession, restitution, and ongoing self-examination.

Some 7,000 OA groups meet regularly in fifty countries. Each group is self-supporting, unaffiliated with any public or private organization, nonpolitical, and independent of any specific religious group. OA also does not promote any particular diet program. The focus is entirely on becoming free of compulsive eating with the support of and accountability to others who are dealing with this problem. Needless to say, one can participate in OA while utilizing other resources to address a weight problem. Indeed, the help a person receives in an OA group may be the key to implementing sound nutritional advice that he or she has known for years but has been seemingly powerless to put into consistent action.

To learn more about this organization, check its Web site at www.oa.org. Other contact information:

Overeaters Anonymous
P.O. Box 44020
Rio Rancho, New Mexico 87174-4020
Telephone: (505) 891-2664
Fax: (505) 891-4320
E-mail: info@oa.org

you need to address the emotional issues in your life—especially those that provoke overeating as a form of comfort or self-medication. A trained counselor can help you gain insight and offer strategies that might take much longer to figure out on your own. Some counselors have special training in handling food-related issues, although such expertise is not mandatory for a counselor to provide useful and compassionate help with a weight problem.

Give this project the time and attention it deserves.
If you get nothing else from this segment, take this thought home: If you have a significant weight problem, and especially if you have fought a losing battle for years, don't sell yourself short by taking a random stab at it now and again. Don't pursue the quick fixes and the magic formulas and the miracle supple-

PROFILE: TAKE OFF POUNDS SENSIBLY (TOPS)

If you're looking for some helpful and inexpensive support for your weight-loss efforts, you may want to look into Take Off Pounds Sensibly. TOPS is a nonprofit, noncommercial international weight-loss support organization founded in 1948 and currently boasting some 200,000 members in 10,000 chapters across the United States, Canada, and a number of foreign countries. Members pay modest annual dues and can attend weekly meetings where an equally modest tab (about a dollar) covers a private weigh-in followed by a motivational program and discussion. One can also become an online member without attending chapter meetings. TOPS encourages members to follow the specific dietary advice of their own physician or dietitian, but it also encourages the use of the dietary exchange system formulated decades ago by the American Diabetes Association and the American Dietetic Association. It also publishes a magazine for its members and sponsors retreats and rallies.

In addition to providing ongoing support for its members, since 1966 TOPS has donated more than $5 million to obesity research at the Medical College of Wisconsin in Milwaukee, where the TOPS Center for Obesity and Metabolic Research opened in 1994.

You can learn more about TOPS and find a local chapter on its Web site at www.tops.org, or by contacting it at:

TOPS Club, International
4575 South Fifth Street
P.O. Box 070360
Milwaukee, WI 53207-0360
(414) 482-4620

ments. They'll waste your time and money, and they can make your problem worse if your weight yo-yos up and down with each passing fad. It takes time to learn the basics of nutrition, to become a smarter shopper, to try new and healthier recipes, to figure out what you're preparing for dinner tomorrow rather than hitting the drive-through, to exercise, to work on your emotional issues, to meet with health professionals who can actually help you. Next to quitting smoking (if you have that particular habit), losing excess weight should be the most important item on your health agenda.

A Brief Tour of Popular Diet Plans

One of the most confusing aspects of the current weight-loss scene is the abundance of contradictory advice about foods you should emphasize—or eliminate. Your local bookstore or library contains literally dozens of diet books that claim to have the inside track on the right and wrong foods, but these tracks go in several very different directions. To list and comment on all of them would be impractical and would bore you senseless. (Besides, there's always a new crop of titles every year.) However, we can gather most of them into a few groups with common themes and characteristics. Armed with some basic understanding of nutrition—read chapter 5 if you haven't already—as well as some perspective on current trends in weight loss and a healthy dose of skepticism, you can decide whether the latest diet best seller or surefire diet plan beckoning from the magazine at the supermarket checkout line is potentially worthwhile or a lot of hype.

Low fat/high carbohydrate

As we discussed in chapter 5, a few decades ago researchers concluded that elevated blood cholesterol was associated with an increased risk for diseased arteries, heart attack, and stroke. Furthermore, foods containing fat tend to be more calorie dense—fat, after all, contains nine calories per gram, while carbohydrates and protein contain four calories per gram. Therefore, if you want to lose weight and avoid having a heart attack, avoiding fat would be a good idea, right?

"Reduce your intake of fat" has in fact been advised for decades, but some have promoted this idea as the main event, the first commandment both for health and healthy weight. The most widely quoted proponent of a fat-restricted diet is Dean Ornish, M.D., founder and director of the Preventive Medicine Research Institute in Sausalito, California, and author of several books, including *Eat More, Weigh Less*. He advocates a very low-fat diet (less than 10 percent of total calories from fat) that is plant based—whole grains, fruits, and vegetables—except for nonfat dairy products and egg whites. All meats, oils, and products that contain oils, nuts and seeds, olives, avocados, and any commercial product containing more than 2 grams of fat per serving are to be avoided or eaten as little as possible. While his 1990 book *Dr. Dean Ornish's*

Program for Reversing Heart Disease gave a green light to nearly any type of carbohydrate, more recently he has discouraged sugar and refined/processed carbohydrates.

His comprehensive program for patients with coronary disease includes moderate exercise, stress management, and group support. He has published controlled studies in reputable medical journals demonstrating weight loss and even reduction of coronary artery disease among patients who adhere closely to his program. How much of their improvement is specifically related to diet (as

DEALING WITH DETRACTORS

You would think that everyone in your circle of family and friends would be excited about your changes in eating habits, especially if one or more of them have been dropping hints about your weight. Think again. Your weight-loss efforts and their results may provoke some responses you didn't expect.

"Don't rock our boat." Ever try to row a boat when three other people in the same boat are rowing in the opposite direction? Some gallant parents (usually moms) struggle to change their eating habits while preparing and serving meals for a houseful of people who aren't interested in changing theirs. With rare exception, this will be a recipe for frustration and failure. Unfortunately, not everyone in the family may be excited if you decide to bypass fast-food restaurants and bring home some healthier items from the store. ("Hey, Mom, when are you going to get off this health-food kick?") You may also get some flak from relatives who equate the amount of food you eat with your love and gratitude. ("I made your favorite apple pie, and you won't eat any. Are you sick or something?")

Your best bet is to have a heart-to-heart with family members, individually or together, in which you explain what you're trying to do and why. If you're embarking on a highly restricted approach—for example, one in which you replace most of your food with special snacks and shakes from a commercial weight-loss program—the adults and older adolescents in your family may have to prepare their own food. A better approach, for many reasons, is to make healthier choices a family project, one in which neither you nor anyone else must endure deprivation.

Remember: Healthy eating patterns shouldn't require spartan, unpleasant, or bizarre food choices. Yes, the junk—the fatty or sugary (or both), highly processed stuff that carries big calorie loads and little else—will need to go or at least be seriously restricted, but that will help everyone live longer. And yes, the overweight person(s) will have to deal with portions and the other dynamics of overeating. But food that is good for a person trying to lose weight is good for everyone else as well, not to mention just plain good in aroma, taste, and

opposed to the other elements of his program) is unclear, although Dr. Ornish advocates forcefully for the entire package.

Another low-fat program was popularized by inventor Nathan Pritikin, who in 1956 discovered that his blood cholesterol level was well above 300. He then failed a stress test, suggesting the presence of significant coronary artery disease. Facing this grim situation at the age of forty-one, he questioned the prevailing medical advice of that time, which in essence said, "Don't exercise, don't climb stairs, take naps, and don't bother changing your diet because you

texture. This sensible-eating approach is definitely preferable if more than one family member needs to lose weight. The chances of success are greatly enhanced if everyone works together, encourages one another to stay the course, and agrees to eat the same types of foods.

"You're making me uncomfortable." If you've been eating out on a regular basis with friends who enjoy feasting, what happens when you shift gears to more sensible fare and smaller portions? Hopefully they'll applaud and encourage your decision. But some may feel uneasy, because they know *they* should do likewise but aren't ready. Or they may even become a little jealous as you begin to look (and feel) better while they remain in the same rut. As harsh as it may sound, rather than being inspired by your example, some will feel better if you *don't* succeed. It's a syndrome as old as sin—as much as we may say otherwise, it's hard to keep envy from rearing its ugly, little green head when someone we know starts doing better in life—especially when he or she worked hard to reach a goal and *especially* when we know we could make similar gains if we put our mind to it. We'll never say it out loud, but it's somehow reassuring when another person slips back to the old familiar routines.

There are all sorts of subtle (and not so subtle) ways that others may undermine your efforts: offering you food, offering you *more* food, encouraging you to "live a little" just for tonight, needling you about being a health nut, and so on. A variation on this theme occurs when the smoker or drinker decides to call it quits: The old gang that enjoys tobacco and alcohol may not want to lose a member. In order to stay on track, you may need to draw some clear but friendly boundaries. Don't back away from having a heart-to-heart with any friends who seem to be pulling you away from your goals. If they really care about you and your health, they'll be willing to support you and perhaps even join you. If they're not willing to back you, it may be time to part company for a while and spend more time with people who will. Whatever you do, don't make a lot of bold claims about what you are going to do and then fail to follow through. No one will take you seriously the next time you make the effort. ■

can't control your own cholesterol." Instead, he embarked on a vegetarian diet and a rigorous program of walking and jogging. By 1960 his cholesterol was a mere 120 and a follow-up stress test was normal.

Encouraged by these results, Pritikin initiated a number of research projects, wrote several books (including *Pritikin Program for Diet and Exercise*), and in 1975 opened the Pritikin Longevity Center. Now located in Aventura, Florida, the Center has hosted some 75,000 guests, who spend one or two weeks in a resort-like setting to initiate lifestyle changes based on Pritikin's dietary and exercise principles. The diet is similar to that advocated by Dr. Ornish, though a single small serving of lean meat is allowed every day. Dozens of research studies in mainstream scientific journals have documented a number of medical benefits, including weight loss, reduced cholesterol and triglycerides, and improved control of diabetes among individuals who have followed this or a similar dietary and exercise approach. After Nathan Pritikin's death in 1985, his autopsy reportedly revealed that he was free of coronary artery disease.

Nathan Pritikin's son Robert now carries his father's low-fat torch, but he has reframed it somewhat in what he calls the Calorie Density Solution. In the book *The Pritikin Principle,* he advocates eating foods that have a low-calorie density—that is, fewer calories per pound—without going hungry or worrying about portions. As you might imagine, fruits, vegetables, beans, and unprocessed grains have much lower calorie densities than highly processed, fatty, and sugary foods. (A pound of broccoli, for example, contains a mere 130 calories, while a pound of chocolate chip cookies packs more than 2,000.) Low-density foods, many of which have a lot of fiber, generally create a sense of fullness (especially if a generous amount of water is part of the meal), and so Pritikin claims that one can eat them freely without worrying about portions or going hungry. The book lists hundreds of foods according to their calorie density, and following the program involves keeping the average calorie density for a meal below a certain level. He also recommends walking thirty miles a week, or more than four miles per day—a worthy goal, but at a brisk pace this represents at least an hour of walking every day.

Advantages: There can be little doubt that someone who perseveres on a diet consisting of vegetables, fruits, unprocessed grains, and very little fat can nearly always expect to lose weight and see improvements in cholesterol, triglycerides, and blood glucose. Add some regular moderate exercise and the results will be even better. From a strictly medical perspective, there is not much to quibble about, and a body of research supports the benefits of this approach. In fact, some research into the role of the hormone leptin adds some weight, so to speak, to the low-fat position (see sidebar: "Leptin, Ghrelin, Yo-Yo, and Low-Fat Diets" on page 236).

Disadvantages: If you're already used to a low-fat diet, you probably don't have a weight problem. For everyone else, maintaining this type of diet requires considerable commitment—indeed, perhaps more than you might be willing to sustain, unless a major heart attack or some other medical crisis precipitated your dietary conversion experience. To shift to daily fare containing less than 10 percent fat represents a rather drastic change for most Americans. Serious makeovers in shopping, food preparation, and eating out need to be learned and practiced. This is one reason why many who launch the Pritikin program do so in a weeklong immersion experience at its Longevity Center. (The calorie-density approach of Robert Pritikin can be eye-opening, but Nutrition Facts labels don't include "calories per pound," and keeping track of these numbers adds another layer to an admittedly challenging task.) While a very low-fat meal, especially one high in fiber, can fill the stomach without a major load of calories, it also won't satisfy hunger nearly as long as a meal with a bit more fat in it. Eating more frequently may result, which may or may not undermine weight-loss efforts, depending on the number of calories involved. In general, many nutrition experts question the wisdom of diets—whether very low fat or very low carbohydrate—that essentially banish an entire class of nutrients. Not all fats are bad for you, and some are essential, as we discussed in chapter 5.

One additional caution: those who embark on Dr. Ornish's comprehensive program should be aware that his approach to stress management reflects a strong commitment to yoga—not merely as a source of stretching and breathing exercises, but as a comprehensive spiritual worldview.[16] The word *yoga* means "yoke" or "union," and the ultimate purpose of yogic practices is to bring about an *experience* of the unity of all things in the universe, a worldview known as *monism*. While adherents generally claim that yoga is compatible with all religious traditions, its premise and purpose flatly contradict the biblical understanding that God is distinct from His creation (including us), and that He alone is God. Needless to say, it is not necessary to adopt an Eastern religious or mystical worldview in order to lose weight using a low-fat program.

Very low or limited carbohydrate

The notion that avoiding or limiting carbohydrates can help you lose weight has been expounded for well over a century, but in the past two decades low-carb diet plans have taken off like a rocket. In case you need convincing, check your neighborhood bookstore or library, where you can find shelves lined with books explaining how to do Atkins, Protein Power, Sugar Busters!, the South Beach Diet, the Carbohydrate Addicts Diet, the Glucose Revolution, the Zone, and a host of others. Many of these have become literal franchises, as the success of an author's first book leads to numerous sequels that provide updated information about the particular plan, new recipes, variations on the diet's basic theme for various groups (kids, adolescents, women, seniors), and so on. The term *Atkins,* once merely shorthand for the stringent low-carbohydrate program created by Robert C. Atkins, M.D., has become not only a brand name attached to a variety of foods but also a part of everyday lingo in phrases such as "on Atkins," or "Atkins friendly."

LEPTIN, GHRELIN, YO-YO, AND LOW-FAT DIETS

You may have heard about **leptin**, a hormone whose discovery in 1994 was initially heralded as the key to curing obesity. Controlled by what is called the obese (or "ob" for short) gene and secreted by fat cells, leptin affects appetite and metabolism. When fat stores become low, leptin levels drop, resulting in increased appetite and a decreased metabolic rate. As fat stores increase so do leptin levels, resulting in decreased appetite and an increased metabolic rate. Mice that lack leptin because of a genetic defect eat like there's no tomorrow and literally look like little furry billiard balls. When injected with leptin, they resume a normal appetite and size. (The word *leptin* comes from the Greek *leptos,* meaning "thin.")

News of leptin's amazing effect on mice led to speculation that obese people were short on this hormone, and that leptin injections would become the breakthrough treatment. (Leptin can't be taken orally because the stomach digests it.) Alas, it has been found that with few exceptions overweight people have plenty of leptin and injecting them with more doesn't curb their appetite or speed their metabolism. Researchers theorize that excess fat leads to a lack of response to leptin, just as type 2 diabetics have plenty of insulin but are resistant to its effects.

Unfortunately for dieters who succeed in losing weight, shrinking fat cells mean less leptin is in circulation, so appetites may increase while metabolism slows down. If they bail out of their weight-loss plan for any length of time, metabolism may not automatically speed up, resulting in the infamous "overshoot" effect—gaining more weight than was lost. Furthermore, when people lose weight, the stomach releases another hormone called **ghrelin**, which increases appetite. These hormones may contribute to the plight of yo-yo dieters, who lose and gain weight several times and find that excess fat seems more difficult to lose with every attempt.

Interestingly, ghrelin levels are less likely to rise when people lose weight on very low-fat diets—an effect that is unique to this dietary approach. (Ghrelin levels also appear to decrease among people who have undergone gastric bypass surgery. These individuals commonly report having less hunger after their operation.)[17] Furthermore, some research suggests that the brain's sensitivity to leptin increases as a person loses weight on a very low-fat diet, so that appetite is less likely to increase even when leptin levels fall. These hormonal perks might help people on very low-fat diets maintain their weight loss—provided, of course, that they are willing and able to stick with this type of cuisine.[18] ■

If a trip to the bookstore doesn't impress you, check the labels at your local food store. In the 1980s and 1990s, when fat was widely proclaimed to be the nutritional villain, thousands of "low fat" and "nonfat" products appeared everywhere in the supermarket. Now food manufacturers have jumped on the low-carbohydrate bandwagon, and products claiming to be "low in net carbs" or "part of your low-carbohydrate lifestyle" are everywhere.

The low-carb books share some basic assumptions:

1. Carbohydrates—especially sugars and refined starches without much fiber—are more rapidly converted to glucose than proteins and fats, causing a rise in

WHAT DOES THE PHRASE *NET CARBS* MEAN ON A FOOD LABEL?

You won't find the term *net carbs* in any nutrition textbook or on the Nutrition Facts label of a product. Used as a marketing tool by food manufacturers, net carbs (sometimes called "impact," "effective," or "active" carbs) refers to the amount of carbohydrate in a given food that is likely to affect blood sugar levels. It is calculated by taking the total grams of carbohydrate in a serving and subtracting the number of grams of fiber and of sugar alcohols such as mannitol and sorbitol that the body generally does not absorb.

When a label says that a food has "low net carbs," does that means it's good for you? Not necessarily.

- While fiber is indeed a useful ingredient, the impact on one's health and blood sugar of large quantities of sugar alcohols (which are often abundant in sweet foods with "low net carbs," where they serve as artificial sweeteners) is unknown.
- While you're busy counting up your net carbs in a food (especially one of those all-purpose food/energy bars), you may overlook the grams of fat and, more important, the total calories in the bar.
- The Food and Drug Administration (FDA) has neither defined what terms such as *low carb* and *carb free* actually mean, nor has it officially addressed what net carbs actually refers to or what (if anything) can be claimed about them. The only information on a product label that is reviewed and regulated by the FDA is what appears inside the "Nutrition Facts" box.

Here's a tip: If you're looking for foods that are naturally low in the type of carbohydrates that impact your blood sugar, head for the produce section. Nutrition bars that boast "low net carbs" may be a convenient snack (or even a meal substitute), and they're likely to be better for you than a candy bar or a bag of chips, but fruits and vegetables are a far better source of nutrients. ■

insulin levels. The intensity of this response is related at least in part to the glycemic index of a food, a concept we described in chapter 5 (see page 138).

2. Insulin not only escorts glucose into cells that need it for fuel but also facilitates storage of extra calories as fat. It also inhibits mobilization of fat as a source of fuel, even when a person is consuming fewer calories. Furthermore, a rapid rise in insulin levels may result in a drop in blood glucose, causing more hunger.
3. All of the advice to eat less fat and more carbohydrates over the past three decades has been misguided and has unintentionally contributed to America's current epidemic of obesity and diabetes.
4. Limiting your intake of carbohydrates will stop the glucose-insulin roller coaster and promote weight loss with much less hunger and hassle than low-fat diets.

The Atkins diet, introduced in 1972 in the book *Dr. Atkins' Diet Revolution* and reintroduced in 1992 in *Dr. Atkins' New Diet Revolution,* takes these assumptions a step further by recommending very stringent carbohydrate restrictions. During the first two weeks on the Atkins plan, total carbohydrate intake is to be reduced to 20 grams per day—the amount in about three cups of salad—primarily in the form of certain leafy green vegetables. Sugars and starchy carbohydrates such as white bread, potatoes, white rice, and pasta from refined grains are banished more or less indefinitely. Larger quantities of carbohydrates are allowed over time depending on the progress of weight loss, although the types to be eaten (including vegetables and fruits) are carefully regulated according to their carbohydrate and fiber content. In dramatic contrast to the very low-fat approaches of Nathan Pritikin and Dean Ornish, the Atkins dieter partakes freely of protein and fat. Meats (including red meat), fish (including shellfish), fowl, cheese, eggs, mayonnaise, butter, and olive oil are all given the green light. For overweight Americans who had been told that they would have to give up so many of their favorite rich foods in order to lose weight, Atkins' regimen sounded like a dream come true.

The paradox of eating rich foods in order to lose weight is explained by a couple of important survival mechanisms. With so little carbohydrate available to serve as fuel, the body taps into its stores of glycogen—the quick-release fuel that we store in limited amounts in muscle and the liver.

Depending on activity levels, glycogen will become depleted within a couple of days, after which the body will begin generating glucose directly from fat. This process releases chemical compounds called **ketones** into the blood, creating a condition called **ketosis** (which, by the way, also develops during starvation or an extended fast). Ketosis has the effect of suppressing appetite—a biochemical mercy when no food is available—thus theoretically preventing the Atkins dieter from overdoing the rich foods.

Not entirely clear on what glucose and glycogen are? See pages 124 and 141 in chapter 5.

When Atkins' first book appeared in 1972, it was greeted with scorn from the nutritional and medical establishments, which condemned it as dangerous and ineffective. His 1992 follow-up was similarly criticized but sold millions of copies. Critics attributed all weight loss solely to water eliminated from the body when glycogen stores were burned. However, this only accounts for a few pounds and could not explain more substantial weight losses—fifty pounds and beyond—experienced by a number of Atkins dieters. Critics described prolonged ketosis as dangerous, and warnings abounded that the diet's substantial protein intake would overwork or otherwise harm the kidneys. But other than producing a unique breath aroma, ketosis is a physiological adaptation rather than a true disease state (unlike **ketoacidosis**, an entirely different and very serious condition that can occur among type 1 diabetics—those who are unable to make enough insulin and must take injections to survive). Furthermore, Atkins repeatedly challenged his critics to document a single case in which his diet had actually caused kidney disease or failure. No such cases have made medical headlines, although it should be noted that people who already have impaired kidney function do need to regulate protein intake.

Few if any of the other popular low-carb diets restrict carbohydrates as severely as the Atkins program, but each puts its own variation on what is essentially the same theme. Most have received a chilly reception from mainstream organizations such as the American Dietetic Association and an initial shrug from doctors in everyday practice who typically have little time to sift through the avalanche of these books and programs. So why have these plans sold millions of books, established a growing cultural niche, and even earned some cautious recommendations from physicians?

- **A reasonable theory.** Unlike many fad and crackpot diets that have come and gone over the years, the basic theory of the low- or controlled-carbohydrate plans actually makes some physiologic sense. Concepts such as the glycemic index, insulin resistance, and the role of insulin in storing fat aren't bizarre or imaginary. ***However:*** In order to entice and energize readers, the popular low-carb books tend to oversimplify and oversell their ideas. The interplay of food, glucose, insulin, hunger, cravings, weight gain, and weight loss is more complex than the picture painted by most of these books. Indeed, much research is underway to clarify these intricate mechanisms.
- **Unimpressive results from low-fat diets.** "Eat less fat" was the dominant advice from nutritional experts (and even doctors) for decades, and yet the nation (including those doctors' patients) not only failed to lose weight but actually got fatter. ***However:*** Much of the "eat less fat" advice was too vague, such that many overweight people shifted to nonfat sweet and starchy/refined grain foods. Indeed, one of the few points of agreement between low-fat and low-carb advocates is that these foods should be significantly restricted.
- **More appealing food.** Meats, eggs, butter, and cheese are agreeable to Western palates, and so sticking with the plan may be easier—at

least for a while. ***However:*** The stricter the ban on carbohydrates, the harder it is to hang on for the long haul. Eventually most people become weary of avoiding foods such as bread, potatoes, and pasta that they enjoyed for years.

- **Encouraging results.** Many physicians (including Arthur Agatston, M.D., the Florida cardiologist who devised the South Beach Diet) gave low-carb diets a more serious look when some of their patients actually succeeded in losing weight while following them. In 2003 studies began to appear in respectable medical journals demonstrating that in controlled experimental conditions people on low-carbohydrate diets (including ketosis-inducing versions) were more successful at losing weight than those on the typical low-fat diets that had been recommended by mainstream health organizations for decades. Furthermore, weight loss on the low-carb diet resulted in lower cholesterol and triglyceride levels, much to the chagrin of those who had argued that the abundant fat in Atkins and similar diets would have the opposite effect. ***However:*** While low-carb diets have performed better than low-fat diets in some research studies for periods of about six months, over longer time frames (one year or more) the differences become less obvious. There are no doubt many reasons for this, but an obvious one was already mentioned in connection with both low-carb and low-fat diets: The more restrictive the plan, the less likely a person will stay with it for the long haul.

Should you follow a low- or controlled-carbohydrate diet if you are trying to lose weight? This type of approach may be useful if you have type 2 diabetes or metabolic syndrome, because with these conditions you're definitely better off limiting the fluctuations in glucose and insulin levels that arise from sugary and starchy foods. Also, many who have struggled with hunger on low-fat diets may experience more success with a controlled-carbohydrate approach. However, you should note the following cautions:

- The approach you choose should not exclude or strictly limit fruits and vegetables (with the exception of potatoes) for an extended period of time. This is the one area in which tightly controlled low-carbohydrate plans may stray from nutritional common sense. If you are being told to avoid the produce section in order to maintain your low-carb lifestyle, you need to find a different plan.
- You do not need to spend a lot of time (or any time) in ketosis to lose weight. The Atkins' plan involves an extended initial period of ketosis brought on by extremely limited carbohydrate intake. The South Beach Diet proposes a two-week induction period with similar limitations and then shifts to a more liberal carbohydrate intake from fruits and vegetables. The Zone diet is less restrictive than either of these, proposing that an ideal dietary blend (which helps put one "in

the Zone" of optimal health and personal performance) is 30 percent protein, 30 percent fat, and 40 percent carbohydrate. Zone authors Barry Sears, Ph.D., and Bill Lawren resist classifying their approach as a low-carb diet. However, like the low-carb plans described in this section, their underlying premise is that the benefits of being "in the Zone" derive largely from controlling the flow of glucose and insulin.

- Maintaining a low-carbohydrate diet is not a license to ignore portions, the fat content of foods, exercise, or the other important components of managing weight.

Fad diets

Fad diets are a diverse group of eating or weight-loss plans with one or more of the following characteristics:

- **A premise that doesn't make scientific or nutritional sense.** Example: Books that claim the right diet for you depends on your blood type, an idea so eccentric that no reputable scientific organization (or even the vast majority of alternative practitioners) takes it seriously.
- **Claims that the diet is "unique," "groundbreaking," "a breakthrough," etc.** Translation: "I thought this up myself."
- **Extreme restrictions or a focus on a single "miracle" food that boosts metabolism, burns fat, etc.** Examples: the grapefruit diet, the cabbage soup diet, the peanut butter diet, the chicken soup diet, and the apple cider vinegar diet. (There's even a chocolate diet!) Any of these may work for a while, based on two principles. First, if you can eat only one or a handful of foods, after a while you don't look forward to eating, except as a way to curb hunger. (Before long, of course, you'll get sick of the whole thing and toss the diet overboard.) Second, some of these diets tell you to eat smaller portions, exercise more, avoid sugary and rich foods, and (by the way) be sure to eat the featured food every day. Guess which component of the diet actually results in weight loss?
- **Diets invented or endorsed by a celebrity.** They may be sensible or silly, but they depend on a basic craving of many overweight people: "If only I could look just like ______________."
- **Diets that involve "food-combining" or other convoluted restrictions.** Example: Diets that claim you shouldn't eat fruits with other types of food, or that you shouldn't combine starches and vegetables at the same meal, or that you *can* combine starches and vegetables as long you don't add fat, and so on. Usually these diets are based on the ideas of some obscure author of a century or so ago, and none are consistent with solid nutritional science. They also tend to imply that following their particular formula is the best (or only) way for us to enjoy good health. Here's a question to ask of all food-combining

diets: *How in the world did the human race survive (let alone lose weight) before this diet was published?*

- **Diets that claim to "detox" (detoxify) your body.** (See sidebar "Should I Do a 'Detox' Diet?" on the next page.)

Paleolithic/raw foods/Bible diets

A number of books on the market advocate a *real* back-to-basics approach to eating. Some might object to grouping these various types of diets together, but they share some common assumptions: First, because of modern agricultural techniques, processing, chemical additives, and environmental pollution, our modern diet and even our basic food supply are deeply flawed. Second, at least some of our ancestors thousands of years ago suffered less disease because they had better (if limited) food supplies, or because they followed God's directives regarding their dietary choices. Therefore, in order to regain or maintain health, we need to restore the dietary practices of ancient—or in some cases, really ancient—times.

The "best" foods will depend on the author's perspective:

- Paleolithic approaches propose that we evolved over millions of years to thrive on the foods available to prehistoric hunter-gatherers—fruits, vegetables, nuts, fish, and wild game. Some insist that human health went downhill with the dawn of agriculture and the herding of animals for food. When ancient civilizations figured out how to grow and harvest grains and then use them as foods, or to eat meat, milk, eggs, and their various by-products from domesticated animals, they were going against the evolutionary grain, so to speak.
- Raw-food enthusiasts insist that the only foods that are fit to eat are uncooked fruits, vegetables, nuts, and seeds, which are often called living foods. Cooking any of these is said to destroy vital nutrients, especially enzymes that are necessary for digestion and other health benefits.
- An emerging genre of diet books are those that look to Scripture for guidance, taking note of the various kinds of foods mentioned throughout the Old and New Testaments, and especially those that were declared clean and unclean in the dietary laws found in Leviticus 11 and Deuteronomy 14. Some extrapolate from various passages to offer a "Bible cure" for diseases such as cancer, arthritis, bowel disorders, and of course excessive weight.

Advantages: If readers of these books are convinced to eat more fresh fruits, vegetables, legumes, nuts, and seeds, as well as to shun highly processed, sugar- and additive-laced concoctions, they will definitely benefit. The foods in these diets are abundant in useful nutrients, including vitamins, minerals, and phytochemicals, and (with the exception of nuts) are not calorie dense.

Because of the amount of fiber present and the time it takes to chew and

SHOULD I DO A "DETOX" DIET?

The prospect of detoxifying the body has a lot of appeal both for people trying to lose weight and for those suffering from fatigue or other chronic complaints. The premise goes something like this: Chemicals that pollute our air, water, seas, and soil have found their way into our food (or they have been put there during modern processing) and have accumulated in our body. Our ability to eliminate them is hampered by poor food quality, stress, and a number of other factors, resulting in weight gain, fatigue, depression, headaches, bowel problems, arthritis, and even cancer. We may be harboring harmful organisms such as *Candida albicans,* which release more toxins into the body. This state of toxicity can be treated by a usually stringent combination of raw fruits and vegetables, a water or juice fast, supplements, herbs, colon cleansing (including enemas), and perhaps other treatments as well, including massage, breathing exercises, aromatherapy, and so on. Words such as *flushing, cleansing, neutralizing, elimination,* and even *scrubbing* (as in, "our product will scrub out your cells") are used frequently, bringing to mind a spring cleaning of the body, after which health and well-being (not to mention weight loss) will follow. All sorts of detox programs are marketed on the Internet, in health-food stores and spas, and via infomercials, often with price tags as impressive as their claims.

Alas, while the detox concept provides some appealing mental imagery, otherwise it is at best vague and at worst mythological. The promoters of these diets and programs never identify, let alone measure, the actual toxins that are supposedly being eliminated. None can offer any reasonable biological explanation of how their diet, supplements, or treatments remove toxins or help the body perform this function. There is no coherent body of research that demonstrates or remotely proves the existence of a detox process as described by these individuals and companies. The words may be different, but the twenty-first-century pitch bears a striking resemblance to the nineteenth-century medicine show, and in both cases the marketing horse is many miles out of the scientific barn.

Bottom line: There's nothing wrong with getting back to basics with some wholesome fruits and vegetables, and cutting back on the processed foods and megaportions. We will feel better, but we don't need to buy into (literally) a lot of supplements, enemas, and half-baked theories to get this result. ■

swallow raw foods, it's difficult to become or remain obese when these are your main source of nutrition. Most proponents of these various diets stress eating organically grown produce, for which the benefit may (or may not) be worth the extra cost. If the diets that include animal products also convince readers to eat more fish (while limiting the top-of-the-food-chain species that may harbor worrisome amounts of mercury) and to seek meats from free-range animals rather than those raised in feedlots, readers may gain additional health benefits.

For more information about mercury in fish, turn to page 153 in chapter 5.

Disadvantages: Most of the problems with these diets arise from what we might call excess baggage: ideas that are eccentric, excessive, or even oppressive.

- **Paleolithic diets:** These are built on speculation—not only leaning on evolutionary theory in general, but also on a dubious assumption that our prehistoric ancestors (some would say humanoids) were healthier than we are. It would be difficult to prove that mankind would benefit from reverting to a hunter-gatherer diet and abandoning grains, which are staple foods for most of the world's population.
- **Raw foods:** The assumption that cooking somehow saps all the vital essence from vegetables or fruits is misguided. (Meats are definitely off the raw-food menu. Some proponents also exclude foods such as corn that do not grow in the wild.) True, you do lose some nutrients if you boil vegetables and toss out the water. But cooking also renders many foods more digestible (not to mention more palatable). Furthermore, the benefits of beta-carotene in carrots and lycopene in tomatoes are enhanced when they are cooked. Also, raw-food enthusiasts need to plan carefully (or take supplements) to get adequate amounts of vitamin B_{12} (found only in animal products), omega-3 fatty acids, calcium, and iron.

  One claim made by many raw-food enthusiasts is that we need the enzymes found within fruits, vegetables, nuts, and seeds to digest them, and that these enzymes are destroyed by cooking. Actually, whatever enzymes are present in food (raw or cooked) are unceremoniously broken down in our stomach and small intestine to provide amino acids to make our own proteins. (As we saw in chapter 5, enzymes are complex proteins that serve as catalysts to speed very specific reactions within plants and animals. Enzymes found in plants serve the plant, not the one eating the plant, except as a source of amino acids.)

  One other caveat—sharing a meal with others is one of the most significant forms of human interaction, and those on raw-food diets need to exercise creativity and finesse to deal with social situations involving eating. A worst-case scenario would be for an individual to adopt an obsessive (or worse yet, judgmental) posture regarding food that would isolate himself or herself from others.
- **Bible diets.** There's nothing wrong, and a lot that's right, with building a diet around the foods mentioned in the Bible, including meats

declared to be clean in the Old Testament. But in many areas such as this, where the Scriptures do not offer clear moral directives for all times and peoples, some cannot resist offering their own particular interpretation or even going beyond what is clearly stated in the biblical texts and then declaring their position to be God's way of doing whatever is under discussion. Such certainty of divine authority puts someone with a different opinion in an awkward position: *If I don't agree with you, are you saying that I'm disobeying God?* This becomes a thornier problem when those promoting the diet throw extraneous and controversial opinions—for example, opposing immunizations or condemning the use of mercury amalgams in dental fillings—into the mix.

One other caution: Some authors can't resist the temptation to promote their own brand of vitamins, supplements, and other items apparently necessary for good health—even if you follow their book's advice. Since it would be a little shaky to claim that God's own diet is inadequate, the usual explanation is that our modern food supply is so compromised that handfuls of supplements are necessary, or at least advisable, for maintaining good health. Unfortunately, linking this type of aggressive merchandising to claims of divine authority brings to mind some individuals who were doing brisk business in the Temple courtyards until a certain Galilean drove them out.

We will look at the safety concerns surrounding immunizations in chapter 11.

Here are some important things to remember when considering diets from these camps. While you can appreciate the authors' desire to improve our dietary habits, it's wise to maintain some healthy skepticism as well. You can certainly pick up some suggestions about the foods they promote (none of which are likely to be harmful), but it's also possible to eat well without becoming rigid or obsessive about your choice of foods or how you prepare them. Finally, remember that books claiming to contain the Bible's or God's detailed advice on all diet and health matters should be taken with a grain of salt—or the seasoning of your choice.

"Middle of the road" or lifestyle approaches

These encompass the weight-loss advice you're likely to get from:

- Mainstream professional and academic organizations, such as the American Dietetic Association, the American Heart Association, the American Medical Association, the American Academy of Family Physicians, the Institute of Medicine, Mayo Clinic, and Tufts University Friedman School of Nutrition Science and Policy
- Commercial weight-loss programs such as Weight Watchers or Jenny Craig
- Books such as *Eat, Drink, and Be Healthy*, by Walter C. Willett, M.D., of Harvard Medical School; *The Ultimate Weight Solution* by Phillip

McGraw, Ph.D., (TV's "Dr. Phil"); and *The Tufts University Guide to Total Nutrition*

- Agencies of the federal government such as the Centers for Disease Control and Prevention, the National Institutes of Health, the Food and Drug Administration, and the U.S. Department of Agriculture

You won't get a lot of surprises, magic formulas, or "breakthrough" revelations about food from these sources. Not all of these are precisely aligned in their approach, but for the most part you'll hear a lot of commonsense advice: decrease your caloric intake and portions, increase exercise, cut the sugar, limit fat to 20 to 30 percent of total calories, eat lots of fruits and vegetables, and so on.

Advantages: These resources avoid the extremes, the fads, and the weird ideas that waste time, money, and even health. They are committed to solid research and conservative recommendations. If you spend much time with them, you are likely to pick up ideas and even inspiration that will help you lose weight and keep it off.

Disadvantages: The only potential drawback is the "familiarity breeds contempt" problem: You may think, *This is the "same old same old." I've heard it all before, and it didn't work for me.* This is a losing (and we don't mean weight) mind-set, much like avoiding church because you tell yourself, *I've heard it all before.* If you have a long-standing weight problem, you may be particularly vulnerable to the lure of the latest quick fix, when in fact what you need most is to figure out how to make the more reasonable advice work in daily life.

Getting the Most from a Nutrition Program or a Weight-Loss Consultant

You've decided that it's time to get some help losing weight. Should you join Weight Watchers, try Jenny Craig, see a dietitian, or check out a local weight-loss clinic that just opened? Here's the bottom line first: Think and evaluate carefully *before* you spend your time and money on a program, a dietitian, a nutritionist, or other weight-loss consultant. What specifically should you be thinking about?

Why am I doing this?

Some good reasons to begin such a program are to establish some basic structure for your food choices and a track to run on for the long haul, as well as to receive troubleshooting, insight, accountability, and encouragement.

Some bad reasons are the desire for a quick fix, a magic formula, rapid weight loss, and a radical and restrictive diet, or simply to achieve short-term goals.

The good reasons involve a mind-set that *you,* not someone else, are ultimately in charge and responsible for your health, and that whatever you do must work for the rest of your life. The program or the individual is providing advice and expertise to assist you in the process. The bad reasons involve a passive but often desperate mind-set: *Do something, anything, to me or for me so that I will lose weight without having to address my daily choices.* They also reflect unrealistic expectations and reliance on exotic food formulas or (worse) expensive supplements, rather than an understanding of why some foods are better than others and what behaviors contribute to weight gain.

What are the components of the program?

Don't sign up for any program without knowing exactly what is included—and what you'll be expected to pay for.

- **Information.** Do you just get a list of dos and don'ts, or does the program provide ongoing *education* about nutrition, foods, preparation, and managing your own behavior? Learning to eat well is an important long-term life skill, and the more you know, the more likely you are to make better decisions in the long run. You shouldn't settle for a no-brainer approach to weight loss.
- **Diet plans.** What exactly is the approach to food while you're losing weight? Is the focus on reduced calories, very low calories, low fat, low carb, high protein, food combining, or some other approach? If the plan is extreme (for example, no fats, no carbohydrates, or just fruits, etc.) or far removed from what you're used to eating, it may seem easier to follow . . . at first. It's like starting a really tight, no-frills budget: There's less to think about, and making a decisive change can feel downright energizing. *Hey, I'm really doing something!* If the eating plan is highly restrictive and doesn't include your usual comfort foods, you'll tend to eat simply to quell hunger and not for pleasure, so the pounds will indeed disappear. This is why virtually any diet plan will work—for a while. But as time passes and the novelty wears off, the old foods will begin to sing their siren song. If the plan doesn't have a contingency plan for your previous habits other than "just say no," in a moment of weakness it may get the heave-ho, along with the money you spent on it.
- **Your food or their food?** Some commercial plans offer to supply some or all of your food, prepared, prepackaged, and ready to eat. The advantage of this is that you don't have to do a lot of thinking or preparation, and as long as you carefully follow the program's guidelines, you'll probably lose weight. Also, eating such prepared foods may give you an idea of what reasonable portions of food actually look like. However, such a plan will be more expensive than preparing your own food, and if you don't care for the program's bill of fare, you'll be tempted to cheat. If you're doing prepackaged foods and hope to succeed, your family will have to fend for themselves in the kitchen; it takes nerves of steel to prepare food for others that you're not supposed to eat. Also, since you're not likely to buy from this "store" for the rest of your life, it's often difficult to make the transition from their food to normal food.

- **Very little food.** Some programs give you "substitute meals"—usually some form of powdered concoction that you stir into cold water and drink like a milk shake (only it's not as enjoyable)—in place of one or two regular meals. (Products such as Slim-Fast that serve this purpose are also available at the store; you don't need to join a program to use them.) Very low-calorie diets (sometimes known as **protein-sparing fasts**) drop daily calorie intake to no more than 800 calories, an approach that should only be undertaken under close medical supervision, if ever. As we said earlier, the more restricted eating plans may be more efficient at helping you lose weight in the short run, but you must eventually address a crucial question: *What am I going to do for the rest of my life?* If you go back to the same eating habits, guess what? The pounds you worked so hard to lose will come back, and they may bring a few friends with them.
- **Medications, shots, or supplements.** Beware—if a program offers diet pills or special injections that will "melt off the fat," your chances of long-term success are poor, and you can count on shelling out a fair amount of money that would be better spent elsewhere (such as on fresh vegetables and fruit). We will look at weight-loss medications in a later section.

Who's running the program, and what are their credentials?

You should review this information before any money changes hands. Ideally, a comprehensive program utilizes the services of one or more physicians, registered dietitians, psychologists/counselors, and physical therapists or trainers, all of whom have special expertise in medicine, nutrition, behavior modification, and exercise as they relate to weight loss. Often such programs are formally affiliated with well-established institutions such as universities, regional medical centers, or even local hospitals. At the other end of the spectrum are storefront clinics run by a self-proclaimed expert with little or no formal training.

Beware: Many "nutritionists" with eccentric or even bizarre notions of dietary health offer worthless but often costly tests that are supposed to determine your individual nutrient needs and deficiencies. Worse yet, they frequently have shelves of expensive vitamins and supplements that they promise will correct whatever is wrong, to the tune of one or two hundred dollars per month, or even more.

Before starting a program, find out what type of formal training the staff members have had. This may be easier said than done. Your own physician, for example, may not have much expertise on this subject. Unfortunately, there is no shortage of bogus nutritional schools and "professional" organizations willing to grant degrees or other credentials to anyone who signs up and pays a fee. Furthermore, while it is possible for any health professional (or for that matter a layperson) to gain solid knowledge of nutrition and weight-management techniques through personal study and continuing education courses, the recognized experts in the field are **registered dietitians** or (**R.D.s**).

The person with an R.D. credential has

- earned at least a bachelor's degree from an accredited university or college, with coursework approved by the American Dietetic Association's accrediting organization, the Commission on Accreditation for Dietetics Education (CADE);
- completed a supervised practice program, usually six to twelve months in length, at a CADE-accredited health-care facility, community agency, or food-service corporation;
- passed a national examination administered by the Commission on Dietetic Registration (CDR), which also awards credentials for dietetic technicians as well as specialists in pediatric nutrition and renal nutrition; and
- maintained the R.D. credential through ongoing professional education.

For an individual consultation, a registered dietitian is nearly always the best bet.

As of 1997, only 25 percent of American medical schools had a required nutrition course in the curriculum, while another 50 percent offered an elective course.[19] More recently, however, a number of medical schools have launched programs to integrate nutritional training into clinical practice.[20]

HOT TIP

To get the most from your visit with a dietitian, bring a one- or two-week food diary in which you have written down everything you have eaten—when, what, how much, and what prompted your eating (hunger, coffee break, boredom, etc.). Whether to save face or because of increased awareness of eating patterns during this exercise, many people consume less food when they're keeping a food diary.

What kinds of long-term *results is the program achieving?*

Do any studies or statistics back up the program's claims? Remember—the fact that many clients are able to lose several pounds over the first few weeks may sound impressive, but how many have been able to maintain substantial weight loss over six months, a year, or longer?

How much is it going to cost?

You may be desperate to lose weight and impressed by what you've heard, but don't overlook the *M* word: money. Most programs charge a basic fee to participate, and then you pay extra for food, meal substitutes, medications (if a physician in the program prescribes them), supplements, vitamins, or other services such as lab tests. All of these extras can cost you, so think carefully about what you really need. If the program wants you to get a fasting chemistry and lipid profile but your doctor recently ran the same tests, there may be no need to repeat them right away. Also, your health insurance may cover such tests if ordered by your physician, but not necessarily if they're done by a commercial weight-loss program.

Speaking of insurance, some visits with a registered dietitian or participation in a program (especially one operated from a physician's office, licensed clinic, or hospital) may be at least partially reimbursed by your health plan. Usually this requires an order from your physician, and the dietary consultation or weight-loss program must be tied to a specific medical diagnosis (for example, type 2 diabetes).

Another option is a maximum-impact, multidisciplinary live-in program in which you turn your focus entirely on weight issues for a specified time, such as one or two weeks. These all-inclusive jump starts are quite expensive, and long-term follow-through is essential to get your money's worth. Otherwise, you know what will happen: It's relatively easy to feel inspired and do the right thing when you're immersed in a culture of healthy eating and the food is carefully regimented. But what happens when you return to your own home and job? You need some new coping skills and someone to call if you're having trouble staying the course, or your investment may be squandered.

Other Approaches to Losing Weight

Medications and supplements

Because losing weight is so often a difficult and demanding process, nearly everyone with this problem has longed for a magic bullet that would

- drastically reduce the appetite,
- reduce or block the absorption of fat or starch,
- rev up metabolism,
- selectively "burn" fat, or
- do all of the above.

The ideal concoction would work without our having to make different choices about food and exercise. Ideally, it would work indefinitely—even during sleep. It also would be completely safe, all natural, and affordable. While we're at it, it would also generate boundless energy, reverse the aging process, and enhance our sex life.

Sound familiar? You have no doubt heard of, and perhaps tried, products that have claimed to do all of this and more. Creative entrepreneurs have utilized all sorts of electrical, magnetic, and mechanical contraptions, not to mention patches, creams, wraps, and shoe inserts, to separate the overweight from their money (but not their extra pounds) and have often made them miserable in the process.

Here's an important bottom line: *At the present time, no nonprescription drug or supplement has been shown to be safe and effective for inducing significant long-term weight loss.* Current federal law allows thousands of nonprescription products to be advertised with all sorts of impressive claims, as long as none of them involve treating a specific disease. Unfortunately, none are evaluated by the Food and Drug Administration (FDA) for safety or effectiveness, although the Federal Trade Commission (FTC) may issue warnings to distributors if they are making blatantly misleading statements about their products. Furthermore, a product will be taken off the market only if it is found to be harmful.

This in fact occurred with **ephedra**, a stimulant found in many weight-loss aids (often in the form of the herb *ma huang*) that has been linked to irregular heart rhythm, high blood pressure, stroke, seizures, and even death. In 2004, the FDA prohibited the sale of supplements containing ephedra, although a few may still be in circulation. Another nonprescription drug that was banned by the FDA is **phenylpropanolamine** (or **PPA**), once found both in cold tablets and in diet aids such as Dexatrim and AcuTrim. PPA raised blood pressure and pulse rate too often to be considered safe, and it was even associated with hemorrhagic (bleeding) strokes.

Unfortunately, as obesity has become more widespread in the United States, hundreds of marketers have taken advantage of the opportunity to make some serious cash by offering quick and easy cures to the frustrated and desperate. There are in fact so many weight-loss products lining the shelves and advertised on radio, TV, and especially the Internet that it would be impossible to list even a fraction of them, let alone analyze them. Instead, we will list a number of red-flag claims that are literally too good to be true and that virtually guarantee that a product isn't worth your hard-earned money. Many are a variation on the magic-bullet wish list we included at the beginning of this section:

- **You'll lose two or more pounds every week for several weeks, no matter what you eat and without exercise.** ***Reality check:*** This is the most common—and the least truthful—claim made for weight-loss products. Unfortunately, this promise is a biological fantasy.
- **The product, with or without additional calorie restriction, will cause pounds to "melt away" at spectacular rates (such as a pound per day) for several weeks.** ***Reality check:*** As we mentioned in chapter 5, those who cut their calorie intake significantly will burn glycogen for fuel, and this can result in the loss of several pounds of fluid. (See page 141.) It's encouraging, but it isn't fat. Since a pound of fat represents 3,500 stored calories, to lose a pound of fat in one day would require one to eat nothing while exercising like a lumberjack from dawn until dusk. It doesn't happen.
- **The weight you lose will be permanent. The pounds will stay off, even if you stop using the product.** ***Reality check:*** You can in fact keep the weight off after stopping the product—by maintaining different eating and exercise habits. In other words, you really didn't need the product in the first place.
- **The product will prevent the absorption of fat, resulting in substantial weight loss.** ***Reality check:*** You can lose a modest amount of weight with Xenical, a prescription drug that interferes with fat absorption, but it's hardly a free ride. (See paragraph beginning at the

A 1912 ad for Dr. Cogswell's Reducing Salve claimed that this product, at $2 per jar, "reduces the unhealthy fat, at the same time acting as a corrective by feeding the nerves and building strong, firm, healthy tissue." Better yet, "reducing salve necessitates no change in one's diet or daily routine of living."

bottom of page 253). The only people who lose substantial pounds by failing to absorb nutrients are those with diseases known as **malabsorption syndromes**, which can pose a serious threat to health.

- **The product will produce dramatic results for anyone who uses it. *Reality check:*** When you're talking about any dietary program, medication, or supplement, remember this important phrase: "Results may vary." Nothing works for everyone.
- **Wearing the product or rubbing it on the skin leads to substantial weight loss. *Reality check:*** There is no medical evidence, or even a rational explanation, to support this type of claim, which is the nutritional equivalent of Bigfoot, Elvis sightings, and the tooth fairy.
- **The product is marketed using testimonials. *Reality check:*** This is the least reliable measure of a product's effectiveness. Talk is cheap, and it can easily be purchased by the marketer. Scientifically valid proof that a product is safe and effective requires careful, controlled studies involving large numbers of people.
- **The product contains a formula that is unique, superior to anything on the market, and not available anywhere else. *Reality check:*** In psychiatry such claims would be called delusions of grandeur. Steer clear of any practitioner who offers a treatment or product that is "the only one of its kind," or who implies that "everyone is wrong but me."
- **The product was developed by a leading expert in the field of nutrition. *Reality check:*** There are countless self-proclaimed experts in nutrition. The professionals who are truly respected in this field aren't hawking products on the Internet.

A 1910 advertisement for Fatoff Obesity Cream claimed that this "massage preparation of peculiar reducing properties, pleasant to apply and most exhilarating in effect" had the ability to remove "surplus flesh at the precise place it troubles you." A full-size jar sold for $2.50; "for double chin, $1.50."

What about prescription medications? Can your doctor prescribe a medication that will help you jump-start a diet plan? Mainstream medical thinking has shifted from viewing obesity as a character flaw to treating it as a significant disorder with important health consequences. Furthermore, pharmaceutical manufacturers are well aware that any product that *really* helps people lose excess weight, and does it safely, will be a literal gold mine. As a result, currently a number of promising medications are slowly wending their way through the laborious and expensive development-and-testing process before getting the FDA's green light to enter the marketplace. (This is drastically different from the unregulated environment in which nonprescription drugs are unleashed upon the public.)

At the time of this book's writing, several medications are available at your local pharmacy that might enhance the results of dietary and exercise efforts, but they are hardly miracle drugs that will zap your appetite or melt away the fat. At best they may contribute to a 5 to 10 percent weight loss over the course of several months. This may not seem spectacular, but it could actually make a significant difference in your cholesterol, triglyceride, or blood glucose levels. This would please your doctor, even if it didn't drastically alter what you see in the mirror. The current crop works in one of two ways: altering neurotransmitters in the brain or interfering with the digestion of fat.

Altering neurotransmitters. In the central nervous system, the biochemical "messengers" serotonin, norepinephrine, and dopamine play important roles in both mood and appetite, and medications that affect their levels can also adjust appetite in either direction. Those that tend to reduce it include:

- **Phentermine** (Fastin, Ionamin, and other brands) and **diethylpropion** (Tenuate and others) are stimulants with a mild appetite-suppressing effect. Like other stimulants, they can increase pulse rate and blood pressure, cause tremors, and create a sense of anxiety or irritability.
- **Amphetamines** (Dexedrine and others) are high-powered stimulants used on a tightly regulated basis for treatment of attention-deficit/hyperactivity disorder (ADHD) in children and adults. Not only can they provoke all of the side effects just listed, but they can also be highly addictive, although this is uncommon among those taking amphetamines for ADHD. For these and other reasons *amphetamines are an exceedingly bad choice for weight control.*
- **Sibutramine** (Meridia) is a newer medication that affects both serotonin and norepinephrine levels in the brain to create a sense of fullness with less food. Taken once daily, the drug usually provokes few if any side effects, although it may raise blood pressure a little and should not be used by women who are or might become pregnant. It also isn't recommended for people who are already taking antidepressants (such as Prozac, Zoloft, Paxil, and others) that affect serotonin levels. Indeed, its effect is rather subtle. In one controlled study, people taking sibutramine for a year lost only seven to ten pounds more than those on the same dietary plan taking a placebo. This modest amount may not be exactly earthshaking (especially when the retail price tag is at the hundred-dollar-per-month level), but it may be enough to push lipids and blood glucose in the right direction.
- **Topiramate** (Topamax) is a prescription drug used to control seizures and also to reduce the frequency of migraine headaches. Like other drugs that affect the central nervous system, it has an effect on appetite—in this case, it often reduces it. However, as of this book's publication it has not received formal approval by the Food and Drug Administration for this use, and whether or not it would have this effect over a long period of time, and to what degree, remains to be determined.

For a closer look at the chaos generated by the misuse of amphetamines, turn to page 461 in chapter 10.

Interfering with the digestion of fat. The prescription drug **orlistat** (Xenical) blocks the action of an enzyme called **lipase** that breaks down fats in the intestine so they can be absorbed. At first glance, this sounds like an ideal way to lose weight. But fats that aren't digested continue floating through the

FEN-PHEN: A CAUTIONARY TALE

In 1973 the drug fenfluramine was released as an appetite suppressant that affected serotonin levels but was mildly sedating. Phentermine, released in 1959 as an appetite suppressant, has a stimulant effect. Neither drug by itself was particularly impressive at promoting weight loss, but in 1992 a study in the medical journal *Clinical Pharmacology and Therapeutics* showed that when taken together these medications had a dramatic effect on appetite while limiting each other's side effects. While the combination of these two drugs, which came to be known as Fen-phen, was never promoted by its manufacturers, word of their combined efficiency at curbing appetite spread like wildfire. Most physicians heard about them from patients who were asking for the two prescriptions, and many who prescribed them were impressed by dramatic weight losses, especially among their most seriously overweight patients. In 1996 alone, 18 million prescriptions for this combination were written, though many were taken by people looking for a quick way to lose a modest amount of weight.

Unfortunately, articles in 1997 from the Mayo Clinic and the *New England Journal of Medicine* reported that some who had taken this combination developed heart-valve abnormalities, although later analysis suggested that the likelihood of being affected was low, especially among those who took the drugs for less than three months. Nevertheless, by mid-September the manufacturer of fenfluramine as well as a newer variation called Redux, or dexfenfluramine, withdrew these drugs from the market. Phentermine was not implicated as a cause of heart-valve problems and remains available by prescription.

What might we learn from this experience? First and foremost, even when a drug appears safe in clinical trials involving hundreds or even thousands of people, unexpected and more uncommon side effects may show up when drugs are taken by hundreds of thousands or even millions of people. Second, the Fen-phen phenomenon demonstrates that a truly effective preparation for weight loss does not need to be advertised, because consistent results speak loudly, and word of mouth takes care of the rest. The next time you hear an ad on the radio or television for a miracle weight-loss supplement, don't be the first on your block to try it. If it's the real deal (which is extremely unlikely), you'll find out soon enough. ■

intestine, where they become very effective at provoking loose, oily bowel movements. The word *provoke* is apropos, because these stools exit with some urgency—as in, "gotta go *right now*." They may even occur unexpectedly and involuntarily—definitely not an ideal event if you're stuck in traffic.

Orlistat users usually begin taking the drug once daily with their largest meal and can increase to three doses per day, one before each meal, as tolerated. Some have used the drug as a way to prevent themselves from eating too much fatty food, which they know will send them scurrying to the bathroom later on. Of course, if they eat a lot of sugary or starchy carbohydrates without much fat, the drug won't have any effect at all. Because some necessary fat-soluble nutrients may not be absorbed when taking orlistat, routine multivitamin supplementation (especially for vitamins A and D) is appropriate. Like the neurotransmitter drugs, orlistat can have a modest effect on weight, but by itself it is not the answer for someone with a significant obesity problem, especially at a cost of more than four dollars per day.

Surgery

Surgery that permanently changes the effective size of the stomach, bypasses part of the small intestine, or both is called **bariatric surgery**. This is *not* the same as **liposuction**, a procedure that involves the literal suctioning of fat from certain parts of the body (typically abdomen, thighs, and buttocks) for cosmetic purposes. Liposuction may alter one's shape, but it does not improve overall health. For the right person, however, bariatric surgery can provide a major benefit to both life and health.

A few decades ago, a common type of weight-loss surgery involved bypassing (or even removing) all but a few inches of small intestine. With so little intestinal surface remaining to absorb food, serious medical complications were common. Contemporary procedures are not only much safer but far more effective. The two most widely used are:

- **Gastroplasty**, in which sutures, staples, or a band across the upper end of the stomach creates a pouch roughly the size of a small egg. As a result, a person will feel full after eating only a very small amount of food.
- **Bypass** surgery, in which food passes from the stomach directly to the **jejunum** (the second segment of the small intestine), bypassing the **duodenum** (the short first segment of the small intestine). This procedure bypasses far less of the intestine than the older procedures, but it still reduces to a modest degree the number of calories absorbed.

When done by itself, the stomach banding or stapling procedure is relatively simple and can be performed in as little as half an hour. However, bariatric surgeons commonly perform a more complex combination procedure called a **Roux-en-Y gastric bypass**, or simply **gastric bypass** for short, which is more time consuming but considered by many to be the current gold standard for weight-loss surgery. In this procedure, a small upper stomach pouch is created and then connected directly to the small intestine, allowing food to bypass the lower segment of the stomach, the duodenum, and part of the jejunum. The rest of the stomach does not receive any food but continues to make its usual secretions. These drain out of the stomach through the bypassed duodenum, which the surgeon plugs into the small intestine several inches past the connection with the stomach pouch. As a result, stomach juices can still participate in digestion. (Sound confusing? It's easier to understand if you check the diagram to the left.)

ROUX-EN-Y GASTRIC BYPASS

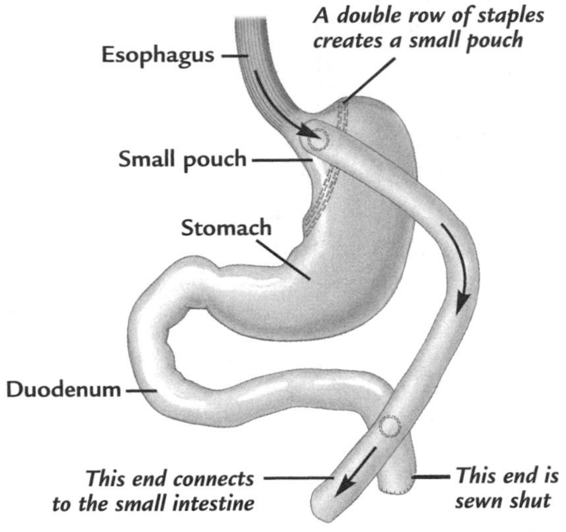

Most of these procedures are performed using **laparoscopy**, in which a few small incisions are made in the abdomen. The surgeon inserts special instruments through the tiny incisions and manipulates them while watching a video monitor. (A number of common procedures, such as gallbladder removal, have been performed laparoscopically since the mid-1980s.) The advantage of this approach is that recovery is shorter and less painful for the patient. As experience and favorable outcomes with these procedures have increased, so have their numbers: from about 25,000 in the United States in 1998 to more than 120,000 in 2004.

The exotic-sounding term *Roux-en-Y* refers to Cesar Roux (1857–1934), a Swiss surgeon, and the Y-shaped connection of small bowel to stomach he devised that is used in gastric bypass surgery.

Bariatric surgery is reserved for people with significant weight problems (the medical term is morbid obesity): those with a body mass index (BMI) greater than 40 or with a BMI of 35 with medical complications such as diabetes, high blood pressure, elevated cholesterol, or sleep apnea. These individuals are typically 80 to 100 pounds or more overweight and have suffered ongoing problems related to weight—emotional, social, and even economic—that affect overall quality of life. In addition, candidates for this type of surgery should meet some additional criteria:

- The weight problem has been chronic and has persisted despite the individual's diligent efforts to lose weight by altering diet, habits, and exercise.
- The individual must be able to understand the nature of the surgery, its potential benefits and risks, and the changes in lifestyle that are necessary for a successful long-term outcome. *This is not a passive, easy, lazy approach to weight loss.* It will seriously impact a person's eating habits, and a lifelong commitment to appropriate food choices and exercise is essential.

- Most bariatric surgeons will operate on properly screened adults between the ages of eighteen and sixty. Under certain circumstances, some will consider operating on adolescents as young as fifteen and adults as old as seventy.
- A person with an ongoing alcohol or drug abuse problem is not a candidate for this type of surgery.
- Conversations with others who have undergone this procedure (often in a support-group environment) are highly recommended, both before and after surgery.

A well-designed bariatric surgery program will include a thorough medical evaluation, consultations with a dietitian (and possibly a counselor or psychologist) before and after the procedure, as well as long-term follow-up. It should also provide detailed instructions, typically in the form of a manual, outlining what to expect, dietary ground rules, warning signs, and so on.

If you are considering this type of procedure, you should ask your primary care physician for a referral to a qualified bariatric surgeon. You can also check the Web site of the American Society for Bariatric Surgery (ASBS) at www.asbs.org to obtain names of members in your area, or contact the ASBS at 100 S.W. 75th Street, Suite 201, Gainesville, FL 32607, phone (352) 331-4900.

While many insurance companies will cover most (or at least some) of the multi-thousand-dollar expenses related to this type of surgery, preauthorization is normally necessary. Various requirements may need to be satisfied and documented before coverage will be authorized. For example, an insurance provider may require evidence that a person has been in a physician-supervised weight-loss program for six months before a procedure is done.

What can a person who has had a gastric bypass procedure expect? The stomach pouch fills rapidly, so that a small amount of food will create a sense of fullness. Eating too rapidly, or taking in more than the pouch can hold, will cause some discomfort or even sudden vomiting. Furthermore, certain types of concentrated carbohydrates (especially sweets) can provoke a "dumping syndrome," characterized by fifteen to sixty minutes of sweating, rapid heartbeat, cramps, diarrhea, or all of the above. Needless to say, these experiences quickly train a person to eat much less, to eat very slowly, and to avoid sweets. As a result of these drastic changes in eating patterns, significant weight loss—typically 70 to 80 percent of excess weight—occurs during the first two years after surgery, with the most rapid loss during the first six months. Some individuals regain 5 to 10 percent of their weight back between the two- and five-year marks, but overall 80 percent of those who have had this surgery will maintain their weight loss for five years or longer—a result markedly better than that typically seen with other weight-loss approaches. Obviously such dramatic weight loss, especially for a person who has struggled for years or even decades with the burdens of obesity, can have profound benefits, providing a literal new lease on life. Furthermore, well before the endpoint of weight loss is reached, important medical risks such as elevated blood glucose, cholesterol, triglycerides, and blood pressure usually show dramatic improvement.

As with any surgery, an individual must acknowledge definite risks before signing on for this procedure. The worst-case scenario—dying in the wake of the surgery—occurs in one out of five hundred to one thousand cases, usually because of a **pulmonary embolism**—a clot that forms in the legs and then travels to the lungs. (It should be noted that a pulmonary embolus is a well-recognized risk after *any* surgery, and a number of measures are routinely taken to avoid it.) Another serious complication, a leak of intestinal fluid from one of the internal connection sites that can provoke **peritonitis** or inflammation of the lining of the abdomen, occurs in about one in two hundred cases among experienced surgeons. Managing a leak may require additional surgery.

Persistent nausea or heartburn may be bothersome but should eventually resolve, although medication may help with this problem. Because of the major reduction in food intake, deficiencies in iron, vitamin B_{12}, calcium, and other nutrients may occur. Follow-up, periodic blood tests, and appropriate supplements can reduce the risk of a nutritional deficiency. In addition, regular exercise is extremely important to maintain muscle mass and overall energy levels.

One important complication of gastric bypass surgery may need to be addressed in counseling before and after the procedure. *This procedure makes it extremely difficult to use food as a primary form of emotional comfort.* This doesn't mean that you can't enjoy eating. On the contrary, you can learn to appreciate taste, texture, and quality, and pay more attention to your companions, as you take your time during meals. But if the way you usually spell relief is e-a-t-i-n-g, and especially if food binges have served as a way to cope with stress and anxiety, you are going to have to make some major adjustments in your life.

A Final Thought: The Bottom Line and the Big Picture

If you flipped to the end of this chapter without reading what came first, hoping to find the single answer that will make your weight problem go away, you will be disappointed. If you have read this material carefully, you'll understand why someone looking for that one bottom line is taking the wrong approach.

There are many reasons why America is in the midst of an obesity epidemic. There are also two important reasons why efforts to lose weight so frequently fail:

1. **We try to make it too simple.** Specifically, we want a quick fix, a miracle cure, a single food (or food group) to eat or avoid that will make our fat go away, without looking carefully at how our life, our habits, our needs, even our hurts affect our eating.
2. **We try to make it too complicated.** We become fixated on whether or not to eat this type of fruit or that cut of meat, or whether we can combine one type of food with another. Some families are divided at the dinner table over

various members' allegiances to a particular dietary school of thought, missing opportunities for intimacy and harmony. Yes, there are clearly ways to eat smarter, but eventually the problem boils down to figuring out how to be satisfied with fewer calories and how to increase the amount of activity we engage in every day.

Before leaving this important topic, we need to look briefly at some important people: those who have lost a significant amount of weight and kept it off. What did they do that was successful? (At this point we are not thinking about the dramatic weight losses achieved through bariatric surgery, which is a solution only for a relatively small proportion of those who are overweight or obese.)

To help answer that question, an ongoing study called the National Weight Control Registry (NWCR) was launched in 1993 by researchers at the University of Colorado, Brown University, and the University of Pittsburgh. The Registry has enrolled more than four thousand adults (eighteen years of age and older) who have lost at least thirty pounds and maintained that loss for a minimum of one year. The NWCR is conducting ongoing studies of these individuals and is also collecting and reporting their stories. What are they doing? What are their habits? What has motivated them? How has their weight loss impacted their lives?

Some interesting—but not terribly surprising—observations about these people have been observed thus far:

- About half of them lost weight without the help of a program, medication, or weight-loss professional. The other half sought and benefited from one or more forms of assistance.
- They lost weight gradually and consistently—sometimes over a period of years—rather than attempting a crash-diet approach.
- They ate smaller amounts of healthier foods and exercised on a regular basis.
- They reduced or eliminated concentrated sweets—cookies, cakes, donuts, etc.
- Nearly all maintain a regular eating pattern of three meals and two snacks every day.
- They identified a highly motivating *reason* for their healthier way of life.
- Here's the most important characteristic, the bottom line if you're looking for one: They have managed to integrate their healthier, lower-calorie eating habits and regular physical exercise into their daily routines. In other words, what they eat and how they stay active *are a way of life*, one that they actually have come to like. Their diet and exercise are not a temporary, unpleasant treatment like a course of medication. Their exact choices of foods and exercise vary considerably, but they have identified what works for *them*.

As you work on your own weight situation, you may want to read some of the stories posted on the NWCR Web site at http://www.nwcr.ws.

The Overweight Child and Teenager

One of the most worrisome developments—indeed, perhaps *the* most worrisome development—in the American weight landscape has been the dramatic increase in the number of overweight children and adolescents over the past forty years. Before we take a look at the unpleasant statistics, however, we need to understand the terms and definitions used by the Centers for Disease Control (CDC) to describe the weight of those between the ages of six and nineteen.

As we described earlier, the body mass index (BMI) calculation for an adult is based on height and weight, without reference to age or sex. We use this number to get a general idea of one's weight status—underweight, normal, overweight, or obese—and this can serve as a useful (if not perfect) tool both for individual assessment and for research. In children and adolescents, however, the significance of a given BMI is much more dependent on age and sex than in adults. The normal amount of body fat not only differs between boys and girls but also changes as they grow and mature. As a result, the CDC has established specific charts of **BMI-for-age** for both boys and girls.

For children and adolescents from two to twenty years of age, the charts show a series of curved lines, each of which represents a certain **percentile** rank. Given a child's height and weight, a BMI can be calculated using the same formula as for adults. But the similarity ends there. By looking at the appropriate chart, one must then determine the percentile rank for that BMI, depending on age. If the child's BMI falls on the 50th percentile curve, it means that half of the children at his or her age have a higher BMI, while half have a lower one. A BMI at the 95th percentile rank means that 95 percent of the children at that age have a lower BMI. As an example, a five-year-old boy with a BMI of 18 would fall on the 95th percentile curve, and this would raise concerns about his weight. But the same BMI for a twelve-year-old boy falls on the 50th percentile curve, indicating a normal combination of height and weight.

Currently the CDC uses the term *overweight* rather than *obese* when referring to excessive weight in children and teenagers, and it uses these two categories:

- Being **at risk for overweight** means that the BMI lands between the 85th and 95th percentiles for age and sex.
- Being **overweight** means that the BMI is more than the 95th percentile for age and sex.

Over the past thirty years, the prevalence of this problem among children and teenagers has increased dramatically. Altogether about 9 million young Americans—children between the ages of six and nineteen—are overweight.

Among children ages two to five and adolescents ages twelve to nineteen, the percentage who are overweight doubled between 1970 and 2000. For children ages six to eleven, that percentage tripled. To make matters worse, today's children who are at the highest percentiles of weight (that is, the ones whose BMI is higher than 95 percent of other children their age) actually weigh more than their counterparts at the same percentile thirty years ago. In other words, you might say that the heaviest children today are heavier than ever.[21]

The 2002 National Health and Nutrition Examination Survey estimated that more than 20 percent of children ages two to five, and more than 30 percent of children and teenagers, are overweight or at risk for overweight (BMI more then 85th percentile). As with adults, Hispanic and African American children are more likely to be overweight: nearly one in four have a BMI over the 95th percentile.[22]

For young people the consequences of being overweight fall into three major categories:

- **Immediate health risks.** As with adults, overweight children and adolescents are at risk for a number of health problems, including insulin resistance, type 2 diabetes, fatty liver disease, orthopedic problems, sleep apnea, and gastroesophageal reflux disease (or GERD). One alarming aspect of the epidemic of obesity in the young is the increasing presence of blood glucose problems normally seen in older adults. An estimated 25 percent of overweight children and adolescents have insulin resistance, and 4 percent have type 2 diabetes.[23] Another sobering finding: 60 percent of overweight children between the ages of five and ten already have at least one risk factor for cardiovascular disease, such as an elevation of cholesterol, triglycerides, or blood pressure. Twenty-five percent have two or more of these risk factors.[24]
- **Long-term weight problems.** The amount of fat in your body reflects both the *size* and the *number* of fat cells, and the number of cells increases most dramatically during late childhood and early adolescence. The overweight child gains more of these cells than his lean counterpart and may begin his teen years with as many fat cells as an adult. When weight is lost, fat cells shrink in size but not in number, and people with more cells regain any lost fat more quickly. As a result, the overweight child or early teen is more likely to become an overweight adult who has difficulty maintaining any weight loss. Furthermore, those who are able to control their weight later in life are still more likely to develop coronary artery disease and arthritis as adults.[26] This is a key reason for dealing thoughtfully and carefully with a child's weight problem. But another is equally important:
- **Emotional and social risks.** For the overweight child or adolescent, whose culture at school (or down the block) rarely overflows with human kindness, every day can be a brutal gauntlet of insults, snub-

In health-care circles you often hear the terms **prevalence** and **incidence**. The prevalence of a disease or health problem refers to the number of people who currently have it, usually expressed as a percentage for a certain population. The incidence of a problem refers to the number of people who develop it during a certain time frame (usually a year).

For background information on insulin resistance and type 2 diabetes, see chapter 3, beginning on page 71. Fatty liver disease involves the accumulation of fat within the liver, which may lead to inflammation and in some cases progressive damage. As many as 75 percent of obese adults, and as many as 25 to 50 percent of overweight children and adolescents, may have this problem.[25] Sleep apnea involves intermittent obstruction of the airway by soft tissue in the neck during sleep, manifested by snoring and pauses in breathing that disrupt sleep. This can cause a number of problems, not the least of which is daytime drowsiness and poor school performance. In children, sleep apnea may be aggravated by enlarged tonsils. (See chapter 15, starting on page 755.) Gastroesophageal reflux disease (GERD) involves a backflow of stomach acid into the esophagus (the tube that carries food from mouth to stomach), causing irritation and discomfort commonly experienced as heartburn.

bing, and loneliness. *This ongoing assault on the heart and spirit may have lifelong consequences,* and preventing or limiting them is one of the most important reasons for parents to take an active role in their children's nutritional health.

Why are so many kids overweight?

The short answer is the same as for adults: Over an extended period of time more calories are going in than are being used, and the body responds by storing the extra fuel as fat. Furthermore, many of the same contributing factors we described earlier for adults—genetics, activity, family and cultural factors, and so forth—are also important in childhood and teenage weight problems. But we need to note some important variations on the adult themes.

When they're not asleep, infants, toddlers, and preschoolers younger than two or three years old, left to their own devices, normally move around *a lot.* Keeping close tabs on one or more of them for a few hours will test the stamina of most adults. Furthermore, very young children will eat almost anything when they're hungry and stop when they're not. There are exceptions, of course, but this default position for activity and eating is a very healthy one. Unfortunately, for too many children it doesn't last. Here are three important reasons why:

Too little physical activity at home. We're not talking about time spent reading books on the back porch. It's all about *screen time*—the explosion of irresistible opportunities to sit (or lie down) in front of a cathode-ray tube monitor, plasma screen, or other video display: dozens of cable channels, movies on DVD or VHS at home or for rent, extremely elaborate electronic games, and the virtually limitless domain of the Internet. Children can become fascinated by video images at a very early age, and time spent watching a screen is time when very little physical activity is going on.

The impact of these enticements on a child's physical fitness will be profound if parents fail to impose some reasonable limits on daily screen time. They will be even more significant if parents themselves are hooked, and especially if they use electronic devices as babysitters and diversions for their kids. More on this later.

Too little physical activity at school. As we describe in more detail in chapter 7, over the past few decades physical education has been phased out of the normal school day in many school districts, especially during the high school years. Furthermore, for too many children and adolescents who haven't developed much athletic prowess or team sports skills, PE can be an ordeal rather than a "user-friendly" class in which they develop habits that maintain fitness for life. We hope that, as communities and schools respond to the challenges of the obesity epidemic, exercise and fitness training during the school day will become a priority.

Changes in family eating habits. Because of busy schedules, long workdays for parents, time pressure, and general fatigue, regular home-cooked meals at which family members sit down and talk with one another have become somewhat of a rarity, a fading memory from the days of *Ozzie and Harriet*. We are not better off as a result, for two reasons. First, meals can and should be a time of sharing (indeed, of intimacy), mutual encouragement, and bonding as a family, not to mention learning about wholesome foods. Second, we have become overly dependent on prepackaged, processed, nuke-and-serve convenience foods or—worse—on trips to the nearest fast-food restaurant, where the fare is cheap, tasty, highly satisfying, and habit forming. It is also marketed aggressively to children, who readily become regular (and sometimes compulsive) customers. While some franchises are making changes for the better, their staple items remain dense in calories, sugars, saturated fats, and trans fats.

How can I help prevent my child or teenager from becoming overweight?

In a way this is like asking, "How can I help prevent my child or teenager from becoming a smoker or a drug user?" Certainly there are defensive measures to consider, but accentuating the positive, including a lot of role modeling of healthy eating and physical activity, is definitely preferable. You may feel as though you don't have a chance against billions of dollars of advertising spent by the food and restaurant industry to influence what your child or teenager eats. But your child's bedroom isn't located in a fast-food restaurant, and soft drinks don't sneak into your cupboard during the night. You have the opportunity and responsibility to decide what foods show up on your table, what drinks chill within your refrigerator, and where your child will have his or her first restaurant experiences.

As with so many other dimensions of parenting, you will need to avoid extremes. You cannot afford to sit back and let marketers and media determine what your family will eat. If nothing else, America's epidemic of obesity, cardiovascular disease, and diabetes should serve as convincing evidence that nutritional "business as usual" isn't an option. Nor can you become an uptight, repressive food dictator with a delusion that you can force your kids to eat exactly what you put in front of them, and nothing more or less. If that's your expectation, you can look forward to a lot of conflict, tears, frustration, and disordered eating patterns once your children are out of your immediate control.

With those general thoughts in mind, here are some specific age-related recommendations.

During infancy. There are many reasons to encourage breast-feeding infants, and one is that a number of studies have shown that this has a modest protective effect against the development of obesity. One aspect of breast-feeding that may contribute to this advantage is that the nursing baby normally will feed in response to his own cues—sucking and swallowing when he's hungry, and stopping when he is full, a sensation that is affected not only by the quantity but also by changes in the fat content of breast milk during the course of a feeding. A baby drinking from a bottle doesn't receive any cues from the content of the formula, and the person holding the bottle may be tempted to continue the feeding session until it is empty. This might lead to overfeeding, at least with some infants.

Remember also that juices should not be substituted for breast milk or formula, and that infants younger than six months should not receive juice at all. There are several reasons for this (and for limiting juice intake in older babies and young children), one of which is to limit their exposure to sweet tastes that could lead to an appetite for sweets later in life. *Soft drinks have no place in the diet of an infant or young child.*

See the chapter 5 sidebar that begins on page 172 for more guidelines about juice for babies and young children.

Among older infants, toddlers, and preschoolers. This is an important period of life for developing eating habits, healthy or otherwise. It is also the time during which children and parents may have more than a few "food fights." Your job is to give your child many opportunities to try a variety of nutritious foods in modest quantities. By her first birthday, if not before, these can be small portions of whatever the family is eating (which hopefully is of good quality). Your child's job is to eat what he wants from what you offer and to stop when he's no longer hungry. (Toddlers will notify you when they aren't hungry by shifting from eating food to examining it or tossing it overboard.) Attempting to force young children, or for that matter older ones, to eat food they don't want is an exercise in futility and frustration.

Whatever you do, don't force a child to sit for hours until he finishes every last morsel on the plate. Showdowns over membership in the "clean plate club" are not only miserable and pointless but also a potential setup for overeating later in life. One of the great challenges of weight management is to listen to hunger as a cue to eat and its absence as a cue to stop. Young children do this instinctively, but by the age of five they're more likely to respond to external cues (what's on the plate) than to internal ones (i.e., *Am I hungry or not?*). The last thing you want to do is attach a lot of guilt and shame to leaving food on a plate.

Another potential trouble spot with toddlers and preschoolers is the highly variable appetite: eating constantly one day, picking at food the next, or displaying both extremes during a single day. Parents observing this erratic intake may worry that their child is going to become malnourished. The situation may become stickier if a child seems to be holding out for one or two favorite foods and seemingly refusing to eat anything else. If you sense that a one-track appetite is developing, it's quite all right to offer lots of healthy alternatives rather than caving in to what might become a form of food extortion: *If I don't get what I want, I won't eat.*

Giving in to a young food faddist can be trouble if she becomes fixated on one or two items that are dense in calories and marginal in nutritional value. If you prepare a plate with a few items from the major food groups and your child turns most of it down, put it in the refrigerator and warm it up for the next meal. When she gets hungry, she'll eat (unless, of course, she gets her hands on a favorite snack between meals). If you're concerned about the amount of food she's getting, write down what she has eaten over a week's time and then discuss her food intake with her physician. If she's active, showing appropriate developmental milestones, and making progress on her growth chart, she's almost certainly getting enough food, even if it seems like she won't eat.

As much as possible, keep your young child away from the fatty, salty, or sugary foods that are aggressively marketed to kids through colorful packaging and TV ads. Fast-food franchises have been spectacularly successful at gaining young customers with kids meals, toys, play areas, highly recognizable characters, tie-ins with animated films, and food items that appeal to their palates. The marketers' goal is to build intense brand loyalty and lots of repeat business that first involves *your* money, and later your children's. What you need to build instead is attachment to the basics—whole grains, fruits, vegetables, lean meats, and so forth. Be careful and conservative about purchasing packaged and processed food items that your preschooler asks (and asks and asks and asks) for in the store, especially those that are geared to young eyes and appetites.

One more caution: Avoid using food to manipulate a child's behavior. If you respond with food to every sign or sound of displeasure from your child (especially when he can't tell you what's bothering him), you may unintentionally teach him to calm himself by eating. Depriving children of food as a punishment—"I heard you and your sister fighting; you're going to bed without your supper!"—or using it to reward their behavior—"If you're good while we're shopping, you'll get ice cream!"—can attach all kinds of unnecessary emotional baggage to eating. There are already plenty of emotional ties to food: it satisfies hunger, first and foremost; it provides pleasant sensations of taste, smell, and texture; it hopefully is associated with times of closeness, connection, and acceptance with family and friends. What small children (and older ones too) do *not* need is to attach their acceptance or worth to the foods that are offered to or withheld from them.

And finally, these are the years when you need to establish limits and expectations regarding TV and video viewing. Current recommendations for prevention and management of excessive weight in childhood call for limiting "screen time" to two hours or less every day. While your toddler won't hound you to watch hours of TV (as he may do when he's older), you may be tempted to use TV and video programs as extended diversions for your child while you try to get other tasks done. Remember—he probably will not become *less* attached to sitting and watching as he gets older, so be very careful about habits you set in motion at a young age.

Among older children and adolescents. Here is where the rubber meets the road, so to speak, because your children or teenagers will be eating more often away from home—at school, with friends, and on their own. Many kids and teenagers bolt out the door without thinking about breakfast and plan to make up the deficit during the "nutrition" break at school. But depending on the policies of your local school district, the offerings on campus (whether in the cafeteria or from vending machines) may be healthy, mediocre, or genuine junk. Unfortunately, in order to supplement sagging revenues, many public schools have made deals with soft-drink, snack, and even fast-food companies to offer their products to the captive audience showing up every day for classes. In high schools that allow students to leave campus for lunch, the only source of a relatively fast meal may be—you guessed it—a local fast-food franchise.

If your children and teens are involved in extracurricular activities, their schedules—and yours—may get so complicated that restaurants, fast-food, and pizza deliveries become your family's primary food suppliers. If media marketers have had their way with your kids, they may become more persuasive about the snack foods and sodas they would like to see in the pantry. Furthermore, interest in computers, the Internet, and video games goes into high gear at this age, not to mention awareness of TV programs and movies that *everyone* seems to be watching. The amount of time spent staring at screens can increase rapidly as a result.

All of these developments can contribute to obesity or, at the very least, a less-than-ideal intake of nutrients. In order to stem this tide, some deliberate steps will be necessary. Ideally, many of these should already be well established as part of your family's culture while your children are growing up.

- Establish a weekly schedule in which several family meals are predictable events. This will take some effort, but older children and teens can and should be involved in the planning, shopping, preparation, serving, and cleanup. Kids won't get this type of hands-on experience at school, and they need to know more about cooking than how to operate the microwave. Ideally these times should introduce and reinforce the value of such staple items as vegetables, fruits, lean meats, and whole grains, as well as some adventurous recipes to complement the old favorites.
- While you're planning the sit-down meals, think through with your kids what they're going to do about breakfast and lunch. Skipping meals (especially breakfast) is common among teenagers but definitely *not* recommended by nutrition experts. You don't need to set up a breakfast buffet every day, but a simple start—juice, fruit, and some cereal (preferably not the presweetened, empty-calorie variety) beats the no-food or grab-a-doughnut approach. While bringing lunch from home also requires some planning, you can usually get more value, both in nutrition and cost, from food items you and your kids assemble than from the cafeteria and vending machines at school. If your children are going to buy lunch at school, do you have any idea what's being served?
- Keep fresh fruits and vegetables available as snacks. (Nuts can be great snacks as well, but remember they are calorie dense. Kids need to learn that a small handful of these constitutes a serving.)

- Phase out the soft drinks and other flavored, sweetened beverages. According to the Institute of Medicine, by age fourteen more than 30 percent of girls and 50 percent of boys are drinking three or more eight-ounce servings of sweetened soft drinks—roughly 300 calories worth—every day. If all of these are excess calories—that is, calories beyond the number needed for normal metabolism and daily activities—they will result in more than thirty pounds of weight gain over the course of a year.
- Limit recreational screen time—TV, videos, and electronic games, as well as computer and Internet activities (including chat rooms) that aren't connected with homework or other productive pursuits—to two hours per day or less. This isn't just a recommendation for the kids, by the way. A profusion of network and cable TV channels beckons adults to sit for hours at a time after work and on weekends. Parents are just as vulnerable as kids to pouring many more hours—including several during the night that would be better spent sleeping—into computer games and the limitless realms of the Internet.
- Encourage all kinds of physical activity. Model it yourself, and brainstorm with your kids about games and activities, whether in the yard or as a family outing, that get everyone moving instead of sitting. We look at this all-important aspect of promoting family fitness in chapter 7, starting on page 308.

What should I do if my child or teenager is overweight?

This is an emotionally charged issue for both parents and kids, and you would be wise to think, pray, and proceed with caution as you address it. The wrong attitudes and approaches can generate a great deal of pain, shame, guilt, anger, and divisiveness among family members who desperately need to be on the same team. In particular, *beware of putting a child or teenager on a "diet"—especially one that involves a significant number of food restrictions—without consulting a professional who is knowledgeable in this area.*

There are some basic questions you need to examine at the outset and then revisit periodically:

Is my child actually overweight? This may sound like a dumb question, but an informed answer usually involves three steps that ideally should be carried out by your child's physician or a dietitian. First, height and weight need to be measured accurately. Second, a body mass index (BMI) should be calculated and then compared to percentile ranks for the child's age and gender, as described earlier in this section. Finally, the current height and weight should be compared with other measurements recorded on your child's growth chart, which hopefully has been set up and maintained at the doctor's office during checkups. This is a form on which height and weight are plotted in relation to percentile curves that provide a comparison of height and weight with those of other children or adolescents of the same age and gender. (If you have moved, or your child has seen more than one physician, you may have to collect height and weight information at different ages from more than one source.)

One important question to address is whether your child's weight and height patterns have been following a certain percentile over a period of years, or if there has been a recent change. For example, if weight has been at the 50th percentile for years (that is, where 50 percent of children of the same age and gender are heavier and 50 percent lighter) and then over a few months it has shifted to the 90th percentile, you might need to consider what was going on during that period of time. (Was there a move? A change in schools? Some turbulence between parents?) On the other hand, a look at the growth chart may demonstrate that a child or adolescent has always been large (often reflecting similar patterns in other family members) and that he or she is merely following a predictable height and weight trajectory.

Whose issue is this? (part 1) Are you primarily intent on maintaining or protecting your child's health and emotional well-being as he grows up and moves into adulthood? If so, good for you. Are you at some level embarrassed by your child's appearance? Are you afraid that his weight problem may reflect badly on your parenting? Do you have difficulty speaking or showing approval for your child because of his weight? Are some of your dreams in jeopardy because your child or teenager isn't turning out the way you hoped? If the answer to one or more of the last few questions is yes, you may be at risk for broadcasting all sorts of critical messages. You may also find yourself owning your child's problem more than he does, thus preventing him from assuming his share of responsibility (and virtually guaranteeing that whatever you have in mind as a solution won't work).

Whose issue is this? (part 2) Is your child or adolescent concerned about her weight, even though she looks perfectly fine to you? At any given time a significant percentage of adolescents are attempting some sort of diet, usually based on unrealistic ideals of physical beauty tied to being thin. Often dedicated athletes or dancers become alarmed over gaining a few pounds, which may in fact be tied to normal development. These situations may seem easy to brush off as adolescent drama, but kids may take drastic (or even dangerous) measures to correct what they perceive to be a threat to their performance.

Assuming that there is a definite problem with your child's weight and its physical and emotional consequences, there are several action items to consider and a number of pitfalls to avoid if at all possible. Many of these will sound familiar if you have read through the section on weight loss for adults. Remember as well that the measures we discussed above for *preventing* obesity in childhood also apply here—indeed, we'll repeat a couple of them for good measure.

1. **Get professional input.** Ideally this should include two evaluations. One should be done by your child's physician to clarify whether there is a weight

problem (and to what degree) and to determine if any other health issues might be present (such as elevated blood pressure, cholesterol, or glucose). The other person to have on your team if at all possible is a registered dietitian who works with children and adolescents. The kind of help you should seek from the dietitian is *not* a lecture about overeating and a highly restricted diet for your child, but rather information for the entire family as well as some positive engagement with and encouragement for the child. If you are dealing with a teenager, a lot of other emotional and social undercurrents will likely need to be addressed. Unrealistic expectations about weight, body image, and dieting may call for some gentle reality checks. A dietitian who works with adolescents should be well aware of these issues and hopefully adept at gaining the confidence of a teenager so that they can be discussed one-on-one in a candid but nonjudgmental way. You need to be open to the possibility that the weight problem is the tip of an emotional iceberg. If the dietitian identifies some personal and family issues that would best be addressed by a qualified counselor, don't ignore this advice.

2. **Do not make a specific restrictive diet the focus of your efforts, except under unusual circumstances involving professional supervision.** In the section on adult weight loss, you may have noticed that we stressed attitude and behavior issues far more than the potential benefits (or drawbacks) of specific diet plans. This orientation is essential for overweight children and adolescents, who respond far better to behavioral change than to diets. Earlier we mentioned that attempting to force a child to eat food items or quantities that he doesn't want is an exercise in futility. The same is true with attempts to force a child to adhere to a strict diet plan, *especially* if it involves spending a lot of time being hungry. Hunger is unpleasant for all of us, and for a child it is particularly unsettling. Even if you are able to enforce this type of approach for a few days at a time, you can count on your child figuring out sooner or later how to get around it. Everyone will lose in the process—the child will overeat in order to compensate (or retaliate) for the ordeal, and you will be at odds with him in an important arena where you should be allies.

3. **At all cost, avoid nagging, name-calling, insults, or other negativity as a tactic to "encourage" weight loss.** It doesn't work for adults, and it absolutely won't work for your child. If she is truly overweight, she is almost certainly getting a heart-wrenching amount of negativity from her peers and perhaps from some thoughtless adults as well. *It is particularly crucial that she understands that her worth as God's child and yours, and His and your love for her, do not change based on what she weighs.* This also means that you'll need to impose a moratorium on wisecracks from other family members (especially brothers and sisters) about her weight. (Indeed, you need to think twice

before making critical remarks about *anyone's* weight problem, because your overweight child will likely apply that sentiment to herself as well.)

4. **Accentuate the positive.** The changes in eating habits that you'll be encouraging for your overweight child or adolescent are *good* for them, in every sense of the word. They are not a punishment or a sign of failure or stupidity. What you are promoting is not endless deprivation but learning to truly enjoy eating. Go out of your way to praise good eating decisions rather than focusing on blocking bad ones.

5. **Everyone in the family should be eating from the same meal plan.** We discussed this earlier with adult weight problems: What's good and healthy for the overweight person(s) should be good and healthy for everyone else in the family. Giving one person a plate of broccoli and carrot sticks while the others are having burgers and fries will guarantee resentment and failure.

   Here are the types of foods to emphasize:
   - Fresh vegetables and fruits.
   - Whole-grain cereals and breads. Try whole-grain pasta, but if it's not to your liking try slightly undercooked regular pasta (al dente style), which is absorbed more slowly.
   - Lean cuts of meat in modest (palm-sized) portions—preferably grilled, baked, or broiled. Steer clear of the deep-fried stuff.
   - Water or milk instead of soft drinks or sweetened and artificially flavored juice drinks.

6. **Gradual changes in eating habits are more likely to succeed than drastic tactics.** If everyone in the family is *really* ready to jettison soft drinks, high-calorie fat/sweet snacks, and fast food, great. If not, it may be better to phase these items out and introduce better choices over time.

7. **While you can't ultimately force an overweight child or teenager not to eat, you can take a number of steps to encourage better habits.**
   - As much as possible, make three meals and two snacks predictable events every day. The object of these is to satisfy hunger and enjoy pleasant food, but also to learn (or relearn) that when the hunger ends, it's time to stop eating.
   - Encourage (and model) eating slowly. This may take a lot of patience, and you may want to create signals to remind your child to slow down without resorting to constant verbal nagging. A silent maneuver such as a referee's time-out gesture might serve this purpose, with an understanding that you're reminding him to put his utensils down, chew and swallow his bite of food, and then silently count to

ten before picking up the fork again. (You could even do a subtle version of this in a restaurant so as not to embarrass him.)

- As part of the "take your time while eating" campaign, you can certainly encourage kids to enjoy their food—but this involves paying attention to it while they're eating. Phase out meals in front of the TV, and by all means don't let it play in the background while you're sharing a meal. (You may of course make an exception for a "TV dinner" on an unusual occasion in which everyone in the family has an interest in the program being televised.)
- If providing predictable meals and snacks clearly means that you don't

THE STOPLIGHT DIET

One teaching tool used by many pediatricians and dietitians to give children a feel for foods to eat and foods to avoid is the Stoplight Diet. This simple approach, devised in the 1970s by University of Buffalo psychologist and childhood obesity expert Leonard Epstein, Ph.D., links various types of foods with the colors of a traffic light:

- "Red" foods are high in calories and low in nutritional yield, and should be avoided as much as possible. These include items such as (you guessed it) cookies, candy, soft drinks, doughnuts, fried foods, and sugary cereals.
- "Yellow" foods are moderate in calories and nutritional yield, and should be eaten in moderate portions. These include starchy foods (such as bread, low-fiber cereal, pasta, rice, muffins, crackers) as well as cheese, butter, and eggs.
- "Green" foods are low in calories and high in nutritional yield, so *go right ahead*. These include vegetables and fruits, whole-grain cereals, lean meats, and low- or nonfat dairy products.

Think of this as a way to prioritize the foods you and your children will eat, perhaps setting a goal of limiting "red" foods to once a day. (Make sure your kids understand that the categories aren't related to the actual color of the food.) If anything, your approach should have a light touch to it, perhaps having a little family fun trying to figure out which foods in the fridge and cupboards belong in which category and planting some appropriately colored stickers on them as a reminder. You might even change the emphasis from the "stoplight"—what should be avoided—to the "go-light."

The point isn't to create a rigid and legalistic system for your family, but rather to help children (especially preteens) get a handle on the foods that will serve them well throughout life.[27] ■

intend for your overweight child or teenager to be hungry, it also means that random eating can be brought to an end. You'll want to remove open boxes, bags, and bowls of snack foods that cue this type of mindless munching, especially while doing other activities. Don't allow food to be taken, scattered, and stashed all over the house.

- As we mentioned earlier, encourage physical activity in which everyone in the family participates—hiking, biking, gardening, backyard games, and so on. As much as possible, lead by example and encourage kids to join you.
- Set a family policy limiting recreational time spent in front of TV, computer, or electronic-game screens. Two hours per day should be the maximum as a general rule (with exceptions for special events, of course), and everyone in the family should abide by these limits.

It will take some time, attention, prayer, and a fair amount of trial and error to figure out the strategies that will work for your child and your family. If you don't seem to be making any progress, by all means regroup with the dietitian (or schedule your first visit, if you haven't done this yet) and figure out what's working and what isn't. Ditto if your efforts to help an overweight child or teenager (and improve the family eating habits) are deteriorating into a lot of arguing and hard feelings. The dietitian will no doubt have many ideas for you to adapt to your own situation, and they may be more meaningful after you've tried a few things already.

Remember that, as with training and molding your children in any area, there is no surefire, detailed plan that works for everyone. There are, however, some fundamental goals and principles (as outlined above) that should give you a basic sense of direction as you work out the specifics for your own family. If you are struggling with one or more children over issues related to food, two books by childhood nutrition expert Ellyn Satter may prove very helpful: *Child of Mine: Feeding with Love and Good Sense* (revised in 2000) addresses in great detail the feeding of infants, toddlers, and preschoolers; and *How to Get Your Kid to Eat . . . But Not Too Much* (1987) deals with eating issues from birth through adolescence.

What about diet pills or even bariatric surgery in children or teenagers?

We saw earlier (see page 250) that prescription diet medications currently on the market offer very limited (if any) help in weight loss for adults, and that nonprescription pills, supplements, and other concoctions sold as cures for obesity serve only to lighten the wallets of those who put their hope in them. None of these are appropriate for children.

The use of prescription medications in overweight adolescents is as unlikely to produce significant results as it is in adults. They should be considered *only* after careful evaluation of the situation by a dietitian and a physician who have special expertise in their use in this age group. Likewise, some bariatric surgery centers are now carrying out gastric banding and bypass procedures on adolescents with severe weight problems. In properly selected teenagers with significant long-standing obesity (especially when medical complications have developed) who have failed ongoing supervised weight-loss efforts, who have reached their adult height, and who have been carefully screened (medically and psychologically), this type of procedure may be health- and even life-preserving. It should only be carried out by surgeons who are highly experienced in performing this surgery on adolescents in the setting of a comprehensive program (most likely in a university or major medical center).

QUESTIONS TO PONDER:

1. If losing weight is an issue for you, what practical steps could you take to begin addressing this issue? For some ideas on positive changes in your food choices and eating habits, see section "So What Can I Do to Lose Weight?" beginning on page 210.
2. If you've tried to lose weight in the past, what worked? What didn't?
3. What positive and negative food habits have you developed? How can you begin to address them?
4. After reading this chapter, do you think your family's eating habits are contributing to or helping prevent a child's weight problem?

Action items: If you are concerned about your weight and would like to determine your body mass index and waist circumference, follow the directions on pages 193 and 195.

If you want to determine what is driving you to eat, begin keeping a food diary. (See sample on page 224.) After one week, review your notes and see if you can begin to identify any patterns as to when you tend to eat too much. Where were you? What time of day was it? What were you feeling? Next, decide what better reaction you can choose the next time you are tempted to overeat in similar circumstances.

Consider setting some family goals to promote better eating habits. For example, you might choose to eat dinner together as a family a certain number of times per week. You might also limit the number of hours your children may watch TV and/or play video or computer games each day.

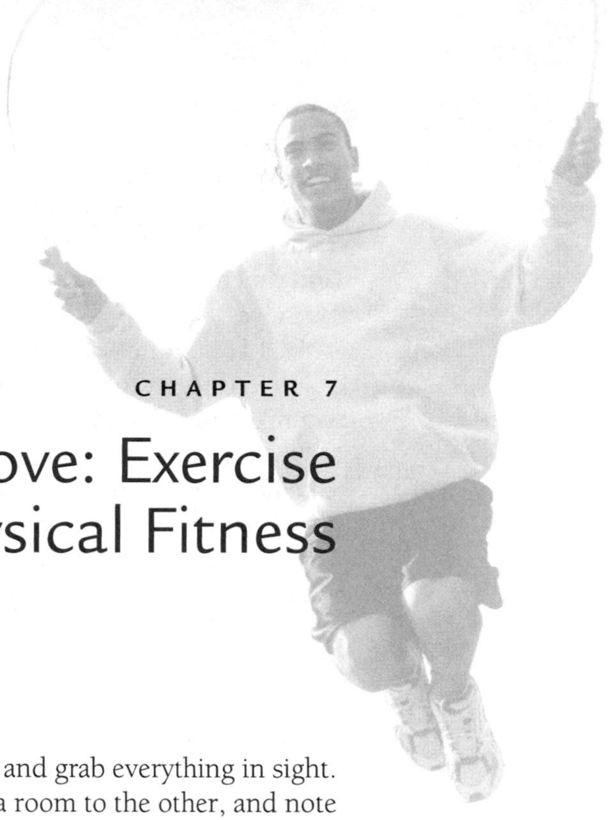

CHAPTER 7

Born to Move: Exercise and Physical Fitness

We were born to move.

Watch a healthy six-month-old kick, wiggle, and grab everything in sight. Follow a toddler as she careens from one end of a room to the other, and note her mother's fatigue after a typical day of keeping this "baby on wheels" out of harm's way. Observe a room full of two-year-olds or preschoolers, and consider how great it would be if we could capture some of their energy and transfuse a little of it to their parents.

Unless significantly impaired or injured early in life, we are born not only with the potential to move ourselves from one place to another, but also with an absolute determination to do so as soon as we develop the necessary strength and coordination. For most of human history, a young child's compulsion to move would usually persist throughout his life, although for a different reason: survival. Gathering, harvesting, or hunting food and finding adequate amounts of water were full-time jobs for our ancestors—and still are in many parts of the world. Even when a culture developed to the point where a smaller number of its members were able to supply the rest with food, other daily labors kept the average person in motion throughout the waking hours—unless, of course, one was wealthy or powerful enough to have others put forth the effort.

But over the past hundred years, the wondrous inventions known as labor-saving devices have given the average American citizen a lifestyle once reserved for royalty. Very few of us grow our own food, chop firewood to heat our homes, and pump water out of the ground or haul it from a nearby creek. Most of us have access to appliances that drastically reduce the amount of effort required to prepare food, clean our dishes, and wash our clothes. Most who are employed outside the home do not need to walk or ride a bicycle to work, and only a limited percentage of our workforce is routinely engaged in physical labor. We use cars to travel even very short distances, and we try diligently to park as close as possible to our destination. We ride elevators and escalators rather than climb stairs. Our most popular forms of recreation involve sitting and watching other people talk, act, or compete in sports, rather than doing so ourselves.

While we often quote statistics and describe health issues in the United States, the same concerns also apply to other developed nations where food supplies and modern conveniences are plentiful.

Of course, not everyone in our country is physically inactive. But recent statistics suggest that far too many of us, including an alarming number of our youngest and oldest citizens, seem determined to avoid moving our muscles. A 1996 consensus statement published by the National Institutes of Health indicated that about one in four adults has what is called a **sedentary** lifestyle. For these people, leisure activity rarely, if ever, includes vigorous or even moderate exercise.[1] This is not to say they are lazy. They may put in twelve-hour (or longer) workdays, diligently care for children, be active in community and church affairs, and feel very short on time. (Indeed, their wall-to-wall schedule may be the primary obstacle to any pursuit of physical fitness.) Another third of the adult population carries on some degree of leisure-time physical activity—but not enough to gain any health benefits.[2]

F.Y.I.

It is important to note that the surveys used to make these estimates of physical activity focused primarily on *leisure-time* activities, and did not take into account the amount of activity involved in housework or an occupation outside of the home, which are more difficult to estimate. Obviously there can be a considerable amount of physical exertion involved in taking care of a houseful of small children, and a lumberjack or ski instructor is going to use much more muscle power during the workday than an accountant.

The statistics appear to be worse in several population groups: women, African-Americans, Latinos, those with less than a twelfth-grade education, those with lower incomes, and senior citizens.[3] Combine this with an abundant supply of food, and we shouldn't be surprised to find ourselves facing a national epidemic of obesity and a host of "diseases of civilization"—heart attacks, strokes, diabetes, and at least some forms of cancer, to name a few.

The word *sedentary* comes from the Latin verb *sedere,* meaning "to sit."

Physical inactivity is not limited to adults. About half of adolescents (young people between the ages of twelve and twenty-one) regularly participate in some form of vigorous physical activity, and about one in four is involved in light-to-moderate activity (such as walking or riding a bike) nearly every day. But one in four never participates in vigorous physical activity, and nearly 15 percent report no physical activity whatsoever—light, moderate, or vigorous. Furthermore, participation in any and all forms of physical activity declines substantially as grade in school increases. Between 1991 and 1999, daily enrollment in physical-education classes declined from 42 percent to 29 percent among high school students, and those classes do not always include a vigorous workout. Fewer than 20 percent of all high school students actually take part in twenty minutes of physical activity during a daily P.E. class.[4]

Why Should I Prefer a Sweat to a Sofa?

We could continue to quote statistics about physical inactivity, but we may succeed only in generating yawns instead of wake-up calls. As with so many health advisories, all of this information ultimately has to provoke a bottom-line question: Why is it important for me and my family to be physically active? As it turns out, a mountain of research over the past few decades has provided a multitude of reasons, which we ignore at our own peril:

Physical inactivity increases your overall risk of dying "ahead of schedule." Several studies have shown that being physically active reduces what the medical literature refers to as all-cause mortality, the likelihood of dying from anything. One important study conducted by the Aerobics Center in Dallas, Texas, showed that men who were at the lowest level of cardiorespiratory fitness lowered their death rate by 44 percent by achieving only a moderate fitness level.[5] After adjusting for other variables, the reduction in death rate from improving fitness actually surpassed the change that would be expected from quitting smoking. Another eye-opening study by Stanford University researchers of more than six thousand men showed that lower peak exercise capacity was a stronger predictor of death than other well-established risk factors, including smoking, high blood pressure, and diabetes.[6] The American Heart Association estimates that up to 250,000 deaths in the United States every year (roughly 12 percent of all deaths) can be attributed to a lack of regular physical activity.[7]

Physical inactivity increases your risk of coronary artery disease. As we described in chapter 3, coronary artery disease—obstruction of blood flow through the arteries that supply the heart—is the leading cause of death in the United States, claiming the lives of two thousand Americans *every day*. Those who are physically inactive roughly double their odds of developing coronary artery disease, a risk comparable to that created by smoking, high blood pressure, or elevated cholesterol.[8] Undoubtedly some of the coronary and life-preserving effects of exercise relate to its tendency to reduce blood pressure and to improve the blend of lipids (fats, specifically cholesterol and triglycerides) circulating in the bloodstream. Also, regular exercise tends to raise the level of HDL cholesterol (the good kind—see page 57 in chapter 3) and to lower triglycercides.

Physical inactivity increases your risk of getting diabetes—and is especially risky if you actually develop this disease. In chapter 3 we described the two types of diabetes and the numerous unpleasant (and all-too-often lethal) complications of this common metabolic disorder. A convincing number of studies suggest that a sedentary lifestyle definitely adds to the risk of developing diabetes during adulthood, when the vast majority of cases occur.[9] The Diabetes Prevention Program, a large clinical trial carried out at twenty-seven medical centers, determined that adults at above-average risk for diabetes reduced their chances of developing it by 58 percent over a three-year period through two straightforward measures: maintaining moderate activity—thirty minutes a day of walking or other moderate-intensity exercise—and losing 5 to 7 percent of their body weight.[10] Furthermore, exercise can delay, or prevent altogether, a number of the most serious complications (involving the heart, eyes, kidneys, and brain, among others) for those who already have this disease.[11]

Physical inactivity increases your chance of developing colon cancer and may increase the risk of developing breast cancer. Cancer of the colon (large intestine) is the third most common type of cancer among both men and women in the United States, killing more than 55,000 every year. More than thirty published studies have shown that physical activity lowers the risk of developing this cancer.[12] In addition, vigorous physical activity during the teen years and early adulthood may reduce a woman's chance of getting breast cancer later in life.[13] Other research suggests that walking seven hours per week at a brisk pace (three to four miles per hour) may over time reduce breast cancer risk by a modest degree (about 20 percent).[14] Thus far, there is no clear indication that exercise helps prevent other forms of cancer, but avoiding colon and breast cancer is well worth the effort.

Physical inactivity increases your risk for osteoporosis (thinning of bone). We will take a closer look at osteoporosis in chapter 13, but for now it is worth noting that this common condition results in about 1.5 million fractures every year in the United States. About 250,000 of these involve the hip, leading to an extraordinary burden of hospitalization, surgery, rehabilitation, long-term care (often in a nursing home or other institutional setting), expense, pain, and, all too often, death. Physical activity of all types—walking and other endurance activities, as well as muscle strengthening—helps develop a healthy bone density during childhood and adolescence, maintain bone density through adulthood, and slow the loss of bone that is so common among women after menopause.

Not everyone is motivated by warnings, and many of us have trouble making changes even when there is clear evidence that our behavior is hurting or even killing us. Furthermore, even after taking a significant step forward in protecting our health—for example, lowering a wayward cholesterol or blood-pressure level—we may not notice any particular difference, other than hearing some encouraging words from a physician or perhaps paying a lower insurance premium. But shifting gears in our level of physical activity is another matter entirely. Exercise changes how we *feel,* not to mention how we look, and its potential benefits for individuals and families are impressive:

Regular exercise increases energy. Chronic fatigue plagues millions of Americans and has many potential causes. But of all of the various measures that might help relieve it, increasing physical activity is usually the one most likely to succeed. Even those who aren't perpetually tired typically notice an invigorating surge of alertness, as if the brain has been swept clean of cobwebs, af-

CHECKING THE EVIDENCE: How Do We Determine Whether Physical Activity Is Good for Us?

Most of what we know about the health benefits of physical activity is based on studies of **endurance** exercise, such as walking, cycling, and jogging. The overall health benefits of **resistance** exercise—the kind that builds up and shapes specific muscles—have not been as well-studied, but its importance is now becoming more apparent, as we will see later in this chapter.

The basic idea of such research is to compare the health of large numbers of people who are physically active with similar numbers of people who aren't. But how do we determine someone's level of physical activity? Very often, researchers must rely on surveys—asking people to recall what they have (or haven't) done over the past week, month, or year—or logs in which people write their day-to-day activities. Obviously, the accuracy of this information depends on the memory, accuracy, and honesty of the people being surveyed. A few studies have classified physical activity based on a person's occupation, assuming that some jobs require more body movement than others. Some researchers actually assess **cardiorespiratory fitness** (also called **cardiorespiratory capacity** or **endurance fitness**), the performance of a person's heart and lungs during exercise. Not only is this more likely to be reliable, but it also directly reflects one's overall activity and exercise habits.

There are two basic ways of comparing the fates of those who are active (however that might be determined) and those who are not. One is called an **observational approach**. Here, the researchers do not try to change anyone's behavior. Instead, they follow large groups of people over months, years, or even decades, and observe who gets what disease(s). They then attempt to sort out any differences—such as dietary and exercise habits, blood glucose and cholesterol levels, and a host of other variables—between those who develop a certain problem and those who don't. From such differences they can often detect connections between various behaviors and health. These often imply (but don't always prove) cause-and-effect relationships.

The most widely recognized measure for cardiorespiratory fitness is called the **maximal oxygen uptake**, or **$\dot{V}O2$ max**, which represents the capacity of the heart, lungs, and circulation system to transport oxygen. Unfortunately, directly measuring one's $\dot{V}O2$ max is no walk in the park. It requires sophisticated equipment and some intense exertion on the part of the person being studied. Fortunately, it is possible to estimate $\dot{V}O2$ max using simpler tests that relate one's heart rate to less strenuous activity.

The other type of study is called a **clinical trial**, which is generally considered to be a more powerful tool. Here the researchers attempt to change the behavior—in this case, exercise patterns—of a group of people, and then determine over time how various aspects of their health compare with a similar group of people who do not change their behavior. As it turns out, both types of studies have supported the idea that an inactive lifestyle is definitely a bad idea. ■

ter a good workout. A number of studies confirm what millions of people know from experience: Regular exercise creates a sense of increased productivity and general well-being. This effect increases with the length of time that we exercise consistently and does not appear to be limited by either age or gender.[15]

Exercise can enhance mood. A sizeable amount of research has confirmed that exercise can improve (and possibly help prevent) anxiety and depression.[16] This may result from changes in biochemical messengers in the brain called **neurotransmitters**, which play an important role in regulating mood. It may also arise from feelings of accomplishment as the conditioning process plays out—*I can do more this month than I could last month!* If you exercise with your family, at a gym, or on a team, camaraderie and interactions with others pursuing similar goals can boost overall mood as well.

We will take a closer look at chronic fatigue in chapter 16.

HOW MANY CALORIES DO I BURN WHEN I . . .

Bicycle 6 mph	240 calories per hour
Bicycle 12 mph	410 calories per hour
Cross-country ski	700 calories per hour
Jog 5½ mph	740 calories per hour
Jog 7 mph	920 calories per hour
Jump rope	750 calories per hour
Run in place	650 calories per hour
Run 10 mph	1,280 calories per hour
Swim 25 yards/min	275 calories per hour
Swim 50 yards/min	500 calories per hour
Play singles tennis	400 calories per hour
Walk 2 mph	240 calories per hour
Walk 3 mph	320 calories per hour
Walk 4½ mph	440 calories per hour

These are estimates for a 150-pound individual. A heavier person burns more calories, and a lighter person fewer, for any given activity, in proportion to weight. (To estimate the amount burned for a 200-pound person, for example, you would multiply the number of calories by 200/150, or 1.33.)

Source: Reproduced with permission from *Exercise and Your Heart: A Guide to Physical Activity* © 2001, American Heart Association

Exercise can improve appearance. Both endurance and muscle-strengthening exercises, as well as a more active lifestyle, burn more calories than sitting still or lying down. Therefore, all forms of physical activity play an important role in losing excess weight. In addition, as we will discuss later, increased muscle bulk (within reason) and tone can make one's body more pleasing to the eye.

Exercise can provide enriching experiences for families. Aside from setting a positive example, parents who join their children in age-appropriate physical activities are able to build some powerful memories. Walks, bike rides, hikes, swims, skiing trips, and other vigorous pursuits in which the entire family participates can provide wonderful opportunities to interact, share good times (and challenges), and forge powerful bonds.

What's Keeping Me from Exercising?

(YOU PROBABLY ALREADY KNOW)

If sports and vigorous daily workouts are as natural to you as breathing, you can skip this part (or read it to help your less enthusiastic spouse, child, or friend). The other 98 percent of you need to read on. Many people do not feel any great affinity for exercise. Perhaps you don't feel particularly coordinated, limber, or muscular. You may have dreaded P.E. in school, or perhaps you were one of the last ones picked when the kids were choosing teams. Maybe you never tried your hand at sports after retiring from Little League. Perhaps you envision a gym, spa, or health club as an alien landscape, populated with intimidating devices and even more intimidating people—sweaty, iron-pumping hunks and shapely young things who apparently spend hours every day toning their musculature while the rest of us try to earn an honest living. Or perhaps you tried your hand (and your legs) at an aerobic pursuit such as jogging or walking, whether on the street or on a treadmill, and found the experience not exactly habit-forming. The "runner's high" that others talked about never showed up, and jogging was not unlike hitting yourself repeatedly with a hammer: It only felt good when you stopped. Walking was more tolerable, but before long it became boring.

Maybe you don't have such a negative opinion of exercise, but you just don't have the time. Getting up before the dawn's early light to sweat and strain may sound about as appealing as a daily root canal. At the end of a long day of work, whether at home or across town, you may have just enough energy left to prepare dinner, help with homework, get kids to bed, and prepare for whatever activities tomorrow's page on the calendar may announce—not to mention attending evening meetings for church, school, or continuing education. Who has the fortitude to hit the streets long after the sun has gone down or when the weather is foul? Who has the energy to climb onto the treadmill or exercise bicycle at the end of a long day, when climbing into bed sounds much more appealing? Obviously some do, but for all too many of us, becoming physically fit looks like a real uphill battle.

You'll be happy to know that you don't need to rearrange your entire life or spend thousands of dollars on fitness hardware in order to benefit from exercise. However, if physical exertion isn't your cup of tea, you may need to make some adjustments in four key areas: your motivation, schedule, creativity, and, yes, self-discipline.

Your motivation. What are *your* reasons to make this effort? It's fine for the Surgeon General or your doctor to announce that exercise is a good idea, but what do you hope to gain? Reviewing the benefits of exercise listed earlier in this chapter is a good starting point, but this needs to be translated into a personal mission statement: "I am ____ [walking thirty minutes, five times per week] in order to ____ [live longer, increase my energy, lose weight, prevent another heart attack, etc.]." Of course, if you have little or no personal experience to confirm that you will see some benefit from this effort, you may have to put a little faith in all of those research studies. Better yet, if you can find someone who is a committed exerciser, ask him or her how this has affected life and well-being. Most likely, you'll get an enthusiastic response.

Your schedule. Without a doubt, this is the point at which you may need to take a stubborn bull by the horns. Until exercise becomes so deeply ingrained in your routine that you feel deprived without it, all of the other demands of your day will usually conspire to exclude it. (By the way, the same principle applies to a regular quiet time with God.) If you can set aside a regular time in the day that will serve this purpose, your job may be easier. More likely, you will need to look through the calendar each week and make some deliberate (and not always easy) decisions. Where will you carve out the twenty, thirty, forty-five or more minutes, allowing time not just for the exercise itself, but for preparations, such as driving to and from another location? What else in the day needs to be adjusted to make this happen? If you lead a busy life, you may have to enter your exercise times in your daily planner as appointments that you intend to keep.

Your creativity. There are many ways to move muscles in order to promote health, and it will be important to figure out which of them might work for you, not only to deal with practicalities and time constraints, but also to find ways to *enjoy* the process. We will make some suggestions momentarily, but they must be adapted to your unique interests and circumstances. Don't forget that it is neither necessary nor desirable to limit yourself to one type of exercise or (worse) one exercise routine. We don't cherish boredom in any other area of our life, and just because some forms of exercise involve repetition doesn't mean that they must be mind-numbing.

Your self-discipline. No matter how convinced you are that exercise is a good idea, there will still be many days when you would just rather not, for any number of reasons. Like many other disciplines—having a daily quiet time, eating sensibly, spending less than we make, and so on—this is an arena of life in which staying the course one day at a time truly pays off. It may be necessary at times (or perhaps most of the time) to do the right thing—in this case, to get moving—when you really don't feel like it.

What Kind of Exercise Should I Be Doing?

As we already mentioned, a great deal of research has demonstrated the health benefits of **endurance** (often called **aerobic exercise**): walking, jogging or running, swimming, and other activities that increase the heart rate for a sustained period (typically twenty to thirty minutes). Any exertion beyond complete rest increases the amount of oxygen we need, primarily to support the metabolic activity of the muscles that are doing the work. Whether we're merely walking to the refrigerator or running several miles, if our heart, lungs, and circulation keep up with this demand for oxygen we are said to be functioning on an aerobic (literally, "with oxygen") basis. During mild activity—a casual stroll, for example—we usually don't notice that this increase in oxygen consumption is taking place.

When the pace picks up, so does our heart rate, and our breathing automatically becomes faster and deeper, the familiar huffing and puffing of exercise. If we meet the increased oxygen demand we can theoretically maintain this higher level of exertion for an extended period of time, until fatigue or some other signal from the body tells us to slow down. But if we cannot keep up with the oxygen demand, as happens relatively quickly during a highly vigorous activity such as a sprint, our muscles shift metabolic gears and function—for a while—on an **anaerobic** (or "without oxygen") basis. When this occurs, we build up what is called an oxygen debt. Sooner or (not much) later, a combination of marked breathlessness, muscle fatigue, and an overpowering feeling that we cannot go any farther will force us to stop and rest, panting as long we need to in order to pay back the oxygen debt.

F.Y.I.

The word *aerobic* was derived from the French *aerobie,* coined in the late nineteenth century by the renowned biologist Louis Pasteur. The term combines the Greek words *aer* (air) and *bios* (life). In the late 1960s, fitness expert Kenneth Cooper, M.D., coined the word *aerobics* to refer to a variety of aerobic exercises that improve cardiovascular conditioning.

Because of the well-documented benefits of aerobic exercise for the heart, medical advisories for decades have viewed overall fitness in terms of our capacity for aerobic exercise. This encompasses not only how much (or little) exertion it takes us to shift from aerobic to anaerobic status, but also how long a given level of aerobic activity can be maintained. Obviously, we would consider someone who can tolerate only a few minutes of very mild exertion to be in very poor condition. And most of us would agree that the marathon runner who can cruise twenty-six miles in less than three hours without turning a hair is extremely fit. But what about the weight lifter whose entire body surface ripples with well-developed muscles? It is possible for that person to look like a Greek god(dess) but have relatively poor endurance if asked to jog or walk at a rapid pace. From a health perspective, the wiry long-distance runner who has a stick-figure physique would appear to be better off than the Charles Atlas look-alike who can't jog a half mile without feeling like a ton of bricks.

But the picture isn't quite that simple. It is, in fact, unwise to look at physical conditioning in all-or-nothing terms, focusing only on endurance exercise or muscle strengthening. Strength training isn't just about "looking buff" to impress someone or scare off a neighborhood bully. More recent research has uncovered a number of health benefits related to building the mass and might of our muscles, especially as we grow older. Strengthening exercises for arms, legs, and trunk improve function and balance in the elderly, even among those who are already frail. Not only can this help maintain independence, but it may also reduce the risk of falling and fractures. (Indeed, it could even be argued that strengthening exercises accomplish more for the elderly than for the young.)

To round out the picture, we have to take note of a third component of physical fitness: flexibility. Appropriate stretching helps to protect and maximize your ability to move, reach, lift, and otherwise do what needs to be done. Ideally, all three components—aerobic conditioning, muscle strengthening, and stretching—should be a regular part of your weekly routine. If you're missing one (or all) of them, it's never too late to start. We'll introduce them now, one step at a time.

First steps (literally)—the basics

The first priority for the person who is exercising rarely or not at all is to *get started on a consistent routine of aerobic activity.* This is the simplest type of exercise to begin and the one most likely to have an immediate impact. Unless you have had a major injury or other physical handicap, for example, it doesn't take any training, experience, or special equipment to begin walking. But how much aerobic exercise—walking or otherwise—should you be doing? This question has been addressed by a number of national organizations (such as the National Institutes of Health, the American Heart Association, and the American College of Sports Medicine) over the past few decades, and the answer has evolved significantly over that time. Recommendations in the 1970s and 1980s reflected the notion that exercise had to be both frequent and strenuous in order to benefit the heart and general health. A more recent consensus, however, is that we can obtain significant health benefits from physical activity that is less intense. The current wisdom may be summarized as follows:

1. Every adult and child should attempt to accumulate thirty minutes of moderate-intensity physical activity on most, if not all, days of the week. We may have different ideas of what constitutes moderate-intensity activity. Is it a couple of laps through the mall? mowing the lawn? running a mile? Current advisories from the National Center for Chronic Disease Prevention and Health Promotion define a moderate amount of physical activity as that which burns approximately 150 calories over the course of a day, or roughly one thousand calories per week. (Several everyday examples are listed in the sidebar "What Constitutes Moderate-Intensity Activity?" on page 285.)

2. It is not necessary for all thirty minutes of activity to be carried out at the same time, nor do they all have to involve the same type of exercise. The benefits of exercise can be obtained through two 15-minute, or even three 10-minute, peri-

WHAT CONSTITUTES MODERATE-INTENSITY ACTIVITY?

There are a number of ways to obtain a moderate amount of activity, and clearly some are more vigorous than others. As the chart below suggests, the more intense the exercise, the less time it takes per session to improve your general health. However, the more vigorous activities on this list (those toward the bottom) may not be appropriate for you because of age, general health, or certain medical problems. If in doubt, you should begin with exercise that's less vigorous (those toward the top), even if it takes more time to obtain the desired results. (See “Risks and Precautions: Is It Dangerous to Get in Shape?” on page 290 for more details.)

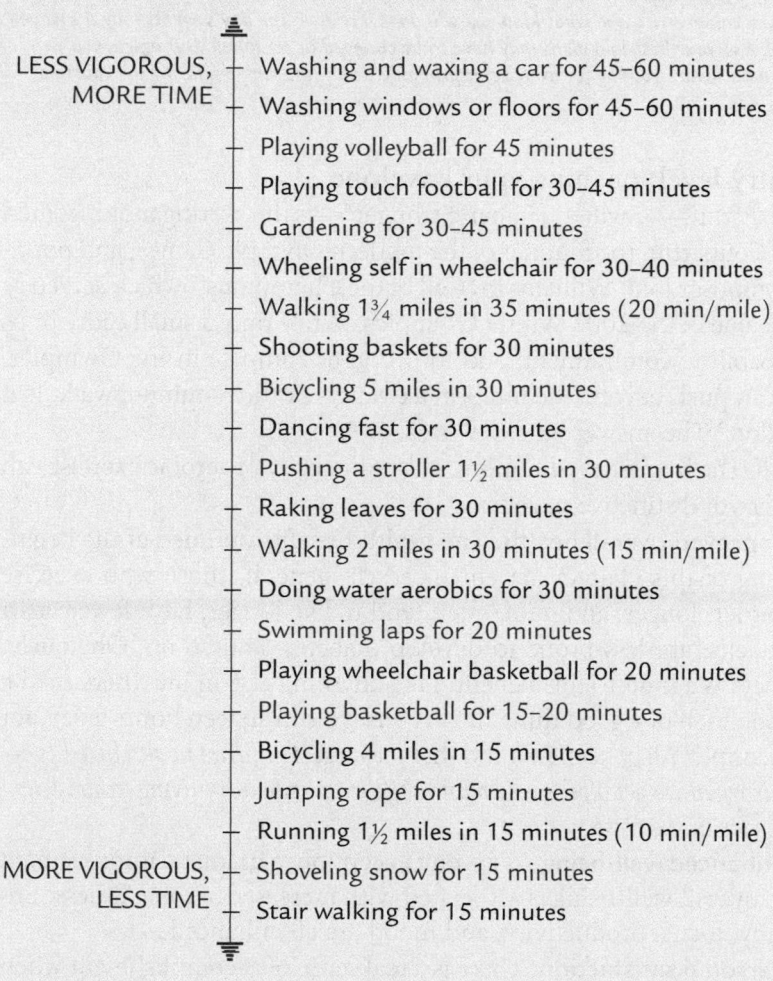

LESS VIGOROUS, MORE TIME

- Washing and waxing a car for 45–60 minutes
- Washing windows or floors for 45–60 minutes
- Playing volleyball for 45 minutes
- Playing touch football for 30–45 minutes
- Gardening for 30–45 minutes
- Wheeling self in wheelchair for 30–40 minutes
- Walking 1¾ miles in 35 minutes (20 min/mile)
- Shooting baskets for 30 minutes
- Bicycling 5 miles in 30 minutes
- Dancing fast for 30 minutes
- Pushing a stroller 1½ miles in 30 minutes
- Raking leaves for 30 minutes
- Walking 2 miles in 30 minutes (15 min/mile)
- Doing water aerobics for 30 minutes
- Swimming laps for 20 minutes
- Playing wheelchair basketball for 20 minutes
- Playing basketball for 15–20 minutes
- Bicycling 4 miles in 15 minutes
- Jumping rope for 15 minutes
- Running 1½ miles in 15 minutes (10 min/mile)
- Shoveling snow for 15 minutes
- Stair walking for 15 minutes

MORE VIGOROUS, LESS TIME

Source: Centers for Disease Control and Prevention

ods of activity. Furthermore, many people prefer to vary the type of exercise they do from day to day, or even within the same day, to prevent boredom.

3. Consistency counts. In order to obtain—and maintain—health benefits, moderate physical activity should be on the agenda every day—or nearly every day. The weekend warrior who shuns exercise during the week and then goes "pedal to the metal" on Saturday, pushing heart and muscles to their limit, is likely to strain, sprain, or break something sooner or later. More importantly, he or she is *less* likely to reap the health benefits of physical activity than the person who puts forth more consistent but less vigorous effort.

HOT TIP

Set a date . . . every day. Before going to bed each night, look at tomorrow's schedule and figure out when you can exercise and what kind you will do. Of course, the day's events may throw you a curveball, and your best-laid plans may have to be changed or scrapped. But unless you've developed a clockwork routine for exercise, it probably won't just happen during the course of the day.

Beyond entry level: pushing your envelope

Citius, Altius, Fortius—"Swifter, Higher, Stronger"—is the stirring motto coined by Baron de Coubertin, the founder of the modern Olympic Games, and popularized by composer John Williams in "Call of the Champions," which served as the official theme of the 2002 Winter Olympics. While only a small cadre of us have the capability, commitment, and fortitude to compete in the Olympics, many of us can push beyond the limits of a twenty- or thirty-minute walk. Is it worth the effort? The answer, in two words, is "Yes, but . . . "

Increasing the frequency, duration, and/or intensity of aerobic exercise can have a number of distinctive payoffs:

- **Improved overall health.** The health benefits outlined at the beginning of this chapter are enhanced. In general, those who exercise harder, longer, and more often tend to live longer, have fewer heart attacks, are less prone to develop diabetes, and so on. Obviously, there is a limit to this benefit. Like anything else in life, there *can* be too much of a good thing. It isn't wise to run sixteen hours a day, for example. Also, keep in mind that *the most significant health benefits occur when we get off the couch and shift from sedentary living to consistent moderate exercise.*
- **Enhanced well-being.** With rare exception, a dramatic improvement in overall well-being is associated with increased aerobic fitness. Energy, focus, productivity, and mood are all enhanced.
- **Personal satisfaction.** There is a real sense of accomplishment when we see some progress, when we reach a goal, when we discover that we can do more than we thought. Ask anyone who has completed a

ARE WE HAVING FUN YET? A Few Ways to Make Exercise More Satisfying (and Consistent)

A highly disciplined person may be willing to submit to a daily exercise routine that he or she truly dislikes. For the other 98 percent of us, it helps if we can make the process as enjoyable as possible. Here are some suggestions:

Exercise with another person. Walk and talk with your spouse; you may find that the opportunity to debrief on a regular basis is habit-forming. Bike, hike, or play vigorously with your kids; to you it may be just a workout, but for them every one of these experiences builds powerful bonds and memories. Set times to exercise with a friend; not only will you enjoy each other's company, but you will be less likely to skip it if you know that someone is waiting for you.

Pay attention to the setting. Is your walking route pleasant and peaceful or polluted and noisy? If you buy a treadmill or a set of weights, do you have to stare at paint cans and boxes in the garage, illuminated by a bare bulb hanging from the ceiling, while you use it? If you're thinking about joining a gym, is it a place you find inviting or a moldy den of sweat strictly for the die-hard bodybuilders? You may not have unlimited options about your surroundings, but you should be able to find a pleasant setting in which to exercise. For example, if there's too much traffic whizzing by, too many unruly dogs running loose, or too many steep hills to climb in the vicinity of your home or apartment, consider driving to a park—or another neighborhood—to go walking or jogging. Many malls open their doors early in the day to offer exercisers a safe, well-lit, and temperate environment.

You don't have to be bored. Some people lose their enthusiasm when their exercise becomes more of a rut than a routine—the same walking path, the same workout video, and so on. As we saw earlier in the chapter ("What Constitutes Moderate-Intensity Activity?" page 285), there are many ways to move your muscles—and that list doesn't even include strengthening and flexibility exercises. Not only can you vary the type of activity, but also the location, time of day, and companion(s): human, animal, or none at all.

You don't have to be bored, part 2. If you're on your own during a workout, the time you spend can be put to use in more ways than one. In the midst of a hectic day, your exercise time may be your one opportunity to think—to process what's going on in your life without distraction. Many people find that their prayer is more focused during exercise, especially when walking or jogging. (If you have enough breath to pray out loud, your train of thought may take even fewer detours.) Portable tape, CD, or MP3 players are now quite inexpensive, and hearing your favorite music while you exercise is a great motivator to keep moving. Better yet, a riveting audiobook can help time pass very quickly. Many public libraries have scores of books on tape or CD, or they can be rented or downloaded for a modest fee from a number of companies. ■

marathon for the first time—no matter how long it took to cover the 26.2-mile course—and you will hear about a rush of emotion at the finish line that far overshadows any sore muscles. Nevertheless, some cautions are worth noting:

1. It is better to do moderate, less taxing exercise consistently (i.e., at least five days per week) than to do more intensive exercise on a hit-or-miss basis.
2. It takes more time and effort to push yourself.
3. There may be some risks involved. These are outlined, along with some basic precautions, in the next section. (See page 290.)

If you have been doing a basic moderate workout (for example, a thirty-minute walk at three to four miles per hour) consistently five days per week and the phrase "Swifter, Higher, Stronger" is starting to reverberate in your brain, keep the following in mind:

1. Get medical clearance if you are a man over forty or a woman over fifty, or if you have risk factors for (or symptoms remotely suggesting) heart disease. (See the next section on risks and precautions for more information.)

2. Make changes gradually in order to prevent injuries, fatigue, and discouragement. If you normally walk for thirty minutes, for example, you may discover some new unhappy muscles if you suddenly jump to sixty minutes. You would be better off increasing the time of your walk by three to five minutes each week. If you are regularly walking two miles in forty minutes and want to speed things up, don't expect to jog or run the entire distance. Instead, after you have warmed up, try alternating jogging and walking every two or three minutes. As your stamina improves, you will be able to increase either the amount of time you spend jogging or your pace, or both. The same principle applies to other aerobic exercise, whether riding a bicycle (moving or stationary), swimming, using a stair-climber machine, and so on. Remember that your purpose is not to push yourself to a near-death experience. If you feel faint, dizzy, or simply unable to press on, *slow down or stop* until you are ready to continue (or, if necessary, call it quits for the day). Ideally you will find a cruising speed at which your breathing can comfortably keep up with your body's increased need for oxygen for longer and longer periods of time.

3. Don't forget to warm up and cool down. This is important for anyone exercising—not merely world-class athletes who are about to compete for a place on the medal platform. In fact, it is particularly important if you have not been exercising consistently (or at all). If your schedule is tight or your day long, you may be tempted to skip these activities, which is definitely a bad idea. Five to ten (or even fifteen) minutes should be spent doing your activity of choice at a more relaxed, comfortable level before shifting gears to begin more serious exertion. If you're going to jog or run, a brisk walk should start your session. If you have just mounted a bicycle, don't begin your ride by storming up the nearest hill. Your heart needs a little time to increase its rate, and your vascular system (your arteries and veins) must divert more blood to muscles that need much more oxygen as they work harder. Those muscles, and the tendons which connect them to bones, are also more prone to tear if they are suddenly called upon to give their all. If you want to stretch before your workout, do it *after* you warm up in order to avoid damaging muscles. Similarly, after a period of vigorous exertion you need to reverse the events that took place during your warm-up. Your heart needs to slow down gradually, and blood needs to be shunted from your muscles to other parts of the body. A sudden shift from "sixty to zero" could cause enough of a drop in blood pressure to make you dizzy or even faint. Some gentle stretching after your cooldown may help prevent cramping and muscle tightness.

4. If you develop chest pain during any workout—even one you have previously tolerated—stop immediately. If the pain does not go away within a few minutes, call 911 or have someone take you immediately to the nearest hospital emergency room. If the pain subsides relatively quickly, talk to your doctor before you resume your exercise program. Not all chest pain is a distress signal from the heart, but this symptom must not be ignored.

5. Use your pulse to guide the pace of your activity. You no doubt know that your heart beats more rapidly during exercise, but how fast should it go? If you have a heart condition or take any medication that affects your heart's response to exercise, you will need guidance from your doctor (or possibly a cardiologist) on this topic. Otherwise, it's useful to know your **target heart rate**, which you can use to estimate how hard this all-important organ is working. Most experts maintain that you benefit most from exercise when your pulse stays between 50 percent and 75 percent of your **maximum heart rate**, which is calculated by subtracting your age from the number 220 (or by using a handy chart such as the table on page 290). You probably won't expend a tremendous amount of energy to reach the lower end of the target zone, and you may feel that you are putting forth Olympian effort to keep it at the upper level. Beginners should stay near the 50 percent mark for a few weeks. They may then gradually increase the intensity of exertion over the next several months until their heart rate approaches the 75 percent level for most of the workout (after an appropriate warm-up, of course). If you've been exercising consistently for six months and have been able to exercise comfortably at the 75 percent level, you may consider pushing up to 85 percent of your maximum rate.

MAXIMUM AND TARGET HEART RATES BASED ON AGE

AGE	TARGET HEART RATE (beats per minute) (50 to 75 percent/max)	MAXIMUM HEART RATE (beats per minute) (220 minus age)
20 years	100–150	200 beats
25 years	98–146	195
30 years	95–142	190
35 years	93–138	185
40 years	90–135	180
45 years	88–131	175
50 years	85–127	170
55 years	83–123	165
60 years	80–120	160
65 years	78–116	155
70 years	75–113	150

Source: Reproduced with permission from *Exercise and Your Heart: A Guide to Physical Activity* © 2001, American Heart Association

Risks and Precautions—Is It Dangerous to Get in Shape?

Every so often we hear an unsettling story of a high school student or even a seasoned athlete who suddenly drops dead during a workout. Jim Fixx, who wrote the best-selling *The Complete Book of Running* in 1977, suffered a fatal heart attack while running his usual ten miles. The great basketball player "Pistol" Pete Maravich, after a distinguished college and professional career, had a cardiac arrest and died while playing an informal game with a few friends. Certainly no one wants to arrive suddenly and unexpectedly at the finish line of life. How can we know if it's safe for us to exercise?

Before we talk about hazards, we need to issue an important reminder: With very rare exception, it is much more dangerous to lead a sedentary life than to embark on a program of regular moderate exercise. Also remember that you are more likely to be injured trying to jump-start your exercise by doing too much too fast, or by trying to cram high-intensity workouts into one or two days per week (or month). With those basic principles in mind, here are some potential exercise risks and some commonsense steps to prevent them.

1. The "big one": heart attack or sudden death. This rare but tragic event usually occurs in one of two ways. As we explained in chapter 3, the common condition known as coronary artery disease can limit the supply of blood (and thus vital oxygen) to one or more areas of heart muscle. When the supply is unable to keep up with the demand, the muscle may generate a sensation of pain, pressure, or other vague discomfort in the chest, with or without sweating, nausea, light-headedness, or shortness of breath. If the muscle is starved of oxygen long enough, it may be

KEEPING TRACK OF YOUR HEART RATE

If you're going to use your pulse as a guide to an appropriate level of exertion, you need to know how to count it. There are two basic approaches:

Low-tech—feel it yourself. With very little practice, you can quickly find the pulse in your wrist (first choice) or your neck (a distant second). The radial artery passes close to the skin near the base of the thumb. Place the tips of the index and middle fingers of your left hand upon the palm side of the right wrist, and then press down until you feel the rhythmic bump of blood flowing through it. (We suggest feeling the right wrist so that you can see your wristwatch. If you wear a watch on the right arm, feel your left wrist.) If you can't detect the pulse, move your fingertips slowly around the area until you find the best spot. To find the pulse in your neck you must locate the carotid arteries, which lie in the broad indentation of the neck on either side of the airway.

It is preferable to use your wrist for this assignment, because undue pressure against a carotid artery could cause the heart rate to slow down. Also, in a susceptible individual, vigorous prodding of a carotid could provoke a fainting episode or (very rarely) even a stroke. However, in some adults the carotid pulse is quite prominent and easier to feel. If your neck serves as your pulse monitor, remember not to push too hard. Don't use your thumb to feel it, and by all means feel only one side at a time.

Once you have become adept at finding your pulse, you need to determine the number of heartbeats per minute. You could, of course, count the number of beats in one minute, but this is rather tedious. Furthermore, if you stop for a full minute during a workout, your pulse rate will start to slow down. You can get a reasonable estimate by counting the beats in fifteen seconds and multiplying by four, or counting for ten seconds and multiplying by six.

High-tech—use a monitor. There is an abundance of electronic gadgets, ranging in price from about forty to three hundred dollars (and up), that can detect your pulse rate and display it on a digital readout. Most of these rely on a light strap that wraps around your chest and transmits your heart rate to the monitor on your wrist. Depending on the amount you're willing to pay and your fascination with the wonders of microcircuitry, you can buy units that do everything but forecast the weather. Available features include time and date, alarms that sound when you drift above or below your target zone, estimates of calories burned during the workout, and the capacity to crunch vast amounts of stored data regarding your performance during one or more sessions. (One unit can recall the particulars of ninety-nine workouts.) A number of monitors download their memory bank into your personal computer so that you can really massage the numbers. Freestanding exercise equipment—treadmills, stationary bicycles, stair-climber machines, and others—may also be equipped to give you feedback regarding your pulse and a number of other variables. ■

damaged, an event known as a heart attack (or a myocardial infarction, in medical terminology). What makes a heart attack so dangerous is that the injured muscle can suddenly set off a chaotic electrical pattern throughout the large chambers (or ventricles) that pump blood to the rest of the body. If this is not reversed, severe brain damage or death is but a few minutes away.

This type of event ended the life of Jim Fixx, who had a strong family history of coronary artery disease. (His father had a heart attack at thirty-five and died of another at forty-three.) He also had an unhealthy, chain-smoking lifestyle before making the changes that began his running career. Fitness experts have speculated that a treadmill stress test, which Fixx was reportedly planning for the week after his fatal run, might well have detected his underlying coronary disease and saved his life. His death serves as a cautionary reminder that the ability to tolerate a long-standing, vigorous exercise program does not guarantee that all is well with the heart.

Sudden death during exercise can also result from certain unusual congenital heart abnormalities that may go undetected until vigorous activity provokes a sudden, fatal rhythm change. This is usually the story behind the headlines when a previously healthy young athlete collapses and dies during a practice or game. Pete Maravich had such a condition, in his case an extremely rare and severe defect in his coronary arteries. (It is actually miraculous that he was able to play basketball as long and as expertly as he did before his cardiac arrest.) More often the problem involves one of the valves within the heart or the system that conducts electrical impulses through the heart muscle.

Reducing the risk of a cardiac catastrophe involves appropriate medical screening, starting at a moderate (or light) level of exercise and advancing gradually, and paying attention to any warning signals. People who should consult with a physician regarding their exercise plans include:

- Anyone with a history of heart disease, including coronary artery disease, congestive heart failure, an irregular rhythm, an abnormal valve, or a congenital (present from birth) abnormality.
- Anyone who has lost a family member who was fifty or younger to a sudden heart-related death.
- Anyone with symptoms that suggest something may be wrong with the heart, including episodes of chest pain or pressure, pounding or fluttering sensations in the chest (called palpitations), faintness, or shortness of breath during mild exertion such as climbing a flight of stairs or walking a short distance. Remember that chest discomfort caused by a heart muscle that is short on oxygen may not even be felt in the chest—it may be noticed in the left arm, jaw(s), or even upper abdomen. This also applies to young athletes. A child or adolescent who develops chest pain, becomes unusually short of breath, or faints during exercise must be evaluated by a physician before participating further in vigorous exercise.

- Men over forty and women over fifty who plan to begin exercising vigorously or who intend to advance from moderate to more intense exercise.

Unfortunately, it is extremely difficult to prevent catastrophic events caused by congenital heart conditions in young athletes, because a sudden, life-threatening abnormal rhythm is usually the *first* sign that anything is wrong. Only rarely will a checkup by a physician uncover one of these problems. In order to detect them, an electrocardiogram (ECG) and an echocardiogram (a sound-wave image of the heart) would have to be performed on every adolescent and young adult participating in vigorous sports, a task that would be monumental in scope and expense. Needless to say, any young athlete who faints or notices pounding in the chest, unusual shortness of breath, or chest pain should be evaluated by a physician before resuming vigorous exercise.

2. Aches and pains, strains and sprains. It should go without saying that exercise involves repetitive movements of muscles and joints, including some we may not know exist until we begin using them. When we ask muscles to work above and beyond their usual levels, we can expect some aching for a day or two. This is usually mild and diffuse, rather than focused in a single area, and shouldn't interfere with normal activities. The aching may actually feel good, an acknowledgment of our recent increase in activity.

More severe pain focused in one area, especially when it causes limping or difficulty moving some part of the body, is a warning that should not be ignored. Strains, sprains, and ruptures (see sidebar "Vocabulary Lesson—Tendons, Ligaments, Strains, Sprains, and Ruptures" on the next page) occur so quickly and create such dramatic pain that the need for medical attention is obvious. Less intense pain may not get our attention right away but is still important.

Inflammation of one or more tendons (or **tendonitis**) is usually caused by what orthopedists call overuse—frequent and/or intense contraction of the muscles to which they're attached. A classic example is so-called tennis elbow, a tendonitis near the elbow caused by repeated gripping and squeezing of the hand (which is powered mainly by large muscles in the forearm and not within the hand itself). Tennis elbow could just as easily be called "suitcase elbow," "jackhammer elbow," "racquetball elbow," or whatever might be the offending activity. (A similar problem has been observed in overzealous Little League pitchers.) **Arthritis**, or inflammation of one or more joints, may be aggravated in some people by repetitive exercises. **Stress fractures**, disruptions of bone that may be too subtle to appear as a clean break on an X ray, may also develop after vigorous exercise. The term **shin splints** refers to a burning, painful sensation along the medial (inner) aspect of the lower leg, usually felt during or after walking, jogging, running, or jumping. The exact origin of the pain has been attributed to a variety of structures: torn muscle fibers, inflamed tendons, and irritation of the covering of bone (or **periosteum**), among others. But there is

VOCABULARY LESSON—TENDONS, LIGAMENTS, STRAINS, SPRAINS, AND RUPTURES

We are all familiar with the muscles that move our arms and legs, fingers and toes, trunk and spine. In order to do so, they must be attached to structures (usually one or more bones) that move in relation to each other. Rather than attaching its fibers directly, each end of the muscle condenses into a tough, fibrous, often cordlike structure called a **tendon,** which concentrates the force of the muscle's contraction into a relatively small area. A few tendons are well-known to us. For example, the Achilles tendon, named for the mythological Greek hero for whom this was a fatal weak spot, attaches our calf muscle to the back of the heel.

When the fibers of a muscle or tendon are stretched beyond their limit or capacity, the result is usually a **strain** (also called a pulled muscle or tendon). Typically this presents itself as a sudden, intense pain in the damaged area, which usually brings the activity to a screeching halt. If enough muscle fibers are torn, blood will ooze into the surrounding tissue, forming a large (and often colorful) bruise. Usually the damage will heal with time, rest, avoidance of activities that hurt, and, when appropriate, physical therapy. If the injury is great enough to separate one end of a muscle from the other or to detach a tendon completely from its moorings, the injury is called a **rupture**. When this occurs, not only is the pain dramatic, but it also becomes difficult, if not impossible, to move the structure to which the muscle or tendon was attached. This is a more serious situation that may require a surgical repair to restore normal function.

A **ligament** is a tough, fibrous band bridging the gap between two adjacent bones. Its function is to limit how far one bone can move in relation to another. When a ligament is stretched forcefully enough to tear, the injury is called a **sprain**. The most familiar of these is the sprained ankle, which typically involves a sudden inward twist of the foot, injuring the ligament connecting the thin, strutlike bone of the lower leg (called the fibula) and the foot. Like strains, sprains usually heal on their own with rest, limiting the amount of weight put on the affected area, and some form of immobilization—splinting or wrapping—to prevent further injury to the ligament. If a ligament is so badly damaged that it can no longer perform its function, a surgical repair may be needed. ■

little doubt that what precipitates shin splints is often overuse—repetitive exercise involving the legs that is either too much, too fast, too long, or that involves inadequate rest between workouts, less than optimal footwear, poor technique, or a combination of these.

Reducing the risk of injury to bones, muscles, joints, tendons, and ligaments (also known as the musculoskeletal system) involves the same commonsense approach we just described for preventing injury to the heart: appropriate medical screening, starting an exercise program slowly and building gradually, and responding to warning signals. You should consult with your primary-care physician or an orthopedist about your exercise plans:

- If you are dealing with pain or swelling in joints that could be affected by the exercise you want to do. The hips, knees, and ankles (known as **weight-bearing joints**) as well as the lower back may be particularly affected by walking, jogging, or cycling.
- If you are at risk for osteoporosis (or thinning of the bones—see chapter 13) and you are involved in **high-impact activities** such as jogging.
- If you repeatedly experience pain somewhere during a particular exercise. This may sound obvious, but we often forget that pain serves the important purpose of warning us when we are causing damage (or are about to) in some part of our body, and it usually guides us in changing our behavior accordingly. Without it, we would literally destroy ourselves at an early age.

There are several other ways to keep the musculoskeletal system happy during and after exercise:

- **Warm up before you open the throttle.** If your exercise includes brisk aerobic activity—running, jogging, fast walking, vigorous dancing, etc.—spend a few minutes at a slower pace before accelerating to your target speed.
- **Similarly, allow a few minutes to cool down when you are done.** We've said it before and we'll say it again: Avoid abrupt transitions not only when starting but also when ending vigorous exercise. This is also a good time to do a few minutes of gentle stretching.
- **If walking, jogging, or running is going to be your primary form of aerobic exercise, invest in a good pair of shoes for that specific activity.** Your bargain-counter sneakers may be okay for everyday chores and relaxing around the house, but when your feet are pounding the pavement for many miles, they need proper support and cushioning. Be sure to try on a few different pairs and move around in them as much as possible at the store. You may want to shop for shoes at the end of the day, when your feet are a little more swollen (thus ensuring that your shoes won't be too tight). Also, wear the type of socks you're likely to use during exercise; athletic socks

are thicker than dress socks, which you aren't likely to wear to a workout. If a pair of shoes isn't comfortable from the moment you try them on, put them back in the box. You can count on spending at least fifty dollars, and most likely a fair amount more, for shoes of reasonable quality. This may seem like a needless expense, especially if you are limiting yourself to walking, but your feet will repay you handsomely for treating them well. (Don't hesitate to look for high-quality shoes on sale, by the way.)

3. Environmental hazards. If your exercise takes you outside or into a pool, it goes without saying that you may encounter a few risks that don't exist in your living room. Nearly all of these can be avoided by taking a few commonsense precautions.

- **Dress appropriately** for current or anticipated weather conditions. In particular, beware of wearing too much clothing when exercising in hot—and especially in humid—conditions. *It is particularly dangerous to do intense workouts in heavy clothing for the purpose of rapidly sweating off excess pounds, because dangerous fluid losses and overheating can result.* (See sidebar "Exercising in the Heat" on page 298.) Similarly, your body temperature may dip to worrisome levels if you exercise in the cold without adequate clothing or swim in cool or frigid water.

RUNNING, WALKING, OR CROSS-TRAINING SHOES?

The notion that you might need different shoes for different activities isn't just an advertising gimmick created by the sporting-goods industry to boost sales. Different activities tend to put predictable stresses on the feet, and footwear engineers have attempted to design shoes for specific activities. For example, because your foot bends more during walking than when running, walking shoes tend to be more flexible. Also, the part of the shoe called the counter, which surrounds the heel, should be firm in a walking shoe, because the heel bears more weight when walking than when running. If you are planning to do a lot of walking over rough terrain, your shoes should have more tread, as well as extra ankle and heel support.

If you participate in a particular sport such as tennis or basketball, you may want to look into shoes specifically tailored for that activity. But for a jack-of-all-trades who participates regularly in a variety of activities, **cross-training shoes** may be best.

If you are new to all of this, don't be afraid to visit a store that caters to runners and walkers. Salespeople in these stores are more likely to be exercise enthusiasts with some personal experience, and because of this, their advice may be more trustworthy. ■

- **Protect your skin from sun exposure.** Don't forget that you can burn just as easily on the sidewalk as at the beach, and that ongoing sun exposure, even without burning, can damage exposed skin. Wear a hat and apply sunscreen if your workout takes you into the sunshine between 10 A.M. and 2 P.M.
- **Be careful on the street.** If riding a bike, invest in a helmet, which absorbs an impact much more successfully than your skull in the event of a fall. If walking or running where there is no sidewalk, you're usually safer going against traffic. If you are out after dark, wear light clothing and consider applying reflective tape to your clothing, shoes, hat (if worn), and bike (if you're riding one). Consider carefully whether you want to walk, jog, or cycle after dark (or any time) through neighborhoods where there may be dogs—or people—with unfriendly attitudes.

4. Special concerns for diabetics. People with type 1 diabetes (who require insulin shots every day) will need to find the right balance between food, insulin, and exercise to avoid hypoglycemic (low blood sugar) episodes. Careful tracking of blood sugar using a glucose monitor—which already should be part of the daily routine for those with this problem—is particularly important to follow a diabetic's response to exercise. For those with the more common type 2 diabetes, a regular exercise program is an extremely important part of the overall strategy for controlling blood sugar and preventing complications. A type 2 diabetic is less likely to become hypoglycemic during exercise unless he or she is using insulin and/or certain types of oral medications; this possibility and appropriate preventive measures should be reviewed with a physician.

Because all adult diabetics, whether type 1 or 2, have a higher risk of developing coronary artery disease, screening for this problem should be discussed with a physician before beginning an exercise program. Properly fitting shoes are also a must for diabetics, whose feet may be more vulnerable to skin breakdown and infection because of poor circulation and reduced pain sensations.

Strengthening Muscles

BUT I'M NOT INTERESTED IN BODYBUILDING. . . .

Before 1990, major health and fitness organizations such as the American College of Sports Medicine and the American Heart Association typically did not include **resistance training** as part of a routine exercise program for the average individual. But times, and thinking, have changed. An ever-growing amount of research supports the notion that making a regular effort to strengthen your body's major muscle groups isn't just an exercise in vanity. What can it do for you?

continued on page 300

EXERCISING IN THE HEAT

We are designed to maintain a body temperature within very narrow limits, but our control systems can be overcome in hot weather, especially when we're exercising.

The results can range from discomfort to disaster. The risk for heat-related illness rises, along with the temperature:

- **When the environment is humid.** We reduce body heat through the evaporation of sweat, which occurs much less rapidly when humidity is high.
- **When you're dehydrated.** During exercise it is possible to become significantly dehydrated before experiencing thirst.
- **Among the very young** (under four years old) **and seniors** (over sixty-five).
- **When certain medications or alcohol are being used.** Several types of antihypertensive drugs—those used to treat high blood pressure—increase the risk of heat illness. Antihistamines, certain medicines called tricyclics and phenothiazines used to treat depression or more severe mental illness, and illegal drugs such as cocaine, heroin, PCP, and LSD (see chapter 10) can also increase the risk.
- **With obesity.**
- **With medical problems** such as fever, heart disease, poor circulation, or sunburn.

The most dangerous heat-related illness is **heat stroke**, in which cooling mechanisms, including sweating, fail and body temperature rises rapidly, often to levels as high as 106° within ten or fifteen minutes. People with impending heat stroke may have a headache; skin that is red, warm, and *dry* (although sweating may be seen in heat stroke brought on by exertion); temperature over 103°; nausea; rapid pulse; confusion; and (eventually) loss of consciousness. Without emergency medical care to bring about rapid cooling, along with other supportive measures, heat stroke can cause permanent damage to multiple organ systems or—in as many as one out of ten cases—death.

Heat exhaustion is a milder type of heat illness that typically involves excess sweating in a hot and humid environment, leading to loss of fluid volume. Many of its symptoms are similar to those of heat stroke: weakness, headache, nausea, and rapid heart rate, among others. But profuse sweating is common, changes in consciousness are *not* seen, and body temperatures do not rise above 105°. Cramping in the arms, legs, or abdomen may be a warning sign of impending heat exhaustion. With rest in a cool area and rehydration, a person with heat exhaustion often feels better within two or three hours.

Heat syncope (fainting) is an episode of dizziness or fainting that occurs after prolonged standing in the heat, or when getting up suddenly after lying or sitting for a while in a hot environment (the light-headed feeling you have when you stand up after sitting at the beach or by the swimming pool on a hot day). Exercising without a cooldown, becoming dehydrated, or exercising without being properly acclimated to a hot environment can also provoke it. Lying down will improve symptoms quickly, and taking fluids will help as well.

Several practical measures will help prevent heat-related problems while exercising:

- Wear loose, light-colored clothing.
- Avoid working out during the hottest time of the day, typically 10 A.M. to 2 P.M.
- Avoid exercising when the temperature is over 85° or the humidity is over 90 percent.
- If you are going to be exercising regularly in the heat, take time to become acclimated. Several less-strenuous workouts with adequate hydration may be required to bring about acclimatization, which helps the body work more efficiently, generate less internal heat, and deal more efficiently with whatever heat is generated.
- Adequate hydration is extremely important. Remember, *significant dehydration can occur before you actually feel thirsty.* If you are going to exercise in the heat, especially for an extended period, you would be wise to *prehydrate* with sixteen ounces of fluid *before* the activity, then consume eight ounces every twenty minutes while exercising. Water or sport drinks such as Gatorade that contain glucose and sodium are appropriate. Drinks containing alcohol and/or caffeine should be avoided because they tend to provoke **diuresis** (an increase in urine output that could result in further loss of fluid).
- If you have any of the medical conditions mentioned at the beginning of this sidebar, or if you take a number of prescription medications, you should exercise in the heat with great caution, if at all—and not before reviewing your plans with your physician.
- Last but not least, if you begin to feel dizzy, faint, nauseated, or otherwise unwell while exercising in a warm environment, *stop immediately,* get into a cool area, and lie down. If possible, take some fluids. If you don't begin to feel better within several minutes, seek medical care right away or ask someone to help you do so. If you do feel better, call off the workout, take it easy for the rest of the day, and contact your physician for further advice before you exercise again. ■

continued from page 297

Enable you to do more. While few of us are called upon to bend steel with our bare hands or leap tall buildings with a single bound, it's a simple fact that those who are strong can do a wider variety of everyday tasks, do them longer, and do them with less risk of strains, sprains, and falls than those who are not. As we will discuss later in this chapter, *this is especially obvious, and particularly important, among the elderly.* The frail person may have difficulty lifting a bag of groceries, moving a stuck closet door, or pulling a toddler out of a crib. Even if you belong to the auto club, it's nice to know that you can change your own flat tire should the need arise. Compared to our ancestors, far fewer of us have jobs that are physically taxing, but even if our loads are lighter, we still need to carry them if we want to live independently.

Enhance weight control. On a pound-for-pound basis, muscle consumes more calories than fat, even while you're resting. Not only do you use extra calories during a workout (whether aerobic or weight training), but whatever muscle tissue you add when exercising will also burn more fuel when you're not. Furthermore, those who are cutting back on food intake in order to lose weight can count on losing not only fat, but muscle as well. Muscle-building exercises (and aerobic activity too) help ensure that if you're shedding pounds, you'll dump your fat and not your form.

Increase bone density. Earlier in this chapter we mentioned the benefits of weight-bearing aerobic exercise (such as walking) on bone density, especially for women who are approaching or have passed menopause. However, not everyone who could benefit from this is able to do it, often because of chronic aches and pains in the back and weight-bearing joints (such as the hips and knees) that are more common in older age groups. Resistance training may offer a solution in that it also builds bone density—in fact, probably more effectively—but with exercises that can be tailored to the individual.

Improve appearance (usually). Let's face it, a flatter stomach, some definition of muscle in certain areas, a straighter posture, and a general appearance of being fit and trim is something we all strive for at some level. We're not talking about the hyperbulked, anatomy-book (or comic-book) physiques seen at bodybuilding competitions, where beauty is definitely in the eye of the beholder. We heartily discourage preoccupation with appearance that becomes an anxiety-ridden obsession or a form of self-idolatry, and we readily acknowledge that our culture is far too willing to assign worth based on physical perfection. That being said, there's nothing wrong with improving the way we look to others, whether in the context of family, vocation, or ministry.

So how do I strengthen my muscles?

The famous phrase "use it or lose it" certainly applies to muscles of all shapes and sizes. If a muscle sits idly or moves against little or no resistance for even a

VOCABULARY—PUMPING IRON AND RELATED PURSUITS

We are all familiar with such well-worn terms as **bodybuilding, weight lifting,** and **pumping iron**, which may bring to mind visions of sweaty gyms, impossibly sculpted physiques, and individuals with nicknames such as Hulk or Spike. But such clichés are overdue for retirement, because improving muscle strength and tone is a worthwhile project for all of us. In recognition of this fact, a different collection of phrases has entered our vocabulary: **strength training, weight training,** and more recently **resistance training** (or **resistance exercise**), reflecting the fact that there are ways to improve our muscles that do not involve moving heavy objects up and down. In this book we will use these terms interchangeably.

You may hear some additional terms related to this type of exercise: **isometric, isotonic,** and **isokinetic**.

Isometric exercises are those in which muscles exert force against something that will not budge (for example, a wall). The muscle tenses but it doesn't contract, so no movement occurs. (The word *isometric* literally means "same measure.") While this might seem to be an exercise in futility, so to speak, isometric exercises may be useful in certain situations. For example, someone recovering from an injury that limits free movement of an arm or leg may be instructed in isometric exercises to strengthen immobile muscles. However, the effect is specific only for the angle at which the force is applied. And while isometric exercises have the advantage of not requiring special equipment, overzealous effort may temporarily increase blood pressure. For these reasons, and their questionable benefit for everyday activities, isometric exercises are not widely recommended for the average person who is attempting to improve overall fitness.

Isotonic exercises are those in which muscles move against a fixed (but moveable) resistance. These include the most familiar types of strengthening exercises, such as lifting barbells, using a weight machine, or doing push-ups. While the word *isotonic* literally means "same tension," more effort is usually expended at the beginning and the end of a muscle's movement against resistance.

Isokinetic (literally, "same motion") exercises require special equipment that can control the speed of a muscle's contraction as it pushes or pulls against resistance through its range of motion. These are normally used by physical therapists who own Cybex, Biodex, or similar machines. ■

few days, it will begin to weaken and shrink in size. (Ask anyone who has worn a cast for a month or more. When the affected arm or leg is freed from captivity, most people are shocked to see how much smaller it has become.) If a muscle is repeatedly called upon to exert force against ever-increasing resistance, the opposite occurs. Furthermore, if muscles become stronger as a result of working against more resistance, they must be *kept* working at that level to maintain their strength. The bad news is that, just as with aerobic fitness, there is no way to improve and maintain muscular fitness without ongoing effort. There is no finish line at which you can proudly announce you are done with the discipline of routine exercise, unless your goal is to become frail and easily fatigued. The good news is that you don't have to spend hours every week handling hardware in order to make some progress.

Current research supports the following guidelines for resistance training in all adult age groups:

How often? Two or three times per week, with one or two days between workouts to allow the muscle groups to rest.

How many muscle groups should be exercised? Eight to ten muscle groups, encompassing the major muscles of the arms, legs, abdomen, and back.

How many repetitions (or reps) of an exercise for a given muscle group? Eight to twelve reps for those younger than fifty to sixty years of age; or ten to fifteen reps, using a lower resistance, for those fifty to sixty or older and for people with heart disease (with the approval of their physician). A greater number of repetitions with lower resistance is less likely to cause injury in the elderly.

How many sets of repetitions? One per workout is appropriate for beginners, for those who are getting started after a prolonged time-out from exercise, or for those interested in basic health maintenance. After several weeks, those who want to enhance strength or performance of some or all muscle groups may consider doing a second set.

How long should this take? Each repetition should involve a steady, controlled movement—typically two seconds to lift the weight and four to lower it, without jerking, grunting, or breath-holding. (Inhale while lifting or exerting against resistance, exhale while lowering or releasing.) A single set of exercises will typically last about twenty to thirty minutes, depending on your familiarity with the exercises and equipment.

How much resistance? That depends on the muscle group, the particular exercise you're doing for that group, your experience, age, and a few other factors. If you are just getting started, it would be wise to go easy. Use a relatively light weight that allows you to complete ten to twelve reps using good form for the particular exercise. When this can be done comfortably and smoothly, the weight can be increased by 5 percent for the next session. You should work toward a level at which the last one or two reps require some effort. Obviously, there is an absolute limit to each person's strength, and you would be wise to avoid increasing the resistance beyond the point where you cannot complete more than a few reps. On the other hand, you will not accomplish a great deal by remaining at a light level of resistance and repeating the same exercise dozens of times. (In order to track the weights or resistance settings you are using for each exercise, you'll need to keep a simple log.)

How do I get started with resistance training?

Most of us can begin an aerobics program with little more than a decent pair of walking shoes and a street. But to do a complete set of resistance training exercises requires at least some equipment and some direction as well. Things you can use to provide resistance include:

- **Your own body.** Push-ups, pull-ups, sit-ups, and knee bends, among other maneuvers, are time-honored exercises that work large groups of muscles. Obviously no purchase is required, and this "equipment" will always be with you. But there isn't much you can do to adjust the amount of resistance, and so progress is usually measured in the number of reps you can do before the muscles involved cry uncle.
- **Elastic bands and tubes.** These are basically pieces of rubber of varying size, shape, and thickness to which handles may be attached, or which may be hooked to a door or other immovable object. They are definitely low-tech, inexpensive, portable, and versatile. Without a hefty investment and without hogging a fair amount of floor space, they can be used to exercise many different muscle groups. However, because no actual weights are involved, it may be difficult to gauge how you're progressing. Also, bands and tubes might raise a healthy welt on an unsuspecting body part if you accidentally lose your grip.
- **Free weights.** These are the familiar dumbbells, which can be gripped by one hand, and barbells, which require two hands to hold a metal bar onto which various-sized weights can be attached at each end. Free weights are not named in honor of their price (which can run several hundred dollars or more for a full set), but because they are not joined via cables, pulleys, or tracks to a machine. They are definitely less expensive than weight machines (see next page), and they can be used to strengthen a wide assortment of muscle groups in the upper body. However, many exercises with free weights involve a learning curve, where one must not only move the weight but also control its flight path to work the appropriate muscle(s) without straining or some other mishap. Also, a number of exercises using free weights require the services of a padded bench, the cost of which should be factored into any decision about buying equipment for use at home.

- **Weight machines.** In well-equipped health clubs and workout rooms you will usually find an array of these devices, which isolate individual muscle groups from one end of the body to the other. They are typically easier to use than free weights because the machine defines the motion; you merely adjust the resistance, sit or recline in the appropriate position, and go to work. For several hundred to a few thousand dollars, you can buy your own home gym that offers the services of several individual resistance machines. Obviously such equipment offers a great deal of convenience—no need to trek off to the health club, hire a sitter, etc.—but like any major investment one should not be purchased before you do some homework. Perhaps the most important question to be addressed—even before "What can we afford?" and "Where will we put it after it's unloaded from the delivery truck?"—is "Will we really *use* this equipment after the novelty wears off?" Like idle treadmills, home gyms make expensive clothing racks or spider hotels.

The specific exercises you do will depend to a large degree on the equipment you plan to use. If you are going to join a fitness center or have one available to you at work, someone who is well-versed in resistance training should

SHOULD I TRY A PILATES CLASS?

First things first: *Pilates* isn't pronounced like the guys who fly airplanes, or the Roman governor named Pontius. It's pronounced *puh-LAH-teez,* named for Joseph Pilates, who developed the technique in the early 1900s and taught it to wounded English soldiers during World War I.

Later it was adopted by famous choreographers such as George Balanchine and Martha Graham as a rehabilitation program for injured dancers.

Pilates exercises emphasize strengthening, posture, balance, and alignment of major muscle groups of the abdomen, back, thighs, and buttocks, referred to as the "core" muscles. Learning the exercises is a long-term process requiring appropriate training, ongoing practice, and a lot of concentration, but those who stay the course are likely to improve their strength, flexibility, and coordination with little risk. Pilates studios offering lessons and classes have appeared in cities from coast to coast, and many health clubs offer Pilates classes as well. Private lessons can be expensive (from forty to two hundred dollars per session). Currently there is not a nationally recognized certification process for Pilates instructors. However, the nonprofit Pilates Method Alliance is engaged in an ongoing effort to establish certification and continuing education standards for those who teach this method. The PMA Web site (http://www.pilatesmethodalliance.org) provides guidance for finding qualified teachers. ■

be available to help you select a set of exercises and orient you to the equipment available. Even if you are going to set up your own program at home, it may be worth hiring a trainer for a few sessions to help you set up a routine and use your equipment properly. For those who do not have access to such resources but want to begin a basic set of strengthening exercises with modest expense (using your own body, a rubber tube, and/or some free weights), we have described and illustrated several options for the major muscle groups in appendix D, beginning on page 929.

Stretching

DO I REALLY NEED TO?

The good news about stretching is that it doesn't require special equipment, membership in a health club, or any investment other than time. The bad news is that after rearranging your schedule to do aerobic activity five times per week and strengthening exercises two or three times a week, you may feel that additional time is an investment you can't afford. But there are a number of reasons to find a few more minutes each week to keep your body in its best possible condition.

Like muscle strength, flexibility is a "use it or lose it" commodity. Over time, muscles and tendons tend to tighten unless they are regularly stretched. We get a small taste of this if we have to spend an hour or two in a cramped space (for example, in the backseat of a small car or the middle seat on a crowded flight): It feels so good to break loose and move around, and it may take a few minutes before we can move as freely as usual. As the decades pass, a similar process may occur in a more gradual and subtle way, resulting in what physicians call **decreased range of motion.** This becomes particularly noticeable in the shoulders, hips, neck, and back, which normally are capable of moving in many directions. The ability to reach upward, pick up an object, look around, or bend forward can become drastically reduced, as occurs all too often among senior citizens. These changes with aging are not inevitable, nor are they attributable solely to arthritis or degenerative changes in the joints.

In order to "preserve, protect, and defend" our mobility, fitness-promoting organizations such as the American College of Sports Medicine now recommend that stretching exercises be included in our weekly routine.[17] Some general ground rules include:

- Do a stretching routine at least two or three times per week, and more often if possible. If you are exercising regularly, stretch *after* your workout.
- If you're going to stretch without doing an aerobic or strengthening workout, don't try to do so when your muscles are cold. You may convert a stretch to a strain—or an outright muscle pull. Warm up first, perhaps by walking briskly while swinging your arms in a comfortable range for a few minutes, and then begin.

continued on page 308

SHOULD MY FAMILY JOIN A HEALTH CLUB?

The answer may be yes if you have fitness goals that you don't think you can reach without the instruction, classes, equipment, and encouragement that a club might provide. This is especially true if you want to do strength training and have concerns about putting together the proper training and equipment on your own.

On the other hand, the answer may be no if the thought of huffing and puffing in plain view of other people turns you off or terrifies you, or if you can't stand exercising indoors. And it certainly *should* be no if you do a soul-searching reality check and can't honestly answer yes to the following question: "If I spend my hard-earned money on a health-club membership, will I actually *use* it on a consistent basis?" Do your current commitments, lifestyle, schedule, and track record with other projects agree with that affirmative answer?

In one respect, health clubs can be a lot like churches: Both have a number of people—sometimes the majority—who claim to be members but don't show up. (Of course, the people who don't come to church regularly usually don't contribute. The health club, on the other hand, already has your money, or will bill you for it, whether you come or not.)

Assuming that you feel inspired to join a health club or fitness center and are convinced that you will go often enough to make it worthwhile, what else should you think about?

Is the location convenient? If you have to add the better part of an hour to your exercise time in order to negotiate distance and traffic, you may not be likely to keep up a workout routine when your life gets hectic.

What hours is it open? If the facility isn't open when you want to use it, you might as well not join. Many communities now have one or more fitness centers that are open literally twenty-four hours a day, which can be wonderful if you have a demanding schedule.

Can you afford the fees? Many clubs have an initiation fee (which may be waived if they're trying to attract new members), and all will have a monthly membership fee. There may be a reduced rate if you're willing to pay in advance for more than one month at a time. Is the price tag compatible with the family budget? Also, are there extra charges for particular classes, child care, parking, or other services?

Do you have to sign a contract? If so, for how long? And what happens if you decide after a few months that you don't want to continue, or if you suffer an injury and *can't* continue? Do you still have to pay the full fee?

HOT TIP

Don't sign for longer than a year at a time. ***Hotter tip:*** *Never buy a lifetime membership. The club may fold, or you may decide to bail out, long before you get your money's worth.*

What does the club offer in terms of equipment? Does it offer aerobic equipment of various types—treadmills, stair-climber machines, elliptical trainers, and so on—as well as machines for strengthening a wide range of muscle groups? What about free weights? Some fitness centers are literal supermarkets of exercise options and may include swimming pools, squash courts, and other elaborate sporting options. Others are much more limited in scope, which isn't necessarily bad. Are there enough machines to use, especially at the time you expect to show up? How does the equipment look? Is it well kept or worse for wear?

HOT TIP

If you're primarily interested in fitness classes, some large churches make these available for various age groups. You might find the costs and the company to your liking.

If you want to work out in a group, are classes scheduled at convenient hours? Are they geared to your level of fitness or experience?

Are you—and your kids—comfortable with the child care offered? Check out the staff-to-child ratio, child-care center hours and activities, and ask how and when the center would summon you if your kids needed you while you were working out. Once you've met the staff, ask yourself whether you'd feel comfortable leaving your children in their care.

Are there other services that might help you? Some centers offer additional services such as children's programming and nutritional counseling.

How does the staff treat you? Are you greeted warmly and courteously? Are they willing to answer questions about the facilities, classes, and fees? What kind of evaluation of *your* fitness and needs do they carry out before setting up your exercise program? Do you see the staff circulating in the facility to help members with the use of equipment? Do you feel like you're being pressured into signing on the dotted line?

What kind of credentials do the staff members have? Ideally one or more employees on the premises have been certified by a professional organization such as the American College of Sports Medicine, the National Strength and Conditioning Association, or the American Council on Exercise.

What about a club that's open only to one gender? Women in particular may feel more comfortable working out in a setting where they don't need to feel self-conscious about the shape of their body. Some national franchises such as Curves cater strictly to women.

How comfortable do you feel in the club or fitness center? Do you sense that the facility is user-friendly and well-maintained and that staff members are professional? Are the sights, sounds, and smells agreeable to you? (Be sure to check the condition of the locker room and shower facilities.) Does the place seem like a giant singles bar without the alcohol, or does it strike you as welcoming all ages, interests, and levels of experience? ■

continued from page 305

- Move into the stretched position slowly, rather then jerking or thrusting toward your goal.
- Stretch to a point of feeling tension or mild discomfort, but not overt pain. (Remember, pain is your body's alarm system. Don't ignore or override it.) Hold the position for ten to thirty seconds and then gradually release. Repeat this cycle for a total of four stretches per muscle group. Don't bounce or jerk at the stretched position or you may injure a muscle or tendon.
- Breathe slowly and comfortably during the stretch. There's no benefit to be gained from grunting and groaning.
- Most of all, try to relax and enjoy the process. Stretching isn't supposed to be an intense, rushed experience. Give yourself permission to slow down for a few minutes as you work through your routine.

What should be stretched? There are a multitude of possible stretching exercises, but ideally a routine will include the neck, upper and lower back, shoulders, front and back thighs (the quads and hamstrings), and calves. You may choose to follow a routine demonstrated in a fitness center or on a video. We have included examples of several useful stretches in appendix D on page 941.

What about doing yoga? We will take a look at this age-old meditative exercise in chapter 17.

Physical Activity in Children . . . and in the Family

As we mentioned at the beginning of this chapter, no one has to encourage toddlers and two-year-olds to be physically active. During most of their waking hours, their agendas involve some form of perpetual motion. But as a child grows and his attention span increases, so does the lure of activities in which minds may be engaged but bodies sit still. TV, video games, and computers can captivate children even before they set foot in preschool, and for many the grip of those electronic devices never loosens. Add to that the demands of school attendance, studying, and homework, not to mention time spent in conversations with friends (whether face-to-face or via phone, cell, or chat room), and far too many of our youngest citizens exit childhood and adolescence overweight and underactive. We already noted the dwindling percentage of children who remain physically active as they continue through high school and the alarming increase in childhood obesity over the past few decades. Unfortunately, any bad habits forged in your home over the years (beginning in preschool) are likely to continue well into adulthood.

How can you launch your children into a healthy trajectory for this important aspect of their lives? Basically in the same ways you promote any value that you care about: by modeling it yourself, by doing it with them, and by encouraging them to do it on their own.

1. Modeling physical activity. You may be convinced that your offspring are hard of hearing when it comes to heeding your advice. But children and teenagers care a great deal about consistency and integrity, and they will rarely take to heart any input from you that implies "Do as I say, not as I do." Throughout this book you will frequently encounter a warning to be careful how you behave, because your sons and daughters are likely to imitate you. (Children who see their parents smoking, for example, are more inclined to try tobacco products—and other harmful chemicals—than those who do not.)

By now it should be clear that you cannot keep your body in shape by exercising once a month. Maintaining physical fitness requires a routine and a measure of self-discipline, and hopefully your children will have the opportunity to see you doing what needs to be done. Should you decide to buy fitness equipment to use at home—a treadmill or a set of free weights, for example—you not only will have the flexibility to exercise at times that suit you, but your children will also be more likely to see you in action. Indeed, when they are old enough to use such equipment safely, you can let them try it as well. But by all means don't let your investment gather dust for weeks on end in your bedroom or the garage. Doing so will waste not only your money but also untold numbers of teachable moments.

You can increase the amount of physical activity in many ways other than participating in designated exercise sessions. If you get in the habit of doing a number of these, you will not only burn extra calories and improve your muscle tone, but you will also set an example for other family members to follow. Some possibilities:

- Take the stairs instead of the elevator or escalator.
- Don't play "chicken" with other drivers for that hotly contested parking space near the entrance to the mall. Deliberately park some distance away (where there are plenty of spaces) and walk.
- If you have to run an errand that isn't too far away, walk or ride a bike.
- Get a cordless phone with a headset so that you can walk around while talking rather than sitting in one place.
- Do your own yard work or at least some of it.
- When socializing with friends, consider options beyond merely talking and eating. Try walking or hiking together or recreational sports such as tennis or golf.
- If you travel on business, try to stay at hotels that have a fitness center or pool, and make use of these amenities.
- For physical, intellectual, emotional, and spiritual reasons, the time your kids spend staring at the television, playing video games, or using the computer for recreation should be limited to two hours per day. The same goes for you.
- Walk while you pray. (Imagine what would happen if we converted half of our TV time to walking and praying.)

2. Doing physical activities as a family. Role modeling is great, but you will definitely get more mileage by involving your kids in activities you do together.

SHOULD MY KIDS DO STRENGTH TRAINING?

Nearly all advisories about physical fitness in children and adolescents—including the ones in this book—emphasize aerobic exercise, such as walking, running, or cycling. While the idea of children pumping iron may seem a little odd, recently organizations such as the American College of Sports Medicine and the American Academy of Pediatrics have suggested that strength training can make a worthwhile contribution to overall fitness in a child or adolescent, with the following provisions:

- Children who are old enough to participate in organized sports programs can also potentially participate in strength training, assuming they can follow directions and use appropriate equipment safely. Children should not participate in competitive weight lifting or bodybuilding, nor should adolescents until they have attained full physical maturity.
- The purpose of strength training should be to improve overall fitness, in conjunction with aerobic exercise. If the goal is to improve performance in a particular sport, practicing and mastering the specific skills for that sport are more likely to be beneficial.
- As with adult strength training for general fitness, children and adolescents can learn basic exercises for eight to ten muscle groups, doing a set of eight to fifteen repetitions for each group, two or three times per week. They should start with a low resistance and an emphasis on proper technique and safety. Weight is added in small increments only when all eight to fifteen repetitions can be performed without strain and with good technique.
- A medical evaluation should be considered before a child or young adolescent begins a strength-training program. If there is any pain, dizziness, or other symptoms in connection with this (or any other physical) activity, a physician should be consulted before the activity is resumed.
- Adult supervision, proper training in the use of equipment, safety precautions, and appropriate expectations are essential. A child should not start strength training for the purpose of building muscles like Popeye (he won't), clobbering a neighborhood rival, or satisfying some other need for recognition or superiority. ■

Not only does everyone reap physical benefits, but also the potential for bonding, communication, and pure fun is virtually unlimited. Young children rarely turn down an opportunity to play a physical game with one or both parents. For older children and adolescents, these activities can play a huge role in establishing their identity as members of your family.

Nearly all of the suggestions in the previous section can be done with one or more children. In addition, consider the following:

- As soon as your children are old enough, have them join you when you walk or jog. Little ones can be pushed in a stroller or carriage. (Some models are specifically geared for greater distances and speed.) Older children who can't keep up with your walking or jogging pace can tag along on a scooter or bicycle.
- Let your children try recreational sports that they can enjoy throughout their lives. Nearly every child enjoys learning to play catch. Tennis, golf, and skiing (both downhill and cross-country) can be enjoyable family pastimes. Backyard games—badminton, volleyball, and even informal softball tournaments (using toy balls and plastic bats that can't cause any damage or injury)—can introduce children to sports that they may take more seriously later on. Remember that if you're going to teach these games to your kids, the object is to have fun and create cherished memories. Impatience, anger, or taking the outcome of a game a bit too seriously can spoil what should be a pleasant experience.
- When you go to the beach or a park, don't just bring blankets and food. Sporting goods stores and variety stores sell all sorts of nifty flying objects (such as plastic discs of various shapes and sizes), as well as ingenious toys that swat or fling balls back and forth and that are fun and challenging for all ages. Playing with them generates a lot of muscle motion.
- Make yard work or gardening a family activity, rather than a solo job for a child or parent, as often as possible.
- Plan vacations that include walking, hiking, swimming, and other physical pursuits, rather than merely sitting (in a car or tour bus) or hanging out at a hotel.

3. Encouraging your kids' physical activity. Aside from your own example and your participation in physical activities with them, there are a number of ways to increase the likelihood that your offspring will move their muscles on their own:

- As we noted earlier, for *many* reasons it is wise to limit your kids to two hours per day (or less) of TV, video games, or recreational computer activities.
- Children arriving home from school should have some time for physical activity rather than plowing directly into homework.

- When buying birthday or Christmas presents, think about gifts that will encourage physical activity. Consider giving a tennis racket or a baseball glove rather than a new computer game.
- Encourage your child's participation in school physical education classes and programs, even if it isn't her strong suit. If she's having trouble keeping up, take an active role in helping her improve her performance. Comments such as, "Oh well, it's just P.E. . . ." may convey an attitude that exercise is a waste of time.

In addition to the above, most children and adolescents at some point participate (at least for a while) in organized team-sports programs such as Little League baseball, softball, soccer, basketball, or football. Others become active in individual competitive sports such as swimming, gymnastics, or skating. In some families, children and teens become involved in archery, bowling, sailing, or horseback riding. There are few athletic or physical skills that children cannot begin to learn during their grade school years, with a few exceptions:

- Collision sports such as football or hockey should be postponed until age twelve to fourteen unless they are specifically noncontact games. Sports with a potential for physical contact such as soccer or basketball may be intimidating for children under age eight. A child who is younger, smaller, or less aggressive than his fellow players may find these activities too intense.
- Because of its potential for causing damage to the brain, boxing should be avoided completely.
- Use discernment if your child or teenager wants to join a martial-arts program. Martial-arts classes are more popular than ever, and they can help build confidence and self-protection skills. But some guidelines are in order. Make sure that the emphasis is on building balance, coordination, and restraint, not on thrashing an opponent. Check out the safety guidelines in the classes. For example, breaking boards should not be part of the curriculum for students under twelve because of the risk of damage to bones, tendons, and ligaments in the hands and feet. Also watch for any religious or mystical component that might be incompatible with your faith.

Participation in sports and competition can have many benefits: developing strength and coordination, acquiring self-discipline, learning cooperation and sportsmanship, and building friendships. But these activities also have the potential to cause physical injury; generate considerable stress or permanent emotional scars; and nourish a host of negative attitudes, including elitism, hostility, and an obsession with winning. To maintain balance and build positive experiences through sports, revisit the following questions on a regular basis:

- Is your child really interested in this activity? You may have loved football, but he may prefer swimming.

- Is your child physically and emotionally ready to practice and compete in the sport?
- Is the proper protective equipment available and used at all times?
- Do the coaches and trainers enjoy working with children or teenagers, including those who are the least skilled? Are they focused on the right attitudes and values (see below), or do they appear driven to win at all costs? Are they competent?
- Do you have the resources and time to support your child or adolescent through the tryouts, practices, and events?
- How heavily is your child's—or your own—self-concept dependent on his success? Does the emotional weather at your home rise and fall with the fortunes of the team or your child's ranking at the last swim meet?
- Are positive values being taught and modeled by all concerned? Is

WHEN IS IT OKAY TO QUIT?

Your daughter begged you to let her begin gymnastics classes, but now her muscles are sore and it's clear that it is hard work–much harder than she thought it would be. Furthermore, she's not as good as the other girls, and more than a couple of times she's landed with a painful thud on the mat. She's had enough, but you've spent ninety-five dollars for a class that will continue for another six weeks. Do you let her bail out or make her continue to the bitter end–perhaps quoting the adage that "winners never quit and quitters never win"?

The answer will depend on your child and her track record. If she has a habit of making enthusiastic false starts and rarely completing a project, she will probably benefit from the experience of struggling to complete the course she started. This reality therapy will be especially important if you have funded the classes after she promised to finish them. In this case, being true to her word is the issue rather than the classes themselves.

When the activity in question is something that other family members enjoy together, such as skiing or skating, positive encouragement to struggle through the learning process in order to enjoy a lifelong payoff would be appropriate.

If she has been consistently involved in other long-term activities but is clearly miserable in this one, you may want to let her quietly retire. Make sure the problem isn't a mismatch with the wrong coach or mistaken placement into a group that is too advanced. At times a change of venue, trainer, or team can make a significant difference. However, if the activity proves to be a dead end, don't berate her for it. Allowing her to maintain her dignity will accomplish far more than any trophy on the family shelf. ■

unsportsmanlike conduct tolerated? Are parents who watch the events behaving themselves?

- Are we having fun yet? The vast majority of young sports participants will not become professional athletes or Olympic contenders, so the experiences of sports and competition should be enjoyed, not endured. If the sport becomes a thorn in your child's side or constantly drains her of energy and joy, reconsider goals and priorities.

QUESTIONS TO PONDER

1. How much moderate-intensity exercise are you getting each week? If you're not currently exercising regularly, what is getting in your way? Is it a busy schedule? dislike of exercise? lack of equipment? a health issue? All of these problems can be overcome. What ideas from this chapter could you use to incorporate more exercise into your schedule?
2. If you are exercising regularly, are you incorporating both endurance and resistance training in your workouts? What new goals can you set for yourself to ensure that physical activity remains rewarding for you?
3. If you have children living at home, do you know how much exercise they get from PE classes, organized sports, and free play? If they aren't active much of the time, how can you encourage them to spend more time in physical activities?

Action items: If exercising consistently is difficult for you, refer to the chart on page 285 for a list of more than twenty activities that qualify as moderate-intensity activity. Choose at least one to work into your schedule a few times this week, and do so again next week and the following two weeks. Soon you may find that this time has become a pleasant—as well as health-building—habit.

Make a date with your spouse, kids, or a friend to try a physical activity that has always appealed to you. If you love watching Olympic skaters, find the nearest ice arena and call to find out their open skating hours. If being outside and enjoying nature is more your speed, check with a local park district or state park for a map of nature trails. And if your kids have begged you to let them play laser tag, now might be the time to try it out—together!

If exercise is already a regular part of your schedule, congratulations. You're probably already aware of the many benefits to your physical and emotional health. After reading this chapter, how might you make exercise safer, more enjoyable, and better balanced between endurance and strength training?

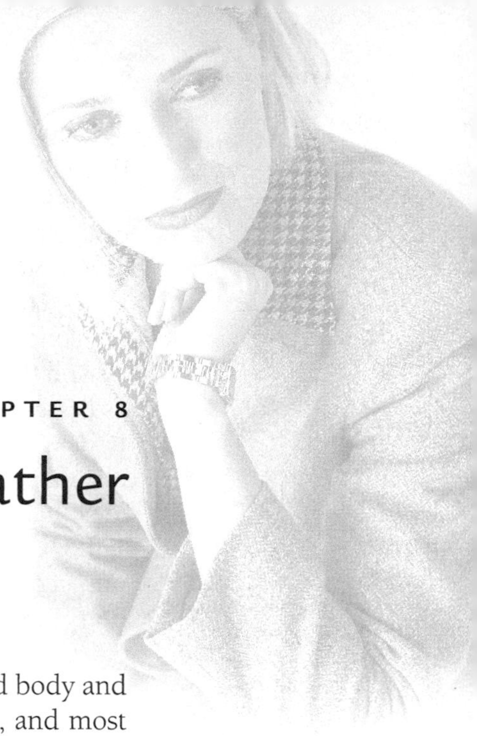

CHAPTER 8

The Emotional Weather

We have gone to some length to describe the importance of a sound body and offer ways to protect and maintain it. But the healthiest, strongest, and most beautiful body is of little use if it is governed by disordered thoughts and emotions. The heart, lungs, and other organs can work perfectly well inside the body of someone who is delusional, suicidal, or a career criminal. Furthermore, we tend to think of what goes on inside our head as somehow disconnected from the rest of the body. But in fact, the brain is also a physical organ, profoundly affected by what goes on from the neck down. Conversely, what goes on in the brain can have powerful effects elsewhere. Hearing an unusual thump outside the bedroom window late at night, for example, can set off an alarm in the mind—based on the concern that a dangerous prowler is lurking outside—that in turn triggers a racing pulse, a rise in blood pressure, and a host of other physical responses.

Ongoing patterns of thought and emotion can affect the functions of other organ systems that are normally beyond our conscious control. Any primary-care physician will testify that a substantial number of any day's patient visits are generated by physical symptoms arising directly from the emotional weather. For example, the symptoms of irritable bowel syndrome (IBS), which affects as many as one in five Americans and accounts for one in ten doctor visits, are frequently provoked and aggravated by stressful events. Furthermore, headaches and pains arising from other parts of the body—especially the neck and back—frequently are intensified by stress, anxiety, and depression.

While there is no doubt that our mental status can affect **physiology** (how things function) throughout the body, can it cause **pathology**, the actual presence of diseased tissue? The answer appears to be a qualified yes, as reflected in the growing body of research connecting depression and important disorders such as heart disease. The "qualified" part of the answer is that the picture is very complex, and teasing out the role of a moving target like emotion from all the other important variables is far easier said than done in a scientific study.

Is it possible to open clogged arteries, shrink cancers, calm inflamed joints, or prolong survival by adjusting your attitude? Some have proposed that such accomplishments are indeed possible through various mental exercises, stress-management techniques, and psychosocial support. Support for this tantalizing concept often comes from anecdotes—provocative stories about individuals and their illnesses. A famous example is the 1979 book *Anatomy of an Illness as Perceived by the Patient* by Norman Cousins, a former editor of the *Saturday Review*, who recovered from a severe arthritic disorder through a combination of rest, improvements in nutrition, and generous doses of laughter. Drawing meaningful conclusions about the mind's impact on healing through well-designed controlled studies is a challenging task, but it is one that continues to be pursued vigorously by researchers in **psychosomatic** (now often called **mind/body) medicine**.

"A sound mind in a sound body, is a short, but full description of a happy state in this world. He that has these two, has little more to wish for; and he that wants either of them, will be but little the better for any thing else."
—JOHN LOCKE
English philosopher
(1632–1704)

Our purpose in this chapter is not to attempt to review that research (which is indeed a moving target). Rather, like the rest of this book, we are looking at the most common disturbances, approaches to preventing them, and strategies for enhancing overall health—except that here we will focus on the realm of the mind and especially the emotions, rather than the heart, lungs, muscles, bones, and all the other organs and systems in the body.

Anxiety and Depression

Anxiety and depression are two common emotional problems to be avoided if at all possible. Does this sound a little familiar? You may recall a similar theme in chapter 3, where we explored three health problems—cardiovascular disease, cancer, and diabetes—that take more lives every year in our country than all other causes of death combined. Because anxiety and depression are both so common, such a great source of distress, and so often misunderstood, we're going to take a look at them in more detail, just as we did with the three disorders in chapter 3.

Anxiety disorders: not just a simple case of the jitters

There are a host of things we are afraid of, or at least have a healthy respect for, and an appropriate amount of anxiety is a God-given emotion that helps keep us and our loved ones out of harm's way. Anxiety keeps most of us from poking a beehive with a stick, driving recklessly, or sticking our hand on a hot stove. It causes us to get up in the middle of the night to see why the baby is crying, to "toddler-proof" our home, to explain bicycle safety to our school-age children, and to warn our teenagers about drinking and driving. Anxiety prompts us to call the doctor when we have a pain or feel a mysterious lump, or to dial 911 when we hear a prowler outside the bedroom window in the middle of the night. All too often, however, anxiety's "still, small voice" isn't heeded, and too many of us experience health problems (or even outright catastrophes) because we have ignored it. Some of us have too *little* anxiety about the tobacco smoke we're inhaling, the rising number on our bathroom scale, or our lack of exercise.

Anxiety also commonly crops up in situations that aren't necessarily threatening to life and limb but are unfamiliar, uncertain, or perceived as potentially threatening to relationships, income, social status, or virtually any other desire or goal. On the positive side, anxiety spurs us to complete our homework assignments, obey the law, show up for work, and pay our taxes. It also gives us sweaty palms during a job interview, on a first date, or when we're about to stand up in front of a group to make a presentation, sing a song, or simply introduce ourselves. The adrenaline rush that occurs during these events may provide a little burst of energy and alertness that enhances our performance—but it can also provoke a wave of nervousness that undermines our efforts.

For some people, anxiety isn't limited to these common occurrences but instead becomes an ever-present and overbearing companion. It can disrupt relationships, work, and school. It can interfere with sleep. It can provoke overeating and obesity, loss of appetite, or a full-blown eating disorder. It can drive habits and rituals that are literally crippling. It can drive a person to seek relief by attempting to self-medicate, especially with alcohol, prescription medications, or even illicit drugs (such as marijuana), in a misguided effort to find temporary relief. In some cases, episodes of severe anxiety known as panic attacks arrive suddenly and unexpectedly, taking off like a runaway train that literally puts every other activity on immediate hold until it ends. When a person has anxiety that is persistent, disruptive, and out of proportion to the actual threats of everyday life, he or she is said to have an **anxiety disorder**.

According to the National Institute of Mental Health (NIMH), an estimated 19 million American adults have an anxiety disorder.[1] There are several types and some variability in the way each of the different disorders manifests itself. At the same time, the symptoms of the various anxiety disorders may overlap. In other words, they don't always fit into neat categories, and it isn't unusual for a person to experience features of more than one type of anxiety disorder. Furthermore, as we mentioned earlier, there are powerful connections between emotions and physical events throughout the body. Because physiological responses normally accompany anxiety, physical symptoms are extremely common in anxiety disorders. Indeed, they are often what drive people with this problem to the physician's office. Some of these include:

- **Pounding of the heart (palpitations).** This sensation is often accompanied by a racing pulse.
- **Shortness of breath.** Often the person with shortness of breath arising from anxiety complains that he or she "can't get enough air" or that "air isn't getting all the way into the lungs." Paradoxically, the complaint is usually more noticeable at rest than during vigorous ex-

ercise. This is very different from shortness of breath caused by asthma, where air flow is impaired both entering and leaving the lung, or by coronary artery disease or congestive heart failure, where shortness of breath occurs with very little exertion.

- **Pain or other discomfort in the chest.** This symptom, along with the others just listed, raises immediate concerns about serious and urgent problems in the heart (in particular, the obstruction of a coronary artery, leading to a heart attack) or lungs (especially a **pulmonary embolus**, in which a clot arising from the deep veins of the leg or pelvis suddenly floats into one of the arteries supplying one of the lungs). Often it will be necessary to rule out one or more of these problems, even when a physician suspects that anxiety may be the underlying cause of the symptoms.
- **Aches and pains.** Headache, neck pain, or tightness of muscles around the head, neck, or upper back is often caused by anxiety.
- **Tightness in the front of the neck.** This sensation often feels like a "lump in the throat" that won't go away. This is called a **globus syndrome** (formerly given the less flattering name *globus hystericus*) and may occur in people who do not feel particularly stressed or anxious. Needless to say, other medical problems are normally ruled out before this diagnosis is made.
- **A variety of intestinal complaints.** These include loss of appetite, nausea, vomiting, indigestion, abdominal pain (often cramping in nature), and diarrhea. Some of these overlap with a common physiological disorder known as irritable bowel syndrome. As with the other symptoms listed above, a medical evaluation is in order before any of these can be classified as a by-product of anxiety. This is particularly important if fever is present or if blood is visible in one or more bowel movements, because neither of these is brought on by anxiety.
- **Difficulty falling or staying asleep.**
- **Menstrual irregularity and discomfort.**
- **Fatigue.**
- **Increased feelings of distress or discomfort from other medical problems**, such as arthritis or chronic pain.

As we will see shortly, not only do anxiety and depression commonly occur together, but many of these physical symptoms (and a few others) also occur among people who are depressed.

Some of the more common forms of anxiety disorders include:

Generalized anxiety disorder (GAD) affects some 4 million American adults. As the name suggests, anxiety is a constant companion for these people. People with GAD worry day and night about literally everything: health, family, job, the state of the nation, the fate of the world, or simply getting through the day. Sometimes they can't pin down exactly what it is they are worried about.

Health-care professionals (including counselors and psychologists) use detailed and specific criteria to diagnose emotional disorders. These are listed in a resource known as the *Diagnostic and Statistical Manual of Mental Disorders* (or *DSM*), published and periodically revised by the American Psychiatric Association. (The fourth edition of the manual, commonly referred to as *DSM-IV,* was released in 1994, and the next edition, *DSM-V,* is due in 2010.) Our purpose here is to provide some basic information about these problems rather than to list all of the diagnostic details. Needless to say, you should be careful about drawing conclusions about a diagnosis in yourself or anyone else based on what you read in this book, the *DSM,* a magazine article, or anywhere else—this should be left to a professional.

They often have trouble relaxing, concentrating, or falling asleep. Sooner or later, they're likely to be called a worry wart or a nervous Nellie—or to apply one of those names to themselves. Although they may realize that their immediate circumstances (or their life in general) don't warrant the constant anxiety, they just can't shake it off or snap out of it. GAD develops gradually and can occur at any stage of life, including childhood, and by definition lasts six months or more. Depression often accompanies this problem.

People with GAD often experience several of the physical symptoms just listed, which in turn generate more anxiety. These symptoms may provoke frequent visits to the doctor's office, where a careful evaluation and a host of tests may be needed to confirm that the symptoms do not reflect a serious disease. In a best-case scenario, the physician will pick up on the clues, provide appropriate medical reassurance, and then carefully broach the subject of an anxiety problem and the possibility of treatment. Unfortunately, the visit(s) may lead to a less productive outcome, especially if the physician concludes that "there's nothing wrong with you" or (worse) "it's all in your head," a verdict that leaves a person feeling no less anxious, and demoralized as well.

Obsessive-compulsive disorder (OCD) weighs down a person with a combination of intrusive and unwelcome thoughts or mental images (the **obsessions**) and a compelling need to carry out certain rituals (the **compulsions**). The recurrent thoughts may focus on primal concerns—safety, health, cleanliness, sexuality, spirituality—or more obscure issues, such as numbers, colors, or the arrangement of items on a kitchen counter. These obsessive thoughts can be likened to a giant boom box playing annoying or alarming programs inside the head day and night. (These are *not* the same, by the way, as the auditory hallucinations or the inner voices heard by people with schizophrenia.) The anxiety these thoughts provoke is relieved (temporarily) by ritualistic behaviors such as washing hands over and over, checking several times to be sure that the door is locked, counting all sorts of obscure items, lining up towels or groceries in the pantry very precisely, and other behaviors that may seem even more bizarre. Adults with OCD generally realize that the rituals are irrational, and they derive no pleasure from them. (Children with OCD, however, do not have the same understanding, and they may believe that their rituals actually affect what happens in the world around them. Health professionals often call this "magical thinking.") They might describe their anxiety as a pressure building inside, like a volcano getting ready to erupt. The rituals somehow relieve at least some of that pressure more effectively than logic, argument, or reasoning.

OCD affects more than 3 million American adults, and it usually begins during childhood, the teen years, or early adulthood. One in three people with OCD can recall symptoms beginning in childhood. Symptoms can wax and wane over time and may reach a point where they thoroughly disrupt life at home, school, or work. Counseling can be helpful—especially in clarifying the nature of the problem and learning coping skills—but OCD usually improves dramatically with medications in the widely used selective serotonin reuptake inhibitor (SSRI) class. When one of these takes effect, a person with OCD often describes the mental "boom box" receding way into the background, where its noise can be ignored or brushed off, and a similar fading of the need to carry out rituals. It is generally accepted that a combination of medication and counseling represents the most effective treatment of OCD.

Panic disorder is a condition marked by recurrent, unpredictable episodes known as **panic attacks**. Those of us who are fortunate enough not to have had one of these may not appreciate how distressing and disruptive they can be. You might think of anxiety as the feeling you get when you see red and blue lights flashing in your rearview mirror and realize that they're meant for you. As you pull over, your heart might speed up a little and your neck muscles might tighten as you wonder, *What did I do?* or *How much will the fine be for the speed I was going?* But compared to a panic attack, your response to getting a traffic ticket would be a stroll in the park. To get a glimpse of what a person with panic disorder experiences, imagine (just for a moment) that you're on an airliner at thirty-five thousand feet when you hear a loud noise you have never heard before and the plane begins listing at a steep angle that you know isn't normal. Your physical response and thoughts—*What is going on? I'm going to die!*—would probably be like nothing you had ever felt before, but they would be similar to what happens during a panic attack.

People having one of these episodes suddenly get a profound and terrifying sense that they are doomed, that death is imminent. They may feel jolted, almost as if by electricity or by some other event that is emotionally shocking, but the sensation persists. Powerful surges of adrenaline usually kick in, so the heart pounds, the chest tightens, and air seems to escape the lungs, never to return. Most of these peak in about ten minutes (which feels like hours), but some last much longer. The first panic attack—and often the second or even the third—usually lands a person in the emergency room, where he or she expects CPR to begin any second, only to be reassured (after things settle down and appropriate tests have been run) that there isn't any medical threat. *You're kidding! What in the world was that? Whatever it was, I don't want it to happen to me ever again!*

Panic attacks are notorious for occurring out of left field when they are least expected—not in the middle of a heated argument or after hearing some terrible news, but while driving to work or walking through the grocery store. Some people have only one in their life, and that's one too many. Most who have experienced a panic attack will tend to avoid the place or circumstances in which an episode occurred, just as anyone else might avoid a place where he or she was mugged or raped. The emotions are that powerful. If the attack occurred in the workplace, the car, or some other location where one normally needs to go, the result can be very disruptive to everyday life. If panic attacks occur over and over and are not properly treated, a person can begin to feel that no place outside of the home is safe, thus leading to the fear of leaving the house. This is known as **agoraphobia**, and it can keep an individual literally housebound. Actually, some don't even feel that safe at home, because episodes can also occur there (even during sleep). Still, most people with panic disorder don't feel quite as helpless when an attack happens at home. Ironically, after the first couple of panic attacks, subsequent episodes can be generated simply by the *fear* of having another one, so that they can become self-perpetuating.

About 2.5 million American adults have panic disorder, and two out of three of these are women. Many also have symptoms of depression or other anxiety-related syndromes. As with OCD, counseling can help clarify the nature of the problem and identify coping strategies, but judicious use of medication is usually needed to rein in the problem. Typically a short-acting **anxiolytic** (anxiety-reducing) medication such as alprazolam (Xanax) is prescribed for use at the onset of a panic attack in order to terminate it or at least reduce its severity. This is critical to restore a sense of control and prevent the helpless feeling of being on a runaway train, which is so distressing during one of these episodes. At the same time, a medication that helps normalize neurotransmitter levels (usually one of the SSRIs) is introduced as a maintenance agent to prevent further episodes, or at least to reduce their frequency and severity. It is important that the person with repeated panic episodes not rely solely on the anxiolytic medication, just as the person with recurrent asthma attacks should not become dependent on a fast-acting inhaler. In both cases, dealing with the underlying cause(s) is critical to gaining containment and control of the problem.

Post-traumatic stress disorder (PTSD) involves a constellation of disabling symptoms that arise after a traumatic event that is perceived as terrifying and life threatening to self or others. Situations that give rise to PTSD include a direct experience of:

- personal assault, such as a mugging, rape, torture, or kidnapping
- a serious automobile, train, plane, or other type of accident
- a natural disaster, such as an earthquake, flood, or tornado
- exposure to combat, especially when seeing others maimed or killed

PTSD can also occur after a traumatic, life-threatening (or fatal) event in the life of a loved one, or after viewing a catastrophe such as a wreck or the victim of a violent death.

Symptoms of PTSD include:

- Reexperiencing the event through intrusive memories, dreams, or powerful **flashbacks**. The latter may be triggered by sights, sounds, or even smells that cause a person to relive a traumatic experience.
- Emotional "numbing" or unresponsiveness to others, including those with whom a person was previously close.
- Some PTSD victims become **hypervigilant** and startle easily. (The

The experiences of Vietnam War veterans were instrumental in classifying PTSD as a specific diagnosis. Interestingly, symptoms identical to those of PTSD have been reported for hundreds of years by historians and journalists chronicling battle carnage. Among soldiers in previous generations, the phenomenon was called battle fatigue and shell shock.

classic example is that of a combat veteran who leaps for cover in response to hearing some nearby firecrackers.)

It is important to note that one's *perception* of an event plays an important role in determining whether PTSD will develop. Someone who survives a horrendous train wreck and then concludes that "it simply wasn't my time to go" may not experience any symptoms. But another person involved in a minor fender bender may experience that event as a near calamity and become convinced that "this world is a dangerous place, and I'm not safe anywhere, at any time." This individual is more likely to develop symptoms of PTSD. Research on this phenomenon is also focusing on biological events within the brain that seem to perpetuate powerful reactions to traumatic events rather than allowing the person's physical and emotional responses to subside.

A number of counselors who have dealt with women struggling with emotional difficulties in the wake of an abortion have noted that, in many cases, symptoms bear a striking resemblance to those occurring in PTSD. Some have coined the term **postabortion syndrome** or **postabortion distress** to refer to this syndrome, although there has been controversy in the professional community regarding its frequency and severity. A detailed look at emotional issues following abortion may be found in the book *A Solitary Sorrow* by Teri K. Reisser.

Over 5 million adult Americans are affected by PTSD. In order to be diagnosed with it, a person must experience a combination of the defining symptoms for at least one month. They typically begin within three months of the traumatic incident (although some surface many months or even years later) and may last for months or even years, often accompanied by depression, irritability, other anxiety disorders, and substance abuse. A variety of treatment approaches are used to help people manage and recover from PTSD.

Social anxiety disorder (also called **social phobia**) creates an extreme and disabling level of anxiety in social situations. A specific situation, such as giving a presentation, interacting with others at school or work, or even attending a party, can provoke trembling, nausea, blushing, difficulty speaking, or other unpleasant reactions. More than 5 million Americans are affected (men and women equally so), and not surprisingly, these individuals may also suffer from depression and other anxiety disorders. They often use alcohol and other drugs as self-medication to better tolerate social situations.

Specific phobias are intense and irrational fears of a particular thing, place, or situation that does not represent a genuine, immediate threat or provoke a similar response in most people. Most of us have heard of (or know) someone who has claustrophobia (fear of closed spaces), acrophobia (fear of heights), or aviophobia (fear of flying). Of course, it isn't unusual to be a little edgy when looking over the edge of a cliff or roaring down the runway in a jetliner. Most of us aren't crazy about snakes and spiders, but few of us have full-blown ophiophobia (fear of snakes) or arachnophobia (fear of spiders). A person with a phobia reacts with very severe anxiety or even a full-blown panic episode in the presence of the thing feared, and will often go to extreme lengths to avoid it. Obviously, when the object of the fear is easy to avoid, a phobia won't be particularly disruptive. But others definitely interfere with life at home or on the job. If your career involves a lot of travel, for example, refusing to fly could cost you your job.

Phobias affect more than 6 million Americans and are twice as common in women as in men. Dozens of specific phobias have been identified, many of which provide a rich source of material for word buffs and quiz shows but are no laughing matter to those affected by them.

Researchers now believe that a combination of genetics and a malfunction of structures deep in the brain (known as the **amygdala** and **hippocampus**) that regulate our responses to threats are the setup for phobias, but it still isn't clear how specific objects or situations trigger extreme reactions. If avoiding the object of the phobia isn't possible, specific types of therapies and desensitization processes can help a person prevent or at least tone down the response. The usual treatment involves approaching the feared object or experience first from afar (even using one's imagination), and then over time increasing exposure gradually enough to avoid an anxiety response, until eventually it provokes little or no reaction.

Have you ever heard of ailurophobia (fear of cats), coulrophobia (fear of clowns), or chionophobia (fear of snow)? Atheists might be prone to homilophobia (fear of sermons), a career pessimist might have euphobia (fear of good news), and some parents could be accused of suffering from ephebiphobia (fear of teenagers).

Depression: more than a case of the blues

Everyone suffers losses. We lose a coin, a key, a ring, or a home. We lose a pet, a friend, a distant cousin, a parent, a spouse. We lose an assignment, a contest, a job, a goal, a dream. We lose our health and eventually our life.

Everyone has a bad day, a bad week, a bad year. No one gets exactly what he wants (or thinks he wants) out of life. For many people on our planet, almost every day is filled with hardship and discomfort. (Indeed, the annoyances that we find grievous—a malfunctioning car or an interruption of Internet service, for example—pale in comparison to what millions suffer every day.)

Sadness, tears, and grief are normal responses to life's losses and reversals. Anger, lost sleep, second thoughts, and regrets are common reactions as well. Often lessons are learned, compassion is discovered, and directions in life are altered for the better as a result. The New Testament refers to losses and reversals as trials and gives them a value we ought to take to heart:

> *Consider it pure joy, my brothers, whenever you face trials of many kinds, because you know that the testing of your faith develops perseverance. Perseverance must finish its work so that you may be mature and complete, not lacking anything.*
> (JAMES 1:2-4)

For a substantial number of people, however, sadness, anger, and other turbulent emotions settle in for a long and unpleasant stretch. Depression—more specifically, symptoms significant enough to be classified as **major depression**—affects more than 15 percent of our population at some point in life and more than 6 percent of American adults at any time.[2] Furthermore, according to the American Academy of Child and Adolescent Psychiatry, at any given time 5 percent of children and adolescents also suffer from depression. (Major depression—also called **major depressive disorder**, **endogenous depression**, and sometimes **clinical depression**—is what we are referring to as "depression" in this segment, unless otherwise stated.) More than two-thirds of those affected with depression have another mood disorder, most commonly an anxiety disorder, which occurs in more than half of those with depression. We're not talking about a bad attitude or a droopy day, but a serious problem that very often has important physical roots and consequences.

Symptoms of major depression

Most of us have an idea of what it means to be depressed, but not everyone appreciates the spectrum of symptoms that can occur with major depression. The two primary ingredients are:

A depressed mood—feeling sad, helpless, and hopeless. Nothing seems right, the future looks bleak, and small challenges look like Mount Everest. A person with depression often cries easily or feels like crying much of the time. Hopelessness can be particularly troublesome among teenagers, because they usually lack the perspective that comes with decades of life lessons and have a limited fund of responses. If they can't see a satisfactory route past the current problem, they may begin to think that their life is over or not worth living. This, combined with an adolescent's susceptibility to impulsive decisions, creates a very real risk for a suicide attempt by a depressed young person.

Loss of interest or pleasure in activities that were once enjoyable. This may be experienced as a pervasive "what's the use?" mentality. Getting out of bed in the morning feels like a major accomplishment. Everyday tasks are carried out purely in response to the call of duty (though with teeth gritted) or are even left undone. You've probably heard the word *hedonist* applied to someone who lives for life's pleasures, but a depressed person can be classified as having **anhedonia**, the loss of the ability to experience pleasure.

In addition to these core problems, several other symptoms commonly accompany depression. Indeed, when a number of these are present at the same time, a person may feel as though he or she is literally falling apart at the seams.

- **Ongoing fatigue.** This is extremely common—indeed, almost universal—with depression. Conversely, unrecognized depression is the single most common cause of chronic fatigue. While a physician will normally attempt to rule out one or more medical problems when a person complains of persistent tiredness, depression should not be overlooked as a possible cause.
- **Sleep disturbances.** Insomnia—difficulty falling or staying asleep—and the opposite, **hypersomnia**, where a person feels like sleeping night and day, often accompany depression.
- **Irritability and agitation.** A depressed person often has a short fuse and seems to become riled over anything and everything. Family members may run for cover or retreat to their room when the depressed person comes through the door, because *nothing* is right and the slightest annoyance leads to an explosion of angry words or even violence. In adolescents, agitation and acting out arising from de-

pression are commonly mistaken for "runaway hormones," "teen drama," or "a lot of lip."

- **Slowing of thoughts or actions.** This characteristic (the technical term is **psychomotor retardation**) is the flip side of agitation. The unusually slow pace of the person's thoughts and actions gives the impression of a videotape playing at too slow a speed.
- **Poor concentration.** Depression can interfere dramatically with focus and decision making. Even little decisions seem like a big deal (*I can't even figure out which pair of socks to wear*). In children and adolescents, this may manifest as poor school performance.
- **A negative self-concept or sense of utter worthlessness.** This is particularly troublesome among adolescents, who normally struggle with identity, self-consciousness, and self-image. When depression is present, these concerns can take a very dark turn.
- **Changes in appetite and weight.** Depression may be associated with decreased or increased appetite and thus with weight loss or gain.
- **Decreased interest in and enjoyment of sex.** Ironically, this particular symptom may be worsened or even brought on by many commonly used antidepressant medications.
- **Thoughts about death.** This sometimes takes the form of an ongoing focus on death and dying or overt suicidal thoughts and plans.

To be diagnosed with a major depression, a person must have a sad mood, a loss of pleasure in activities (especially those that were previously enjoyable), and three of the other symptoms listed above nearly every day (for most of the day) for more than two weeks. **Minor depression**, as the name suggests, involves fewer symptoms—either a sad mood or a loss of interest, as well as one to three of the other symptoms—for at least two weeks. Minor depression may resolve on its own or progress to major depression and may play a role in many ongoing physical complaints such as chronic pain.

Very often a major depression seems to come literally out of nowhere. (Indeed, that's often a clue to internal or **endogenous** origin of the problem.) In fact, someone may be dismayed by the apparent lack of reason for his or her dark mood: *I don't get it; everything is going so well in my life, so why am I crying all the time? I must be going crazy!*

Endogenous means "originating from within," reflecting the fact that neurotransmitters (chemical messengers) within the brain play a significant role in this process.

We have already mentioned that anxiety disorders frequently accompany depression. Furthermore, one or more of the physical symptoms that are common in anxiety disorders may be present as well. To make matters more complicated, depression is also associated with some chronic medical conditions:

- About 25 percent of people being treated for cancer have symptoms of depression, and depression among cancer patients has been associated with impaired immune function.
- About 20 percent of people with cardiovascular disease have major

depression, and another 20 percent have minor depression. Similar percentages have been found for patients following a stroke. Depression may precede the appearance of heart disease, and once coronary artery disease has developed, depression increases the likelihood of heart attack, hospitalization, and especially heart-related mortality in the future.

- There appears to be a relationship between depression and diabetes, with the first preceding the second by several years.
- About half of those with Alzheimer's disease have symptoms of depression, and 5 percent to 15 percent have major depression.

We take a closer look at Alzheimer's disease in chapter 14, beginning on page 692.

Some connections between disease and depression might seem obvious: Who wouldn't be depressed if faced with a threatening, debilitating disease and its frequently unpleasant treatments? Perhaps people who are depressed are more likely to develop heart disease and diabetes because they don't take care of themselves or because they resort to alcohol or tobacco to improve their

SUICIDE: DON'T IGNORE THE WARNING SIGNS

Few things in life are more devastating than losing a loved one or good friend to suicide. More than thirty thousand Americans end their life this way every year, leaving behind a horrific wake of grief, rejection, and guilt among those who cared about them. Women are more likely than men to attempt suicide, but men are four times more likely than women to succeed in their attempt—often because they resort to violent means, such as using a gun or leaping from a building, rather than a less drastic method such as taking an overdose of medication (from which recovery is more likely).

When the victim is a child or adolescent, the loss is even more profound. Suicide is the third leading cause of death among those between the ages of ten and twenty-four, claiming the lives of almost five thousand people in this age group every year in the United States. The number may actually be higher, because many accidents (such as drug overdoses, drowning deaths, or fatal automobile crashes involving a lone teenage driver) may in fact be suicides. Many people broadcast clues that they are thinking about ending their own life, but these are often overlooked or ignored. Here are some warning signs:

- **Talking or joking about suicide or "not being around."** Comments like "You'd be better off without me" or "I just don't want to be here anymore" or "Nothing matters" should be taken seriously and should prompt a careful conversation about how the person is feeling.
- **Putting one's affairs in order.** A depressed person may write a will—not

mood. Both of these possibilities and many others no doubt play a role, but the picture becomes more complex (and intriguing) as research uncovers more about the connections between mind, body, and disease. For example, symptoms of depression are common among those with Parkinson's disease, deficiencies in folic acid and vitamin B_6, autoimmune disorders (syndromes such as rheumatoid arthritis in which the immune system attacks a person's own tissues), and hypothyroidism—that is, too little thyroid hormone in circulation. (Hyperthyroidism—too much thyroid hormone in circulation—is more often associated with symptoms of anxiety.)

Recognizing the potential connection between mood and disease can be beneficial if it leads to appropriate treatment. In some situations, however, patients and occasionally practitioners arrive at a conclusion that can be either helpful or potentially harmful: *If I get rid of my mood problem, my heart disease [or cancer or diabetes] will improve.* There is undoubtedly at least some truth to this idea. Depression can definitely lead to poor self-care, and we have yet to un-

a bad idea, but a red flag when in this emotional state—or begin giving away prized possessions or saying farewell to friends, as if going on a long trip. Giving away clothing, an entire CD collection, or other valuables is particularly common among teenagers who are planning suicide.

- **Marked agitation and sleeplessness for several days.**
- **Withdrawal and isolation from family and friends.**
- **A previous suicide attempt or a history of suicide in the family.**
- **Acquiring a gun or another weapon.** Anyone who is depressed should not have access to weapons, especially firearms. This is especially true for adolescents, among whom guns are the most common means of committing suicide.

If you believe that a family member or friend might commit a self-destructive act, it is critical not only that you express your concern but also that you help that person seek assistance immediately. You may want to contact your (or their) physician for advice or referral. If anyone in your family has met with a counselor, this individual may be the appropriate initial contact. Many communities have a mental-health center that offers on-the-spot assessment of an individual's suicide risk. Some even send an assessment team to homes. If you feel that there is an imminent risk of self-harm, *stay with the person* (or make certain that he or she remains in the company of a responsible adult) until you have reasonable assurance from a qualified individual, along with a clear commitment from your friend or loved one, that he or she will not attempt suicide. When that assurance cannot be obtained, the suicidal individual may need to be hospitalized for safety, further assessment, and the initiation of treatment. You will also need to take appropriate safety precautions, including removing any guns from the home and controlling access to medications. ■

ravel the breadth and depth of biochemical connections that might also aggravate many chronic medical conditions. But some jump to less reasonable, or even agonizing, conclusions:

- *If I just straighten out my mood, or even visualize myself as healthy, my mind will cure my body.*
- *If I don't get better, it must mean that I really don't want to be well.*
- *The disease I have is a message from my "inner self" about a problem in my life.*
- *I brought this disease on myself—it's entirely my fault.*

Some popular authors stress this type of mind-body interaction and propose all sorts of mental and meditative exercises to help readers get in touch with their "inner guide," visualize their white blood cells attacking a cancer, and so forth. All of this sounds intriguing and even reassuring, not to mention more pleasant than treatments like chemotherapy. But it can also lead to false guilt and even despair, especially among cancer patients who may turn themselves inside out trying to figure out what metaphor or message the disease represents. (*If this is a lesson from my "inner teacher," I want a substitute!*) In fact, while depression is common among cancer patients, it is unwise to jump to potentially distressing conclusions about the role of mood in the cause and progression of this disorder, which involves complex biochemical, genetic, and immunologic mechanisms.

Types of depression

Just as there are a number of anxiety disorders, there are also different types of depression. We have already described the characteristics of major and minor depression, the two most common forms of this disturbance. In addition, there are a number of other conditions that can involve a depressed mood.

Adjustment disorder is an episode in which significant and disruptive emotional symptoms develop within three months of one or more stressful events, such as a divorce, loss of a job, or death of a loved one. Obviously, grief, sadness, and even anger are common—indeed, normal—responses to these events, and the grieving process is not the same as a depression. But some people do not seem to come to an emotional equilibrium after their losses, or they experience a response that is more extreme and disabling than would normally be expected. (Obviously, determining what is "normal" grieving and what is an adjustment disorder may be easier said than done and may require input from a person with professional training.) By definition, an adjustment disorder does not persist for more than six months. If it does, a different disturbance (for example, major depression) most likely is present.

Dysthymia (also called **dysthymic disorder**) is a chronic, low-grade depression that waxes and wanes for years. In fact, the diagnosis is based on having a depressed mood and two or more associated symptoms with mild to moderate severity for at least two years. Indeed, dysthymia is so insidious that people with this problem may have become accustomed to their mood and believe it to be normal. (A person with dysthymia who responds to treatment may actually ask, with some surprise, "Is this what *normal* people feel like?")

Seasonal affective disorder (abbreviated, appropriately enough, **SAD**) is a condition in which symptoms of depression, along with lethargy, sleep problems, and headaches, develop during the fall and winter months. It appears to be related to the amount of available sunlight and its effects on the **circadian rhythm**, the body's biological clock that regulates a host of internal functions.

As you might expect, SAD is more common in northern climates. Treatment for this problem is unique among depression and anxiety disorders: about one to two hours of daily exposure (usually in the morning) to a special light source that is many times brighter than ordinary indoor light can improve symptoms in as many as 80 percent of people with SAD.

We will look at circadian rhythm in more detail in chapter 15, which deals with sleep.

Premenstrual syndrome (PMS) and **premenstrual dysphoric disorder (PMDD)** are mood disturbances that are related to the menstrual cycle. We mention them here because they appear to be linked to the same neurotransmitter disturbances that play a role in depression and anxiety disorders (and they respond to the same medications). We explore these in detail in chapter 13, beginning on page 619.

Postpartum depression is actually an episode of major depression that begins within a few weeks of delivery. As many as 70 to 85 percent of women experience depressed mood, irritability, and difficulty with appetite and sleep, commonly called the baby blues, after delivery. This normally resolves on its own within seven to ten days. Postpartum depression, which may affect as many as one out of ten new mothers, involves more serious symptoms that continue for more than two weeks and can jeopardize the health (and occasionally the life) of both mother and infant. Poor self-care and neglect of the baby, difficulty in bonding between mother and infant, and even developmental problems in the baby may result. Risk factors for postpartum depression include a history of depression or another psychiatric condition, poor spousal or family support, a poor outcome for the baby, and one or more previous episodes of postpartum depression.

Unfortunately, a woman—especially a first-time mother—who has been through the rigors of delivery and is short on sleep because of the round-the-clock feeding needs of the newborn may not realize that her crying, poor concentration, and fatigue are abnormal. She may even chastise herself for being a "bad mother," and family members who are unaware of postpartum depression may do likewise, compounding the problem. A woman who develops a persistent depression or other significant mood issues that last more than two weeks after delivery should be evaluated by her physician immediately. This is particularly critical if she manifests any delusional thinking (for example, believing that the baby is demon-possessed or trying to kill her), which is a manifestation of a much less common (one in five hundred to one thousand births) but far more serious condition known as **postpartum psychosis**.[3] This is a psychiatric emergency requiring immediate evaluation and treatment because of the very real risk of harm to both mother and infant.

Bipolar disorder (also called **manic-depressive disorder**) is a less common but more complex mood disturbance in which a person experiences not only depression but also one or more episodes of abnormally elevated mood called **mania** or **hypomania**. (Because the other types of depression manifest symptoms only on one side of the mood spectrum—the "down" or depressed side—they are referred to as **unipolar**.) Bipolar disorder affects more than 2 million adults in the United States, appearing during adolescence or early adulthood and persisting throughout life. The depressive side of a bipolar disorder involves symptoms we have previously listed, sometimes to a severe degree. During a manic episode, a person may appear to have inhaled rocket fuel or consumed a hundred cups of coffee. He may need little sleep and appear impossibly energetic, outgoing, enthusiastic, and extremely confident. Thoughts race, and speech is often rapid or even pressured, such that others may have difficulty getting a word in edgewise. On the downside, concentration can be impaired. He may make decisions such as business deals, high-risk investments, or expensive purchases that show poor judgment or are even reckless. It's common for someone in a manic episode to become irritable or even agitated. During a hypomanic episode, which is similar in many ways but less intense and disruptive than mania, a person will also be very energetic and outgoing, and because judgment is typically not impaired, even highly productive. Some who are informed of their diagnosis may be reluctant to take medication that might stabilize it because they don't want a hypomanic (or even manic) episode to end.

The frequency and severity of depressive and manic episodes can vary greatly. Some people, for example, have only one manic episode, while others (called rapid cyclers) may have four or more manic episodes in a year. Some people who appear to have a unipolar type of depression actually have bipolar disorder, but the diagnosis may not be clarified for months or even years. Several clues suggest the possibility of a bipolar disorder (but by no means make the diagnosis). These include

- Early onset and multiple episodes of depression (that is, in childhood or adolescence)
- Abrupt onset and improvement of depressive symptoms
- A tendency toward irritability and agitation
- A highly variable or unstable mood during a depressive episode
- Failure to respond to medications that normally improve depression, or worsening symptoms when these drugs are taken
- A family history of bipolar disorder—more than half of those with this disorder have a family member who is also affected

While symptoms of bipolar disorder may be triggered by stress or traumatic events, the underlying disturbance is biochemical, and treatment—especially the stabilization of manic episodes—involves medication regimes that nearly always require the expertise of a psychiatrist. Counseling can be very helpful in coping with this problem and managing its fallout, but it should be done in conjunction with appropriate medical management.

Eating disorders arise from a complex interaction of anxiety, depression, issues of life, and concern over body image that converge into compulsive and often highly dangerous behaviors. According to the American Psychiatric Association, at any given time, roughly a half million people in the United States are affected with an eating disorder. Of these, about 90 percent are young women between the ages of twelve and twenty-five; most are from middle- or upper-income families. (These conditions are rarely seen in developing countries.) Athletes, models, dancers, and others in the entertainment industry are at particular risk, usually because of intense concern over maintaining an often unrealistic appearance or level of performance. The two most common eating disorders are anorexia nervosa and bulimia nervosa.[4]

Anorexia nervosa is a condition of self-imposed starvation that eventually leads to a body weight at least 15 percent below the expected level for an individual's age and height. It is characterized by an extreme fear of gaining weight and a striking disturbance of body image; the anorexic who appears grossly emaciated will look in the mirror and see herself as overweight. This distorted perception typically is stubbornly resistant to feedback from families, friends, and health professionals, even in the face of serious physical and medical consequences.

As more weight is lost, the fear of gaining weight intensifies rather than diminishes, leading to nonstop preoccupation with eating and weight. Behaviors common to those with obsessive-compulsive disorder often attend this disorder as well. What little food is eaten will usually be derived only from "safe" low-calorie sources, often measured out in precise quantities and then consumed in an exacting, almost ritualistic manner. Food might be cut into tiny pieces and then arranged and rearranged on the plate to give the impression that some of it has been eaten. Anorexics often obsess over the number of calories they might ingest from obscure sources such as the coating of a medication or from licking a postage stamp. Often they carefully monitor body measurements such as upper-arm circumference. The fervor with which calories are restricted is frequently applied to burning them as well, and an anorexic individual will sometimes exercise vigorously for hours every day. Other efforts to rid the body of calories include "purging" behaviors, such as self-induced vomiting, which are seen more commonly in bulimia nervosa.

It should come as no surprise that medical consequences, most arising from the body's attempt to conserve energy, become more serious as starvation and weight loss continue. With loss of fat and circulating estrogen, the intricate hormonal interplay of a woman's monthly cycle shuts down. (The absence of three consecutive menstrual periods is one of the diagnostic criteria for anorexia nervosa.) This, combined with an ongoing inadequate intake of nutrients and calcium, leads to loss of bone density, which can cause stress fractures, especially during intense exercise.

Starvation leads to reduced capacity of the stomach and delays in its emptying of food, as well as constipation, all of which may be falsely interpreted by the anorexic as weight gain. Dry skin, thinning of the scalp hair, and development of a fine hair growth on the body called **lanugo** typically occur. Loss of fat stores and metabolic energy conservation lead to a lower body temperature, often causing the anorexic to wear more layers of clothing to keep warm. More serious complications arise from the heart, which typically slows its contraction rate and decreases in size in an effort to conserve energy. Heart rhythm might become irregular, sometimes to a life-threatening degree, especially in the presence of purging behavior, which can deplete the body of potassium.

For all these reasons, anorexia nervosa should be considered a very serious condition with lethal risks. Between 5 and 20 percent of anorexics die from starvation, cardiac arrest, or suicide. (The higher death rates are observed among those with a long duration of anorexia, more severe weight loss, poor family support, and multiple relapses despite treatment.)

Bulimia nervosa is characterized by behavior known as binging and purging, which may continue for decades. During a binge, an individual quickly consumes an enormous amount of food containing many thousands of calories, often without even chewing or tasting it. The resulting physical and emotional discomfort will then provoke a purge, usually involving self-induced vomiting. Bulimics often use laxatives and diuretics (so-called water pills, medications that increase urine output)—sometimes in dangerous quantities—in a misguided belief that these medications will somehow help rid the body of the food that isn't lost through vomiting. The binging and purging cycles may occur a few times a week or, in severe cases, several times daily.

Bulimia is much more common than anorexia, but it frequently goes undetected because most episodes take place in secret and typically do not lead to significant weight loss. (However, some individuals with anorexia may engage in binge-and-purge behavior.) Nevertheless, bulimia can have many serious medical consequences. The repeated exposure of teeth to stomach acid (during vomiting) erodes enamel, causes a yellowish discoloration, and sometimes leads to decay. The throat and esophagus may become chronically inflamed, and the salivary glands—especially the parotid glands that lie directly in front of the ears—can become enlarged in response to continuing episodes of vomiting. Repeated use of laxatives often leads to severe constipation, while heavy diuretic use may have an adverse effect on kidney function.

Potentially dangerous disturbances in heart rhythm can arise from the repeated loss of potassium from vomiting, as well as from excessive ingestion of diuretics and laxatives. Other equally serious (but fortunately uncommon) events include bleeding and even rupture of the esophagus or stomach from frequent vomiting. Food aspirated into the airway during vomiting can cause choking or pneumonia.

What causes such seemingly unrewarding and even dangerous behaviors? While each case is unique, potential contributing factors include the following:

- *Cultural factors.* In developed countries, advertisements, films, videos, and TV programs continually display images of bodily perfection, especially for females. Those who are shapely, sleek, and most of all thin are seen as successful, sophisticated, desirable, and apparently free of emotional or personal pain. A vulnerable individual who desperately desires these attributes but cannot attain them through normal means may engage in unhealthy and extreme behaviors.
- *Personality and psychological factors.* A typical anorexia patient is a perfectionistic, high-achieving, adolescent female. She may be seen as a compliant "good" girl by her parents (one or both of whom might be perfectionistic also), and she usually does not rebel or even have much of a social or dating life. While excelling in many areas, she may berate herself over any performance that falls short of perfection. Some researchers theorize that refusing to eat may serve as a form of rebellion or that it may represent the single area of her life over which she can exercise total control. Bulimics, on the other hand, are less predictable in personality and attributes, although alcohol or drug abuse may be a concurrent issue. In nearly all individuals with either type of eating disorder, anxiety and depression play a significant role.
- *Biochemical factors.* Chemical messengers in the brain called neurotransmitters are known to be associated with mood, emotional stability, appetite, and sleep. As we will discuss later, many people are genetically vulnerable to changes in neurotransmitter levels that can lead to depression and anxiety disorders, including obsessive-compulsive disorder (OCD). Neurotransmitter imbalances appear to play a role in the origin of eating disorders, and many features of anorexia bear a striking resemblance to those of OCD.

Because eating disorders can put health and even life in serious jeopardy, they should be taken very seriously. Initiating treatment can be difficult for the bulimic, who hides so much of her disordered behavior, and for the anorexic, who may stubbornly deny that she needs help or may undermine therapeutic efforts. In order to be effective, treatment must address a variety of issues and will often require a team approach. A thorough medical evaluation is extremely important and will sometimes reveal a variety of problems that need attention. Counseling is necessary on a long-term basis and should involve the entire family. Antidepressant medication that normalizes neurotransmitter levels can help stabilize mood, relieve depression, and reduce the obsessive component of anorexia. A dietitian should also be involved to provide nutritional input and accountability. Pastoral counseling can help the patient work through issues of guilt and shame and begin to look at life from God's perspective. In severe cases of anorexia, hospitalization and medically supervised refeeding may be necessary to prevent a fatal outcome.

Where do anxiety and depression come from?

No one can say for certain why a person develops a problem with anxiety or depression. Nevertheless, we can say with some confidence that a number of factors play a role in the onset and persistence of these disturbances and that they interact in complex ways.

Many if not most cases appear linked to imbalances (for lack of a better word) in chemical messengers within the brain known as **neurotransmitters**.

HOW PARENTS CAN HELP PREVENT EATING DISORDERS

Eating disorders commonly begin during the teen years (in some cases, even earlier), and while it is impossible to predict who might develop an eating disorder, parents can help reduce the risk in the following ways:

- Beware of perfectionism, especially in regard to weight or physical appearance. Your child must understand that her worth and your acceptance of her are not based on physical beauty or perfect performance but are, in fact, unconditional.
- Beware of demands on an adolescent to "make weight" for an athletic team, slim down for cheerleading or ballet, or subject the body to stringent dietary restrictions for any other reason. Help your child understand that body shape and build have a strong genetic basis and that few women are capable of attaining cover-girl status, even with intense effort.
- Eliminate—from your own and your family's conversations—jokes or other demeaning comments about the appearance of others.
- Point out to your children how advertising and other media put forth images of beauty and body image that are out of reach for nearly everyone.
- Be a good role model in your own eating and exercise habits, and be careful about openly criticizing your own body appearance.
- Focus on relationships and building emotional intimacy in your family, rather than on food-related issues. Be aware of the purposes—beyond relieving hunger—that food might be serving in your home. Is it used for comfort or reward? Is it used to relieve boredom? Be careful not to use food as a substitute for hugs and saying "I love you." ■

These compounds move in and out of the microscopic gaps between **neurons** (nerve cells) throughout the nervous system, allowing for interaction between cells in a rapid and extraordinarily complex manner. There are many different neurotransmitters, but those that are prominently linked to mood include **serotonin**, **norepinephrine**, and **dopamine**. Altered (usually depleted) quantities of these compounds between neurons in certain areas of the brain are associated with mood disturbances. How exactly they affect mood, why they become abnormal, and to what degree they are the cause versus the result of the mood problem remain mostly unanswered questions. But their importance is confirmed by the dramatic effect of medications that adjust neurotransmitter levels in people with anxiety or depressive disorders.

Genetic factors appear to play a role in a person's vulnerability to anxiety and depression. Many times, the same disturbance (for example, obsessive-compulsive disorder) will appear in multiple members and generations of the same family. This appears to be biologically driven, not merely the result of parenting patterns or children imitating behaviors they see in a parent.

Physical illness and medications, as we noted earlier, can also provoke episodes of anxiety and depression. Among women, changes in hormone levels during the menstrual cycle, after delivery of a baby, and during the years surrounding menopause appear to affect neurotransmitters and can trigger mood disturbances.

Stressful life experiences, both during childhood and later on, appear to interact with one's genetic predisposition to bring on or sustain anxiety and depression. Abuse during childhood (physical, emotional, sexual) may be a setup for trouble later in life.

Lifestyle can be an important component. Lack of sleep, inadequate exercise, and poor dietary choices may all contribute to a mood disorder. A frantic, overcommitted schedule, especially one accompanied by a constant sense of urgency or low-level threat, may play a primary role in provoking a mood disorder, may aggravate one already underway, or may interfere with a person's efforts to take corrective action. Substance use and abuse—specifically tobacco, alcohol, and illicit drug use—have long been recognized as forms of self-medication for people attempting to relieve anxiety and depression. But these ultimately perpetuate the problem (or may make it worse) because of their own impact on neurotransmitters and overall health.

Bad choices (for lack of a better word) may arise directly from a mood disorder (for example, the poor judgment exercised during a manic phase of bipolar disorder). But whether related to neurotransmitters, inadequate upbringing, lack of internal values, poor self-control, or all of the above, they definitely make the problem worse. Poor work habits, overspending, sexual misadventures, gambling, inappropriate comments or outbursts, disregard for the law and the rights of others, disorderly conduct, and general carelessness all complicate life and are guaranteed to make a person more miserable. The book of

Proverbs in the Old Testament aptly identifies these behaviors as foolish, catalogs them in some detail, and also efficiently describes their consequences.

What about stress (and distress)?

You don't need to have a full-blown anxiety disorder to feel stressed. Over the past few decades, stress has been blamed not only for emotional disturbances but for a host of physical ailments as well, including coronary disease, cancer,

MOOD DISORDERS VS. THOUGHT DISORDERS

We have discussed anxiety and depression in some detail because these problems are common, cause a great deal of suffering, generate millions of medical visits every year, are definitely treatable, and are to some degree avoidable. Since this book is not an encyclopedia of psychological disorders (any more than it is a handbook of medical illnesses), we are not going to delve into the length and breadth of other mental and emotional disturbances. But it is important at this juncture to clarify the difference between **affective** (mood) and **thought disorders**.

Anxiety, depression, and related disorders are called affective disorders because they are problems involving mood, emotions, or (to use the everyday term) feelings. A person with an affective disorder may be panicked or despairing, but his or her grip on reality—what's real and what isn't—is intact. You can carry on a conversation with such a person and sense that you're both processing the same information about the world around you. But there is another type of disturbance known as a thought disorder (the technical term is **psychosis**) in which that is not the case. **Schizophrenia**, in all of its variations, is the most common and chronic of these, although they may crop up in other situations as well.

Earlier, for example, we mentioned postpartum psychosis, which occurs after a woman gives birth. Certain medications (for example, high doses of steroids) can provoke a psychotic episode in susceptible individuals. As we will discuss in chapter 14, delusional thinking sometimes accompanies disorders of aging such as Alzheimer's disease. Psychotic features may also arise as a part of an anxiety disorder or a depressive episode (especially in bipolar disorder).

During a conversation with a person suffering from a thought disorder, you will begin to realize that his basic grip on reality is definitely loose. He may have delusions—that he is on a mission from God or that the FBI is monitoring his thoughts or that persons unknown (and usually unseen) are trying to harm him through invisible rays or other secret weaponry. He may have hallucinations, which are frequently auditory—he'll hear voices within his head or from the TV that is turned off or through the walls, often accompanied by accusing, threatening, or even obscene commentary. Very often the delusions and hallucinations involve God or

A common misunderstanding about schizophrenia is that it involves a split personality or **multiple personality disorder** (as depicted, for example, in the film *The Three Faces of Eve*). The latter phenomenon, now called **dissociative disorder**, is unrelated to schizophrenia in origin, manifestations, and treatment.

headaches, intestinal disturbances, and many others. (Needless to say, some of these claims are more accurate than others.) Books, tapes, and seminars dealing with the identification and management of stress have become an industry in the United States and other developed countries.

Before we can have a meaningful discussion about this topic, we need to clarify what exactly we mean by *stress*. The word commonly refers to four different entities:

Jesus Christ in convoluted scenarios. Some people with thought disorders manage to adapt and function adequately in daily life. More often, however, the various manifestations become disruptive and may be accompanied by emotional disturbances, especially anxiety and agitation, which can become extreme.

There are two other significant differences between affective and thought disorders that are worth noting. First, people with an affective disorder are nearly always able to recognize that they have a problem and are often willing to explore possibilities for treatment. A person with obsessive-compulsive disorder, for example, will acknowledge that there is no rational reason to wash her hands every ten minutes, but nevertheless she will become very uncomfortable if she doesn't. For a person with a thought disorder, however, the delusions and hallucinations are so compelling that he will usually be neither able to acknowledge that they are unreal nor willing to discuss the possibility of treatment. Ironically, it is not unusual for a person with an affective disorder to question his or her sanity ("I don't understand these mood swings; I think I must be crazy!"), while the person with a thought disorder rarely if ever will do so. Even the most gentle and loving reality check—"You know, John, I know this feels very real to you, but it really isn't possible for the CIA to read your thoughts"—is likely to be met with disbelief, resistance, and resentment. The person may even clam up, keeping his thoughts to himself because those around him won't accept them as valid.

Second, mood disorders can be addressed in a variety of ways. Counseling, medication (where appropriate), and spiritual disciplines all play important roles. But a thought disorder is at its core a biochemical issue and must be treated as such if it is going to improve. Attempting to engage a psychotic individual in cognitive (talk) therapy is nearly always an exercise in futility. A counselor or pastor *can* play a critical role in recognizing the disorder and then lovingly but firmly guiding that person toward an appropriate medical (in nearly every case psychiatric) consultation. The good news is that medication can be highly effective in controlling the delusions and hallucinations, as well as the emotional distress that commonly accompanies them. Because psychotic individuals may be less than enthusiastic about taking their medications (especially on a long-term basis, which is usually necessary), caring family members and friends may need to provide encouragement and assistance for them to do so. ■

- **External events.** Bad things that happen to people—losses, illness, abuse, or simply a pileup of inconveniences—are often called stressors. When people say "I'm really under stress," they usually mean that a lot of unpleasant things are going on in their life at that moment. As we will see momentarily, "good" things such as a promotion, a windfall of income, or getting married can also be stressors.
- **An internal response.** The emotions we feel when things aren't going the way we'd like—annoyance, anxiety, or even a sense of being overwhelmed—are often referred to as stress, as in "I'm so stressed out about my mom's operation."
- **The body's response.** When confronted with a challenge demanding some action, our body activates several physiological mechanisms that are collectively called the stress response.
- **The results of ongoing stress responses.** Disturbed bodily functions (for example, chronic headaches) or even outright physical damage (for example, cardiovascular disease) have been linked to chronic stress, which itself is often described as a disease.

The most accurate definition of *stress*, and the one we will use here, is *any situation that requires a person to act or change*. The situation may be trivial (answering the phone), profound (fighting off an attacker), pleasant (gaining an inheritance), or unpleasant (being criticized by an employer). The **stress response**, on the other hand, is a relatively stereotyped series of physiological events that enable us to deal with any of these situations.

The stress response typically involves a rise in blood pressure, increase in heart rate and muscle tone, shunting of blood to the brain and skeletal muscles (which propel the body into action), and a diversion of blood from the intestinal tract, which doesn't need as much at that particular moment. Much of this is directed by the powerful hormones **adrenaline** (also called **epinephrine**) and **cortisol**, which are secreted by the adrenal glands that sit atop the kidneys. The sympathetic nervous system, a division of the autonomic nervous system that regulates many body functions, also kicks into gear. Together they focus our attention, rev up our reaction time, and increase our strength in preparation for what is known as the fight-or-flight reaction (that is, we're ready either to fight off a threat or run away from it). "Fright" (freezing up) may be a variation of this response. When the challenge, whatever it is, has been met, the body is designed to issue a physiological "all clear" signal and return to its baseline state. We've all felt an adrenaline rush after a near miss on the freeway, but we may not be aware that a milder form of this response is necessary to meet routine, everyday challenges as well.

Two kinds of problems can develop from this system by which the body reacts to stress. One occurs when an individual becomes what might be called a "hot reactor," responding physiologically to everything in life as if it were a four-alarm fire. A phone call, a traffic jam, or even playing a game provokes a significant jump in pulse and blood pressure, even if the person doesn't feel particularly upset. Whether this is a genetically programmed or a learned response is unclear.

The other stress problem is more common, more insidious, and probably unique to contemporary lifestyles. A series of challenges occurs in a rapid-fire sequence throughout the day: the alarm clock doesn't work, the kids aren't ready for the car pool, the phone won't stop ringing, the dog makes a mess on the carpet, traffic is terrible, the boss isn't happy, and so on. The result is an ongoing activation of the stress response without an opportunity to recover—partly because the pace of life doesn't allow it, and partly because we can't unleash an all-out fight-or-flight reaction in the store or at the workplace without causing more trouble, so we just stuff it.

Nonstop exposure to increased levels of adrenaline and cortisol (and probably other substances as well) not only provokes unpleasant symptoms but can also potentially lead to actual damage in the body through a variety of mechanisms:

- Increased blood pressure, which is a risk for coronary artery disease and stroke
- Altered immune function, which could affect not only responses to infection but could also trigger flares of autoimmune disorders such as lupus or psoriasis
- Provocation of asthma attacks
- Increased acid secretion in the stomach and the potential damage to the stomach and duodenum (the first segment of the small intestine) that may result
- Weight gain, either as a direct response to cortisol or an indirect (but all too common) result of overeating as a self-calming behavior

In addition, through mechanisms yet to be unraveled, the ongoing stress response may trigger neurotransmitter disturbances that in turn lead to anxiety and depression.

As with all of the topics we have discussed in this chapter, individual responses to stress can vary enormously. Some people appear genetically programmed to a calm disposition, unfazed by whatever comes their way. Others seem destined to have a jittery response to nearly everything that crosses their path. Mothers can detect the difference between calm and jittery babies soon after birth (or even before birth), although behavior during infancy isn't always a predictor of temperament later in life. All sorts of experiences, family dynamics, security or rejection during childhood, learned reaction patterns, and—very importantly—spiritual outlook can affect how the body and emotions respond to stress. Needless to say, a number of strategies for promoting emotional and spiritual health have also been found to help with stress management. We will look at a number of these both in this chapter and the next.

Dealing with anxiety and depression

What should you do if you or a loved one is showing signs of anxiety that are disruptive or symptoms of depression that are clearly more than a transient case of the blues? There are three basic approaches to these common problems, all of which are very important, although their application and emphasis will vary from person to person. They are: (1) addressing the medical and physiologic component; (2) addressing the issues of life, past and present, including thought and behavior patterns; and (3) addressing spiritual issues.

Depending on their vantage point (and sometimes other agendas), physicians, therapists, counselors, pastors, conference speakers, or even your friends and relatives may focus on one of these as the ultimate solution while downplaying or ignoring the others. You may hear:

- "Anxiety and depression are physiological problems. All you need to do is get on the right medication [or supplement or diet] and your troubles will be over."
- "Anxiety and depression arise from the issues of life—what happened in your past, your current conflicts, and how you feel about yourself. All you need to do is spend enough time in therapy, and your troubles will be over."
- "Anxiety and depression are manifestations of a spiritual problem. All you need to do is read your Bible, pray more fervently, deal with unconfessed sin, and straighten out your relationship with God, and your troubles will be over."

All of these are correct except for the "all you need to do" part, because you may need to address more than one area in order to feel better in the short run and improve in the long run.

We will discuss all of these in the order listed above, although not necessarily in the order of importance. However, in many cases, stabilizing the medical/physiological status may help a person address issues in the other arenas much more effectively.

Medical management encompasses two tasks: checking for any medical cause for the problem and prescribing medication where and when appropriate.

A physician's evaluation is necessary to determine whether any other underlying condition might be responsible for the mood disturbance and to evaluate physical symptoms that are almost invariably part of the equation. A number of medical problems might provoke a mood disorder:

- **Thyroid disease.** Abnormal levels of thyroid, both low (hypothyroidism) and high (hyperthyroidism), can lead to mood disturbances.
- **Neurological disorders** such as Parkinson's disease, Alzheimer's and other dementias, multiple sclerosis, stroke, tumors (although rarely), or other physical disturbances in the brain can affect mood.
- **Cancer.** We noted that a significant percentage of people under treatment for cancer deal with depression, but in addition, certain types of tumors (such as cancer of the pancreas) specifically affect mood.
- **The onset of menopause** (or premature ovarian failure) may have

an impact on mood. (For more information about menopause, see "When the Cycles End: Menopause and Its Aftermath" starting on page 653 in chapter 13.)

- **Medications.** In some individuals, certain blood pressure medications, cortisone, hormonal preparations (such as birth control pills), and even one class of antibiotics (called **fluoroquinolones**) can cause transient mood problems.

As we will discuss in chapter 14, in some seniors the loss of cognitive (thinking) ability isn't the cause of depression, but the result: Depression causes an apparent loss of mental capacity, and treating the depression restores it.

Interestingly, only a small percentage of people with anxiety or depression have some other medical problem that, when treated, solves the problem. Furthermore, no specific blood test or brain scan makes a definitive diagnosis of anxiety or depression. There is no specific test for neurotransmitter levels in the brain. In almost every case, the assessment involves a careful review of the history of the problem, the current complaints, and a look at one's general health.

If the medical evaluation suggests that a neurotransmitter problem is likely playing a role in a significant mood disturbance, a trial of medication may be a reasonable option. When there is a disturbance involving one or more neurotransmitters, working on the issues of life or spiritual concerns may be far more difficult, somewhat like trying to swim across a lake with weighted boots clamped to your feet. It takes so much energy just to keep your head above water that forward motion is nearly impossible. Normalizing the physiology in the brain is like getting rid of the boots: you still have to do the swimming, but at least you don't feel like you're drowning every minute, and you can eventually get across the lake.

Antidepressants are not addictive or even habit-forming. They do not induce a tolerance for higher and higher doses or a craving for themselves, as do narcotics. Claims (on the Internet or elsewhere) that antidepressants are addictive are untrue, but they may be fueled by a phenomenon known as a **discontinuation syndrome** that occurs in some individuals when certain of these medications are stopped suddenly. Symptoms such as vertigo, fatigue, and odd "electric shock" sensations in the head may occur, and they will disappear if the medication is restarted. This occurs more commonly among antidepressants such as venlafaxine (Effexor) and paroxetine (Paxil) that have what is called a short **half-life**, meaning that their activity in the body declines more rapidly when they are stopped. Fluoxetine (Prozac), in contrast, has such a long half-life that it rarely, if ever, provokes discontinuation symptoms. Unlike withdrawal symptoms induced by long-term use of narcotics, antidepressant discontinuation symptoms are by no means universal and can be avoided by gradually reducing the dose of the drug. (This is unnecessary with lower entry-level doses.) Needless to say, changes in these medications should be made only under the supervision of the prescribing physician.

Antidepressants do not create an artificial high, but instead they stabilize the emotions. (One of the most common responses to successful treatment is "I feel like myself again.") Their use does not represent some sort of Band-Aid that avoids addressing the real problem, but rather facilitates more effective work with a therapist or pastor. Furthermore, a person who does *not* have a neurotransmitter problem is very unlikely to notice any particular improvement in mood or undergo a personality makeover as a result of taking one of these medications.

Contrary to sensationalistic news stories, the antidepressants that are most commonly used today do not provoke senseless acts of violence or suicide. Obviously, the possibility of self-harm is always a concern when someone is depressed, especially when someone *isn't* treated. That being said, when *any* antidepressant is started (whether one of the older medications—the tricyclics and the MAO inhibitors—or one of the newer agents) there is a remote possibility that a depressed person may be lifted out of a state of lethargic inactivity before the mood actually improves. A suicide attempt is indeed a risk at that point, and thus careful follow-up of any suspicious statements or activities is important whenever an antidepressant is started. However, millions of people have been started on these medications without incident.

The most widely used antidepressants are called **selective serotonin reuptake inhibitors** (or **SSRIs**). Introduced in the late 1980s, this class of medication revolutionized the medical treatment of mood disorders because of markedly improved safety profiles, fewer side effects, and effectiveness for both major depression and a broad spectrum of anxiety disorders. They have also been helpful for many women with significant premenstrual distress. One other feature that has made these medications useful in treating depression is that they are not likely to harm if taken in an overdose. SSRIs currently available include fluoxetine (Prozac, the first of these on the market), sertraline (Zoloft), paroxetine (Paxil), citalopram (Celexa), and escitalopram (Lexapro). Venlafaxine (Effexor) and the newer agent duloxetine (Cymbalta) affect both serotonin and norepinephrine levels.

While SSRIs are less likely to cause serious toxicity than older (tricyclic) antidepressants, *any overdose, whether deliberate or accidental, is a serious event that requires immediate medical evaluation.* SSRI overdose, for example, can provoke a central nervous system disturbance called **serotonin syndrome** that requires careful medical observation. Also, overdoses often involve multiple medications, which in combination can be hazardous.

Mirtazapine (Remeron) affects serotonin and norepinephrine levels, but by a different mechanism from the SSRIs. Bupropion (Wellbutrin) affects dopamine and norepinephrine but not serotonin, and it may be taken along with an SSRI in some individuals. Both of these tend to have far fewer sexual side effects (such as decreased libido or a blunted sexual response) than the SSRIs.

Older antidepressants that are still in use (though less commonly) include the **tricyclics** (such as amitriptyline, doxepin, and norpramin) and the **MAO inhibitors**. Both classes of medications can have significant side effects, and MAO inhibitors are used infrequently because of the possibility of serious reactions when taken with certain other medications and foods. Both types of medication are also much more dangerous if an overdose is taken. A variety of **mood stabilizers** are used in the treatment of bipolar disorder, and several classes of medications known as **antipsychotics** are used to manage thought disorders, although they may be helpful in bipolar and some atypical depression syndromes as well.

The specific uses, profiles, doses, and side effects of these various agents are beyond the scope of this book and should be discussed in detail with the prescribing physician. There are, however, a few important considerations to keep in mind.

First, antidepressants do not work immediately. In some cases, the first signs of improvement may be noticeable within a few days, but more commonly, benefits evolve gradually over a few weeks. If one agent does not seem to work or causes side effects, it is not at all unusual for a physician to try another. Since there is no way to know for certain which medication will work best for a given individual, some trial and error may be necessary, much like trying different keys in a lock.

Also, antidepressants are not like antibiotics that are taken for a few days and then stopped. If a medication appears to be working well, it is important to continue taking it for an extended period of time—typically at least six to twelve months. If the medication is stopped too soon, symptoms are likely to return. For many individuals, mood disorders related to neurotransmitters are a chronic or recurring problem, and long-term use (sometimes years) may be necessary to maintain the beneficial effects.

While benefits may take a few weeks to evolve, side effects are often noticed right away. Some—for example, a mild upset stomach or a sense of fatigue—resolve within a few days. Others—for example, sexual side effects with SSRIs—may be very persistent. Any problems with these medications should be discussed promptly with the physician prescribing them, who may adjust the dose, try another drug, or discontinue medication(s) altogether. Patients should avoid stopping a medication or adjusting the dose on their own.

It is important to contact the prescribing physician immediately if an antidepressant *worsens* symptoms of anxiety or depression. Responses such as increased anxiety, irritability, agitation, or increased suicidal thinking are particularly worrisome and warrant an immediate reevaluation of the medication (and possibly the diagnosis).

One other type of medication was mentioned earlier in this chapter and bears noting again here. Some anxiety disorders are so disruptive that immediate relief is needed. A physician may prescribe an anxiolytic (anxiety-reducing) medication to provide some immediate (and at times crucial) relief while an antidepressant is taking effect. Usually this will be one of the **benzodiazepines**, which have been used for many years for this purpose. Examples are alprazolam (Xanax), clonazepam (Klonopin), lorazepam (Ativan), and diazepam (Valium), among others. All tend to be sedating to some degree, and the choice and dose of medication is usually based both on duration of action (the length of time the drug works after a dose is taken) and the severity of the anxiety being treated. (Some are even prescribed to promote sleep in people who are not necessarily anxious, as we will describe in chapter 15.) Alcohol intensifies the effects of these drugs, so it should not be consumed when a person is taking them. Dosage guidelines should be followed carefully, and the prescribing physician should explain clearly whether this type of medication is to be used around the clock or only as needed. If a person is extremely depressed or

WHOM SHOULD I SEE FOR PROFESSIONAL HELP?

During many of life's trials, the support and counsel of family, friends, fellow church members, or pastoral staff are extremely important, and no paid professional can substitute for what they do. However, there are times when it is wise—and in some cases, critical—to consult with professionals who have special training and experience in helping people deal with emotional or thought disorders, interpersonal conflicts, and crises such as catastrophic losses or traumatic experiences. Who provides this type of service?

Primary-care physicians, whether family practitioners, internists, obstetrician/gynecologists, or pediatricians, as well as physician assistants and nurse practitioners are often the "first on the scene" with anxiety, depression, and other mood or thought disturbances. One reason is that such problems are usually accompanied by physical complaints; indeed, the symptoms are often the presenting problem, and it may be a physician who helps clarify the connection between two types of disturbances. (Many people are far more comfortable going to their own doctor with a complaint of fatigue or insomnia than calling a psychiatrist to discuss anxiety or depression.) In addition, when appropriate many primary-care physicians will prescribe one or more medications for anxiety and depression and monitor the results. While they rarely have the time or training to do formal cognitive therapy—the extended conversations that go on for weeks with a therapist—they often can provide straightforward and timely counsel that definitely helps a person move in the right direction. In addition, the primary physician can make referrals to appropriate consultants when expertise and formal counseling are needed.

Psychiatrists are physicians with special training and expertise in diagnosing and treating mood and thought disorders. Unlike the old caricature of psychiatry—the bearded, pipe-smoking analyst muttering "Uh-huh" and "Mmmm" and "Tell me about your mother" while the patient lies on a couch, free-associating endlessly about his childhood—contemporary psychiatry tends to focus primarily on medical management. (The old-school Freudian psychoanalytic approach had enormous influence during the first half of the twentieth century but is now practiced by a very small cadre of psychiatrists.) Because primary-care physicians are able to diagnose and successfully treat many people with anxiety and depression, psychiatrists are frequently called upon to manage problems that are more severe or complex. While some

potentially suicidal, someone else should be in charge of dispensing this and all other medication. Furthermore, if benzodiazepines are used regularly for a number of weeks, discontinuation should be done gradually under the physician's supervision in order to prevent withdrawal effects such as tremors, insomnia, or even seizures. One other medication that specifically targets anxiety

emphasize psychotherapy, most psychiatrists focus on prescription medications rather than extended counseling sessions on life issues. This is not necessarily bad: When someone is extremely depressed or agitated, unresponsive to basic interventions, or is manifesting overtly delusional thinking, the skillful use of medication can definitely help restore order. Very often psychiatrists refer their patients to other types of therapists for cognitive (talk) therapy or will even partner with therapists in their own office for this type of work.

The nonmedical approach to anxiety, depression, and other problems in life (especially marital strife)—call it counseling, psychotherapy, or simply talk therapy—can be carried out by different types of professionals.

Clinical psychologists have a doctorate in psychology and may be involved in a variety of endeavors, including research, testing, and therapy. **Marriage and family therapists (MFTs)** provide both short- and long-term counseling. Depending upon state requirements, they typically take two or more years of postgraduate classes after earning a bachelor's degree and then spend another two or more years accruing a required number of hours counseling under the supervision of a licensed therapist. Some **social workers (MSWs)** also do individual therapy. All three types of counselors are licensed by state regulatory agencies, and qualifications vary from state to state.

Some churches also train **lay counselors** who work part- or full-time with individuals within their congregations. Normally they have referral arrangements with local licensed practitioners for situations that are more serious.

Before beginning a formal relationship with a counselor, you should definitely consider asking about his or her training, credentials, and license status, as well as clarifying who is supervising the counselor if that person is accruing hours while in training. Think twice before receiving (and paying for) counseling from someone who is unwilling to offer this information. You should also proceed with caution before seeking counseling online. Proponents of this expanding arena of Internet activity note that it may offer help for people who have difficulty accessing or paying for qualified counselors. But much of the benefit of counseling derives from the conversational interaction between two people, which is impossible to duplicate through e-mail or chat room interactions. Furthermore, there is significant potential for problems with confidentiality, inadequate follow-through, or even misrepresentation on either side of the computer keyboard. ■

is buspirone (BuSpar). It differs from the benzodiazepines in that it is typically not used as needed, but rather on an ongoing basis.

Before we discuss counseling and the spiritual aspects of dealing with anxiety and depression, a few other avenues for dealing with these problems are worth mentioning:

Exercise has been well established as valuable in dealing with mood disorders of all kinds. The last thing anxious and especially depressed people (who are typically very tired as well) may want to do is go out and move their muscles, but doing so daily will go a long way toward improving symptoms. Even a ten- or fifteen-minute walk will help.

An adequate amount of restorative sleep—or the lack of it—can have a major impact on emotional health. The Green Bay Packers' legendary coach Vince Lombardi famously remarked that "fatigue makes cowards of us all." We would add this corollary: Lack of sleep makes us irritable and depressed. While insomnia is a common by-product of anxiety and depression (and may have biochemical roots), burning the candle at both ends and trying to get by with very few hours of sleep will invariably erode our ability to cope with life's demands. During prolonged sleep deprivation, concentration deteriorates, and irritability and mood swings become a virtual certainty. As we describe in chapter 15, dealing with insomnia might require some help from your physician or even a specialist in sleep disorders, but the necessity of sleep for emotional well-being must not be overlooked.

Diet and supplements. Despite all of the extravagant claims you might find in books, magazines, ads, and Web sites, no specific diet can reliably be considered a cure for any mood disorder. Obviously, a person who is so depressed that he or she is eating very little, or one who is consuming vast amounts of high-calorie junk food in response to anxiety or daily stresses, may develop other health problems and certainly won't feel any better in the long run. Eating an appropriate amount of good-quality foods, as discussed in depth in chapter 5, will help combat any type of disturbance, emotional or otherwise. That being said, some dietary adjustments and supplements can help, though they should not necessarily be considered the primary treatment.

- **Folic acid (folate).** Some research suggests that low blood levels of folic acid may be associated with both depression and a poor response to antidepressant therapy. Aside from eating plenty of leafy green vegetables and legumes, which are abundant in folic acid, a person who is depressed might consider an additional 400 to 800 mcg of folic acid daily, either as a specific supplement or in a multivitamin. (Tablets containing more than 1000 mcg require a prescription and are used for purposes other than helping a depressed mood.)
- **Vitamin B_6** supplements have been widely promoted as a treatment for depression because of this vitamin's role in converting the amino

acid tryptophan into serotonin. Depression is a symptom of overt vitamin B_6 deficiency, and alcohol abuse accelerates its loss from the body. While research supporting the efficacy of B_6 as a specific treatment for depression is not compelling, taking some in the form of a multivitamin (most contain the daily value of 2 mg) is reasonable if you are dealing with depression. Taking more than 50 mg per day is unwise, and high doses (500 mg or less) are associated with toxic side effects.

- **Omega-3 fatty acids** that are abundant in fish oils are known to be beneficial to the heart, blood vessels, and central nervous system. They may help stabilize mood as well. For most people, eating a three- to four-ounce serving of fish twice weekly—especially fatty, cold-water fish such as salmon, mackerel, lake trout, albacore tuna, herring, and sardines—is a reasonable way to obtain adequate dietary omega-3 fatty acids. People with known coronary artery disease are often advised to take up to 3 grams per day, which can be obtained from an omega-3 supplement (usually derived from fish oils). It is possible that doing so might also be beneficial (although not in itself a cure) for those who are depressed. We discuss these nutrients in chapter 5, starting on page 152.
- **Specific nonprescription dietary supplements for depression** are touted as "all natural" and some may be beneficial, but keep in mind that once an herbal substance is concentrated into a pill or tonic, it is no more natural than any prescription drug. **St. John's wort** has been used widely in Europe to treat mood disorders, and in a number of studies its effectiveness has compared favorably with prescription agents for mild depression.[5] However, it is unregulated by the FDA. It may interfere with the action of certain medications used to treat AIDS and should not be taken with other antidepressants without explicit approval of a knowledgeable physician. Also, it normally requires three-times daily dosing to be effective, which is a significant disadvantage compared to once-daily prescription agents. **SAM-e**, pronounced "sammy," short for S-adenosylmethionine, is a compound used to treat depression in Europe (by prescription) and sold in the United States as a nonprescription dietary supplement. It may increase levels of serotonin and dopamine in the brain, and research now under way in the United States will help clarify its effectiveness and safety (or lack thereof). For the time being, use of SAM-e with other antidepressant medications is not recommended.

Counseling—also referred to as psychotherapy or simply talk therapy—has been a mainstay of treatment for anxiety and depression for decades. Like contemporary psychiatry, it usually bears little resemblance to the lengthy probing of the subconscious devised by Sigmund Freud and his followers in the early twentieth century. In fact, therapists use a number of approaches to address mood disorders and other issues of life, but most are purposeful and oriented toward problem solving (as opposed to less directed explorations of a person's life). While a look at those approaches is beyond the scope of this book, most will address to some degree the following concerns:

- *Current symptoms.* What are the characteristics of the problem? What kinds of emotions and thought processes are going on? How are they affecting family and other significant relationships, work, sleep, and other dimensions of life?
- *History.* What happened in the past that might have played a role in the development of the mood problem? This might involve exploring what occurred during childhood and adolescence (sometimes called "family of origin" issues), the history of other significant relationships such as marriage(s), and major life events—especially serious losses, trauma, or other stressors.
- *Current sources of stress or support.* Especially important are conflicts within the family (involving spouse, children, or parents) or on the job.
- *Behaviors*—especially habitual ones—and beliefs that may be contributing to the problem.
- *Spiritual orientation and beliefs.* Is religious faith part of the current equation? Is it helping or making things worse?
- *Strategies* for changing thoughts, behaviors, relationships, or all of the above.

Exploring the relevant issues may involve sessions (typically weekly, but in some situations twice weekly) extending over several weeks, months, or even years. An extended time of history-taking may be necessary to understand the depth and breadth of the problem. Techniques such as journaling may be employed to help track, express, and clarify thoughts and feelings. With the individual's permission, other family members may be asked to provide input or enter into ongoing discussions. Relational conflicts (especially within a marriage) will often need to be sorted out. A well-trained therapist should be able to recognize and suggest medication that may be appropriate and can help make an appropriate referral to a psychiatrist or a primary-care physician who is qualified to prescribe it.

Because the conversations are prolonged, often intense or even painful, and may involve very personal details about past and current life events, it is critical that a person feel comfortable and safe with a therapist. In addition, because core values and spiritual concerns usually enter the discussion, it is wise to choose a therapist who is not only appropriately qualified but also shares one's spiritual perspective. (In most cases, a compatible worldview is more important when working with a therapist or counselor than when consulting with a psychiatrist, who nearly always focuses primarily on the choice and management of medication.)

If you seek counseling and can't find a therapist whose core values and faith are basically aligned with yours, it is important that whomever you see at least acknowledges and respects your views. Professionals in this field, regardless of their personal faith or lack thereof, are trained and expected to be sensitive and supportive of a client's religious orientation, and it is unlikely that one would deliberately attempt to erode your faith or corrupt your moral values. (In the event that this does occur, you would be wise to seek help elsewhere.) However, since one's understanding of God plays an important role in addressing anxiety and/or depression, it is indeed helpful if your therapist has both an active faith and a working knowledge of the Scriptures. (Don't disqualify a counselor as not being "spiritual enough" if she doesn't open your session with prayer or quote from the Bible throughout the session. She may be deliberately holding back in this area while determining what best serves you.) Your pastor or a member of your church staff can usually refer you to a local therapist who is both professionally competent and spiritually well-grounded. Focus on the Family (800-A-FAMILY) also maintains a referral list of qualified counselors, as does Focus on the Family Canada (800-661-9800).

What if an anxiety disorder or depressive episode responds dramatically to a medication and a person seems to be restored to normal within a few weeks? Is it really necessary to spend weeks or months in counseling if that occurs? In fact, a certain percentage of people have a mood problem that is almost purely biochemical. They are basically well-adjusted, stable, productive people who function well at home, school, work, and church but are genetically vulnerable to a neurotransmitter imbalance. At some point in life, or perhaps periodically, dark emotional clouds roll in and won't leave. These people may experience a sudden panic attack. They may feel as though they're going crazy because they can't understand where the turbulence is coming from. They're not necessarily in denial about some deep, dark issue or conflict lurking in the subconscious mind. When they take an antidepressant, the dark mood clears and things return to normal. Should these people visit a therapist?

Anyone who has a significant mood disturbance—even one that responds spectacularly well to medication—would be wise to spend some time in counseling. Previously, we described the complex interaction of genetics, physiology, and the events of life in the genesis of anxiety and depression. Everyone has some sort of baggage—issues from the past, current conflicts, habits, and persistent beliefs, to name a few—that might trigger or feed a mood disorder or stand in the way of recovery. Also, the mood disturbance is likely to affect family members, coworkers, and others, or there may be damage to relationships from previous episodes that needs to be repaired. These are all worth addressing, along with formulating strategies to help prevent future episodes. It should come as no surprise that research into how best to manage mood disorders consistently shows a greater likelihood of improvement when one uses medication and cognitive therapy together rather than one or the other by itself. Furthermore, a number of people with mood problems do not need or respond to medication at all.

When dealing with the **spiritual dimensions** of anxiety and depression, there are two extremes to avoid. One is to leave God out of the equation entirely and assume that the problem is wholly the result of disordered neurotransmitters, personal conflicts, or lack of self-esteem. This is a critical defect of a purely secular worldview, which unfortunately pervades our culture. The other extreme is to decide that a mood problem is strictly the consequence of lack of faith, unconfessed sin, inadequate time in prayer or Bible study, disobedience, or some other offense that has caused a rift in one's relationship with God. The latter opinion is unfortunately all too common in some churches and parachurch organizations. Obviously, taking steps to restore one's relationship with God if it has been neglected or abandoned (or to begin one if it has never been clearly established) is crucial, as we will see momentarily. But two very flawed assumptions often underlie the "you only need more faith" position: (Flaw #1) If you are rightly related to God, you will be happy all the time, and (Flaw #2) If you're not currently happy, you must not be rightly related to God.

These beliefs are not only wrongheaded but also heap unnecessary guilt on a person who already feels miserable. Even under normal circumstances, there are always peaks and valleys in life, times when life is rich and full and others when it seems bland or even barren. It is the reality of life on this fallen planet, and the Bible is full of stories and laments of people who walked with God and yet were suffering, anxious, or even depressed for a time. Furthermore, neurotransmitter disturbances, like other physical ailments, afflict both the godly and the unbeliever. (It's unlikely that any of us would rebuke a friend for having pneumonia or cancer, claiming that the illness is the consequence of unconfessed sin or lack of faith.) Even people who have been faithful and disciplined in their spiritual affairs may find themselves immersed in depression or the persistent grip of an anxiety disorder, simply because the level of one or more neurotransmitters in the brain has sagged.

What is both common and cruel about these disorders is that they can cause a person to feel as though God has literally disappeared. Prayers seem to hit the ceiling and bounce back with a "return to sender" stamp. Reading the Bible generates about as much inspiration as reading the phone book. Such people certainly need to maintain and in fact persevere in their spiritual disciplines—not to woo God back into their life, but to remind themselves that He has never left their side. But those efforts may be far more arduous if an underlying biochemical problem isn't addressed as well. (Imagine trying to have a quiet time with a freshly broken leg or gaping wound. We could and should cry out to God under those circumstances, but we probably wouldn't engage in tranquil meditation or a thoughtful study of the Scriptures until someone helped us relieve the pain.)

Nonetheless, there may be some important spiritual issues to be addressed when a person is dealing with anxiety and depression. As a starting point, we will consider a few of the many passages in the Bible that relate to this problem.

This meditation from David is a beautiful portrait of a tranquil mind, and it certainly communicates the heart's desire of someone with an anxiety disorder:

The Lord is my shepherd, I shall not be in want.
He makes me lie down in green pastures,
he leads me beside quiet waters,
he restores my soul.
He guides me in paths of righteousness
for his name's sake.
Even though I walk
through the valley of the shadow of death,
I will fear no evil,
for you are with me;
your rod and your staff,
they comfort me.
You prepare a table before me
in the presence of my enemies.
You anoint my head with oil;
my cup overflows.
Surely goodness and love will follow me
all the days of my life,
and I will dwell in the house of the Lord forever.
(PSALM 23)

The person struggling with depression probably has some difficulty identifying with these sentiments:

Sing to the Lord a new song,
his praise in the assembly of the saints.
Let Israel rejoice in their Maker;
let the people of Zion be glad in their King.
Let them praise his name with dancing
and make music to him with tambourine and harp.
For the Lord takes delight in his people;
he crowns the humble with salvation.
Let the saints rejoice in this honor
and sing for joy on their beds.
(PSALM 149:1-5)

Rejoice in the Lord always. I will say it again: Rejoice!
(PHILIPPIANS 4:4)

The apostle Paul summarizes an emotional and behavioral mind-set that sounds far removed from the realm of anxiety and depression: "The fruit of the Spirit is love, joy, peace, patience, kindness, goodness, faithfulness, gentleness and self-control" (Galatians 5:22-23).

Since God is interested in our emotional weather and intends that it be sunny and calm rather than dark and stormy, what could be wrong if a person is anxious or depressed? We've already noted several biological and behavioral conditions that increase the likelihood of developing a problem with anxiety and depression. Later in this chapter, and for most of chapter 9, we will describe spiritual orientations and disciplines that promote healthy emotions (not to mention physical well-being). But for a moment, it's worth considering some spiritual risk factors for anxiety and depression.

No relationship with God. If this world is truly all there is, if "life is hard and then you die," if we're nothing but a collection of chemicals that randomly assembled themselves into living entities over billions of years, if no one is keeping score, then anxiety and depression could be considered the only emotions that make any sense. Skeptics claim that human beings concoct religion because they can't deal with the truth of their meaningless existence. But the universe, the world around us, the spectacular complexity of living systems, the remarkable testimony of the Old and New Testaments, and the life and teachings of Jesus Christ instruct us otherwise, in ways that are too numerous and compelling to recite here. Needless to say, establishing a relationship with God—to be more exact, becoming reconciled to God and experiencing spiritual birth—is the most critical step toward wholeness that you will find in this entire book. If you have not taken that step or are not certain how to do so, go to page 399 in the next chapter before you read any further.

A relationship with God disrupted by our choices. We can be born into God's family and experience the benefits of this new relationship (described in the New Testament as becoming a "new creature"). But as long as we live in our present physical body, we will have to contend with an old nature that wants its own way rather than God's. That struggle can generate a considerable amount of distress, as powerfully described by the apostle Paul in his letter to Roman believers:

> *When I want to do good, evil is right there with me. For in my inner being I delight in God's law; but I see another law at work in the members of my body, waging war against the law of my mind and making me a prisoner of the law of sin at work within my members. What a wretched man I am! Who will rescue me from this body of death?*
>
> (ROMANS 7:21-24)

Our capacity to do what is wrong and to resist doing what is right inevitably leads us to commit what are called "sins of commission" and "sins of omission," which disrupt our relationship with God. How long that disruption continues significantly affects our emotional well-being.

Unwillingness to restore the relationship. Maintaining our relationship with God requires an ongoing process of acknowledging wrongdoing and experiencing the forgiveness that He has provided. The New Testament calls this confession, and it needs to be done on a regular basis—as often as we find sin in our life. We get into trouble, emotionally and otherwise, when we become careless about this process or resist doing it altogether. Denying, making excuses, deluding ourselves, and blaming others (or even God) will keep us from enjoying the refreshment of a restored relationship: "If we claim to be without sin, we deceive ourselves and the truth is not in us. If we confess our sins, he is faithful and just and will forgive us our sins and purify us from all unrighteousness" (1 John 1:8-9).

A shallow, compartmentalized relationship with God. We can be law-abiding citizens and civil in our behavior, but on our own terms. We can give God a tip of the hat while saying grace or make the right noises at church but then live the rest of life as if He doesn't exist or is off tending to business in some other corner of the universe. (*Catch you later, Lord. . . . I've got stuff to do.*) Sooner or later this lack of spiritual depth and breadth will lead to problems, especially when we are buffeted by life's inevitable troubles. The process of growth in our relationship with God involves a number of disciplines that we will discuss in the next chapter.

Distorted understandings of God's character. The Scriptures refer to God with names that describe various aspects of His character, but the one we hear most often is Father. Comparison or even identification of our heavenly Father with our earthly one is almost inevitable, for better or worse, and this may implant negative and inaccurate ideas about God deep into our emotional core. These may not be what we *say* we believe, but they are often what we actually *feel* that God is like. If we sense that God is testy, critical, perfectionistic, distant, even cruel, we may need to do some Scripture- and soul-searching to revise our perceptions.

Guilt, true and false. God has dealt with our *true* guilt, if we have accepted His offer of complete forgiveness through Christ. (As noted in the first of these spiritual risk factors, if you have not taken this step, turn now to page 399 in the next chapter.) Even after beginning a relationship with God, we may continue to feel pangs of guilt over past or recent thoughts and actions. If these lead to genuine repentance, confession, and changes in behavior, then they serve a useful purpose. Some guilt, however, arises from the unreasonable expectations of other people that pull at our heartstrings. This guilt may also arise from perfectionism or from legalistic teachings about God that base a person's spiritual status on adhering to a long list of dos and don'ts that do not necessarily cause one to grow closer to God or love other people.

A classic and enlightening book dealing with false assumptions about God's character is *Your God Is Too Small* by J. B. Phillips (New York: Touchstone, 1997).

Bitterness. This is literally a cancer of the emotions, one that is almost guaranteed to provoke or aggravate depression if left untended. Jesus went to some length to describe how we are to forgive others, just as we are forgiven—indeed, He gave His life so that we could have that privilege. Ongoing bitterness against an individual, a group of people, a government, or even God Himself—an ironic posture, given what He has done for us—accomplishes nothing except to erode the emotional well-being of the one who clings to it. (It should come as no surprise that scientific research is now validating the benefits of forgiveness.) Forgiving someone does not, by the way, mean that a person must feel warm and fuzzy toward that individual or group, nor is forgiveness necessarily an instantaneous response after a particularly grievous offense. It also doesn't mean that someone who has harmed you through an illegal act should be exempt from the consequences of the law. Instead, it primarily involves releasing hostile emotions and giving up the desire to extract personal revenge. For someone with very intense, deep-seated, or long-lasting bitterness, it may be necessary to work through the process of forgiveness and release over time with a counselor or pastor.

Spiritual warfare. This is a delicate subject for a book such as this that has the utmost respect for solid scientific research and evidence. Much harm has been done over the centuries by those who believed that various physical or emotional disorders—for example, epilepsy or schizophrenia—result from demon possession. Nevertheless, Jesus explicitly acknowledged the existence and activities of evil entities within the spiritual realm and dealt decisively with them when necessary. We are told in Scripture that they exist, that they can and do afflict human beings, and that dealing with them requires discernment and prayer. It is unwise either to assume that they are directly involved with any and all problems we might face (emotional or otherwise), or at the opposite extreme to ignore them entirely. We are also clearly instructed not to traffic with any spiritual entity other than God Himself—for example, by attempting to contact the dead or "spirit guides" through various techniques—and for good reason. In so doing, a person opens himself to being influenced by forces with which human beings are not equipped to interact. Someone who has been involved with this type of activity and is now experiencing anxiety or depression should consider consulting with a mature pastor or counselor who has experience and discernment in this troubling arena.

Habits That Promote a Healthy Mind and Emotions

We've made it abundantly clear throughout this book that maintaining good physical health requires some deliberate decisions and disciplines. For many of us, "doing what comes naturally" often leads to overeating, underexercising, and the pursuit of all sorts of transient pleasures that ultimately erode health and shorten life. The same principle applies to our emotional, cognitive, and spiritual health. Even if we're not fighting an uphill battle to overcome the effects of neurotransmitter problems or hardships in life, it's all too easy to drift into a mental landscape that is stale, stagnating, or stormy. Maintaining a vibrant outlook on life, stable but responsive emotions, satisfying relationships, and ongoing contentment requires cultivating some habits that may not be among your autopilot settings but aren't out of reach either.

Spiritual health

Spiritual and emotional health are so closely intertwined that it is almost impossible to talk about one without considering the other at the same time. We will look at a number of disciplines that build spiritual health in the next chapter, but for now we need to focus on an extremely important concept. Indeed, it is the ultimate foundation of your emotional health.

There is a sense of deep, abiding, unshakable contentment that lies at the heart of emotional health and satisfying relationships. It comes from knowing—not as a doctrinal belief, but in the core of your soul—that you are loved, accepted, and cherished by God and that your relationship with Him is a settled certainty. The implications of this understanding are profound. If we are the beloved sons and daughters of the eternal God who created, owns, and rules the universe and everything in it, that relationship overshadows every other concern we have during our life on this planet. Whatever we accomplish or earn not only pales by comparison but also ceases to become the currency on which we place our value or significance.

What this knowledge accomplishes is both deep and far-reaching. It is the basis for a contentment that is independent of circumstances. It short-circuits the need to acquire wealth for the sake of power or status and at the same time releases an individual to use money and possessions as a tool to benefit others. When we know that we belong to God, we are free to enjoy whatever recognition we get, even if it's none at all, for a job well done. We are freed from the need to fret over whether we are first or last, at the head of the line or bringing up the rear. It is the reason that the apostle Paul could write these words while imprisoned: "I have learned to be content whatever the circumstances. I know what it is to be in need, and I know what it is to have plenty. I have learned the secret of being content in any and every situation, whether well fed or hungry, whether living in plenty or in want" (Philippians 4:11-12).

The world at large, and all of us to some degree, seek this contentment in the wrong places—wealth, possessions, fame, approval, romance, sex, among others—fueled by a pervasive (though often unspoken) assumption: "If I could just have ____, then I'd be happy." Most of our economy and virtually all of its marketing strategies are driven by this premise. Magazine ads and TV commercials are skillfully crafted to create desire or outright craving for whatever product the company is selling. A little everyday experience readily exposes the myth that contentment comes from having whatever the "if only" might be, but taking that idea to heart and reacting to situations accordingly is a lifelong process.

Much has been written over the past few decades about the importance of self-esteem and how lacking it leads to all kinds of emotional and relational problems. When properly understood, that notion is indeed correct. All of us have met people who are highly anxious about interacting with others or who see themselves as so worthless that they allow habitual abuse by others (or pour it upon themselves). We have all encountered people who seem to have so much self-esteem—indeed, who are so full of themselves—that it is a relief to get away from them. Their inflated egos may actually arise from insecurity, or they may genuinely position themselves at the center of their universe.

Ironically, the person who is self-abasing and the one who is self-inflating actually have very similar problems: they're both overly self-conscious and self-centered. Healthy self-esteem, perhaps better expressed by the term *healthy self-concept,* is a state of security and serenity based on one's relationship with God in which the status of self no longer is a concern. C. S. Lewis described this quality beautifully in *The Screwtape Letters*:

> [God] wants to bring the man to a state of mind in which he could design the best cathedral in the world, and know it to be the best, and rejoice in the fact, without being any more (or less) or otherwise glad at having done it than he would be if it had been done by another. [He] wants him, in the end, to be so free from any bias in his own favour that he can rejoice in his own talents as frankly and gratefully as in his neighbour's talents—or in a sunrise, an elephant or a waterfall. He wants each man, in the long run, to be able to recognize all creatures (even himself) as glorious and excellent things. He wants to kill their animal self-love as soon as possible; but it is His long-term policy . . . to restore to them a new kind of self-love—a charity and gratitude for all selves, including their own; when they have really learned to love their neighbours as themselves, they will be allowed to love themselves as their neighbours.[6]

Establishing, maintaining, and being transformed by an intimate relationship with God is ultimately the most important item on your health agenda because it is the foundation on which every other type of health—physical, emotional, and relational—is based. We discuss this subject in more depth in chapter 9.

Physical health

A primary theme of this chapter is that body and mind are not separate entities and that the way one is working will have a significant effect on how the other functions and feels. Your emotions have a better chance of being stable and harmonious if you're tending to the following, all of which are discussed elsewhere in this book:

- Eating high-quality nutrients (chapter 5)
- Maintaining a healthy weight (chapter 6)
- Exercising regularly (chapter 7)
- Avoiding tobacco, excessive alcohol intake, and illicit drugs (chapter 10)
- Getting restorative sleep (chapter 15)
- Taking steps to avoid cardiovascular disease, cancer, and diabetes, and when possible to detect their presence before they cause serious harm (chapters 3 and 4)

Healthy relationships

The seventeenth-century poet John Donne wrote the famous statement, "No man is an island," and we would propose an amplified version: "No man, woman, child, or infant is an island." From the moment of birth—some would argue before that moment—our health and development are profoundly dependent on the touch and sounds of others. This reality was tragically demonstrated on a colossal scale after the Romanian dictator Nicolae Ceausescu was deposed and then executed in December 1989. A spectacularly misguided effort to double the country's population within one generation, combined with a cultural acceptance of turning unwanted children over to state-run orphanages, led to a situation that some have described as a "gulag for children": Some 150,000 children were housed in facilities in which caretakers could not or would not do much more than feed them and change their diapers. Infants and toddlers would lie in cribs untouched and untended, and even the bottles they were given were propped in place so that the adult personnel did not have to interact with them during feedings.

Journalists and medical personnel who first entered these facilities were shocked to find warehouses full of babies and children who were malnourished, suffering from a variety of medical problems, and most notably, displaying striking delays in physical, intellectual, and emotional development. Two- and three-year-olds were not walking or talking. Children were withdrawn and anxious. When offered food, they refused it or ate too much. They rocked back and forth, studying their hands and fingers, or they lay in cribs or beds without attempting to signal that they were awake. Researchers who followed Romanian orphans adopted into nurturing homes found that they eventually resolved most of their medical and developmental deficits, but that the emotional, behavioral, and social problems were much more difficult to overcome.

The Romanian tragedy graphically demonstrates that in order to thrive, infants and children desperately need not only food, clothing, and shelter, but also touch, emotional nurturing, and interaction with caring adults. Unfortunately, we may lose sight of the fact that *all* of us need these—not only as children, but throughout our adult lives—if we are going to be truly healthy. A growing body of medical research continues to confirm what might seem obvious: that a sense of belonging, a network of friendships, and emotional intimacy—in other words, healthy relationships in which we both give and receive affirmation and support—result in improved health. Longer life, fewer symptoms, less illness, and faster recovery have been demonstrated for a variety of medical problems among those who feel cared for and supported, whether in satisfying marriages or other friendships. On the flip side, a variety of adverse health outcomes have been demonstrated among those who feel isolated or abandoned or who are entrenched in hostile or abusive relationships, marital or otherwise.

We were built for reciprocal love and intimacy. For some who were brought up in a loving and secure environment and who are blessed with a knack for interacting with others, meeting people and building close friendships seem almost second nature. For others, perhaps because of inherent shyness or awkward experiences growing up, developing and maintaining relationships is a struggle. Some who have endured rejection or abuse from those they should have been able to trust come to the bitter conclusion that emotional isolation is the safest course for survival. Wherever you find yourself on this spectrum, keep one basic thought in mind: *Just as maintaining and improving physical health requires time and deliberate effort, so does the building and enhancement of healthy—and health-sustaining—relationships*. Because an entire book could be devoted to this subject (and many have been), here we can only point you in a few important directions.

If you are married, tending to that relationship must be your highest priority after tending to your relationship with God. In a best-case scenario, your spouse is your soul mate, your best friend, your lover, your number-one cheerleader, your companion for life, and the person with whom you feel safest. If he or she is indeed all of these, you are truly blessed, and you have probably also figured out by now that this doesn't happen by accident. Like a garden, a solid marriage that gets consistent and careful attention from each member grows in beauty, provides a sweet fragrance, and becomes a place of refreshment and restoration for others. What waters and nourishes that garden?

- Daily expressions of love, appreciation, and respect
- Time allotted regularly for debriefing—finding out what is going on in the other person's life and thoughts
- Individual and mutual commitment to God and to spiritual growth
- Unexpected gifts, cards, flowers, notes, calls, e-mails
- Time spent away from the daily routine—a dinner out, a weekend away, even breakfast on the back porch
- Learning the other person's "love language"—what words and deeds communicate your love for that person (and what don't)—and making the conscious decision to "speak" that language
- Learning how to resolve conflicts in ways that are mutually respectful
- Talking about and exploring ways to enhance physical intimacy

FOUR QUESTIONS TO ASK YOUR SPOUSE

Here are four important questions that a husband and wife should ask each other on a regular basis (at least weekly, if not more often). They should then listen carefully to the answers:

1. ***What was the high point of your week (or day)?***
2. ***What was the low point?***
3. ***What are you most worried about right now?***
4. ***Is there anything I can do right now to help you with what you are worried about (or anything else)?***

HOT TIP

Alas, far too many marriages are like gardens that are regularly bulldozed, overgrown with weeds, strewn with trash, barren, neglected, or abandoned. It is very possible that the first priority for your own health and that of your family will be to declare a cease-fire from criticism and harsh comments between you and your spouse—with an *immediate and final* end to any physical combat or abuse—and to engage in counseling with a qualified therapist or pastor.

Even if your marriage isn't turbulent, it can always be enhanced. Some excellent resources that you might want to explore include

- A marriage-enhancement weekend sponsored by your church or an organization such as Marriage Encounter (http://www.marriage-encounter.org, or 800-828-3351) or FamilyLife (http://www.familylife.com, or 800-FL-TODAY)
- A small-group or individual study such as the *Focus on the Family Marriage Series Group Starter Kit* (http://www.family.org/resources, or call 800-A-FAMILY)
- Books on marriage enhancement (and protection), such as *The Marriage Masterpiece* by Al Janssen, *Love and Respect* by Emerson Eggerichs, *His Needs, Her Needs* by Willard F. Harley, and *Love for a Lifetime* by Dr. James Dobson.

If you have children or teenagers living at home, tending to your relationship with them must be your highest priority after tending to your marriage (or if you are a single parent, after tending to your relationship with God). Only you can be the father or mother to your children. Providing a stable, loving, secure environment for them, teaching values and life skills, and launching them into responsible adulthood are the most important and rewarding projects on the planet. Again, as with your spouse, if you are experiencing difficulty with one or more children, you should seek help from a qualified counselor, your pastor, or your child's physician. Whether your parenting journey is currently smooth or turbulent, you should strongly consider consulting some useful resources, including

- The Focus on the Family *Complete Book of Baby & Child Care*. If one or more of your children are teenagers, the Focus on the Family *Parents' Guide to Teen Health* contains an updated version of the first book's content specifically geared to parents of adolescents.

- The Focus on the Family *Parents' Guide to the Spiritual Mentoring of Teens* and *Parents' Guide to the Spiritual Growth of Children.*
- Parenting books such as *The New Dare to Discipline*, *The New Strong-Willed Child,* and *Bringing Up Boys* by Dr. James Dobson; *Making Children Mind without Losing Yours* by Dr. Kevin Leman; and *The Family Compass: Practical, Intentional Ways to Pass Godly Values on to Your Child* by Kurt and Olivia Bruner.

Beyond the borders of your immediate and extended family, you should cultivate—in a healthy way—a broader circle of relationships. This is especially but not exclusively important for those who are not married or rearing children. You may be anxious to find companionship or the love of your life, and you might even be tempted to "look for love in all the wrong places." We don't want to sound like a greeting card or a platitude-quoting relative, but there are a number of fruitful ways to build relationships:

- Get involved in one or more groups for those who share a common interest. Your church is a good place to start, especially in a small-group setting where it's possible to know and be known by others. Another great way to form bonds is to participate in group projects where the focus is on a specific goal rather than on one another, a scenario that may make conversation much easier than at parties or dating situations. People who serve together on a short-term mission project, work detail, drama team, or other ministry often create lasting friendships.
- Volunteer in your community or church, at your local hospital, senior center, soup kitchen, or animal shelter. Most communities have nonprofit centers that help women with crisis pregnancies explore alternatives to abortion, and they (and their clients) can always use help. Service clubs offer numerous opportunities to enhance communities and socialize as well.
- Get to know your neighbors.
- Don't wait for other people to call you. Take the initiative to invite one or more neighbors or friends to join you for coffee, a meal, or a concert in the park.
- Be a good listener. Not only will others think you are wise and thoughtful, but you will be amazed how often actively listening to someone else is therapeutic for both of you. (An added bonus is how much you learn as you come to understand another person's history, occupation, interests, and passions.)
- Beware of looking, sounding, or acting too needy, even if you feel that way. Some people may be willing to spend time with you out of kindness, but after a while their forbearance may wear thin, especially if they sense that you are clingy or even demanding of their attention.
- Ask yourself this question: *Do I tend to be critical, cynical, sarcastic, or pessimistic?* If so, could this be interfering with lasting friendships?

An organization that provides this type of service may be called a pregnancy resource center, crisis pregnancy center, pregnancy care center, or women's resource center. Your church may already be involved with a center, or you can check with umbrella organizations such as Care Net (703-478-5661 or http://www.care-net.org), or Heartbeat International (888-550-7577 or http://www.heartbeatinternational.org).

That's just the way I am, might be your response, but it's also the language of the lonely and isolated.

- Find a healthy balance in your relationships. Some of us tend to be good at striking up surface relationships and may have lots of them. But we also need a few people with whom we feel safe to candidly discuss difficult experiences from the past and deeper concerns of the present. On the other hand, some of us are prone to wear our heart on our sleeve, sharing personal information too freely, perhaps with people who haven't yet earned our trust (and may be turned off as well). If you have difficulty getting past the surface or get into difficulties because you release too much information too quickly, you might wish to explore these topics with a counselor to find out why this happens and what to do about it.

As important as relationships may be to our overall health, they are not a foolproof, guaranteed means of creating emotional health. No one can make another person happy. A pessimistic, miserable, self-centered single person who gets married will become a pessimistic, miserable, self-centered married person. The unfortunate spouse who believes that he or she is responsible for another person's mood will eventually become sick of it or sick because of it. A great marriage or friendship—one with deep bonds, strong communication, shared interests and goals, and unshakable mutual respect—can take a person a long way toward emotional health and contentment. A bad relationship can do exactly the opposite. It can be toxic, draining joy, health, and even life out of both who are unfortunate enough to be bound in it. Here are some characteristics of disordered relationships:

- **Excessive neediness.** Relationships in which one person is intensely dependent on the other, and thus clingy and smothering, are draining and ultimately a turnoff. Even within a marriage, a sense of one's own identity and an appropriate level of independence is not only necessary but attractive.
- **Excessive control.** Respectful accountability in a close friendship, especially in a marriage, is healthy. Trying to control everything that someone else does, buys, watches, or thinks is *not.*
- **Isolation from others.** Whether arising from neediness, control issues, or both, beware of the person who wants you all to himself. Obviously, within marriage, romantic and physical affection must be mutually exclusive. But the person who wants to isolate another from friends, acquaintances, or even family members has serious problems.
- **Pressure for sex.** In a nonmarital relationship, a man who suggests, begs, haggles, or pushes for sex lacks respect for the boundaries and welfare of his would-be partner. If the woman is doing the asking, there are other issues involved (usually arising from her own physi-

cal boundaries being compromised at an early age), especially a mistaken sense that sex can serve as a bargaining chip in a relationship. In a marital relationship, begging, bargaining, and even demanding sex are symptoms of disrupted dynamics, sexual and otherwise, that need to be addressed with an experienced counselor (more on this in chapter 12).

- **Emotional roller coasters.** Passionate expressions of love one day, fighting like cats and dogs the next, crying and making up over and over (often with sex as part of the reconciliation) is immature, distracting, and draining.
- **Disrespect.** The toxicity of insults, name-calling, and verbal abuse can never be underestimated. It is indeed tragic that couples who promised to love, honor, and cherish one another at the altar so often become careless with their words within a few weeks or months.
- **Physical or sexual abuse.** Nonmarital relationships in which physical or sexual abuse occur must be terminated immediately. When it occurs within marriage, it is imperative that the couple separate until appropriate counseling occurs and other measures are established to guarantee safety.

If one or more of these patterns are occurring in a nonmarital relationship, you would be wise to end it. Keep in mind that abuse in a premarital relationship will not improve (and will probably worsen) after the knot is tied. If these problems are characteristics of your marriage, counseling with a qualified therapist or pastor and accountability to a mentor couple with a stable marriage are important to help you learn how to implement some necessary changes.

Don't overlook the emotional benefits of a relationship with a four-legged friend. A growing body of research suggests that pets—usually dogs, cats, and even birds—can provide emotional support, especially for those (such as the elderly) who live alone. Many hospitals now allow carefully trained (and extremely well-groomed) dogs to be brought into selected patients' rooms by their handlers as a way to brighten everyone's day. Similar and more lasting effects have been noted in nursing homes where residents are allowed to handle well-behaved pets on a regular basis. Obviously, an emotional attachment to an animal shouldn't override or displace relationships with family members and other humans. Also, pets may not be an option when the health of someone who is allergic to animal dander would be compromised by a pet in the home. But otherwise, an ongoing connection with "man's best friend" (or other creatures that make decent companions) may be worth the time and effort.

Create "margin"

You've just completed your physical exam, and the moment of truth has arrived. Your doctor takes another look through her notes and your lab results, clears her throat, and delivers the verdict: "First the bad news. Your blood pressure, cholesterol, triglycerides, blood sugar, and weight are all too high. You're on the verge of developing diabetes, and by the time it appears, your arteries probably will already be damaged.

"Now the good news: I can give you some medications that will reduce your risk of having a heart attack or a stroke. The most important steps, however, are ones that you can take yourself—in fact, no one can do them for you. They can correct most, perhaps all, of the abnormalities that I just mentioned. They will not only reduce your risk of a premature death, but they will help you feel better than you have in years. Want to know what they are?"

You nod enthusiastically.

"Okay, here's what you need to do." She takes out a pad of paper and gives it to you to take notes as she continues: "Lose fifteen pounds over the next three months and continue losing a pound per week for another three months. You'll need to do some reading about nutrition and also prepare more meals at home using fresh ingredients, especially fruits and vegetables.

"Walk two miles every day. It may take you about forty minutes when you start, but as you become conditioned you should be able to cover this distance in a half hour or less.

"Get eight hours of sleep every night.

"Spend a half hour every day being quiet—praying, reflecting, or reading something that is meaningful or inspirational to you.

"You're focused on your job, in one way or another, seven days a week. You must have one day every week during which you lay those responsibilities aside and instead focus on worship, enjoying your family, and other activities (including perhaps an afternoon nap) that refresh and restore you."

You put down the pen and lean back in your chair, considering these recommendations.

What would be your first response?

a) "Okay, Doc, I'll do whatever it takes!"

b) "That all sounds well and good, *but I just don't have the time. . . .*"

If your answer is *a,* your doctor might faint on the spot. If your answer is *b,* your doctor would probably not be surprised.

Do you have too little time to get eight hours of sleep, a half hour of exercise, a half hour of quiet time, and at least one unhurried meal shared with family or friends every day? most days? some days? If so, your greatest obstacle to good health may not be a family history of heart disease or cancer, a love for fatty food, or even a tobacco habit. It may be your calendar.

Wall-to-wall commitments, a frantic lifestyle, two or three jobs (or one job with the demands of two or three), constant noise, too much stuff, mounting debt, a nonstop current of messages flooding your mental in-box, and with them a constant state of fatigue and anxiety—these are manifestations of living without margin, which Richard A. Swenson, M.D., describes in the classic book *Margin:* "Margin is the space between our load and our limits. It is the amount allowed beyond that which is needed. It is something held in reserve for contingencies and unanticipated situations. Margin is the gap between rest and exhaustion, the space between breathing freely and suffocating."[7]

As futurists living in the first half of the twentieth century observed rapid developments in technology and the mass production of labor-saving devices, they confidently predicted twenty- to thirty-hour workweeks and a bounty of leisure time for everyone in the second half of that century. Instead, at the dawn of the twenty-first century, we are dealing with the fallout from exponential increases in complexity. We're working harder than ever, and our "leisure time" (if we can find any) may be anything but relaxing or restorative. We have a hundred channels instead of seven, twenty screens at the multiplex that replaced the single-screen movie house, dozens of e-mails to read every day, voice-mail messages piling up if we don't pick up the phone, cell phones going off night and day, and faxes coming in from parts unknown. We have places to go, people to see, things to do, and we're exhausted.

Most of us who are marginless would protest that our calendars are crowded with good and useful things, and indeed they probably are. There are daily responsibilities, making a living, paying the bills, and for those with older children at home, overseeing not only the daily flow of schoolwork but also lessons, sports, practices, and rehearsals. (Those with toddlers and preschoolers have their hands full *before* any other activities enter the picture.)

We may serve in several ministries at church, belong to a service club, and take part in community events. But all of these activities, like possessions, have a way of accumulating. Few of us, upon accepting a new responsibility, deliberately choose to give up another to make allowance for it. We don't want to disappoint anyone. We may feel flattered when someone asks for our help or nominates us to lead a project. It's easy to believe, *No one can take care of this problem but me.* We make a commitment and write a fateful notation on the calendar, without making an honest evaluation of the time and effort required to fulfill that obligation.

Eventually we begin to feel out of control as the "activity debts" arising from promises we've made outstrip our time and energy, and even collide with one another. When we talk about being under stress, we may in fact be describing overcommitment that we ourselves set in motion. Indeed, the default setting for our internal throttle isn't just "full speed ahead," but "hurry up!" Life becomes a relentless series of brushfires, with the hottest and the closest flames getting the most attention. As the heat rises, guess what gets pushed aside? Those "expendable" items in our lives, such as exercise, sleep, quiet reading and reflection, nourishing food, meaningful conversations, and listening to those we care about (including God). If we're not careful, we'll also push aside spiritual growth, the relationships we care about, any semblance of contentment, and sooner or later our health.

Changing a marginless lifestyle is not an easy task, and for some it will be a lifelong challenge. One cannot reclaim blocks of time without experiencing (and causing others) serious repercussions. The process requires motivation, planning, accountability, and time. Reading (or rereading) Dr. Swenson's book *Margin* would be a good place to start. (A revised edition was released by NavPress in 2004.) In the meantime, here are some ideas to think about.

1. **Take a careful and prayerful inventory of your current activities, and evaluate them in light of your core values and goals.** You may need to begin by clarifying what exactly those values and goals are, especially if they have been forgotten or neglected during years of frantic living. This may require a weekend away with your spouse or a trusted friend, perhaps at a retreat center, to devote some unhurried (and uninterrupted) time to this project. As you think through your list of activities, commitments, and responsibilities, consider:
    - **Is this something that only I can do?** Many functions in our life for which we believe we are indispensable are in fact just functions, things others can do just as well (or better). There are actually only a limited number of things that only *you* can do, and the most important of these involve your own body and soul and the people you care most about. Only you can exercise your body, pray your prayers, journal your thoughts, be your child's father or mother, and so on. If you are buried in activities that someone else could do—even ones that are worthwhile—and as a result are neglecting those that *only you* can do, you may need to make some changes.
    - **Does this pass the "end of life" test?** Imagine yourself near death, reflecting on your life. Will you be glowing inside as you consider all the meetings you attended or pining over the extra hours you could have spent at the office? Will you ask your children to bring your diplomas and your portfolio to the bedside so that you can gaze upon these objects one last time? You get the idea. As you approach your final breath, what matters most will be the God you served and the people you blessed.
    - **Does it pass the eternal significance test?** You may have heard the familiar admonition, "One life to live; t'will soon be past. Only what's done for Christ will last."[8] Remember that the most mundane activities can be carried out with the attitude of serving as an ambassador for Christ on this planet. Reassuring your child at bedtime about his place on earth and in heaven, or reading to a shut-in, or doing a host of other things that involve loving God and serving other people may have far more lasting significance than running a corporation or writing the great American novel. Beware, however: The sentiment of the couplet above can also be used as leverage to pressure you into accepting one more assignment at church that pushes your load past

your limits. Remember that Jesus didn't heal every sick person in Judea. He also frequently retreated from the crowds that desperately wanted the benefits of His touch. During His walk on this planet, He recognized His physical limits, and so must you.

2. **Learn to say (respectfully) the two-letter word that toddlers love.** When someone asks you to add another commitment to your life or entry on your calendar (even something as benign as coming for dinner), reply with the all-important phrase "I'll get back to you shortly," and then ask yourself some serious questions. What will be involved in this commitment? Is it important? Are the basics that I care about (especially my relationship with God and family) going to suffer as a result? Do I need to give up something else if I do this? Is this something I really want to do, or am I merely trying to avoid someone else's disapproval? Most important, have the courage to say no when it's appropriate. If you are marginless and have trouble saying this word, make a pact with your spouse or a mature friend: Before agreeing to any new activity or commitment, you will give this person permission to grill you with the above questions and provide input regarding your decision. Realize that you can't possibly do all the wonderful things you would like to do. Drawing boundaries is an act of humility, not laziness.

3. **Become free of financial bondage.** TV screens, magazines, catalogs, and computer monitors overflow with items that not only can satisfy our basic needs for food, clothing, and shelter, but also offer all sorts of experiences, prestige, and stimulation. Once upon a time, most people stopped buying when they were out of money. Unfortunately, most of us today have ways to bypass that inconvenience, usually involving credit cards or other types of loans that give us the illusion of having money in the bank. As a result, too many of us must devote a great deal of time and energy trying to earn money to support our lifestyle (or "debt-style"), not to mention juggling bills, racing to the bank, answering unpleasant calls from creditors, and arguing with spouse and children about finances. (Obviously, not everyone who struggles to make ends meet has been careless with credit cards and loans. Layoffs, rising costs of living, unexpected needs for funds—such as a sudden health problem or a car repair—can create a lack of financial margin for the most diligent individuals and families.)

   Getting out of debt involves many of the same principles as losing excessive weight, a process we discussed in depth in chapter 6. Like attaining and maintaining a healthy weight, acquiring financial health is an ongoing process rather than a quick fix. It involves a lot of course corrections, attitude adjustments, new habits, changes in the way we relieve stress and experience contentment, and regular acknowledgment that God ultimately owns all of our earthly goods. Exploring the details is well beyond the scope of this book. Even if you don't have issues with your financial margin, we highly recommend the resources of Crown Financial Ministries, especially the ten-week small-group study that many churches offer on an ongoing basis. For more information you can check http://www.crown.org on the Internet, call (800) 722-1976, or write to Crown Financial Ministries at P.O. Box 100, Gainesville, GA 30503-0100.

Healthy boundaries

Healthy boundaries are crucial for emotional and physical health, but like margin, the concept of boundaries is often misunderstood or oversimplified as a sort of relational "just say no" campaign. Unlike margin, which deals with how much (if any) time and energy you hold in reserve to prevent overload and physical exhaustion, setting boundaries involves determining what are—and what aren't—appropriate obligations within a relationship. In a nutshell, when you have secure boundaries, you understand clearly what you are (and are *not*) responsible for. Once you can recognize where these lines are drawn, it becomes much easier to make healthy choices when interacting with others.

Imagine that you and everyone you know are sitting inside the boundaries of large circles marked on the floor of a huge room. Each person is in charge of everything that goes on in his or her circle. You decide whether to keep your belongings neat or strewn about. It is your decision whether you stretch out or sit cross legged in your circle. You may not enter someone else's circle uninvited, and no one else can intrude into your space without your consent. If someone wants something from your circle, he or she must ask permission, and you may not impose on someone else's space without permission.

The circle, of course, represents your life. As an adult, you are ultimately in charge of yourself, your belongings, and your schedule. However, as we discussed earlier, it isn't healthy or satisfying to live in isolation. We *do* cross boundaries and enter each other's circles to varying degrees (hopefully with their permission), and other people enter our circles (hopefully, but not always, with our consent). The tricky part comes in developing a clear understanding of what we are responsible for in another person's life and what they are responsible for in ours. Problems arise when people have differing, unhealthy, or nonexistent understandings about each other's boundaries. For example:

- Newlyweds (or even long-married couples) may have problems with the role of either person's parents in the new household they've established. What are the boundaries for advice, influence, and even financial support?
- Parents who persist in doing for their children what they can and should do for themselves are developing a boundary problem, which may become more serious when the parents repeatedly bail older (or even adult) children out of the consequences of their own irresponsibility.
- People who are unable to say no to any request or demand for their

time have not only a major boundary problem but will eventually have a margin (and fatigue) problem as well.

- People who feel responsible for another's mood have an impossible boundary problem, especially when the other person (for example, a spouse, adolescent child, or aging parent) is demanding, irritable, or subject to outbursts of anger.
- Pastors are at risk for personal burnout and family breakdowns when they cannot establish reasonable boundaries with members of their congregation who want and expect access on a 24-7 basis.

The concept of boundaries must not only be learned but also adjusted for various situations. Obviously a mother will have few boundaries with her newborn infant. An individual may voluntarily lay aside a number of boundaries in order to care for an aging parent. We have a different set of boundaries at home, school, work, and church, and need to be clear which is which. (For example, employees who cannot leave their personal issues at home may be cheating their employers out of the work for which they have been hired. Employers who demand that employees repeatedly suspend their personal lives after hours to complete job assignments are overstepping their boundaries.) We also need to understand how healthy boundaries mesh with our commitment to serve God and others within our community of faith.

These are all important issues that are aptly discussed in a series of books by Henry Cloud and John Townsend. The first of these, simply called *Boundaries,* is an essential book for personal growth. Others in the series—*Boundaries in Dating, Boundaries in Marriage,* and *Boundaries with Kids*—are also highly recommended.

Guarding the mind

In a day when consumers read product labels and strive to keep themselves free from additives and pollutants, we often demonstrate an impressive lack of selectivity about what enters our eyes, ears, and minds. Members of the baby boom and the preceding generation are well aware of the startling changes in popular media that occurred between the 1950s and 1970s and that have progressed (too often downhill) ever since. We will not recite the gory details of those events here, but needless to say, over the course of a single decade (the 1960s) unprecedented language, violence, and sexuality were suddenly "now playing at a theater near you." Over the same period of time, popular music turned its attention from teen romance to celebrating drugs, "free love," and general rebellion.

Today's "family hour" of network TV programming routinely explores themes that would have knocked the tube's first generation of viewers out of their chair. For decades, popular music has contained blistering language and themes of sexual anarchy, violence, nihilism, and despair, and now video games played for hours on end by the young do likewise. Pornography is a mouse click away or available at the flick of the remote at home or in most hotels. Newspapers and TV newscasts earn their keep by informing us, with a few exceptions, what went wrong yesterday, what's wrong today, and what will go wrong tomorrow.

A steady diet of this material eventually takes a toll on the human mind and spirit. We can't and shouldn't live with our heads firmly embedded in the sand, and serious looks at real problems are a necessary part of responsible citizenship, not to mention the stimulus for earnest prayer. But the content and tone of materials to which we subject our mind—and especially those of our children and teenagers—need ongoing review.

Media and the family

Electronic media are now so varied and pervasive in our culture that words and images that are jarring, value eroding, discouraging, and generally inappropriate for kids of all ages (not to mention grown-ups) can literally flood a home unless parents and other responsible adults take deliberate defensive measures. And while you may be careful about what you allow your family to see and hear, your neighbors up the street may be careless about the music they play, the images flickering on their TV screens, or the material they download—not to mention who is in the room to see and hear them.[9]

To make matters worse, school-age children and teenagers are intensely curious about "adult" matters and consider it a badge of honor to get a look at something you've declared off-limits. And while violent or sexually explicit sights and sounds can create profoundly strong and disturbing memories, repeated exposure has a desensitizing effect that can seriously warp attitudes and erode respect for the human body—and life itself. Unless you cut your family off from civilization altogether, you will need to be vigilant about the material your son or daughter sees and hears, and you should be ready to deal with objectionable content that leaks past your defenses. In doing so, you'll be guarding your family's hearts and minds and creating a healthy emotional environment for everyone. More importantly, you need to do this in a way that prepares your children to make mature, informed decisions about their listening and viewing habits after they leave home. They won't watch *Sesame Street* reruns forever.

Where and how do you draw the line?

With respect to music, the primary issue is content (and its repetition), not style. There is simply no way that relentlessly negative and destructive lyrics can pound into anyone's mind without making an impact. But some music that is grating to your ears may actually contain lyrics that challenge the listener to a better lifestyle or tell a cautionary tale. If you hear something throbbing through the walls or headphones that turns you off, call for a joint listening session. Get the liner notes if possible (and a magnifying glass to read them), then review the CD or the download together with your teenager. Talk about what the lyrics are saying, and how she feels when she listens to them. (You may hear, by the way, an argument that "I just like the beat and the music. I don't listen to the words." Don't buy it. More often than not, she can recite lyrics without missing a beat.)

You'll need courage to separate your older child or adolescent from music that is toxic, an open mind to endure the stuff that isn't, and wisdom to know the difference. You should also be prepared to suggest alternatives. For families with a Christian commitment, there is plenty of contemporary music available in a breadth of styles—including pop, rock, rap, metal, and alternative—that specifically (if noisily) promotes positive values. In addition, a little research will uncover secular music that, while not including overtly biblical phrases or themes, combines high-quality musicianship with family-friendly themes. *Plugged In* magazine, published by Focus on the Family (http://www.family.org) does an excellent job reviewing new releases, both secular and Christian. (You can subscribe and view archived reviews online at http://www.pluggedinonline.com. You can also subscribe to the print edition by calling 800-A-FAMILY.)

When dealing with TV, movies, DVDs, video games, and the Internet, you have several options. First, you might take a simple but austere approach: no TV, movies, DVDs, video games, or Internet. If everyone will go with this flow and you can provide plenty of other forms of stimulation (such as reading, music, games played between human beings, and good, old-fashioned, interesting conversation), you may bring up the smartest and most literate kids in town. But they may also be a little clueless about the culture in which they live, an attribute that may not serve them well if they are to be informed and responsible adult citizens later on. Furthermore, if you take too rigid an approach, including strict social restrictions to maintain your rules, rebellion is inevitable. It is virtually certain that sooner or later your preteen or teenager will secretly seek and find some rotting forbidden fruit and then ingest it without your knowledge or input. Also, Internet access is increasingly important for students completing research projects—not to mention for adults completing routine functions in most jobs and homes. Remaining unplugged is becoming about as realistic as refusing to ride in an automobile.

At the other extreme is a hang-loose, anything-goes mentality that abdicates important responsibilities. Some parents become so intimidated by the swarm of media mosquitoes that they shrug their shoulders and don't bother to put up any protective netting. This is about as foolish as turning children loose to play with power tools and caustic chemicals in the garage.

Somewhere in between lies a guided-access approach, which demands time and energy but is potentially rewarding. In this case, the various media are regarded as neutral tools through which either positive or negative material may flow. In order to protect your children's hearts and minds—and emotional health—it's important that you set specific standards for individual members based on age and maturity. Viewing should be planned and limited, both in time and content. Previewing and choosing material that children (and their parents) watch is an important part of the process. Most worthwhile are the opportunities to discuss what has just been seen and to teach some critical thinking. What take-home lessons were depicted? What positive values were portrayed? If negative material was present, what was wrong with it? (As with music, *Plugged In* magazine is an extremely useful resource for evaluating films in current release and on DVD, as well as tracking trends on television. Reviews of current films are posted online almost immediately after the movies are released, and an extended library of reviews is maintained at http://www.pluggedinonline.com.)

With respect to TV, remember that too much time watching even wholesome and nourishing material is detrimental. TV watching is physically and mentally passive. Young and old viewers alike who sit for hours are not moving muscles in any meaningful way (unless doing so at the same time is a requirement for TV viewing in your home). Obesity and poor physical fitness are common among avid TV watchers. Furthermore, as images, sounds, and ideas generated by programmers and marketers pour into a viewer's mind, thinking, reasoning, imagining, or creating come to a screeching halt. TV watching can become the centerpiece of family life, and group staring can replace talking, working, playing, eating, or praying together.

To prevent the tube from becoming the center of gravity in your family, set specific ground rules for everyone:

- Preplan how much, when (after homework and other responsibilities are done), and what will be viewed.
- Use videocassette recorders, DVD players and recorders, and time-shifting technologies (such as TiVo and others). Material can be recorded, rented, purchased, or even borrowed from the library, allowing you more control over content and scheduling.
- Think twice before installing a TV in your child's or teenager's room. You'll lose control of the viewing activity, and your son or daughter will be isolated from the normal flow of family life.
- Think carefully before subscribing to a cable or satellite service that includes access to unedited films. You'll not only be more likely to waste hours watching something obnoxious that just happens to be on, but your kids will also find it all too easy to tune into objectionable material when you aren't around.

With respect to motion pictures, conflicts may arise when "everyone" has seen a certain PG-13 or R-rated film, and your child or adolescent wants to watch it too, either at the theater or on DVD. You will need to set and maintain your own family's standards, but at some point you may want to introduce him to more grown-up subject matter under your supervision. Do some homework and read the write-ups (especially in family-oriented magazines). Sometimes an otherwise excellent film receives an R rating for a brief spurt of bad language or for one or two quick sequences that can be bypassed using the fast-forward button on the remote control. Likewise, a film bearing the milder PG or PG-13 rating may actually be loaded with obnoxious and offensive material. Whatever you and your child or teenager see, talk about tone and content. Is this film or program selling a viewpoint, and if so, what is it? If something struck you as offensive, why? Was there a positive message involved? What was it? Before your teenager is finally living on his own, he's going to need to learn discernment. Otherwise, while you may succeed in keeping every scrap of offensive material off his mental radar screen while he's in high school, he's eventually going to be exposed to it, but without your preparation or guidance.

Three excellent resources for families who want to watch and discuss movies together are *Movie Nights for Kids*, *Movie Nights*, and *Movie Nights for Teens* (Focus on the Family). Each provides commentary and discussion questions on twenty-five films—the first book geared toward children, focusing on films such as *Babe* and *The Black Stallion*, while the second two are intended for teen viewers, covering films such as *Remember the Titans* and *Apollo 13*. These books are available from Focus on the Family at http://www.family.org or (800) A-FAMILY.

Video games (whether played on a home computer or on a dedicated game system) are enormously popular with all age groups and can consume vast amounts of time and money. Whatever platform you might have available at home, *everyone* needs specific limits on the time spent playing with them. Kids aren't the only people who can become hooked on electronic games. Adults can spend hundreds of hours playing solitaire or become hopelessly entrenched in complex virtual worlds where they interact with thousands of other players on the Internet. (Believe it or not, marriages have been threatened or even broken apart when one member becomes so immersed in an online game that he or she neglects basic responsibilities at home.) Even if you have a good grip on the time factor, be careful about the content of games you or your kids buy, borrow, rent, or play at the local arcade. While many are good, clean fun, some consist of nonstop fighting, and a few contain harsh language, vivid images of carnage and sex, or overtly antisocial themes. Sometimes these show up at advanced or deeper levels of the game, so once again you need to read up on the current electronic fare.

On a related note, you must supervise your child's or adolescent's use of the Internet at least as carefully as you monitor his film, video, or TV viewing. *Don't leave him alone in his room for hours on end playing with a computer and a modem.* You might be pleased to think that your budding genius is becoming proficient with modern communications technology, but he could be tapping into extraordinarily explicit and perverse sexual material, antisocial and violent text and images, and chat rooms where the online conversations get very raunchy and inappropriate.

Make it clear that your child or teen should not give her name, address, phone number, or any other personal information to someone online or agree to go somewhere to meet any new "friends" she might have spoken with by modem. (Sexual predators and other criminals have discovered online services to be fertile ground for finding unsuspecting targets.) Most online services have mechanisms that allow you to limit your child's access to certain areas, and new software can to some degree serve as an electronic "nanny" that will terminate inappropriate material. But these tools are imperfect, and you would be wise to require that all your child's online activities take place only when you are home and only on a computer you can directly monitor.

While you want to encourage reading as an alternative to TV watching, pay attention to the books your adolescent brings home from the library or bookstore. Much of what lands on current best-seller lists is truly pulp fiction, laced with vivid scenes of horror, violence, and sex that are far more explicit than the contents of most R-rated films. Even the so-called romance novels, whose covers are emblazoned with bare-chested hulks looming over bodice-busting sirens, generally contain an abundance of vivid and immoral sexual material. If your teenager is engrossed in a steady diet of books focused on bloodletting, body counts, and bawdy situations, offer some alternatives of better content and quality. (By the way, what books are on your nightstand?)

A more dangerous influence—one that encompasses a variety of media, including books, magazines, and videos—is pornography. We will look at this plague in more detail in chapter 12.

The bottom line is this: Like so many areas, images and sounds that are negative often seem to come into our life automatically. More often we have to seek out the things that refresh and renew our outlook and thus our emotional health. The apostle Paul's advice deserves our consideration on a daily basis: "Whatever is true, whatever is noble, whatever is right, whatever is pure, whatever is lovely, whatever is admirable—if anything is excellent or praiseworthy—think about such things" (Philippians 4:8).

Surroundings

We have stressed repeatedly that contentment is an "inside job," that no one person or thing can make you happy, and that the world is full of people who are wealthy enough to live in comfortable and beautiful surroundings every day of the year but are emotional wrecks. That being said, we do react to our surroundings, which in a sense speak to us, sometimes very loudly. While we don't need to live in palatial splendor to lift our spirits, we can certainly tend to our immediate environment, no matter how humble or elaborate, as a way of caring for our emotions. Specifically:

Keep it clean. Obsessive spotlessness isn't next to godliness, but dirt, stains, and debris everywhere—on sinks and counters, walls and floors, showers and (gasp) toilets, cars (inside and out), and of course on our own skin and hair—announce to others and ourselves that we're not taking care of some basic needs.

Keep it uncluttered. One of the great plagues of Western civilization is the endless flow of *stuff* into our life. Even people of very modest means can manage to accumulate piles of purchases, gifts, trinkets, magazines, mailings, and various knickknacks that seem to explode over every surface in the house, yard, garage (which for many of us has become a storage bin, not a place for the car), and even automobile. Our closets are full of clothes that don't fit or that we haven't worn in months (or years). Few children are born with a knack for or interest in neatness, so left to their own devices, they will contribute mightily to the chaos.

For many people, one of the most important steps toward tranquillity is to begin a fearless campaign of decluttering. The trash bin—or if you're really serious, a rented dumpster—can become your new best friend as you jettison the stuff that's busted, rusted, never used, or just plain ugly. If you haven't worn it in a year, get rid of it. That pile of old magazines that you "might get around to some day," and even books that you've enjoyed but aren't likely to read again, need a new home. If any of these items are usable or wearable by someone else, by all means donate them to a thrift store or other charity, where they can help generate some income or be given to those in need.

Equally important is developing the discipline of not acquiring *more* stuff that we really don't need. The fact that something looks attractive or happens to be on sale doesn't necessarily mean that it belongs in our home or on the wall. Do you really need all those catalogs and magazines? What about giving experiences like tickets to a concert or a restaurant gift certificate to family members as a gift rather than another object that takes up space they may not have?

If you're a compulsive shopper or garage saler, or you can't keep your eyes off the shopping channel or your Web browser off eBay, a little soul-searching may be in order: *Why* do you feel the need to buy something you don't really need or even want? There may be some other need that should be addressed, and you may want to have an honest conversation with God, your spouse, a mature friend, or even your pastor or counselor about this issue.

Control the noise. Wherever there's life there will be sound, hopefully most of it pleasant. Sometimes, however, we can become immersed in noise, especially from a TV or radio that is left on day and night like a guest long overstaying his welcome. If no one's really listening, consider turning it off. Also, if younger family members are prone to play their favorite music night and day, and it's rattling both walls and your brain, consider having a calm discussion about reducing volume levels. (If they use headphones, by the way, make sure they're not turned up too loud. Long-term exposure to loud noise, whether recreational or work-related, can eventually cause hearing loss. If someone in your home is wearing headphones and you can hear the music across the room, the volume is probably way too loud.) You might consider designating an hour or two of noise-free time every day for quiet conversation, reading, or thinking.

Add a little beauty. How about setting some fresh flowers or a bowl of fresh fruit on your table? Think about creating a small "reserve" in your home or yard where you can sit and gather your thoughts at the beginning of the day, decompress at the end, or have a quiet conversation. A small garden or some inexpensive plants and flowers on a porch can provide a refreshing area of respite and beauty.

A few miscellaneous ideas to reduce stress

The most basic and important concepts for managing the stresses of life have already been presented in this chapter or will be set forth in the next. But there are a few additional nuggets that we would like to leave as parting gifts at the end of this chapter.

1. **Don't allow everyone and everything to "push your buttons."** If errant drivers, slow lines at the bank, cranky customers, rude coworkers, or even misbehaving public figures get you upset, you've unwittingly given far too many people and things permission to rock your emotional boat. (Remember: No one can make you mad unless you allow him or her to do so.)

2. **Practice the "brain tumor" exercise.** When someone who is particularly rude, obnoxious, unreasonable, or unruly crosses your path, ask yourself, *How would I react if I knew that the person had a brain tumor that was causing his behavior?* After a moment's reflection, you will probably let whatever he said or did roll off you rather than get steamed up about it.

3. **Engage your senses.** Whenever you have an opportunity to study a flower, view a sunset, gaze at the stars on a clear night, or look over a park or grassy field, allow yourself a few minutes to experience it with as many senses as possible. Touch the grass. Listen to the wind. Smell the flower. This may sound like greeting-card mush, but it can be highly relaxing and a way to appreciate both the senses that God gave us and the incredible world He created for us to enjoy.

4. **Study the universe.** Speaking of stars, take some time to learn about the size of the universe, the number of stars and galaxies it contains, and the mind-boggling events that are happening on a colossal scale beyond the limits of our vision. With inspired insight, the psalmist wrote that "the heavens declare the glory of God; the skies proclaim the work of his hands. Day after day they pour forth speech; night after night they display knowledge" (Psalm 19:1-2). It doesn't take much information about the universe to inspire awe at God's handiwork and to put our affairs into perspective.

5. **Count your blessings.** Every day write down three things (or more) for which you are thankful. Be sure to thank God for them. While you're at it, if any of these involve people, let them know as well. Gratitude is very therapeutic for both giver and receiver.

6. **Take a break from the news.** Since most of the news in the paper or broadcast on TV, radio, or the Internet is unsettling at best, try taking a time-out from it for a day or even a week. If something truly earthshaking happens,

you will definitely hear about it. Otherwise, you'll be impressed with how little has changed the next time you turn on the news or open the paper.

7. **Observe a Sabbath day every week.** This is a reminder from the section on margin. When Jesus said that "the Sabbath was made for man, not man for the Sabbath" (Mark 2:27), He was speaking both practical and theological wisdom. Working seven days per week is a surefire way to become exhausted, irritable, and burned out. Ideally, one day every week should be set aside for worship, refreshment, and recharging your batteries. If personal responsibilities (for example, caring for one or more infants or small children) do not allow you to take an entire day off, it is important to arrange for at least a few hours every week during which you can be off duty from the needs of others or your own to-do list of tasks. If you think this is being selfish, think of it as a way to ensure that your service to others is regularly invigorated and sustained.

8. **Learn to meditate/contemplate/get quiet.** Much research has demonstrated the physiological benefits of regular periods of quiet alertness. This should not be dismissed as a pop-psychology gimmick or an entrée into Eastern mysticism but an important discipline for personal health and spiritual growth. We will discuss it further in the next chapter.

QUESTIONS TO PONDER:

1. Do you have any specific physical symptoms (such as headaches or abdominal cramps) that seem related to anxiety or stress? Do you have any recurring physical symptoms that affect your mood? If either of these patterns is disruptive in your life, have you thought about getting some help from a physician or counselor to address them?
2. Does your mood depend on what is going on around you? If your emotional weather and general contentment seem to be determined by your immediate circumstances (good or bad), what attitude adjustments might help your mood become more stable and less affected by life's inevitable ups and downs?
3. While almost everyone feels anxious or has a bad day or the "blues" once in a while, have you or a loved one experienced some of the longer-lasting mood problems and symptoms described in this chapter that might indicate an anxiety disorder or depression?
4. Do you have strong opinions about mood problems that might affect whether you or a loved one seeks help for anxiety or depression? (For example, do you feel that someone who is

depressed should just "snap out of it," or that anxiety is primarily a manifestation of lack of faith in God, or that counseling is a waste of time, or that antidepressant medications are a cop-out?) Has reading this chapter changed any of those perspectives?

5. Does your lifestyle counteract the negative emotional impact of media messages in our culture? Do you need to make any changes in order to model more consistently the values you want others (especially your children or grandchildren) to follow?
6. Do you feel stressed much of the time? What are your current sources of stress? Have you thought about steps you could take to change circumstances that you find stressful? Are there some things you could do (such as the stress management ideas that start on page 375) that would adjust your reaction to those circumstances?
7. Are you aware of the connection between your spiritual well-being and your emotional health? Do you take time for any specific practices that might impact your emotions, such as prayer or meditating on biblical passages that are meaningful to you?
8. Do you believe God loves you? Do you think He likes you? Did you hesitate for a moment in response to either question (especially the second one)? What experiences in your life have affected your understanding—not only your beliefs, but your actual feelings—about God's attitude toward you?
9. How much margin do you have in your current lifestyle? Do you feel as if you (and your family) are constantly in a hurry or running on empty? If so, why do you think this is happening, and what might you do to change it?
10. Do you observe a true Sabbath once a week? Do you have a day during which you take a real time-out from the usual demands of your life so that you can focus on God and the people you care about? Do you spend some time on this day in activities that are truly refreshing and restorative? What might you change so that this might happen?

Action items: If you are seeing your health-care provider about one or more physical symptoms (or if you're getting a checkup), be sure to bring up any current mood issues you might be experiencing. This is important information for any medical evaluation.

Become familiar with the manifestations of anxiety disorders and depression described in this chapter, as well as the warning signs of suicide listed on page 326. While you should not attempt to diagnose these conditions in your loved ones, friends, or even yourself, your awareness may help guide someone you care about toward the help he or she needs—and may save a life.

If you are married, pick two of the items that were listed on page 358 as ways to nourish your relationship with your spouse and implement them over the next month. In addition, find a time every week for each of you to ask and answer the "Four Questions to Ask Your Spouse" listed on page 359.

Look over the list of healthy ways to cultivate relationships (beginning on page 360) and pick one of these items to work on over the next few months.

If you are struggling with a lack of margin in your life, carefully review the ideas for dealing with the problem (starting on page 362). Consider reading the book *Margin* by Richard A. Swenson as well. Talk with your spouse, or a mature and trusted friend if you are unmarried, about the steps you might take to deal with this issue.

Schedule an "unplugged day" for your family (or at least for yourself) during which you abstain from TV, radio, the Internet—even the newspaper. Spend the time enjoying good conversation, reading, exercise, prayer, and perhaps a family game that involves interacting with one another. If you enjoy this experience, try it on a regular basis.

Make a list of all of the things for which you are thankful. Look at it and update it every week, and be sure to give thanks to God on a frequent basis for His good gifts.

Be sure to read the next chapter in this book ("More Than Molecules"), which deals with spiritual health—a critical component to your emotional health.

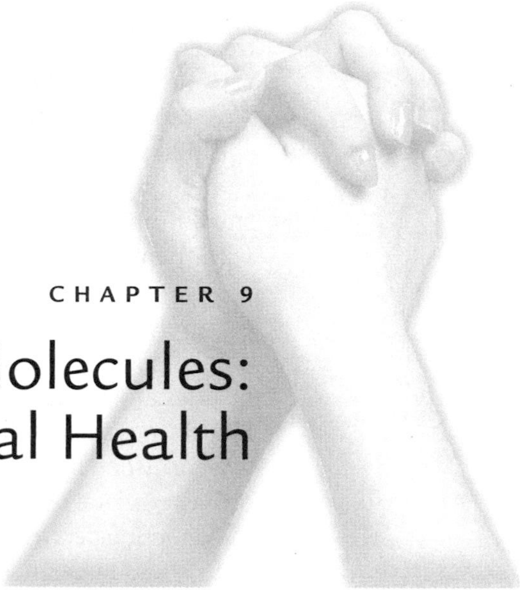

CHAPTER 9

More Than Molecules: Spiritual Health

Are our lives on this planet merely "ashes to ashes, dust to dust"? Are we more than physical structures animated by extraordinarily complex biochemical reactions? Is our health influenced by any forces other than the laws of chemistry and physics? Does our faith affect our physical well-being? If we or those we love become ill, will recovery be affected by our prayers?

We've become so used to relying on scientific research and sophisticated technologies that, when faced with an illness or an emergency, our first call is nearly always to the doctor's office (or 911)—and not to a pastor. As a result, most of us are only dimly aware that throughout the majority of human history, and in a number of cultures today, the role of healer has nearly always been filled by a priest, shaman, or medicine man. A scientific approach to medicine that does not specifically seek to engage spiritual forces is a relatively new concept. Nevertheless, in Europe, North America, and developed countries throughout the world it gained such preeminence over the last few hundred years that for all practical purposes health care became a purely secular enterprise by the second half of the twentieth century.

Even so, most people are not entirely comfortable with an approach to wellness that ignores the spiritual dimension. Scientific inquiry still has not answered many fundamental questions about the way we tick, and it probably never will. Science and technology have no inherent moral values but instead merely serve the purposes of those who employ them. They can devise vaccines that save millions of lives—or create weapons that can kill millions.

Furthermore, we generally don't see ourselves merely as elaborate biochemical machines, and we don't want to be viewed as such by a physician or anyone else. Most of us sense that there is more to us, and to our health, than the interactions of atoms and molecules in our bodies, and we want to be treated accordingly. Polls of American adults consistently demonstrate that a very high percentage—typically 90 to 95 percent—believe in God.[1] Surveys have repeatedly found that more than 70 percent of patients would like to have spiritual issues or needs addressed as part of their medical care or would welcome a conversation about faith with their physicians, yet only a relatively small number (10 to 20 percent) report that their doctors discuss these issues with them.[2]

During the closing decades of the last century, a groundswell of resistance to purely mechanistic medicine and a desire for health care that addresses the whole person—body, mind, and spirit—grew among patients and many health-care providers. This sentiment blossomed in the 1970s with the **holistic health** movement, whose worthy objective of dealing with the "whole person" was tarnished by its embrace of eccentric therapies and the fervent promotion of Eastern/New Age mysticism as its essential worldview. The holistic health movement faded from public view during the 1980s but was reborn, and now flourishes, under the banner of **complementary and alternative medicine** (often abbreviated **CAM**). We will look at CAM in more detail at the end of this book, but for now it is important to note that Eastern (that is, Taoist and Hindu) understandings of spirituality are deeply entrenched in many of its popular therapies, especially ancient Chinese medicine and traditional East Indian medicine known as *ayurveda*.

In the 1970s and 1980s, some proponents of health care that addressed a broad range of concerns (including spirituality) from a Judeo-Christian perspective used the term *wholistic*—spelled with a *w*—to distinguish themselves from "holistic" practitioners who so often promoted Eastern/New Age worldviews. Today, however, the particular choice of spelling does not necessarily identify the spiritual orientation of a practitioner or clinic.

A very different response to the purely materialistic, mechanistic approach to medicine has been spearheaded by researchers such as Harold G. Koenig, M.D., of the Center for Spirituality, Theology and Health at Duke University Medical Center; Michael E. McCullough, Ph.D., of the University of Miami; Dale A. Matthews, M.D., of Georgetown University School of Medicine; and the late David B. Larson, M.D., founder and president of the International Center for the Integration of Health & Spirituality. These individuals, and many others, have both conducted and compiled studies on the impact of religious attitudes and practices on health, amassing a convincing body of evidence that religion is very likely to enhance both physical and mental well-being. The *Handbook of Religion and Health* (New York: Oxford University Press, 2001), written by Drs. Koenig, McCullough, and Larson, is the definitive resource on this subject. At seven hundred–plus pages, it is far less a handbook than a comprehensive analysis of more than twelve hundred research studies and four hundred research reviews dealing with the interaction of religion and a vast array of physical and mental health conditions. (Dr. Matthews's book *The Faith Factor* covers some of this ground on a more informal basis.)[3]

As you might imagine, designing scientific studies on the health benefits of religion presents significant challenges. For one thing, how do you measure a person's religious commitment? There is no blood test for spirituality, nor any guarantee that activities such as attending church necessarily correlate with the depth of one's relationship with God. (As the old saying goes, sitting in church doesn't make you spiritual any more than sleeping in the garage makes you a car.) Many of these studies are observational, attempting to correlate specific religious activities (such as going to services) or spiritual orientation (as reflected in responses to surveys on belief or attitudes about God) with specific health outcomes such as length of life, frequency of illness, length of time to recover from surgery, blood pressure, and so on. Obviously, it is impossible to do a true controlled experiment along these lines. You can't take five hundred people who lack any spiritual commitment, instruct half of them to "get religion," and then compare the two groups a year or two later to see what happened. Nevertheless, well-constructed observational studies can provide useful information. It was this type of study, after all, that established the link between smoking and a host of health problems.

For those who are concerned about research methodology, the *Handbook of Religion and Health* ably addresses the related issues as well as the strengths and weaknesses of the studies it reviews. An attempt to summarize the findings of this immense work (and other research completed since it was published) would be far beyond the scope of this book, but we can offer a few general conclusions of studies in this field. In general they indicate that religious commitment and activity—manifested in a variety of ways, including involvement in a faith community, regular prayer, and affirmation that a relationship with God is an aspect of life—are associated with:

- longer life span
- decreased likelihood of cardiovascular disease, stroke, and cancer
- better ability to cope with illness
- more rapid recovery from illness
- less anxiety and depression
- more rapid recovery from depression
- decreased likelihood of alcohol and drug abuse[4]

Not every study in this field supports these conclusions, although systematic reviews suggest that the vast majority of studies (over 80 percent) find religious commitment and activity beneficial to health.[5] We should briefly consider some of the reasons why this would be likely:

- Most religious faiths discourage activities such as tobacco use, drug and alcohol abuse, sexual promiscuity, and other forms of reckless behavior that are likely to endanger health.
- Communities of faith typically offer opportunities to socialize, build close relationships, and develop a sense of identity or even family ties, as well as provide ongoing emotional and practical support in times of illness or other setbacks. All of these can benefit both physical and emotional well-being.
- Most religious faiths promote a sense of purpose, meaning, and optimism that helps to prevent or counter anxiety and depression.

- Giving, sharing, practicing forgiveness, and volunteering to help those in need can also have positive effects on outlook and overall health.
- Certain practices such as quiet meditation or contemplation can have beneficial effects on human physiology (see page 384).
- God may intervene directly to bring about physical or emotional healing.

We also need to consider a number of cautions about conclusions we might draw from research supporting the idea that religion benefits health:

- It is unrealistic to assume that a consistent walk of faith *guarantees* good health. People who are deeply committed to God and to serving Him still develop health problems sooner or later, and all will eventually die.
- It is unwise to treat one's faith as a quid pro quo (something for something) arrangement where the question "What's in it for me?" is always in the foreground.
- For a person who believes that religious commitment is supposed to yield good health, an illness could provoke a crisis of faith: *If I'm sick, I must be lacking faith or somehow displeasing God.*
- Not all religious ideas and groups promote emotional and physical health. The teachings or leaders of some groups, sects, or cults promote guilt, shame, abuse, agitation, violence, and even murder. A history of world religions is hardly a tale of universal sweetness and light.
- An ongoing personal religious struggle could have a negative effect on health. One study involving more than four hundred hospitalized patients at the Duke University Medical Center found that those "who believed that God was punishing them, had abandoned them, didn't love them, didn't have the power to help, or felt their church had deserted them experienced 19 to 28 percent greater mortality during the two-year period following hospital discharge."[6]

While acknowledging these cautions, we want to take a moment to accentuate the positive: This body of research provides important (and not particularly surprising) "news we can use" about life, faith, and health. Prayer, spiritual commitments, and connection with a faith community are generally associated with living longer and better. As we focus on improving the overall quality of our health—paying attention to our food choices, exercising more consistently, getting enough sleep, eliminating harmful habits such as tobacco use, and so on—we also need to look at our relationship with God and our involvement with others who share our commitments. Our physical, emotional, and spiritual health are intimately connected, and we cannot isolate them, nor should we attempt to do so.

For the remainder of this chapter we are going to look at a number of critical aspects of spiritual health: (1) important questions about the definitions of spirituality, meditation, and prayer; (2) how to establish a relationship with God—the *most* important step in one's spiritual health (and indeed in all of life); and (3) the concept of spiritual growth and practices known as *spiritual disciplines* that are a crucial part of that process.

If these topics are new or unfamiliar to you, it is vitally important that you read on. Even if you feel you are firmly established in your relationship with God and well-seasoned in the activities that maintain that relationship, we would encourage you not to skip or merely glance through this chapter. We believe that a careful reading will reward you with a few (or more) ideas that will enhance your ongoing journey.

What Do We Mean by *Religion* and *Spirituality*?

We need to take a moment to address the inevitable question about the meaning of the terms *religion* and *spirituality* in connection with this type of research. Typically *religion* refers to formal, structured, organized systems of belief and practice relating to God (or gods) or other concepts of a Supreme Being, higher power, or other transcendent intelligence. The term *spirituality* is often used to refer to a much broader concept that encompasses not only formal religion but almost any endeavor that touches on life's meaning and values. One description of spirituality from *American Family Physician,* the journal of the American Academy of Family Physicians, reads as follows:

> Spirituality is a complex and multidimensional part of the human experience. It has cognitive, experiential and behavior aspects. The cognitive or philosophic aspects include the search for meaning, purpose and truth in life and the beliefs and values by which an individual lives. The experiential and emotional aspects involve feelings of hope, love, connection, inner peace, comfort and support. These are reflected in the quality of an individual's inner resources, the ability to give and receive spiritual love, and the types of relationships and connections that exist with self, the community, the environment and nature, and the transcendent (e.g., power greater than self, a value system, God, cosmic consciousness). . . .
>
> Many people find spirituality through religion or through a personal relationship with the divine. However, others may find it through a connection to nature, through music and the arts, through a set of values and principles or through a quest for scientific truth.[7]

Considering the breadth of this definition, it should not be surprising that the notion of what constitutes "spirituality" varies enormously in research studies or in medical school training programs. One significant trend in medical education is that more than half of U.S. medical schools (as opposed to a handful in the early 1990s) now offer or require courses dealing with the interaction of spirituality, illness, and medical care. Some training programs teach medical students, interns, and residents how to take a spiritual history or inventory. This can help to assess the role that a patient's faith might play in lifestyle, emotional support, resources, decision making, and overall outlook, all of which can affect the management and outcome of health problems. A number of medical schools address spirituality within courses or clinical work in complementary and alternative medicine. Some alternative therapies, especially those involving altered states of consciousness or manipulation of invisible energy fields, specifically purport to interact with nonphysical/spiritual realms.

Meditation and Relaxation Techniques

One area of research in which definitions of spirituality and religion become blurry involves the impact of various types of **meditation** on physiology and health. Meditation has been an integral component of Eastern religious practices (Hinduism, Taoism, and Buddhism) for thousands of years. It is also extolled in the Bible, and for centuries it has served as a spiritual discipline for Christians, though with significantly different purposes. We will discuss these later in this chapter.

During the 1970s, thousands of Americans and Europeans alike became acquainted with meditation through the efforts of Maharishi Mahesh Yogi, who successfully promoted Transcendental Meditation (TM) as a simple, supposedly nonreligious technique to manage stress, improve concentration, and enhance overall health. For a fee of about one hundred dollars, individuals learned a simple process of sitting quietly and repeating a special word, or *mantra,* over and over for twenty minutes twice daily. (Like the cost of all other services over the past few decades, the fee for TM instruction and initiation has increased significantly since 1970.) Skeptical investigators eventually determined—and ex-TM teachers confirmed—that the mantras were actually the names of Hindu deities and that the initiation ceremony involved an invitation to worship Guru Dev, the Maharishi's deceased teacher. These and other revelations not only contradicted TM's claim to be nonreligious but also derailed plans to teach the technique in public schools and other taxpayer-funded institutions. Aside from its endorsement by celebrities (including the Beatles), one of TM's selling points was that scientific studies had demonstrated that this practice could produce favorable physiological responses such as reduced blood pressure and pulse rate.

Eventually, however, researchers such as Harvard cardiologist Herbert Benson, founder of Harvard's Mind/Body Medical Institute, determined that the TM mantras were neither unique nor necessary for inducing these physiological responses, and that any word or phrase chosen by an individual could be used in a simple technique to induce both physical and emotional relaxation. Dubbed the "relaxation response," this exercise involves repeating a word or phrase over and over for ten to twenty minutes once or twice daily while sitting in a comfortable environment. In Benson's 1975 book, *The Relaxation Response,* and a 1996 follow-up titled *Timeless Healing: The Power and Biology of Belief,* he describes how regular practice of this approach produces a predictable series of physiological events associated with relaxation, including reductions in pulse, breathing rate, blood pressure, and muscle tension.

The relaxation response has been found to be beneficial for a number of conditions, including high blood pressure, chronic pain, anxiety, mild to moderate depression, and insomnia. While the technique has no implicit religious overtones, Benson has found that when given a choice between a secular and a religious word or phrase to repeat, 80 percent of participants choose phrases that are spiritually meaningful to them, such as "The Lord is my shepherd" or "Hail Mary, full of grace." Furthermore, one in four described a feeling of "increased spirituality" while practicing this technique.[8]

Dr. Benson's relaxation response is only one of hundreds of techniques intended to empty the mind of normal, conscious thought for a short time on a regular basis. Most involve focusing on one's breathing, staring at complex visual patterns (called *mandalas*), doing repetitive body movements and exercises (including yoga), and other rituals. A number of these have been studied using technologies that not only monitor pulse and blood pressure but also evaluate detailed patterns of electrical and metabolic activity within the brain. Some research has observed changes of electrical patterns in the brain that may in part explain a sensation that has long been described as a goal of Eastern-based meditation: experiencing a dissolving of the boundaries of the physical body and feeling "one with the universe." This experience, however it is brought about, is said to enlighten a person as to the true nature of self, universe, and God, and clearly represents a more profound event than entering a simple state of relaxation. But is such an experience enlightening or misleading?

The notion that "all is one"—that there is no distinction between ourselves and other humans, animals, trees, the entire universe, or, for that matter, God—is called **monism**. It is the core understanding of Eastern mystical teachings and traditions, but it is not validated by normal waking consciousness. It also contradicts the explicit teaching of the Old and New Testaments, which present a Creator definitely distinct from what (and whom) He has created. (One can only speculate whether the concept of monism actually arose from brain functions altered by intense meditative techniques.) Needless to say, if you are considering using this type of relaxation or meditative technique, you should consider carefully its roots and connections: Is this merely a relaxation exercise, or is it meant to begin a systematic overhaul of your understanding of God? As we mentioned earlier, we will look further at meditation later in this chapter as we consider the biblical understanding of this activity.

Research on Prayer and Healing

Another arena of spirituality and health in which definitions assume enormous significance involves studies of prayer as a specific treatment for illness. This has become an active area of research over the past few decades, and one that has also generated considerable controversy. The fact that people pray specifically about health (especially when they or someone they love is ill) is, of course, no great revelation. Those who pray for the sick, whether occasionally or as an ongoing ministry, do not need research articles in medical journals to convince them to continue doing so.

Medical expertise certainly can help to determine whether a healing following prayer might be considered miraculous, or at least out of the ordinary. But can prayer on behalf of self or others realistically be subjected to the rigors of scientific experimentation? Is it reasonable to set up experimental conditions in which one group of people (or, for that matter, animals or plants) with a particular medical problem receives a specified amount of prayer while another group under similar conditions does not, and then compare the results? Many researchers evidently think so, as does the United States government, which spent $2.3 million funding various types of prayer research between 2000 and 2004.[9] Private organizations, such as the John Templeton Foundation, have spent much larger sums supporting this type of experimentation. Have they succeeded in bridging the gulf between scientific methodology and the supernatural?

Before we address that question, we need to look at some of the thorny issues raised by prayer research. One of the most basic tasks of such studies is to define what is meant by prayer, but unfortunately this is not done consistently. Some researchers provide a clear definition of prayer as intercession that beseeches God on behalf of individuals with a particular condition. But even those who adopt that definition have used intercessors with a variety of backgrounds and beliefs. A 1999 study of prayer for patients in a coronary-care unit involved participants from a number of Christian denominations who were asked only to agree to this minicredo: "I believe in God. I believe that He is personal and is concerned with individual lives. I further believe that He is responsive to prayers for healing made on behalf of the sick."[10] Another project studying the effects of various alternative therapies on patients undergoing invasive heart procedures (specifically, angiography to evaluate coronary arteries and angioplasty to open areas that are obstructed) has used intercessors from a variety of religious groups, including Buddhists in Nepal, Sufi Muslims and Roman Catholics in America, and Jews at the Western Wall in Jerusalem.[11]

Many studies that purport to evaluate the effects of prayer actually involve a variety of activities that are referred to as **distant healing**, **spiritual healing**, **mental healing**, or even the older term **psychic healing**. Here the individual may meditate or make some other conscious mental effort to benefit another person's physical or emotional health from a distance. Unlike intercessory prayer, this is not an attempt to influence God or any other supernatural intelligence to act on someone else's behalf. Rather, the assumption is that a person's thoughts and consciousness are "nonlocal," extending well beyond the limits of his or her brain and are capable of affecting another without limitations of distance or even time. Popular author Larry Dossey, M.D., has written extensively and enthusiastically about this type of activity, both as a mode of healing and a subject for scientific study.[12] While he routinely uses the term *prayer* to refer both to intercessory petitions to God and to every form of nonlocal healing efforts, some critics have objected to his universal application of this word as misleading.[13]

Despite popular claims that scientific research has "proven" the power of prayer to be effective in improving health, there is little if any solid research that supports this conclusion *in the setting of controlled experimentation.* Comprehensive reviews of studies involving both distant healing techniques and intercessory prayer have consistently found that no meaningful conclusions can be drawn about prayer as a healing modality from this type of research.[14] The studies that have appeared to show a definite benefit have been discredited under careful scrutiny because of flaws in methodology or analysis. There are in fact good reasons why this "underwhelming" result has been the norm thus far and will almost certainly continue to be so in the future.

First, the studies dealing with distant healing are attempting to demonstrate the efficacy of a human capacity—for lack of a better term, a form of psychic power—that has been widely dramatized in novels, movies, and supermarket tabloids but *never* demonstrated with any credibility in a controlled setting. If such a capacity for healing exists in gifted individuals or the human race at large, it has yet to be convincingly documented.

Second, studies dealing with intercessory prayer repeatedly tread on thin ice, both scientifically and theologically. Remember the basic concept: One group of patients in the hospital, undergoing a particular procedure or dealing with a certain type of illness, receives prayer from designated intercessors. The other (control) group does not. The problems that arise in designing such a study are numerous and profound:

- What is a valid measure of a person's response to prayer? A complete healing would be ideal, but how much improvement would be convincing?
- How do you monitor the amount of prayer people receive when they are ill? You can't prevent others (not to mention the patients themselves) from praying for those in the "control" group (that is, those who are not assigned to receive prayer as part of the experiment).
- Should you inform patients that they are being prayed for? (Some studies have been criticized for not doing so.) If you do, would that by itself cause them to feel better?
- Is there a "dose effect" with prayer? Does the number of prayers—or the number of pray-ers—affect the outcome?

Illusionist James Randi, who has for years debunked numerous claims of psychic abilities, has been offering a monetary prize since 1964 "to anyone who can show, under proper observing conditions, evidence of any paranormal, supernatural, or occult power or event." The prize is now one million dollars. While hundreds have applied, no one has passed a basic preliminary test of a claim for a supernatural ability. Details about the test, and an interesting list of frequently asked questions, may be found at http://www.randi.org/research/.

- Which deity are the intercessors praying to? Jehovah? Allah? Krishna? A nonspecific higher power? Should the study control for this, or should any prayer to any supernatural entity be allowed?
- What would we conclude if our study shows that the people who receive intercessory prayer do worse than those who don't? Would we conclude that God was malevolent? Would we advise against prayer for the sick?
- Assuming that the intercessors are beseeching God as He is revealed in the Old and New Testaments—God Almighty, Creator of the universe, and Lord of all that dwell on earth and in heaven—can we presume to design a test that will help us understand how He will behave under a given set of circumstances?

The insurmountable problem with experiments attempting to demonstrate the effect of intercessory prayer is not that prayer lacks efficacy. As we will discuss later in this chapter, prayer accomplishes a great deal—indeed, very often much more than the person who is praying might have in mind. But assessing the impact of prayer (both on the object of the intercession and the one doing the praying) in a controlled experiment is an enterprise built on the deeply flawed assumption that God might be reduced to the status of a variable in a research study.

An insightful quote from C. S. Lewis (written nearly fifty years ago, but with impressive foresight) deserves some careful consideration:

> I have seen it suggested that a team of people—the more the better—should agree to pray as hard as they knew how, over a period of six weeks, for all the patients in Hospital A and none of those in Hospital B. Then you would tot up the results and see if A had more cures and fewer deaths. And I suppose you would repeat the experiment at various times and places so as to eliminate the influence of irrelevant factors.
>
> The trouble is that I do not see how any real prayer could go on under such condition. . . . You cannot pray for the recovery of the sick unless the end you have in view is their recovery. But you can have no motive for desiring the recovery of all the patients in one hospital and none of those in another. You are not doing it in order that suffering should be relieved; you are doing it to find out what happens. The real purpose and the nominal purpose of your prayers are at variance. In other words, whatever your tongue and teeth and knees may do, you are not praying. The experiment demands an impossibility. . . .
>
> The very question "Does prayer work?" puts us in the wrong frame of mind from the outset. "Work": as if it were magic, or a machine—something that functions automatically. Prayer is either

> a sheer illusion or a personal contact between embryonic, incomplete persons (ourselves) and the utterly concrete Person. Prayer in the sense of petition, asking for things, is a small part of it; confession and penitence are its threshold, adoration its sanctuary, the presence and vision and enjoyment of God its bread and wine. In it God shows Himself to us.[15]

Lewis has in a few words described one of the boundaries past which scientific experimentation cannot legitimately explore (though many will no doubt continue to try). Science can tell us how various attitudes and behaviors related to religious commitment appear to correlate with physical and emotional health. It can help us understand some of the physiology associated with relaxation and other mental states, including prayer. As we noted earlier, it can give us some insight into whether an individual's recovery in response to prayer (or some other intervention) might be considered out of the ordinary, even miraculous.

But these inquiries and insights cannot define the character of God or the terms on which we relate to Him. Indeed, as we saw earlier in the quote from *American Family Physician,* medical research into this realm usually takes the approach that spirituality encompasses the tenets of any and every religion, or none at all. It assumes that spirituality can involve seeking and hearing from God, gods, cosmic consciousness, an inner teacher, or any sort of nonphysical entity. Or it may even entail a quest to prove that nothing exists beyond the material universe. Researchers may seek to evaluate how any of these approaches affect the emotional and physical health of their adherents, but their studies do not attempt to determine whose map of the spiritual realm is actually correct. Indeed, their methodology cannot do so. If we are going to discuss spiritual health, which map should we use?

Unrolling a Map toward Spiritual Health

It is at this point, therefore, that we must depart from the realm of statistics and scientific journals as we continue to explore the all-important topic of spiritual health. Here we will not take our direction from the National Institutes of Health, the American Academy of Family Physicians, or any other professional medical organization. We also will not follow the mandate of our culture, which would insist that we consider any and all approaches to spirituality as having equal validity. Indeed, claiming (or even hinting) that one worldview has a better or more coherent grasp of the truth about the spiritual realm and the human condition than another has become very unfashionable.

Nevertheless, throughout this book we make such a claim on behalf of the content of the Old and New Testaments. This is not based on our own wisdom or cleverness and is certainly not done in a spirit of pride or arrogance. Indeed, for one who grasps the most basic biblical teaching about what God has accomplished on our behalf, conceit would be a foolish and irrational response. More appropriate is an attitude like that of a starving beggar who has been revived by the most delicious and nourishing bread, and then with joy and gratitude simply wants to explain to anyone who will listen where it can be found.

The Bible consists of sixty-six books written over some fifteen hundred years, containing a variety of literary genres including history, poetry, biography, and explicit expositions of God's dealings with humanity. A review of its reliability from the standpoint of archaeology and manuscript analysis is beyond the scope of our efforts here, but it is certainly a rewarding area of study. However, we can make one observation about the Bible's reliability from both scientific and medical perspectives. Critics of religion and of the Bible in particular have often charged that faith and biblical teachings stand in opposition to reason and scientific progress. That is inaccurate—in fact, the opposite is true.

The Bible clearly teaches that the physical universe is not all there is and all there ever will be, as a purely materialistic scientist might proclaim, but it also describes a world whose workings are stable, discoverable, and knowable. Furthermore, this information can be verified by anyone with the capacity and desire to do so, with or without acknowledging the One who designed it. The Scriptures invite us to study the created order and stand in awe of God's ingenuity. The psalmist did not have access to telescopes, but he wrote:

The heavens declare the glory of God;
the skies proclaim the work of his hands.
Day after day they pour forth speech;
night after night they display knowledge.
There is no speech or language
where their voice is not heard.
Their voice goes out into all the earth,
their words to the ends of the world.
(PSALM 19:1-4)

This proclamation both undergirds and encourages scientific investigation. When scientists have been motivated and guided by biblical admonitions to serve others and alleviate suffering, their work has led to the most significant advances in combating disease in human history.

This is not the case with the basic assumptions of many other ancient and modern spiritual philosophies. Much of Eastern mysticism and its contemporary variations make the assumption that the physical world we inhabit is an illusion (often referred to as *maya*), a prolonged dream that we all have somehow conjured and persist in accepting. Altered states of consciousness achieved through meditative techniques (or by taking a chemical shortcut with mind-altering drugs) are designed to lift the veil from this "unreal" realm that we experience during our normal waking state. When enlightened by these experiences, we supposedly not only can experience our true identity as "one with the cosmos" (or God) but also can eventually learn to alter our physiology, cure disease, or even defy the laws of physics. Such notions may sound tantalizing, but they are in fact profoundly antiscientific, standing squarely in the way of learning how the world around us operates. Why try to discover the principles of physics, chemistry, and biology that govern an illusion?

That being said, we would hasten to point out that the Bible's primary focus is on our spiritual well-being. For those who are not familiar with the Bible's contents, the following three sections—"Our terminal condition," "The cure," and "What shall we do?"—will present a brief but vitally important synopsis of its basic message. Even if you are well versed (no pun intended) in the Bible, we

INSPIRED SIMPLICITY

Why doesn't the Bible contain more specific details about how the human body works? We get an interesting perspective when we consider ancient Chinese medicine and its East Indian counterpart (*ayurveda*), two of today's most popular alternative therapies. Based on the worldviews of Taoism and Hinduism, both claim a complex system of invisible energies (called *Ch'i* and *prana*) that are said to flow through equally invisible structures (called *meridians* and *chakras*). Furthermore, they presume that health and illness are the direct result of the quality of this flow, and their therapies involve complex formulas that purport to manipulate it. But centuries of scientific and technological advances have failed to provide any objective evidence that these invisible entities—*Ch'i, prana, meridians,* and *chakras*—actually exist. Furthermore, no meaningful understanding of the causes and treatment of important diseases or public-health measures that might prevent them arise from these elaborate systems.

By comparison, the Bible's virtual silence regarding human anatomy and physiology could be construed as compelling evidence of divine inspiration. The Scriptures contain dietary and public-health admonitions that were important to the well-being of the nation of Israel. They also admonish us regarding prudent behavior that, if universally followed, would save the world untold disease and suffering. One biblical statement that refers to a specific body function is the repeated claim in the first books of the Old Testament that "the life of a creature is in the blood" (Leviticus 17:11, for example), a statement that is entirely correct from a physiologic perspective. Any tissue deprived of a steady flow of blood (and thus of life-sustaining oxygen) will die within minutes. Had these passages declared that "the life is in the bile" or "the life is in the urine," contemporary believers would have a lot of awkward explaining to do. ■

encourage you to continue reading. It's never a waste of time to take another look at the basics, and hopefully you'll gain a fresh insight or two. These sections lead into a discussion on spiritual growth and maturity, which are important concepts, even for those who are familiar with the Bible.

Our terminal condition

The sweeping arc of the Bible tells the story of the relationship between God and the human race—not only as a group, but as individuals—that was lost but can be restored. The world we know and the bodies we inhabit do not function as they were originally intended. The wonderfully straightforward biblical account of Creation tells us that disease and death, and the terrible hurt that human beings inflict on one another, were not originally present on this planet. We were designed to live in harmony not only with one another, but also with the animals, the world around us, and most importantly with God.

It is crucial to understand that our relationship with Him was not designed to be one of a master and a pet, or an inventor with a sophisticated talking doll. If our love for God and desire to communicate with Him are to have any meaning, it is necessary for us to *choose* to love Him, not be compelled by force or some sort of hardwiring within the brain. You can program your computer to say "I love you" every time you turn it on, but this expression of electronic affection would be meaningless. Even a toddler can learn to say those words, hopefully mimicking what he hears from loving parents and other nurturing adults. But this cannot compare to the experience of having your child or another adult look you in the eye and say "I love you" when you know that he or she understands what it means and that it is a spontaneous and genuine sentiment.

For God, allowing human beings the freedom to choose to love Him meant accepting the possibility of our ignoring Him or deciding to rebel against Him. According to the opening chapters of the Old Testament, the first humans enjoyed a perfect environment and direct communication with God, but they made a deliberate, fateful, and ultimately fatal decision to disobey Him. The bitter result of their action permanently affected not only their lives, but ours as well (see Romans 5:14-18; 1 Corinthians 15:21-22). The Old Testament prophet Isaiah gives us a poignant sense of what we have been missing in his description of life at a future time on a "new earth" where God's order will be restored:

> *"Never again will there be in it*
> *an infant who lives but a few days,*
> *or an old man who does not live out his years;*
> *he who dies at a hundred*
> *will be thought a mere youth. . . .*
> *No longer will they build houses and others live in them,*
> *or plant and others eat.*

For as the days of a tree,
so will be the days of my people;
my chosen ones will long enjoy
the works of their hands.
They will not toil in vain
or bear children doomed to misfortune;
for they will be a people blessed by the Lord,
they and their descendants with them.
Before they call I will answer;
while they are still speaking I will hear.
The wolf and the lamb will feed together,
and the lion will eat straw like the ox,
but dust will be the serpent's food.
They will neither harm nor destroy
on all my holy mountain," says the Lord.
(ISAIAH 65:20, 22-25)

Even more profound a consequence of that original rebellion is the grim fact that every human born since (with one notable exception—Jesus) has also had a lifelong bent toward rebellion against God, played out in a spectacular number of ways. The New Testament uses the phrase *sinful nature* to describe this rebellion, and we use the word *sins* for its specific manifestations. Of all the teachings in the Bible, this is one for which ample proof can be found every day in every newspaper of every city of the world. Human beings, no matter what their culture or background, have always done horrific things to one another. Even when we abide by rules, mores, and manners, we engage in put-downs, gossip, outbursts of temper, shading the truth to suit our interests, and a host of other behaviors that serve ourselves. No organization or home, no matter how lofty its goals, escapes the impact of human sin. One of the most common Greek words used to refer to sin in the New Testament is *hamartia,* which means "missing the mark." In our culture, where standards of morality shift like sand, it is possible to lose sight of the fact that there is a Creator to whom we are accountable, and that He has standards against which our thoughts and behaviors are measured. God provides a definitive list of these standards in the Ten Commandments, and Jesus summarizes them even more concisely:

One of [the Pharisees], an expert in the law, tested him with this question: "Teacher, which is the greatest commandment in the Law?"

Jesus replied: "'Love the Lord your God with all your heart and with all your soul and with all your mind.' This is the first and greatest commandment. And the second is like it: 'Love your neighbor as yourself.' All the Law and the Prophets hang on these two commandments."

(MATTHEW 22:35-40)

In a presentation much like that of a prosecuting attorney making his case before a tribunal, the apostle Paul in the opening chapters of his monumental letter to the Romans makes it abundantly clear that "all have sinned and fall short of the glory of God" (Romans 3:23). Should there be any doubt that we have all "missed the mark" with respect to God's standards, the apostle James makes this unsettling pronouncement: "Whoever keeps the whole law and yet stumbles at just one point is guilty of breaking all of it" (James 2:10).

Where does that leave all of us? *Guilty as sin,* as the old phrase goes, but that's not all. In numerous places the Scriptures describe our condition as walking in darkness or as being slaves, blind, lost, and dead. The apostle Paul writes, "Once you were dead because of your disobedience and your many sins. . . . All of us used to live that way, following the passionate desires and inclinations of our sinful nature. By our very nature we were subject to God's anger, just like everyone else" (Ephesians 2:1, 3, NLT).

To make matters worse, we are incapable of meeting God's standards or restoring our standing with God through our own efforts, however painstaking or sincere. For millions (perhaps billions) of people, religious activity is an attempt to solve this problem by "doing the right thing"—striving to obey the Ten Commandments or some other set of rules, doing good works, searching the soul in an effort to root out destructive attitudes, even engaging in sacrificial service for others—all in an effort to make the grade. These enterprises may be praiseworthy and helpful to humankind, but they still fall far short of God's standard. Paul writes, "Those who depend on the law to make them right with God are under his curse, for the Scriptures say, 'Cursed is everyone who does not observe and obey all the commands that are written in God's Book of the Law.' So it is clear that no one can be made right with God by trying to keep the law" (Galatians 3:10-11, NLT).

Is there any cure for this terminal condition? We can, of course, attempt to deny its reality, staking our hope on any number of other explanations for whatever mess we have made of our lives and our world. Here are just a few common justifications:

Perhaps we're really not so bad. "After all, I'm only human" is a timeworn excuse for bad behavior, but it only confirms our sorry state. Some religious outlooks and philosophies make the case that we're endowed with an inner core of pure goodness that can shine through if we shed baggage from the past or repeat positive affirmations. But much of this (wishful) thinking represents an effort to deny what all of us realize when we take a hard, honest look at our motivations and desires, as well as the dark places they so often take us. In case we need any confirmation, Jesus did not paint a particularly rosy picture of what resides in our heart of hearts: "What comes out of a person is what defiles him. For from within, out of the heart of man, come evil thoughts, sexual immorality, theft, murder, adultery, coveting, wickedness, deceit, sensuality, envy, slander, pride, foolishness. All these evil things come from within, and they defile a person" (Mark 7:20-23, ESV).

An even more unflattering statement was made by the prophet Jeremiah in the Old Testament: "The heart is deceitful above all things, and desperately sick; who can understand it?" (Jeremiah 17:9, ESV).

Perhaps God doesn't really take all of those standards seriously, or maybe they were intended for another time in history. We defer to the explicit statements of Jesus—whose unique authority we will discuss momentarily—on this particular point. In the Sermon on the Mount, He declares, "Do not think that I have come to abolish the Law or the Prophets; I have not come to abolish them but to fulfill them. I tell you the truth, until heaven and earth disappear, not the smallest letter, not the least stroke of a pen, will by any means disappear from the Law until everything is accomplished" (Matthew 5:17-18).

Perhaps there isn't anyone to whom we're accountable. If the material universe is all there is, then the only standards we need to be concerned about are those that represent whatever culture we live in or those guidelines that work for us and maximize our pleasure. That might sound reasonable—until we start talking about justice, or we attempt to explain why genocide, slavery, torture, sexual abuse, prejudice, and a host of other evil and destructive behaviors are in fact *wrong.* If we don't like the concept of a God who has absolute standards and cares deeply about what we do, we need to ponder the alternative: What if there are *no* standards and no ultimate justice in the world? What if the only thing that determines whether something is right is the will and brute strength of the person or group holding that opinion?

The cure

If and when we realize the futility of these justifications, we must finally face the awful truth of our sinfulness, our separation from God, and our utter inability to bridge that gulf through our own efforts, religious or otherwise. But acknowledging this diagnosis, this terminal condition, is in fact the first step toward finding the cure.

Ultimately the only remedy for our desperate condition comes from God Himself—indeed, it *is* God Himself. The primary focus of the Bible is the account of our rescue, with the Old Testament setting a long and very detailed stage and the New Testament telling and elaborating on the good news that God directly entered human history as a human being. His name is *Yeshua,* a Hebrew word literally meaning "the Lord saves," but He is known to us as Jesus of Nazareth. The narratives of His life and teachings in the New Testament, known as the four Gospels (from the Old English *godspel*, a shortened form of *good-spell,* meaning "good news"), are remarkable in more ways than we can enumerate here. You may best appreciate their impact simply by reading them in a reliable modern translation. Let the story and Jesus' words speak for themselves, without allowing preconceptions or cultural baggage to dilute their impact. When this is done, several points become apparent.

First, Jesus' teachings and parables are at once arresting, surprising, and challenging. They address both everyday concerns and sweeping themes about God and humanity. Jesus often frustrated His followers because He told stories rather than making outright pronouncements. He also behaved in a way that upended the religious establishment of His day. He socialized with prostitutes and crooked tax collectors and was criticized for hanging out with such notorious "sinners." (For a contemporary point of reference, imagine Jesus having dinner with porn stars and drug dealers.) He outwitted efforts by the proud and pious to trip Him up on points of doctrine, and He repeatedly exposed their hypocrisy.

What most confounded Jesus' contemporaries were His claims about Himself, and these continue to perplex many today. Over three years, before small groups of followers and assembled multitudes, in intimate conversations and heated arguments, He described Himself as the Bread of Life, the Light of the World, the Son of God, the resurrection and the life. He told people that their sins were forgiven, a bold statement that shocked observers: *Who can forgive sins but God alone?* they asked themselves (see Mark 2:7). To one of His followers, Jesus made a statement that has raised spirits, eyebrows, and hackles for two thousand years: "I am the way and the truth and the life. No one comes to the Father except through me" (John 14:6). On numerous occasions He either implied or claimed outright that He was God. Announcements that "I and the Father are one" (John 10:30) or "I tell you the truth . . . before Abraham was born, I am!" (John 8:58) provoked violent responses from the religious establishment of His day.

When Moses encountered God in a burning bush and received orders to lead the Israelites out of Egypt, he asked, "Suppose I go to the Israelites and say to them, 'The God of your fathers has sent me to you,' and they ask me, 'What is his name?' Then what shall I tell them?" This was God's answer: "I AM WHO I AM. This is what you are to say to the Israelites: 'I AM has sent me to you'" (Exodus 3:13-14). Jesus' enemies made the connection immediately when He said "Before Abraham was born, I am!" and were ready to stone Him on the spot for blasphemy (see John 8:59).

Jesus' teachings were riveting and His claims provocative, but what drew throngs to Him were His healings. These did not involve subjective, equivocal improvements in symptoms that are so often proclaimed to be miracles by contemporary healers. If Jesus relieved some headaches and back pain, these accounts didn't make it into the Gospels. Instead, we read about sight restored to eyes blind from birth, withered hands returned to normal, paralytics able to walk, lepers touched and cleansed, even the dead brought back to life. These are healings that required no X rays or committees of clinicians for validation. They were readily apparent, undeniable, and indisputable. Jesus even performed some of them on the Sabbath—a day that had become associated with strict regulations regarding work that was to be avoided, even including healing—to demonstrate that works of mercy were more important to God than rules and regulations. The healings certainly got people's attention, and word of them spread wildly through whatever region Jesus visited, drawing crowds from near and far.

Over the centuries, critics have attempted to tease out of the Gospels what they call the "historical" Jesus—that is, His teachings and deeds minus the healings, His other miracles (such as feeding thousands from an initial supply of a few fish and loaves of bread), and His claims to divinity. They suggest that these details were added some years after the fact by zealous followers and the hierarchies that developed after them, all intent on expanding the story (and perhaps their own power as well). Aside from the presumption inherent in these demythologizing efforts, such arguments trample on the inherent logic of the Gospel narratives. Vast crowds and the authorities' strong reaction to Jesus don't make any sense if all He did was wander around Judea uttering a few niceties about loving your neighbor. In a famous and blistering rebuttal to such a viewpoint, C. S. Lewis dismisses this idea:

> A man who was merely a man and said the sort of things Jesus said would not be a great moral teacher. He would either be a lunatic—on a level with the man who says he is a poached egg—or else he would be the Devil of Hell. You must make your choice. Either this man was, and is, the Son of God: or else a madman or something worse. You can shut Him up for a fool, you can spit at Him and kill Him as a demon; or you can fall at His feet and call Him Lord and God. But let us not come with any patronising nonsense about His being a great human teacher. He has not left that open to us. He did not intend to.[16]

When reading the Gospels, we cannot ignore how much they emphasize the final week in Jesus' life. In his thought-provoking book *The Jesus I Never Knew,* Philip Yancey notes

> Of the biographies I have read, few devote more than ten percent of their pages to the subject's death—including biographies of men like Martin Luther King Jr. and Mahatma Gandhi, who died violent and politically significant deaths. The Gospels, though, devote nearly a third of their length to the climactic last week of Jesus' life. Matthew, Mark, Luke and John saw death as the central mystery of Jesus.[17]

Amidst all the escalating conflict, the tender farewells, the betrayal, the accusations, the religious and political schemes, the shifting loyalties, and the appalling torture and death that Jesus endured, one message comes through: Jesus was neither caught off guard nor caught up by forces He didn't understand. He knew exactly what was going on and what He was doing. He was going to, as He put it, "give his life as a ransom for many" (Mark 10:45). At His last meal with His disciples, in words and gestures rich with symbolism from the Passover feast, Jesus told them that His body, broken like the bread they would eat, would be given for them, and that His blood would be "poured out for many for the forgiveness of sins" (Matthew 26:28). After enduring hours of unspeakable pain in arguably the cruelest form of execution ever devised, He cried out, "It is finished" (see John 19:30). He was not merely announcing that His life was moments from ending. The word He used, *tetelestai,* was the Greek term for "to complete."

It is an astonishing notion that this horrendous crime—the trial and execution of Jesus—would be the vehicle by which God Himself would pay the price of—and suffer for—human rebellion. But this passage from the prophet Isaiah, written more than seven hundred years before Jesus endured the scourge and nails, states it plainly:

> *He was despised and rejected by men,*
> *a man of sorrows, and familiar with suffering.*
> *Like one from whom men hide their faces*
> *he was despised, and we esteemed him not.*
> *Surely he took up our infirmities*
> *and carried our sorrows,*
> *yet we considered him stricken by God,*
> *smitten by him, and afflicted.*
> *But he was pierced for our transgressions,*
> *he was crushed for our iniquities;*
> *the punishment that brought us peace was upon him,*
> *and by his wounds we are healed.*
> *We all, like sheep, have gone astray,*
> *each of us has turned to his own way;*
> *and the Lord has laid on him*
> *the iniquity of us all.*
> (ISAIAH 53:3-6)

Yet the story does not end here. All four Gospel accounts, the history that follows in the book known as the Acts of the Apostles, the exposition of the other New Testament writers, and the witness of centuries of repaired lives proclaim that Jesus did not remain entombed. His final breath on the cross was not in fact final. Before two days had passed, His followers not only discovered that His burial cloths and tomb were empty but that He was alive and very well. Multiple conversations and appearances convinced startled witnesses that they were not dreaming, that Jesus was not an apparition, that He was in fact who He had claimed to be all along—and most importantly, that the crushing weight of both sin and death had been forever overpowered. Before departing from them in a startling manner (see Acts 1), Jesus commissioned His followers to tell His story not only in their own communities but also throughout the world. And that they did, with a speed and joyful determination (even in the face of fierce opposition and martyrdom) that itself validated their claim that "He is risen indeed."

Seven weeks after Jesus exited His tomb, on what is called Pentecost, an earthquake occurred, with benevolent aftershocks that spread throughout the ancient world. Its epicenter was in Jerusalem, where visitors from many countries suddenly heard Jesus' followers tell His story—not only with unexpected boldness but also in the listeners' own languages. Even more surprising was the voice of the apostle Peter, who had completely lost his nerve on the night Jesus was captured, addressing the crowd that had gathered. With eloquence uncharacteristic of an uneducated Galilean fisherman, he reminded them of Jesus' deeds, quoted liberally from the Old Testament prophet Joel and from the Psalms, and then confronted them about what had happened fifty days earlier: "Therefore let all Israel be assured of this: God has made this Jesus, whom you crucified, both Lord and Christ" (Acts 2:36).

Those who heard were "cut to the heart" (Acts 2:37). They responded with the most important question one must ask when confronted with this information: *"Brothers, what shall we do?"* (v. 37, emphasis added).

What shall we do?

Once we truly grasp the nature of our predicament and what is at stake—that we are estranged from God not only by what we do (sin) but by what we are (sinners), that we cannot restore our relationship with God by our own efforts, that we deserve death, that when Jesus died He took the entire penalty for our sin—the answer to that question matters above all others.

Peter gave the answer to the crowd: "Repent and be baptized, every one of you, in the name of Jesus Christ for the forgiveness of your sins" (Acts 2:38).

We don't see or hear the word *repent* very often today, and many people think of it only as the word scrawled on the sign of a street preacher brandishing a bullhorn. It is in fact a term rich with meaning: Turn around. Give up. Wave the white flag. Abandon the idea that you're in charge, the master of your fate. Stop trying to gain God's favor by being religious. Stop trying to ignore Him by claiming you're "not religious." Stop justifying your ego, your betrayals, your gossip, your harsh words, your lust, your bitterness. Stop making excuses. Stop trying to prove that you're not so bad after all. Stop denying what you know in your gut when you can't sleep at three in the morning.

Turn toward home. Let your Father embrace you. Accept the pardon. Take the gift of forgiveness and life that was so costly—the one that only Jesus, and not you, could pay for. Thank Him for enduring what you deserved. Thank Him for rescuing you. Put Him in charge of your future. Let Him have your relationships, your job, your stuff, your time. Give Him access to the breadth and depth of your mind and emotions. Give Him permission to haul out the junk, to make repairs, to restore, to redecorate.

This can be done now—right now—if you haven't done so already. You don't need a pastor or a priest, a heavenly chorus, or a ceremony. Stand, sit, kneel, or fall on your face. Talk to God using your own words, aloud or silently. No special verbiage, no thees or thous are needed. Just be sure that it's *you* saying what you mean, not someone else putting words in your mouth or you trying to come up with words that you think God wants to hear. This is the most important step you will ever take, and no one can do it for you. Others may have tried to pressure you to do so in the past, but God will not. The door is open, with warmth and light on the other side, and it's up to you to decide to walk through it.

Once you have taken this step, nothing is the same. At that moment, you may feel profound relief, joy, gratitude, or nothing in particular. It is literally like saying "I do": One moment you're single and the next you're married, even if it took you months or years to arrive at the altar. Jesus described it as being born a second time. A new life begins, and it never ends, even when the physical body wears out. The apostle Paul describes a person who has taken this step as being "in Christ" and writes that "if anyone is in Christ, he is a new creation; the old has gone, the new has come!" (2 Corinthians 5:17). The word *Christian,* meaning "one who belongs to Christ," now genuinely applies to that person, whether or not he or she understood its meaning before.

According to the book of Acts in the New Testament, the word *Christian* was first used to describe those who brought this message about Jesus to Antioch, the third largest city in the Roman Empire. Whether the word was one they devised themselves or a term of derision coined by their opponents, it is an apt description of the status of one who has repented and yielded the reins of his or her life to Christ. (The word *Christ* literally means "the Anointed One" and is the Greek translation of the Hebrew word *Messiah.*)

The apostle Peter told his listeners to "repent and be baptized." What about the second part of that statement? Is baptism necessary? God's forgiveness, the second birth, the new and eternal life—all are gifts, received strictly by faith in the Giver, without additional requirements, because all of the requirements were completely beyond our reach and all were met by Jesus. But there is no way anyone else can know that you have taken this step, other than by what you say and do thereafter. (No wings will sprout from your back, for example, nor will a glow suddenly emanate from your head.) Baptism is not a requirement for receiving the gift of God's pardon, but it is commanded for those who have done so, and it serves as a wonderful way to acknowledge publicly what has happened. From the Greek word meaning "to dip," baptism typically involves a very brief immersion in water (or a sprinkling of water on those who physically cannot be immersed), symbolizing the death of the old self and the birth of the new, as well as identification with Jesus' death and return to life. It can be done in a church, in the ocean, in the Jordan River, or in a backyard pool. It may occur immediately after your encounter with Christ or at some time in the future.

In the ancient world *baptize* also referred to the process of dying cloth, which gave the word additional meaning: As a cloth was immersed, the dye would permeate it and change its color. The "baptized" cloth would be permanently altered by its encounter with the dye. Immersing someone in water beautifully symbolizes the permanent change that occurs as a result of being reconciled to God.

While baptism is a powerful and joyous event, it is only one of many experiences that can and should follow on the heels of the life-changing and eternity-changing decision to accept God's gift of forgiveness. In the remainder of the chapter we will look at several others.

Growing Healthy and Strong

If we think of the decision to repent as a spiritual birth, as Jesus clearly described it, then we must also come to grips with the fact that the transition from spiritual newborn to mature adult does not occur overnight. Like physical and cognitive development, spiritual growth is a process; unlike them, it is not automatic or predictable. It may occur rapidly and consistently, in fits and starts, or it may not develop beyond infancy or toddlerhood. The Bible is a rich and essential source of guidance for this process, and provides explicit directives to follow, examples to emulate, and cautionary tales warning of choices to avoid. All of these tell us that growth requires several ingredients.

Before we describe a number of these elements, however, it is critical that we understand what is—and isn't—the ultimate goal and manifestation of spiritual growth. It is not committing vast amounts of Scripture to memory or having an unerring command of biblical teaching. It is not perfect church attendance. It is not putting money in the collection plate every week, singing in the choir, volunteering for multiple committees, or traveling to distant lands to tell others about the life that Christ has made available. Many of these activities are highly worthwhile and may well be manifestations of spiritual health, but they are not an end in themselves.

In addition, spiritual growth is not necessarily demonstrated by avoiding behaviors that may be unhealthy or that someone might consider imprudent. The list of "rules and regulations" that have been considered essential to spirituality by one group or another over the past two thousand years is virtually endless. (Emphasizing a list of dos and don'ts as the centerpiece of spiritual growth is known as legalism, and it is highly effective in driving people away from a vital relationship with God.)

Why can't we view religious activities and prudent behavior as clear-cut evidence of spiritual health? Here's a hint: Many of us have known people who could make all the right noises in church and yet be chronically critical, ornery, or even abusive everywhere else. This brand of would-be spirituality can even become a vehicle for one person to inflict his or her appetite for control over others. Jesus reserved His most searing indictments for the externally righteous (and self-righteous) religious leaders of His day. They were meticulous in their observance of a host of laws and customs, yet so lacking in mercy, justice, and even faith that He called them snakes, sons of vipers, hypocrites, whitewashed tombs, and blind fools, among other colorful epithets.

Throughout history, religion in general and Christianity in particular have often been used as an excuse to intimidate, harass, torment, and even kill others who didn't toe a particular line. If you have been harmed by such behavior, you need to know that it is a complete misrepresentation of God's character and purposes.

The twenty-third chapter of the Gospel of Matthew consists almost entirely of one of these blistering addresses, delivered publicly and directly to the Pharisees.

If religious activity isn't necessarily a manifestation of spiritual growth and health, what is? Jesus gave us a wonderfully succinct answer, one that we quoted earlier in this chapter but that bears repeating: "'Love the Lord your God with all your heart and with all your soul and with all your mind.' This is the first and greatest commandment. And the second is like it: 'Love your neighbor as yourself.' All the Law and the Prophets hang on these two commandments" (Matthew 22:37-40).

The apostle Paul expanded on this theme in a famous and eloquent passage that is frequently read at weddings but in fact applies to every aspect of life. It expresses nothing less than the heart of spiritual health and spiritual growth:

> *If I speak in the tongues of men and of angels, but have not love, I am only a resounding gong or a clanging cymbal. If I have the gift of prophecy and can fathom all mysteries and all knowledge, and if I have a faith that can move mountains, but have not love, I am nothing. If I give all I possess to the poor and surrender my body to the flames, but have not love, I gain nothing.*
>
> *Love is patient, love is kind. It does not envy, it does not boast, it is not proud. It is not rude, it is not self-seeking, it is not easily angered, it keeps no record of wrongs. Love does not delight in evil but rejoices with the truth. It always protects, always trusts, always hopes, always perseveres.*
>
> *Love never fails. But where there are prophecies, they will cease; where there are tongues, they will be stilled; where there is knowledge, it will pass away. For we know in part and we prophesy in part, but when perfection comes, the imperfect disappears. When I was a child, I talked like a child, I thought like a child, I reasoned like a child. When I became a man, I put childish ways behind me. Now we see but a poor reflection as in a mirror; then we shall see face to face. Now I know in part; then I shall know fully, even as I am fully known.*
>
> *And now these three remain: faith, hope and love. But the greatest of these is love.* (1 CORINTHIANS 13:1-13)

The essence of spiritual growth—what is also called transformation or spiritual formation—is loving God and people more. It is that simple, but it's also impossible to do through willpower alone. We can certainly make many changes under our own steam in response to guilt and pressure or in an effort to enhance our reputation. Indeed, it is actually easier to make some external adjustments in behavior than to renovate what lies at the core, where our deepest urges and instincts take us when we're not paying attention. But sooner or later the circumstances of life and the foibles of those around us will break through the surface or get to us, and our true colors will be evident for all to see. Or, just as often, an appetite we can't seem to satisfy or contain—for food, alcohol, sex, possessions, risk taking, recognition—will get us into trouble.

What is both fascinating and reassuring about the Bible is how accurately it assesses this universal human condition. With the exception of Jesus, even biblical heroes—Abraham, Moses, David, the twelve disciples, and many more—had feet of clay, and the Scriptures give unvarnished accounts of both their faith and their failures. The apostle Paul describes every person's struggle to "do the right thing" when our instincts take us elsewhere: "I know that nothing good lives in me, that is, in my sinful nature. For I have the desire to do what is good, but I cannot carry it out. For what I do is not the good I want to do; no, the evil I do not want to do—this I keep on doing. Now if I do what I do not want to do, it is no longer I who do it, but it is sin living in me that does it" (Romans 7:18-20).

After a lengthy description of this conflict comes a cry of exasperation: "What a wretched man I am! Who will rescue me from this body of death?" And then immediately the answer: "Thanks be to God—through Jesus Christ our Lord!" (Romans 7:24-25). The lifelong solution, it turns out, was promised by Jesus to His disciples (and all of us) before His death.

> *I will ask the Father, and he will give you another Counselor to be with you forever—the Spirit of truth. The world cannot accept him, because it neither sees him nor knows him. But you know him, for he lives with you and will be in you. . . .*
>
> *But when he, the Spirit of truth, comes, he will guide you into all truth. He will not speak on his own; he will speak only what he hears, and he will tell you what is yet to come. He will bring glory to me by taking from what is mine and making it known to you. All that belongs to the Father is mine. That is why I said the Spirit will take from what is mine and make it known to you.*
>
> (JOHN 14:16; 16:13-15)

Once again God provides—and is Himself—the solution and the source of our deepest and most meaningful change. Paul elaborates, describing how our efforts to comply with God's standards (as spelled out in the law of Moses) on our own are doomed to failure:

> *The law of Moses was unable to save us because of the weakness of our sinful nature. So God did what the law could not do. He sent his own Son in a body like the bodies we sinners have. And in that body God declared an end to sin's control over us by giving his Son as a sacrifice for our sins. He did this so that the just requirement of the law would be fully satisfied for us, who no longer follow our sinful nature but instead follow the Spirit.*
>
> *Those who are dominated by the sinful nature think about sinful things, but those who are controlled by the Holy Spirit think about things that please the Spirit. So letting your sinful nature control your mind leads to death. But letting the Spirit control your mind leads to life and peace.*
>
> (ROMANS 8:3-6, NLT)

What Paul is describing is so mind-boggling that it is difficult to grasp. We cannot make ourselves more loving. We cannot transform our nature or replace our self-serving instincts. Only God can, but He cannot (and will not) force us to love Him or others. The life and peace that we so desperately want, and that evades our best efforts, God Himself—the Holy Spirit—will provide. This definitely goes against our do-it-yourself, self-help, rugged individualist, master-of-my-fate grain. (But then again, so does the entire biblical message of sin, repentance, and forgiveness.) And yet, paradoxically, relying on God to bring about these changes does not resign us to a life of passivity, plodding along in our usual routine until He decides to speak through a burning bush in our front yard, write instructions for us in the clouds, or take control of us like a hand in a sock puppet.

If we are going to grow, to become spiritually healthy, we need to do some things on a regular basis—not because God will love us more if we do them, not because we're trying to earn His approval or heavenly gold stars, not because they will make us "better" than someone else, but because they put us in the place where God can transform us into people who love Him and love others. These activities, these things *we* can do, are often called **spiritual disciplines**—not in the sense of punishment or harsh restrictions, but rather in keeping with the original meaning of the word *disciple:* a learner. Spiritual disciplines, in a variety of ways, allow us not just to learn about Him but in fact to *know* Him, to build a relationship with Him of such depth and intimacy that it truly transforms us. They also expand our capacity to love and serve others in our immediate family, workplace, neighborhood, and—of utmost importance—community of faith. The latter is critical because it is extremely difficult to experience spiritual growth when isolated from others who share your faith.

Before we look at some of these activities, two analogies are worth considering. Throughout this book we have described a host of activities that can, if done consistently, improve physical and emotional health. We may forget, as we do them day in and day out, that we have very little control over their specific effects on our body. With nourishment, for example, several times every day our job is to put food in our mouth, chew it, and then swallow it. We do not manage, let alone even comprehend, all of the complex mechanisms that digest and absorb the components of our food, before using it in thousands of ways everywhere from the brain to the toenails. With exercise, our job is to put one foot in front of the other for a half hour or more. We do not control how this activity builds muscle fibers, conditions the heart and lungs, or improves the status of our arteries. With sleep, our job is to lie down and close our eyes when we become tired at the end of the day. We can barely understand, let alone direct, the restorative activities within our brain that occur during the night.

The fact that the jobs we must do to maintain health are relatively simple does not at all ensure that we will do them consistently or well. Many different foods will relieve hunger, for instance, but not all will keep our body in optimal condition. But if we learn more about these activities and practice them regularly, we become more proficient and can even make adjustments for specific purposes. If we're planning to run a marathon, for example, our exercise in preparation for that twenty-six-mile task will need to be very different from the half-hour daily walk we might do for general fitness. When we practice proper techniques in strength-training exercises, we do them more effectively. So it is with spiritual disciplines. We cannot, for example, predict exactly what God will do as a result of our prayer or how He will interact with us during a time of meditation. But we can learn from our experiences (especially if we keep track of them in a journal) and become proficient in these activities as we practice them. Like the marathon runner who undergoes specific training for an upcoming race, we may also need to adjust our spiritual "exercise" level in anticipation of a particular challenge that lies ahead.

Another analogy may be even more helpful, and this we owe to pastor and teacher John Ortberg. In his engaging look at spiritual disciplines, *The Life You've Always Wanted,* Ortberg reminds us that Jesus compared the effects of God's Spirit to those of the wind: "The wind blows wherever it pleases. You hear its sound, but you cannot tell where it comes from or where it is going. So it is with everyone born of the Spirit" (John 3:8). Ortberg then likens our spiritual progress to catching the wind when sailing:

> Consider the difference between piloting a motorboat or a sailboat. We can run a motorboat all by ourselves. We can fill the tank and start the engine. We are in control. But a sailboat is a different story. We can hoist the sails and steer the rudder, but we are utterly dependent on the wind. The wind does the work. If the wind doesn't blow—and sometimes it doesn't—we sit still in the water no matter how frantic we act. Our task is to do whatever enables us to catch the wind.[18]

Practicing spiritual disciplines is like becoming more proficient at sailing. Even the most expert sailor cannot control the wind, but by logging time in a sailboat in various locations, conditions, and seasons, a person becomes more attuned to the wind and more capable of maneuvering his or her boat in response to it. Skills can also be enhanced by reading about sailing, taking classes, and interacting with experienced sailors. However, if you're going to get anywhere in a sailboat, you eventually have to climb aboard, raise the sails, and wait for the wind. Sitting at the dock, watching other people sail (and judging their performance), or simply floating along with the currents is no substitute.

What we want to communicate with these illustrations is that spiritual growth—loving God and loving people, and behaving accordingly—isn't brought about by our trying to generate a feeling of being loving toward God and people. We are unlikely to be consistently successful at being patient, kind, humble, and so on by gritting our teeth and attempting to generate these virtues. Instead, the spiritual disciplines represent things that we *can* do, activities during which God can meet us, mold us, and change us. They prepare and hoist our sails, so that the Wind can take us where it will. Is the trip worth the effort? Absolutely! If you believe that God wants to limit your horizons, squash your individuality, and consign you to a life of boredom, you need to revise your understanding of "him who is able to do immeasurably more than all we ask or imagine" (Ephesians 3:20).

The spiritual disciplines have inspired enough books to fill entire libraries. Here we will focus specifically on three disciplines—prayer, study, and meditation—that establish and maintain our conversation with God. We will also mention several others and provide some recommendations for further reading and exploration. Overall, we want to extend an invitation to "taste and see that the Lord is good" (Psalm 34:8). Like nutrition and physical exercise, you can only learn so much about spiritual health by reading about it. At some point (hopefully early in the process) you must shift from being an observer to being a participant.

Prayer: the essential conversation

We will start with prayer, which we hear about so often in Scripture and in other settings that we may forget what a privilege it represents. The Bible repeatedly exhorts us to pray—indeed, to do so continually (see 1 Thessalonians 5:17)—and teaches a startling idea: The Creator of the universe actually wants to hear from us. We don't need special credentials, protocols, or representatives to act on our behalf. Imagine being able to pick up the phone and speak directly with the president of the United States or the prime minister of another country without an appointment or prior authorization and then having that person's undivided attention. Only an immediate family member would have that right. When we pray, we enjoy a similar status, that of sons and daughters of the One who has far more authority than any head of state. Furthermore, God attends to what we say and responds personally. No prayer goes unanswered, although the response may not necessarily be what we expect, and it may not occur (or be recognized) in the time frame that we would prefer.

Many of the biblical advisories on prayer—especially those from Jesus, who was uniquely qualified to address this subject—are disarmingly straightforward, using analogies to everyday conversations, especially those between parents and children. All too often, however, our conversations with God become bogged down by habits that interfere with direct, honest communication. As a mental exercise, think of the most meaningful discussions you have ever had with a close friend or with your own child. Ask yourself if the following ways of conversing might hamper that sort of heart-to-heart communication between two people, and then consider whether they might have the same effect on your conversations with God.

Unnatural language. Some people pray as if God were unable to comprehend modern English. If thou findest that this enhanceth heartfelt communication with God, by all means continue doing so. All kidding aside, for some using everyday phrases seems disrespectful when addressing God, and framing prayer in more formal language (at least on some occasions) may enhance one's sense of worship and awe. But this might also risk putting some distance between you and God, as if He were a foreign dignitary who also happens to be about four hundred years behind the times. Pop quiz: Do you think God understands how the Internet works? If you hesitated, even for a second, you need to grasp the reality that the Ancient of Days has no problem comprehending our twenty-first-century lives and language.

Same old, same old. For many of us, our prayer life is limited to a well-worn tip of the hat to God before the first bite of dinner and perhaps a longer acknowledgment before the Thanksgiving turkey is carved. Imagine how you would feel if your child said nothing to you all day except "Thanks for breakfast!" "Be nice to me today!" or "I'm hungry! Where's my food?" God is actually interested in hearing from us about the length and breadth of our lives—not merely as a mindless habit before a meal, and not just on special occasions, but all day, every day.

Blah, blah, blah. An unproductive alternative to "same old, same old" is endless, repetitive, and often meaningless verbiage directed at God, as if He is impressed by word counts. Jesus assures us that He isn't: "When you pray, do not keep on babbling like pagans, for they think they will be heard because of their many words. Do not be like them, for your Father knows what you need before you ask him" (Matthew 6:7-8).

Giving a speech. Jesus warned against "grandstanding" prayer, especially one that is meant to impress or influence others. He said: "When you pray, do not be like the hypocrites, for they love to pray standing in the synagogues and on the street corners to be seen by men. I tell you the truth, they have received their reward in full. But when you pray, go into your room, close the door and pray to your Father, who is unseen. Then your Father, who sees what is done in secret, will reward you" (Matthew 6:5-6).

It doesn't make any difference. If we don't believe that prayer actually accomplishes anything, our interest in praying may be seriously crimped. This may arise from thinking of our world in strictly material terms and dismissing apparent answers to prayer as mere coincidences. Perhaps we have trouble understanding how God could possibly pay attention to all the prayers arising at any given moment from all corners of the world and then orchestrate His various responses. Or it may stem from seeing God's purposes as immutable and any attempts to influence Him as being futile. But the Bible contains plenty of evidence that prayer is anything but an exercise in talking to oneself. Jesus made a famous statement about prayer in His Sermon on the Mount: "Ask and it will be given to you; seek and you will find; knock and the door will be opened to you. For everyone who asks receives; he who seeks finds; and to him who knocks, the door will be opened" (Matthew 7:7-8). If we have difficulty grasping how God could deal with all of this asking, looking, knocking, and seeking, we need to remember that we are finite creatures, and God is our infinite Creator. Speaking through the prophet Isaiah, He made this abundantly clear: "'For my thoughts are not your thoughts, neither are your ways my ways,' declares the Lord. 'As the heavens are higher than the earth, so are my ways higher than your ways and my thoughts than your thoughts'" (Isaiah 55:8-9). We don't need to understand how our digestive system works before eating, and we don't need to comprehend how God responds to us in order to interact with Him.

"When I pray, coincidences happen, and when I don't pray, they don't."
—WILLIAM TEMPLE (1881–1944), Archbishop of Canterbury

Command performance. The flip side of believing that prayer is futile is the conviction that God *must* grant the request of one or more people who are claiming a specific answer. This often occurs with prayer for healing of a serious illness, and it has the potential to paint everyone into a very uncomfortable corner. If the sick person does not recover, the "do or die" intercessors are left to deal with some very unpleasant explanations. Either God let them down—He didn't care or He didn't have the power to bring about the healing or other desired outcome—or else there was a fatal lack of faith on someone's part. (A variant explanation is that the patient or someone who was praying harbored a covert sin that prevented God from taking action.) Those who are praying (including the person who is ill) may become stuck in denial and ultimately feel isolated from one another because no one wants to be the first to acknowledge that things are not improving (and thus admit a "lack of faith"). Unless they acknowledge that God could say no and still be loving, those facing a loss may also feel guilty or estranged from God rather than drawing close to Him for comfort.

Like our conversations with others we care about, meaningful prayer is not limited to a particular time, place, subject, or duration. Indeed, the more often we pray, the more meaningful our dialogue is likely to become. We can pray standing, sitting, walking, kneeling, lying in our bed, or flat on our faces. We can pray with our eyes shut or open, head bowed or raised, hands folded or lifted to the sky. We can pray at home, at work, at school, at church, or at play. We can pray silently or out loud, by ourselves or with others. Many people find that praying aloud while others listen is so distracting that they prefer to stay silent in groups and pray audibly only when alone. Others find their mind wandering during silent prayer and maintain better focus while talking to God out loud, or even writing out their prayers.

Some prayers are like a quick telephone call to a loved one while we're engaged with other responsibilities—"Just wanted to stay in touch." But like any relationship in which we desire openness and intimacy, we need regular time to talk with God that is quiet, undistracted, unhurried. Couples who do not regularly set aside time to connect with one another will see their marriage grow stagnant and distant. The same can happen with God if our conversations with Him are only quick, superficial "hi-bye" exchanges, or the equivalent of leaving a short message on His voice mail.

Supplication

Just as there are many times and situations in which to pray, so there are many subjects that we might bring up. Perhaps the most common of these is the request (or what is called **supplication** in more formal language). Many of us go to God in prayer primarily when we want something, need something, or are in dire straits. We should be relieved to know that God actually invites us to be completely open with Him—in other words, to tell Him what we're actually concerned about, rather than simply recite all the noble sentiments we think He wants to hear. One of the most profound statements about not holding back anything from God is this: "Do not be anxious about anything, but in *everything*, by prayer and petition, with thanksgiving, present your requests to God. And the peace of God, which transcends all understanding, will guard your hearts and your minds in Christ Jesus" (Philippians 4:6-7, emphasis added). There is no prequalification for how "spiritual" the request might be, and there's also no guarantee that any specific request will be granted. But there is a wonderful promise of peace that transcends all understanding, which results from trusting God and not necessarily from gaining whatever we want.

Indeed, many of us can recall praying to God for something we desperately wanted—for a romantic relationship to work out, for example, or for a particular job to become available—and years later, with the advantage of hindsight, we were thanking Him with equal fervor for declining that request. If we have children, we will hear a stream of requests for everything from a drink of water to a new car. We will grant many of those requests and also decline many, based on our more mature (though not always perfect) judgment. Jesus assures us that God has both perfect wisdom and our best interests in mind as He responds to our petitions: "Which of you, if his son asks for bread, will give him a stone? Or if he asks for a fish, will give him a snake? If you, then, though you are evil, know how to give good gifts to your children, how much more will your Father in heaven give good gifts to those who ask him!" (Matthew 7:9-11).

As much as we might enjoy hearing what our children want and thoughtfully satisfying many of their desires, it could also become wearisome if we only heard from them when they wanted something from us. Most parents look forward to the time when an older or grown child will sit across the kitchen table and ask, "Mom, how are you doing?" or "Dad, what do you think I should do in this situation?" Life becomes truly interesting and exciting when we move beyond "God, here's what I want" to "God, what do *You* want?" There are, indeed, a number of other elements in addition to requests that can and should be a part of regular times of prayer. These include confession, thanksgiving, and adoration and praise.

Confession

Regularly acknowledging actions, inactions, and thoughts that we know violate God's standards is important if we are to maintain a healthy relationship with God. "If we confess our sins, he is faithful and just and will forgive us our sins and purify us from all unrighteousness" (1 John 1:9), writes the apostle John. A powerful example of a heartfelt prayer of confession may be found in the Old Testament in Psalm 51, which was penned by David, who is described in the

Bible as "a man after [God's] own heart" (see 1 Samuel 13:14). Having been anointed king of Israel and blessed with unique gifts of courage, leadership, and spiritual insight, David nevertheless experienced a disastrous moral failure. After observing a beautiful woman bathing, he ordered her to be brought to his palace and began an adulterous affair with her. Upon learning that she was pregnant, David began a cover-up that eventually led to his order that her husband be killed in battle. When confronted by a prophet about what had happened, David acknowledged both his wrongdoing and the One he had ultimately offended: "I have sinned against the Lord" (2 Samuel 12:13). He later recorded his thoughts as breathtaking poetry:

For I know my transgressions,
and my sin is always before me.
Against you, you only, have I sinned
and done what is evil in your sight,
so that you are proved right when you speak
and justified when you judge.
Surely I was sinful at birth,
sinful from the time my mother conceived me.
Surely you desire truth in the inner parts;
you teach me wisdom in the inmost place.
Cleanse me with hyssop, and I will be clean;
wash me, and I will be whiter than snow.
Let me hear joy and gladness;
let the bones you have crushed rejoice.
Hide your face from my sins
and blot out all my iniquity.
Create in me a pure heart, O God,
and renew a steadfast spirit within me.
Do not cast me from your presence
or take your Holy Spirit from me.
Restore to me the joy of your salvation
and grant me a willing spirit, to sustain me.
Then I will teach transgressors your ways,
and sinners will turn back to you.
(PSALM 51:3-13)

Note David's passionate desire to restore his relationship with God. Note also his acknowledgment that God desires "truth in the inner parts." This is the essence of confession: giving up excuses, lies, and denial, and having a relationship with God built on the truth about ourselves and what we do. Our experiences with other people readily confirm that a relationship in which one or both parties are dishonest will be crippled or doomed. If you are a parent, at some point you no doubt have watched with a mixture of amusement and sadness as your child has attempted to lie his way out of an uncomfortable situation. You don't love him any less, but as long as he persists in the dishonesty, the basic fabric of your relationship will be compromised. We cannot expect a vibrant relationship with God under similar circumstances.

Thanksgiving

Gratitude, like honesty, is another necessity of a healthy relationship with God. It acknowledges the reality that we cannot take credit for all the good things in our life: our very existence, the gifts of spiritual birth and an unending relationship with Him that we ourselves could not earn, family and friends—even each heartbeat. From one end to the other, the Scriptures exhort us to give this acknowledgment. "Give thanks to the Lord, for he is good; his love endures forever," says the psalmist numerous times (see, for example, Psalm 118:29 and 136:1). "Pray continually; give thanks in all circumstances, for this is God's will for you in Christ Jesus," says the apostle Paul in 1 Thessalonians 5:17-18. The lyrics to an eighteenth-century hymn offer a wonderful perspective on the length and breadth of our dependence on God and our need to acknowledge all of His good gifts:

We plow the fields, and scatter
The good seed on the land,
But it is fed and watered
By God's almighty hand;
He sends the snow in winter,
The warmth to swell the grain,
The breezes and the sunshine,
And soft refreshing rain.

We thank Thee, then, O Father,
For all things bright and good,
The seed time and the harvest,
Our life, our health, and food;
No gifts have we to offer,
For all Thy love imparts,
But that which Thou desirest,
Our humble, thankful hearts.

[Refrain]
All good gifts around us
Are sent from heaven above,
Then thank the Lord,
O thank the Lord
For all His love.[19]

Thanking God for daily needs is, in the language of nutrition, a minimum daily requirement. Thinking beyond life's necessities to thank Him for everyday delights—a sunset, a child's laugh—is refreshing and therapeutic. Thanking Him for life itself—physical and spiritual—is music to His ears.

Adoration and praise

When we praise and adore God, prayer enters a realm where our communication is no longer about us at all—not what we've done, what we want, or even thanksgiving for what we experience. It is instead about making an effort to grasp what we can of God's essence, His character, who He is, and what He does. The Psalms are a rich source of expressions of adoration and praise that may blend worship with another spiritual discipline and may be used when alone or with other people. They may provoke singing, dancing, or even shouting. The last of the 150 psalms proclaims:

Praise the Lord!
Praise God in his sanctuary;
praise him in his mighty heavens!
Praise him for his mighty deeds;
praise him according to his excellent greatness!
Praise him with trumpet sound;
praise him with lute and harp!
Praise him with tambourine and dance;
praise him with strings and pipe!
Praise him with sounding cymbals;
praise him with loud clashing cymbals!
Let everything that has breath praise the Lord!
Praise the Lord!
(PSALM 150, ESV)

The idea of giving God praise may seem a little abstract (or perhaps overly emotional), but in fact we have similar experiences at much less sublime occasions. We cheer and chant in the stands as we root for our favorite sports teams. Popular singers and rock groups generate such adulation among their fans that these objects of affection are routinely called idols.

And speaking of objects of affection, the language with which lovers woo one another (or at least the words they once used) is often that of praise and adoration. Popular song lyrics, old and new—"You send me," "You light up my life," "You are the wind beneath my wings"—are expressions of "praise and adoration" for another person. Simpler statements such as "I love you" or "I appreciate you" still speak volumes as well. (Unfortunately, in too many long-term relationships this type of communication doesn't continue.)

In human relationships, praise and adoration usually arise from a starry-eyed and often unrealistic understanding of the object of one's attention. With God, the opposite is the case. "God, help me!" is often the regular prayer of the spiritual newborn. "God, You are awesome, amazing, incomparable" is the prayer that emerges as a person logs time studying and meditating on God's character and comes to appreciate His handiwork throughout the universe and in human lives.

Study and meditation: learning to listen

Study and meditation are two different disciplines with a similar purpose: hearing from God. Becoming familiar with the Bible's contents is as essential to spiritual growth as food is to physical functioning. Before He began His public ministry, Jesus spent forty days in the desert without food. When tempted to turn rocks into bread, He quoted from the book of Deuteronomy: "Man does not live on bread alone, but on every word that comes from the mouth of God" (Matthew 4:4). The message is profound: as critical as nourishment might be for a man who has not eaten for more than a month, feeding on God's words is actually more important. The psalmist describes God's Word as a "lamp to my feet and a light for my path" (Psalm 119:105), a simile we might appreciate more fully after attempting to walk through unfamiliar terrain in the pitch dark. A frequently quoted passage in the New Testament confirms that the Scriptures are not a collection of manuscripts whose contents might be dismissed as historically interesting but otherwise irrelevant to the daily affairs of a twenty-first-century reader: "For the word of God is living and active. Sharper than any double-edged sword, it penetrates even to dividing soul and spirit, joints and marrow; it judges the thoughts and attitudes of the heart" (Hebrews 4:12).

The discipline of **study** involves taking the Bible seriously enough to learn about it and know its contents in detail. Study should always involve asking questions: Who wrote these sixty-six books in the Bible? Where did they come from? What stories do they tell, and what was their significance? Who were the patriarchs? What happened to the nation of Israel over the hundreds of years covered in the Old Testament? Who were the prophets and what was their mission? Who wrote Psalms and Proverbs, and what messages do these books of poetry contain? How does the Old Testament both predict the coming of a Messiah and give clues about His identity? What was going on in the ancient world when Jesus was born and during His public ministry? What did He teach? What did He say and do that stirred such controversy? What happened during the final week of His life? How did the news of His death and resurrection spread? What were the conflicts that developed among the first believers?

The study of the Scriptures should be an inquiring, active, challenging pursuit, not a passive, dumbed-down, rote learning experience (although memorization can certainly be a part of it). It should be focused on one or more reliable contemporary translations, such as the New International Version (NIV), the *New American Standard Bible* (NASB), the English Standard Version (ESV), or the

New King James Version (NKJV). (While the original King James Version is a landmark of both biblical translation and English literature, its four-hundred-year-old expressions may not communicate as effectively to a modern reader as the language in a contemporary translation.) Each Bible translation has numerous study editions, which contain detailed introductions, maps, and textual notes and explanations of challenging passages.

An overview of the Bible or an exploration of a particular book by a qualified teacher or pastor is also an excellent way to study the Scriptures. Many churches also offer ongoing small-group studies, which can serve a dual function of exploring the Bible and being involved with other people. These should be active, thoughtful, and hopefully interactive experiences. If a passage (or its explanation) doesn't seem to make sense, *ask about it* and investigate it further.

Meditation can occur at the same time as study and can certainly be propelled by it, but it is a different process—one by which the words and ideas in the Scriptures are assimilated into our thoughts, emotions, and behavior. This may involve a variety of activities:

- Reflecting on a particular passage—or even a single verse, turning it over and over in your mind throughout the day, pondering it, and considering how it applies to your life *now*.
- Vividly imagining a scene or a story. For example, after reading about Jesus' healing of the man blind from birth in the ninth chapter of the Gospel of John, imagine yourself in the middle of this situation. What would it be like to be blind from birth? How would that feel? What would it be like to be healed but then scorned by the religious rulers as a result?
- Committing single verses or entire passages to memory.
- Contemplating God's character, His attributes, and their specific expression in the life of Jesus. For example, consider this incident recorded in the Gospel of Mark:

> *People were bringing little children to Jesus to have him touch them, but the disciples rebuked them. When Jesus saw this, he was indignant. He said to them, "Let the little children come to me, and do not hinder them, for the kingdom of God belongs to such as these. I tell you the truth, anyone who will not receive the kingdom of God like a little child will never enter it." And he took the children in his arms, put his hands on them and blessed them.*
>
> (MARK 10:13-16)

What does this passage tell us about God's priorities? about how He views children? What is it about the children's faith that He appreciates? How does that compare to our attitude toward children and to the nature of our own faith? This brief paragraph contains a wealth of food for thought.

The Bible is full of advisories to meditate on God, His Word, and His precepts, and it is rich in descriptions of the benefits of doing so. The first Psalm offers this description of one who is truly blessed:

> *His delight is in the law of the Lord,*
> *and on his law he meditates day and night.*
> *He is like a tree planted by streams of water,*
> *which yields its fruit in season*
> *and whose leaf does not wither.*
> *Whatever he does prospers.*
> (PSALM 1:2-3)

Psalm 119, the longest single chapter in the entire Bible, is an extended review of the benefits of meditating on, delighting in, and internalizing God's Word and principles. These benefits include happiness, encouragement, freedom, comfort, restoration of joy and health, wisdom, and peace.

Needless to say, this type of meditation is quite different from the mind-emptying exercise of Eastern traditions and even from the relaxation response we discussed earlier. This is not ridding the mind of thought, but rather focusing one's thoughts on the Creator. Practicing meditation may be challenging, however, because our days tend to be saturated with noise from all directions. (Even our church services tend to be programmed down to the minute, such that a few minutes of silence for quiet reflection would seem like a giant stretch of dead air.) In order to meditate, we need to be very deliberate about setting a regular time, finding a quiet place, shutting off any potential sources of interruption (such as our phone), and sitting quietly for even a few minutes—or perhaps longer—to contemplate God's character or a passage of Scripture in one of the ways suggested on the previous page. This, of course, can be a time for prayer as well, but it is worth making a specific effort to *listen* for God's leading during this special time.

Other spiritual disciplines

A number of other disciplines are specifically mentioned in Scripture and have been practiced over the millennia by followers of Christ who have earnestly sought spiritual growth. We will mention several of them here and then recommend some excellent resources for further exploration of this important subject. Remember that these are not meant to become part of a burdensome to-do list or to generate a sense of nonstop guilt and inadequacy. Consider this frequently quoted but profound promise of Jesus—indeed, one that would be an excellent subject for contemplation: "Come to me, all you who are weary and burdened, and I will give you rest. Take my yoke upon you and learn from me, for I am gentle and humble in heart, and you will find rest for your souls. For my yoke is easy and my burden is light" (Matthew 11:28-30).

Fellowship

We mentioned in the previous chapter that isolation is not good for emotional health, and it is also not conducive to spiritual health. From infancy, our physical and emotional growth and development are profoundly affected by our interactions with those around us. We are meant to be raised in a loving and secure family. The same is true after spiritual birth. We cannot experience authentic spiritual growth and maturity in isolation.

The apostle Paul writes at length that the followers of Christ are very much like a physical body, where the abilities and gifts of the various parts are all necessary for the proper function of the whole. We need to commit ourselves to spending time around others in the setting of a local church for mutual encouragement, teaching, prayer, and opportunities for service. It is in this setting that we can also find a "learning laboratory" of sorts, where we will interact with people whom we may find congenial or disagreeable. This will provide opportunities for (and challenges to) spiritual growth in the all-important arena of loving people. Indeed, the way we deal with conflict within our own spiritual family can and should serve as a model for settling disagreements graciously within our extended families and wider communities. Furthermore, a number of important spiritual disciplines, including service, worship, and celebration, involve interacting and bonding with others, as we will see.

Worship

Worship encompasses elements of prayer, meditation, and fellowship and may involve music, celebration, or complete silence. We usually think of worship as occurring in the context of a structured service for which people have gathered for that specific purpose. However, it is possible to sit through a "worship service"—or many of them—while feeling unmoved, distant from God, and unaware of God's presence. It is also possible to have a profound experience of worship while watching a sunrise, taking a walk in the park, or driving to work. Worship, like the other spiritual disciplines, involves some deliberate decisions and practice. While an experience of worship may occur as a joyful surprise in an unexpected setting, we shouldn't wait passively for worship to happen to us.

Years ago Bob Dylan wrote the song "Gotta Serve Somebody," which made a cogent point: No matter what you do or who you are, "you're gonna have to serve somebody." We could make the same point about worship: Rich or poor, powerful or weak, young or old, everyone worships something or someone. Whatever drives us, stirs us, draws us, will be, in a very real sense, the object of our worship. We may not be conscious of holding the possessions, pursuits, or people in our life in such esteem, but to the degree that they capture our emotions and devotion, we give them *worth*—the root of the word *worship.* As we grasp who God is, what He has done for us, and how much He loves us, the only sensible response is to make Him the object of our worship. Worship is not meant to be limited to one hour each week; learning to worship God on a daily basis is a lifelong pursuit.

Worship can certainly occur while we pray, and it can be inspired by reading and meditating on Scripture (especially the psalms). Singing and listening to music that glorifies God can often usher us into an experience of worship. We can also make the most of a weekly worship service by *preparing* for it. We can pray that God will meet us there. We can strive to get a good night's sleep before a morning service. We can allow enough time to get ourselves and our family members ready, so we arrive without feeling hurried and harried.

We also need to remember that worship doesn't always involve an emotional experience. It is indeed more of a decision and an attitude than a particular set of emotions. Worship that occurs when we're not feeling particularly inspired or when we feel like we're in a spiritual dry spot may bring about more growth than worship that occurs in a state of great enthusiasm.

Some excellent resources that explore the role of worship in our life are *Worship* (Chosen Books, 2003) and *Worship His Majesty: How Praising the King of Kings Will Change Your Life* (Gospel Light Publications, 2000), both written by Jack Hayford.

Fasting, solitude, and silence

These three disciplines are relatively foreign in Western culture, where food is abundant, socializing is celebrated, and conversation is normal and usually nonstop in our lives. Obviously, there is nothing wrong with eating and interacting with others. Indeed, these are vital to our physical and emotional health. But planned, limited spans of time during which we abstain from one of these necessities for the specific purpose of drawing near to God may have a profound effect on the quality of our relationship with Him. There are many potential benefits, but two are worth noting: grasping God's sufficiency in any and all circumstances and coming to grips with our dependence on all the stuff that surrounds us (and releasing it). The apostle Paul, writing while in captivity, summarizes a mind-set that would be a worthy objective for all of us: "I have learned to be content whatever the circumstances. I know what it is to be in need, and I know what it is to have plenty. I have learned the secret of being content in any and every situation, whether well fed or hungry, whether living in plenty or in want. I can do everything through him who gives me strength" (Philippians 4:11-13).

A fast need not be a marathon lasting days or weeks to have an impact on spiritual growth. In fact, small steps taken on a regular basis are the most appropriate way to approach this practice. For example, you might bypass one or at most two meals on a day chosen each week for this purpose, while taking enough water to remain hydrated. The idea is not to earn a merit badge from God (or anyone else) for being miserable but rather to remain cheerful and focused on God's adequacy through the day. Jesus issued a caution about appearances and purposes for this activity: "When you fast, do not look somber as the hypocrites do, for they disfigure their faces to show men they are fasting. I tell you the truth, they have received their reward in full. But when you fast, put oil on your head and wash your face, so that it will not be obvious to men that you are fasting, but only to your Father, who is unseen; and your Father, who sees what is done in secret, will reward you" (Matthew 6:16-18).

A specific focus for the time spent without food is appropriate—perhaps prayer for one's children or community, or listening to God for guidance about a current issue at home or work. It is also fruitful to record your thoughts and reactions to the process, especially as it is practiced over time.

Because fasting could have medical implications for some individuals, we want to add a few cautions regarding this practice. Fasts lasting more than one or two days are best carried out after gaining some experience with shorter fasts, after some study on the subject, and ideally after input from someone experienced in this practice. Individuals with chronic medical problems such as diabetes, heart disease, or cancer, as well as people taking multiple medications, should carefully review any fasting plans with their physician. Pregnant women and nursing mothers should explore practices other than fasting for spiritual growth. For those with eating disorders (bulimia or anorexia, described in the previous chapter), eating appropriate amounts of food on a regular basis—and *not* fasting—is a critical discipline for both physical and spiritual health, as is ongoing accountability to a counselor and a dietitian.

F.Y.I. **A popular but unfounded notion holds that any discomforts one might feel in the early days of a prolonged fast result from the body ridding itself of accumulated "toxins" acquired from the environment or poor eating habits. There is no reasonable scientific evidence to support such a claim.**

It is worth noting that we can also grow by "fasting" from items other than food. We might benefit, for example, by fasting for a day, a week, or even longer from television, newspapers, or the Internet (especially chat rooms, games, or random browsing), which may be soaking up a lot of our time without yielding much benefit to mind, emotions, or spirit. Diverting that time to studying the Scriptures, meditating, praying, or serving others could prove so rewarding that a fast—or at least a limit on how much time we spend with media—might become a long-term habit. Other useful fasts might include a decision to abstain for a day or more from complaining about circumstances, criticizing others (especially family members), gossiping, or other forms of negativity. If these are long-standing habits, curtailing them—even for a few hours at a time—may be very challenging. But doing so can serve as an opportunity to rely on God on a moment-by-moment basis.

Solitude and silence, like fasting, do not need to be undertaken in epic lengths to have an impact on spiritual growth. A morning or afternoon once a month, for example, might be set aside to spend time alone with God—to think, pray, listen, read, and reflect on Scripture and write down some thoughts. Longer periods of time—a weekend or more at a retreat center, for example—require more planning and preparation, as well as appropriate provision for the well-being of other family members.

Some excellent suggestions for the implementation of these practices may be found in a contemporary classic on spiritual disciplines, *Celebration of Discipline* by Richard J. Foster (HarperCollins Publishers, 1978, 1988, 1998).

Service and secrecy

These related disciplines can help loosen the grip of our need for influence and recognition. Prior to His last meal, Jesus carried out a remarkable object lesson for His disciples, who had repeatedly argued with one another over which of them was the greatest:

> *Jesus knew that the Father had put all things under his power, and that he had come from God and was returning to God; so he got up from the meal, took off his outer clothing, and wrapped a towel around his waist. After that, he poured water into a basin and began to wash his disciples' feet, drying them with the towel that was wrapped around him. . . .*
>
> *When he had finished washing their feet, he put on his clothes and returned to his place. "Do you understand what I have done for you?" he asked them. "You call me 'Teacher' and 'Lord,' and rightly so, for that is what I am. Now that I, your Lord and Teacher, have washed your feet, you also should wash one another's feet. I have set you an example that you should do as I have done for you. I tell you the truth, no servant is greater than his master, nor is a messenger greater than the one who sent him. Now that you know these things, you will be blessed if you do them.*
>
> (JOHN 13:3-5, 12-17)

A passage in the New Testament that was probably an early hymn describes a mind-set that is anything but intuitive for us:

> *Your attitude should be the same as that of Christ Jesus:*
> *Who, being in very nature God,*
> *did not consider equality with God something to be grasped,*
> *but made himself nothing,*
> *taking the very nature of a servant,*
> *being made in human likeness.*
> *And being found in appearance as a man,*
> *he humbled himself*
> *and became obedient to death—*
> *even death on a cross!*
> (PHILIPPIANS 2:5-8)

Both of these passages stress that Jesus carried out these remarkable acts with full awareness of His position as Teacher, Lord, and God Himself, yet He didn't need or demand human recognition. The continuation of the latter passage tells us where the only meaningful recognition comes from:

Therefore God exalted him to the highest place
and gave him the name that is above every name,
that at the name of Jesus every knee should bow,
in heaven and on earth and under the earth,
and every tongue confess that Jesus Christ is Lord,
to the glory of God the Father.
(PHILIPPIANS 2:9-11)

We are not, of course, eligible to receive the honor that belongs to Christ alone, nor should that be our primary concern. Nevertheless, God makes it clear that His rewards are the only ones that have any lasting value, and that all of the possessions and recognition we so diligently seek—what He calls our treasures—are all destined to become landfill. "Do not store up for yourselves treasures on earth, where moth and rust destroy, and where thieves break in and steal. But store up for yourselves treasures in heaven, where moth and rust do not destroy, and where thieves do not break in and steal. For where your treasure is, there your heart will be also" (Matthew 6:19-21).

Many of these permanent treasures accrue not just from acts of service and obedience to Him, but from the attitude and posture with which they are carried out. Just as Jesus warns against making a public display of prayer and fasting to get recognition, He warns against showy acts of service:

Be careful not to do your "acts of righteousness" before men, to be seen by them. If you do, you will have no reward from your Father in heaven.

So when you give to the needy, do not announce it with trumpets, as the hypocrites do in the synagogues and on the streets, to be honored by men. I tell you the truth, they have received their reward in full. But when you give to the needy, do not let your left hand know what your right hand is doing, so that your giving may be in secret. Then your Father, who sees what is done in secret, will reward you. (MATTHEW 6:1-4)

The disciplines of service and secrecy can often be linked in a powerful way. Acts of service involve gifts of our time and resources in arenas where there is no direct payback. There is nothing wrong with earning a wage for the work we do, of course, but there also is much to be gained from serving those who have little or nothing to offer in return—the poor, the weak, the severely handicapped, the imprisoned, the elderly, the unborn—the "least of these" as Jesus called them. Every community has an unlimited supply of opportunities for service, whether carried out with others (such as through a church or service organization) or on our own when a need comes to our attention—for example, helping out a single parent next door or at work who is ill, or visiting a nursing-home resident for whom family members or friends are in short supply. In chapter 8, you can pick up several ideas for service in the section dealing with cultivating a broader circle of relationships (see page 360).

Ideally, whatever we do arises from genuine concern (perhaps even a direct "tap on the shoulder" from God) and will prove to be satisfying in and of itself. We can, of course, perform acts of service for all sorts of reasons that are not particularly conducive to spiritual growth, including guilt, pressure from others, and (quite commonly) the desire for approval from others whose opinions we value. This is where the discipline of secrecy may enter the picture.

We all tend to avoid taking responsibility for something we have done wrong, and we *really* find it hard not to get credit for what we have done right—especially if it has involved considerable effort or even sacrifice. Yet we are told that if our primary reason for our acts of service is to gain recognition from others, then whatever we get now will be all there is—a paltry sum in God's economy. The discipline of secrecy involves a deliberate decision to carry out virtuous acts without others knowing about them. This doesn't mean, of course, that we can't enjoy the recognition of others for a job well done or shouldn't graciously acknowledge it. (It also does not mean that we should withhold praise and recognition from others, especially within our own family.) The purpose of the discipline of secrecy is to become free of a constant need and striving for approval from others.

In a wonderful chapter on this discipline in *The Life You've Always Wanted,* John Ortberg provides some concrete examples of ways to practice this discipline:

> The opportunities for practicing secrecy are all around. Pick someone in your life and immerse that person in prayer—and don't tell anyone. Make a lavish donation to an organization, or send a sacrificial gift to a person in need—and keep it anonymous. Live so deeply with a portion of Scripture that it becomes etched on your mind and heart—and don't tell anyone you have memorized it. Mow your neighbor's lawn. Follow the bumper sticker that says, "Commit random acts of kindness and senseless beauty."[20]

It should come as no surprise that acts of service, especially those done secretly, may not always come naturally or easily. Like any other discipline, we learn as we take steps (even little ones) in the right direction and see what happens. Indeed, we can learn a lot from our mistakes and failures. What matters most is keeping the big picture in mind—allowing God to change us through these actions so that we can love Him and others more freely and consistently.

Celebration

An important reminder: Spiritual disciplines are activities that are meant to bring growth and freedom, not repression and added burdens. Furthermore, they are not intended to be joy killers or fun regulators. Jesus said, "I have come that they might have life, and have it to the full" (John 10:10). He didn't say that His purpose was to make life drab, shallow, or humorless, although some of His followers over the centuries have sadly made that their mission.

To provide a unique perspective on spiritual matters, C. S. Lewis wrote the incisive (and quite witty) classic *The Screwtape Letters,* in which a senior demon, Screwtape, attempts to instruct a junior tempter on preventing and later derailing a man's relationship with God (whom Screwtape refers to as "the Enemy"). In one letter he laments about the demons' limitations in using pleasure as a weapon:

> Never forget that when we are dealing with any pleasure in its healthy and normal and satisfying form, we are, in a sense, on the Enemy's ground. I know we have won many a soul through pleasure. All the same, it is His invention, not ours. He made the pleasures: all our research so far has not enabled us to produce one. All we can do is to encourage the humans to take the pleasures which our Enemy has produced, at times, or in ways, or in degrees, which He has forbidden. Hence we always try to work away from the natural condition of any pleasure to that in which it is least natural, least redolent of its Maker, and least pleasurable.[21]

Much of our culture's understanding of celebration is that of partying, which all too often can become a mindless and meaningless exercise in excessive alcohol, noise, and even shallow sexuality. This, as Screwtape describes, does little more than steer straightforward pleasures—diversion from work, music, laughter, and friendship—into dark and even dangerous territory.

But celebration can and should actually draw us closer to God and those around us. We can celebrate God in a worship service, an informal gathering for singing, or a concert. We can honor events in Jesus' life: not only His birth, which requires some effort to keep in focus amidst the other December traditions, but also the events leading to His death and, most importantly, His triumph over death. We can celebrate other national holidays such as Thanksgiving (which has an obvious focus on God's generosity), Independence Day, Memorial Day, and the birthdays of presidents and heroes by enjoying festivities and food while honoring God's role in these events. We can show our appreciation for those we love at birthdays, weddings, anniversaries, and even memorial services. Jesus' first public miracle involved turning more than a hundred gallons (around four hundred liters) of water into wine at a wedding—a clear indication that He was hardly one to put a damper on a celebration. Indeed, He was attacked by His glum and irritable critics for attending feasts and banquets (especially when they were hosted by the "wrong" sort of people).

Laughter—not ridicule—should be present and accounted for at these events (even the more serious ones). It is a gift from God, serving both to lighten our load and prevent us from taking ourselves too seriously. In another of his diabolical letters, Screwtape describes joy, fun, and laughter as quite detestable:

> I divide the causes of human laughter into Joy, Fun, the Joke Proper, and Flippancy. You will see the first among friends and lovers reunited on the eve of a holiday. . . . Laughter of this kind does us no good and should always be discouraged. Besides, the phenomenon is of itself disgusting and a direct insult to the realism, dignity, and austerity of Hell.
>
> Fun is closely related to Joy—a sort of emotional froth arising from the play instinct. It is very little use to us. It can sometimes be used, of course, to divert humans from something else which the Enemy would like them to be feeling or doing: but in itself it has wholly undesirable tendencies; it promotes charity, courage, contentment, and many other evils.[22]

Earlier in this chapter we quoted Psalm 150's admonition for us to sing, dance, shout, and play musical instruments to honor God. We will close this chapter with a reminder from another Psalm that we have our own cause for celebration: He has rescued us, restored us, welcomed us, and turned despair into rejoicing: This is the essence of spiritual health, and it brings joy that can transcend whatever circumstances of life or conditions of physical health we might experience during our brief time on earth.

> *You turned my wailing into dancing;*
> *you removed my sackcloth and clothed me with joy,*
> *that my heart may sing to you and not be silent.*
> *O Lord my God, I will give you thanks forever.*
> (PSALM 30:11-12)

FOR FURTHER READING

THE PURPOSE-DRIVEN LIFE
by Rick Warren
(ZONDERVAN, 2002)
Provides a straightforward look at the basics of spiritual growth and health. It's written in forty short chapters that lend themselves nicely to daily, step-at-a-time reading.

MERE CHRISTIANITY
by C. S. Lewis
(HARPERCOLLINS, 2001)
A classic and compelling explanation of the foundational teachings of the Bible.

THE LIFE YOU'VE ALWAYS WANTED
by John Ortberg
(ZONDERVAN, 1997)
An engaging and irresistible introduction to the spiritual disciplines.

CELEBRATION OF DISCIPLINE
by Richard Foster
(HARPERCOLLINS, 1978)
This classic book provides a more comprehensive look at twelve key disciplines.

THE SPIRIT OF THE DISCIPLINES
by Dallas Willard
(HARPERCOLLINS, 1988)
For those wanting even more substance, Willard's book provides deeper underpinnings for these practices.

QUESTIONS TO PONDER:

1. Before reading this chapter, had you ever considered the relationship between spiritual issues and your physical health?
2. Have you ever discussed spiritual issues with a health-care provider? Do you wish such discussions were included as a regular part of your care? If your spiritual, moral, or ethical values have been discussed in connection with some aspect of your health care, did your physician affirm, ignore, or belittle your views?
3. Scientific research and statistics aside, can you point to an instance in which you (or a loved one) recovered from or were healed of a physical illness or injury, which you personally attribute to answered prayer or divine intervention?
4. Where would you consider yourself on your own spiritual journey? A skeptic? An inquirer? An observer? A beginner? A seasoned explorer? What factors are propelling—or inhibiting—your beginning a relationship with God, if you haven't done so already?
5. As you think about the illustration of spiritual growth as learning how to sail (see page 405), where would you place yourself in that analogy? Are you drifting with the currents? Are you making any effort to "raise your sails" on a regular basis? Are you studying how and where the wind blows? Do you become impatient waiting for the wind and take matters into your own hands? (In this analogy, are you like someone putting an outboard motor in the water so that you can go where and when you want?)
6. How does the idea of sitting quietly for a half hour a few days every week to read Scripture and meditate on God's character strike you?
   a. A nice idea, if I just had the time.
   b. A nice idea, if I just had a quiet place to sit.
   c. A nice idea, if my mind wouldn't wander.
   d. A nice idea, if my kids would leave me alone for two minutes.
   e. A waste of my precious time.
   f. I'm willing to give it a try.
   g. I'm already doing this, and it's making a difference in my life.

   What would it take for you to move from one of the first five answers to one of the last two?

Action items: Look again at the second of the "Questions to Ponder" on the previous page. If you sense that your health-care provider is not supportive of your spiritual, moral, or ethical values and that this is affecting important medical decisions, set a time to discuss your concerns, or perhaps express them in a letter.

If you have not already taken the steps listed in this chapter to begin the journey of spiritual life and health, review that section of the chapter and seek counsel from a trusted, mature Christian or church leader. If you have more questions or are just now taking that step, you can also obtain some helpful information by calling (800) A-FAMILY.

If you have already begun your spiritual journey, choose *one* of the three spiritual disciplines that were emphasized in this chapter—prayer, study, or meditation—that you feel you need to learn more about or perhaps deserves more of your time or attention. What's the first step you could take to begin practicing that discipline regularly?

Of the other disciplines mentioned in this chapter—fellowship, worship, fasting, solitude, silence, service, secrecy, and celebration—consider which one (or more) of these might be most useful for promoting your spiritual growth. You can learn more about them (and a number of others) in the excellent books on spiritual disciplines listed on page 423.

Speaking of excellent books, consider making a commitment to read the books mentioned in this chapter over the next year or two. (No need to rush—take the time to ponder and absorb their content.)

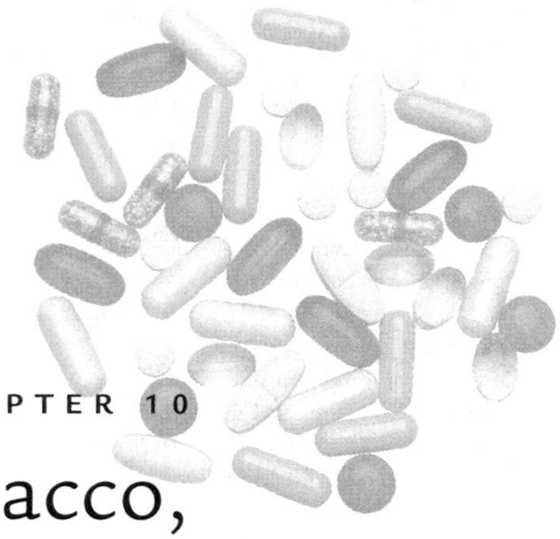

CHAPTER 10

Bad Habits: Tobacco, Alcohol, and Drugs

From time immemorial, young and old alike have found that certain items offer a pleasant experience when chewed, swallowed, drunk, inhaled, smoked, or (with advances in technology) injected into the body. Very often, the escape from pain, stress, a sad mood, normal emotions, or reality itself leaves a lasting impression . . . and a desire to repeat the experience. The more intense the pleasure (or relief), the stronger the attraction—and the more likely that the source of pleasure will become a ball and chain. As the substance, whatever it is, washes through the brain again and again, a hook is set, and a person begins to feel uneasy (or miserable) until the next dose arrives. More often than not, the longer this cycle continues, the more the whole body suffers—or even dies prematurely.

In this chapter we will take an unpleasant but necessary look at some products that cost all of us dearly, even if we don't use any of them. People in every country on earth spend vast sums of money purchasing tobacco, alcohol, and drugs (legal and otherwise) that all too often prove to be habit-forming, damaging to body and mind, and disruptive to families, communities, and entire nations. Many billions (in every currency) are spent on health care, counseling, and rehabilitation. Untold amounts disappear through lost productivity, crime, legal fees, welfare payments, and programs intended to combat the distribution of these substances and prevent their use. All in all, it is heartbreaking to ponder the extent of these losses and the misery that accompanies them. It is also staggering to consider what might be accomplished if all of the resources these substances drain could be put to other uses.

This chapter is for anyone who struggles with a substance problem or knows someone who does (even if he or she doesn't acknowledge it). In other

Substance abuse in the United States is estimated to cost its citizens more than $484 billion per year. Of this staggering amount, $138 billion is related to smoking, $185 billion to alcohol abuse, and $161 billion to illegal drugs. One out of four deaths in the United States every year can be linked in some way to these substances.[1]

words, it is for everyone. Most people who have become ensnared by tobacco, alcohol, and/or addictive drugs—often more than one substance is involved—will need more than a book to set them free. They will need, to varying degrees, encouragement, accountability, prayer, counseling, and perhaps even medical attention. Our purpose isn't to wring our hands or wag our finger at them, but rather to acknowledge the gravity of the problem, provide some motivation to change, suggest some beginning steps, and offer direction toward additional resources that could be helpful or even lifesaving. In addition, we will make a strong case for the ounce of prevention: taking positive steps to keep children and teenagers away from substances that could require many pounds of cure later on.

Tobacco: Big Business, Bigger Costs

Let's start with a little history.

Many centuries before Europeans arrived in the New World, leaves of the tobacco plant were used by indigenous peoples throughout Central and South America as a medicine, mood elevator, accompaniment to religious ceremonies, and appetite suppressor when food was in short supply. Like the potato, tomato, and eggplant, tobacco was native to the Americas and unknown in other parts of the globe before 1500. Christopher Columbus and his crew were offered tobacco leaves (along with other valuables) by natives upon their arrival in the Americas in 1492, but the sailors, apparently finding no use for them, tossed them overboard. As European exploration continued, however, more voyagers and merchants became aware of the pleasurable effects of tobacco, and by the mid-1500s, it had been introduced and dispersed throughout the continent and England. Within a hundred years, it had been taken to every corner of the globe. The first English colonists carried tobacco back to North America, where its cultivation grew to enormous economic importance in mid-Atlantic and Southern states. It was in fact a literal cash crop, serving as currency in many areas for nearly two hundred years.

Native Americans had long believed in tobacco's curative powers, and many European physicians of the early 1600s proclaimed that it could cure everything from cancer to broken bones and could even prevent bubonic plague. No doubt their enthusiasm flowed from having few reliable treatments for any serious health problem, combined with the key factor that has kept tobacco so popular for more than five hundred years: Once a first-time user overcomes the body's natural resistance to inhaling smoke, sniffing a foreign substance, or chewing something that lacks the taste appeal of any food, tobacco offers a payoff that is usually irresistible: a unique combination of relaxation and stimulation. If it could help someone feel better rather quickly, as it often did, one might conclude that it must be good for "whatever ails ya."

Of course, not everyone embraced tobacco use. A number of rulers and governments felt it necessary, for various reasons, to decree tobacco use a punishable offense: the pope in 1624, Massachusetts in 1632, Czar Alexis of Russia in 1634, China in 1638, New Amsterdam (soon renamed New York) in 1639, among many others. All of these prohibitions were eventually repealed because of tobacco's spreading popularity among leaders and commoners alike. Some doctors, however, began to notice serious health problems among its users. In 1761 English physician John Hill warned snuff users that they were at risk for cancer of the nose. Some thirty years later, Sammuel Thomas von Soemmering of Maine described lip cancer in pipe smokers. In the late 1790s, America's most famous eighteenth-century doctor, Benjamin Rush, wrote not only about medical hazards connected with tobacco but identified what would be called the gateway effect two centuries later: Smoking or chewing tobacco, he warned, led to drunkenness. Nicotine was identified in 1826, and within two years German researchers described it as a dangerous poison.

F.Y.I.

The scientific name of the most widely cultivated tobacco plant is *Nicotiana tabacum,* from which we derive two common words. *Nicotiana,* the source of the word *nicotine,* comes from the name of French ambassador Jean Nicot. In 1560, Nicot sent some tobacco to Catherine de Medicis, who had been the queen of France. *Tabacum,* the basis for the word *tobacco,* probably hearkens back to the Arabic word *tabaq,* a euphoria-producing herb.

By 1900 Americans were purchasing about 2.5 billion cigarettes every year, even as legislators in four states outlawed their sale. By 1902, the Sears, Roebuck and Company catalog featured a "Sure Cure for the Tobacco Habit," and before the end of the decade fifteen states had outlawed cigarettes. The first medical paper to suggest that smoking was linked to lung cancer appeared in 1912. The disease was relatively rare, with only 371 cases reported in the United States in 1914. In 1930, 2,357 cases were reported, and in 1956, the number of lung-cancer deaths reached 29,000.[3] (Today lung cancer's annual death toll in America exceeds 160,000, and more than 170,000 new cases are diagnosed every year.)[4] Nevertheless, during the first half of the twentieth century many physicians were slow to recognize that tobacco might be harming their patients (and themselves). In the early 1950s free cigarettes were passed out at medical conventions, and some ads went so far as to show doctors happily puffing a particular brand or recommending it to patients as "easier on the throat."

Evidence of tobacco's connection to cancer accumulated relentlessly through the 1950s. A 1956 study involving forty thousand physicians, for example, demonstrated that those who smoked more than twenty-five cigarettes per day were twenty times more likely to die of lung cancer than nonsmokers. But there was no shortage of new customers as tobacco companies skillfully began to use television to market cigarettes. The first U.S. Surgeon General's report on cancer risks related to smoking appeared in 1964, the same year that the "Marlboro Country" ad campaign was launched. Another report from the Surgeon General showing that heart disease was even a greater risk to smokers

GREAT MOMENTS IN TOBACCO ADVERTISING

"I'd walk a mile for a Camel!" (Slogan launched in 1921 multi-million-dollar ad campaign)

. . .

Philip Morris originally sponsored the phenomenally popular sitcom *I Love Lucy* when it debuted in 1951. Because Lucky Strike cigarettes were Philip Morris's leading competition, the sponsor would not allow the word *lucky* to be used on the show.[2]

than cancer did not appear until 1979. By then, however, smoking had been successfully promoted to women as a means of demonstrating independence and sophistication. "You've got your own cigarette now, baby—you've come a long, long way," claimed one famous jingle. A long way, indeed. Smoking among women increased dramatically between 1940 and 1960, and so did the number of women suffering from lung cancer. According to the Centers for Disease Control and Prevention (CDC), in 1950 lung cancer accounted for 3 percent of all deaths from cancer in women; by 2000 it was 25 percent.

GREAT MOMENT IN TOBACCO ADVERTISING
Marlboro is introduced in 1924 as a cigarette for women that is "mild as May."

How much tobacco do we use?

In terms of pure consumption, the success of the tobacco industry over the past century has been nothing less than spectacular. According to the World Health Organization, in 1900 about 50 billion cigarettes were smoked around the world. One hundred years later, at the dawn of a new millennium, 5.5 *trillion* cigarettes were consumed—a mind-boggling 15 billion every day, or about one thousand cigarettes every year for every man, woman, and child on the planet. China, whose citizens smoke more than 1.64 trillion cigarettes every year, is the world's leading tobacco customer, followed by the United States, where consumers inhaled more than 388 billion cigarettes (roughly 1,800 per person) in 2004.[5] Americans also buy more than 100 million pounds of so-called smokeless tobacco every year.[6]

F.Y.I. In 1900, the use of cigarettes averaged about fifty per person per year in the United States. In 1963, the all-time-high per capita consumption rate was reached: more than 4,300 cigarettes for every American. This number has steadily declined since that year, although the total number of cigarettes consumed in the United States peaked at 640 billion in 1981.[7]

CDC figures indicate that as of 2003, 21.6 percent of American adults over eighteen (or about 45.4 million people) were current users of cigarettes. Sadly, the highest rates were among the youngest adults: Nearly 24 percent of eighteen- to twenty-four-year-olds and 26 percent of twenty-five- to forty-four-year-olds were smokers.[8] Even worse: More than 11 percent of pregnant women were smoking in 2002.[9] Worse yet: As of 2004, 22.3 percent of high school students identified themselves as current smokers, although rates have been slowly declining since 1997. Among ninth graders the smoking rate was nearly 24 percent; for twelfth graders, it was more than 35 percent.[10] More than 80 percent of habitual smokers started before the age of eighteen—in many cases, at a much younger age—and more than five thousand adolescents try their first cigarette every day. The CDC estimates that more than 6.4 million children alive today will die prematurely because of a decision to try smoking before they reach adulthood. One alarming trend among teenagers is the rising popularity of inexpensive fruit- and candy-flavored cigarettes called bidis and clove-containing cigarettes called kreteks.

Cigarettes represent well over 90 percent of tobacco sales.

F.Y.I.

The term *current smoker* in most reports indicates a person who has smoked at least once during the past thirty days. More than half of those who identify themselves as current smokers in such surveys smoke more than fifteen cigarettes per day.[11]

Rates of smokeless tobacco use vary considerably by age and sex. CDC statistics suggest that about 3.5 percent of adults in the United States are current users of smokeless tobacco, but men outnumber women by a ratio of nearly thirteen to one. The use of smokeless tobacco has nearly tripled in the past twenty years, with a dramatic increase among adolescents. In a 2004 survey, nearly 11 percent of boys and 1.4 percent of girls in grades nine through twelve reported smokeless tobacco use at least once during the previous month. This rate is significantly higher than among adults.[12] Usage rates are even higher in many Native American populations.

GREAT MOMENTS IN TOBACCO ADVERTISING

"Not a cough in a carload!" (Long-standing slogan for Old Gold cigarettes, introduced in 1926)

. . .

"20,679 physicians say Luckies are less irritating." (1930 magazine ad)

What is tobacco use costing us?

Tobacco manufacturing in the United States is big business, involving a cash flow of nearly $24 billion every year.[13] Even with a ban on TV and radio advertising, U.S. cigarette manufacturers spent almost $12.5 billion in 2002,

WHAT ARE BIDIS AND KRETEKS?

Ever heard of a bidi? In India, 70 percent of tobacco is sold in the form of these small, inexpensive, sweet-tasting cigarettes that are rolled in leaves rather than paper. With flavors such as chocolate, vanilla, fruit, and root beer, an exotic appearance resembling a marijuana joint, and a popular misconception that they are additive free and somehow safer than regular cigarettes, bidis have caught on with American teenagers as well. They are especially popular in urban areas where they can be easily purchased in ethnic grocery stores, tobacco emporiums, and "head shops" catering to drug users. (Most grocery or convenience stores don't sell them, but that merely adds to their mystique.)

The Centers for Disease Control estimates that 2 to 5 percent of teenagers—up to 40 percent in some cities—have tried bidis at least once. Yet in spite of their candy flavoring and lower tobacco content, bidis actually pump more tar, nicotine, and carbon monoxide into young bodies than conventional cigarettes, both filtered and unfiltered. As a result, they pose a higher risk for causing tobacco addiction and long-term health consequences.

Kreteks are Indonesian cigarettes containing two-thirds tobacco and one-third clove. They're sold with or without filters and typically are wrapped in brown paper or even cornhusk. In some American cities, they are more popular than bidis. Unfortunately, they also come loaded with two to three times the nicotine of a regular cigarette. ■

promoting their products in newspapers, magazines, billboards, at sporting events, and by other means, such as giveaway promotions.[14] (Smokeless-tobacco producers spend quite a bit less but still pay well over $200 million per year for advertising and other promotions.)

But aside from the money spent manufacturing, marketing, and purchasing tobacco products, how much does our national tobacco habit cost us? A 2005 Centers for Disease Control summary of the price of cigarette smoking for the years 1997 to 2001 is eye-opening.

- Smoking was responsible for approximately 438,000 premature deaths annually, making it the leading preventable cause of death in the United States. The body count included more than 123,000 deaths from lung cancer, more than 90,000 from chronic lung disease, and nearly 87,000 from heart disease.[15]
- Cigarette smoking was calculated to be responsible for a total of 5,566,046 years of potential life lost among adults (3,349,072 combined years lost for men; 2,216,974 years lost for women). Men lost

GREAT MOMENT IN TOBACCO ADVERTISING

TV Guide's Commercial of the Year for 1950 is Lucky Strike's "Be Happy, Go Lucky," featuring cheerleaders singing, "Yes, Luckies get our loudest cheers / On campus and on dates. / With college gals and college guys / A Lucky really rates!"

TWO BIG REASONS WHY TOBACCO USE AMONG THE YOUNG IS A SERIOUS PROBLEM

First, almost every long-term smoker begins to light up during adolescence. Over the past two decades, the average age at which tobacco use begins has dropped from sixteen to twelve. The younger one becomes nicotine dependent, the more cigarettes one will smoke as an adult. The tobacco industry's annual multibillion-dollar advertising budget is supposedly intended to encourage adults to switch brands, but the cartoon characters, sexy young couples, macho men, and liberated women in cigarette ads have clearly been shown to influence children and adolescents. Heavy visibility of these ads at sporting and cultural events also sends definite signals that tobacco is hot stuff. Warnings issued in health-education classes pale in comparison. In one survey of high school smokers, more than 95 percent said they were aware of health risks, but 70 percent claimed they were not concerned enough to stop.

Second, cigarettes keep very bad company. Smoking is associated with significantly poorer school performance and a higher likelihood of sexual activity. Because the use of alcohol and marijuana is significantly greater among adolescent smokers, tobacco is identified as a gateway drug—one that increases the odds of a person using even more dangerous substances. It is the last of these points that should sound the alarm for parents of adolescent smokers. If your teenager is smoking cigarettes, he is seven times more likely to be using illicit drugs[16] and eleven times more likely to be drinking heavily than his nonsmoking counterparts.[17] ■

an average of 12.9 years of life because they smoked, while women smokers lost an average of 12.4 years.[18]

- Smoking was responsible for losses of $92 billion in mortality-related productivity and $75.5 billion in personal medical costs every year: a whopping $167.5 billion total.[19]
- Each pack of cigarettes sold in the United States costs our country an estimated $8.61 in medical-care expenses and lost productivity.[20]

And where does all this loss come from? A number of the key reasons are printed on every pack of cigarettes and every ad promoting them in the United States, which by a 1984 federal law must carry one of the following four warnings:

1. SURGEON GENERAL'S WARNING: Smoking Causes Lung Cancer, Heart Disease, Emphysema, and May Complicate Pregnancy.
2. SURGEON GENERAL'S WARNING: Smoking by Pregnant Women May Result in Fetal Injury, Premature Birth, and Low Birth Weight.
3. SURGEON GENERAL'S WARNING: Cigarette Smoke Contains Carbon Monoxide.
4. SURGEON GENERAL'S WARNING: Quitting Smoking Now Greatly Reduces Serious Risks to Your Health.

Forty years after the first Surgeon General's report to sound the alarm about the link between smoking and lung cancer, the twenty-eighth report, issued in May 2004, warned: "Smoking harms nearly every organ in the body." Its blunt conclusion: "Smoking remains the leading cause of preventable death and has negative impacts on people at all stages of life. It harms unborn babies, infants, children, adolescents, adults and seniors."

These statements reveal the tip of a mammoth iceberg of health problems that have been linked to cigarette use. One-half of all continuing smokers will die as a direct result of their habit, which kills more people in the United States than automobile accidents, homicides, suicides, AIDS, alcohol, and illegal drug abuse combined.[21] The risks include

- **Cancer** of the lung, mouth, throat, larynx (vocal cords), and esophagus. More than 85 percent of all lung cancers, the most lethal form of cancer, are caused by cigarette smoking. Men who smoke are twenty-three times more likely and women smokers thirteen times more likely to develop lung cancer than nonsmokers.[22] In addition, smoking has been linked to cancers of the bladder, kidney, cervix (the opening of the uterus), pancreas, and stomach.[23]
- **Cardiovascular disease.** Cigarette smoking is widely acknowledged to be the most important of the six known modifiable risk factors—that is, ones we can change—for clogging of arteries, and especially for coronary artery disease, the leading cause of death in the United States.[24] (The others are high blood pressure, elevated cholesterol, obesity, diabetes, and lack of exercise. Age, gender, and family history are the nonmodifiable risk factors.) Cigarettes also magnify the effects of the other risk factors and increase the odds that a heart attack will provoke life-threatening or fatal rhythm disturbances. Women who smoke and use oral contraceptives are much more likely to suffer a heart attack or stroke than their nonsmoking counterparts. In addition, cigarette use increases

Coronary artery disease, heart attack, and stroke are reviewed in detail in chapter 3.

GREAT MOMENTS IN TOBACCO ADVERTISING

In 1964 "Marlboro Country" ads introduce the "Marlboro Man" cowboy, using the heroic theme from *The Magnificent Seven.* In October 1995 Marlboro Man David McLean dies of lung cancer.

. . .

In 1968 Philip Morris introduces a new Virginia Slims ad campaign using the slogan "You've come a long way, baby." The ads portray smoking as a sign of sophistication and liberation for women. Six years later, the rate of smoking among twelve-year-old girls has increased more than 100 percent.[29]

. . .

In a vintage black-and-white TV commercial, cartoon characters Fred Flintstone and Barney Rubble puff on prehistoric cigarettes and declare that "Winston tastes good, like a cigarette should!"

the risk both for stroke and for clogging of the arteries of the legs, which can lead to disability or even amputation.

- **Chronic obstructive lung disease.** This affects 15 to 30 million Americans and kills nearly 125,000 annually (the fourth leading cause of death in the United States). Habitual cigarette use is implicated in 80 to 90 percent of cases.
- **Other health problems.** Smoking may provoke or aggravate peptic ulcer disease, heartburn, Crohn's disease (a form of inflammatory bowel disease),[25] osteoporosis in women, impotence in men, infertility in both sexes, dry and wrinkled skin,[26] and periodontal (gum) disease.[27] Indeed, hardly a month passes without an announcement of new research linking smoking to yet another malady.
- **Harm to unborn children.** Smoking before, during, and after pregnancy causes a host of problems for the preborn/newborn infant, as the nicotine, carbon monoxide, and other toxins found in Mom's cigarettes alter the baby's blood and nutrient supply. Cigarette use during pregnancy is associated with an increased risk of stillbirth, miscarriage, premature delivery, and a low birth-weight infant.[28] To make matters much worse, smoking during and after pregnancy is clearly implicated as an important factor in **sudden infant death syndrome (SIDS)**.
- Smoking harms more people than the one doing the inhaling. A growing body of research has implicated **environmental tobacco smoke (ETS)**, also called **secondhand smoke** or **passive smoking**, as a hazard to those exposed to it, whether arising from cigarettes smoldering in an ashtray or exhaled from someone else's lungs. Chronic exposure to ETS not only increases a nonsmoker's risk of developing lung cancer but also can provoke headaches, nausea, and eye irritation. The increased risk of sudden infant death syndrome in a smoking environment has been already mentioned. In addition, babies and children in smoking households—and especially those stuck with smoke in a confined space such as the inside of a car—are more prone to colds, ear infections, and asthma.[30] The American Lung Association estimates that every year in the United States secondhand smoke causes 150,000 to 300,000 bronchial and lung infections among children younger than eighteen months of age, resulting in 7,500 to 15,000 hospitalizations.[31]

What about cigars and pipes?

A generation ago, cigar smoking was generally viewed as an eccentric and annoying (because of the disagreeable odor) behavior of political bosses, noisy middle-aged male sports fans, poker players, and a few historical figures.

WHAT IS CHRONIC OBSTRUCTIVE LUNG DISEASE?

The phrase *chronic obstructive lung disease* (widely known as chronic obstructive pulmonary disease, or COPD for short) refers to a variety of problems that result in persistent difficulty exhaling air from the lungs. Normally air flows freely through a series of branching tubes called **bronchi** and **bronchioles** (the smaller branches) into millions of tiny air sacs in the lungs called **alveoli**, where oxygen enters the blood and carbon dioxide passes from the blood into air that will be exhaled. The bronchial tubes are lined with cells whose surface is covered with microscopic hairlike projections called **cilia**, as well as glands that produce mucus. Normally the cilia move in a coordinated pattern that moves mucus and debris (such as dust and microorganisms) upward toward the larger airways, where they can be cleared out. The structure of the bronchial tubes also contains a layer of muscle that can contract and tighten their diameter.

- In **chronic bronchitis,** the bronchial tubes become inflamed and damaged. The mucus cells work overtime and the cilia don't function properly, resulting in a pileup of mucus and debris. This provokes coughing, which may be particularly impressive in the morning (the so-called smoker's cough). Bacteria can gain a toehold more easily, resulting in more frequent and severe infections.
- In **asthmatic bronchitis,** the muscles surrounding the bronchial tubes are unusually twitchy, and their spasmodic contractions can dramatically narrow the diameter of large and small airways, resulting in wheezing. Extra mucus in the airway aggravates the problem.
- In **emphysema,** the alveoli (air sacs) are broken down, resulting in a loss of surface area for exchanging oxygen and carbon dioxide with the blood. (Think of a sponge in which all of the holes are large, preventing it from holding much water.)

Most people with COPD have all of these problems to varying degrees. The common feature is that air can enter the airways and lungs but has difficulty leaving. Symptoms can include ongoing coughing, shortness of breath (especially with exertion), wheezing, abnormally low oxygen levels, and high levels of carbon dioxide in the blood. The last of these can be a sign of respiratory failure, an ominous development if it cannot be corrected or at least stabilized. Needless to say, cigarette smoke, with its vast collection of irritants and carbon monoxide (which binds tightly to red blood cells, reducing the amount of oxygen they can carry), provokes and aggravates all of these conditions. ■

Vocabulary update: The word *bronchus* comes from the Greek word for "airway," and the suffix *-itis* means "inflamed," so the common term *bronchitis* thus means "inflamed airway." The word *emphysema* comes from the Greek for "bellows" or "bladder," suggesting the hollowed-out appearance of affected lung tissue. The word *alveolus* literally means "little hollow" or "little belly," a descriptive picture of an air sac.

By the way, we didn't mention pneumonia, which refers to inflammation of a segment of lung tissue, usually caused by bacteria or viruses, although other irritants (such as chemicals or even stomach contents that are accidentally inhaled) can cause it as well. Pneumonia is not a component of COPD, but it can certainly make a person with COPD much worse. Smoking hampers the body's recovery from either.

F.Y.I. Bearing the responsibility for an estimated three thousand nonsmoker lung-cancer deaths every year, environmental tobacco smoke has been formally recognized by the U.S. Environmental Protection Agency as a known (group A) human carcinogen (that is, cancer-causing agent).[32]

Over the past decade or so, however, cigar smoking became chic and hip (much like drinking gourmet coffee or microbrew beer) among thousands of younger enthusiasts, including many females. Because most cigar smokers don't inhale—the smoke, after all, is more irritating—many mistakenly believe that their favorite stogies are a relatively safe alternative to cigarettes. As a result, the sales of all forms of cigars—large and small, regular and premium, machine- and handmade, domestic and imported—have risen dramatically over the past two decades.

The most famous photographic portrait of Winston Churchill portrays him with a scowl, reportedly provoked when the photographer suddenly took away his cigar.

F.Y.I. The term *stogie* is an abbreviation for Conestoga, a valley in Lancaster County, Pennsylvania, and the famous wagons that originated there. Conestoga drivers were known for creating and smoking long, thin cigars made from the local tobacco.

Unfortunately, cigars can wreak the same type of havoc as their smaller, paper-wrapped counterparts. Regular cigar smokers (those who smoke one or more per day) are particularly prone to cancer of the lip, mouth, tongue, throat, larynx (vocal cords), and esophagus. Those who inhale are at a higher risk for all of these, and can add lung, pancreas, and bladder cancer to the list of dangers. Cigars appear to be as hard on the gums as cigarettes.[33] Respiratory and heart disease, as might be expected, are also more likely among cigar smokers (especially those who inhale) than nonsmokers, although not to the degree seen in cigarette users. However, as with cigarettes the likelihood of trouble increases with the number of cigars smoked every day and the duration of use. Furthermore, the impact of environmental tobacco smoke from cigars on nonsmokers may be worse than that from cigarettes. Cigars contain more tobacco than cigarettes, they burn much longer—up to two hours for a large specimen, compared to about seven minutes for a typical cigarette—and their smoke contains a higher concentration of toxic chemicals.[34]

And what about pipes? Despite whatever air of distinction or quaintness might be associated with pipe smoking, all of the health risks associated with regular cigar use also accrue with the daily puffing and inhaling of tobacco burned in a pipe. (Pipe smokers actually face a higher risk of developing cancer of the lip.) As with cigars, more frequent use and inhalation are associated with greater risk. The risk of occasional use of cigars or pipes, on the other hand, is less certain. But no one can say how much (or little) smoking might be considered safe.

What about smokeless tobacco?

Smokeless tobacco is the generic term for all forms that are not set on fire and inhaled into the throat or lungs. In bygone days these included dry powdered snuff that was sniffed up the nose, but today the term **snuff** usually refers to a form of finely ground tobacco, usually sold in cans, that is typically placed between the lower lip and gum. The classic chewing (or "chaw") tobacco comes in loose-leaf, plug, or twist forms, and a large wad may be kept in the mouth for hours at a time. Some health educators feel that the phrase smokeless tobacco is too dignified, noting that tobacco companies coined the term in order to give the impression that these products are somehow safer than cigarettes. To counter this trend, these educators use the less attractive term *spit tobacco.*[35]

The literal sniffing of snuff tobacco up the nose isn't extinct but is definitely more common in Europe than in the United States.

In 1986 the United States Surgeon General announced in no uncertain terms that using smokeless tobacco is not a safe alternative to smoking, and for good reason. Ongoing contact with tobacco wads irritates and damages the inside of the mouth. After as little as a week of regular use, and certainly within a few months, white patches called **leukoplakia** may become visible inside the mouth. Up to 6 percent of these become cancers, and tobacco chewers definitely bear an increased risk for developing tumors anywhere inside the mouth: lip, gums, tongue, inner surface of the cheeks, floor, or roof, not to mention larynx, throat, and esophagus. Smokeless tobacco is also hard on the teeth and gums, contributing to a variety of ailments including receding gums, tooth decay and loss, and thinning of the bone in the jaw. Staining of teeth and bad breath are other "bonuses" to be expected from habitual use. In addition, the various chemicals (including nicotine) absorbed from tobacco parked inside the mouth can increase the risk of high blood pressure, heart attack, and stroke.[36]

F.Y.I.

The risk for cancer of the cheek and gum may be as much as fifty times higher among smokeless tobacco users compared to nonusers. Sadly, surgical treatment for oral cancer can disfigure the face or jaw, and half of those who develop it do not survive more than five years.[37]

What exactly makes tobacco so bad for you?

Tobacco is not an agricultural product like an apple or a carrot that is simply harvested and then consumed in a pure form. Tobacco leaves must be **cured** or dried (to remove the sap from them), then aged for two to three years, during which time a chemical change called **fermentation** improves its aroma and taste. Various additives are used for a variety of purposes:

- To create a particular flavor
- To keep the tobacco moist
- To make the smoke easier to inhale (for example, menthol)
- To make secondhand smoke less objectionable
- To adjust the amount and speed of the nicotine effect in the smoker or chewer

GREAT MOMENT IN TOBACCO ADVERTISING

In exchange for $42,000, the makers of the 1981 movie *Superman II* included twenty-two exposures of the Marlboro logo. Lois Lane, who never smoked in fifty years as a comic-book character, chain-smokes Marlboro Lights in the movie.[38]

Tobacco industry documents supplied to the U.S. Department of Health and Human Services in 1994 listed 599 ingredients—not including nicotine, which is native to the tobacco plant—that may serve as additives in cigarettes.[39] (Manufacturers of smokeless tobacco products provided 562 on their list.)[40]

When processed tobacco leaves, additives, and wrapping paper are set on fire and inhaled, some four thousand chemical substances stream into the mouth, airways, and lungs. The particle residue of this material is called tar, in honor of its sticky brown appearance wherever it accumulates, whether on teeth, fingers, or in the lungs, where it is known to be especially harmful. Not surprisingly, a good number of tobacco-related compounds are not fit for consumption. They include

- **Carcinogens**—chemicals that are known to cause cancer. At least sixty have been identified in tobacco smoke and twenty-eight in smokeless tobacco.[41] A potent group of carcinogens, tobacco-specific nitrosamines (or TSNAs), are particularly abundant in cigars and smokeless tobacco.
- **Poisonous gases**, including **hydrogen cyanide**, **nitrogen oxides**, and especially **carbon monoxide**, the lethal odorless gas normally associated with car exhaust and malfunctioning heaters. Carbon monoxide binds strongly to hemoglobin in red blood cells, reducing the amount of oxygen they can carry and contributing to tobacco's harmful effects on the heart.
- **Nicotine**—the compound that gives tobacco both its primary appeal and its major addictive hook. Depending on the amount and speed of delivery, nicotine has the unique capacity to be stimulating and relaxing at the same time. Many consider it to be as physically and psychologically addictive as heroin or cocaine. (Indeed, it is not uncommon for people who have been successfully treated in alcohol and drug treatment programs to remain hooked on cigarettes.)

Smokers who attempt to reduce their cancer risk and tobacco dependence by switching to light or mild cigarettes that contain less tar and nicotine rarely accomplish their goal. Instead, the vast majority compensate (subconsciously or otherwise) by inhaling more deeply and frequently, or simply smoking more often, to absorb as much nicotine from their light brand as they were before. The bottom line is that smoking *any* brand, light or otherwise, is a health risk.

Tobacco worsens the quality of life for users and those around them in a number of other ways.

- The stale, rank smell of smoke permeates homes, cars, clothes, hair, and breath.
- The impaired sense of taste and smell hampers enjoyment of food.
- Clothes and upholstery are damaged from accidental tobacco burns.
- Ashes, cigarette and cigar butts, and wads of tobacco and saliva spit out by chewers create a foul mess.
- Major damage and loss of life results from fires set by people who fall asleep while smoking or who toss a burning cigarette into dry brush.
- Personal financial costs, such as the price of the tobacco product (over $2,900 per year for a two-pack per day smoker, assuming a tab

F.Y.I. According to the National Fire Protection Agency, smoking materials are the leading cause of fatal fires in the United States, resulting in approximately 830 deaths, 1,770 injuries, and more than $386 million in property damage every year.[42]

of $4.00 per pack) and increased life and health insurance premiums, are high.

- Smokers face increasing social isolation, as smoke-free environments become the rule rather than the exception in the United States.
- Smokers set a bad example for children and teenagers. Children of adults who smoke not only suffer exposure to health-robbing secondhand smoke but are more likely to use tobacco themselves.
- The gateway effect: Children and adolescents who smoke are not only more likely to use alcohol and illegal drugs but also to carry weapons, get involved in fights and high-risk sex, and attempt suicide.[43]

GREAT MOMENT IN TOBACCO ADVERTISING
In January 1971, cigarette ads are banned from television and radio.

How can a person become free of a tobacco habit?

Mark Twain once quipped, "Quitting smoking is easy. I've done it a thousand times." His wry observation speaks volumes about the iron grip that a tobacco habit so often exerts on its users. More than a century later, a detailed U.S. Public Health Service Clinical Practice Guideline entitled *Treating Tobacco Use and Dependence* pointed out:

> It is a testament to the power of tobacco addiction that millions of tobacco users have been unable to overcome their dependence and save themselves from its consequences: perpetual worry, unceasing expense, and compromised health.[44]

Why is this? A typical cigarette contains only about one milligram (mg) of nicotine, but delivers it directly from the lungs into the bloodstream with remarkable efficiency, rivaling that of an injection directly into the veins. (A 60 mg dose of nicotine, if consumed all at once, would be lethal.) Each cigarette delivers several hits of nicotine that stimulate receptors in the brain associated with pleasure, establishing a physiological reward pattern that frequently becomes a compulsion—*especially when smoking begins at an early age.* A few regular smokers have a "take it or leave it" relationship with cigarettes, smoking one now and then at a social gathering. The vast majority, however, burn through ten to forty per day, often in rituals tied to other events: having a cup of coffee in the morning, reading the paper, picking up the phone, starting the car, watching a favorite TV program or sports event, pouring a cocktail before dinner, and so on. Nicotine from cigars and smokeless tobacco enters the bloodstream more slowly, but often in greater quantity. A cigar may contain the amount of nicotine found in three or more cigarettes, as can a dip or chew of tobacco. A smokeless tobacco user who takes eight to ten doses per day will have the same nicotine exposure as a two-pack-per-day smoker.

Take the brain's response to nicotine, combine it with dozens of daily routines, add sensations of touch, taste, and smell that many find pleasant, mix them together thousands of times and you have a habit that won't go away without a fight. The battle is intensified because tobacco use, and cigarette smoking in particular, becomes a rapid and reliable calming agent, a stress reliever, a brief vacation during a tough day (or life). The icing on this powerful confection is the unpleasant collection of withdrawal symptoms that can arrive within hours of the last dose of nicotine. These include:

- Physical discomforts: headache, fatigue, increased appetite, insomnia
- Mood disturbances: irritability, depression, restlessness
- Poor concentration
- Above all, craving for another smoke or chew

Withdrawal symptoms typically reach their peak at two to three days but may last for several more.

These formidable barriers to quitting can lead to startling behaviors. Most of us know at least one person who has continued to smoke in the face of dire consequences: a diagnosis of lung cancer, a heart attack, the amputation of a foot or leg that lost its blood supply, shortness of breath, and even ongoing oxygen use (which exposes the smoker to the risk of fire or explosion). One stomach-turning antismoking ad shows a woman inhaling a cigarette through a hole in her neck created by surgeons after her cancerous larynx has been removed.

U.S. Public Health Service data indicate that about 70 percent of all current American smokers have tried to quit at least once, and nearly 50 percent try to quit each year. Sadly, only about 7 percent of those who make an attempt remain abstinent from tobacco after one year.[45] Such dismal success rates can discourage not only smokers and chewers but also their physicians, who may feel that repeated attempts to warn long-term users about the hazards of tobacco are an exercise in futility. But current research supports a different perspective: Tobacco dependence should be viewed as a chronic disease, and users are vulnerable to relapse after weeks, months, or even years of quitting. This conclusion has three important implications:

1. No single approach to quitting will work for everyone.
2. Success should not be defined in "all or nothing" terms, in which anything short of permanent abstinence from tobacco use is seen as a failure.
3. Those who are trying to quit, and those who want to help their loved ones quit, should be prepared for a multidimensional struggle. For some, it is more like a war with several fronts.

If you want to become free of tobacco products, here are some important ingredients of any serious attempt:

First and foremost, identify *your* reasons to quit, write them as personal statements, and review them often. They should all be meaningful, at least some should be emotional, and most importantly they should be *your* reasons. If you are a habitual user, smoking or chewing isn't a casual, "take it or leave it" activity. Your original decision to start didn't involve a thoughtful weighing of the benefits and risks, and what drives the ongoing habit is a combination of intense physical and psychological impulses that seem to bypass the rational mind. Most adult and teenage tobacco users have heard an earful about the health risks of tobacco. Those who haven't experienced any problems (especially the young) may be convinced that "it won't happen to me," and, as we have just noted, many who have suffered serious consequences keep smoking or chewing anyway. Some, however, get a wake-up call from a chest pain, a persistent cough, or even a trip to the coronary-care unit, and decide to take action.

Some of the most powerful reasons for quitting involve a deep commitment to another person, combined with a sober assessment of the ongoing threat:

- "I don't want my children to grow up without me."
- "I want to see my grandchildren."
- "I don't want my wife to be a widow."
- "I want to set a good example for my children."
- "I don't want to harm my baby growing inside me."

The last of these statements is particularly potent, as many women who might not quit for any other reason will abandon tobacco products for what they know to be a clear and present danger to a son or daughter they will meet in the delivery room. On the other hand, reasons such as "I want my wife/husband/kids/doctor to stop nagging me" reflect someone else's priorities, and probably won't help a person hold the line when the going gets tough.

Examples of some other potentially meaningful statements:

- "I want to take better care of the body that God has given me."
- "I want to stop coughing every morning."
- "I want to be able to walk/run/dance without feeling out of breath."
- "I'm ready for my house/car/clothes/breath/hair to smell normal again."
- "If I weren't spending money on cigarettes (and extra cleaning bills), I could afford to ______."
- "I don't want any substance to have a choke hold on my life."

Second, set an actual quit date. This needs to be more specific than "someday this year (or next)," because "someday" isn't on any calendar. The date may have some significance—such as New Year's Day (a perennial favorite), a birthday, anniversary, graduation, or even a vacation that will allow for some distraction and relaxation. The quit date might even coincide with a

GREAT MOMENT IN TOBACCO ADVERTISING

In 1987, the Joe Camel ad campaign is introduced. In 1991, a study published in the *Journal of the American Medical Association* indicates that 91 percent of six-year-olds can identify the product Joe Camel advertises, and that he is as familiar to preschoolers as Mickey Mouse.

R. J. Reynolds discontinues the ads in 1997, after the Federal Trade Commission accuses the company of illegally targeting children and youth with this ad campaign.

loved one's birthday and might prove to be a very meaningful gift to that person. It's all right for this day to be a little way in the future, in order to gear up and make any preparations, if needed.

Third, make the decision and the date a public event. In other words, let as many people know as possible, and ask for their support in various ways, such as:

- Encouragement and prayer from nonsmoking family and friends
- Information and possibly medication (see page 444) from your doctor
- Accountability to a few trusted individuals who have permission to ask pointed questions about your staying the course
- A wide berth from family and friends who *are* tobacco users, and a commitment from them not to offer you tobacco or invite you to smoke with them

COLD TURKEY OR SLOW TAPER?

Rather than setting a formal quit date when tobacco use will cease completely, some prefer to phase out their habit over an extended period of time, gradually using less and less over a period of weeks or even months. Experts on tobacco dependence, however, generally recommend that smoking or chewing end on a specific day, for several reasons:

- The quit-date approach is more decisive and specific. Tapering off has a tendency to become a little vague: "I'm cutting back" sounds respectable and may keep the doctor at bay until the next visit, but what exactly does it mean? Some people have been "cutting back" for years.
- Tapering off tends to drag out the unpleasant symptoms of withdrawal. Why not get it over with?
- Ongoing use of tobacco is not recommended while using any of the nicotine substitutes, which can be very helpful in quitting.
- Many of the important benefits of quitting don't kick in until smoking or chewing is finally over. Even one cigarette per day, for example, can make your heart more irritable or impair the ability of your airways to clear mucus and bacteria.

Those who find the prospect of eliminating tobacco in one day too daunting and want to move more slowly should try to be both specific and definite about the approach they will take. If today's smoking habit is twenty cigarettes per day, start tomorrow with an allocation of nineteen—and no more. The drop to eighteen can take place in three or four days, or even a week, but then make it stick. Map it out on the calendar, and enlist the support of others to help you stay with it. Later on, as the number dwindles to a few per day, you may find it simpler (and easier) to stop completely. ■

In addition to the help and (hopefully) reduced temptation that can result from this action, a public declaration creates another barrier to tobacco use: the risk of embarrassment and the discomfort of making excuses to others when the promise of a tobacco-free life has been broken.

Fourth, consider using medication to help you through this process. When appropriate, most authorities recommend using one of the nicotine-releasing products currently on the market, or the drug bupropion (Zyban, Wellbutrin), or both to ease the physical symptoms of withdrawal. While none of these delivers the relaxing hit of nicotine to the brain that comes with a cigarette or the sensory pleasures of tobacco use (which are definitely an acquired taste), they help temper the unpleasant response that many experience when quitting.

F.Y.I.

Between 70 and 90 percent of smokers identify nicotine-withdrawal symptoms as their main obstacle to quitting. Furthermore, the vast majority (between 84 and 95 percent) who attempt to quit for at least six months without using some type of medication support are unsuccessful, often because of withdrawal symptoms.[46]

Fifth, tap into any other resources that can help you. You're not the first person who has faced an entrenched tobacco habit, and you might as well take advantage of the experience and expertise of those who are well versed in the struggle. These could include

- A friend or relative who has successfully quit and maintained a tobacco-free life for many months (or better yet, years).
- A stop-smoking program organized by a local hospital, your church, the health department, or a professional organization such as the American Cancer Society or American Lung Association.
- A local Nicotine Anonymous group, if one is available in your community. These apply the principles of Alcoholics Anonymous to tobacco addiction.
- Quitlines, which are free counseling services available by phone in more than thirty states. Counselors are trained to help individuals map out their own quitting strategy and can provide ongoing support, which may be more convenient to access than a meeting. Information about accessing a quitline can be obtained from the American Cancer Society at (800) 227-2345 or at the North American Quitline Consortium Web site at http://www.naquitline.org.
- Most importantly, rely on God, who is well acquainted with human weakness in general, and yours in particular. Bring your struggle to Him in prayer as often as necessary, which may be dozens of times per day.

The approach used by Alcoholics Anonymous and other twelve-step groups is reviewed in detail later in this chapter, starting on page 480.

Sixth, as much as possible separate yourself from opportunities to use tobacco, and alter the cues (or your response) that lead to smoking or

continued on page 446

MEDICATIONS THAT MAY EASE THE QUITTING PROCESS

Does it make sense to use nicotine or an antidepressant to help overcome a tobacco habit? Unless there are other reasons to avoid them, the answer is usually yes. While a number of helpful products are available without prescription, you should review all of the options with your doctor. These include:

1. **Nicotine replacement therapy**, which deposits nicotine into the bloodstream at a controlled rate via the skin, mouth, or nose. This type of treatment should not be used if you are pregnant or have heart or circulatory disease, unless you and your doctor have determined that the benefits outweigh the risks. (This is because nicotine, with or without the toxins found in tobacco, can raise blood pressure, increase the pulse rate, and constrict blood vessels.) Also, nicotine replacement should not be used by someone who is still smoking or chewing tobacco, because the combined dose from the two sources of nicotine could be hazardous (not to mention expensive—most forms of replacement cost at least as much as a pack of cigarettes per day). Available forms of nicotine substitutes include:
   - **Nicotine patches** deliver a steady dose of nicotine through the skin over sixteen to twenty-four hours. The patch is applied every morning to an area of dry skin between the neck and waist. Typically one will begin with a higher dose (15 to 22 mg) for a few weeks and then use one or more lower doses (5 to 14 mg) for a few more weeks. While eight- to twelve-week courses of treatment are common, some people use patches for months. The steady influx of nicotine can ward off withdrawal symptoms, and twenty-four-hour patches can prevent morning withdrawal symptoms (though they may disrupt sleep). Depending upon individual sensitivity and the type of patch used, possible side effects can include skin irritation, headache, rapid heartbeat, disturbed sleep, or upset stomach.
   - **Nicotine gum** allows a person more control over the amount of nicotine taken through the course of the day. When feeling the urge to light up, a smoker chews a piece of gum until noticing a "peppery" flavor, after which the gum is parked inside the cheek until the taste fades. (Newer forms of nicotine gum offer more agreeable flavors.) More chewing and parking continues for about twenty to thirty minutes. The larger (4 mg) size is recommended for those who smoke more than a pack per day, while lighter smokers may want to try the 2 mg dose. Some nicotine-gum users establish a routine in which they chew a piece every thirty to sixty minutes to ward off cravings. Others use it as needed. Whichever approach is chosen, no more than twenty pieces should be chewed over the course of a day. Nicotine gum may irritate the mouth and cause bad breath. Also, swallowing the saliva, or the piece of gum itself, should be avoided because doing so may upset the stomach.

Some researchers have obtained favorable results by combining patch and gum treatments. A twenty-four-hour patch delivers a steady level of nicotine throughout the day, and a piece of gum up to four times daily serves as a backup to battle cravings.

· **Nicotine inhalers** and **nasal sprays** have been introduced more recently and, unlike the patches and gum, require a doctor's prescription. Both take advantage of more rapid absorption—the inhaler through the mucus membranes of the mouth (not through the lungs, like a cigarette), and the nasal spray through the lining of the nose. The oral inhaler uses a cartridge that dispenses nicotine in a vapor when the user puffs on it, an action that resembles the act of smoking. Not surprisingly, either can be irritating to the throat and nose.

All nicotine substitutes are intended to be used for a limited time, typically only three to six months, with the tobacco user presumably weaning off over time. In reality, many feel the need to continue much longer. The long-term safety of nicotine replacements is not entirely certain, but presumably any of them would be preferable to the toxic effects of tobacco.

2. **Bupropion** is a prescription antidepressant that has been available for many years as Wellbutrin, as well as in sustained-release forms called Wellbutrin SR and Wellbutrin XL. Since mid-2000, a sustained-release form of bupropion has also been available under the name Zyban as an aid to quitting smoking. (Despite their different names and appearance, Wellbutrin SR and Zyban are identical in all respects.) Bupropion affects some of the same receptors in the brain that are stimulated by nicotine, and it can reduce withdrawal symptoms when a user quits. Typically a person begins taking bupropion for one or two weeks before the quit date. Once tobacco has been discontinued, any form of nicotine replacement can be added as well. One important point about bupropion: *It does not give a person the desire to quit using tobacco.*

Bupropion can cause nausea, difficulty sleeping, jitteriness, and high blood pressure (especially when used with nicotine replacement). It is not recommended for use during pregnancy, primarily because there is very limited experience with it in pregnant women. It has also been associated with seizures in one out of one thousand people taking 300 mg per day (the recommended dose for helping with tobacco withdrawal). The odds of this happening are higher for certain people:

· Those who have had one or more seizures in the past.
· Those abruptly stopping the use of alcohol or sedative medications.
· Those with an eating disorder (anorexia or bulimia).
· Those who take a higher dose of bupropion, whether by using more than the recommended dose or unknowingly taking the two forms of this drug at the same time. (For example, a person already using Wellbutrin to treat depression should not also take Zyban to help quit smoking.)

Fortunately, most people who use bupropion tolerate it very well. Side effects (such as nausea), if they occur, tend to be mild and fade over several days or weeks. While significant side effects are very uncommon, *this medicine should only be used under the supervision of a doctor* who knows a person's history, medical conditions, and *all* current medications (including nonprescription supplements). ■

continued from page 443

chewing. Biblical admonitions to flee temptation (2 Timothy 2:22, for example) definitely apply to addictive substances. To put it simply, it is a lot easier to deal with the desire to use tobacco when none is immediately available. Also, the tobacco user—especially the cigarette smoker—frequently has connected lighting up with a host of innocent daily activities, such as reading the paper or pouring a cup of coffee. Strategies for this part of the process include the following steps:

- When the quit date arrives, get rid of everything connected with tobacco use: cigarettes (or whatever the product), lighters, ashtrays, perhaps (gulp!) even a favorite chair if it has a strong association with smoking. Don't merely stash these items in a closet where they can be retrieved. Bury them in the trash.
- If anyone else living with you is going to continue smoking, politely but firmly insist that smoking be done elsewhere, far enough away that you cannot see or smell it. (Even a whiff of someone's cigarette in the backyard may be irresistible to the struggling ex-smoker indoors.)
- As much as possible, stay away from places and situations where tobacco is routinely used.
- Stock up on gum, carrot and celery sticks, or other low-calorie items to substitute for the oral gratification of smoking or chewing. If you need to do something with your hands, try knitting or doing needlework, squeezing a rubber ball, stroking or brushing a pet dog or cat, giving your spouse a foot massage, doodling or drawing, and so forth.
- Plan for some healthy alternatives to relieve stress or unwind at the end of a tough day: a brisk walk, a hot bath, shooting some baskets with one of the kids, playing a musical instrument, praying, talking or writing to a family member or friend, journaling, watching a half hour of vintage comedy (or even classic cartoons) on videotape or DVD. (The evening news may not provide the diversion you need.)

Seventh, think of quitting as a "one day at a time" process. For many tobacco users (especially those who have longstanding habits), the thought of *never* smoking or chewing again may generate apprehension ("I don't think I can do it") that can stall the decision or create overconfidence that can be badly shaken by a slipup. Either problem may be avoided by taking the process a day at a time. Some smokers, for example, are able to declare that "I'm not going to smoke today"—and then "not smoke today" for years on end. If a moment of weakness leads to an episode of backsliding, getting back on track doesn't have to be such a colossal process.

SELECTED SOURCES OF INFORMATION AND HELP WITH TOBACCO ADDICTION

AMERICAN CANCER SOCIETY
(800) 227-2345
www.cancer.org

AMERICAN HEART ASSOCIATION
(800) 242-8721
www.americanheart.org

AMERICAN LUNG ASSOCIATION
(800) 586-4872
www.lungusa.org

NATIONAL CANCER INSTITUTE (Cancer Information Service)
(877) 448-7848
www.nci.nih.gov/cancerinfo/tobacco

NICOTINE ANONYMOUS
(415) 750-0328
www.nicotine-anonymous.org

OFFICE ON SMOKING & HEALTH
National Center for Chronic Disease Prevention and Health Promotion
(800) 232-1311
www.cdc.gov/tobacco

Alcohol: Relaxing—and Dangerous

Unlike tobacco, which did not circle the globe until about five hundred years ago, alcoholic beverages have been concocted from all manner of fruits, cereals, and grains by every civilization that has ever existed on this planet. No one knows who first drank the juices of fermented fruits and discovered their intoxicating effects. The first reference to drunkenness in the Bible occurs early in the book of Genesis, where Noah is described as a "man of the soil" who planted a vineyard after his tour of duty with the ark was completed. He then became drunk on its wine, with unfortunate consequences for one of his sons (Genesis 9:20-27).

F.Y.I.

Wild elephants have been observed swaying and staggering after eating large quantities of fermented fruit, and some have speculated that observing such a phenomenon in animals may have inspired early humans to try the fruit themselves.

The brewing process for beer was probably well developed in Sumeria before 3000 B.C., while the ancient Egyptians made wine from pomegranates, figs, and dates, as well as from grapes. One of the last gods to be added to the ancient Greek pantheon was Dionysus, the god of wine, whom the Romans later adopted as Bacchus. The annual festival honoring him (known as the Bacchanalia) became so notorious for inciting sexual and criminal misbehavior that the Roman Senate outlawed it in 186 B.C. The process of distillation, which significantly increases the alcohol content of a beverage (and thus creates hard liquor), was not widely used in Europe until the twelfth century, although it had probably been developed in India by 500 B.C.

According to Greek mythology, Dionysus was the god who granted King Midas his ill-fated wish to turn anything he touched to gold.

If people in every culture have enjoyed the aromas, tastes, and temporary euphoria created by alcoholic beverages, they have also been well acquainted with the grief and destruction that can accompany them. The book of Proverbs contains a colorful description of the general chaos in the life of an alcohol abuser, and the disorientation and hallucinations that can occur during alcohol withdrawal:

> *Who has woe? Who has sorrow? Who has strife? Who has complaints? Who has needless bruises? Who has bloodshot eyes? Those who linger over wine, who go to sample bowls of mixed wine. Do not gaze at wine when it is red, when it sparkles in the cup, when it goes down smoothly! In the end it bites like a snake and poisons like a viper. Your eyes will see strange sights and your mind imagine confusing things. You will be like one sleeping on the high seas, lying on top of the rigging. "They hit me," you will say, "but I'm not hurt! They beat me, but I don't feel it! When will I wake up so I can find another drink?"*
>
> (PROVERBS 23:29-35)

The alcohol content of a beverage is often expressed as proof, a number that is twice its alcohol percentage. Eighty-proof rum or tequila, for example, is 40 percent alcohol.

What we normally call alcohol is actually **ethyl alcohol**, a simple molecule that is a member of a much larger class of chemical compounds with a distinctive molecular structure. In nature, ethyl alcohol (which we will refer to as alcohol from here on) is a by-product of the action of bacteria or yeast on simple sugars—glucose, fructose, maltose, and lactose—that are found in honey, fruits, grains, and even milk. Beer typically contains 3 to 5 percent alcohol; wine, 10 to 12 percent; and distilled spirits, as much as 40 to 50 percent alcohol.

How much alcohol intake is safe?

As we will see later in this section, for many people the answer to that question is *none*. These include:

- Pregnant women
- Children and adolescents under the age of twenty-one
- Anyone who has struggled with alcohol dependence (alcoholism), or who has a family history of this problem
- People taking medications that are sedating—for example, drugs used to treat anxiety, such as alprazolam (Xanax), clonazepam (Klonopin), or diazepam (Valium)
- People taking medications whose effects may be altered by the presence of alcohol, or which may combine with alcohol in a way that could be hazardous

F.Y.I. **Few people realize that the common pain reliever acetaminophen (Tylenol and many other brands) can have toxic effects on the liver when taken in excessive doses. Even when used within recommended guidelines, multiple daily doses of acetaminophen and alcohol on an ongoing basis could be harmful to the liver.**

- Anyone about to drive an automobile, pilot an airplane, or operate any equipment for which safety is a concern
- Anyone with acute or chronic liver disease—especially hepatitis

Other groups of people should be very careful not to drink alcoholic beverages beyond current recommended limits, if they partake at all:

- The elderly, for whom alcohol may aggravate ongoing health problems or interact with prescription (or nonprescription) drugs. (Seniors are generally more likely to be taking more medications than younger adults.)
- Women, for whom differences in the metabolism of alcohol not only lead to higher blood levels than occur in men taking in the same amount, but also create a narrower margin between safe (or beneficial) and harmful amounts.
- Anyone with high blood pressure (hypertension), because this problem becomes more unpredictable and difficult to control in the presence of high levels of alcohol.

- Anyone with lipid (cholesterol or triglyceride) levels that are elevated beyond recommended levels, because excessive alcohol intake can further raise them.
- Anyone who has had problems related to alcohol use in the past: family, school, or work conflicts; an accident or injury while intoxicated; an arrest for driving under the influence (DUI); etc.
- Anyone in a situation in which alcohol use could cause someone else to have a problem (or, to use the biblical term, "to stumble"), or could send the wrong message to a child or teenager. For example, having a drink with a dinner companion who has struggled with alcohol dependence or having multiple drinks when young people—especially one's own children—are watching could be inviting trouble.

For details about problems related to lipids, see chapter 3: "Three Health Problems You Want to Avoid."

For an otherwise healthy adult, under appropriate circumstances, current research suggests that there may be health benefits to what is called moderate alcohol consumption, defined as *one or two drinks per day for men, and one per day for women.* Consuming this amount of alcohol may be associated with an improved cholesterol profile (with more of the HDL or "good" component present) and a decreased risk for both coronary artery disease and heart attack. Risk for stroke, clogged arteries in the legs, and even Alzheimer's disease may be reduced as well. (Until recently these benefits had been attributed only to wine, but they probably occur with other alcoholic beverages as well.)

WHAT CONSTITUTES A "DRINK"?

Since moderate and high-risk alcohol use are defined in terms of number of drinks per day, exactly how much is one drink? It is defined as the amount of a beverage that contains 14 grams (or about 0.6 ounces) of pure alcohol. This is the amount of alcohol in:

- 12 ounces of beer or 8 to 9 ounces of malt liquor
- 5 ounces of wine or 3 to 4 ounces of fortified wine (such as sherry or port)
- 2 to 3 ounces of aperitif, liqueur, or cordial
- 1½ ounces of brandy
- 1½ ounces of distilled spirits (e.g., 80-proof rum or vodka)

Note that malt liquor may be sold in bottles that can contain 16, 22, or even 40 ounces—the latter being the equivalent of five drinks. A typical wine bottle contains about 25 ounces, the equivalent of five drinks. For mixed cocktails, the amount of alcohol will depend upon the particular concoction and the inclinations of the bartender. Keep in mind that 1½ ounces of distilled spirits, the amount that constitutes one drink, is the quantity contained in a single jigger. ■

How much alcohol is considered unsafe?

There is, unfortunately, a narrow gap between the amount of alcohol per day that might be considered safe for an adult (assuming that he or she should not be abstaining for one or more reasons) and the amount that is potentially harmful. The following drinking patterns are considered to be risky:

- For men: more than fourteen drinks in a typical week, or more than four drinks in one day.
- For women: more than seven drinks in a typical week, or more than three drinks in one day.

A person who drinks below these levels has less than a one in one hundred chance of having an alcohol disorder (and essentially zero risk if he or she doesn't drink at all, or has fewer than twelve drinks in a year). But when one exceeds these limits, the odds change drastically. The male partygoer who downs five or more drinks on a Saturday night (or a female who consumes four or more drinks) has a one in fourteen chance of having an alcohol problem. If this happens once per week or more, the odds change to one in seven for a man and one in six for a woman. About three in ten Americans engage in risky drinking behavior.[47]

How does excessive use of alcoholic beverages cause trouble?

Intoxication. The vast majority of alcohol users aren't drinking to quench their thirst or to savor the taste of wine, beer, or spirits. As the blood alcohol level rises, a person may experience a feeling of relaxation, decreased anxiety, mild euphoria or "buzz," a lifting of the spirits (hence the optimistic term *happy hour* for the late afternoon cocktail service at many bars and restaurants), and an increased willingness to socialize. As the brain goes further under the influence, a host of familiar effects may be seen:

- Loss of inhibition (verbal, physical, sexual)
- Changes in personality: the reserved person becomes more outspoken, or the civil person becomes more hostile or abusive
- Impaired thought processes, memory, coordination, and reaction time
- Confusion, drowsiness, stupor, and (at high enough levels) coma

"Alcohol is necessary for a man so that he can have a good opinion of himself, undisturbed by the facts."
—FINLEY PETER DUNNE

F.Y.I. Passing out—going unconscious because of the sedating effects of a large dose of alcohol—is different from experiencing a blackout. A blackout does not involve loss of consciousness, but rather is an episode in which a drinker simply does not remember what happened over several hours. This occurs at a much lower dose of alcohol and is an important symptom of alcohol dependence.

It is while people are intoxicated, of course, that accidents and mishaps of all kinds are more likely to happen: automobile and motorcycle crashes, falls, unplanned sexual contacts, daredevil stunts, fights, criminal acts, and suicide attempts.

WHAT DETERMINES HOW DRUNK A PERSON GETS?

The factors that most impact how a person responds to alcoholic beverages are the **blood alcohol concentration (BAC)** and individual tolerance. Once it arrives in the small intestine, alcohol is absorbed relatively quickly, and its effects may be felt within ten minutes, peaking at about forty to sixty minutes. Absorption is faster on an empty stomach and slower when food (especially if high in fat content) is present. Alcohol is metabolized by the liver, but at a limited rate. If the drinks are consumed faster than the liver can handle their alcohol content, BAC will rise. BAC is measured in grams of alcohol per 100 ml of blood, and for most people, an increasing level results in more profound effects on body and mind.

The following symptoms are typical of the blood alcohol concentration noted:

- BAC of 0.10—slurred speech
- BAC of 0.20—impaired motor control
- BAC of 0.30—confusion
- BAC of 0.40—stupor
- BAC of 0.50—coma
- BAC of 0.60—suppression of breathing and death

Alcohol is distributed exclusively through the fluid volume of the body. A woman has less fluid than a man of the same weight, which accounts for the higher blood alcohol level that she develops.

The blood alcohol level rises more slowly in heavy than in slender people, and a woman will generally develop a higher blood alcohol level than a man of equal weight in response to the same amount of alcohol.

Most states set the legal definition of intoxication at a blood alcohol concentration of 0.08 to 0.10, regardless of the behavior being manifested. However some driving functions are affected by a blood alcohol level as low as 0.02. As a point of reference, a 160-pound man can be expected to develop a level of 0.04 one hour after drinking two 12-ounce beers on an empty stomach.[48] Some people have an inborn or acquired tolerance for alcohol, which causes them to show surprisingly little response to amounts that would drastically affect more susceptible drinkers. These have typically been characterized as people who can hold their liquor. In fact, the person with a high tolerance is at higher risk for alcohol dependence, because he or she has to drink much more to feel any effect. ■

Alcohol abuse occurs when someone repeatedly drinks enough to create problems for self or others. These could include any of the following:

- Absences or other problems at work or school
- Neglect of personal or family responsibilities
- Reckless behavior, such as driving, swimming, or in some other way risking life and limb while drinking
- One or more arrests for driving under the influence of alcohol (DUIs)
- Fighting or other acts of violence while intoxicated
- Physical injury or medical problems that are brought about or aggravated by alcohol
- Continued drinking even in the face of problems arising from alcohol use

WHAT IS A HANGOVER, AND WHAT ARE THE "DT'S"?

Last night at twelve I felt immense,
Today I feel like thirty cents.
My eyes are blurred, my coppers hot,
I'll try to eat, but I cannot.
It is no time for mirth and laughter,
The cold, gray dawn of the morning after.
—GEORGE ADE, FROM 1903 COMIC OPERA *THE SULTAN OF SULU*

Depictions of the morning after, in which someone had one (or several) too many the night before and is miserable, have been the subject of comedies and cartoons for decades. So have visions of pink elephants and other strange creatures haunting the alcoholic. But neither is a laughing matter.

The common hangover is an unpleasant mixture of symptoms that occur after alcohol has been consumed and then fully metabolized. The drinker is no longer intoxicated but feels rotten, usually with a strong headache and often with nausea, diarrhea, shakiness, and fatigue. It is actually not a form of alcohol withdrawal and, in fact, is much more common in light to moderate drinkers than in heavy drinkers. Typically the downing of at least five to six cocktails (fewer for women) over several hours will set a hangover in motion, although the severity of symptoms doesn't always correlate with the number of drinks. Dehydration, lack of food, increased physical activity while drinking, and poor sleep tend to worsen the symptoms. In addition, compounds called **cogeners** that are present in wine, brandy, whiskey, and other dark liquors are known to increase not only the likelihood of getting a hangover but also its severity. Rum, vodka, gin, and other clear liquors cause far fewer hangovers, which may explain why people with long-term, heavy alcohol dependence more frequently consume them.

While conventional wisdom holds that hangovers primarily punish overzealous partygoers, they also exact a significant cost to others. Poor work performance and

An alcohol abuser may not necessarily be intoxicated (or even drinking) on a daily basis. He or she may have little or no alcohol during the workweek, for example, but then consume much larger amounts on weekends. Alcohol abuse encompasses a spectrum of trouble and strife, ranging from a few abnormal lab tests at the doctor's office (which might herald bigger problems in the future) to behavior that creates chaos and misery for months or years on end.

Alcohol dependence—known also by the more familiar term **alcoholism**—has four basic features:

- **Tolerance**: Larger and larger quantities of alcohol become necessary to achieve intoxication, or merely to feel normal.
- **Craving**: An intense desire to drink, even in the face of serious conse-

absenteeism caused by hangovers waste billions of dollars every year. Furthermore, hangover sufferers aren't merely uncomfortable. Their dexterity and perceptual skills are impaired long after alcohol is no longer measurable in the bloodstream, a fact that has been demonstrated experimentally in pilots, drivers, and skiers.[49] People who are not intoxicated but experiencing a hangover should therefore think twice about driving, flying aircraft, operating heavy machinery, or engaging in other activities where life and limb depend upon being in top form. While literally hundreds of remedies have been suggested to prevent or treat hangovers (including "taking the hair of the dog that bit you—"that is, drinking more alcohol), the only approach that is known to work is the obvious one: drinking in moderation, if at all.

Delirium tremens ("shaking delirium"), otherwise known as the "DT's," is a serious, potentially life-threatening form of alcohol withdrawal that is more common among those who are heavy users (in the range of eight to ten drinks or more per day) for an extended period of time (typically ten or more years) and who have had symptoms of withdrawal in the past. It may be precipitated by an illness, lack of food (especially following a prolonged binge), or a hospitalization during which the patient has not disclosed his or her drinking habits to the hospital staff. Symptoms typically begin about seventy-two hours after the last drink, although they may be delayed as long as seven to ten days. Central-nervous-system symptoms can be particularly severe, including not only the irritability, nausea, and anxiety seen during withdrawal, but also agitation, disorientation, hallucinations (especially visions of animals such as bugs and snakes), and even seizures. Fever, dehydration, and heart rhythm disturbances may be present as well. Needless to say, their surprise appearance in a hospitalized individual can cause considerable commotion and may provoke an elaborate evaluation if their cause is unknown. Even after the diagnosis is made, aggressive medical care is needed to prevent serious consequences, including death. ■

quences. Alcohol is no longer a "take it or leave it" accompaniment to a meal or a party, something that can be put aside with a little willpower. The drive to obtain it can be as intense as that for water or food and may cause a person to cut down or give up other activities that used to be important or enjoyable.

- **Loss of control**: An inability to limit how much alcohol one consumes on a given occasion, either drinking more or drinking longer than intended. A person with alcohol dependence may want to cut down or stop, and may even have tried many times, but finds it difficult or impossible to do so.
- **Withdrawal symptoms**: Tremor, anxiety, nausea, sweating, in some cases seizures, or a more dangerous syndrome called **delirium tremens** (or the DT's), when alcohol intake stops.

Note that it is possible to abuse alcohol—to drink in such a way that an adverse consequence occurs at least once in a year—without being alcohol dependent. The reverse is true as well, although (not surprisingly) more than half of those who are alcohol dependent also meet diagnostic criteria for alcohol abuse.

During pregnancy. In the early 1970s, the term **fetal alcohol syndrome (FAS)** was coined to describe a collection of behavioral and neurological problems among children born to women who consumed alcohol during pregnancy. Now recognized as the leading known preventable cause of mental retardation, FAS is characterized by certain facial abnormalities, growth retardation, and brain damage that can cause both intellectual difficulties and behavioral problems. Estimates of the number of children affected in the United States range from less than one in three thousand to as high as three in one thousand. While FAS is uncommon among women who consume five or fewer drinks per week, *no safe level of alcohol consumption during pregnancy has been established,* other than *none at all.*[50]

In some cases brain damage is seen without other abnormalities in a child born to a mother who used alcohol during pregnancy. This condition is called **alcohol-related neurodevelopmental disorder (ARND).**

In the young. Alcohol use by those under twenty-one is illegal in all fifty states for several good reasons. It is by far the most dangerous of the gateway drugs. Alcohol causes more deaths among adolescents than any other substance. It is involved in approximately half of all automobile crashes involving teenagers (the leading cause of death in this age group), and frequently plays a role in adolescent deaths from other causes, including homicides, suicides, drownings, and motorcycle and bicycle accidents. It is also linked to up to two out of three sexual assaults and date rapes, and plays a prominent role in high-risk sex among the young. In most instances, the first sexual encounter for a teenage girl involves the use of alcohol. The fact that putting alcohol into a young body frequently leads to reckless, dangerous, violent, and lethal outcomes

COLLEGE DRINKING: A NOT-SO-VENERABLE TRADITION

Landlord, fill the flowing bowl until it doth run over,
For tonight we'll merry, merry be, tomorrow we'll be sober.
—TRADITIONAL COLLEGE DRINKING SONG

Keggers, beer busts, tailgate parties, frat-house parties, spring-break revels, and drinking songs (often set to four-part harmony) are an age-old tradition on college campuses, seemingly as much a part of the campus landscape as ivy-covered buildings and football games. But recently the destructive effects of student intoxication have become a matter of national concern. According to a sobering report published in April 2002 by a special federal task force of the National Advisory Council on Alcohol Abuse and Alcoholism, *every year* alcohol use by American college students eighteen to twenty-four years of age leads to the following incidents:

- Under the influence of alcohol, 500,000 are unintentionally injured, and of these 1,400 die.
- Students who have been drinking are responsible for 600,000 assaults on other college students.
- About 100,000 students report having sex while too intoxicated to remember whether or not they consented to do so.
- Alcohol contributes to 70,000 students becoming victims of a sexual assault or date rape.
- About 150,000 develop a health problem related to alcohol.
- At least one percent report having attempted suicide because of drinking or drug abuse.
- More than 10 percent report damaging property while intoxicated.
- Over 2 million report driving while under the influence of alcohol.
- More than 100,000 are arrested for an alcohol-related offense (including driving under the influence).
- More than 30 percent meet diagnostic criteria for alcohol abuse and more than 5 percent could be classified as alcohol dependent, based upon questionnaire responses about their drinking habits.[51]

The report, entitled "A Call to Action: Changing the Culture of Drinking at U.S. Colleges," recommends a coordinated effort by college administrators, parents, student leadership, and communities surrounding college and university campuses to bring about significant changes in the drinking habits of students. ■

Approximately 11 million children and adolescents drink—half of them to excess. The average age for a first drink among boys is eleven; for girls, thirteen. According to the American Academy of Pediatrics, about one in five fifth graders has experienced alcohol intoxication. Twenty percent of twelve- to twenty-year-olds report binge-drinking episodes (in which they consume at least four drinks at a time).

is not breaking news. Recent research, however, has added an ominous new concern: Underage alcohol use damages both the hippocampus, an area of the brain involved in memory and learning, and the prefrontal area, which undergoes major changes during adolescence and plays a role in shaping an individual's behavior and personality as an adult.[52] The human brain undergoes important transformations during adolescence and is more vulnerable to damage from alcohol before age twenty-one than at any time later in life. The underage drinker who is sowing wild oats may in fact be reaping long-term—or even lifetime—problems with learning and relationships.

F.Y.I. Obviously, not everyone who turns twenty-one becomes a model of responsibility where alcohol is concerned. Too many young adults (and older ones too) lose any semblance of judgment under the influence of alcohol.

Long-term effects on health. Aside from problems with relationships, work, the law, or bodily injuries caused by alcohol, those who drink to excess on a long-term basis are at risk for a number of health problems. Because of gender differences in the metabolism of alcohol, women are more prone to alcohol-related health problems than men. They also progress more rapidly toward alcohol dependence.[53]

The word *cirrhosis* comes from a Greek word meaning "tawny," referring to the color of the diseased liver.

- **Alcoholic liver disease.** Alcohol is processed by the liver, and over time large amounts of it provoke inflammation, known as **alcoholic hepatitis**, throughout this all-important organ. The effects are more pronounced if there is any other factor causing inflammation, such as a smoldering case of hepatitis B or C. Over time, the liver may develop extensive scarring called **cirrhosis**. As liver functions gradually fail, a host of awful (and eventually lethal) consequences can develop. (See sidebar on pages 458–459.) About 2 million Americans have alcohol-related liver disease, and 10 to 20 percent of heavy drinkers will develop cirrhosis. Alcoholic hepatitis may resolve if drinking stops; the scarring of cirrhosis, on the other hand, is a permanent fixture, although abstaining from alcohol increases the odds of survival.

F.Y.I. Like any type of liver inflammation, alcoholic hepatitis causes the release of certain enzymes from the liver into the bloodstream. Elevated levels of these enzymes are often picked up on routine screening tests as part of a physical exam or during an evaluation for symptoms such as fatigue.

- **Cardiovascular (heart and blood vessel) disease.** While modest amounts of alcohol may reduce the risk of coronary artery disease, excessive use can raise blood pressure, cholesterol, and triglycerides, and increase the risk for stroke. In addition, alcohol can be toxic to heart muscle itself, and excessive intake may lead to a condition called **alcoholic cardiomyopathy**, in which the heart's ability to pump blood is greatly impaired.

- **Cancer** of the mouth, throat, esophagus, and larynx (vocal cords) is more common among long-term heavy alcohol users. Some research suggests that women who consume between two and a half and five drinks per day have a 40 percent higher risk for developing breast cancer compared with nondrinkers. Furthermore, the risk for breast cancer increases with the amount consumed on a daily basis.[54]
- **Pancreatitis** is an acute or chronic inflammation of the pancreas, the large organ in the upper abdomen that manufactures both digestive enzymes and insulin. Acute pancreatitis causes a great deal of abdominal pain, along with nausea, vomiting, and a host of potential complications that can be fatal. Chronic pancreatitis can cause ongoing pain, diarrhea, and weight loss due to poor digestion and absorption of food. Both are related to heavy drinking.
- **Neuropathy**, or nerve damage, brought on by excessive alcohol use can cause chronic, unpleasant sensations—especially pain or tingling—in various parts of the body, especially the feet.
- **Nutritional and vitamin deficiencies** may be seen in severely alcohol-dependent people whose primary source of calories every day is their favorite beverage.

Insulin is the all-important hormone that escorts glucose (blood sugar) into cells throughout the body. Detailed information about insulin and diabetes can be found in chapter 3, starting on page 70.

How do I know whether I have an alcohol problem . . .

A common characteristic of the problem drinker is denial, the seeming inability to recognize or acknowledge that his or her alcohol use is an issue. Two straightforward sets of screening questions can help make the diagnosis:

"Actually, it only takes one drink to get me loaded. Trouble is, I can't remember if it's the thirteenth or fourteenth."
—GEORGE BURNS

1. Quantity and frequency:
   a. How many drinks do you have in an average week?
   b. What is the maximum number of drinks you had on any given day during the past month?

   You are definitely at risk for alcohol-related problems if the answer to the first question is more than fourteen for a man or more than seven for a woman, or if the answer to the second question is more than four for a man or more than three for a woman.

"An alcoholic has been lightly defined as a man who drinks more than his own doctor."
—ALVAN L. BARACH

2. The CAGE (an acronym for the italicized words below) questions:
   During the past year:
   a. Have you ever felt that you should *cut down* on your drinking?
   b. Have people *annoyed* you by criticizing your drinking?
   c. Have you ever felt *guilty* about your drinking?
   d. Have you ever had an *eye-opener* drink first thing in the morning to steady your nerves or get rid of a hangover?

If you answered yes to more than two of the CAGE questions, you are probably alcohol dependent. If you answered yes to even one of the questions, you need to be concerned about alcohol abuse or dependence.

F.Y.I. Studies have shown that using either the quantity-frequency questions or the CAGE questions alone will identify 60 to 70 percent of people with alcohol abuse or dependence problems. When both are used, 80 percent will be identified.[55]

. . . and if I do, can I just cut down, or do I have to quit?

For the alcoholic (that is, the person who is dependent on alcohol) attempting to cut down rarely if ever is successful. Eliminating alcohol use altogether is the appropriate course of action, though one that rarely can be taken without ongoing support. Some alcohol abusers who have been drinking irresponsibly but are not dependent on alcohol may be able to limit their use of alcohol to a level that does not threaten their health or create problems for themselves and others. But if a person is unable to stay within these relatively narrow bounds, abstinence is the appropriate goal.

ALCOHOLIC LIVER DISEASE: NOT A PRETTY SIGHT

Weighing in at three to four pounds in an adult, the liver is the largest internal organ in the human body. It is, in fact, a giant metabolic factory, carrying enormous responsibility for our well-being with more than five hundred metabolic functions. These include handling most of the nutrients transported to it from the intestinal tract; processing and detoxifying chemical substances (including medications and alcohol); manufacturing clotting factors and cholesterol; and secreting bile, which flows into the small intestine and assists in the digestion of fat.

Although we typically think of cirrhosis of the liver as an end product of alcohol abuse, it can have a number of other causes. These include chronic hepatitis B and/or C infection, inherited disorders, inflamed or blocked bile ducts (which normally drain the liver), and ongoing exposure to toxins.

No one who has observed at close range the fallout of a scarred, failing liver can ever see chronic alcohol overuse in quite the same light. Some of the more dramatic problems associated with a damaged liver include:

- **Bleeding.** Blood returning to the heart from the intestines, spleen, and pancreas normally passes first through the liver via a large blood vessel called the **portal vein**. When the liver is scarred by cirrhosis, blood cannot easily pass through it and must return to the heart by other routes. This can lead to the formation of enlarged (varicose) veins elsewhere, especially in the stomach and lower esophagus. These vessels have thin walls that are not designed to carry blood under increased pressure. If an enlarged vein in the esophagus or stomach ruptures, the results are spectacular and horrifying. Without warning, a person may suddenly feel ill and throw up a huge amount of blood. Alcohol overuse can also cause erosions of the esophagus and stomach, and these can bleed as well. To compound the problem, the diseased liver is unable to manufacture several important clotting factors, thus making it even more difficult to stop the bleeding.

Either way, just about everyone who decides that it's time to square off against an alcohol problem will need some help, and usually a lot of it. Needless to say, recognizing, acknowledging, and treating alcohol abuse and dependence are very important topics that we will address later in this chapter beginning on page 478.

Trouble from the Drugstore: Prescription-Drug Abuse

Prescription drugs that relieve pain, calm anxiety, or treat attention deficit hyperactivity disorder (ADHD) can occasionally become a bigger problem than the condition they are intended to treat. The 2003 National Survey on Drug Use and Health reported that, within the month prior to the survey, an estimated 6.3 million people (about 2.7 percent of the population age two and over) had used prescription drugs for nonmedical reasons—intentionally taking them in quantities or for purposes beyond what the prescribing physician intended. Some of these

- **Fluid accumulation.** Chronic liver disease can cause the accumulation of large amounts of fluid in the legs (called edema) and the abdomen. Over time, huge amounts (literally gallons) of this liquid can collect in the belly, potentially creating an uncomfortable bulge that eventually can interfere with breathing.
- **Kidney failure.** As if experiencing sympathy pains, the kidneys may also shut down as liver failure progresses, a condition called **hepatorenal syndrome.**
- **Brain malfunction.** Accumulation of toxic by-products in the bloodstream can damage the brain. One in particular—ammonia, arising from the breakdown of protein—can cause **alcoholic encephalopathy**, a malfunction of the brain that can cause confusion, altered mood, delirium, and even coma.
- **Jaundice.** The liver normally processes bilirubin, which is produced from the breakdown of the protein hemoglobin from red blood cells that have been removed from circulation or destroyed for any reason. Bilirubin is present in bile, the fluid secreted by the liver into the intestinal tract to help in the digestion of fats. (Bilirubin flowing through the intestine gives stool its normal brown color.) When bilirubin accumulates in the blood, a person develops a characteristic yellow color of the skin and the whites of the eyes, known as jaundice. This is often associated with an annoying, widespread itching.
- **Osteoporosis** (thinning of the bones) is more common among those with chronic liver disease, because the liver processes calcium and vitamin D, which play an essential role in the maintenance of bone density.
- **Cancer of the liver** can be a complication of any form of cirrhosis. Unfortunately, this tumor usually has a poor prognosis. ■

Bilirubin that cannot exit the body via the liver may be excreted by the kidney, giving the urine a dark amber color. At the same time, stool, which contains less bilirubin than normal, turns grayish.

individuals are virtual "career" abusers, people who will go to great lengths to obtain their drug(s) of choice and who may consume them in quantities that would put the average person into a stupor. Drug seekers may obtain these prescriptions from multiple doctors, clinics, or emergency rooms, complaining of painful ailments (that usually defy a clear diagnosis) and visiting several pharmacies a month. A few unscrupulous physicians make a comfortable living writing hundreds of prescriptions for "patients" who are happy to pay for them, usually in cash. Too often, however, drug problems develop one step at a time, as a person who needs help with difficult issues receives one or more habit-forming prescriptions from doctors who sincerely want to offer some relief.

What kinds of prescription drugs are most often abused?

Opioids (also called **narcotics**) are extremely effective painkillers that have been used and misused for more than a hundred years. **Morphine** and **codeine** are the prototypes, but physicians in all specialties commonly prescribe newer variations of these drugs—especially **hydrocodone** (Vicodin, Lortabs, Norco, and others), **oxycodone** (Percodan, Percocet, OxyContin, and others), and **propoxyphene** (Darvon). **Hydromorphone** (Dilaudid) and the synthetic **meperidine** (Demerol) are used in the hospital or emergency department more often than in office settings.

F.Y.I. Many preparations of opiates, such as Vicodin and Darvocet, include variable amounts of **acetaminophen**, the pain reliever used in many nonprescription remedies. In overdose situations involving one of these combination drugs, treating the medical consequences of the excessive acetaminophen dose, which can cause severe liver damage, may be more difficult than dealing with the narcotic.

The vast majority of prescriptions for these drugs are written appropriately for pain management, and their use—even when on a long-term basis—does not routinely lead to abuse or addiction. But in some people they create a general sense of well-being and relief from emotional distress, such that a short-term solution to a pain problem evolves into long-term use and dependence. This inevitably involves two developments: **tolerance**, in which higher and higher doses provide less and less relief, and **symptoms of withdrawal**, if a day—or even a few hours—goes by without a dose. These symptoms typically include restlessness, sweating, cramping, diarrhea, and vomiting. In a worst-case scenario, these features become powerful forces in full-blown, and sometimes full-time, drug-seeking behavior.

Sedatives and **hypnotics** are medicines that in appropriate doses relieve anxiety or insomnia. A few decades ago, physicians commonly prescribed **barbiturates** as sedatives and sleeping pills. Because of problems with overdoses, abuse, and withdrawal, few doctors now recommend them. **Benzodiazepines** (Valium, Librium, Xanax, Tranxene, Klonopin, and others) are widely prescribed to treat anxiety, usually (but not always) on a short-term basis. More sedating forms (Dalmane, Restoril, and Halcion) are often used to induce sleep. These drugs are not commonly sold on the street, but legitimate prescriptions can be misused or overused and lead to dependence.

Prolonged use of barbiturates or benzodiazepines usually leads to psychological and physical dependence. High doses of these medications, particularly when combined with other drugs (especially alcohol), can produce stuporous intoxication, depressed breathing, coma, and even death. Depending upon the particular drug, dosage, and length of use, sudden withdrawal can be uncomfortable or even hazardous, with symptoms including anxiety, tremors, panic, and, in extreme cases, seizures.

Stimulants have been more widely prescribed by physicians over the past several years because of their usefulness in helping many children and adults with attention deficit disorder (ADD). These include various forms of amphetamines (Dexedrine, Adderall, and others) and methylphenidate (Ritalin, Metadate, Concerta, and other preparations). Strattera, introduced in 2002 to treat ADD, does not have stimulant properties. Amphetamines and less potent stimulants (such as phentermine) have also been prescribed as weight-loss aids (with marginal success) because of their tendency to decrease appetite. Because stimulants can increase alertness and energy, lift one's mood, and decrease the need for sleep, they have significant abuse potential.

OXYCONTIN ABUSE

OxyContin is a time-release prescription painkiller containing oxycodone, a potent derivative of codeine that for many years had been available only in short-acting (four- to six-hour) preparations (such as Percodan, Percocet, and Tylox) that typically contain 5 mg of oxycodone combined with aspirin or acetaminophen. OxyContin tablets, however, can contain much larger amounts of oxycodone: 10, 20, 40, 80, or 160 mg, which when swallowed are gradually released over twelve hours. When properly used, this drug can provide safe and very effective relief for a variety of serious pain problems.

Unfortunately, soon after its introduction in 1996, drug abusers began chewing OxyContin tablets, crushing them and inhaling the powder, or (worst of all) dissolving crushed tablets in water and injecting them by vein. When misused in any of these ways, a very large dose of oxycodone can enter the bloodstream, producing effects ranging from euphoria (much like that obtained from heroin) to sedation, respiratory depression, and even death. Addiction, illegal sales, pharmacy theft, and crime related to OxyContin have become a significant drug-abuse problem, especially in the eastern United States.

Needless to say, OxyContin tablets should never be chewed or otherwise tampered with, and their use should be carefully supervised by both the prescribing physician and responsible caregivers. ■

F.Y.I. Widespread use of Dexedrine, Ritalin, and related drugs in treating attention deficit disorder (ADD) has placed more of these stimulants in circulation, thus increasing the likelihood of potential misuse. However, those who receive proper doses of these drugs appear to have little risk of addiction to them.

When taken in excessive doses or used inappropriately (i.e., smoked or injected), stimulants can rev up the central nervous system and produce a sense of energy, excitement, and invincibility. But with these come a number of serious risks and consequences. Increased blood pressure, rapid heart rate, and irregular heart rhythm may occur. Excitement may deteriorate into excitability, irritability, paranoia, delusions, and even violent behavior. Profound fatigue and depression are common when these drugs wear off. Tolerance results in a need for higher doses, and addiction is not unusual. Chronic abuse can lead to physical deterioration caused by malnutrition (from decreased interest in food) and loss of sleep. Heavy use can result in permanent brain damage, stroke, or heart attack.

F.Y.I. Contrary to popular belief, prescription antidepressants such as Prozac, Zoloft, Paxil, Effexor, Wellbutrin, and others are not habit-forming, are not controlled substances, and do not have any potential for abuse.

Preventing prescription-drug abuse . . .

Misuse and abuse of legal prescription drugs can create medical, personal, and even legal problems as serious as those associated with illegal drugs. Many of these difficulties can be avoided by following some straightforward guidelines:

- If you are going to receive a prescription from any physician, clinic, or emergency department, be certain that the physician has a list of *all* medications (both prescription and nonprescription, including herbal supplements) that you are currently taking. Also be sure to give the physician accurate information about your use of alcoholic beverages, which can interact dramatically with many medications—especially painkillers and sedatives.
- Be sure that you understand (ideally from written directions) why, when, and how your medications are to be taken. If you have some flexibility (for example, the medication is to be taken "as needed" for pain or anxiety), stay within the physician's guidelines. More is not necessarily better, and some drugs cause problems if you abruptly stop taking them.
- Find out if any new medication—especially one for treating pain or anxiety—can be habit-forming.
- *Do not share your medications with anyone.*
- If you are taking a narcotic painkiller or other medication with known abuse potential, be sure to keep it where it won't be found by children, teenagers, or anyone else who might be tempted to try, "borrow," or steal it.

- Have the courage to tell your physician if you have had any problem in the past with drug abuse or addiction. An honest conversation about what happened will be extremely helpful in choosing the best medication(s) for you.

. . . and dealing with it when it occurs

A person who is abusing or addicted to prescription drugs may be involved in a complex dance with multiple physicians, pharmacies, and family members, none of whom may have a complete picture of what is actually going on. Furthermore, rather than seeking drugs purely for the pleasurable experiences they provide, prescription-drug abusers often have a list of medical problems and symptoms that can prevent or delay dealing with the drug problem, often for years. There's always another headache (usually severe), another bout of abdominal pain that can't be pinned down, another round of disabling back spasms, even an injury or two, that take center stage in the doctor's office or emergency room. Facing the drug problem can become sidetracked because

- Most physicians want to help their patient feel better as soon as possible, and painkilling or sedative drugs are definitely effective for that purpose, at least for a while.
- Until a clear pattern of drug-seeking has become evident, doctors generally give their patients the benefit of the doubt. They also typically feel the need to rule out virtually every possible cause of the patient's distress (which may take weeks or months) before entertaining the possibility that the addictive need for painkillers or other drugs is part (or all) of the problem.
- Confronting a patient about a drug problem is unpleasant, often emotional, and nearly always very time-consuming. In the middle of a frantic day at the office, it's usually easier for a doctor simply to renew the drug rather than negotiate with an unhappy or argumentative patient, who often insists on picking up a prescription *today*.

As a result, getting a person who is abusing prescription drugs into appropriate treatment can be an extremely difficult and contentious process. Not only do abusers of prescription drugs frequently deny or lie about their problem, they also generally resent others' concern. ("But I'm in such pain all the time! I'm not a pill-popper! I wouldn't take all of these drugs if I didn't need them.") Very often a planned confrontation (or "carefrontation") involving the physician and concerned family members is necessary to convince the drug taker that he or she needs help specifically to deal with the medications themselves. And even that effort may be unsuccessful if the user refuses to acknowledge that his or her prescriptions are a problem. The basic principles involved in addressing and treating prescription-drug abuse and other substance problems are presented in the section "How Are Alcohol and Drug Problems Treated?" beginning on page 478.

Toward the Abyss: The World of Illegal Drugs

Marijuana—inhaled intellectual impairment

Baby boomers who experimented with **marijuana** during the 1960s may not be terribly concerned about this drug. But ongoing research suggests they should think again. Today's average batch is likely to contain a good deal more of its primary mood-altering chemical—delta-9-tetrahydrocannabinol, or THC for short—than what flower children were inhaling nearly four decades ago. According to the Office of National Drug Control Policy, the average THC content for all types of marijuana has been steadily rising.

What is it? Marijuana is a shredded mix of various parts (leaves, stems, seeds, flowers) of the hemp plant *Cannabis sativa.* Ordinary marijuana contains an average of 5 percent THC. Sinsemilla (Spanish for "without seed") is a more potent form of marijuana (averaging 12 percent THC) made from the buds and flowers of unpollinated female plants. Hashish (the Arabic word for hemp) is the sticky resin of the female plant flowers, containing an average of 10 percent THC (or as much as 28 percent).[56]

F.Y.I. The word *cannabis,* the generic name for the hemp plant, is also used to refer to all of the mood-altering concoctions made from it: marijuana, sinsemilla, hashish, and hash oil. The word *sativa* means "cultivated," no doubt reflecting its cash-crop status in many parts of the world.

What are some of its street names? *Pot, grass, weed, herb,* and *Mary Jane,* among others. Some strains of marijuana have been given "brand" names such as Texas tea, Maui wowie, and Bubble gum.

F.Y.I. Those who are unfamiliar with illicit drug culture will have a jaw-dropping experience at any Web site that offers a dictionary of street names for these substances. An extensive collection, entitled "Street Terms: Drugs and the Drug Trade," can be found at the Office of National Drug Control Policy site (http://www.whitehousedrugpolicy.gov/streetterms/default.asp). More impressive (and alarming) than the multiplicity of creative names is the number of ways in which hazardous drugs are combined.

How many people are using it? Marijuana is the most commonly used illegal drug in the United States. According to the 2004 National Survey on Drug Use & Health, over 14 million people twelve years old and over reported using it during the previous month, and more than 96 million have tried it at least once. The 2004 Monitoring the Future survey indicated that 11.8 percent of eighth graders, 27.5 percent of tenth graders, and 34.3 percent of twelfth graders had used marijuana at least once during the previous year.[57] From the 1960s to the late 1970s, there was a steady increase in the number of twelfth graders who had used marijuana during the previous year, reaching a peak of 51 percent in 1979. The percentage then declined to a low of 22 percent in 1992, followed by a steady rise through the 1990s.

Since 1975, the Monitoring the Future study has consistently found that between 83 and 90 percent of high school seniors said they could obtain marijuana easily if they wanted to.

How is it used? Marijuana is most commonly smoked, whether rolled into a cigarette, packed into a pipe, or stuffed into a cigar from which tobacco has been removed. Crack cocaine or other dangerous drugs may be added to the mix to be smoked, with or without the user's knowledge, sometimes with unpleasant results. Marijuana can also be added to foods or drinks (or even brewed as tea), though much more THC is delivered to the brain when the drug is inhaled. When smoked, its effects are felt almost immediately and typically last one to three hours. In food or drink, effects are delayed by thirty to sixty minutes but may last as long as four hours.

WHERE DO WE GET STATISTICS ABOUT SUBSTANCE ABUSE?

The most widely quoted statistics about the use and abuse of tobacco, alcohol, and drugs in the United States (especially among the young) come from three ongoing surveys that are funded by various agencies of the U.S. Department of Health and Human Services.

The National Survey on Drug Use & Health (formerly called the National Household Survey on Drug Abuse) has been conducted periodically since 1971, and annually since 1990, by the Substance Abuse and Mental Health Services Administration (SAMHSA). The survey is the primary source of information on patterns of tobacco, alcohol, and illegal drug use among the U.S. general population ages twelve and over. Past and current survey data are available at http://www.oas.samhsa.gov/nhsda.htm.

The **Monitoring the Future Survey** has been conducted by the University of Michigan's Institute for Social Research since 1975. Funded by the National Institute on Drug Abuse (NIDA), one of the twenty institutes comprising the National Institutes of Health (NIH), this survey focuses on the use of tobacco, alcohol, and drugs among eighth, tenth, and twelfth graders, as well as their perceptions and attitudes about these substances. Some fifty thousand students are surveyed in approximately four hundred schools across the United States, and a sample of each graduating class receives follow-up questionnaires for several years. Current information, survey results, and discussions can be found at http://monitoringthefuture.org.

The **Youth Risk Behavior Surveillance System (YRBSS)**, funded by the Centers for Disease Control and Prevention (CDC), is a school survey that studies a variety of health-related risk behaviors, including drug use, among ninth through twelfth graders. The first YRBS was conducted in 1990, and subsequent studies have been carried out every other year. The most recent findings can be found at http://www.cdc.gov/HealthyYouth/data_stats/index.htm. ■

F.Y.I. Additional slang: a marijuana cigarette is a joint; a water pipe used to smoke marijuana, a bong; and a marijuana cigar, a blunt. A blunt smoked while downing a forty-ounce bottle of malt liquor is called a B-40.

What's the attraction? Marijuana users are seeking a sense of euphoria, a relaxed high, which may be accompanied by an increased sensitivity to sights, sounds, and smells. Time may seem to pass more slowly, and minor goings-on or conversations among friends may seem extremely interesting or funny. Increased thirst or hunger ("the munchies") isn't uncommon. After the drug effect has worn off, the user may feel sleepy or even depressed. Depending on the preparation, additives, and mind-set of the user, unpleasant emotions such as anxiety, paranoia, or even panic can also occur. The presence of other drugs in the mix may cause unexpected and even serious reactions.

What are the health risks? The casual attitudes about marijuana in our culture and the media over the past thirty-five-plus years would suggest that this is basically a harmless diversion whose risks are overblown by law enforcement and government "fun regulators." But to the contrary:

- Marijuana smoke is more irritating to the mouth, throat, airway, and lungs than tobacco smoke, and it contains 50 to 70 percent more cancer-provoking hydrocarbons. The tendency to inhale deeply and hold one's breath while smoking aggravates this tendency. Long-term marijuana smokers, like their tobacco-puffing counterparts, are thus at higher risk not only for developing chronic lung disease but also cancer of the upper respiratory tract and lungs.
- People at risk for heart attack should think twice before inhaling marijuana, which causes a temporary rise in blood pressure and pulse rate. One study has suggested that an individual's risk for a heart attack increases fourfold during the first hour after smoking marijuana.

What about other consequences? Marijuana's greatest drawback, especially in light of its widespread use among the young, is that it impairs intellectual function—concentration, memory, and judgment—as well as motor skills. During the teen years a child should be learning how to think and act more maturely, but frequent marijuana use can derail that process. Short-term fallout can include injuries and death from motor-vehicle accidents or other trauma, as well as sexual misadventures resulting from loss of inhibition and rational thinking. A number of research studies also have demonstrated that impairment of memory, learning, and concentration continues for days or weeks after the immediate effects of the drug wear off.

Long-term users are known for an amotivational syndrome in which goals and self-discipline (especially in school and work performance) literally go up in smoke. One study demonstrated lower scores on standardized verbal and mathematical tests among twelfth-grade marijuana smokers compared to their nonsmoking peers, even though both groups had performed equally well during the fourth grade. Other research has associated marijuana use with overall poorer job performance, including increased tardiness, absenteeism, accidents, and workers' compensation claims.[58]

Finally, marijuana keeps very bad company. For adolescents and young adults alike it can be a gateway drug, introducing them to the harrowing world of illegal drugs and the criminals who produce and distribute them.

What happens when a user quits? While marijuana is not widely perceived as highly addictive, some long-term users will continue to smoke it compulsively even though it is clearly having a negative impact on school, work, and relationships. Long-term regular users who quit may experience anxiety, irritability, and sleeplessness. According to the National Institute on Drug Abuse, for more than 1.7 million admissions to publicly funded drug treatment programs in 2003—about 15 percent of all admissions—marijuana was the primary drug of abuse. Sadly, nearly half of these were under twenty years old, and more than half had started using by age fourteen.

Inhalants—cheap (and dangerous) thrills

More than a thousand different products that can be purchased at the supermarket, hardware store, or hobby shop—or that are simply sitting in the garage—can end up in the hands, lungs, and brain of a child or adolescent who is looking for an inexpensive intoxication, with potentially disastrous results.

What are they? Four types of products are inhaled by (mostly) young thrill seekers:

- **Solvents** or solvent-containing products, such as paint thinner, lacquer, degreaser, model glue, contact cement, gasoline, felt-tip marker fluid, and dozens of other volatile products can have mind-altering effects if inhaled deeply.
- **Aerosols** that contain solvents and propellants, such as hair sprays, deodorants, and spray paint.
- **Gases** present in household products such as whipped-cream dispensers, butane lighters, and propane tanks.
- **Nitrites**, which primarily dilate blood vessels and relax muscles. Examples are cyclohexyl nitrite, found in room deodorizers, and amyl nitrite, which has been used as a treatment for angina (pain caused by inadequate blood flow to the heart).

What are some of their street names? These include *air blast* and *poor man's pot.* Inhalant use is known as bagging or glading. Nitrites go by a variety of names on the street, but poppers and snappers are perhaps the most common, because they are often dispensed in small glass vials that have to be snapped open before use.

How many people are using them? With the exception of nitrites, inhalant use typically starts in childhood or early adolescence. The age of peak use is typically twelve to fourteen, with first experiences occurring as early as six to eight years of age. In the 2004 Monitoring the Future study, 10.9 percent of twelfth graders, 12.4 percent of tenth graders, and 17.3 percent of eighth graders reported using an inhalant at least once in their lifetime.[59] The National Survey on Drug Use & Health (formerly called the National Household Survey on Drug Abuse) has documented a disturbing and persistent increase in new inhalant users over the past two decades. There were an estimated 410,000 new users in 1985; 618,000 in 1994; and 857,000 in 2004.[60]

How are they used? Solvents, gases, or aerosols are either inhaled through the nose (sniffing) or by mouth (huffing), either directly from the container, from plastic bags containing the fumes and held over the mouth and nose, or from a cloth that has been sprayed or saturated with the material.

What's the attraction? Depending upon the substance used, several deep inhalations bring on a sense of euphoria—frequently with hallucinations—as well as stimulation and loss of inhibition, which may lead to other high-risk behavior. Drowsiness and sleep may follow. Nitrites are used primarily in an attempt to enhance sexual experiences.

What are the health risks? Given the huge variety of toxins that are being abused through inhalation, it should come as little surprise that a host of serious medical consequences have been observed. A number of products can be lethal during or after a single use. One disastrous consequence known as **sudden sniffing death syndrome** can occur in a previously healthy user, especially when butane, propane, and aerosols are inhaled. (This may result from an increased sensitivity of the heart muscle, and it is possible that an abrupt adrenaline surge in response to being startled can provoke a lethal irregular heart rhythm.) Users can also die by asphyxiation, when the inhaled substance interferes with oxygen exchange within the lung, or from suffocation, when a plastic bag is pulled over the head.

The most serious by-product of chronic inhalant use is permanent damage to the brain and nervous system, causing loss of intellectual function and coordination. Depending upon chemical structure and the number and intensity of exposures, inhaled substances can also damage the tissues of other internal organs. Toluene, for example, found in glue, spray paint, and gasoline, can cause brain damage (including actual loss of tissue), disturbances of gait (walking) and coordination, vision and hearing loss, and injury to the liver or kidney.

Nitrites are most commonly inhaled as a party drug (especially among homosexual men) in an attempt to enhance sexual performance and pleasure, often in situations where sexual activity is anything but safe and the likelihood of becoming infected with a sexually transmitted disease high. Ironically, in animal research these drugs impair immune function, which would be an obvious disadvantage for someone who is at risk for acquiring a potentially serious infection—or already has one.

What about other consequences? Like other drug users, solvent and aerosol inhalant abusers may display erratic behavior, poor self-care, and declining school performance. Parents may notice specific clues such as the aroma of the inhalant (which can persist in the breath for several hours), stains and odors in clothes, and an unusual stash of products (such as gasoline or aerosol cans) in a child's room. An adult who discovers children or adolescents in the act of inhaling should avoid surprise tactics or a sudden confrontation that might cause a startle reflex, since this could precipitate a dangerous heart-rhythm disturbance.

Club drugs—the death of the party

A number of unrelated substances have been grouped under this title because they are used by teenagers and young adults at dance clubs and bars, and especially at raves and trances—all-night dance parties held in clubs, warehouses, or even outdoors, for groups ranging from a few hundred to several thousand. While rave and trance culture is focused primarily on the driving music and the physical and emotional release of dancing for hours with an exuberant crowd, many who attend try to enhance the experience with one or more drugs, sometimes with disastrous results. The most common include **MDMA (Ecstasy)**, **Rohypnol**, **gamma hydroxybutyrate (GHB)**, **ketamine**, and the not-so-golden oldie of the 1960s, **LSD**. (Methamphetamine, a relative of MDMA that has been an abused drug for many years, shows up at the rave scene as well.) Obviously, this cast of characters is subject to change without notice, and those interested in staying current on this phenomenon may want to get an update at http://www.clubdrugs.org, a service of the National Institute on Drug Abuse.

MDMA (Ecstasy): Love and brain damage

What is it? MDMA is a synthetic drug with a chemical structure resembling both methamphetamine (a stimulant) and mescaline (a hallucination-generating drug). Originally intended to be an appetite suppressant, MDMA was used in psychotherapy during the 1970s to help individuals open up and discuss their emotions. This practice was discontinued in the mid-1980s when researchers found that MDMA causes brain damage in animals.

What are some of its street names? *Ecstasy* is the most widely used name. Others include *XTC, E, hug drug, love drug,* and *disco biscuit.*

How is it used? MDMA is nearly always swallowed as a pill, although more adventurous (and foolhardy) individuals may crush pills and then snort the powder or inject a solution containing it. Occasionally MDMA is taken in suppository form.

What's the attraction? This drug supplies energy to dance the night away. Users may feel relaxed, and they may experience a sense of increased awareness and deep feelings of love for others. While MDMA does not cause florid hallucinations, it can alter one's perception of time.

What are the health risks? Like other stimulants, MDMA can raise the pulse and blood pressure, and may interfere with temperature regulation. In hot, stuffy, tightly packed club settings, the combination of MDMA and the ongoing intense exertion of dancing can lead to **hyperthermia**, a marked increase in body temperature that can cause muscle breakdown and kidney failure. Also, as is typical with stimulants, ongoing use is associated with anxiety, depression, insomnia, and paranoia—just the opposite of the good feelings that are its primary appeal.

Perhaps the most worrisome aspect of MDMA use is the finding that it causes long-term brain damage in animals and produces changes in brain scans (using positron emission tomography) in humans. MDMA appears to damage and deplete cells that release serotonin, an important chemical messenger, in areas of the brain involved in memory. Some research suggests MDMA users score more poorly on memory tests than their nonusing counterparts, but whether such changes are permanent is unknown.

Rohypnol and gamma hydroxybutyrate (GHB): Predator tools

Both Rohypnol and GHB have become notorious as date-rape drugs. Accounts of sexual predators using them to incapacitate victims led Congress to pass the Drug-Induced Rape Prevention and Punishment Act of 1996, increasing federal penalties for the use of any controlled substance in a sexual assault.

What are they? Rohypnol (flunitrazepam) is a sedative in the class called benzodiazepines, to which familiar medications such as **diazepam** (Valium) and **alprazolam** (Xanax) belong. Originally introduced as a sleeping aid in Europe in the 1970s, it was found to cause short-term loss of memory and profound drowsiness, especially when mixed with alcohol. It has never been approved for use in the United States, but it is available in more than sixty countries.

Gamma hydroxybutyrate (GHB) was sold in health-food stores until the early 1990s and touted as an aid for weight reduction and bodybuilding. It is in fact a central nervous system depressant, especially when mixed with alcohol.

What are some of their street names? Rohypnol is called *roofies, rope, ropies, forget me drug,* and the more blunt epithet, *the date rape drug.* GHB also goes by the names *liquid ecstasy, G, soap, goop,* and variations on its initials, such as *Georgia home boy* and *grievous bodily harm.*

How are they used? Both drugs are taken orally: Rohypnol is taken as a pill or ground into powder, and GHB as a powder or liquid. They are both colorless and odorless, but GHB has a soapy or salty taste.

What's the attraction? When taken voluntarily, Rohypnol is used to induce sleep and GHB is used to create a sense of relaxed euphoria (usually mixed with alcohol). But more often sexual predators slip one of these drugs into an unsuspecting victim's drink. Rohypnol causes a rapid onset of deep sleep and amnesia for whatever happens during the next few hours—and thus serves as the rapist's best friend. It obliterates the victim's ability to resist or remember who did what. Similarly, when slipped into a victim's drink, GHB can incapacitate a victim against resisting a sexual assault.

What are the health risks? Long-term users of Rohypnol are likely to develop physical and psychological dependence, and may have withdrawal symptoms (including an increased risk for seizures) when the drug is stopped. Depending on dose and other drugs being taken, GHB's sedative effects can be extreme, leading to unconsciousness, coma, and even death. By far the most grievous damage related to these drugs, however, is the fallout from a sexual assault: the physical and emotional trauma, as well as the possibility of pregnancy and/or a sexually transmitted disease.

LSD: Checking out of reality

LSD (lysergic acid diethylamide) was first synthesized in 1938 by Swiss pharmaceutical chemist Albert Hofmann, who was looking for medical remedies among variations on lysergic acid, a compound derived from a fungus called ergot. One day he accidentally swallowed a tiny amount of this chemical and was startled when objects all around him appeared distorted, grotesque, and threatening. Far from finding this an entertaining or enlightening experience, he was terrified that he could not stop "these demonic transformations of the outer world" and "the dissolution of my ego."[61] He recovered, and for a while the drug was considered a possible candidate for treating schizophrenia.

For many years drugs derived from ergot (such as Cafergot) were a mainstay of migraine-headache therapy. The initials *LSD* come from the German name for this compound: Lyserg-Säure-Diäthylamid.

In the early 1960s, Harvard professors Timothy Leary (who coined the phrase "Tune in, turn on, drop out") and Richard Alpert (later to become New Age philosopher Ram Dass) helped put LSD on the cultural map, after which it became a countercultural icon of the turbulent 1960s and early 1970s. Long after bell-bottoms and psychedelic artwork became faded relics, LSD has continued to find new consumers among the children of baby boomers, especially in the rave culture.

What is it? LSD is known as a hallucinogen, with properties similar to drugs such as mescaline (found in the cactus peyote, for example). These have been used for centuries in many cultures to induce visions and departures from reality, often in pursuit of religious or mystical experiences. Hallucinogens alter the action of the neurotransmitter **serotonin** in certain key areas of the brain that process and interpret sensory input from the outside world. Uncontaminated LSD is an odorless and colorless powder, sold as small tablets (called microdots), or more commonly dissolved and applied to absorbent paper, which is then cut into quarter-inch individual doses.

What are some of its street names? *Acid, dots, Lucy in the Sky with Diamonds, window pane, Elvis,* and *mellow yellow* are a few of its slang names.

What's the attraction? Depending upon the dose, setting, and other (usually unpredictable) variables, LSD produces both hallucinations and changes (especially increased intensity) in colors, sounds, and smells that can feel both pleasant and fascinating. Users are often intrigued by **synesthesia**—the blending of sensations in which a person "hears" colors and "sees" sounds. Some claim to have profound insights into themselves, the universe, and God while under the influence of LSD and other hallucinogens. With repeated use of LSD, tolerance can develop, such that higher doses may be needed to produce the same effect. This disappears after stopping the drug for several days, and ongoing use of LSD is not associated with physical withdrawal symptoms or overt addiction.

What are the health risks? Like its discoverer, Albert Hofmann, LSD users may experience more than they bargained for when the drug induces a "bad trip" that can generate profound anxiety, panic, confusion, despair, or even self-destructive behavior. Helping and supporting such a person through the mental and emotional turbulence may keep friends, family, or health-care providers occupied for several hours until the drug wears off. If the LSD is taken with one or more other drugs—a "Frisco special," for example, is the combination of heroin, cocaine, and LSD—all bets are off and more elaborate medical or psychological care may be needed.

What about other consequences? Two long-term problems may plague LSD users for years after their last dose: The first, and most serious, is a **drug-induced psychosis**, a persistent mental disorder involving not only mood disturbances (including both mania and depression) but also disorganized and irrational thinking, as well as recurrent hallucinations. The second is the so-called LSD flashback, now more formally known as **hallucinogen persisting perception disorder**, or **HPPD**. This is usually a replay of one or more of the visual disturbances that the user experienced on LSD, which occurs spontaneously and often repeatedly for years. (One common manifestation is seeing a colorful "trail" behind a moving object.) Aside from being annoying, these may cause some alarm *(Am I having a stroke?)* and generate a potentially expensive medical evaluation to rule out a neurological disorder.

Dissociative drugs: Ketamine and phencyclidine (PCP)

What are they? Ketamine and its older and more toxic sibling PCP (which is not a common rave drug) are injectable medications originally developed as anesthetics for both humans and animals. As it wears off, PCP causes so many problems, especially delirium and severe agitation, that it is only used in veterinary medicine. Ketamine, introduced in 1963 to replace PCP, is used for both humans and animals, although 90 percent of sales are to veterinarians.

What are some of their street names? Ketamine is known as *K, Vitamin K, Special K, cat Valium, jet.* PCP is referred to as *angel* with various names attached (*angel dust, angel hair, angel mist,* etc.), as well as *super weed, super grass* (when mixed with marijuana), *zombie, hog, rocket fuel, animal trank.*

How are they used? Ketamine comes in a liquid form that can be directly injected or evaporated into powder that is swallowed, snorted, or smoked. PCP is taken as a pill or ground into powder to be snorted or smoked (after being sprinkled on tobacco, marijuana, or even parsley).

What's the attraction? Both of these drugs produce a sense of detachment from reality, as if floating or being out of the body altogether. Ketamine's effects are shorter, milder, and less likely to be violent than PCP's.

What are the health risks? PCP is notable for its unpredictable and often violent side effects. Elevations in pulse, blood pressure, and temperature occur at all doses, and a large dose can cause seizures, stroke, extreme elevations of body temperature (hyperthermia), coma, and death. Involuntary and uncoordinated muscle contractions can be so intense as to cause breakdown of muscle fibers or even bone fractures. PCP's behavioral effects are its most dreaded calling card, however. Users may experience not only detachment but also overt hallucinations, fear (or outright panic), paranoia, a sense of invulnerability, and decreased awareness of pain. A nightmare (and a highly dangerous problem) for law-enforcement or emergency-department personnel is to be confronted with a disoriented, agitated, violent PCP user who seemingly has superhuman strength and no apparent sense of pain.

Ketamine, as noted above, is less likely to induce the unpredictable and severe behavioral reactions seen with PCP, although it can generate most of the other medical side effects, especially at higher doses. An unpleasant and frightening sense of complete sensory detachment caused by ketamine has been dubbed the K-hole.

What about other consequences? Because ketamine is tasteless and can induce temporary memory loss, it is also part of the sexual predator's bag of evil tricks.

What happens when a user quits? Regular users of PCP may go through withdrawal when they stop, and in addition they may experience long-term problems with depression and memory loss. Repeated ketamine exposure may also interfere with memory and learning on a long-term basis.

Methamphetamine—speed trap

What is it? A derivative of amphetamine and chemically similar in some respects to MDMA, **methamphetamine** is a potent central nervous system stimulant. When first synthesized it was used as a nasal decongestant and asthma treatment. Today it is still prescribed occasionally to treat narcolepsy (a disorder in which an individual suddenly falls asleep without warning) and ADD. Unfortunately, it is relatively easy to manufacture in home "laboratories" using store-bought ingredients, making it the most commonly synthesized illegal drug in the United States.

What are some of its street names? These include *speed, meth, poor man's cocaine, ice, crank, crystal,* and many others.

How many people are using it? The 2004 National Survey on Drug Use & Health indicated that almost 12.4 million people over the age of twelve have tried methamphetamine at least once. High school students represent a large portion of users, as seen in the percentage that have ever used methamphetamine: 7.6 percent, according to the 2003 survey of the Youth Risk Behavior Surveillance System.[62]

How is it used? Methamphetamine is taken in tablet form, dissolved in water or alcohol, smoked, snorted, or injected. Yaba, a tablet containing methamphetamine and caffeine, has been popular in Southeast Asia and has begun to appear in Asian communities on the West Coast.

What's the attraction? Like other stimulants, methamphetamine creates a temporary feeling of increased energy and well-being, and a decrease in appetite. Taken orally, its effects are noticeable within a half hour or less, and the pleasurable response may last for several hours. Smoking or injecting it, on the other hand, produces a more intense rush within a few minutes. Many of the drug's effects last for the better part of a day, but the pleasurable component fades well before that. This and the inevitable tolerance that develops (that is, more drug is needed to produce the same effect) may induce methamphetamine users to go on binges to try to maintain their drug-induced high.

What are the health risks? Methamphetamine stimulates not only the nervous system but also the rest of the body, raising the pulse rate (and the likelihood of irregular heart rhythms), blood pressure, and body temperature. Heart attack, stroke, hyperthermia (dangerously elevated body temperature), seizures, and death are all possible consequences. Users who inject methamphetamine, like users of any drug shot into a vein, run the risk of acquiring HIV/AIDS and hepatitis B or C from shared needles or other equipment, not to mention bacterial infections of the skin, bone, or heart.

Long-term use is likely not only to lead to addiction but also to induce long-term, or even permanent, changes in the central nervous system. (Some evidence suggests that damage to nerve endings in the brain may occur after a single dose.) Intense emotional and behavioral turbulence—agitation, anxiety, insomnia, and violent behavior—are not uncommon. Psychosis, with delusions, hallucinations, and paranoia (including homicidal or suicidal thoughts), can occur.

What happens when a user quits? Depression, fatigue, anxiety, and an intense craving for another dose occur. Methamphetamine users may embark on a desperate run in order to override their tolerance for the drug, injecting large quantities every few hours over several days in a sleepless binge.

Cocaine—a fast track downhill

What is it? Cocaine, the most powerful stimulant occurring in nature, is one of the most addictive drugs on the street and in many ways the most dangerous. Coca leaves, the source of cocaine, grow in the highlands of the Andes in South America, primarily in Colombia, Bolivia, and Peru. They have been chewed for thousands of years for their stimulant and hunger-reducing effects. In the late 1800s pure cocaine hydrochloride was extracted from coca leaves and found to be useful in medical procedures involving the nose and eyes because of its ability to reduce pain and constrict blood vessels. It was also incorporated into hundreds of patent medicines, tonics, cigarettes, and wines. Crack cocaine (also called freebase) is a form in which the hydrochloride has been removed, creating a form of the drug that can be smoked. The crackling sound that occurs when cocaine is heated during this preparation gives the final product its name.

F.Y.I.

The coca bush bears no relation to the tropical cacao tree, from which we obtain chocolate and cocoa. While some people consider themselves chocoholics, these everyday temptations have nothing in common with cocaine.

What are its street names? *Coke, blow, nose candy, snow,* and *C* (and numerous words that begin with this letter: *Cecil, Charlie, coconut*) are just some of the dozens of street names.

How many people are using it? Cocaine use peaked during the mid-1980s when 5.7 million people, or about 3 percent of the population, were classified as current users (defined as having used it during the previous thirty days). Levels of use then declined until 1992; since then they have remained relatively stable. According to the 2004 National Survey on Drug Use & Health, more than 34 million Americans ages twelve or older had tried cocaine at least once; 5.7 million had used it during the previous year; and 2 million were current users. Young adults (ages eighteen to twenty-five) had the highest rate of use. During 2004, an estimated one million Americans became new cocaine users, with an average age of twenty. According to the 2004 Monitoring the Future Survey, more than 5 percent of twelfth graders have used cocaine within the last year.[63]

How is it used? Cocaine nearly always is inhaled (snorted), entering the bloodstream via the inner linings of the nose; injected into a vein; or smoked. When inhaled, its high lasts about ten to fifteen minutes—much shorter than that seen with methamphetamine. When injected or smoked, the effects are felt immediately but may last only a few minutes. Cocaine is also injected with heroin (a combination known as a speedball, among other names), smoked with tobacco or marijuana, or combined with virtually any other mind-altering drug. Powdered cocaine may be diluted with cornstarch, talcum, or sugar.

What's the attraction? Dopamine, one of several important chemical messengers between nerve cells, plays an important role in the activation of certain areas in the brain associated with pleasure. Cocaine causes a temporary pileup of dopamine in these areas, resulting in a sense of energy and euphoria well beyond anything a person has experienced before. This may be accompanied by increased alertness; mental focus; sensitivity to light, sound, and touch; and decreased need for food and sleep. Because tolerance to cocaine can develop rapidly, a person's first experience with this drug may be the most intense, especially if it's smoked or injected. The desire to repeat this ecstatic event again and again is frequently overwhelming, but many users never experience as much pleasure as they did with their first dose.

What are the health risks? There are many, and they're serious.

- Cocaine's powerful jolt to the central nervous system also triggers a rapid heart rate, constricted blood vessels, and elevated blood pressure. Even in young, well-conditioned bodies, these events can cause stroke, seizures, or cardiac arrest. Cocaine precipitates more emergency-room visits than any other illegal drug.
- All of cocaine's routes of entry into the body pose unique hazards. Snorting cocaine up the nose can lead to destruction of the septum (the structure separating the two nasal passages) and eventual collapse of the bridge of the nose. Injecting cocaine into the veins can transmit dangerous microorganisms, including the viruses that cause hepatitis and AIDS, when needles or syringes are shared with other users. Allergic reactions to injected cocaine, or one of the additives mixed with it, can be severe or even fatal.
- When cocaine and alcohol are used at the same time (not an uncommon event), the liver may convert them to a compound called **cocaethylene**, which is more toxic than either drug alone. According to the National Institute on Drug Abuse, cocaine and alcohol are the two drugs that, when used together, are most likely to result in death.
- Multiple doses of cocaine taken in a binge—often involving increasing doses because tolerance has resulted in a diminishing effect—can lead to increasing restlessness, paranoia, or psychosis, complete with delusions and hallucinations.

What happens when a user quits? When the drug wears off, cocaine users become anxious, irritable, depressed, and desperate for the next dose. Bigger and more frequent doses are needed to produce the desired effect, and the progression from first use to desperate addiction can be rapid. (With crack, addiction frequently begins with the first dose.) Money becomes important solely as a means to obtaining more cocaine, and huge sums may be spent, borrowed, or stolen to buy it. Exchanges of sex for drugs enhance the spread of HIV/AIDS, hepatitis, and other infections.

Heroin—no way to live

What is it? Heroin is the most highly addictive narcotic and the scourge of any individual, family, or neighborhood affected by it. Though by no means the most widely used illegal drug, heroin generates medical problems, crime, and general chaos that more than make up for its fewer number of users. A derivative of morphine, heroin was first synthesized in 1874 and, like cocaine, was widely used by physicians at the turn of the century before its powerful potential for addiction was recognized.

What are some of its street names? *Horse, smack, Big H, Dr. Feelgood,* and *thunder* are a few, but there are many more, including names for combinations of heroin and other drugs.

How many people are using it? According to the 2004 National Survey on Drug Use & Health, more than 3.1 million Americans over the age of twelve have tried heroin at least once, and almost 400,000 have used it within the previous year. The United Nations Drug Control Program estimates that there are some 8 million users worldwide.[64]

How is it used? For decades heroin has most commonly been taken by direct injection into a vein. Because of increasing supplies of purer and cheaper heroin, however, more users now smoke or sniff it.

What's the attraction? Injected directly into a vein, heroin proceeds within seconds to the brain, where it is converted to morphine and binds to special sites called **opioid receptors**. The result is an immediate rush that first-time users find overwhelmingly pleasurable. When sniffed or smoked, this occurs more slowly (over ten to fifteen minutes) and with less intensity (but no less potential for addiction). After the initial euphoria, users will feel relaxed and sedated for hours—and then want to find another dose.

What are the health risks? As with cocaine, there are many, and they are serious, especially for the user who is injecting it.

- Veins that are repeatedly invaded by needles and nonsterile materials become scarred, and bacteria accidentally shot into the bloodstream can infect heart valves, bone, and other tissues.
- Heroin sold on the street doesn't go through quality control. Dealer profits are increased when the drug is diluted (or "cut") with other substances such as sugar, cornstarch, powdered milk, other illegal drugs, or even strychnine (which is often used as a rodent poison). Some of these materials do not dissolve in the blood and may obstruct small arteries, leading to tissue damage in vital organs such as

the lungs, liver, kidney, or brain. These damaged areas are in turn more vulnerable to bacteria introduced during injections.

- Sharing needles and other paraphernalia is a highly efficient means of spreading life-threatening (and life-ending) viral infections, including HIV/AIDS and hepatitis B and C. The National Institute on Drug Abuse estimates that a third of all HIV infections and half of hepatitis C infections are transmitted in this way. These then can be spread to sexual partners and from infected mothers to their babies.
- The chaotic lifestyle, poor self-care, malnutrition, and general squalor that characterize the life of a hard-core addict set them up for even more infections, such as tuberculosis, pneumonia, and skin ulcers.
- Heroin users rapidly develop tolerance—bigger doses are needed to bring about a pleasurable effect—and physical dependence, such that without a steady supply of the drug, the user experiences an unpleasant withdrawal within several hours.
- Variations in the quantity and purity of heroin can result in a user getting a much bigger dose than expected. Heroin overdose puts the brain into a stupor or flat-out unconsciousness and depresses respirations. If the dose is big enough, and especially if the user has ingested other sedating drugs (such as alcohol), any injection could lead to the morgue.

What about other consequences? Like cocaine, heroin can rapidly draw a user into a full-time pursuit of the next dose and the funds necessary to acquire it. Wages (if there is a job), savings, and possessions are likely to be consumed by this addiction. Theft, dealing one or more drugs, prostitution, or simply trading sex for the next dose often become part of a grim way of life.

What happens when a user quits? With increasing tolerance leading to bigger doses of heroin, physical dependence is virtually inevitable. Once this hook is set, the user will begin to feel uncomfortable within a few hours of the last dose. If no drug is forthcoming, by twenty-four to forty-eight hours life becomes a miserable mix of sweats, cramps, shaking, nausea, vomiting, and diarrhea. For most users these symptoms subside within a week, and as rotten as they may feel, an adult in reasonable health will survive this ordeal even without any medical support. (This may not be the case, however, for the unborn child of a pregnant woman undergoing withdrawal.) Unfortunately, a user may crave this drug and stumble back into its enslaving grip months after withdrawal symptoms have completely disappeared.

How Are Alcohol and Drug Problems Treated?

While the specific approaches must be tailored to individuals, a few key elements are nearly always a part of the recovery process—and they all involve working with other people. Of course, sobriety can only be maintained by those with the substance-abuse problem. No one else can do it for them. And there are, to be sure, some people who decide one day to plant their feet, set their jaw, square off against the bottle or the drugs, and "just say no." But they usually soon find themselves embroiled in a war that has a lot of intense fronts: altered brain and body chemistry that generate intense cravings; very unpleasant withdrawal symptoms; personal issues and crises that are stressful; anxiety and discontent; friends or family members who may be drinking or using drugs (and thus not terribly supportive of the decision to become and remain sober); activities and surroundings full of cues and triggers that set off the desire to drink or use drugs; and an internal voice arguing that one drink or just another dose can't hurt that much. Here or there one of these "lone rangers" may succeed, but for the vast majority the first step toward freedom is acknowledging that there really *is* a problem and then seeking all the help they can get.

Apart from a direct, miraculous intervention from God, recovery is never a quick fix for those who are abusing and addicted to alcohol and drugs, but rather it is often a lifelong process. Furthermore, even with appropriate treatment, counseling, and support, many struggle with relapses, even after years of being clean and sober.

Those users who admit their problem and are willing to seek help can draw on several resources:

1. **Medical care.** Alcohol and drugs often have such an iron grip on individuals that any attempt to cut back or stop provokes a highly uncomfortable or even dangerous physical response. Such people are candidates for a medically supervised withdrawal or detoxification ("detox" for short), which may require hospitalization to be carried out safely. Medications are available that reduce cravings, anxiety, agitation, nausea, and even the risk of a seizure during the early stages of withdrawal. Long-term heavy drinkers or drug abusers often have a number of other medical problems that need attention as well, such as malnutrition, infections (including such serious opponents as tuberculosis, hepatitis, or HIV), and malfunctioning organs such as the liver, kidney, or pancreas.

   Once withdrawal has been accomplished, other medications are sometimes used as part of a multifaceted approach to help maintain abstinence. **Disulfiram** (Antabuse), which has been available for many years, can be a powerful deterrent to drinking: People who take it regularly will feel genuinely rotten if they drink so much as a nip of alcohol. **Naltrexone** (ReVia) can be useful in treating alcohol and/or narcotic addictions and can reduce cravings for alcohol. Narcotic addicts may be started on methadone maintenance, which can provide some semblance of stability and help them steer clear of more dangerous and destructive drugs.

   In addition, many substance abusers have mood disorders (especially anxiety and depression) for which alcohol and drugs may have served as a form of self-treatment. These conditions may have a biochemical origin, and medical treatment that helps stabilize them can make a big contribution toward preventing a relapse. Needless to say, the use of *any* medications during withdrawal and recovery—whether prescription or nonprescription drugs, vitamins, or supplements—must be closely supervised by a knowledgeable physician.

Chapter 8 includes a detailed look at anxiety and depression, including their biochemical, relational, and spiritual dimensions.

2. **Personal and family counseling.** No alcohol or drug problem occurs in a vacuum, and a skilled counselor can expedite the process of sorting out past and present conflicts that contributed to or were created by it. Both users and family members may have to face some tough issues as they grapple with the fallout from abuse or dependence, and as they adopt new roles and behaviors. Life with users is anything but pleasant and orderly. Most often it is unpredictable, chaotic, anxiety-ridden, or even violent. This is one arena in which **accountability**—a very important commodity in recovery—can be maintained. And as we will discuss later, in order for people in recovery to succeed, it is vital that their family be actively involved in the process, which requires much more than "fixing" the drinker/user.

3. **Group work.** One cornerstone of achieving and maintaining sobriety is ongoing participation in a group in which people with drinking and/or drug problems can find encouragement, support, and especially accountability. This is such an important area, in fact, that we will look at it in some depth.

   The oldest and best known of these groups is **Alcoholics Anonymous (A.A.)**, founded in the mid-1930s in Ohio by Bill Wilson, a stockbroker, and Bob Smith, a surgeon. Both men had long-standing and seemingly unsolvable drinking problems, but they found that their compulsion to drink was significantly reduced as they exchanged their stories and feelings with others who were dealing with the same problem. Presently more than 100,000 A.A. groups meet in 150 countries, serving over 2 million members. All groups are self-supporting via "pass the hat" donations at each meeting. There are no fixed dues or fees, and no contributions are sought or accepted from nonmembers. A.A. is nonsectarian, nondenominational, and nonpolitical, and the only requirement for membership is a desire to stop drinking. Meetings occur in all types of settings: churches, synagogues, schools, hospitals, community centers, and private homes, among others.

   The centerpiece of A.A.'s approach to recovery is in the Twelve Steps. When the original members of what would become known as Alcoholics Anonymous analyzed the process that had led to their success at becoming and staying sober, they identified twelve specific steps. An initial impulse to codify them into twelve "commandments" for others to follow shifted to a basic history of "what we did." The steps were first described in 1939 in the

Information about A.A. and the location of local groups can be found at its Web site (www.alcoholics-anonymous.org) or by calling (212) 870-3400.

organization's basic textbook, entitled simply *Alcoholics Anonymous* but also widely known as the *The Big Book.* Since then these twelve steps have been adopted and adapted by recovery groups dealing with other addictions: Narcotics Anonymous, Cocaine Anonymous, Overeaters Anonymous, Gamblers Anonymous, and so on. These are often labeled self-help groups, but in fact the central theme of the steps is the utter powerlessness of the individual to overcome the addiction, and the need to turn the reins of one's life over to God. (*Mutual help,* referring to the assistance and accountability among group participants, is perhaps a more accurate term than *self-help*.)

The Twelve Steps read as follows:

1. We admitted we were powerless over alcohol—that our lives had become unmanageable.
2. Came to believe that a Power greater than ourselves could restore us to sanity.
3. Made a decision to turn our will and our lives over to the care of God as we understood Him.
4. Made a searching and fearless moral inventory of ourselves.
5. Admitted to God, to ourselves, and to another human being the exact nature of our wrongs.
6. Were entirely ready to have God remove all these defects of character.
7. Humbly asked Him to remove our shortcomings.
8. Made a list of all persons we had harmed and became willing to make amends to them all.
9. Made direct amends to such people wherever possible, except when to do so would injure them or others.
10. Continued to take personal inventory and when we were wrong promptly admitted it.
11. Sought through prayer and meditation to improve our conscious contact with God, as we understood Him, praying only for knowledge of His will for us and the power to carry that out.
12. Having had a spiritual awakening as the result of these Steps, we tried to carry this message to alcoholics, and to practice these principles in all our affairs.[65]

The Twelve Steps embody strong themes of repentance, submission to God, confession, restitution, ongoing self-examination, and spreading the word to others. While references to God are nonspecific (i.e., to "God as we understand Him"), these themes stem directly from biblical teachings, and thus many A.A. and other twelve-step groups have been formed or comfortably hosted within churches or synagogues. On the other hand, in order to make the twelve steps as inclusive as possible, some have interpreted the notion of God or a higher power very broadly indeed—He or it might be any supernatural personage, force, the A.A. group, or even the twelve steps themselves. (More about this later.)

Below are some other basic elements of A.A. and other twelve-step programs that follow its model:

- Frequent attendance at meetings (in various locations) is encouraged in order to build a habit of sobriety. Unlike service-club gatherings or Sunday church services, A.A. isn't considered a once-weekly proposition, especially in the beginning. Newcomers may hear about "ninety meetings in ninety days," a daunting challenge that can nevertheless help make some serious changes in one's lifestyle.
- Even though they are not issued as commandments, working through the Twelve Steps is intended to be a serious undertaking. Simply nodding in agreement won't cut it. The process involves a lot of soul-searching, remembering, writing, talking with others in A.A. and elsewhere, making amends to those who have been harmed, and continuing self-examination.
- Identifying a sponsor—someone in a group who has maintained sobriety for no less than two years and who will serve as a one-on-one coach and mentor through the recovery process—is very important. This person should ideally be friendly, available (including a willingness to respond to an SOS call in the middle of the night, if necessary), objective, compassionate, but also tough. The sponsor needs to be able to ask hard questions ("Did you drink or use last week?" "Did you think about doing it?" "Did you come close?"), to insist on honest answers, and to attempt to see through and confront a person about any answers that are less than truthful.
- A.A. and other twelve-step groups understand that maintaining sobriety requires ongoing vigilance and effort. Those abstaining from their substance or behavior problem are said to be in recovery, not recovered. "One day at a time" is the operative phrase, not "I'm never going to drink/use again."

A.A. and its Twelve Steps have provided (and still remain) the preeminent road map for recovery from addiction. But times, and a lot of cultural attitudes, have changed since the late 1930s, and it should come as no surprise that those who do not like the Twelve-Step model have become increasingly vocal. Since the 1980s a countermovement known as secular recovery has gathered adherents who consider the Twelve Steps cumbersome and reliance on God unnecessary and irrelevant to the recovery process. One group, LifeRing Secular Recovery, states that "over time, and with work, the desire to stay clean and sober that lies within us can grow into the actual power to do it. We see 'Higher Powers' . . . as redundant at best to the recovery process."[66]

Another secular movement, Rational Recovery (RR), takes an even more radical departure from the principles of A.A. and other twelve-step groups, which it considers counterproductive. RR proposes "immediate self-recovery" and "planned permanent abstinence" for people dealing with alcohol and drug problems, using a mental process called the Addictive Voice Recognition Technique. There is no Higher Power involved, no groups, no meetings, no sponsors, no steps, and no moral inventory. Those who have already experienced twelve-step groups are encouraged to state a "Declaration of Personal Independence"—"I will never, ever attend another meeting of Alcoholics Anonymous or any other recovery-group organization, nor will I obtain professional services of any kind, for the purpose of ending my addiction."[67]

At the other end of the recovery spectrum are Christian groups that have used or adapted the Twelve Steps to move beyond "God as we understand Him" to God as He is revealed in the Old and New Testaments. The International Association of Christian Twelve Step Ministries (or IACTSM), an umbrella organization for several networks and resources for recovery, acknowledges and honors the Twelve Steps, noting that they are "a kind of spiritual kindergarten. Think of it as Introduction to Spirituality 101. It is the introductory course (with laboratory required!)." In stark contrast to the "captain of my fate and master of my soul" mentality of the secular recovery, one of the basic shared principles of IACTSM is that "there is a God . . . and we're not Him."

In its Statement of Shared Principles, IACTSM says:

> When we are active in our addictions, we are our own God. Whether we are aware of it or not, we have chosen ourselves to be our "Higher Power." The first baby-step in early recovery involves learning that we have made a very poor choice. Recovery begins when we recognize that we are not a suitable candidate for "Higher Power" and we agree to let somebody or something other than ourselves be God. . . . From this humble beginning we have, over a period of time, come to believe that the God of the Bible, who is revealed most clearly in Jesus, is the real power behind all recovery and is, therefore, the only fully appropriate choice for Higher Power.[68]

One increasingly popular approach, Celebrate Recovery, uses eight Recovery Principles that are derived from the Beatitudes, the "Blessed are . . ." statements of Jesus that begin the Sermon on the Mount in Matthew, chapter 5. While encompassing the central elements of the Twelve Steps, Celebrate Recovery explicitly emphasizes the importance of a personal

F.Y.I.

The first principle of what Celebrate Recovery calls "The Road to Recovery" reads, "Realize I'm not God: I admit that I am powerless to control my tendency to do the wrong thing and my life is unmanageable." This statement comes from the Beatitudes: "Happy are those who know they are spiritually poor." (Adapted from Matthew 5:3)

commitment to Jesus Christ, spiritual growth, and small-group interactions. Originating at Saddleback Community Church in Southern California, this program has been reproduced in hundreds of churches and is applicable to a broad range of personal issues.

Secular critics notwithstanding, it makes perfect sense to base a recovery process upon biblical principles. Alcohol and drug addiction is essentially a fast-track version of what the Bible declares to be the universal problem of human self-will. We are all bent on being in charge and finding contentment and pleasure on our own, without acknowledging and acquiescing to the Creator who fashioned and loves us. We may achieve a pinnacle of learning, acquisition, achievement, and sensual experiences, as did King Solomon, only to discover that "everything is meaningless!" (Ecclesiastes 12:8). We may plow—or plod—through life assuming, or even proclaiming, that we don't need God to live a good life, thank you very much. People whose lives are careening out of control because alcohol and drugs are in fierce command may never find freedom before their last breath is drawn—or, like the Prodigal Son, they may come to their senses after residing for a while, hungry and miserable, in the pigsty. Their recovery begins when they acknowledge their condition for what it is, repent, gratefully receive God's forgiveness, and submit their life on a day-to-day basis to the One who made them.

But that is precisely what the Bible says we all desperately need to do, whether rich or poor, sophisticated or simple, drinkers or teetotalers. People who have hit bottom because of alcohol and drugs may actually have an advantage over their sober peers, because they have come to the end of their frayed rope more quickly. They may understand more clearly where their appetites can take them; their capacity for denial, lying, and excuses; their personal bankruptcy; and their inability to climb out of the hole on their own. They may be more likely to take their faith seriously, to act on the "action items," to be disciples rather than dilettantes, and to put on the hiking shoes and set forth down the road rather than sit on the sidelines and critique those who are walking by. When they go to an A.A. or similar twelve-step meeting, they are not likely to find distinctions based on bank account, occupation, age, or color. They may also, alas, find more acceptance there, more of the sense that "we're all in this together," than at their neighborhood church. The International Association of Christian Twelve Step Ministries, in its Statement of Shared Principles, notes that:

> The acceptance, honesty, safety and mutual support found in most Twelve Step meetings often comes as a shock to Christians when they first attend. They wonder why it feels safe to talk about what is real on Thursday nights in the recovery group but it does not feel safe to talk about what is real on Sunday mornings. Why,

they wonder, does it feel like you have to already be a good Christian before you feel comfortable at church? We think this is a good question. People in the Twelve Step community have a lot they can learn from the church. But the church also has a lot it could learn from the Twelve Step community if it had the spiritual humility to pay attention. We believe it is God's intention for Christian fellowships to be safe places to be people-in-process. It is our collective prayer that the Christian community will learn something from A.A. and other Twelve Step fellowships about how to be a safe, supportive fellowship that welcomes people who are struggling with the most difficult of life's problems.[69]

How do I help someone with a substance problem?

Obviously those who enjoy alcohol and drugs, or feel rotten without them, may not be interested in changing their habits, let alone seeking help. Unless treatment is mandated by a court order or suddenly imposed by a medical problem (such as an admission to the hospital, where alcohol or drugs are no longer available), the decision to enter into some form of treatment lies with the users alone.

F.Y.I.

To avoid a lot of complicated sentences, we frequently designate the person with a substance problem as the "user." By this we mean someone who has an abuse or dependence problem with alcohol, prescription medications, illegal drugs, or all of the above.

Unfortunately, denial that a problem exists is common among those who are alcohol and drug dependent. Furthermore, family members and friends may be unwilling or unable to deal with the problem, for any number of reasons:

- They may be afraid of rocking the boat—disrupting whatever peace may exist at home or risking the breakup of a relationship.
- They may be intimidated or even terrorized by a user who is verbally or physically abusive.
- Users may repeatedly express remorse over their behavior, and loved ones desperately want to believe that "it won't happen again."
- Family members or friends may also have a drinking/drug problem.
- Family members—for example, mothers with young children—may not have the funds or support to go elsewhere if users refuse to stop.
- Access to treatment resources may be limited.

In a misguided attempt to support their substance-abusing or dependent loved ones, family members may repeatedly clean up the mess, so to speak, by covering, making excuses, or otherwise shielding them from the consequences of their behavior. Unfortunately, this process, commonly called enabling, perpetuates the problem. In some families a subtler scenario undermines any meaningful change: nonusers (usually a spouse) may adopt a role (usually that of the victim or martyr) that, consciously or not, serves other purposes within

CHRISTIAN RECOVERY RESOURCES

INTERNATIONAL ASSOCIATION OF CHRISTIAN TWELVE STEP MINISTRIES
www.iactsm.com

CELEBRATE RECOVERY
25422 Trabuco Road
#105-151
Lake Forest, CA 92630
(949) 609-8305
www.celebraterecovery.com

CHRISTIAN RECOVERY INTERNATIONAL
P.O. Box 215
Brea, CA 92822-0215
(714) 529-6227
www.christianrecovery.com

OVERCOMERS OUTREACH
P.O. Box 2208
Oakhurst, CA 93644
(800) 310-3001
www.overcomersoutreach.org

TEEN CHALLENGE
P.O. Box 1015
Springfield, MO 65801
(417) 862-6969
www.teenchallenge.com/usa

Resource list continued on next page

THE NATIONAL ASSOCIATION FOR CHRISTIAN RECOVERY
P.O. Box 215
Brea, CA 92822-0215
(714) 529-6227
www.nacronline.com

AMERICAN ASSOCIATION OF CHRISTIAN COUNSELORS
P.O. Box 739
Forest, VA 24551
(800) 526-8673
www.aacc.net

the relationship. For example, as long as users continue the problem behavior, nonusers may feel a sense of being on the moral high ground, which can deflect the need to look at their own shortcomings.

If a loved one's or friend's behavior is harming you and your family, what specific steps can you take to encourage change? You'll need to consider all of the following critical elements:

F.Y.I. In this segment we are talking about dealing with an *adult* with a drinking or drug problem. Later (starting on page 494) we will look at the approach to an adolescent in the family with a substance problem.

First, you, as the spouse, child, parent, or close friend of the user, need to address your own issues. With rare exception, it is naive to think "everything would be just fine if only [fill in name] would stop drinking/using drugs." Yes, a lot of things would be more tolerable if the alcohol or drugs would disappear. Unfortunately, this problem doesn't occur in a vacuum, but rather within the context of many relationships. Usually those closest to the user have made all sorts of adjustments, adopted a lot of behaviors, altered their lifestyle, and shaped the ways in which they talk to (and often argue with) one another. Strong emotions—anger, anxiety, outright fear, frustration, confusion, shame, and many others—have been experienced, sometimes for years. If the user is going to get well, *everyone's* life and issues need to be sorted out. (In fact, if this doesn't happen, there is a strong likelihood that the recovery process will unravel.) This will mean going to a pastor, counselor, or other support group *for yourself,* not merely to learn how to "fix" someone else.

Second, it isn't necessary for the user to be willing to get help, or even to acknowledge that there's a problem, for you to start making some changes. You cannot control what a person will or won't do, but you can begin to change what *you* do in a calm, deliberate, and, yes, loving manner. It doesn't require a giant confrontation, for example, to decide to stop lying on behalf of the other person, but the impact can be dramatic. Remember, however, that you probably will need ongoing support to become and stay comfortable with these new behaviors.

Third, you are going to be working on a process—not usually a single event—of helping the person with the alcohol or drug problem understand a nonnegotiable bottom line: It's time to get whatever help is necessary to become and stay sober. This process is called **intervention**, and to do it effectively you should seek input from others who have experience with this type of situation. These may include

- **Your pastor** or, if available, someone in your church who is involved in a recovery ministry.
- **A professional counselor.**

- **The drinker's/user's physician.** Note that confidentiality laws may not allow a doctor to give you any feedback about your loved one's medical status. That does not, however, prevent you from sharing your concerns—and possibly providing information that could affect important medical decisions.
- **An Al-Anon group. Al-Anon** was started in 1951 by two women, one of whom was the wife of Bill Wilson, the cofounder of A.A. Al-Anon's purpose is to help the families and friends of alcoholics. Its structure and philosophy mirror those of A.A. **Alateen** is a part of the Al-Anon fellowship and is specifically geared to family members nineteen and younger. Altogether more than 26,000 Al-Anon and Alateen groups meet in 110 countries. While people who attend are able to share their experiences and feelings in a nonjudgmental setting, Al-Anon and Alateen meetings are far more than gripe sessions. They can be instrumental not only in helping a person understand a family member's or friend's dependence (whether on alcohol or other drugs) but also in making constructive changes in one's own thinking and behavior. They may also provide referrals for counselors or other professionals who can guide a more formal intervention, if necessary. (For information, including times and places of meetings, call (888) 4AL-ANON or go to http://www.al-anon.org.)

Hopefully the input you receive will guide you in broaching this subject, which is not likely to be comfortable. Nagging, whining, browbeating, finger-wagging, begging, pleading, and other forms of manipulation, by the way, are rarely productive. (Even if you have tried these, don't give up on trying a more measured approach.) Pray about what you want to say, gather your thoughts, write them down, and discuss them with one or more people who have experience with this process. Basically, you want to communicate

- Your sincere love/affection/regard for the person.
- Your concern over what you see happening.
- How the problem is affecting *you* (and, when appropriate, others, especially when children are suffering as a result of the substance problem). Generalizations (such as "You always ________.") should be avoided, as should "Why?" questions ("Why do you drink so much?") that tend to provoke defensive or hostile responses. Specifics are critical. For example, you might say, "Last Wednesday, when you came home drunk and angry, the kids and I were really frightened."
- Your unwillingness to cover, make excuses, or prevent any consequences that might arise from using alcohol and/or drugs.
- The step(s) you are asking the user to take. These might include

seeing a counselor, making (or keeping) a doctor's appointment, starting A.A. or another recovery process, or even entering a formal detoxification program. You should have specific information available, by the way, about where (and when) the next steps are to be taken.

- What will happen if the drinking/using continues. This should be thought through very carefully, because you must be willing and able to follow through with it.

This conversation may take place one-on-one, but it is highly advisable that it occur in the presence of one or more other people—a pastor, counselor, physician, friend, family members, or any and all of the above. Not only will the impact be stronger, but also it is less likely that the user can outtalk, manipulate, or overpower (verbally or otherwise) more than one person. (Needless to say, it should *not* take place when the person is under the influence of any substance.) Timing is important as well. Broaching such an important topic may not be wise at the end of a long day or after an intense discussion of another issue. And unless children are specifically going to participate, think twice before starting this conversation if they are present or within earshot.

In some cases, a person who is experienced in initiating the recovery process may be asked to conduct a formal intervention, a surprise attack of sorts that is intended to provoke enough "shock and awe" in the user to lead him or her into immediate treatment. Typically this occurs early in the morning, with the person awakened from sleep and brought into a room where several people are gathered, each of whom tells how the user's behavior is affecting him or her. The objective is usually to convince the person that the next step—to be taken *right now*—is to get into the car and go directly to a center where arrangements have already been made to begin treatment.

This type of intervention must be carefully planned and prayed over, and its purposes clearly understood. Because it has the potential to become an emotional free-for-all, the person who conducts it needs the experience and ability to keep things under control. This is not an occasion to lash out, humiliate, or retaliate for past grievances, although the impact of specific offenses will need to be spelled out. ("Dad, last month you promised you would take me to the father-daughter banquet. I bought tickets and got all dressed up, but you didn't come home until late, and you were drunk. Now I can't believe anything you tell me.") The purpose is not to stomp the user into the ground but to break through all of the denial and to bring into stark focus how the person's behavior is impacting those who are closest, and most vulnerable, to him or her.

One other aspect of an intervention such as this must be carefully planned. What will you do if the user refuses to cooperate? You need to give clear notice of the consequences of not cooperating in advance, and you must be prepared to carry them out. An empty bluff here will be disastrous and will seriously undermine any efforts to make changes in the future. If this situation involves a friend, then the consequence may be an end to further contacts until the user begins treatment. More often, a spouse may need to remove himself or herself (and often one or more children) from a user who is threatening the stability, sanity, and safety of the family. If the user won't start treatment, then he or she will need to face living alone until further notice. Obviously, a warning of this magnitude must be issued with arrangements made for a place to go, in case the answer is no.

Substance Abuse in Youth: Resisting the Epidemic

It is a sad reality that the vast majority of people who become addicted to tobacco, alcohol, and drugs take their first puff, chew, sip, snort, or injection when they are young—often, very young. Worse, in recent decades substance abuse has become more widespread among preteen children. Like the scourges of old, this epidemic spreads without regard to economic, racial, geographic, educational, religious, or family boundaries. While containing it in our nation and our communities is an important priority, we can't rely solely on government, law enforcement, education, or even church programs to prevent it from moving across our own doorstep.

No child is immune from the drug epidemic. (Throughout this section, unless otherwise stated, the words *drug* or *drugs* will be used to indicate any potentially harmful substance—tobacco, alcohol, prescription medications, or illegal drugs.) You must work diligently over the years to "drug-proof" your children. This project involves various tasks that cannot be tackled haphazardly. First, you must understand what draws kids toward drugs. You also need basic information about the substances that are currently prevalent in your neighborhood. You should become familiar with the signs that a drug problem might be developing in your home. Finally and most importantly, you must be prepared to take long-term preventive measures and to respond appropriately if one or more of these toxins should breach your family's defenses.

Why do kids—and for that matter, adults—start (and continue) using drugs?

Several factors can exert a significant influence on who will and who won't try drugs:

- **Attractiveness of drugs.** Smoking and drinking are widely promoted as habits enjoyed by sophisticated, fun-loving, attractive, and sexy people—what most adolescents long to become. Illegal drugs are "advertised" by those using them in an adolescent's peer group.

- **The high induced by drugs.** If drug use wasn't pleasurable, it would be relatively easy to keep kids and harmful substances separated. But the reality is that many kids enjoy the way they feel on drugs—at least for a while.
- **Attitudes of parents toward tobacco, alcohol, and other substances.** Children learn what they live. Smoking, drinking, and other drug-related behaviors among parents will usually be duplicated in their children.
- **Availability of drugs.** Finding drugs is not difficult for children and adolescents in most communities, but tougher local standards can help keep drugs out of less-determined hands.
- **Peer pressure.** Peers play a huge role at each stage of a child's or adolescent's drug experience—whether resisting them, experimenting, becoming a user, or confronting withdrawal and recovery. The need for peer acceptance is especially strong during the early adolescent years and can override (or at least seriously challenge) a young person's values and commitments. "Just say no" may not mean a whole lot when smoking, drinking, or taking drugs determines who is included among the highly esteemed ranks of the inner circle. There are three obvious implications: First, it is important that kids find their niche in the right peer group(s), among friends who are not only committed to positive values (including a drug-free lifestyle) but also involved in worthwhile and enjoyable pursuits. Second, you may have to intervene if your adolescent (especially in the early teen years) is hanging out with the wrong crowd. Finally, children and adolescents with a healthy, stable identity and an appropriate sense of independence will be more resistant to peer pressure.
- **Curiosity.** Unless your family lives in total isolation, your child will be aware of smoking, alcohol, and drug use well before adolescence from discussions at school, watching TV and movies, or direct observation. Some curiosity is inevitable: *What do these things feel like?* Whether this leads to sampling will depend on the individual's mind-set; whether an experiment progresses to addiction will in turn depend on the physical and emotional responses to the particular substance.
- **Thrill-seeking.** This desire for excitement is in all of us to some degree and is what propels us toward certain activities: skydiving, roller coasters, movies (where sights and sounds are bigger than life), firework displays, sporting events, and so on. Some of these are more risky than others, but none require chemical alteration of the senses to be satisfying. Unfortunately, many children and adolescents seek

drug experiences to produce thrills that normal life and consciousness can't duplicate. Some observers have argued that this desire to alter consciousness is universal, wired into humans much like the desire for food, and that trying to prevent it is as futile as sweeping back the ocean with a broom. Assuming this is the case (which is certainly debatable) does not mean, however, that any and all forms of thrill-seeking should be given free rein. A number of other human instincts are no less universal, but hardly virtuous: pride, greed, hunger for power, the desire to dominate other people, lust, selfishness, and so on.

- **Rebellion.** Wayward children may engage in smoking, alcohol, and drug use as a show of independence from family norms and values.
- **Escape from life/relief from pain.** For many people—indeed, for most people in the world—life is just plain tough, and normal waking consciousness brings a constant stream of unpleasant sights, smells, sounds, and sensations. The prospect of a chemical "time-out" may look very attractive. Furthermore, even when a person has plenty of creature comforts, the prevailing emotional weather can still be turbulent: kids and teens often feel anxious, angry, depressed, oppressed, stressed, bored, unfulfilled. Whether one is down and out or rich and famous, drugs that bring about relaxation, stimulation, or pure escape can be appealing. The strongest resistance to drug abuse therefore arises from an ongoing sense of joy and contentment that transcends circumstances. These attitudes are usually acquired, not inborn. Early positive experiences in the family and an active, wide-awake relationship with God play the most important roles in molding such attitudes.
- **A conviction that "it can't happen to me" or that the consequences don't matter.** Many teenagers and young adults are prone to assume their own invulnerability or immortality, make shortsighted decisions, or shrug off the most fervent warnings about life's pitfalls and perils with a smirk or the defiant pronouncement "I don't care." Shedding this perspective, learning to weigh consequences, and adopting a long-range view of life are normal parts of maturing into adulthood. Unfortunately, some who become deeply involved in drug use remain stuck in an immature, self-destructive mind-set.

Stages of adolescent substance abuse

Experts in adolescent substance problems have identified a common progression of alcohol- and drug-related behaviors that moves from bad to worse. While it is not a foregone conclusion that everyone who experiments with drugs will progress to the worst stages of involvement, a child can incur a lot of damage before parents or others notice that something is wrong. Secretive adolescent behavior and skillful lying, combined with parental denial ("No one in our family could have a drug problem!"), may delay identification of the problem. While paranoia and daily inquisitions around the breakfast table are counterproductive, wise parents will keep their eyes and ears open and promptly take action if they see any signs that a problem may be developing.

Stage one: Experimentation—entering the drug gateway

CHARACTERISTICS:

- Use is occasional, sporadic, often unplanned—weekends, summer nights, unsupervised parties.
- Use is precipitated by peer pressure, curiosity, thrill-seeking, desire to look and feel grown-up.
- Gateway drugs are usually used—cigarettes, alcohol, marijuana, possibly inhalants.
- A drug high is easier to experience because tolerance has not been developed.

PARENTS MAY NOTICE:

- Tobacco or alcohol on the breath or intoxicated behavior.
- Little change in normal behavior between episodes of drug use.

Stage two: More regular drug use—leaving the land of the living

CHARACTERISTICS:

- Alcohol and other drugs are used not only on weekends but also on weekdays, and not only with friends but when alone.
- Quantities of alcohol and drugs increase as tolerance develops; hangovers become more common.
- Blackouts—periods of time in which drugs or alcohol prevent normal memories from forming—may occur. "What happened last night?" becomes a frequent question.
- More time and attention are focused on when the next drug experience will occur.
- Fellow drinkers/drug users become preferred companions.

PARENTS MAY NOTICE:

- A son or daughter will be out of the house later at night, overnight, or all weekend.
- Unexplained school absences and deteriorating school performance.
- Outside activities such as sports are dropped.
- Decreased contact with friends who don't use drugs.
- Disappearance of money or other valuables.
- Withdrawal from the family, and an increasingly sullen and hostile attitude.
- The user is caught in one or many lies.

Stage three: Waist deep in the mire of addiction—and sinking

CHARACTERISTICS:

- Alcohol and drugs become the primary focus of attention.
- Becoming high is a daily event.
- A willingness to try more dangerous drugs or combinations of drugs.
- More money is spent each week on drugs. Theft or dealing may become part of drug-seeking behavior.
- Increasing social isolation and loss of contact with non-drug-using friends. More drug use in isolation, rather than at parties or with other users.

PARENTS MAY NOTICE THE BEHAVIORS LISTED ON THE PREVIOUS PAGE, PLUS:

- Escalation of conflicts at home.
- Loss of nearly all control of the adolescent.
- Possible discovery of a stash of drugs at home.
- Arrest(s) for possession of and/or dealing drugs or for driving while intoxicated.

Stage four: Drowning in addiction

CHARACTERISTICS:

- Constant state of intoxication. Being high or stoned is routine, even at school or a job (if the user even bothers to attend).
- Blackouts increase in frequency.
- Physical appearance deteriorates, with noticeable weight loss, infections, and overall poor self-care.
- Injectable drugs may be part of the user's routine.
- Involvement in casual sexual relationships, at times in exchange for drugs.
- User will likely be involved with theft, dealing, and other criminal activity.
- Guilt, self-hatred, and thoughts of suicide increase.

PARENTS ARE LIKELY TO DEAL WITH:

- Complete loss of control of adolescent's behavior and escalation of conflict, possibly to the point of violence.
- Ongoing denial by the user that drugs are a problem.
- Increasing problems with the law and time spent with police, attorneys, hearings, court officials, etc.
- Other siblings negatively affected because the family is preoccupied or overwhelmed by consequences of the drug user's behavior.

This descent into drug hell is a nightmare that no parent envisions while rocking a newborn baby or escorting an eager five-year-old to kindergarten.

But it can happen in any neighborhood, any church, any family, even when parents have provided a stable and loving home environment. In fact, it is often in such homes that a drug problem goes undetected until it's reached an advanced and dangerous stage. *This can't be happening; not in my house!* But if it does, parental guilt, anger, and depression can undermine the responses necessary to restore order.

Reducing the risk for substance abuse

Drug abuse is so widespread in our culture that you cannot expect to isolate your child from exposure to it. However, as with diseases caused by bacteria and viruses, you can institute "infection-control measures" by taking specific steps to reduce the likelihood of contact with drugs and to build your child's immunity to using them. These measures should be ongoing, deliberate, and proactive.

1. **Model behavior you want your children to follow.** When it comes to drugs, two adages are worth noting: "Children learn what they live" and "What parents allow in moderation their children will do in excess." While not absolute truths, these maxims reflect the reality that kids are looking to their parents for cues as to what is acceptable behavior, while at the same time developing the discernment required to understand what moderation is all about.
    - If you smoke, your offspring will probably do likewise. But it's never too late to quit, and your decision to give up cigarettes will make an important statement to all the members of your family—especially if you are willing to hold yourself accountable to them.
    - If you consume alcohol at home, what role does it play in your life? Does it flow freely on a daily basis? Do you need a drink to unwind at the end of the day? Is it a necessary ingredient at every party or family get-together? If so, your children will get the idea that alcohol is a painkiller, tension reliever, and the life of the party, and they will likely use it in a similar fashion. For their sake (and yours), take whatever steps are necessary to live without alcohol.
    - If you drink modestly—an occasional glass of wine with dinner, a beer every other week, a few sips of champagne at a wedding—think carefully about alcohol's role in your family. Many parents decide to abstain while rearing their children in order to send an unambiguous message to steer clear of it. Others feel that modeling modest, nonintoxicated use of alcohol (while speaking clearly against underage drinking, drunkenness, driving under the influence, and other irresponsible behaviors) equips children and teenagers to make sensible decisions later in life.
    - Each family must weigh the options carefully and set its own stan-

dards. But if you or any blood relatives have a history of alcohol addiction (or any problem caused by drinking), make your home an alcohol-free zone and warn your adolescent that he or she may have a genetic predisposition toward alcoholism.

- Also think about the impact of your family's habits on visitors or guests, including your teenager's friends. What might be perfectly harmless for you could prompt someone who has a potential for alcohol addiction to make a bad decision. All things considered, nothing is lost and much can be gained by abstaining.
- What about the medicine cabinet? If you are stressed, upset, or uncomfortable, are d-r-u-g-s the way you spell r-e-l-i-e-f? Have you accumulated prescription narcotics and tranquilizers that you use freely when the going gets tough? Kids aren't blind. If they see the adults around them frequently taking legitimate drugs to dull their pain, they wonder why they can't use their own drugs to do the same.
- Finally, if you use marijuana and other street drugs, whether for recreation or because of an addiction problem, you are putting the parental stamp of approval not only on the drugs but also on breaking the law. For your own and your family's sake, seek help immediately and end this dangerous behavior.

2. **Build identity and attitudes that are resistant to drug use.** This is an ongoing process, beginning during the first years of your child's life. Specifically:
    - Create an environment that consistently balances love and limits. Children and teenagers who know they are loved unconditionally are less likely to seek pain relief through drugs, and those who have learned to live within appropriate boundaries will have better impulse control and self-discipline.
    - Instill respect and awe for the God-given gift of a body and mind—even one that isn't perfect.
    - Help children and adolescents become students of consequences—not only in connection with drugs but with other behaviors as well. Talk about good and bad choices and the logic behind them. "Just say no" is an appropriate motto for kids to learn, but understanding *why* it is wrong to use harmful substances will build more solid resistance.
    - Build a positive sense of identity with your family. This means not only openly affirming and appreciating each member but also putting forth the time and effort for shared experiences that are meaningful and fun. A strong feeling of belonging to a loving family builds accountability ("Our family doesn't use drugs") and helps prevent loneliness, which can be a setup for drug experimentation.
    - Encourage church-related activities (and family devotions) that build a meaningful, personal faith. Reliance on God is the cornerstone of

effective drug-treatment programs, and it makes no sense to leave the spiritual dimension out of the prevention process. A vibrant faith reinforces the concept that the future is worth protecting, stabilizes the emotions during turbulent years, and provides a healthy response to the aches and pains of life. In addition, an awareness of God's presence and a desire not to dishonor Him can be strong deterrents to destructive behavior.

3. **Begin talking early about smoking, alcohol, and drugs.** Because experimentation with drugs and alcohol commonly begins during the grade-school years, start appropriate countermeasures in very young children. A five-year-old may not be ready for a lecture about the physiology of cocaine addiction, but you should be ready to offer commentary when you and your child see someone smoking or drinking, whether in real life or in a movie or TV program. When intoxication is portrayed as humorous (as in the pink-elephant sequence in the movie *Dumbo,* for example), don't be shy about setting the record straight.

4. **Keep talking about smoking, alcohol, and drugs as opportunities arise.** Make an effort to stay one step ahead of your child or adolescent's knowledge of the drug scene. If you hear about an athlete, rock star, or celebrity who uses drugs, be certain that everyone in the family understands that no amount of fame or fortune excuses this behavior. If a famous person is dealing with the consequences of drug use (such as being dropped from a team or suffering medical or legal consequences), make sure your kids hear the cautionary tale.

   Be aware of current trends in your community and look for local meetings or lectures where abuse problems are being discussed. Find out what's going on—not only from the experts but also from your kids and their friends. If you hear that a group of kids are smoking, drinking, inhaling, or injecting drugs, talk about it. What are they using? What consequences are likely? Why is it wrong? What help do they need?

   All this assumes that you are available to have these conversations. Be careful, because the time when you may be the busiest with career or other responsibilities may also be the time one or more adolescents at home most need your input. If you're too overworked, overcommitted, and overtired to keep tabs on the home front, you may wake up one day to find a major drug problem on your doorstep.

5. **Don't allow your child or adolescent to go to a party, sleepover, or other activity that isn't supervised by someone you trust.** Don't blindly assume that the presence of a grown-up guarantees a safe environment. Get to know the parents of your kids' friends. Make certain your children know you will

pick them up anytime, anywhere—no questions asked—if they find themselves in a situation where alcohol or drugs are being used. And be sure to praise them for a wise and mature decision if they call you for help.

6. **Have the courage to curtail your child's or adolescent's contact with drug users.** The epidemic of drug abuse spreads person to person. Whether a recent acquaintance or a long-term bosom buddy, if one (or more) of your teenager's friends is known to be actively using alcohol and/or drugs, you must impose restrictions on the relationship. You might, for example, stipulate that your adolescent can spend time with that person only in your home—without any closed doors and only when you are around.

   However, even with these limits in place, you will need to keep track of who is influencing whom. If your family is reaching out to a troubled adolescent and helping to move him toward healthier decisions, keep up the good work. But if there is any sign that the drug-using friend is pulling your teenager toward this lifestyle, declare a quarantine immediately. By all means, if your teenager feels called to help a friend climb out of a drug quagmire, don't allow him to try it alone. Work as a team to direct that person toward a recovery program.

7. **Create significant consequences to discourage alcohol and drug use.** Teenagers may not be scared off by facts, figures, and gory details. Even the most ominous warnings may not override an adolescent's belief in her own immortality, especially when other compelling emotions such as the need for peer acceptance are operating at full throttle.

   You can improve the odds for your child by making it clear that you consider the use of cigarettes, alcohol, or illegal drugs a very serious matter. Careful judgment regarding punishments will be necessary, of course. If your adolescent confesses that she tried a cigarette or a beer at a party and expresses an appropriate resolve to avoid a repeat performance, a heart-to-heart conversation and encouragement would be far more appropriate than summarily grounding her for six months.

   But if your warnings repeatedly go unheeded, you will need to establish and enforce some meaningful consequences. Loss of driving, dating, or even phone privileges for an extended period of time may be in order. You can make the bitter pill less threatening by pointing out the following:

   - He can easily avoid the penalty by staying clear of drugs and the people who use them.
   - Consistent responsible behavior will lead to more privileges and independence. Irresponsible behavior will lead to decreased independence and more parental control.
   - The drastic consequence can be used as a reason to get away from a bad situation. If a friend starts to exert pressure on your child to

smoke, drink, or use drugs, he can say, "Sorry, but I don't want to be stuck without transportation for the next six months."

What if a problem has already developed?

Even closely knit families with strong values and ongoing drug-proofing have no guarantee that substance abuse won't affect one or more of their children. The problems may range from a brief encounter with cigarettes to an episode of intoxication (perhaps with legal consequences) to an addiction. As you begin to cope with one or more chemical intruders in your home, keep the following principles in mind:

1. **Don't deny or ignore the problem.** If you do, it is likely to worsen until your family life is turned inside out. Take the bull by the horns—but be sure to find out exactly how big and ugly the bull is. The marijuana cigarette you discovered may be a one-time experiment or the tip of the iceberg. Talk to your child or adolescent about it—but also talk to siblings, friends, and anyone else who may know the extent of the problem. You may not like what you hear, but better to get the hard truth now than a ghastly surprise later.

2. **Don't wallow in false guilt.** Most parents assume a great deal of self-blame when a drug problem erupts in their home. If you do carry some responsibility for what has happened (whether you know about it immediately or find out later on), face up to it, confess it to God and your family, and then get on with the task of helping your child. But remember that young users must deal with their own responsibility as well.

3. **Seek help from people experienced with treating drug problems.** Talk to your physician and pastor. They should be part of your team, even if in a supporting role. It is likely that you will receive a referral to a professional who is experienced in organizing a family intervention. This may include educational sessions, individual and family counseling, medical treatment, and long-term follow-up. When the user's behavior is out of control and he is unwilling to acknowledge the problem, a carefully planned confrontation by family members and others affected may need to be carried out under the supervision of an experienced counselor. The goal is to convince the drug user in a firm but loving way of the need for change—now. The confrontation should include specific alternatives for the type of treatment he will undergo and clear-cut consequences if he is not willing to cooperate.

4. **Be prepared to make difficult, "tough love" decisions.** If you have a drug-dependent adolescent who will not submit to treatment and insists on continuing drug use and other destructive actions, you will need to take the stomach-churning step of informing him that he cannot continue to live in

your home while carrying on this behavior. This will be necessary not only to motivate him to change but to prevent his drug-induced turbulence from destroying the rest of your family.

If you must take this drastic step, it would be helpful to present him with one or more options. These might include entering an inpatient drug-treatment center, halfway house, boot-camp program, or youth home, or staying with a relative or another family who is willing to accept him for a defined period of time. More ominous possibilities may need to be discussed as well, such as making him a ward of the court or even turning him over to the police if he has been involved in criminal activity. If you continue to shield him from the consequences of his behavior or bail him out when his drugs get him into trouble, he will not change and you will be left with deep-seated anger and frustration.

5. **Don't look for or expect quick-fix solutions.** It is normal to wish for a single intervention that will make a drug problem go away. But one conversation, counseling session, prayer time, or trip to the doctor won't be enough. Think in terms of a comprehensive response encompassing specific treatment and counseling and the gamut of your child's life—home, school, friends, and church.

6. **Remember the father of the Prodigal Son.** Tough love means allowing the consequences of bad decisions to be fully experienced by one who is making them. It also means that your child knows a parent's love for him is so deep and secure that it will never die. Never give up hope, never stop praying, and never slam the door on reconciliation and restoration when your child comes to his senses.

QUESTIONS TO PONDER

1. If you use tobacco in any form, what are the reasons *you* need to quit? There is a lot of bad news about tobacco in this chapter, but not all of it may impact you personally. What are the risks of tobacco use that make you uncomfortable? Write these down and review them before your next smoke or chew.
2. If you drink alcoholic beverages, ask yourself the following:
   a. Are your drinking habits within medically safe limits? (See pages 448–449.)
   b. Complete the CAGE questionnaire on page 457. Do your answers reveal a need to change any habits or seek help?
   c. Does your use of alcohol ever make others uncomfortable—or tempt them to drink when they shouldn't?
   d. Do you need to consider taking a time-out from alcohol use until your children become adults?
3. If you have children, what messages have you been giving them about tobacco, alcohol, and other drugs (whether by your own use of these substances or in discussions you have about them)?
4. If someone in your family is abusing alcohol or drugs, are you enabling his or her behavior in any way?
5. Does your church participate in any recovery programs? If getting involved in this type of ministry interests you (or scares you to death), check the Celebrate Recovery Web site (http://www.celebraterecovery.com) for more information and inspiration.

Action items: If you are smoking or chewing any form of tobacco and are convinced that you need to end this habit, get out a calendar and set a quit date—ideally with family and friends as witnesses and accountability partners. If you aren't convinced, go back and reread pages 428–439. If you still can't bring yourself to quit, make a commitment that you will use tobacco *only* where nonsmokers (especially your children) or others who are trying to quit will have zero exposure to your smoke.

Refer to "Reducing the risk for substance abuse" on pages 494–499 for ideas on how to talk with your children about the dangers of drugs and alcohol. Don't wait until there is a problem before discussing these issues—if your children are school-age, begin talking simply and at an age-appropriate level about the dangers of tobacco, alcohol, and other drugs.

If you realize you are dependent on any drug, seek help now. The list of Christian recovery programs on pages 485–486 is a great place to start.

If a family member is abusing drugs, don't suffer in isolation. *Reach out for help.* This chapter contains many recommendations on how to confront this difficult issue with the assistance and support of others. Check out pages 479–489 for practical tips.

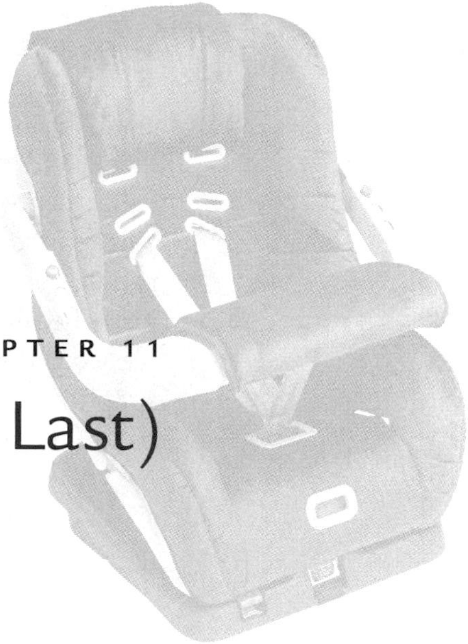

CHAPTER 11

Safety First (and Last)

PREVENTING ACCIDENTS AND INJURIES

Much of what we have presented in the last ten chapters has dealt with preserving or improving health by taking action to prevent three major disorders: cardiovascular disease (specifically heart attack and stroke), cancer, and diabetes. In chapter 3 we described these conditions, and then in chapter 4 we examined some screening tests that can help detect them—hopefully before they threaten well-being (or life itself). In chapters 5, 6, and 7 we looked at the health benefits of eating properly, losing excess pounds, and exercising regularly, and in chapter 10 we went to some lengths to warn against tobacco use and the abuse of alcohol and drugs. We noted that all of these worthwhile efforts help to prevent—guess what?—cardiovascular disease, cancer, and diabetes.

Why do we keep mentioning these problems? Because they cause or contribute to the vast majority of deaths in the United States every year. But there's an important fact you need to know: Most of these deaths occur in older age groups. *If you're younger than forty-five, the greatest threat to your life* right now *is an accidental injury,* the leading cause of death for those between one and forty-four years of age. Every year in the United States more than one hundred thousand lives are lost to accidents, which consistently rank as the fifth overall leading cause of death.[1]

In addition to one hundred thousand deaths from accidents, more than thirty-one thousand lives are lost to suicide and more than seventeen thousand to homicide in the United States every year.

Accidents cost the U.S. economy over $600 billion annually, including medical bills and lost productivity. They also result in 29 million emergency room visits.[2] Even among survivors, unintentional injuries exact a high toll: More than 5 million people live with chronic disabilities as a result of accidents.[3]

Why Can't We Prevent More Accidents?

The suffering caused by accidental injuries is even more tragic because so many could be prevented by modest safety measures, most of which are simple, quick, and incur little or no expense. So why do so many people fail to implement them? The answer lies in the complex constellation of personal beliefs, perceptions, and habits that surround risk-taking and risk avoidance. Often people don't bother to take basic steps to reduce the likelihood of common injuries because of some irrational (but all too common) attitudes. As an example, consider some of these refrains, and how a number of them impact the simple but effective safety measure of "buckling up" in the car. Do any of these strike a familiar chord?

- *Bad things happen to other people . . . not to me.* This brand of foolhardy optimism is particularly common among teenagers, who are notorious for believing in their own immortality. Unfortunately, it also extends to older age groups as well.
- *When my time's up, there's nothing I can do about it.* In a survey conducted by the National Highway Traffic Safety Administration (NHTSA), more than a quarter of respondents agreed with the statement, "If it is your time to die, you'll die, so it doesn't matter whether or not you wear your seat belt." Among drivers who rarely or never wear seat belts, the percentage of people with that attitude climbed to 61 percent.[4] This fatalistic conviction that there is little one can do to avoid injury or death may stop people from taking steps that *would* help them avoid injury and death.
- *The Lord knows when my time is up, and He won't call me home until then.* This is essentially a spiritualized version of the fatalism just described and a misunderstanding regarding God's knowledge of "the number of our days."
- *If I'm walking in God's will, He'll protect me even if I take some risks.* Sometimes answering a call to serve God in a primitive or unstable part of the world will put someone in harm's way. But even those who walk into such situations by faith can still exercise reasonable precautions (such as obtaining vaccinations and medications to prevent illness). Taking careless and reckless chances with the presumption that God will offer protection from harm could represent "putting God to the test"—a practice that both the Old and New Testaments warn against.
- *It's such a hassle. . . .* One study showed that 43 percent of motorists who wouldn't buckle up felt that these restraints were uncomfortable, inconvenient, or unnecessary.[5]
- *A lot of "safety tips" really aren't that safe.* Again looking at seat belts, 38 percent of respondents to a NHTSA survey agreed somewhat or

strongly with the statement, "Seat belts are just as likely to harm you as help you," even though research has consistently demonstrated that they are highly effective in reducing fatalities and injuries in motor-vehicle crashes.[6]

- *I just forgot. . . .* We hear this excuse from kids a lot ("I forgot to put on my helmet before I got on my bike"), but forgetfulness is also one of the most common reasons adults give for not taking safety precautions.[7] In our fast-paced society, it's easy to allow preoccupied minds and busy schedules to distract us from doing the things that could preserve our lives and those of our loved ones.

If you take the time to read this chapter (and we hope you will), you may become a little glassy-eyed as you look over what may seem like a multitude of recommendations. You may think, *If I follow through with all of these safety precautions, I won't have any time to live my life.* That isn't true, of course, and it's important for us to consider honestly why we might be unwilling to take certain safety measures—and whether we might need some attitude adjustment. Many who have invested a good deal of time and money on medical consultations still struggle with the consistent use of medications that would reduce their risk of disease and death (for example, by lowering blood pressure and cholesterol). Furthermore, as the number of drugs increases, the likelihood of long-term compliance with the doctor's advice decreases. Yet it may be even more challenging to begin and maintain safety habits, such as wearing bike helmets or using seat belts, which are often perceived as matters of personal preference rather than of life and death.

Nevertheless, all of the reasons to pursue good health set forth in chapter 1 apply just as much to avoiding injury as to avoiding disease. One of these—the fact that our health is a gift for which we have some stewardship responsibilities—applies not only to our relationship with God but also to our responsibility for the well-being of our loved ones, and indeed to any who are in our sphere of influence. This means (using seat belts as an example again) that even if we don't feel an overwhelming urge to buckle up every time we get in the car, we should at least do it for those we love—not only to preserve our own health but also to serve as an example. This modeling aspect of safety is crucial. Children and teens have a remarkable ability to calculate the value that Mom and Dad place on safety (or anything else) based on their behavior rather than on any lectures they might deliver. The command to "do as I say and not as I do" always falls on deaf ears . . . as it should.

While safety for ourselves and others is something we all should take seriously, we want to stress that chronic anxiety (or routine panic) and hypervigilance are not appropriate alternatives to a careless attitude about risk. Obviously, there are an unlimited number of ways we might be injured from the minute we wake up ("Don't cut your finger while slicing that bagel") until we fall back into bed ("Don't slip on the throw rug when you put out the cat").

Alarming reports about everyday hazards greet us regularly in the morning paper and the evening news. When we watch our kids exploring their world, whether as toddlers or teenagers, we can easily become anxious, worrying about head-bonks—or head-on collisions. We might begin to think that it isn't safe to get out of bed, except that being bed-bound carries its own very real risks, as any caregiver in a convalescent home can tell you.

What we need is a commonsense approach that looks at the likelihood of certain accidents and hazards and then takes levelheaded precautions to reduce those risks. For this reason, we'll narrow our focus to safety concerns that are both part and parcel of everyday life and also potentially serious (if not life threatening). An important note: many accidents occur on the job, where safety hazards vary enormously depending on the work environment. These should be addressed regularly at the workplace as part of the employer's compliance with federal and state regulations. We'll restrict our discussion here to injuries that are generally associated with the home, the car, and certain types of recreation.

For more information about on-the-job safety and ergonomic injuries—that is, those related to the work environment, whether an office cubicle or a steel mill—visit the Occupational Safety and Health Administration's Web site at http://www.osha.gov.

Safety in and around the Home

The word *home* usually evokes thoughts of a place of both comfort and safety. Many people make great investments—in furniture or entertainment systems, for example—to create comfort in their homes, but often safety is an afterthought. Sadly, every year millions of people are injured by accidents in the home, and more than thirty-three thousand lose their life.[8] The majority of these injuries arise from a relatively small number of causes. The good news is that a number of simple precautions can dramatically reduce their likelihood.

Fire and smoke

Fire is perhaps the most dramatic and devastating hazard that we might encounter in the home, with a terrifying capacity to destroy property and lives. There are more than four hundred thousand residential fires in the United States each year, causing more than 3,100 deaths, 14,000 injuries, and almost $6 billion in damage.[9]

Depictions of fires on television and in movies often show firefighters and other heroes running through blazing buildings in which there is surprisingly little smoke. For your own safety, you need to understand the difference between a fire created by Hollywood special-effect technicians and the genuine article. Real fires can progress rapidly from a small flame to an uncontrolled conflagration, and within minutes an entire building can be filled with disorienting black smoke, reducing visibility to inches at best. After a few more minutes, a house can be completely engulfed in flames.

The temperatures generated by an average house fire may surprise you. At ground level the temperature generated by a fire can be around 100°F. At eye level, it rises to 600°F—hot enough to singe hair, melt clothing onto skin, and scorch lungs that inhale air heated to this temperature. As deadly as the heat itself can be, the main cause of injury and death in residential fires is not flaming infernos, but the inhalation of smoke and toxic fumes. All too often, sleeping victims of fire are overcome by smoke before they ever wake up.

Protecting yourself and your family from fire

Fire safety in the home begins by recognizing the common causes of residential fires. These include:

- *Cooking.* Three out of ten residential fires start in the kitchen, and thus cooking has the dubious honor of being the leading cause of both home fires and home-fire injuries. Most cooking fires are caused by food left unattended on the stove or other human error, as opposed to a malfunction of cooking equipment. Spattering grease is particularly good at starting fires that can burn out of control if not caught and extinguished quickly.
- *Smoking.* While cooking is the cause of most home fires and home fire injuries, smoking is the cause of most home-fire deaths. Falling asleep while holding a lit cigarette and throwing smoldering cigarette butts into the trash are the main triggers of smoking-related fires. Not surprisingly, mattresses, bedding, upholstered furniture, and trash are the most common items that initially catch fire. A disproportionate number of fatalities in smoking-related fires occur among older adults, with 40 percent of victims age sixty-five or older.
- *Heating equipment.* The second leading cause of residential fires is heating equipment, including kerosene heaters, gas heaters, electric heaters, fireplaces, and woodstoves. Not surprisingly, more of these occur during winter months. Many of these fires occur when combustible materials are placed too close to the source of heat, or involve accidents with liquid or gas fuel. Additionally, if chimneys and stovepipes are not cleaned regularly, they can become coated inside with creosote. This flammable residue can ignite, weakening or deforming chimneys and pipes and ultimately causing a house fire.
- *Electrical wiring and equipment.* Wiring, switches, outlets, cords and plugs, circuit breakers, and lighting fixtures all can cause fires if they are faulty, improperly used, or not maintained. According to the National Fire Protection Association, electrical wiring and equipment is the third leading cause of residential fires and the second leading cause of fire fatalities. Electrical wiring and equipment can start fires when circuits are overloaded, causing them to overheat. Loose electrical connections can lead to a discharge of electricity between two points (called an arc) that can ignite nearby combustibles.
- *Children playing with fire.* Most kids are naturally curious about fire. Children playing with fire accounted for nearly fourteen thousand

While not considered accidental, arson accounted for a significant number of residential fires and more than three hundred deaths in 2003.

structural fires and more than two hundred deaths in 2002. Tragically, most of these fatalities are among children age five and younger. About two-thirds of all fires started unintentionally by children involve matches or lighters, but candles, fireworks, stoves, and cigarettes in young hands also cause many fires.[10]

Recognizing and avoiding these common causes of residential fires are the first steps to keeping your family safe. In addition, you should take several steps to prepare your family in the event of a fire.

Stop fires before they start. Never leave food cooking on a stovetop unattended. Make sure that the area around any cooking surface is clear of combustibles such as pot holders and dish towels, and avoid wearing loose clothing that can dangle onto hot surfaces and catch fire. When cooking, turn handles of pots and pans inward so that young children cannot pull scalding food or hot grease down on themselves.

Smoking is always a bad idea, and if you aren't convinced of tobacco's numerous ill effects you should review pages 433–439 in chapter 10. It is especially foolish, however, to smoke while in bed or while dozing. If you can't or won't part company with tobacco, at least make a firm pledge that you will put out your cigarette, cigar, or pipe before you lie down. And take care not to dispose of a lit cigarette butt or hot ashes in a trash can containing flammable materials.

You can avoid fires related to heating equipment by having furnaces and heaters inspected by a qualified professional each year or as recommended by the manufacturer. Have your fireplaces or woodstoves inspected yearly as well, and have chimneys cleaned as often as recommended by whoever does the inspection. Keep space heaters at least three feet from flammable objects. Use kerosene heaters only in well-ventilated areas, and add only the appropriate type of fuel (never use gasoline). Wait until the heater is cool before you add fuel. Never leave a portable space heater unattended.

When buying electrical devices, choose items that have been tested and certified by an independent laboratory such as Underwriters Laboratories. Repair or replace frayed or worn electrical cords on all electrical devices, and do not overload electrical outlets: Overloaded circuits can get dangerously hot.

Finally, keep matches, lighters, fireworks, and anything else designed to ignite out of the hands of small children. Teach children that matches and lighters are to be used only by adults, and impress on them the dangers of playing with fire.

Know the best way to respond to a fire. You can contain some fires in your home if they are small and you have the means to handle them. Others may be well out of your league even before you discover them. First and foremost, remember that people are infinitely more important than property. Before you battle even a small blaze, see to it that others have made their way out of the house (or are on their way out). Also, make sure that the fire department has been called or is being called. This might seem like overkill if you've got a fire on the stovetop, but the adage "better safe than sorry" certainly applies in this case. Even if a fire is small and appears that it can be easily contained, it is crucial to understand that not all fires are created equal. Knowing how to respond to a fire based on its characteristics is essential to extinguishing it safely and quickly.

If you have a small fire contained in a pan on top of the stove, put on an oven mitt and carefully place a lid on the pan to smother the flame. Small fires can also be extinguished by sprinkling them with baking soda, but be careful not to burn yourself or toss the baking soda too vigorously, which can accidentally spread the fire. Never douse a grease fire with water or discharge a fire extinguisher directly at it at close range. These actions can unintentionally (but quite effectively) spread the fire.

Electrical fires pose unique dangers beyond those of their flames. *Don't throw water on an electrical fire,* because water is an excellent conductor of electricity. The current can travel to you instantly through the stream of water and deliver a harmful shock. Use only a multipurpose fire extinguisher, which can be used on all types of home fires.

Use smoke alarms. *Smoke alarms save lives.* The good news is that 96 percent of homes in the United States now have at least one smoke alarm. The tragic news is that half of home-fire deaths occur in the 4 percent of homes that have no smoke alarms. Here are some suggestions for the installation and maintenance of residential smoke alarms:

- Install at least one smoke alarm on each floor of your home, positioned near each sleeping area.
- Use the test button to check your smoke alarms each month. In one survey of households that had had a house fire, the alarms had not worked in one out of four homes equipped with smoke alarms.[11]
- For battery-operated smoke alarms, replace the batteries at least once each year. Several safety organizations suggest designating a day each year to replace all of the smoke detector batteries in your home. (New Year's Day or July 4—holidays often celebrated with the discharge of fireworks, legal or otherwise—would be easy to remember.) Smoke alarms are designed to "chirp" repeatedly when battery levels are low. This is meant to be annoying, and you must resist the foolhardy urge to remove the battery simply to stop the chirping. (This is about as clever as covering a warning light on your dashboard with duct tape so that you won't have to look at it anymore.) Once the chirping starts, don't remove the battery until you're about to replace it—and do so promptly.
- Because their efficiency decreases over time, you should replace your smoke alarms every ten years.
- If you or someone in your home is hearing impaired, install smoke alarms with strobe lights.
- Some electronic home-security systems include smoke detectors and

will notify a monitoring service, or the fire department directly, if the detector is activated. (These allow a short window of time to cancel this notification in case of a false alarm.) To ensure that this type of automated system continues to work properly, be sure to follow the testing guidelines of the security service, and be sure to keep current on any ongoing fees.

Know how to use a fire extinguisher. You should have a multipurpose fire extinguisher—the kind that can be used on all common types of house fires—for each floor of your house. Acquainting yourself and others with its proper use before a fire occurs is an important part of your fire-preparedness strategy. A fire extinguisher is used primarily when a fire is contained to a small area (such as a wastebasket) and not spreading. Again, before you begin to put out a fire, make sure that others in the house have been evacuated and that the fire department has been notified.

When using an extinguisher, remember the acronym **PASS**:

- Pull the pin. Release the locking mechanism with the nozzle pointed away from you.
- Aim low. Point the nozzle of the extinguisher toward the base of the fire.
- Squeeze the lever, applying slow and even pressure.
- Sweep the nozzle from side to side.

Have an escape plan. Arming yourself with a fire extinguisher—and knowing how to use it—is a good idea. But there are situations in which you and your extinguisher may be completely outgunned. If a fire is too big or growing quickly, the only thing to do is to make sure that everyone gets out *fast*. Few families, though, ever devise and practice a fire-escape plan.

To keep your family safe, draft an escape plan using these tips from the National Fire Protection Association:

- Draw a floor plan of your home, marking the locations of all exits from each room (including windows). Also note the location of each smoke alarm.
- Make sure that everyone recognizes the sound of the smoke alarms and understands what to do when they hear an alarm sound. Make sure that no escape routes are blocked, that windows open easily, and that adults and children alike know how to open them.
- If you have windows covered by security bars, make sure that they have quick-release mechanisms on the inside, and that everyone in the house knows how they operate.
- If you have a multistory home—especially one with upstairs bedrooms—invest in one or more chain ladders and learn how to deploy them for a window escape if a fire prevents use of the stairs.
- Practice your escape plan at least twice a year.
- Agree on a meeting place that is far enough away from your house to

be safe. In case of a fire, everyone should go immediately to that place after getting out of the house so that you can be certain that all have been safely evacuated.

- If you live in an area where 911 service is not available, make sure that everyone in your house memorizes the local emergency response phone number. Get everyone out of the house before you stop to call the fire department.
- If you live in an apartment building, know your building's evacuation plan and the location of emergency exits. During a fire, use the stairs, not the elevator.
- Remind everyone to stay low to the ground when smoke is present and to avoid opening any doors that are hot to the touch.
- Explain to younger children what firefighters may look like in their full gear. Unless prepared ahead of time, children might be frightened by their bulky shapes, face masks, axes, and other tools. Hiding from them could be disastrous.
- Make sure your house number is clearly visible from the street, and consider having the number painted on the curbside as well.

Carbon monoxide: the silent threat

While fire and smoke in the house are obvious signs of combustion gone out of control, carbon monoxide can arise from heating equipment or other appliances that seem to be working well. A colorless, odorless, but extremely dangerous gas, carbon monoxide is produced when fuels are incompletely burned and can be generated by any equipment that burns gas, coal, wood, charcoal, kerosene, or oil. This includes nonelectric furnaces, stoves, fireplaces, grills, and space heaters, as well as water heaters and clothes dryers that use natural or propane gas.

The major products of efficient combustion are (along with heat) water vapor and carbon dioxide (CO_2). When ventilation is poor, combustion occurs less efficiently, and carbon monoxide becomes more prevalent among the combustion products. Carbon monoxide can also build up to dangerous levels when combustion occurs in a confined space where exhaust products are not allowed to dissipate (for example, when a car is running in a closed garage).

Carbon monoxide is dangerous because of its strong affinity for hemoglobin, the compound that carries oxygen within red blood cells. Carbon monoxide binds to hemoglobin two hundred times more efficiently than oxygen.[12] As the level of carbon monoxide in the air increases, it competes powerfully against oxygen for binding sites on the hemoglobin molecule, leaving less hemoglobin available to carry oxygen. This biochemical asphyxiation eventually generates a host of symptoms including dizziness, blurred vision, nausea, headache, shortness of breath, weakness, disorientation, confusion, fatigue, sleepiness, and eventually unconsciousness and even death. The abrupt onset of headache and nausea may suggest food poisoning or flu, making the diagnosis difficult in the early phases of the illness. The very young, the elderly, and those with underlying medical conditions such as chronic heart or lung disease are particularly vulnerable, and a person who is in a deep sleep or intoxicated may die of carbon monoxide poisoning before symptoms develop.

F.Y.I. Beware if a number of people in your home simultaneously develop severe headache and nausea. This may indicate the presence of carbon monoxide exposure, and you should *immediately get everyone outside into fresh air*. Then call your fire department or local gas company to have your home checked for carbon monoxide before anyone goes back inside. If this gas is detected, everyone who was in the house should be evaluated without delay at the nearest emergency department.

Each year an estimated three hundred people die in the United States from accidental carbon monoxide poisoning. (Sadly, more than two thousand die every year by intentional self-poisoning with carbon monoxide.) About 40 percent of the accidental deaths are caused by consumer products such as heating and cooking equipment, while the rest result from motor-vehicle exhaust.[13] The good news is that with a few precautions you can easily protect your family from this invisible threat.

Keep your heating and cooking equipment maintained properly. Have your furnace, fireplace, or other heating equipment inspected each year by a qualified professional to see that they are working according to the manufacturer's specifications. Verify that heating equipment is properly vented to the outside with exhaust systems that do not leak.

Make sure that heating and cooking equipment is properly ventilated. Have fireplace flues and chimneys cleaned each year. When using a fireplace or woodstove, be sure the flue is open. An open flue creates an updraft that carries exhaust gases out and pulls fresh air in to feed the combustion. A closed flue allows buildup of dangerous exhaust fumes. Charcoal grills, hibachis, and camp stoves are meant to be used in the great outdoors—not inside your house, camper, or tent, where they pour carbon monoxide into the air you breathe. Other pieces of equipment, including many types of space heaters, are designed to be used indoors but need to be used in well-ventilated areas. Do not use unvented kerosene or gas space heaters in enclosed spaces.

If you buy a "vent-free" or "ventless" fireplace setup, make sure it is properly installed—and don't burn wood logs or other material in it. These heat-generating fireplaces combine nonburning "logs" and other decorative materials with natural gas to produce a pleasant facsimile of a log fire, but without smoke, ashes, or carbon monoxide. As a result they can "burn" safely without an open flue. However, they must be installed correctly and, very importantly, they are *not* meant to burn real logs or other materials with a closed (or nonexistent) flue. Doing so will generate both smoke and dangerous carbon monoxide gas.

Use the right fuel. Use of improper fuels in space heaters can increase output of carbon monoxide.

Do not idle your car in the garage. Even when a garage door is wide open, exhaust fumes can be drawn into the house. If you need to warm up your car on a cold morning, open the garage door, start the car, pull it out of the garage, then close the garage door so that exhaust will not seep back inside your home.

Do not idle your car if the tailpipe is close to a snowbank, or while digging your car out of snow. If snow or other material is blocking your tailpipe, the exhaust—and carbon monoxide with it—could back up and accumulate in the passenger compartment.

Install carbon monoxide detectors. Although the best way to deal with the risk of carbon monoxide poisoning is to take preventive measures, carbon monoxide detectors are a good supplementary approach. They are relatively inexpensive and can be purchased as combination smoke alarm/carbon monoxide detectors.

Like smoke alarms, carbon monoxide detectors should be installed on each level of the home near sleeping quarters according to the manufacturer's instructions. They should not be installed directly above a fuel-burning appliance, since these appliances normally emit a small amount of carbon monoxide after being turned on. Replace the battery according to manufacturer's instructions. Most detectors contain a carbon monoxide sensor that must be replaced every five years.

If a carbon monoxide detector alarm sounds, immediately open windows and doors to get fresh air into your home. Get everyone out of the house and call a qualified appliance or furnace technician who can pinpoint the source of carbon monoxide emissions. (Some utility providers offer this service free of charge.) If anyone in your home is experiencing any symptoms of carbon monoxide poisoning, call 911 or your local fire department.

Poisons around the house

There are nearly 2.4 million poison exposures each year,[14] and poisoning ranks as one of the top ten causes of nonfatal injuries in the United States each year.[15] Poisoning can occur at any age, but two groups of people are at particular risk: older adults and young children. Among seniors, poisoning usually involves one or more medications (prescription or otherwise) in one of these situations: inadvertently overdosing, ingesting the wrong type of drug, or combining medications in some way that produces adverse effects. We will talk more about the problems of medication among older adults in chapter 14, starting on page 713.

Young children have the highest poisoning risk of all age groups, and it's not hard to see why. Babies and toddlers experience the world with their hands and mouth. If an interesting object within reach will fit in their mouth, into their mouth it will go. This unsettling capacity for oral exploration can result in contact with hazardous objects and toxic substances. Likewise, preschoolers and older children, curious about items that smell or look attractive (and even some that don't), or perhaps imitating the grown-ups around them, are apt to swallow pills, liquid medications, or other hazardous substances that they might discover. More than half of all poison exposures (approximately 1.2 million cases each year in the United States) involve children age five or younger.[16]

One of the most common drugs on which children accidentally overdose is the familiar acetaminophen (Tylenol and many other brands). While benign and helpful at proper doses, acetaminophen can cause serious liver damage after an overdose if not treated in a timely manner.

Symptoms of poisoning

In young children, indications that your child has swallowed a toxic substance (or an overdose of medication) can include any of the following:

- Sudden illness for no apparent reason
- Close proximity to a potentially toxic substance such as a household cleaning product or a medication—especially if the container is open and pills or liquid are spilled
- Unusual behavior
- Unusual liquids, stains, or powder on the skin, clothing, or around the mouth
- Dizziness, weakness, stupor, confusion, or coma
- Blurry vision, double vision, or a change in the normal size of the pupils
- Rapid heart rate
- Fever, headache, irritability
- Rash or changes in skin color (blue, flushed, or pale)
- Depression or unusual shifts in mood
- Coughing, chest pain, or difficulty breathing—with or without increased noise during breathing
- Nausea, vomiting, abdominal pain or cramping, or diarrhea
- Twitching muscles or unexplained muscle pain or cramping
- Excessive saliva
- Inability to control urine or bowel movements
- Loss of appetite
- Abnormal breath odor

Protecting young children against poisoning

Make your home a safer place for children by keeping dangerous substances, whether household cleaning supplies, medicines, vitamins, or other chemicals, locked away and out of sight of young ones. A variety of cabinet locks are available to keep inquisitive children out of household chemical-storage areas. Finish all medications as prescribed and safely dispose of any leftover or unused medications. Keep medications stored in child-safe containers, and do not take medicine in front of young children, since children imitate adult behavior. Never refer to medicine as candy or call it anything other than what it is. Teach children never to eat or drink anything unless it is given to them by an adult they know.

In the garage, keep paint, pesticides, fertilizers, and other dangerous chemicals in a locked cabinet. Place gasoline and kerosene high and out of reach.

Keep toxic chemicals in their original containers, and never transfer them to containers that were once used for food or beverages.

What to do if you suspect poisoning

Post the poison control center number on your refrigerator or next to your telephone: (800) 222-1222. This number is a nationwide access number that will route your call to the poison control center closest to you.

A child who has ingested a toxic substance or an excessive amount of a medication may or may not be able to tell you what has happened. This will depend on the child's age, his condition after the episode (that is, alert, drowsy, or unconscious), and his emotional state.

If the situation indicates that poisoning may have occurred, take the following treatment steps:

- Check the ABC's—airway, breathing, and circulation—and begin rescue breathing or CPR if necessary. If CPR has been initiated, have someone call 911. (If you are alone, call 911 and then begin CPR. If possible, use a portable or cell phone so that you can communicate with the dispatcher as you continue to assess and administer CPR, if needed.)
- If CPR is not needed, call the poison control center number: (800) 222-1222.
- If the child is having seizures, protect him from injury by positioning him on his side and placing something soft, such as a pillow, under his head. Do not place anything in his mouth.
- If the child vomits, try to protect the airway. Position him on his side so that whatever is vomited will exit away from the mouth and not accidentally be inhaled into the airway. If necessary, gently remove any remaining material from his mouth.
- If the exposure was a skin contamination, remove all contaminated clothing and wash skin, hair, and nails with lots of tap water.
- If he has been exposed to fumes, remove him from the area in which the fumes are present.
- If the material went into the eye, irrigate the eye area thoroughly with copious amounts of tap water.
- Take the substance and its container with you to the doctor's office or emergency room and be prepared to answer some questions: Where was the child found? What and how much was ingested? When did symptoms (if any) begin? Did symptoms begin gradually or abruptly? What treatment was done at home and when?
- *Do not* wait for dramatic signs of illness before seeking medical assistance.
- *Do not* give anything as an antidote or attempt to neutralize a poison

unless you have been told to do so by a physician or poison control center.

- *Do not* attempt to give the child anything by mouth if he is unconscious.
- *Do not* induce vomiting unless directed to do so by a physician or a poison control center. Some poisons can cause more damage if regurgitated.
- *Do not* rely just on the label of a medication or other substance to tell you whether or not it is potentially hazardous.[17]

Protecting Little Ones in Your Home

If you have or will have infants, toddlers, and young children living in your home (or stopping by for visits), you need to look at your living areas with a

WHAT ABOUT IPECAC AND ACTIVATED CHARCOAL?

Common sense would seem to dictate that if a child swallows something poisonous, the best thing to do is to have him immediately purge the toxic substance by vomiting. For decades, **ipecac**, a medicine that induces vomiting, was sold to parents for just that purpose. However, the home use of ipecac has come under increased scrutiny by medical professionals, who warn that inducing vomiting may cause harm after the ingestion of a host of materials and objects, including:

- Alkaline materials: detergents, drain cleaners, oven cleaners, bleach, and flat circular batteries. Chemical names to look for include lye, sodium hydroxide, potassium hydroxide, ammonia, calcium oxide, trisodium phosphate, and wood ash.
- Acids: automobile battery fluid, toilet-bowl cleaners, soldering fluxes, antirust compounds, and slate cleaners. Chemical names include sulfuric, hydrochloric, phosphoric, hydrofluoric, and oxalic acids.
- Petroleum products: cleaning fluid, gasoline, kerosene, coal oil, fuel oil, or paint thinner.
- Sharp or solid objects: glass, nails, razors, and thermometers.

The number of times in which ipecac has been recommended by poison control centers has declined dramatically in recent years. In 1985, poison control centers in the United States recommended that parents administer ipecac to their children in 15 percent of their consultations. That percentage has decreased each year, to less than half a percent in 2004.[18] Based on the lack of clear evidence that children receiving ipecac at home have better outcomes than those not receiving it, the American Academy of Pediatrics recommends

new set of eyes. Odds and ends that look perfectly innocent on your floors, tables, and shelves could prove hazardous or even lethal to little ones in ways you might never imagine. We'll list a number of important safety tips, and with them in mind you should get down on your hands and knees to take a child's-eye tour of any room that a child may be exploring. Some of these may duplicate material you have seen elsewhere in this chapter (or in this book), but there's no harm in a little repetition when something as precious as a child's safety is at stake.[21]

In the nursery

In chapter 15 we will discuss sleep-related concerns and review sleeping arrangements that reduce the risk of sudden infant death syndrome (SIDS). You can read more about important guidelines for sleep beginning on page 770. In addition, there are important safety precautions to consider when a baby sleeps in a crib.

that ipecac *not* be used routinely as an intervention at home following accidental ingestion of a toxic substance.[19]

The fact that home use of ipecac is now frowned upon by medical organizations has prompted interest in other means of "gastric decontamination." One alternative that has been used in emergency departments for many years is **activated charcoal**, a form of charcoal that has been treated to make it highly porous, thereby vastly increasing its surface area and thus its capacity for binding chemicals. When placed in a liquid, activated charcoal can adsorb large quantities of organic and other compounds, effectively filtering them out of the liquid. (This is why aquarium filters often utilize it.) When placed in the stomach of someone who has ingested certain poisons, activated charcoal may prevent the poisons from being absorbed into the digestive tract and introduced to the bloodstream.

The idea behind using activated charcoal to decontaminate the stomach of a poisoning victim is sound, and activated charcoal stands as a preferred means of decontamination in hospital emergency rooms. Unfortunately, some very practical issues prevent this from being a useful home remedy. In hospitals, charcoal is administered through a nasogastric tube—a flexible tube passed into the stomach by way of the nose. Needless to say, the familiar phrase "don't try this at home" definitely applies to nasogastric tubes, so children at home would have to swallow activated charcoal. Good luck. Young children frequently gag on this stuff and vomit it up, negating its benefits and creating a spectacular mess (with some very tough stains). Furthermore, research studies have failed to demonstrate that children swallowing activated charcoal at home are likely to do better than those who receive it in the emergency room. As a result, the American Academy of Pediatrics does not support the routine use of activated charcoal in the home after the accidental ingestion of a toxin.[20] ■

Did you catch the words *adsorb* and *absorb* in the above paragraph? They're not typos. Activated charcoal *ad*sorbs toxins, meaning that these substances bind to its surface. The intestine *ab*sorbs, or takes in, nutrients and other chemical compounds.

A crib can be the newborn's sleeping place from day one and typically will be in use for two to three years. Since your baby will spend time in a crib without direct supervision, this must be a completely safe environment. In order to prevent falls and other types of accidents, crib manufacturers in recent years have had to comply with a number of safety requirements. If your baby is going to be using an older model, you will need to check the following:

- The slats in the crib should be no more than two and three-eighths inches apart.
- Unless they are supporting a high canopy, corner posts that extend above the rails are a potential hazard because they may entangle loose clothing. They should be unscrewed or cut off.
- Paint on an old crib may contain lead, and any flakes of paint accidentally swallowed by a curious baby could cause lead poisoning. When in doubt, sand off the old coat (taking care not to inhale it yourself) and apply some high-quality enamel in its place.
- The headboards and footboards should be solid and without decorative cutouts that could trap a head, hand, or foot.

In addition, you should check the following before you place your baby in any crib, new or old:

- The mattress pad should fit snugly into the frame. If you can wedge more than two fingers between the pad and the crib side, the mattress pad is too small. Remove any extraneous tags and thin plastic wrappings. If you use a mattress cover, be sure it is made of thick plastic that can be zipped around the pad. Don't place pillows or any soft bedding material other than a fitted sheet under the baby. Her head or face might become accidentally buried in the soft folds, especially if she happens to be facedown, which could lead to suffocation. Sheepskin, down mattresses, feather beds, and wavy water beds pose similar risks.
- Bumper pads, securely tied in place, should line the inside of the crib. When your baby can pull up to a standing position, the pads should be removed, since they can assist a baby's attempts to climb over the rail. The same is true of large stuffed animals that a toddler might use as a soft step or launching pad for a trip over the side.
- The side rails should latch securely in place, with the release mechanism out of reach of exploring fingers. When fully raised, the rails should extend at least twenty inches above the top of the mattress. As your baby grows and eventually stands up, the mattress will need to be lowered.
- If you hang a mobile above the crib, be sure it remains out of reach when your baby begins to move toward (and grab for) interesting objects.
- For many reasons—sun exposure, shades, cords, and, worst of all,

the possibility of a disastrous fall—never put a crib next to a window, whether open or shut.

One other important piece of equipment in the nursery is the changing table, which can be a convenient one-stop location for diaper duties at home. But it is also notorious for being the place from which a baby takes her first fall. If you use a changing table:

- Never step away, turn around, or otherwise divert your attention from the job at hand unless you pick up the baby to do so. Babies seem to choose the moment you're not looking to show off their new ability to roll over—and then take a fast trip to the floor. Never answer the phone or the door if it means walking away from your baby.
- To reduce the likelihood of such a fall, make sure you have all the changing gear—new diaper, wipes, etc.—within reach before you start.
- The table should have a two-inch guardrail around its edge and a safety strap to help you secure the baby. However, these should not be considered a substitute for your undivided attention when your infant is on the changing table.
- Don't distract an older baby by letting her handle a container of baby powder (which she might accidentally unload into her or your airspace), play with a disposable diaper (whose plastic liner she might rip off and choke on), or suck on some other miscellaneous object on the changing table.

Some safety reminders for parents of younger infants

- ***Don't leave your baby alone on any high surface, including a kitchen counter or sofa.*** He will invariably pick that moment to demonstrate his ability to roll over.
- ***Don't leave your baby unattended even for a few seconds while he is in water, whether bathing in the sink, infant tub, or adult bathtub.*** He can drown in an inch or two of water.
- ***Everyone in your house, including young children, should know how to dial 911 in case of an emergency involving the baby.*** All adults and children over twelve should be trained in infant CPR. Local hospitals normally conduct CPR classes on a regular basis.
- ***Be extremely cautious about leaving one of your older children in charge of your baby, even for a few minutes.*** This assignment should be considered only for a responsible sibling more than twelve years of age who has been observed handling the baby appropriately for a number of weeks. Your older child must have explicit information about your whereabouts, instructions about what to do if the baby cries or has any other type of problem, and names and phone numbers of people to call for help if needed.

- ***Always buckle your baby securely into his car seat, no matter how short the ride.*** Until he weighs twenty pounds and reaches his first birthday, he will still be sitting backward. The center of the backseat is the safest location for him; thus you should avoid putting him in the forward passenger seat. This means that, should he start to fuss, you will have to resist the temptation to turn around and tend to him while your vehicle is in motion. If your car has a passenger-side air bag, you should never place your baby in the forward passenger seat. If the air bag inflates during an accident, it could cause serious or even fatal injuries to a baby. (For more information on car seats, see page 532.)
- ***Never carry your baby while you are also holding a cup of hot liquid.*** One strong wiggle could result in a scalding injury to one or both of you.
- ***Keep a watchful eye for small objects scattered around your living space.*** These include older children's LEGOs, marbles, action figures, and other toys that might come within your baby's reach and therefore go into his mouth. If your baby is going to spend time on the floor, put your face at his level and scan the horizon. Look for stray coins, paper clips, pieces of dry pet food, plastic wrappers, electrical cords, or unstable objects that might fall on your baby if given a gentle shove.
- ***Beware of parking your baby in an infant swing or doorway jumper and then turning your attention elsewhere.*** After four months, a baby with enough wiggle power may be able to squirm out of a swing or even bring the whole thing down.
- ***Keep your baby out of walkers, which are responsible for thousands of accidents every year.*** This device will not teach your child how to walk or speed up his motor development. Instead, it gives your active baby the opportunity to propel himself to the edge of the stairs, investigate whatever is sitting on your coffee table, or flip the walker over when he bumps into an obstruction.
- ***Extremely vigorous play (such as tossing a baby a few inches into the air and catching him) is not a good idea for young infants.*** Rapid accelerations and changes in direction, however playful, can have the same effect as shaking a baby, risking injury to his neck and brain.
- ***A baby's skin may become sunburned after as little as fifteen minutes of direct exposure to the sun.*** Don't allow your baby to have prolonged exposure to direct sunlight (even on a hazy or overcast day), especially between 10 A.M. and 3 P.M. This is particularly important at higher altitudes or around lakes and seashores, where the sun's ultraviolet light can reflect off sand and water.

  If your baby is going to be outside for any length of time, try to avoid the time of peak intensity, keep him in the shade as much as possible, and use appropriate clothing (as well as a hat or bonnet) for protection. An explorer who is going to be in and out of sunlight will benefit from a sunscreen with a **sun protection factor (SPF)** rating of at least fifteen, applied an hour before he ventures forth. If you are going to take him with you into the pool, use a waterproof formula and reapply it after you are done. Occasionally a baby will react to the common UV-protecting ingredient known as **PABA**, the most commonly used ultraviolet-absorbing ingredient in sunscreens. If your baby has very sensitive skin, you might take your sunscreen for a "test drive" by applying some to a small area of his skin (an inch or so wide) for several hours to see if any reaction develops.

Furthermore, sunscreens containing PABA shouldn't be used on your baby's skin before he is six months old. You may, however, wish to use a PABA-free sunscreen specifically for babies if sun exposure is unavoidable. If you take your baby outdoors for any length of time, keep him in the shade or use an umbrella and make sure his skin is covered with appropriate clothing (including a hat or bonnet) even if he is in the shade.

Safety around the house for crawlers and toddlers

By nine months of age, your baby's curiosity will be insatiable. She will not be content merely to inspect items within her reach. She will be aching to get her hands on all those interesting shapes that she's been seeing from across the room. Her intense curiosity will become a driving force in advancing her motor skills.

This normal—and necessary—development will generate extra work and worry for everyone in your baby's life. Her explorations should be encouraged, but they will inevitably require some adjustment of your living arrangements. You'll need to balance your baby's healthy curiosity against her need for a safe environment and your need for some semblance of order.

It's important to avoid extremes. Confinement for hours on end in a playpen, which might be convenient for the grown-ups, will impair the flow of information to your baby's developing brain. But giving her unlimited access to all parts of the home without some thoughtful preparation is an invitation to harm or disaster. Furthermore, attempting to train a baby at this age by subjecting her to a nonstop torrent of "no's" and hand-slapping while she is merely trying to find out what's what in her world will make everyone miserable and exhausted.

Some reasonable baby-proofing and commonsense precautions will spare everyone a lot of toil and grief.

Take a child's-eye tour of whatever living space is available to your crawler/cruiser/walker. Are there any top-heavy items—chairs, tables, floor lamps, bookshelves—that might fall if pulled by your baby? any electrical cords or outlets within reach? (Install plastic plugs to block unused outlets from inquisitive fingers.) Do you see any wires with frayed insulation? These are a hazard to everyone, not just the baby. What about cords dangling down from a curling or steam iron resting on a counter or ironing board? A yank on one of these could cause not only a hazardous bump on her head or body but also a very painful burn.

Are there any small objects lying around that she could choke on? Your vigilance regarding small objects will be a daily concern if you have older children at home, because their toys and games tend to have lots of tiny parts and pieces that have a way of dispersing throughout your home. How about cords attached to draperies and blinds? These should be looped or tied on a hook well out of reach to prevent your baby from getting tangled in them.

Don't leave your prized china or other valuable breakables within reach of a newly mobile baby and then demand that she not touch them. She will have no concept of the difference between a cup made by Wedgwood and one brought home from Wendy's, except, perhaps, the sound they make when they hit the floor. Your expensive collectibles should be displayed (or stored) out of reach during this season of your child's life.

While some recommend that your kitchen be kept off-limits to little explorers, this will probably not be a realistic option. Most parents and older children traverse the kitchen many times each day, and dealing with a barricade every time is a major nuisance. Lots of family interactions take place in kitchens, and your baby will not want to be left out.

This will mean, however, relocating cleaning compounds and other chemicals to higher ground. Bleach, furniture polish, and drain cleaners are particularly hazardous, and automatic-dishwasher powder can be extremely irritating if it gets into the mouth. Sharp objects, which of course are abundant in kitchens, must also be kept out of reach at all times. If you have an automatic dishwasher, be sure to keep the door latched when you are not loading or unloading it. A wide-open dishwasher door is not only an irresistible climbing spot but also a gateway to all sorts of glassware and sharp utensils.

Many families set aside a low cupboard for "baby's kitchen stuff"—a collection of old plastic bowls, cups, spoons, lids, and other safe unbreakables that the baby can examine and manipulate to her heart's content. (By the way, she will probably spend a fair amount of time moving the cupboard door back and forth on its hinge.) You may want to steer her toward this particular cupboard and away from the others (this will take lots of repetition) or make the arrangement more formal by installing plastic safety latches on the cupboards and drawers that are off-limits.

While kitchens are difficult to barricade, bathrooms are another story. Like kitchens, they are full of potential hazards: medications, cleaners, and most important, bodies of water. Any medications (prescription or over-the-counter, including vitamins and iron) and cleaning substances must be stored well out of reach and returned to their secure spot immediately after each use.

Never leave a baby unattended in the bath, and be certain to empty the tub as soon as you're done with it. Open toilets are an irresistible destination for a cruiser. The possible consequences of a baby's investigation of an unflushed toilet are both unsafe and stomach-turning. Even more dangerous is the possibility that a top-heavy toddler might lean over far enough to fall in.

Never leave hair dryers, curlers, or other electrical devices plugged in after you use them. For that matter, no one should be using any of these items when the baby (or anyone else) is in the bathtub, unless you have a very large bathroom with a lengthy distance between appliance and water. If your baby or an older child tries to take the hair dryer for a swim, even if it's turned off but plugged in, the resulting shock could be lethal.

Unlike most kitchens, bathrooms have doors that can be shut to prevent unsupervised entry. If an enterprising explorer learns to turn door handles, an additional high latch may need to be installed.

Survey your home for "what's hot and what's not." Radiators, heaters, floor furnace grills, and fireplace screens can all become surprisingly hot, and a protective barrier between these surfaces and little fingers will be needed, at least at some times of the year.

Some stoves have exposed knobs that babies and toddlers might twist and turn. If these are easily detachable, you may want to remove them between meals. You can also buy safety covers at a hardware store. Be sure the handles of pots on hot burners don't extend over the edge of the stove, since one healthy pull could result in a severely scalded child. A similar reminder applies to hot liquids such as soups and gravies near the edge of your dining table, especially if they sit on a tablecloth that could be pulled from below.

Set your hot water heater temperature below 120°F to minimize the risk of an accidental scald from the tap.

What about those houseplants? Infants and toddlers can be quite adept at pruning your prized houseplants if they are within reach. A more worrisome possibility is that these young children might choose to sample the leaves and stems, which may be irritating to the lining of the mouth or even overtly toxic. Now is the time to move the plants out of reach, unless you know for certain that they are nontoxic and you don't care if they get mangled sometime during the next few months. In order to prevent your explorer from playing in the dirt of any plants that remain at floor level, cover the soil with screen mesh.

Finally, think about your baby's introduction to the great outdoors. When the weather's nice and the family gathers in the backyard, what interesting but hazardous items might cross her path? Once again, make a baby's-eye survey of any area that she might reach (if she's a skilled crawler, keep in mind how fast she can move while your attention is diverted).

If you have a swimming pool, make sure that a childproof fence surrounds it. (Some states have a law requiring this safety barrier.) If your yard contains a spa, it should be securely covered when not in use. Pool and hot-tub drain covers should be checked periodically to make sure they are properly in place. If not, a child's hand or even hair could be pulled into the outlet by the suction created by the pump, and he might be unable to break free. Children have drowned in such circumstances. As a backup precaution, make sure that the pump's on-off switch is readily accessible.

Check the lawn for mushrooms, and if you are not absolutely certain they are nontoxic, get rid of them, because anything your baby finds at this age is likely to go straight into her mouth. Are there any garden tools, insecticides, fertilizers, or other unfriendly items lying around? The more potential dangers you can eliminate from her immediate access, the more you can enjoy your time outdoors with her.

Parental vigilance

Many of these guidelines represent passive restraints—fixed barriers between children and potential hazards. But you cannot anticipate every possible risk or create enough safeguards for a 100 percent safe environment, unless you want to turn your home into a padded cell. You will need to take more active measures as well, including your own surveillance and some basic training for your baby.

From your standpoint, perpetual vigilance is the price of child rearing, at least for now. You must develop an ongoing sense of your child's whereabouts,

SOME SAFETY REMINDERS REGARDING FOOD AND FEEDING

Do not feed honey to babies under twelve months of age because of the risk of **infant botulism**, a form of food poisoning that can cause serious damage to the nervous system and in very rare cases is even fatal. (Honey should also not be added as a sweetener to infant formula, or anything else, for infants in this age group.) Corn syrup has also been found to cause infant botulism.

Avoid feeding babies without teeth any foods that might cause choking—small and hard items such as seeds, nuts, small candies, uncooked peas, and popcorn. Also keep your baby away from foods that are sticky, chewy, stringy, or small and round. Peanut butter and hot dogs are off-limits, along with grapes, uncooked vegetables, raw apples, and dried fruit. In a nutshell, foods that can't be smushed by gums or easily dissolved in saliva or that might fit snugly into a small airway don't belong in your baby's mouth.

As your baby begins to eat more solid foods, you may find it easier to feed him in a high chair. As with all baby equipment, a few simple precautions will help prevent unpleasant or even serious accidents.

- As with bathtubs and car seats, never leave your baby unattended while he is sitting in a high chair.
- Make certain that his chair has a broad base so it cannot be easily tipped over. Grandma's high chair might be a venerated family heirloom, but if it doesn't sit rock solid on the floor, use a newer one. If you use a chair that folds, make sure it is locked into place before your baby gets in.

a third eye and ear that are tuned in to him, even when he is in a confined and seemingly safe space such as his crib. You will need to monitor his activities constantly to see what new perils might cross his path in the immediate future.

The riskiest times will be those when you are distracted, frazzled, or just plain weary. You may be in the middle of a project involving hazardous tools or materials—a long overdue deep cleaning, for example. Suddenly the phone rings, or someone is at the door, or another child cries out in another room. Before you drop everything to attend to the new situation, look at what might be open, exposed, or available to your baby. Could he get to any of it? You may have to delay your response for a few moments while you ensure there is no way your baby in motion can get his hands on something dangerous.

Beware of those times in the day—especially the late afternoon—when your energy may be low, your mind preoccupied, and your patience short. One or more other children may be irritable at this time, competing for your attention. But don't lose track of your youngest crawler/cruiser/toddler, who may have just discovered something interesting that was dropped under the kitchen table.

Sometime in your parenting career, you may reach a point of such sheer ex-

- Take a few extra seconds to secure your baby with the chair's safety straps. This will prevent him from wiggling and sliding out of position or standing up to survey the horizon, both of which could result in a serious injury.
- Before your baby is seated, make sure the chair is a safe distance away from the nearest wall or counter. Otherwise, a healthy shove from your young diner might topple her and the chair to the floor.
- Don't let other children play under or climb on the high chair.
- Clean food debris off the chair and tray after each meal. Your baby may have no reservations about sampling any leftovers—in various states of decay—that are within finger range.

If you use a portable baby seat that clamps onto a table when you travel or eat out, observe a few additional precautions:

- Make sure the table is steady enough to support both chair and baby and that the chair is securely clamped to the table before your baby gets in. Card tables, glass tops, tables supported only by a center post, and extension leaves are not strong or stable enough for this job.
- Position the chair so your baby can't push against one of the table legs and literally "shove off" for a voyage to the floor.
- The chair should attach to the bare surface of the table, not to a tablecloth or place mat that can slide off.
- Don't let older children play under the table or seat, since they might accidentally bump and dislodge the seat. ■

haustion that you just have to lie down for a little while. Do you let an older child watch the baby or let your toddler roam around your bedroom while you close your eyes for a few precious minutes? Think hard before you stretch your safety boundaries. An older child is more likely to become distracted by a friend or toy, and a major problem could develop during a few moments of inattention. If you are really that tired, see if a trusted adult such as a friend, neighbor, or relative might relieve you for one or more hours' respite.

Some additional cautions for two-year-olds and preschoolers

While children in this age group can understand more sophisticated verbal cautions (such as "Don't chase your ball into the street"), their impulse control and judgment have a long way to grow. Your child will also be unlikely to comprehend the ultimate risks of violating your warnings. To make matters worse, if she's in a limit-challenging mood, she may decide to create a contest over one of your safety rules. Therefore, constant vigilance must be maintained, with particular attention to the following areas:

- *Traffic hazards.* Because she can run more swiftly and dart into the nearest street, she must be monitored at all times when she is in an area where there are no barriers separating her from traffic.
- *Harmful substances.* Medications must remain completely inaccessible, especially if they happen to be liquid and pleasantly flavored. Not only is she more skillful with the use of her hands, but her pretending games or imitation—new and important behaviors at this age—may include scenarios of playing doctor or taking medicines to get well.
- *Car-seat struggles.* She may become more vocal in protesting the use of her car seat, or she may actually figure out how to get out of it at some choice moment. Don't give an inch on your insistence that the seat be used for every ride in the car, no matter how short.
- *Dangerous "grown-up toys."* Never underestimate her ingenuity in getting her hands on appliances, tools, or other hardware that she has seen you use. Imitation may come into play here as well.
- *The bathtub.* She is still too young to be left in a bathtub unsupervised. The physical prowess that now makes shallow water seem less hazardous also enables her to turn on the faucet, leading to a possible scalding injury or even an overflowing tub. (Setting the temperature of your water heater below 120°F will reduce the risk of this type of injury.) She might also decide to see what happens when she jumps up and down in the water—and in so doing, slip and fall.
- *Water hazards.* Nonstop watchfulness is an absolute necessity whenever your two-year-old is near a swimming pool or any other body of water. Curiosity is abundant and caution scarce at this age, and a child can make a beeline toward a body of water in just a few mo-

ments while you are distracted with something else. If your child is playing in water, she must be observed by a responsible individual—ideally by someone who is in the water with her—at all times. Do not rely on an inner tube, water wings, or other flotation device to keep your child safe.

Firearms

There are more than 200 million privately owned firearms, including 65 to 70 million handguns, in the United States. Approximately 60 to 65 million of us, comprising 45 percent of American households, own guns.[22]

Whether the sale and ownership of firearms should be more (or less) tightly regulated is an ongoing, hotly contested political issue. Regardless of where you stand on the gun-control debate, however, there is one truth that everyone can agree on: When improperly used or stored, firearms represent a serious safety risk. The discharge of firearms was the second leading cause of injury deaths in the United States in 2002, accounting for more than 30,000 lives lost, or 19 percent of injury deaths. The actual number of deaths caused by *accidental* discharge of firearms was much lower—762 during the same year—but this represents 762 accidental deaths too many. Some research indicates that the availability of firearms in the home increases the risk that a suicide attempt will be lethal. All things considered, this should not come as a surprise. Suicide accounted for about 57 percent (or more than 17,000) of firearm-related deaths in 2002, and firearms claim more suicide victims than all other methods of self-harm combined.[23]

The mere fact that firearms pose such a deadly risk has prompted a number of mainstream medical organizations (such as the American Academy of Pediatrics) to assert that the most effective way to deal with the risk of firearms is to remove them from the home entirely. The logic is straightforward: Since firearms are not an absolute necessity and yet pose a real danger, why have them around at all?

For many Americans, however, hunting and shooting sports have long been a part of family recreation and culture, and getting rid of firearms would not be an option. For these families, firearm safety in the home rests squarely on the shoulders of the parents. If you own a gun—especially if young children live in or visit your home—it is imperative that you take the following precautions:

- Store all firearms unloaded, locked away, and out of sight.
- Keep ammunition locked away separately from the firearm.
- Use trigger locks.

Some who keep a handgun at home for protection might think these safety measures defeat the purpose of owning a firearm, but avoiding a tragic accident (especially where small children are concerned) should be the highest priority. Young children can have difficulty distinguishing reality from make-believe. Whether you own a firearm or not, you should teach your child that guns are not

continued on page 528

LOWER BACK INJURIES

Unlike the other safety issues mentioned in this chapter, lower back injuries usually do not result from contact with an external hazard. Instead, most of these arise from repetitive everyday activities, wear and tear, poor posture, overuse, and improper lifting behavior.

As a result, they are a common injury: According to the American Academy of Orthopaedic Surgeons, four out of five adults will experience significant lower back pain sometime during their life. Even though back injuries are the most common occupational hazard, many back injuries occur at home or at play as well.

The causes of lower back pain include:

- *Sprains and strains.* The vertebrae (the bones that make up the spinal column) are connected by tough fibrous bands called ligaments that define and limit how two adjacent bones move in relation to each other. Like other ligaments in the body, those attached to vertebrae can become weak or stiff when underused or overworked. Rapid, forceful movements can stretch them enough to cause a tear called a sprain. The muscles of the lower back can also be stretched beyond their capacity when subjected to intense forces, resulting in an injury called a strain. This is more likely to occur when muscles are poorly conditioned.

For more information about sprains, strains, and other injuries, see "Vocabulary Lesson—Tendons, Ligaments, Strains, Sprains, and Ruptures" in chapter 7 on page 294.

- *Wear and tear.* As we age, cumulative wear-and-tear damage to the joints of the vertebrae is inevitable. Most of us go about our business for decades without significant pain or loss of function. For some, however, the damage can become more severe, resulting in pain and stiffness. Wear-and-tear damage aggravated by arthritis may lead to bone spurs and inflammation that can irritate nerves as they exit one or more levels of the spinal column. This can cause pain not only in the back but also in one or both legs.
- *Fractures.* As we age we tend to lose bone density. This is particularly troublesome for many women after menopause, but it can affect men as well. Substantial bone loss, a condition called osteoporosis, can render the vertebrae vulnerable to damage from falling, lifting heavy items, or merely supporting the weight of one's own body. A common injury of the spine is a **compression fracture**, which involves a literal collapse of the main body of one of

the vertebrae accompanied by a significant amount of pain. Multiple compression fractures can lead to loss of height and deformity of the spine. Until recently, treatment involved only bed rest and pain relievers. Now, however, spine surgeons as well as specially trained radiologists can perform a relatively simple procedure that restores a collapsed vertebra to its original shape, with a marked reduction in pain.

- *Bulging disks.* The vertebrae that comprise our spinal column are separated by fibrous disks that provide cushioning and allow flexibility. As we age, these disks may develop cracks and tears, which not only cause pain but also may allow the softer inner portion of the disk to push outward. This condition is called a **herniated** or **slipped disk**. If a protruding disk presses against a nerve exiting the spinal column, it can cause pain or even weakness in the area (usually part of the leg) supplied by that nerve.[24]

How can some of these problems be avoided? First, stay in shape. As we described in detail in chapter 7, one of the many benefits of exercise is that, when done properly, it can help prevent some of the stiffness, aches, and pains that many people accept as normal parts of aging. Some basic exercises for the back muscles can help maintain strength and flexibility. Stretching before beginning a repetitive activity such as raking or shoveling may be helpful as well.

Maintaining proper posture can also reduce stress on the back. If you are overweight, the extra load—especially if a good deal of it is in the abdomen—can put considerable stress on back muscles, day in and day out. A chronic backache may provide some motivation to lose excess pounds.

When lifting, make sure you use proper form and motion. Place your feet shoulder-width apart for proper balance. Lift with your legs, never your back, and bend at the knees and hips, not at the waist. Avoid twisting your body while lifting, and position the load close to your body.

One final note: According to the American Academy of Orthopaedic Surgeons, smokers experience a higher incidence of back pain than nonsmokers. If you smoke and are suffering from chronic lower back pain, you now have one more reason to quit. ■

We review osteoporosis and its treatment in detail in chapter 13, starting on page 661.

Some basic strengthening and stretching exercises can be found in appendix D beginning on page 929. As an alternative, you may want to consult with a physical therapist or a trainer to develop your strengthening and stretching routine, especially if you are having ongoing back problems.

Many people rely on "back belts" while lifting to help them avoid injury. Unfortunately, reliable studies have shown that frequent use of back belts may not reduce the incidence of back injuries.

The best advice to prevent injury is to rely on proper lifting technique rather than back belts.[25] Use proper form and motion when lifting *any* low-lying object, whether it weights five ounces or fifty pounds. If something is too heavy for you to lift alone, get help.

continued from page 525

toys and that they can kill. Also, teach them what to do if they find a gun, either in the house or away from home. Under no circumstances should your child touch a gun or get near it. He should leave it where it is and immediately find a parent, a teacher, or some other responsible adult to report where the firearm was found.

One final note: Even if you have had firearms in your home for generations and are fastidious with safety measures, you should strongly consider removing them entirely if anyone in your home—especially a teenager—is dealing with depression. A person who swallows a handful of medication in a moment of despair will nearly always recover fully if discovered within a reasonable time frame. But a person who turns a firearm on himself in that moment of despair will almost certainly die, or at best sustain a terrible injury.

Avoiding Injuries Outside the Home

There are countless ways we might be injured once we walk out the front door or pull out of the garage. In this book, we focus on those that cause the most deaths and injuries, that involve everyday activities or common recreational pursuits, and most importantly that can be avoided by taking reasonsable precautions.

On the road again: staying safe in the car

Hurricanes, tornadoes, and floods always make big news, but every year motor vehicle accidents kill more Americans than all forms of natural disasters combined. The good news is that ongoing advances in automobile design (such as passenger restraint technologies) as well as newer regulations (such as mandatory seat-belt laws) have made a significant dent in the annual rate of injuries and fatalities due to traffic accidents over the past few decades.

Nevertheless, much remains to be done if we are to stem the flow of losses from motor vehicle accidents. Almost 2.8 million people were injured and more than 42,000 lost their life in motor vehicle crashes in 2004. According to a National Highway Traffic Safety Administration (NHTSA) report, the economic costs associated with traffic accidents in the year 2000 totaled over $230 billion, including lost productivity, property damage, and medical expenses.[26]

As with all hazards, the best approach is to avoid motor vehicle accidents. Unfortunately, no one can foresee what events on the road might conspire against you and your vehicle, and you certainly cannot control what other drivers do. It's crucial, therefore, to think beyond measures to avoid an accident and consider also what will protect you and your loved ones in case the unexpected happens. The two major areas over which you have the most control are your vehicle and your behavior.

Vehicle safety

When it's time to shop for a new or used car, what influences your purchasing decision? Manufacturers and advertisers frequently try to manipulate you with ads suggesting that driving their vehicle is a sensual, empowering, ego-boosting experience. More practical matters often take center stage when reality (i.e., the family budget) enters the picture: Is this car dependable, durable, and a good value? But in addition to the tug-of-war between your desire for that dream car and the payments you'll have to make every month, you need to think about one other concern: safety features. Does this vehicle have both driver- and passenger-side air bags? What about side-impact air bags? How did it rate in crash tests? What about rollover tests? Does it have antilock brakes? Does it have shoulder belts that can be adjusted for shorter passengers? If any of these questions will affect your choice of vehicle (and they should), make sure that you get some meaningful answers. For most vehicles you can find answers to these questions at NHTSA's safety Web site, http://www.nhtsa.dot.gov/cars/testing/ncap/index.cfm.

You don't have to buy a new or late model car to make sure you have a safe one. While safety issues arising from automotive design flaws and defects have garnered lots of media attention, many lower profile problems can be addressed or eliminated with proper vehicle maintenance. Here are just a few items that should be on your checklist:

- *Tires.* Your vehicle should ride on tires that are appropriate for the weather conditions you are likely to face. If you live in an area where winter routinely brings ice and snow, install snow tires or all-season tires that provide adequate traction on snowy roads.

  Check your tire treads. Badly worn treads reduce your ability to control your vehicle, especially when the road is wet or snowy. For just a few dollars, you can buy a tire-tread depth gauge to tell you exactly how much of your tread is left. In most states, tires are considered by law to be worn-out if they are at a tread depth of one-sixteenth of an inch or less. At this point you must replace them. However, if rainy roads are a concern to you, consider replacing your tires before they get to one-sixteenth of an inch. At two-sixteenths of an inch, tires are much more prone to hydroplaning (skimming over a layer of water) on wet surfaces. Tires lose their traction on snowy roads when tread depth is below three-sixteenths of an inch.

  Check your tire pressure once a month to make sure your tires are inflated as recommended in your vehicle's owner's manual. Improperly inflated tires not only result in uneven tread wear but present other safety risks as well. Underinflated tires can diminish your steering control and also cause your car to hydroplane (skim over wet surfaces). Overinflated tires are more easily damaged by road debris or potholes. Always maintain the vehicle manufacturer's recommended tire pressure, not the pressure stamped on the tire's sidewall. The number on the tire represents the upper pressure limit at which the tire should perform without posing an immediate safety hazard, not the pressure for optimal function.

An inexpensive and low-tech approach to checking your tread depth is to use a coin. Insert a penny into your tire's tread with Lincoln's head upside down; if all of Lincoln's head is visible above the tread, your tread depth is less than one-sixteenth of an inch. If you insert a quarter into the tread and can see Washington's head without obstruction, you still have two-sixteenths of an inch of tread. If you insert a penny into the tread with the Lincoln Memorial upside down and find that the top of the building is below the tread, you still have three-sixteenths of an inch left.

Don't forget to check the pressure in your spare tire when you check the other four.

- *Brakes.* We take it for granted that a little pressure on the brake pedal will slow and eventually stop our car. But we don't really appreciate the job our brakes do until we have the heart-pounding experience of seeing a child dart into the street in front of us or the car ahead of us suddenly screech to a stop. While driver inattention is often the cause of accidents, faulty brakes contribute to a large number of disastrous collisions.

  In order to bring you to a safe stop, your car's brakes must convert a serious amount of kinetic energy (from your moving vehicle) into heat (from friction). To do this, the brake system relies on parts that are exposed to intense wear and tear. To keep your brakes working (and to avoid the "life flashing before your eyes" situation in which your brakes *don't* work when you need them), you must maintain them properly. Have your brakes checked at least once every year, and be on the lookout for signs of wear. These include squealing or grinding noises when you apply the brakes, pulling of your car to one side when braking, or an ominous "spongy" feeling when you press on the brake pedal. Antilock brakes are designed to pulse in order to keep wheels from skidding, especially on slippery surfaces. If your vehicle is not equipped with antilock brakes but you feel the brake pedal pulsing when you step on it, have the brakes checked as soon as possible.
- *Lights.* Your lights not only allow you to see objects in the road when it gets dark, but they also allow you to be seen by other motorists and pedestrians. To check your lights, turn them on and walk around your vehicle, making sure they all work. Specifically, make sure that each headlight and taillight is as bright as its mate on the opposite side of the car and that there is no water on the inside of the lenses. Ask someone to help you check the turn signals, emergency flashers, brake lights, and back-up lights. If any of these are out of order, repair them immediately.

  One recent safety advancement has been the advent of daytime running lights (DRLs), a headlight system that turns on automatically when the ignition is started and is overridden when the regular headlights are activated. DRLs increase vehicle visibility, and numerous studies have shown a decreased risk of crashes in cars equipped with them.[27] While not required by law in the United States, all new cars sold in Canada must be equipped with them. Some safety experts have recommended that drivers of vehicles without DRLs turn on their headlights during the daytime. While not a legal requirement, you may wish to consider making this a habit as an additional safety measure.
- *Wipers.* Visibility is always compromised when it rains, and the last

thing you need on a stormy day is a pair of wipers that makes things worse by smearing your windshield. If your wiper blades are brittle, cracked, or unable to clear water from the windshield, by all means replace them—preferably before the next storm clouds gather.

- *Horn.* Some drivers seem to believe that the horn is just another way of expressing anger or venting frustration. It's not. Your horn is an important tool for alerting pedestrians or other drivers that the potential for danger exists. Keep your horn in good working condition.

Driver and passenger behavior

"What's the most dangerous part of a car?" asks the old riddle.

Remember the answer? "The nut that holds the wheel!"

You may have the best-engineered and maintained vehicle on the block, but those virtues offer only limited protection when its occupants are behaving irresponsibly. You can improve your chances of surviving your next trip to the store (or across the country) by following these recommendations:

Wear a seat belt. Three-point restraints (consisting of a lap and shoulder belt) are a highly effective safety feature, distributing the force of a collision to the strongest areas of your body—the bones of the hips, shoulders, and chest. The alternative isn't pretty: a high-speed trip through the windshield or head and upper body crushed against the steering wheel or dashboard. (Note: Wherever we mention seat belts in this segment, we are referring to the combination lap and shoulder restraint.)

Safety belts have been shown to reduce the risk of dying in an accident by 48 percent. The good news is that seat belts save an estimated 14,000 lives each year, and have saved approximately 109,000 lives between 1991 and 2001.[28] The heartbreaking news is that roughly 7,000 people die every year because they do not buckle up.[29]

Even though these life-and-death statistics are well established, many people neglect to wear a seat belt consistently (or at all) because of false optimism, fatalism, laziness, or forgetfulness, as we noted at the beginning of this chapter. Some consider seat belts annoying, uncomfortable, or ineffective. Others offer the following wrongheaded reasons for staying unbuckled:

- *I'm only driving a short distance.* Fact: 75 percent of injury-causing accidents occur within twenty-five miles of home.[30]
- *I don't drive fast enough to need a seat belt.* Fact: An estimated 80 percent of all accidents occur at speeds under 40 miles per hour.[31]
- *Seat belts are a hazard.* Have you ever heard (or thought), "If I get in an accident and my car bursts into flames, a safety belt would probably trap me inside"? Or how about, "Without a seat belt I would be safer, because I would be more likely to be thrown clear of the accident"? Wrong on both counts. Fact: Fewer than one in two hundred accidents involve fire, and wearing a seat belt would *increase* your

likelihood of surviving and escaping a vehicle that is on fire or under water.[32] Why? Because if you're wearing proper restraints you're less likely to be stunned or knocked unconscious. Additionally, your chances of death or serious injury are many times greater if you are ejected from a vehicle, since this may involve a high-speed flight of a hundred feet or more and a very hard landing.

Given the advantages of seat belts and the research supporting their effectiveness, it is not surprising that almost all state or provincial governments across North America have passed laws requiring their use in passenger cars. All Canadian provinces and every U.S. state except one (New Hampshire, whose state motto is "Live Free or Die") have enacted seat belt statutes, although specific requirements and enforcement policies vary. Some states mandate that all vehicle occupants wear a seat belt, while others require only that they be worn by those in the front seat. In some states you can be pulled over and cited specifically for lack of belt usage, while in others, the ticket for seat belt nonusage is given only as a "bonus" after being pulled over for another violation.

Regardless of the seat-belt laws where you live—or their enforcement—you should always buckle your seat belt and check to make sure that others in your car are protected as well. This is an absolute necessity with young children, but don't be shy about insisting (respectfully, of course) that your adult passengers are buckled up before the car leaves the driveway. A reminder for pregnant women: The lap portion of your seat belt/shoulder restraint should lie across the lower abdomen *below* the uterus, in order to avoid trauma to that organ that could endanger both mother and child.

Use appropriate child seats and restraints. In 2002, 459 infants and children under the age of five were killed in motor vehicle accidents. About 40 percent of those killed were completely unrestrained. In that same year it is estimated that 376 lives were saved by use of proper child restraints, and that hundreds more could have been saved had they been used.[33]

It is imperative that *each* infant, toddler, or young child be properly secured in an appropriate car seat *every* time he rides in a car—*no exceptions*. If you are holding a baby or child in your lap in an accident, even if you are wearing a seat belt, he may be crushed between you and the dashboard (unless he is thrown through the windshield first).

The NHTSA recommends a variety of child restraints, the choice of which depends on the height and weight of your child. **Rear-facing child-safety seats** are appropriate for children from birth to at least one year of age and twenty pounds in weight. **Convertible seats** can be used facing the rear or front of the vehicle. Babies under twenty pounds or under one year of age *must* be in the rear-facing position, while children between one and four years of age who weigh between twenty and forty pounds can face forward. **Forward-facing-only seats** are available for children between the ages of one and four who weigh between twenty and forty pounds, as are **high-back booster seats**. For young children ages four to eight who are less than fifty-seven inches tall, a high-back booster seat or a **belt-positioning booster seat** may be used.[34]

It is crucial that infants face the rear of the vehicle. With limited (or in newborns, nonexistent) head control, a forward-facing infant could experience a potentially dangerous rapid forward movement of the head during a sudden stop or collision. The backseat is the safest place for all children age twelve and under, and they should ride there whenever possible. If your vehicle has a passenger-side air bag you should *never* place a young child in the front passenger seat.

Child auto seats must be used properly if they are to provide their full benefits, yet research shows that many adults do not secure children appropriately, or at all. One report revealed that as many as 14 percent of children aged fourteen and younger ride unrestrained. Nearly a third of all children observed in that study were wearing the wrong restraints for their size and age.[35] Another report found that as many as two out of three infants travel in forward-facing car seats.[36]

All fifty states require that children be properly restrained when riding in a car, although the age at which they may begin to use adult seat belts varies by state. In Canada, infants must be restrained in a rear-facing infant safety seat, while children under forty pounds must be restrained in a child booster seat. If you have any questions about the types of car seats, their use, or whether the one you have is safe and appropriate for your child, ask someone who is trained in child-restraint safety. Many local or state police departments and fire departments offer child-seat inspection services, as do some auto insurance companies. To find a safety-seat inspection station near you, visit http://www.nhtsa.dot.gov/nhtsa/whatis/regions/index.cfm?fitting=yes. For more information about the various types of child safety seats, see NHTSA's child passenger safety Web site at http://www.nhtsa.dot.gov (select "Traffic Safety" and then "Child Passenger Safety"), or the American Academy of Pediatrics' online guide to safety seats at www.aap.org/family/carseatguide.htm.

Ride safely with your vehicle's air bags. Air bags are credited with saving more than ten thousand lives in the United States since becoming widely available in automobiles in the late 1980s.[37] These are designed to inflate from the steering column (or from the dashboard, in vehicles with passenger-side air bags) and then to deflate, all within a fraction of a second after a sensor in the car detects a collision roughly equal to that of hitting a solid barrier (such as a tree or a brick wall) at 8 to 14 mph, or a parked car at about 28 mph.[38] When everything works as planned, the bag delivers a few abrasions (and a bit of a surprise) while preventing the head and upper body from slamming into the steering wheel, windshield, or other unyielding objects in the case of a moderate to severe collision. Air bags are supplemental safety devices, meaning that they are not intended to be a passenger's primary protection during a crash. They provide optimal protection when used in conjunction with seat belts.

Per U.S. federal requirements, all passenger cars built since 1998 have included both driver-side air bags and air bags for the right front passenger position. Driver-side and passenger-side air bags have been included in all light trucks, including pickup trucks and minivans, since 1999. In most older cars, you can determine if there is an air bag by looking on the steering wheel or dashboard for the letters *SRS*, which stand for supplemental restraint system.

Air bags are designed to expand rapidly—at roughly 200 miles per hour—

toward the chest of an adult occupant of average height positioned ten or more inches away from the steering wheel or dashboard. While this design has proven safe and effective for the overwhelming majority of adults when used properly, it is not the safest design for everyone. In the late 1980s, shortly after air bags became common in new vehicles, it came to public attention that the speed and trajectory of air-bag deployment (inflation) caused a number of deaths among adults of short stature as well as average-sized adults who were not using seat belts properly. Even more troubling was the fact that a number of those killed upon air-bag deployment were children, some of whom were properly buckled into child restraints (although in the front seat). As of January 2003, in the United States there were 140 confirmed cases of children killed upon deployment of air bags.[39]

Air bags can thus be a double-edged sword, putting some lives at risk while saving many more. However, by following a few basic guidelines you can drastically reduce the risks to your children that are associated with air bags.

- Infants in rear-facing safety seats should *never* be placed in the front seat of a vehicle with a passenger-side air bag. *Doing so puts the baby at an extremely high risk for a serious injury or death if the air bag deploys.*
- Small children should always ride in a rear seat, properly secured in a child safety-seat approved for their age and size.
- Children twelve and younger should always ride buckled up in a rear seat.
- If a child older than one year must ride in the front seat with a passenger-side air bag, secure the child appropriately for his age and size—in a front-facing child safety seat, a booster seat, or with a properly fitting lap/shoulder belt—*and* move the seat as far back as possible. Note: Most vehicles that lack a rear seat, or that have a rear seat that will not accommodate a child-safety seat, are equipped with an on-off switch that allows you to disable the passenger-side air bag. If you have a child twelve or younger in the front seat, NHTSA recommends that the air bag be switched to the off position.

The following safety tips apply to adults:

- Driver and front passenger seats should be moved as far back as possible, allowing both for driver control and rear-seat passenger comfort.
- Adults should buckle up with both lap and shoulder belts on every trip.[40]

Why are these guidelines for adults so important? Remember that the air bag is intended to protect a driver or passenger whose breastbone (the bone in the center of the chest) is at least ten inches from the steering wheel or dashboard. Serious injuries may occur if that air bag hits someone who is sitting much closer to it. If you're not wearing a proper lap and shoulder belt when the brakes slam on before a crash, where do you think you'll be when the air bag goes off? *Right next to it.*

F.Y.I.

If you want to learn more about air bags, how they work, and how to be safe if they deploy in your car, an informative brochure entitled "What You Need to Know about Air Bags" is available at the National Highway Traffic Safety Administration's Web site: http://www.nhtsa.dot.gov/people/injury/airbags/airbags03/.

Watch your speed. Whether impatient, behind schedule, showing off, or simply not paying attention to the speedometer, a driver whose right foot gets a little too heavy is much more likely to be in an accident. Speeding—whether racing, driving too fast for prevailing weather and road conditions, or simply exceeding the posted speed limits—accounted for nearly 31 percent of fatal crashes in 2003, with a death toll of more than 13,300 people.[41] Speeding is the most common type of driver error in fatal crashes.[42] You don't need to be a rocket scientist or an automotive engineer to understand why "speed kills."

Lead-footed drivers have less time to react to emergency situations, such as a child dashing out into the street or an obstacle in the road. They also need more room to maneuver, make a turn, or come to a stop. These driver-response problems increase dramatically as the speedometer climbs. So does the severity of a crash, because the energy of an impact increases not directly *with* but rather *by the square* of the collision speed. For example, the speed of a crash at 60 mph is double that of a crash at 30 mph, but the energy of impact is *four* times greater. As a result, the risk of dying in a crash *doubles* for every 10 mph over 50 mph. You may enjoy tooling down the highway at 80 mph, but at that speed your risk of dying in an accident is *eight times higher* than at 50 mph.

Here's a philosophical question: Are the few minutes (or more commonly, seconds) that you might save by driving at high speeds really worth all of the extra risk?

Never drink and drive. Of all the consequences associated with the misuse of alcohol, the fallout from driving under its influence is arguably the most dramatic. In 2002, alcohol played a role in an estimated 258,000 crashes and more than 17,400 motor vehicle deaths, more than 40 percent of the total number that year.[43] If you do the very sad math, *that's more than forty-seven people killed each day.*

As we described in chapter 10, the amount of alcohol in the bloodstream or blood alcohol concentration (BAC) is measured in grams of alcohol per 100 ml of blood. In most states, intoxication is legally defined as a BAC of 0.08, although some states have set lower thresholds at which operating a motor vehicle is illegal. At a BAC of 0.08, almost all drivers experience significant impairment of the skills and abilities needed to drive safely, including response time, judgment, braking, steering, lane changing, and attentiveness. The risk of being involved in a crash is eleven times greater for drivers with a 0.08 BAC than it is for drivers with no alcohol in their system.[44] It is important to note, however, that for some people, driving ability can be impaired at a BAC level as low as 0.02.

Sadly, all of the sobering statistics and horrifying consequences of drunk driving (publicized for decades by organizations such as Mothers Against

Drunk Driving) still don't prevent some people from drinking and driving. NHTSA's 2001 National Survey of Drinking and Driving Attitudes and Behaviors found that 22 percent of individuals sixteen and older had driven within two hours of consuming an alcoholic beverage during the previous year. It is estimated that each year these drivers make a total of between 800 million and one billion driving trips within two hours of taking a drink, and that about 10 percent of these trips are made by people with a BAC of 0.08 or greater.[45] While you can't control what other drivers have been sipping before starting the ignition, it is critical that *you* not join the ranks of the drinker-drivers. If you're going out to eat at a restaurant or a private home where alcohol will be served and you decide to partake, be sure you're with a designated driver who has made a commitment not to drink any alcoholic beverage.

If you have teenagers at home, talk frankly about the hazards of combining alcohol and automobiles. Even if you know they're committed to avoiding alcohol, impress on them the dangers of traveling with others who have been drinking or using drugs. Let your teen know that she can call you for a ride—no questions asked—if she is ever in a situation where she or her driver has taken a drink. (Since her safety and survival are on the line, you don't want her to avoid calling out of fear of getting a tongue-lashing in the car. There will be plenty of time for a calm discussion later on, once she is safe and both of you are in the right frame of mind.) Consider a parent/teen contract that helps set expectations for both of you. You can find a sample at MADD's Web site, http://www.madd.org. By the way, don't forget that your example speaks volumes. If you use alcohol in social situations, let your teens know that you always designate a nondrinking driver and that you are committed to calling a taxi or a family member (including one of them) if necessary to get home safely.

Stay awake and alert. Driving while fatigued or drowsy may seem like a modest safety risk compared with drunk driving, but the statistics tell a different story. Every year in the United States, one hundred thousand crashes, seventy-one thousand injuries, and more than fifteen hundred deaths occur because drivers fall asleep. These figures only scratch the surface of the problem, however, because they only take into account crashes with all of the following characteristics:

- The accident occurred between midnight and 6 A.M.
- It involved a single vehicle driven by a sober driver.
- The vehicle left the roadway, and there was no indication that the driver attempted to correct its off-road trajectory.

These statistics do not include accidents occurring during daylight or early evening hours, or those involving multiple passengers, multiple vehicles, or alcohol. Without question, driving while drowsy is a widespread problem. A survey by the National Sleep Foundation in 2005 discovered that 60 percent of all adult drivers that year had driven a vehicle while feeling sleepy, and 37 percent of drivers admitted they had actually fallen asleep while driving.[46]

Anyone can be involved in a driving accident while drowsy, but several factors increase a person's risk. Because of the way their job schedule usually interferes with sleep routines, shift workers are at a significantly higher risk of an accident. Similarly, people who get only six to seven hours of sleep per night are twice as likely to be involved in a crash as those who get eight hours of sleep or more.[47] Others at higher risk include individuals with sleep disorders such as sleep apnea or insomnia, and people who regularly use sedating medications or alcohol.

To state the obvious, the best way to avoid an accident due to fatigue is to get the sleep you need. Even if you are getting an adequate amount of restorative sleep (see chapter 15 for more information on this important subject), you may have to make adjustments in your driving habits if you take medications (prescription or otherwise) that cause drowsiness. Prescription medications now routinely come with an intimidating printout listing dozens of potential side effects, many of which are highly uncommon. Pay close attention, however, if drowsiness or sedation is on the list, and be very careful if a "May cause drowsiness" sticker is on the bottle. Also, don't forget that many nonprescription drugs—especially the older antihistamines such as diphenhydramine (Benadryl, and various combinations whose name often includes "PM")—can impair a driver's skills as much as an alcoholic beverage.[48]

If you are feeling tired or sleepy while driving—you find your head nodding or your vision blurring, you begin yawning frequently or drifting out of your lane, or you find you are forgetting scenery or missing traffic signs or exits—*take corrective action immediately*. Find the first safe place where you can pull over or exit the highway, get out, and walk around. If it's late and you've got a long distance ahead, seriously consider finding a motel where you can stop for the night. If that's not an option, try to find a safe, well-lit place where you can try to get some rest. (Use caution, however, if traveling alone.) Even a short nap can restore some wakefulness. Caffeine or "energy drinks" may provide a short burst of alertness, but they sometimes require up to half an hour to take effect. Other activities such as rolling down the window or blaring the radio are not very effective at keeping drowsy drivers awake. If you have a companion in the car who can drive and isn't sleepy, by all means let him take the wheel, or at least ask him to keep you engaged in conversation.

Avoid distractions. Most of us heard in driver-training class that operating a motor vehicle is a "full-time" job. Most of us are also guilty of allowing our mind and body to be engaged in one (or several) other pursuits while behind the wheel, whether in heavy traffic or cruising the open road. Some distractions beckon from outside—street signs, billboards, scenery, and wildlife (animal and human), among others. But all too often we're drawn into other activities inside our own vehicle—eating, sipping a beverage, talking with passengers, adjusting the radio, changing CDs, applying makeup, reading a map, and that most popular pastime, talking on our cell phone. These may sound perfectly harmless, but according to the NHTSA, driver distraction is implicated in an estimated 11 percent of fatal crashes and 25 to 30 percent of crashes involving injury or property damage.

Speaking of cell phones, in 2002 more than 60 percent of the drivers in the United States reported owning a cell phone, and nearly one in three used their phone while driving.[49] How many accidents are actually caused by cell-phone users? It's difficult to say exactly, but some reports suggest that using your cell phone in the car quadruples your risk of having an accident at any given time.[50] As a result, some states have outlawed the use of handheld cell phones while driving. While these bans reduce the distraction caused by using one hand (or a shoulder) to hold a phone, they don't address what some researchers feel is the main hazard of cell phones: driver inattention. In fact, one study comparing drivers using handheld or hands-free cell phones showed that both groups missed traffic signals twice as often—and took longer to react to the signals they did see—while engaged in phone conversations.[51]

Obviously, the safest time to use a cell phone is when you are not moving. Yes, we all like to multitask and take care of those phone calls while we're running errands or driving to work, but none of those conversations are worth the hassle—or the tragedy—that could arise from a collision. If you are driving and feel you need to use a cell phone, think first about your safety and that of your passengers and other drivers. Is there anyone else who could drive while you make your calls? If not, consider the driving conditions before using the phone, and avoid calling while in heavy traffic, hazardous conditions, stormy weather, or any circumstance that *really* demands your full attention. Also, remember that it's quite all right to resist the impulse to fumble frantically through your purse or pocket to answer that insistent electronic chirp. Whoever is calling can leave a message, and you can return it when the car is stopped. Finally, consider a hands-free phone configuration for use in your car. While this doesn't eliminate all the distraction that accompanies cell-phone usage, it does allow you to talk while keeping both hands on the wheel.

Besides taming your cell-phone use in the car, there are several simple and practical ways to minimize other distractions while driving. Most involve a little forethought, a bit more patience, and generally a lot less hurrying:

- Adjust mirrors, seat position, the radio, and the heating or air-conditioning *before* you start driving.
- When on the road, resist the temptation to take care of business that would best be done when the car is parked: rifling through the glove compartment, cleaning the inside of your car, applying makeup, giving a bottle to the baby in the backseat, or checking your PDA for that next appointment.
- If you must refer to a map, pull out of traffic first.
- If a pressing matter in the backseat demands your attention—a crying infant, for example, or a full-blown fistfight between squabbling siblings—*don't* turn around and attempt to restore order while driving. Pull over and stop in a safe place before you address the problem.

Bikes, scooters, and skateboards

Long before children grow up and discover the pleasures (and pains) of driving an automobile, many experience the joys of another source of mobility —pedal power. The freedom to ride a bicycle to the park, the store, or a friend's house produces in many children a sense of independence not unlike that felt by many teens when they first start to drive a car. Skateboards are another fun and fast way for kids to get around, as are scooters. By the way, the term *scooter* has been used to describe a multitude of devices, from electric-powered wheel-chair-type vehicles to motorized bikes that look like undersized motorcycles

FOR PARENTS OF TEENAGE DRIVERS

Driving is one of the most momentous steps that a teenager will take toward personal independence. Being able to drive provides mobility, the gratification of not having to rely on parents or friends for a ride, and a definite sense of prestige (even if the vehicle involved is the family fixer-upper). Like every other new freedom that beckons the adolescent moving toward adulthood, there are a number of risks—and responsibilities—that must be acknowledged and addressed. Because of the safety issues that accompany taking the wheel for the first time, new drivers and their parents should prepare for this next phase of life with the utmost diligence.[52]

If you're a little apprehensive about your teenager becoming a driver, your concerns are not unfounded. (The fact that automobile insurance rates are greatly increased for adolescent drivers—especially for males—is no accident, so to speak.) Motor-vehicle accidents are the leading cause of death of young people ages fifteen through twenty, killing more than five thousand youths in America each year.[53] Even though this age group comprises less than 7 percent of the driving population, it accounts for 14 percent of vehicle-related fatalities. Over the past decade, over sixty-eight thousand teens have died in car crashes.[54]

Inexperience is a major risk factor for teens involved in accidents. Driving is, after all, an amazingly complex task. New drivers must learn to control their vehicle and its speed, while at the same time detecting and responding to hazardous driving conditions and emergency situations. The vast majority of teens are not lacking in the motor skills and coordination necessary to be an excellent driver. (Indeed, they're probably better equipped in this regard than Mom and Dad.) But what isn't fully developed is their judgment, decision-making ability, or a healthy respect for the unexpected—and their own mortality.

Indeed, an important factor contributing to accidents involving teens is their willingness to engage in risky behaviors. Speeding is a factor in about 30 percent of all traffic fatalities, and putting pedal to the metal is a major temptation for teenage drivers—especially males.[55] Alcohol is involved in more than a third of all traffic deaths for young people ages sixteen through twenty.[56] One

FOR PARENTS OF TEENAGE DRIVERS ***continued on page 540***

(think Vespa or Honda gas-powered scooters). When we talk about scooters in this section, we are talking about the type most favored by children and teens. These generally consist of a short platform between two low-friction wheels similar to those found in in-line skates, with a handlebar attached to the front. Like a skateboard, these scooters can be propelled by foot (kick scooters) or by a small gasoline or electric engine.

Beyond their usefulness as modes of transportation, bikes, skateboards, and scooters also provide recreation, physical activity, exercise (except in the case of motorized scooters), and even a sense of community (as in the case of skateboarders).

FOR PARENTS OF TEENAGE DRIVERS *continued from page 539*

survey found that at least 12 percent of high school students reported driving after drinking alcohol, and more than 30 percent of teens had ridden with a driver who had been drinking.[57]

Teenagers love to hang out and drive around with their friends, but for a sixteen-year-old driver having one other passenger in the car increases the chance of being killed by 39 percent. If there are two riders, the likelihood of a fatal accident is 86 percent greater, and for three or more passengers it is 282 percent higher than if that teenager is driving solo (or with a parent).[58] Eighteen percent of high school students report that they never or hardly ever use a safety belt when riding in a car driven by someone else.[59] All of these behaviors increase the odds of a teenager being involved, injured, and/or killed in an automobile accident.

After reading such discouraging information, some parents may vow never to let their children sit behind the wheel of a car until they are in their twenties and living on their own. Aside from being unrealistic, such a mind-set is counterproductive and insulting to teens who really want to learn to drive safely. A more constructive outlook is to view the adolescent years as a time when adults can teach safe driving habits and influence a young driver's behavior for life, imparting skills and knowledge that will perhaps save lives many years in the future. Becoming an expert driver requires years of experience, and overseeing the first few years of that experience is a wonderful, though at times ulcer-generating, privilege.

As a parent you can pass on a wealth of driving wisdom in many ways. First, be patient with your teen. His learning to drive may be nerve-racking for you, but it's much more so for him. (Giving all instructions calmly and clearly will help.) Second, as with other behaviors they want their children to adopt, parents must model safe driving habits. For better or worse, children will imitate their parents. Also, parents should not only learn the traffic laws for their state but also be prepared to enforce additional limits and expectations based on their adolescent's attitude and skill.

Recognizing that driver-education courses by themselves are not a complete preparation for novice motorists, most states have instituted graduated driver licensing for teens. Such a system is designed to phase teens into full driving

Skateboards and scooters are almost exclusively the province of young people. There are more than 11 million skateboarders in the United States,[60] and millions of scooters have been sold in North America, mostly for children and teenagers. Bicycles, on the other hand, are popular with people of all ages. One study found that 57 million people ride bicycles, including 17 percent of individuals ages fifty-five to sixty-five, and nearly 9 percent of people older than sixty-five.[61] While this type of equipment doesn't have the weight and speed that can make automobile (and motorcycle) accidents so harmful, the sheer number of people riding bikes, skateboards, and scooters on the

privileges by allowing them to mature and develop their driving skills in steps. Each state's system is different, but the typical graduated-licensing model involves three stages. Beginners must remain in the first two stages for a minimum amount of time, demonstrating a mastery of basic skills under less challenging driving conditions. (For example, the stage-one teenage driver might not be allowed to drive after dark, while in stage two he might be allowed to drive at night, but only with adult supervision.) Even if your state has not yet enacted graduated licensing, you may wish to grant your teen's driving privileges in a similar manner, which allows him to acquire the experience he needs while reducing some of the risks. For example, you might require that your teen driver be accompanied by a parent or other responsible licensed adult driver at all times for a set period of time. You may also wish to set specific ground rules, such as limiting the number of passengers he may have in the car or restricting driving to daylight hours, until he has demonstrated responsible driving behavior for a number of weeks or months.

Always require your teen to buckle up before the engine is started, whether driving or riding. (This is an area where your example speaks louder than your words.) Your adolescent should never drive if he is drowsy. Additionally, while there are many good reasons for him to abstain from alcohol and drugs, don't fail to drive home the message that drinking kills thousands of people every year—many of them teens. Not only should your teenager never drink and drive, but he should also never get into a car if the driver has been drinking. And no matter how strongly you might feel about the use of alcohol, let your adolescent know that he can *always* call you for a ride in order to avoid being in a car with an intoxicated driver—whether himself or someone else.

Unfortunately, no matter how calmly and rationally you explain the conditions you are placing on your teen, he may see these restrictions as unreasonable. If he protests your limitations, stand your ground. And if you see unsafe driving patterns or habits that your adolescent refuses to correct, don't let him have the keys. The first commandment for would-be drivers to learn (and burn deep in their consciousness) is that driving is a privilege, not a right. Your first priority is not to win a popularity contest. It's to keep him (and others on the road) alive and well while he learns to operate an automobile safely and skillfully. ■

road, in parks, or on bike paths, creates a significant potential for injury. There are, however, a number of practical ways to reduce the risk of getting hurt while enjoying these pastimes.

Bicycles

Most fatalities in bicycle accidents involve collisions with motor vehicles. In 2004, more than 700 bicyclists were killed and another 41,000 were injured after colliding with cars and trucks.[62] The injury rate due to all causes (falls, collisions with stationary objects, etc.) is even higher, with nontraffic bicycle-related injuries accounting for approximately 459,000 emergency-room visits in 2003.[63] How can you keep yourself and your loved ones from becoming statistics?

- ***Wear a helmet.*** Helmets are designed to absorb the impact of a direct blow to the skull, and they do their job well. Research shows that wearing a helmet can reduce the risk of sustaining a head injury by 85 percent and the risk of brain injury by up to 88 percent.[64] When choosing a bicycle helmet, select one that meets or exceeds standards set by the U.S. Consumer Product Safety Commission (CPSC). A sticker inside the helmet should provide this information.

  A bike helmet should fit securely and squarely, and should not tilt toward the back of the head. The strap should fit comfortably but not loosely under the chin. Bicycle helmets contain a foam lining that compresses to absorb the force of a head impact. Once the foam is compacted, the helmet loses much of its ability to absorb further impacts and is unsafe to use. Replace your helmet if you ever get in a crash.

  Wearing a helmet when riding a bicycle is important—and not just for children. Adults need to wear a helmet when riding, too, both for their own safety and to model this behavior for younger ones. Like wearing a seat belt while riding in a car, wearing a helmet is one of those behaviors that is caught more than taught. When children see parents strap on a helmet, they will be much more likely to do likewise.
- ***Obey traffic rules.*** Teach your children these rules as well. On the roadway, cyclists must obey the same regulations that govern motorists. In other words, cyclists should stop at red lights and use hand signals when making turns. Look left, then right, then left again when turning or crossing a street.
- ***Ride with traffic.*** Riding against traffic can be dangerously distracting to both the cyclist and oncoming motorists. Additionally, pedaling in the direction of oncoming traffic increases the relative velocity at which a potential collision might take place. Always ride in the same direction as the flow of traffic. If you are riding with a friend, proceed in single file.
- ***Be alert.*** Keep an eye out for anything that might cause an accident: a car door about to open in front of you; gravel, broken glass, or soft

road conditions that might cause you to lose control. Sewer gratings or uneven surfaces can also catch a tire and cause you to fall.

- ***Be visible.*** Make sure that your bicycle is equipped with a red rear reflector and a white front reflector. Wear bright-colored or reflective clothing, especially when riding on dark or overcast days. If you must ride at night, wear reflective clothing and use a bright headlamp. It is wise, however, not to allow children to ride at night.

Skateboards

According to Safe Kids Worldwide, skateboarding accidents resulted in more than 50,000 emergency room visits in 2003 among children ages five to fourteen.[65] Half of all skateboarding injuries occur in this age group.[66]

Fortunately, deaths associated with skateboard accidents are rare, but concussions and internal injuries account for 5 percent of skateboarding injuries, and fractures and dislocations represent another 31 percent.[67] The following advisories will help the skateboarders in your family avoid accidents and injuries:

- ***Wear a helmet.*** As with bicycling, anyone moving at faster-than-running speed and trying to maintain balance while on wheels should be equipped with head protection.

  Although a bicycle helmet might seem like a natural choice for protecting a skateboarder's head, the dynamics of skateboarding are a bit different from those of cycling. Skateboarders tend to fall more frequently than cyclists, and they travel at lower speeds. For that reason, skateboarding helmets are designed to withstand a greater number of hits although at a somewhat lower impact intensity. When shopping for a skateboarding helmet, look for a sticker indicating that it meets skateboarding standards (ASTM F-1492 standard). Some manufacturers make multisport helmets that meet or exceed standards for both bicycling and skateboarding.
- ***Wear protective gear.*** Elbow pads, knee pads, and protective gloves or wrist braces can help prevent abrasions and even the occasional broken bone that occur with skateboarding spills. Wear shoes with nonskid soles.
- ***Use the right skateboard.*** Some boards are built to carry riders of a certain weight. Others are designed for particular styles of riding, whether freestyle, slalom, or speedboarding. If you're not into skateboarding but your child or adolescent is showing a lot of interest, you may need to educate yourself on these matters to help him choose the one that fits his style. Also, the skateboard should have regular safety checks to make sure no parts are loose.
- ***Know the terrain.*** The best places to skateboard are evenly paved, without loose gravel or other surface irregularities. Riding in the street should be avoided.

- ***Practice makes perfect.*** Part of the allure of skateboarding is that expert skateboarders make difficult tricks look easy. Many young people may be unaware that what makes these feats seem effortless is a lot of practice. Those who want to learn complicated tricks should be properly equipped and should practice carefully in specially designated areas.
- ***Play it safe with crowds and cars.*** Skateboarders should avoid riding in pedestrian crowds and should never hitch rides on car bumpers.
- ***Learn how to fall.*** Anyone who rides a skateboard *will* fall, and when this happens it's almost instinctive to extend the arms in order to break the fall. However, slamming the palms on a hard surface can cause fractures of the hands or wrists (especially if one isn't wearing protective gear). On a skateboard it is wiser to try to absorb the impact of a fall by landing on the fleshier, more padded parts of the body and then rolling. Bending the knees if a fall appears imminent may also help, since there will be less distance to fall.
- ***Don't let little ones go it alone.*** Because young children generally lack well-developed judgment skills with regard to safety, traffic, or their own abilities, the American Academy of Pediatrics recommends that children under ten not be allowed to skateboard without adult supervision.

Scooters

When a new generation of scooters became popular and began to proliferate a few years ago, accidents involving scooters did likewise, prompting an estimated 43,900 emergency room visits in 2003 among children ages fourteen and under.[68] While the popularity of scooters has ebbed somewhat and the number of injuries has declined, it's clear that even the simple scooter is best ridden with some basic safety precautions:

- ***Wear a helmet.*** Is this starting to sound familiar? Because of the speeds at which scooters are ridden, riders should wear a helmet that conforms to CPSC standards for bicycle helmets. A helmet is far better equipped than the skull to absorb the impact of a head hitting pavement.
- ***Wear pads.*** Knee and elbow pads can prevent deep and painful abrasions from falls.
- ***Check the scooter regularly*** to make sure that no parts are coming loose.
- ***Know where you are riding.*** Like skateboards, scooters should be ridden on smooth, paved surfaces. Avoid gravel, dirt, or other surfaces that can cause an accident.
- ***Avoid risky situations.*** Do not ride at night. Avoid riding in the street,

and never ride in traffic. Use caution when riding on pedestrian walkways.

- ***Obey the rules.*** Make sure children understand that they should follow commonsense guidelines that govern bike riding, including stopping at red lights and looking left, then right, then left again when crossing a street. Also, find out if there are any local laws governing scooter usage. These might require helmet use or restrict scooters from being used in certain places.
- ***Watch the kids.*** Children younger than eight should use scooters only with adult supervision. Because of the speeds they can achieve, children twelve and under should not ride motorized scooters at all.

Other recreational vehicles: ATVs, snowmobiles, and Jet Skis

Recreational activities involving fast-moving vehicles aren't limited to machines with wheels that travel on streets and sidewalks. Lakes, oceans, sand dunes, remote trails, and snowy fields are all accessible to motorized equipment whose operation isn't always tightly regulated by state and local statutes. As you might imagine, when you combine speed, equipment that may not be as user-friendly as the family sedan, unfamiliar terrain, youthful enthusiasm and inexperience—and in some cases alcohol—accidents, injuries, and fatalities are all too often part of the equation:

- According to the American Academy of Pediatrics, between 1985 and 2000 accidents involving three- and four-wheeled all-terrain vehicles (ATVs) killed nearly 2,800 people and prompted between fifty thousand and one hundred thousand annual emergency-room visits. More than one in three deaths, and nearly half of the injuries, involved children and teens sixteen years and younger.[69]
- There are more than 1.5 million snowmobiles and at least 4 million snowmobilers in North America. Between 1990 and 1998 snowmobile accidents involving children and teenagers led to nearly twenty-five thousand injuries (about one in five) and seventy-five fatalities. Two-thirds of the deaths were caused by head and neck injuries.[70]
- Jet Skis and their variations (formally known as personal watercraft, or PWC) have become very popular, with about one million now in use. As might be expected, injuries (some twelve thousand emergency-room visits in 1995) and fatalities (eighty-three in 1997) have increased steadily with the number in use. More ominous is the impact on younger riders. In California, the American Academy of Pediatrics reported in 2000 that children younger than eighteen years accounted for 14 percent of all boating accidents, 18 percent of all boating injuries, and 5 percent of boating fatalities—but *93 percent* of these incidents involved personal watercraft.[71]

Hopefully you noticed a theme in these otherwise grim statistics: While all of these motorized devices can be a lot of fun when used properly, *none of them should be operated by children under the age of sixteen.* Here's another no-brainer: *No one should operate any of these items under the influence of alcohol.* Furthermore, along with a thorough understanding of the proper use of whatever recreational motorized equipment you might own or rent, there are numerous safety precautions that can help prevent a fun outing from turning into a trip to the ER . . . or the funeral home. Here are some of them:

ATVs (whether two-, three-, or four-wheeled)

- Anyone not old enough to have a driver's license is not old enough to drive an ATV.
- Take a training course before operating an ATV.
- Three-wheeled ATVs are particularly unstable on hard surfaces. If you have one of these, seriously consider trading it in for a four-wheeler.
- Your four-wheeled ATV should have a roll bar and a seat belt.
- Don't ride double. Passengers are frequently injured on ATVs, and so the only person in an ATV should be the driver.
- Wear protective clothing and equipment, including a helmet (one designed for motorcycle rather than bicycle use), eye protection, pants, boots, and gloves.
- ATVs should not be ridden at night, even if they have headlights. Headlights on an ATV should be turned on (even during the brightest hours of the day) to make the vehicle more visible to others.
- Speaking of visibility, flags and reflectors are also helpful for increasing an ATV's visibility.

Snowmobiles

- Snowmobiles should be operated only by people sixteen and older. Children under the age of six may not have the strength and stamina to be passengers, and thus should not ride.
- Snowmobiles should carry no more than one passenger in addition to the driver.
- Be cautious with speed, *especially* in unfamiliar terrain. Stay on designated trails and away from roads, railroad tracks, and pedestrian traffic.
- Avoid snowmobiling on ice unless you are absolutely certain that it is thick enough to support your vehicle.
- Head injury, frostbite, and hypothermia are among the most common causes of emergency-room visits related to snowmobiling. Be sure to wear a helmet, goggles, and waterproof protective clothing, including gloves and rubber-bottomed boots.

- Snowmobilers should travel in groups of two or more and carry a first-aid kit, survival kit with flare, and (where service is available) a cellular phone.
- Don't use a snowmobile (or any other vehicle for that matter) to tow someone riding a sled, skis, tube, tire, or snow saucer.
- Do not under any circumstances operate a snowmobile while under the influence of alcohol.

Jet Skis

- Once more for emphasis: No one under sixteen should operate a Jet Ski.
- Always wear a Coast Guard–approved flotation device.
- Most Jet Ski injuries occur among inexperienced riders (especially renters), and most involve collisions with docks, tree stumps, or other watercraft. The vast majority of deaths related to a Jet Ski are not from drowning but from trauma.
- Make sure you understand the dynamics of a Jet Ski, which behaves differently than other vehicles (including boats). In particular, remember that a Jet Ski has no brakes, and you can only slow down by cutting the throttle and coasting. Unfortunately, you can only steer a Jet Ski when its throttle is open. The only way to avoid an obstacle is to maintain your speed and steer away from it.
- A Jet Ski should not be operated after dark.
- Observe speed limits and no-wake zones (where you travel slowly enough to avoid generating a wake behind you).
- Stay away from areas where swimmers are in the water.
- Need we say it again? Don't operate a Jet Ski under the influence of alcohol.

Water safety

Safety in and around water is affected by a number of factors, including age, swimming ability, water conditions, the use of alcohol, and the use of protective devices. But regardless of which of these factors come into play, it is important to recognize the fact that *anyone*—even the most experienced swimmer—can drown. In 2000, more than 3,200 drowning deaths were reported in the United States, and one-fourth of those were among children ages fourteen and younger.[72]

Drowning usually occurs in one of three settings: swimming, boating, and indoors. Each of these situations has specific drowning risks and preventive measures.

Swimming safety

Swimming is a pastime enjoyed by people of all ages as a means of exercising and cooling off during hot weather, but it is not without risks. Most children who drown do so in residential pools. Here's how to make swimming a safer activity:

- ***Learn to swim.*** Learning to swim is the best way to prevent drowning and water-related injuries, and yet about a third of adults in the United States report not being able to swim a standard pool length (twenty-four yards).[73] If you and your family plan on spending any recreational time in or around water, invest in swimming lessons. Your local YMCA and most city park and recreation departments offer swimming courses for both children and adults.
- ***Learn first aid and CPR.*** Everyone who supervises children by the pool, including relatives and babysitters, should know first aid and CPR. Your local Red Cross can provide information about training classes in your area.
- ***Exercise caution in and around the water.*** It takes neither gross neglect nor much time for a water-related tragedy to occur. One study found that most children ages four and younger who drowned in swimming pools were out of adult sight for less than five minutes and were last seen inside the house. Most were in the care of one or both parents at the time of drowning.[74]

To reduce the likelihood of a disaster, *never* allow young children to go near a swimming area unless they are accompanied by an adult (preferably one who knows how to swim). When supervising kids who are swimming, avoid distractions (reading, talking on the telephone, etc.) that take your attention away from them. If using a public pool, do so at times when a lifeguard is on duty.

Teach your children always to swim with a buddy, never alone. Let them know that horseplay, shoving others into the water, and jumping on others are strictly forbidden. Also teach them never to dive into a pool or swimming area if the water is less than nine feet deep or if they are unsure of the depth.

Make your swimming area as safe as possible. If you have a swimming pool, it should be completely surrounded by fencing. The fence should be at least four feet high, should not be climbable, and should have a self-closing and self-latching gate. The gate should lock so that toddlers cannot gain access to the pool by themselves.

Gate alarms, pool alarms, and automatic pool covers can also reduce the risk of accidents. Pool alarms sound whenever someone or something enters the water; these alarms can sound inside the house as well. Automatic pool covers consist of tarpaulin-like material that can extend over a swimming pool in a matter of seconds, and can support the weight of one or more adults. When considering a pool cover as a safety device, look for one that meets ASTM standards. An important note: A solar pool cover is a thin covering designed to reduce heat loss and evaporation—but it is *not* appropriate as a safety measure.

Keep safety devices such as personal flotation devices (PFDs), life preservers, and shepherd's hooks close to the pool. A telephone should also be kept near the pool in case of emergency. Remove toys from the pool after everyone is out to keep little ones from accidentally falling into the water while reaching for a toy.

Boating safety

Each year more than 70 million people participate in recreational boating. In 2002, more than 4,000 were injured in boating accidents, and 750 people died. Of these, 525 deaths were from drowning.[75] In most cases, drowning can be prevented if boaters follow these recommendations:

- ***Use personal flotation devices.*** PFDs include life jackets and vests as well as throwable devices such as floating seat cushions and life preservers. U.S. federal regulations require all recreational boats to carry one wearable Coast Guard–approved PFD for each passenger. Most boats longer than sixteen feet also need to carry at least one throwable PFD.[76] Life jackets and vests must fit the passenger. Many states also have statutes concerning PFD use.

  Even though the need for universal PFD use has been widely publicized, many people still do not use them. The folly of that choice is revealed by the fact that about 80 percent of those who drown in boating accidents are not wearing a life jacket.[77] Many choose not to wear a life jacket because they're not going far from shore or because they know how to swim. Yet many who drown in boating accidents know how to swim, and many times drowning occurs within feet of safety.

  Make sure you put on a life jacket *every* time you get in a boat, and model this lifesaving behavior for your children and teens.
- ***Don't mix boating and alcohol.*** Alcohol is involved in nearly 40 percent of boating fatalities, many of which result from intoxicated individuals capsizing or falling out of their boat and drowning.[78] Boating under the influence can sometimes be more dangerous than driving under the influence. In a boat, the constant motion, engine noise and vibration, sun, and wind all combine to produce fatigue that compounds and hastens the physical and mental impairments produced by alcohol.
- ***Operate your boat safely.*** Know and practice the essentials of safe boating. You can learn these by taking a boating-safety education course, available through the National Safe Boating Council (http://www.safeboatingcouncil.org) or the U.S. Coast Guard. Some courses can even be taken online. Also, perform a regular check of your boat for any structural, mechanical, or safety problems.

MORE SAFETY INFORMATION

For further information on how to reduce your family's safety risks, contact the following organizations:

INSURANCE INSTITUTE FOR HIGHWAY SAFETY
1005 N. Glebe Rd., Suite 800
Arlington, VA 22201
(703) 247-1500
www.iihs.org

NATIONAL CENTER FOR INJURY PREVENTION AND CONTROL
Centers for Disease Control and Prevention
Mailstop K65
4770 Buford Highway NE
Atlanta, GA 30341-3724
(770) 488-1506
www.cdc.gov/ncipc/

NATIONAL FIRE PROTECTION ASSOCIATION
1 Batterymarch Park
Quincy, MA 02169-7471
(617) 770-3000
www.nfpa.org

NATIONAL HIGHWAY TRAFFIC SAFETY ADMINISTRATION
400 7th St. SW
Washington, D.C. 20590
(888) 327-4236
www.nhtsa.dot.gov

NATIONAL SAFETY COUNCIL
1121 Spring Lake Drive
Itasca, IL 60143-3201
(630) 285-1121
www.nsc.org

U.S. CONSUMER PRODUCT SAFETY COMMISSION
Washington, D.C. 20207-0001
(800) 638-2772
www.cpsc.gov

INFECTIONS AND IMMUNIZATIONS

In previous chapters we have described how many common health problems develop from interactions of genetics (the strengths and vulnerabilities we have inherited), lifestyle (diet and exercise habits, for example), and environmental factors (such as tobacco smoke, whether from our own or someone else's cigarette). There is another realm of diseases and disorders that arise when microorganisms—viruses, bacteria, fungi, or parasites—gain a foothold in the body and cause disturbances that can range from a minor annoyance (a drippy nose from a cold virus, for example) to overwhelming and fatal illness. These are known as **infectious diseases**.

There are many types of microorganisms that can invade our body and many more ways in which those invasions might affect our health. While a catalog of our potential foes is well beyond the scope of this book, you should be aware of the basic types of infectious agents that can cause trouble:

You may hear the word *germ* used to refer to virtually any type of infectious organism, but the term has no specific meaning scientifically or medically. (It's about as accurate as saying, "I think I'm getting a bug" when you wake up with a runny nose.)

Viruses are by far the smallest invaders, visible only under sophisticated electron microscopes. They are also the most primitive, usually consisting of only a packet of DNA or RNA—the chained molecules that transmit genetic instructions in all forms of life—wrapped in a coat of protein. Left to their own devices, viruses cannot reproduce. But viruses have the uncanny capacity to hijack the genetic machinery within living cells (and bacteria) to manufacture billions of copies of themselves. The type and number of cells that are disrupted determine the characteristics and severity of the illness.

Diseases caused by viruses include the common cold, influenza, infectious mononucleosis, measles, mumps, chickenpox, polio, hepatitis, and HIV/AIDS, among many others. Various forms of the human papillomavirus (or HPV) not only cause garden-variety warts but also are strongly linked to cancer of the cervix (the opening of the uterus) in women. Familiar antibiotics such as penicillin have no effect on viruses, although certain other medications (known, appropriately enough, as **antivirals**) can slow or stop the reproduction of some types of viruses.

Bacteria are much larger than viruses, visible under conventional microscopes and capable of reproducing by *fission* (or dividing) under all kinds of conditions—within and on the surface of living (and dead) animals and plants, in bodies of water, in the soil, in food, and elsewhere. They are not necessarily harmful. In fact, the human skin, nose, mouth, intestinal tract, and vagina are colonized by more than two hundred species of bacteria, whose number and type vary with age, sex, diet, and nutritional status. Many of these play a variety of beneficial roles, such as preventing harmful microorganisms from gaining a foothold on or in our bodies, as well as stimulating immunological responses against more harmful bacteria.

There are more bacteria in your intestinal tract than there are normal cells in your entire body.

Other bacteria, however, cause disease by generating toxins that damage tissue or disrupt normal body functions. Sometimes the body's immune response to invading bacteria is damaging in itself. Illnesses caused by bacteria include many forms of pneumonia, tuberculosis, streptococcal ("strep") throat, sinusitis, whooping cough (pertussis), bladder and kidney infections, abscesses, gonorrhea, syphilis, and many others. The development of antibiotics that can selectively disable or kill bacteria without destroying normal cells was one of the most important breakthroughs of the twentieth century.

Fungi are single- or multi-cellular organisms, distinct in a number of ways from both plants and animals, that can gain an annoying toehold on the surface of the body (including the toes) or may invade and cause life-threatening infections, especially among those with a compromised immune system. Common fungal infections include athlete's foot, ringworm, "jock itch" in the groin, and unsightly disruptions of toenails (or, less commonly, fingernails) known as **onychomycosis**. The common "yeast" organism *Candida albicans* can cause a number of itchy and irritating conditions, including some diaper rashes, vaginal discharge, an oral infection called **thrush**, and rashes in wet and warm areas where skin folds come together, especially among those who are overweight.

A widely disseminated notion that *Candida* is also responsible for a host of other ailments, including chronic fatigue, depression, headaches, and intestinal disturbances, is not only unproven but also highly implausible.

Parasites encompass a wide variety of organisms that live within (or sometimes on) a larger organism (called the **host**) in a relationship that benefits the parasite and may harm—or kill—the host. Most that affect humans are protozoa (single-celled organisms, such as amoebas, that can move on their own) and various types of worms, many with complex life cycles involving not only people but also other animals.

In developed countries, public health measures have rendered most parasitic infections relatively uncommon, but you still might encounter diarrhea caused by *Giardia lamblia* (from contaminated water supplies, including untreated stream and springwater), anal itching from pinworms, vaginal discharge arising from *Trichomonas vaginalis*, the more dangerous toxoplasmosis (from a protozoa that can be acquired via cat litter), and even lice and scabies. In many parts of the world, parasitic infections such as malaria, amoebic dysentery, tapeworm, trichinosis, roundworm, and African sleeping sickness are scourges that cause disease and death among young and old alike.

Even with today's high-powered antibiotics and other medical treatments that would have seemed miraculous to previous generations, our primary defense against infection is our own immune system. In a moment we will take a closer look at this fabulously complex and ingenious system that works 24-7 behind the scenes to keep us from being overrun by all kinds of microorganisms. But for now, understand that even the most sophisticated medical management cannot substitute for intact immunity, as anyone who suffers from full-blown acquired immune deficiency syndrome (AIDS) can testify. As a result, the only treatment for many infections is to relieve symptoms (or if necessary provide other support) while the infection runs its course. A familiar example of this process is the common cold, which astute physicians have long observed lasts a week if you leave it alone—and seven days if you treat it. What we do is rest, drink chicken soup and other liquids, and perhaps procure some nonprescription remedies for aches, stuffy nose, and cough. What our immune system does is mount an astonishing response that brings the illness to a conclusion.

We can now assist the immune system in fighting a number of infections with medications that inhibit or kill the specific organisms that are causing a disturbance. For hundreds of years a variety of chemicals were used (with marginal success) to treat certain infections. Sulfur was known to be effective against scabies, for example, and mercury served as an unpleasant remedy for syphilis from the sixteenth to the twentieth century. The problem with these types of treatments was that they were not specific in their toxicity: While they killed the infectious agent, they also poisoned the patient.

The first synthetic antimicrobial chemical was a derivative of arsenic called Salvarsan (the name derived from Latin words for "save health"), discovered in 1909 by the German physician Paul Ehrlich as a treatment for syphilis. Salvarsan required multiple painful injections over an extended period of time before effecting a cure—not exactly a "magic bullet," but definitely more effective than anything that had preceded it. The discovery and implementation of sulfa drugs in the 1930s, followed by the widespread deployment of penicillin during the 1940s, revolutionized the treatment of several common bacterial infections, including pneumonia, soft tissue infections, syphilis, and gonorrhea.

Today, a veritable arsenal of antibiotics (from natural and synthetic sources) is available for fighting infection, but in recent years there has been an alarming increase in the number and types of bacteria that have developed resistance to several of these drugs. One reason is that for decades antibiotics were often inappropriately prescribed by physicians (often at the request of their patients) to treat common respiratory infections such as colds, acute bronchitis, and influenza that are caused by viruses. Another reason has been the frequent (though more appropriate) deployment of broad-spectrum antibiotics in hospitals, where repeated exposure of bacteria to these agents has led to the development of resistant strains. In recent years the Centers for Disease Control and Prevention (CDC) and other professional organizations have been actively educating doctors and patients alike about the importance of avoiding antibiotics to treat viral infections, for which they are ineffective.

It should go without saying that a highly effective way to deal with infectious diseases is simply to avoid coming in contact with the organisms that cause them. Much of our freedom from infections that plague other parts of the world can be attributed to basic sanitation measures that ensure the safety of food and water and that deal safely with human waste. As individuals, we can avoid a number of infections by simple measures such as washing our hands, cooking meat and poultry thoroughly, and avoiding the sharing of utensils, cups, and toothbrushes used by family members who are ill. More extreme measures, such as isolating carriers of certain disease through quarantine, are used less commonly in the United States.

Protecting Yourself from Foodborne Illness

The term **foodborne illness**, often (but usually inaccurately) called **food poisoning**, refers to disease arising from an infection or (less commonly) an actual toxin in something we eat or drink. More than 250 specific types of foodborne illness have been described. This is not the same as food allergy or intolerance, in which a person reacts to a constituent of a food that otherwise is tolerated by most people. In this segment we won't focus on plants that are inherently toxic, such as certain types of mushrooms, or foods that have been literally poisoned, accidentally or otherwise. Instead, we'll examine illnesses caused by viruses, bacteria, and parasites that could wind up in food or fluids you and your family might enjoy today and regret tomorrow. Infectious organisms cause the vast majority of foodborne diseases, and because they usually do most of their dirty work in the gastrointestinal tract, it is common for them to cause nausea, vomiting, and diarrhea—sometimes to an alarming or even life-threatening degree.

Most of us have heard of the severe illnesses such as cholera and typhoid fever that ravage many parts of the world, especially after a disaster such as a flood or earthquake. We are blessed with widespread standards of sanitation, waste disposal, and food preparation that allow us to eat just about anywhere—at restaurants or at our own kitchen table—without worrying about contracting a major intestinal upset. Yet the CDC estimates that every year in the United States there are some 76 million cases of foodborne illness, requiring 325,000 hospital admissions and causing 5,000 deaths. It is impossible to know exactly how many actual cases of foodborne infection occur every year, because many consist of acute bouts of vomiting and diarrhea from which a person recovers without specific treatment, without a diagnosis, and without the illness being reported. As you might imagine, the most serious problems tend to arise among the very young, the very old, or those with compromised immunity.

The three primary ways that foods become contaminated are (1) improper preparation, (2) inadequate cooking, and (3) improper storage.

The foods most likely to become contaminated by unsavory organisms (usually bacteria) are perishables, especially meat and other animal products, fresh fruits, and vegetables. A lot of foodborne illness occurs because

- hands aren't washed enough
- fruits and vegetables aren't washed enough
- meats aren't cooked long enough
- stored foods aren't kept cold enough

Here's a basic list of dos and don'ts to reduce your risk of getting sick from food and drink:

1. Wash your hands with soap and water before you prepare food—especially if you're going to handle meat, poultry, fish, shellfish, or eggs. If you use the toilet, play with a pet, or change a diaper during the course of preparing food, *wash your hands again*. By the way, if *you* have diarrhea or some other intestinal illness, play it safe and let someone else prepare the food.

2. **Wash your utensils, cutting board, and other surfaces** with hot, soapy water after you have prepared food (especially when they include meat, dairy, and egg products). This helps prevent **cross-contamination**, in which organisms from one food are accidentally transferred to another. Also, avoid using wooden cutting boards for meat. Pores in the wood can harbor dangerous bacteria.
3. **Keep your raw meats, poultry, fish, and shellfish out of contact with other foods.** (This is another measure to prevent cross-contamination.) Ideally, these various animal products should be bagged separately at the grocery store, kept in sealed bags or containers so that their juices don't drip onto other foods or surfaces, prepared on separate cutting boards, and placed on different plates.
4. **Wash raw fruits and vegetables in running water** before enjoying them—especially those that are not going to be cooked. Once they're washed, don't put them back into the package or container from which they came.
5. **Cook your meat, poultry, and eggs thoroughly.** Because contaminated food can look and smell normal, experts recommend the use of a food thermometer to help you gauge what's hot enough—140° to 180°F, depending on the food—and what's not. The U.S. Department of Agriculture recommends the following *internal* temperatures be reached in order to kill potentially harmful bacteria:
    - Beef, veal, and lamb: 145°F for medium rare (the rarest you should allow, by the way), 160°F for medium, and 170°F for well-done. Fresh pork: The same, except it should not be eaten medium rare.
    - Poultry: 180°F for whole birds, legs, wings, and thighs; 170°F for breasts.
    - Ground meat: 160°F for ground beef, pork, veal, and lamb; 165°F for ground poultry.
    - Ham: 160°F if fresh, 140°F if previously cooked.
    - Fish and shellfish: 145°F for at least fifteen seconds.
    - Egg dishes: 160°F (cook eggs until the yolks are firm).
    - Casseroles, stews, and leftovers: 165°F.
6. **Room temperature isn't good for perishables** (but bacteria love it).
    - Put your perishables in the refrigerator or freezer within two hours of purchase or preparation (and within one hour if you're having a heat wave and room temperature is 90°F or more). This includes the doggy bag from the restaurant containing the food you—or your dog—want to enjoy the next day.

Undercooked ground beef can harbor the bacteria *E. coli,* and in particular a toxic strain known as *E. coli* 0157:H that can cause bloody diarrhea and cramps lasting five to ten days. In a small percentage of cases, usually in small children or the elderly, this infection leads to a form of kidney failure called **hemolytic uremic syndrome**. More than 170,000 cases, 2,800 hospitalizations, and 80 deaths are caused by foodborne *E. coli* every year.

Infected eggs are a common source of infection with *Salmonella*, a type of bacteria responsible for an illness (consisting of four to seven days of fever, diarrhea, and abdominal pain) that affects 1.3 million people in the United States every year, resulting in 15,000 hospitalizations and more than 500 deaths.

- Make sure your refrigerator maintains a temperature of less than 40°F and your freezer less than 0°F.
- Beef, veal, lamb, or pork should go in the freezer if you're not going to eat it for three to five days. Ground meat, fish, shellfish, and poultry go in the freezer if you're not going to use it within two days.
- Toss refrigerated leftovers after four days.
- Don't let prepared perishables sit at room temperature for more than two hours. If you're having a get-together where food needs to be available for a longer time, keep the hot foods hot with a warming tray or chafing dish and the cold foods on ice.
- Thaw your frozen meat in the refrigerator or microwave, not on the kitchen counter. At room temperature, the outer portions can become hospitable to bacteria long before the center portion has thawed.
- Marinate your meat in the refrigerator, not at room temperature.

7. **Think twice before you eat, or serve your family, any of the following:**
   - raw, rare, or undercooked meat, poultry, fish, and shellfish
   - unpasteurized milk or juices
   - raw sprouts, such as alfalfa, clover, or radishes
   - uncooked eggs, or foods containing them
   - uncooked hot dogs or other lunch meats
8. **Don't drink water directly from streams and lakes.** They may look cool and clear, but they are notorious for harboring the parasite *Giardia lamblia,* which can cause a chronic diarrhea.
9. **If in doubt, throw it out.**

Raw oysters and clams are well-known for transmitting **norovirus**, one of the two types of viruses that can cause **acute gastroenteritis**—a miserable but (usually) mercifully brief illness notable for repeated episodes of vomiting and diarrhea over one or two days.

Raw sprouts themselves are a healthful food, but they have been associated with outbreaks of illness caused by *E. coli* and *Salmonella*. They're grown in a humid environment, and they can harbor bacteria if they are exposed to contaminated water or harvesting equipment.

A Primer on Immunity and Vaccinations

Though we cannot isolate ourselves from every conceivable infectious agent, our body has the ability to develop an immune response as a defense against potential invaders. Immunity to a disease is frequently acquired naturally, as when a child develops chickenpox and then is no longer susceptible to it, even if exposed later to others with the disease. Immunity can also be acquired artificially by purposefully introducing a weakened or killed **pathogen** (a disease-causing agent such as a virus or bacteria), or portions of the pathogen, into the body. Like a microbiologic wanted poster, this process primes the immune system to recognize and mount an efficient defense if the infectious agent makes an appearance.

Like so many other intricate biological structures and mechanisms about which we have much to discover, the immune system speaks eloquently of a Designer. It consists of two basic divisions: innate immunity and acquired immunity. **Innate immunity** is provided by organs, tissues, and cells that act as a first line of defense against invading microorganisms, though one that is not specific against any particular type. For example, our skin is a component of our innate immunity in that it minimizes access of bacteria, viruses, and other microscopic assailants to our body. **Acquired immunity**, on the other hand, is based on the responses of cells of the immune system to specific **antigens**. Antigens are large molecules present on the surface of all microorganisms (and on human cells as well) that are capable of eliciting two basic types of responses from the immune system. **B lymphocytes** (or **B cells**) are stimulated to multiply and produce **antibodies**, proteins that bind specifically to particular antigens and allow other cells of the immune system to destroy them. **T lymphocytes** (or **T cells**) directly attack the antigens—or the cells on which they reside—and also offer a measure of control to the immune response. Exposure to an antigen results in the creation of a pool of "memory" cells, B cells and T cells that when challenged with the antigen again can help mount a swift and robust response. This allows the immune system to rally a quicker, more powerful defense when a pathogen is encountered after an initial infection, and it is this mechanism that provides future immunity against an infectious disease once the disease has been contracted.

F.Y.I.

Almost all cells in the human body are covered with **human leukocyte antigens (HLA)**, also known as **histocompatibility antigens**. Each individual has unique HLA molecules (except perhaps in the case of identical twins). It is this antigenic difference that causes the immune system to attack transplanted organs, leading to a biological rejection. (To prevent this, organ recipients must take a regimen of immunosuppressant drugs, usually for life.) HLA molecules usually do not provoke an immune response within our own body because the immune system is designed to differentiate between self and non-self antigens. However, sometimes the immune system malfunctions and attacks a person's own cells as if they were invaders. This can cause a variety of disorders (known as **autoimmune diseases**) such as rheumatoid arthritis and type 1 diabetes that can range from relatively mild to life-threatening.

The body can encounter a pathogen or its antigens naturally (through infection) or through artificial means. Since intentional introduction of a dangerous pathogen is obviously unwise, scientists have devised ways to introduce weakened or killed forms of certain pathogens, small portions of them, or the toxins they produce. These preparations are called **vaccines**, and once introduced they can stimulate the immune system to recognize pathogens (or their toxins) in the future and destroy them before they cause full-blown disease.

Vaccination was first developed in 1796 by English physician Edward Jenner, who noted that milkmaids who had contracted cowpox (a mild disease passed from infected cows to humans) did not contract smallpox, a highly contagious and often deadly and disfiguring disease. When Jenner took some material from a cowpox sore and scratched it into the arms of patients, they became immune to smallpox.

The word *vaccine* derives from *vacca,* the Latin word for cow.

We now know that the virus that causes cowpox contains antigens that are very similar to those of the smallpox virus. The initial challenge with the cowpox virus thus allowed the body to build an immune response that was also effective against the smallpox virus. Since Jenner's discovery, a host of other vaccines have dramatically reduced suffering and death caused by a number of diseases around the world—and in your neighborhood:

- **Measles** is a viral infection that causes fever, severe coldlike symptoms, and a conspicuous red rash. In adults, measles symptoms are usually more severe. Complications from the disease include ear infections and, in rare cases, diarrhea, pneumonia, and encephalitis, an inflammation of the brain. In some cases, measles encephalitis can lead to death.
- **Mumps** is marked by a painful swelling of the salivary glands below the ears. It can also cause inflammation of the ovaries or testicles and, in rare cases, may cause sterility. In extremely rare cases mumps can cause encephalitis or permanent hearing loss.
- **Rubella (German measles)** is sometimes referred to as **three-day measles**. Rubella is a viral infection that causes a distinct red rash and is less severe than measles except in one respect: If a woman contracts rubella while pregnant, especially during the first trimester, she is at a higher risk of having a miscarriage or delivering a child with **congenital rubella syndrome**, a combination of serious birth defects that may include deafness, blindness, and mental impairment.
- **Diphtheria** is a serious bacterial infection in which a thick membrane forms in the nose, throat, or airway. The membrane attaches to underlying tissues, so that attempting to remove it causes bleeding. Diphtheria bacteria within the membrane produce a toxin that can damage heart, liver, kidney, and nerve tissue. Paralysis and death may result.
- **Tetanus** results from a toxin produced by a specific type of bacteria that can enter the body through contaminated wounds. The toxin causes painful, spasmodic contractions of muscles (which gave rise to the colloquial term *lockjaw* for this disease) and can lead to death.
- **Pertussis (whooping cough)** is highly contagious and causes severe bouts of coughing, often to the point of choking, that can last for months. It is particularly rough on infants and small children and can lead to pneumonia and death, as well as long-term consequences including brain damage, seizures, and mental retardation.
- **Hepatitis B** is a viral infection of the liver that is usually self-limited, but in a few percent of cases becomes a chronic condition that can eventually lead to cirrhosis or liver cancer. Hepatitis B virus is most commonly transmitted in three ways: from an infected mother to her infant, through sexual contact with an infected person, or by exposure to infected blood. However, a large number of cases occur without a history of any of these events, which is one reason health officials recommend universal vaccination against this virus.

The term *diphtheria* comes from a Greek word meaning leather—a vivid reference to the thick membrane created by this disease.

- **Polio** is a viral infection that damages the central nervous system, resulting in mild or serious paralysis. Between 5 and 10 percent of cases are fatal.
- ***Haemophilus influenzae* type B** is a type of bacteria that can cause, among other things, pneumonia and meningitis (an infection of the membranes that enclose the brain and spinal cord). Since the introduction of *H. influenzae* B vaccines, the number of cases of meningitis in young children caused by this bacteria has dropped dramatically.
- **Pneumococcal infection** is an important cause of bacterial meningitis in the United States, although it has become much less common since vaccination has been more widely utilized. Pneumococcus can also cause ear infections (an estimated 5 million cases each year), pneumonia, and sepsis—a serious illness in which large numbers of the bacteria are present in the bloodstream. Children under two years of age are at the greatest risk for significant infection. Unfortunately, many strains of pneumococcus have become resistant to antibiotics that were once effective in treating it. As a result, prevention of pneumococcal infection has become increasingly important, especially in young infants, who now routinely receive an immunization called the pneumococcal conjugate vaccine (or PCV) at ages two, four, six, and twelve to fifteen months.
- **Chickenpox** is caused by the varicella-zoster virus. The hallmark of the disease is an itchy rash consisting of small red spots that evolve into blisters. Chickenpox is usually a mild disease, but in rare instances it can involve the lungs or the brain with potentially serious consequences, including death. (Bacteria can also infect skin through the blisters.) After a chickenpox infection, some of the varicella-zoster virus can survive within nerve cells and then reactivate at a later date, causing a painful condition called **shingles**. This is characterized by the appearance of groups of blisters involving an area of skin supplied by one nerve root (and thus always only on one side of the body). The rash is accompanied by sharp, stabbing pains (called **neuralgia**), which in a small percentage of cases (usually in the elderly) may continue for months or even years.
- **Influenza**, or **flu** for short, is a common respiratory infection that can cause fever, chills, sore throat, headache, and body aches. More than just a really bad cold, influenza can have deadly complications including pneumonia, dehydration, and worsening of chronic conditions such as cardiovascular and lung diseases (including asthma). Complications are most serious among young children, older adults, and those with weakened immunity. All children ages six months to twenty-three months, and those older than twenty-four months who have a chronic illness, should be vaccinated against the influenza vi-

You may have had "stomach flu," an abrupt and unpleasant bout of nausea, vomiting, and diarrhea that usually lasts only a day or two. This is nearly always **acute gastroenteritis**, which is usually caused by one of two types of virus (rotavirus and norovirus) that have nothing to do with influenza.

rus. Since the strains that are likely to cause trouble change from year to year (and new strains may appear as well), a new vaccine must be developed and millions of doses distributed on an annual basis—a phenomenal accomplishment that we may take for granted as flu shots are distributed during the fall and winter.

The immunizations for some of the diseases listed here are available only as individual vaccines, but several can be obtained in combinations. For example, the vaccines for measles, mumps, and rubella are available in a combination known as MMR; the vaccines for diphtheria, tetanus, and pertussis are supplied in a combination called DTaP. Newer combinations on the market combine DTaP, hepatitis B, and polio vaccines in a single injection. A great benefit of these combinations is that they decrease the number of actual injections a child must receive, while increasing the likelihood that more children will get the appropriate number of recommended immunizations. Most of the vaccines a child receives today are given during their first two years, with a second important round at age four or five before entering kindergarten.

The *aP* in *DTaP* refers to the *acellular* form of the pertussis (whooping cough) vaccine, which contains only a part of the bacterium that is essential for an immune response. It is considered safer (and causes fewer reactions) than the older vaccine that contained the entire (killed) pertussis bacterium.

The Advisory Committee on Immunization Practices (ACIP) is a panel of experts in the United States that recommends which immunizations should be given (and when) to children, adolescents, and adults. Because ACIP's recommendations (including guidelines on how to make up one or more missed immunizations) may change slightly from year to year, and because new combinations of vaccines become available periodically, you should review your child's (and your) immunization status with your own physician.

F.Y.I.

To check the most current immunization recommendations, you can visit http://www.cdc.gov/nip/ACIP.

The risks of vaccination

Like virtually every other form of medical treatment, vaccinations sometimes cause unpleasant side effects, although the vast majority of these are minor. Low-grade fever; rash; irritability; and redness, swelling, or soreness at the spot of injection are the most common side effects of vaccination. The risks of more serious events, such as high fever and body aches, are much lower, and the chances of a life-threatening allergic reaction to an immunization are less than one in a million doses. Other severe but extremely rare occurrences after vaccination include:

- long-term seizures and brain damage after DTaP
- encephalitis, deafness, and long-term seizures after MMR
- pneumonia after varicella (chickenpox)

These devastating events are so rare that it is often difficult for experts to be sure whether or not they are caused by the vaccine.

Vaccine safety has been and continues to be a high priority for health-care professionals and regulatory agencies, and vaccines deemed to be unsafe or whose benefits are outweighed by their risks are removed from the recommended immunization schedule. One example was the removal of **oral polio vaccine (OPV)** from the list of recommended immunizations. OPV contained a weakened but live form of the polio virus that in rare cases (one in 2.4 million) could actually *cause* polio. Today the chances of getting polio naturally are so low that the risks posed by OPV are regarded as unacceptably high in comparison, and despite the higher cost, the **inactivated polio vaccine (IPV)** (given by injection) is the only form currently in use in the United States.

It should be noted that there are instances in which a health-care provider might postpone immunization of a child. If he or she is given a vaccine while ill, for example, it might be difficult to determine whether subsequent symptoms, especially fever, are due to the vaccine or part of the natural history of the illness. Likewise, a severe illness might prevent a child from developing an adequate immune response to a vaccine, rendering it less effective than if the child were healthy. Also, some vaccines contain live (but weakened) viruses that are considered unsafe for children with suppressed immunity—for example, those who have HIV or are undergoing certain cancer chemotherapies.

Despite the dramatic effectiveness of vaccines in curbing the spread of serious diseases and saving lives over the past two centuries, in recent years some have strongly questioned their safety, especially in young infants. Seeing them as a greater threat than the diseases they are designed to prevent, some parents refuse to have their children immunized. Concerns about vaccine safety certainly need to be addressed, but they should be evaluated in light of the overall threat from the diseases against which they offer immunity.

Why we need to vaccinate

Given the potential side effects, why would a parent want to vaccinate a child? That question is best answered by looking at the odds of suffering a serious side effect from a vaccine compared to the odds of suffering serious consequences from a disease. The answer parallels the situation described earlier in this chapter: One of the arguments some people make for not wearing a seat belt is that it might trap them in a burning or submerged vehicle. Yet decades of research demonstrate beyond a doubt that passengers who wear a seat belt are much more likely to walk away from an accident than those who don't wear one. Also, the odds of escaping a vehicle on fire or under water are better for those who are restrained—and thus less likely to be knocked unconscious—during the accident.

Some parents use the same line of reasoning with vaccinations: "With all the side effects, it would be better not to vaccinate my child." This reaction often arises from hearing horror stories about reactions to immunizations without appreciating the potential hazards of the diseases against which children are immunized. (Ironically, this is largely due to the success of vaccines.) Today's parents of young children were not around when these diseases regularly cut a wide swath of destruction across North America. Nevertheless, it's worth considering the damage once wrought by just a few of these infections.

- Before the widespread availability of vaccine, paralytic polio affected 13,000 to 20,000 people (mostly children) every year in the United States. During the 1950s many parents refused to let their children participate in activities such as swimming at public pools during hot summer months because of the fear that they would contract this disease and become permanently dependent on crutches, braces, and wheelchairs.[79] Pictures of rows of children confined to iron-lung machines because of paralysis caused by polio were a familiar sight in newspapers and magazines.
- Measles infected nearly everyone in the United States prior to routine immunization. Most recovered uneventfully, but some developed diarrhea, pneumonia, and encephalitis, and an average of 450 people died each year because of this infection.
- In 1964 and 1965, before immunization against rubella became common practice, approximately 20,000 children were affected with deafness, blindness, mental impairment, and other birth defects as a result of congenital rubella syndrome. Rubella infections also caused 2,100 neonatal deaths and over 11,000 miscarriages.
- Only senior citizens are likely to have any memory of the misery and loss inflicted by diphtheria before a vaccine was developed in 1923. In 1921, 206,000 cases and 15,520 deaths were reported in the United States. While only two cases were reported in the United States in 2001, diphtheria is not uncommon in other parts of the world. In the former Soviet Union, a breakdown in public health services (and specifically a lack of vaccination) led to an epidemic with more than 150,000 cases that claimed 5,000 lives between 1990 and 1999.
- Before the *Haemophilus influenzae* type B (Hib) vaccine became widely available, this bacteria caused more than 20,000 serious infections among infants and children in the United States every year. Two out of three of these cases were meningitis, and the rest were a variety of other life-threatening diseases including pneumonia, sepsis (invasion of the bloodstream), and epiglottitis (a highly dangerous inflammation of the flap that covers the airway when swallowing). *H. influenzae* B meningitis took the lives of 600 children every year and left many more with neurological impairments, including seizures and mental retardation. Since the introduction of the vaccine in 1987, the annual incidence of serious *H. influenzae* infection in the United States has dropped 98 percent.
- Prior to the availability of immunization, pertussis (whooping cough) affected between 150,000 and 260,000 individuals and caused as many as 9,000 deaths each year. Currently more than 9,000 cases are reported each year in the United States. While modern medical care has reduced the death rate compared to that seen in

Before the *H. influenzae* vaccine was developed, pediatricians and family physicians routinely cared for infants and small children with *H. influenzae* B meningitis. Now the vast majority of residents training to be physicians in these specialties finish their training without ever seeing a case, while seasoned practitioners recollect (with no fondness whatsoever) the not-so-recent bygone days of lumbar punctures (spinal taps) in sick infants, intensive antibiotic regimes, and parents agonizing over their critically ill children. If you are still unconvinced of the historical benefits of immunizations or need a wake-up call regarding their importance now, check the CDC Web page entitled "What Would Happen If We Stopped Vaccinations?" at http://www.cdc.gov/nip/publications/fs/gen/WhatIfStop.htm.

prior generations, eighteen lives were lost in 2002—all among infants younger than one year of age.

- Even chickenpox, commonly thought of as a harmless childhood ailment, was responsible for 11,000 hospitalizations and about 100 deaths annually during the years prior to vaccination.[80]

The incidence of these diseases has been significantly reduced in most industrialized nations because of vaccination campaigns, but ongoing immunization is crucial because the diseases still exist elsewhere in the world. The one exception is smallpox. The smallpox vaccine was discontinued after the disease was determined to have been eradicated from the world—an astonishing accomplishment given the devastating impact of this infection for hundreds of years. The last cases occurred in the wild in 1977 and in a laboratory in 1978, and eventually the risk of complications from the vaccine became far greater than the likelihood of contracting the disease.

A risky but unfortunately necessary aspect of current preparations for potential terrorist attacks has been the reinstitution of smallpox vaccination for certain military and medical personnel who might be at risk for exposure to smallpox as a biological weapon.

Polio is another disease that has nearly been extinguished. The last case of wild polio in the Western hemisphere was seen in 1991, although hundreds of cases of the disease still crop up each year in other parts of the world, because individuals in some countries entertain misconceptions about the vaccine and refuse to allow themselves or their children to be immunized. As a result, one international airline passenger could reintroduce polio to North America if vaccination coverage in the United States and Canada dipped too low.

Pertussis (whooping cough) remains in circulation even in areas where children are widely vaccinated. Parents who withhold immunizations from their children may be chagrined to find themselves dealing with a very sick child who has an intense and very persistent cough. Tetanus is always a threat to someone who has never been immunized (or whose immunizations are not up-to-date), because the bacteria that cause it are ever-present in soil and on other materials, ready to populate a puncture wound and generate the toxin that causes an extremely unpleasant and often fatal illness.

Several other diseases are rare in North America (and thus often seen as inconsequential) but are still in full swing elsewhere in the world. While the number of new measles cases reported in the United States in 2001 was under 120 with no reported deaths, in the same year there were 30 to 40 million new cases worldwide and a staggering 745,000 deaths.[81] We need to remember that while we don't see too many of the childhood diseases against which we vaccinate, they are still quite capable of causing a massive health crisis unless we remain vigilant in immunizing against them.

Some individuals have never been vaccinated and yet have not contracted measles, mumps, or other diseases for which immunizations are given. The fact that these people remain disease-free might seem to argue against the necessity of vaccination, but their good health is really evidence of the benefits of **herd immunity**, a phenomenon that provides a buffer of immunized individuals between infected persons and unvaccinated ones. For example, someone with an infectious disease may encounter many individuals in his community during the course of his or her infection. If most people in the community are immunized against the disease, the chance of it being spread throughout the community is lower than it would be if many people were not immunized. (Because tetanus is not spread from person to person, herd immunity offers no protective benefit for this disease in an unvaccinated individual.)

Herd immunity requires that a large number of people in the community be immunized. In regions where vaccination rates drop, herd immunity decreases and the incidence of disease rises. Pertussis (whooping cough), for example, is notorious for reappearing wherever vaccinations against it wane in popularity. In eight countries where immunization declined, cases of pertussis soared to ten to one hundred times the infection rate seen in other countries where vaccinations rates remained stable.[82] A well-publicized and sad example occurred in Japan in the 1970s, when concerns over the safety of the older pertussis vaccine caused the vaccination coverage rate to drop from about 80 percent in 1974 to 20 percent by 1979. As a result, a pertussis epidemic occurred in 1979, resulting in thirteen thousand cases of whooping cough and forty-one deaths.[83] When vaccination rates subsequently climbed, the incidence of pertussis once again dropped.

Refusing immunizations not only puts the unvaccinated individual at risk but also increases the risk of disease for others in the community. This is of special concern for individuals who, because of chronic illness or suppressed immunity, cannot be vaccinated and therefore rely on herd immunity.

Vaccine safety controversies

We have already noted that the vast majority of vaccine side effects are minor, and that significant adverse events such as pneumonia or encephalitis occur very rarely. In recent years, however, other serious reactions have been attributed to vaccines, and those claims have caused many parents to opt against immunizing their children. We will look at three specific controversies surrounding vaccines that have generated a great deal of concern in recent years:

- Does MMR cause autism?
- Does the mercury preservative used in some vaccines lead to learning or developmental disabilities?
- Do multiple vaccinations in a short time span overwork an infant's immune system and cause harm?

MMR and autism

In 1998, a team of British researchers published a preliminary report based on their examinations of twelve children, all of whom showed symptoms of both inflammatory bowel disease and developmental regression.[84] Nine of these children were diagnosed with autism. From this report, the parents of these children concluded that there must have been a connection between the onset of these problems and their immunization with the MMR vaccine. The authors of this study suggested only the possibility of an association between the MMR vaccine and some cases of autism, and they clearly stated that there was not enough information to establish any definitive link. Nevertheless, their report received wide media attention, and the notion of a connection between MMR and autism has persisted (especially on the Internet)—even after ten of the study's thirteen authors issued a statement in 2004 retracting their original interpretations and reaffirming that there is insufficient evidence to establish a causal link between autism and the vaccine.

Since the 1998 study was published, several other reports have investigated a possible connection between autism and the MMR vaccine, and so far no such association has been established. For example, researchers in the United Kingdom and the United States have found that increases in the number of newly diagnosed cases of autism had occurred in places where MMR coverage had remained relatively consistent over the same time frame, indicating that the vaccine was not a factor.

Reputable professional organizations such as the American Academy of Pediatrics and the Institute of Medicine have extensively (and independently) reviewed this and other research, and they have reached the same conclusion: The available evidence indicates no relationship between the MMR vaccine and autism.

Mercury

Since the 1930s, a mercury-containing preservative called **thimerosal** has been added to some vaccines to inhibit bacterial or fungal growth in the preparations. A number of parents of children with ADHD, speech or language delays, or neurological and developmental problems questioned whether vaccines containing thimerosal were responsible for these conditions.

In 1997, the Food and Drug Administration performed a comprehensive review of vaccines containing thimerosal and found that the amount of mercury a child might receive under existing recommended vaccine schedules was within acceptable FDA limits. However, depending on the vaccine formulation administered and the weight of the infant, it was determined that during the first six months of life a child could possibly be exposed to a level of mercury higher than that recommended by the Environmental Protection Agency. As a precautionary measure, the CDC and the American Academy of Pediatrics issued a joint statement (later affirmed by the American Academy of Family Physicians) calling upon vaccine manufacturers to eliminate or greatly reduce the amount of thimerosal used in vaccines.

Although data from several studies indicated that toxicity from thimerosal did not occur until the level of exposure reached *one hundred to one thousand times* that found in vaccines, it was nonetheless considered prudent to urge the reduction of mercury content to as low a level as possible. (It should be noted that thimerosal had never been used in many routine vaccines, including inactivated polio, MMR, varicella, and two common formulations of DTaP.) Today, with the exception of some influenza vaccines, all vaccines on the recommended childhood immunization schedule appear in either thimerosal-free or thimerosal-reduced forms (with only trace amounts of this compound). Influenza vaccines are also available in thimerosal-reduced forms.

Too many vaccines

Some parents have expressed concerns that their infant's immune system might be weakened as a result of getting too many vaccines at one time. Currently, some vaccines are administered in combination (such as the MMR and DTaP vaccines), and infants often receive several vaccines during a single office visit. This means fewer office visits, which not only saves time and money for the parents but also is less traumatic for the child. Research indicates that this multiple vaccination strategy offers no increased risk of adverse reactions compared to the administration of single vaccinations over a course of many office visits.

Part of the concern over multiple immunizations is that they might overload a child's immune system. However, a child's immune system is capable of responding to antigens even before birth. Since an infant's immune system has never encountered some of the viruses or bacteria that cause serious diseases (and therefore cannot defend against them), it is important that immunizations be given at this time when children are most vulnerable.

The total number of immune challenges given during vaccinations is negligible. Over the entire recommended immunization schedule, a child's immune system is exposed to 126 or fewer antigens.[85] That is tiny compared to the number of immune challenges a child experiences every day. A viral respiratory infection introduces between four and ten antigens, while a case of strep throat can introduce between twenty-five and fifty.[86] Furthermore, thousands of bacteria are present on a baby's skin and in a baby's intestinal tract, mouth, and nasal passages.

While some parents suggest that, just to be safe, children should receive only one vaccine per visit and that vaccines should be given one component at a time rather than in combination, most medical professionals and child-health advocates, including those in national leadership roles, disagree. Spreading immunizations over a longer period of time is cumbersome for parents and ultimately more unpleasant for the child. Furthermore, it decreases the likelihood that a child will stay up-to-date on his immunization schedule and may leave him vulnerable to disease during the intervals between vaccinations.

A final word about childhood immunization

Earlier in this chapter we discussed a number of ways in which parents can protect the health and safety of their children: making sure that seat belts are buckled during *every* ride in the car, maintaining smoke detectors, and storing poisonous chemicals out of reach, among many others. Immunization, like these safety measures, is a reliable way to safeguard your children's health and protect them from the dangers of infectious disease.

While nearly all credible experts recognize that it is in the best interest of every healthy child to be immunized in accordance with current schedules, obviously parents or guardians are responsible for ensuring that this task is actually carried out. If, after reading this section, you still have doubts about whether it is safe and appropriate to immunize, we recommend that you confer with your child's doctor and make decisions prayerfully based on sound information.

Adult Immunizations

You may be young at heart, but the fact that you're no longer a child does not mean that you have outgrown the need for vaccinations. The Centers for Disease Control and Prevention recommends several routine immunizations for adults for the purpose of preventing disease, based on vaccine history and potential for exposure.

When determining which vaccines an adult might need, health-care providers do not rely on an age-based schedule as they do with children. (An exception is the tetanus-diphtheria, or adult Td, immunization, which should be given to adults every ten years.) Instead, they consider a number of variables that may be summarized using the simple acrostic **HALO** to help decide which immunizations may be appropriate:

- Health factors: chronic disease, history of sexually transmitted disease, immunocompromised status (i.e., cancer, HIV), pregnancy
- Age factors: adolescent or young adult, age fifty or above, age sixty-five or above
- Lifestyle factors: illicit injectable drug use, birthplace outside the United States, men who have sex with men, more than one sex partner in the past six months, international travel, body piercing, tattooing
- Occupational factors: college student, health-care worker, day-care provider, sewage worker, prisoner

Adult immunization recommendations

A brief summary of common immunizations to be considered for adults is outlined below. As is the case with childhood immunizations, there may be specific health reasons (such as pregnancy, immunodeficiency, or a previous allergic reaction) that would make a particular vaccine inappropriate for certain individuals. Before you receive any vaccine, it's important to review not only your own health history, but also pertinent information about the immunization and any potential side effects that might occur. (Since you are likely to have received immunizations from more than one office or clinic over the course of your lifetime, keeping your own vaccination record can save you and your health-care provider a lot of time and energy.) If a significant side effect should occur, you should contact your doctor—not only to determine what treatment (if any) is needed, but also to make note of the reaction in your health record. (You should also note it in your own record.)

1. **Influenza vaccine** is given annually, usually in October or November, although it may be given at any time during "flu" season, which typically extends from December through March.

   Who should receive the influenza vaccine?
   - Adults who are fifty years or older
   - Individuals with chronic diseases, or people living with individuals with chronic disease
   - Women who are or expect to be pregnant during flu season
   - Health-care workers
   - Individuals in institutional settings (dormitories, nursing homes)
   - Travelers
   - Individuals who wish to reduce the likelihood of becoming ill during flu season
2. **Pneumococcal pneumonia vaccine (PPV)** is given to prevent infections caused by *Streptococcus pneumoniae*. This organism causes (among other diseases) a common and intense form of bacterial pneumonia, one that the CDC reports kills more people in the United States each year than all other vaccine-preventable diseases combined. As noted previously, infants now receive a form of pneumococcal vaccine to prevent not only pneumonia but also meningitis and sepsis. Healthy adults usually need only one dose, but there are certain medical situations in which a repeat dose should be given.

   Who should receive PPV?
   - Adults who are sixty-five years or older
   - Individuals with chronic diseases
   - Individuals who have had their spleen removed or are "functionally asplenic" (meaning that an ongoing disease such as sickle cell anemia has markedly reduced the spleen's immunologic functions)
   - Alaskan and certain Native American populations
   - Prisoners
   - Pregnant women who are at high risk for infection
3. **Hepatitis B vaccine** is available for all age groups, and since the early 1990s it has been given to children as a routine vaccine series. Any adolescent or adult who has not previously received this three-part vaccine series is a potential candidate for it. Hepatitis B vaccination confers lifelong immunity.

Who should receive the hepatitis B vaccine?

- All adolescents who did not receive the vaccine as a child
- Individuals with a history of sexually transmitted diseases or more than one sex partner in the past six months
- Immunocompromised patients (i.e., those with cancer or HIV)
- Users of illegal, injectable drugs
- Health-care and public-safety workers (such as police and firefighters) who are at risk for exposure to blood
- Individuals with developmental disabilities and their caregivers
- Certain international travelers
- Prisoners

4. **Hepatitis A vaccine.** Hepatitis A is caused by a virus that is transmitted by the fecal-oral route, meaning that it is present in the feces of infected individuals and can accidentally contaminate food or water that is ingested by another. (Infected food handlers are a common source.) This infection is preventable by immunization, hand-washing before handling food (especially after using the restroom), and proper food preparation, as discussed earlier in this chapter. There are many areas in the world where hepatitis A infection is relatively common. The two-part vaccination series confers lifelong immunity.

   Who should receive the hepatitis A vaccine?

   - Any individual (over two years old) at high risk for hepatitis A
   - Those who travel to places where this infection is common
   - Patients with liver disease and certain chronic diseases
   - Patients with clotting factor disorders (hemophilia)
   - Users of illicit drugs
   - Men who have sex with men
   - Individuals with potential occupational exposure (e.g., sewage workers or laboratory workers working with the virus)

5. **Tetanus-diphtheria (Td) vaccine** prevents both of these infections and renders immunity for approximately ten years before a repeat dose is needed, though there are some circumstances in which it may be necessary to repeat the vaccine prior to ten years.

   Who should receive Td?

   - After an initial primary series has been completed, all adolescents and adults every ten years.
   - In the event of a contaminated wound, Td may be given if the previous update was received more than five years before. (Ideally, the vaccination should be given within forty-eight hours of receiving the wound.)

6. **Measles, mumps, rubella (MMR) vaccine** is normally given during childhood, but some adults are also candidates.

   Who should receive MMR?

- Individuals born after 1957 who have never received a dose of MMR or have no documented proof of immunity
- Health-care workers
- Day-care providers
- College students without proof of immunity or who were not previously vaccinated
- All women of childbearing age who do not have documented proof of rubella immunity
- Individuals born outside the United States
- International travelers

7. **Varicella-zoster (chickenpox) vaccine (VZV)** is now commonly given to children one year and older. Adults who have had neither the disease nor the vaccination should consider being immunized as well, because this illness can be much more severe in adults than in children. A blood test that detects antibodies to varicella-zoster virus can help guide vaccination decisions for those who are unsure of their immune status.

   Who should receive VZV?
   - All susceptible adolescents and adults, especially those who are (or care for people) at high risk of developing chickenpox
   - People who are immunocompromised
   - Health-care workers
   - Day-care providers
   - Teachers
   - Residents or staff in institutional settings
   - Nonpregnant women in their childbearing years
   - Military personnel
   - Individuals born outside the United States
   - International travelers

8. **Meningococcal vaccine** protects against meningococcal meningitis, an acute and often rapidly fatal infection of the linings of the brain and spinal cord caused by the bacteria *Neisseria meningitidis*. While uncommon, certain groups of people—most notably freshman college students living in dormitories—are statistically at slightly higher risk than others. A newer form of the vaccine, approved by the ACIP in early 2005, is believed to confer long-term if not lifelong immunity.

   The ACIP recommends that eleven- to twelve-year-olds receive the vaccine, as well as teens entering high school (approximately fourteen to fifteen years of age) who were not vaccinated earlier. Others who should be vaccinated if they were not previosuly vaccinated include:
   - First-year college students living in dormitories
   - Military recruits
   - Individuals with sickle cell disease or other medical conditions that affect the function of the spleen

- International travelers to areas where meningococcal disease is prevalent at higher-than-average levels or is epidemic

In addition to these immunizations, in the near future you may hear about pertussis (whooping cough) vaccination updates for adolescents and adults. Why would this be advisable? Because immunity from childhood vaccinations does not last for a lifetime and appears to need boosting in order to prevent adult infection. Not only does pertussis cause a significant number of cases of chronic cough in adults, but these individuals are also potential sources of infection that could affect young, unvaccinated infants who are far more vulnerable to this disease.

Immunizations for travelers

There are several vaccinations and medications available to individuals who will be traveling to areas of the world where certain infections (such as malaria, cholera, or typhoid fever) are common. Travelers may be required to fulfill certain immunization requirements determined by the health authorities of different countries prior to entry. The CDC provides informative and useful information on international travel at http://www.cdc.gov/travel or by calling (877) 394-8747. Private- and public-health clinics in many cities can help international travelers obtain appropriate vaccinations prior to departure. Seeking information well in advance is advisable, because some vaccines may require more than one dose (sometimes a month or more apart) in order to provide immunity.

For further information

Your health-care provider may provide additional information about vaccines. In addition, the American Academy of Pediatrics' Web site (http://www.aap.org) and the CDC's National Immunization Program's Web site (http://www.cdc.gov/nip) can answer many questions you might have about immunizations. You can also call the National Immunization Hotline at (800) 232-2522. The Immunization Action Coalition also provides valuable immunization information online at http://www.immunize.org.

QUESTIONS TO PONDER:

1. Can you think of any excuses that you or your family members routinely use to explain any unsafe behaviors? (See page 502 for some of the most common.) After reading this chapter, are you prepared to rethink any of these rationalizations?
2. Do you or your family members need to change any habits to prevent the possibility of a house fire?
3. If young children live in or visit your home, do you have all poisonous substances stored safely away? Are you prepared to deal with a poisoning emergency should it occur? (If you're not sure, see page 513.)
4. What additional driving safety habits should you develop?
5. What steps could you and family members take to be safer while enjoying the following recreational activities:
   - hunting
   - biking
   - skateboarding
   - snowmobiling
   - swimming
   - boating or riding a Jet Ski
   - ATV riding
6. Do you know whether your children's immunizations are current? If you have chosen not to immunize your child, have you weighed the risks—both to your child and the larger community—of not immunizing your child?

Action items: Is your home equipped with smoke alarms, carbon monoxide detectors, and fire extinguishers? If not, acquire these items as soon as possible. If you have them, be sure they are working—and set a date to check them each year.

Review fire-safety tips with your family and then develop a fire escape plan.

If you have young children, or if they regularly visit, take a child's-eye tour of your home to see if you need to do any additional child-proofing.

Complete a safety check of your vehicle. (Not sure where to start? See page 529.)

If your family uses one or more car seats, have them inspected by a local fire or police department to be sure they are in good condition and are installed properly.

Using the tips on pages 542–544 be sure all family members have properly fitting helmets for bike and scooter rides, skateboarding, and other recreational activities.

During your (or your child's) next checkup, ask your physician if immunizations are current. If you haven't already done so, create and then maintain a list for each family member showing his or her vaccinations and the dates they were given.

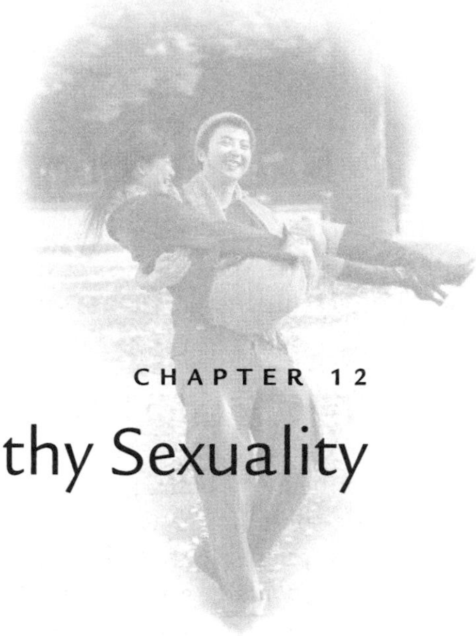

CHAPTER 12

Healthy Sexuality

Sex and sexuality present us with some profound paradoxes:

Sex creates life. All of us are here because of it. We tell our kids, when they're ready to hear about it (which is usually earlier than we think), that sex is the way babies are made. We refer to sexual organs and functions as the **reproductive system**, the part of us that brings new human beings into the world. (We also refer to the physical equipment involved in reproduction as **genitals** or **genitalia**, words derived from the Latin for "beget.") Yet much of our cultural preoccupation with sex ignores—and can even be hostile to—that primary and breathtaking function.

Everyone is interested in sex, though not everyone will admit it. (Did you jump to this chapter before you read about nutrition or exercise? Did you check to see if anyone was looking?)

Films, TV, radio, books, and magazines intended for general consumption contain material about sex that would have been considered shocking fifty years ago. Yet despite all of this apparent cultural openness about sexual matters, few of us are comfortable discussing our *own* sexuality with anyone, even our spouses.

Our language has an elaborate slang vocabulary for sexual organs and for sex itself. (By comparison, how many slang terms can you think of for your ears or toes?) The coarsest word for sexual intercourse, an act intended to be the epitome of love and intimacy, has dozens of colorful variations that serve as offensive expletives and curses.

Sexual intimacy can create the most sublime pleasure and bonds of affection between a man and a woman. Sex can also occur between two people who literally can't stand one another. It can be a profound experience or one devoid of any thought or meaning. It can be affirming or abusive, tender or harsh, a cherished gift between a husband and wife or a vicious crime perpetrated on a helpless victim.

Films depicting various types of sexual activity are called "adult" movies, yet they are uniformly stupid and shallow. There is more sophistication and intelligent dialogue in the average Bugs Bunny cartoon than in any adult film.

The Bible is frequently characterized as disapproving or ashamed of sex, as if God averts His eyes whenever a couple enjoys physical intimacy. But in fact the Scriptures discuss sexuality plainly, celebrate its physical and emotional pleasures, and even use sexual union as a powerful spiritual metaphor.

Two Bottom Lines about Sex

We all have to eat, and we can either provide our bodies with high-quality fuel or health-robbing junk and excess. We all move our muscles, and the way we do so can make us well-conditioned or weak. We are all sexual beings, and we can express our sexuality in ways that are fulfilling and life affirming, or destructive and even deadly. There are, in other words, healthy and unhealthy ways to experience sex.

When it comes to this important subject, we believe that with sex (and indeed with the rest of our lives as well) we should go by the Book. The teachings of the Scriptures on this subject are straightforward and unambiguous. They are medically, emotionally, and spiritually unassailable. If everyone on the planet (or even in one community) followed them explicitly, an untold amount of distress and disease would be avoided. The Bible's insights can be summarized as follows:

1. Sexual activity is intended to be experienced between a man and a woman within the bounds of a mutually exclusive marital relationship. The ideal (and healthiest) situation involves a man and woman who have reserved sexual activity for their wedding night and the years that follow, and who maintain emotional and physical fidelity to one another. For those who have had sexual experiences outside of the marital relationship, a decision to preserve all future sexual activity exclusively within the bounds of marriage is the wisest and healthiest course of action, not to mention the one that God has established as His standard *for our benefit.*

2. Within the security of a marital commitment, sex is to be enjoyed, explored, and cherished in ways that manifest mutual respect. It can involve playfulness, passion, and extraordinary pleasure. It can supply emotional superglue, a powerful bond that helps maintain a marriage through decades of the inevitable ups and downs of life. And it can begin the remarkable experience of bringing a new human being into the world.

Volumes have been written on the topic of sexuality from every conceivable perspective, and we will not attempt to do so again here. Rather, our goal will be to elaborate on the conclusions just stated above, by addressing the following questions:

1. *What are the physical, emotional, and spiritual reasons for preserving sexual activity for marriage?* If you think this is an unrealistic, uptight, overly restrictive view of sexuality, be sure to read on.

2. *How can sexual satisfaction be maximized and sustained over the long haul of a marriage?* The fact that two people are married and free to enjoy sexual intimacy certainly doesn't mean that they won't have issues in this area. While we're not intending to create a manual of sex therapy (there are excellent resources available for that task, some of which we list later), we will provide a map of the terrain and potential trouble spots.

Part One: Preserving the Gift of Sex

This section will lay the groundwork for an important principle: *It is appropriate, wise, and potentially lifesaving to preserve sexual activity for marriage.* While this principle applies to all age-groups, it is particularly important that parents, educators, and health-care professionals communicate it to children and adolescents. Sex is a wonderful, extraordinary, and powerful gift that deserves to be treated with respect. In the context of a permanent and public commitment, it can be savored, explored, and nurtured without guilt or fear of serious consequences. But at the wrong time with the wrong person, sex can bring disappointment, disease, and drastic changes in life—especially in a young life. Adolescents and adults alike need a clearheaded understanding of the benefits and risks of sex in order to make a meaningful decision to experience it within the boundaries of marriage. Even then, maintaining such a commitment isn't easy.

Why is it so challenging to preserve the gift of sex for marriage?

Inner drives. Normal adolescents and adults have sexual interests and feelings. No one passes through his or her teen and adult years devoid of sexual urges and then suddenly switches them on as soon as the minister says, "I now pronounce you man and wife." We are created in such a way that we become sexually and emotionally attracted to others and drawn toward physical intimacy, although there are some significant differences between men and women in the way that this takes place. Indeed, if we didn't experience sexual interest and desire, the human race would die out for lack of new members. We also deeply need love and affirmation. These attractions and needs are powerful, and yet many of us act naively—and at times, carelessly—in the way we deal with them. Learning to manage our sexual thoughts, desires, and actions in a healthy way is an extremely important and challenging task.

Preserving the gift of sex isn't about pretending that our desires don't exist or beating ourselves up because they do, but rather instituting some basic disciplines and realistic strategies to channel them appropriately. This will almost certainly involve setting boundaries and resisting temptations to see or do things that will undermine or violate our commitment. Unfortunately, our culture doesn't provide much help for us in this area.

Provocative images. Sex sells everything from beer to burgers, from cars to chewing gum. For men, who are particularly impacted by what they see, tantalizing images are everywhere: department-store lingerie ads in the newspaper, catalogs that arrive in the mail, the *Sports Illustrated* swimsuit edition, covers of magazines in the supermarket checkout line. More explicit sexual content is readily available on mainstream cable television channels, on pay-per-view in your hotel room, or on millions of Web sites that are but a few mouse clicks away from the home page of your favorite search engine.

Changing standards. A half century ago, Western societies generally supported the concept that marriage was the appropriate arena for sexual activity. During the late 1960s, however, a cultural upheaval sometimes called the **sexual revolution** assaulted traditional sexual ground rules. Virtually all popular media (movies, TV, music, books, magazines) as well as educational, health-care, and governmental organizations were affected by this moral free fall. As a result, unless you live in a strictly controlled or isolated environment, it is difficult to escape exposure to a pervasive philosophy regarding sexuality that might be summarized as follows:

- Sex is okay in any way and with anyone, as long as there is mutual consent, no one gets pregnant (unless she wants to), and no one gets hurt.
- Sex is usual and customary if you are attracted to someone. *Everyone* is doing it.
- Sex unrelated to marriage is normal, natural, expected, and inevitable, so always carry a condom.
- If you are postponing sex until marriage, you must be incredibly unattractive, a social disaster, or a religious fanatic.

This "anything goes" and "everyone's doing it" message can be particularly difficult for teenagers to sort out. But under the assault of these messages, single adolescents and adults alike—even those who are committed to preserving sex for marriage—may begin to feel as if they are completely out of step and missing out on some normal pleasures.

Lack of accountability or (for teenagers) supervision. It's easier to refrain from sexual misadventures when we know someone else whom we respect cares about what we do and has permission to ask us about our behavior. Yet, as we mentioned earlier, it's a lot easier to banter about sex in general than to be open with a trusted friend about our own personal and sensitive concerns. For teenagers, appropriate adult oversight can provide a powerful restraint to youthful passions. But because of fragmented families, complex parental work schedules, easier access to transportation, and even carelessness among adults who should know better, adolescents today are more likely to find opportunities to be alone together for long stretches of time. In such circumstances, it can be much more difficult—even for teens who have made a commitment to wait for sex until their wedding night—to keep their promises to God, to themselves, and to their future spouse. (A small number of parents actually allow their teenage children to engage in sexual activity at home, based on the foolish notion that this makes "safe sex" more likely.)

An overbearing, rigid upbringing. Adolescents who feel smothered in a controlling, micromanaging, suspicious environment are strong candidates for sexual rebellion once the opportunity arises. When restraints are tightly enforced in an atmosphere of ongoing mistrust, kids may be tempted to become sexually involved simply to "get it over with," to see what all the fuss is about, and to assert their independence. Parents can set appropriate boundaries while still entrusting adolescents with increasing responsibility to manage themselves and their sexuality.

Peer pressure. This ever-present influence comes in three powerful forms and impacts teenagers and adults like. Resistance to nonmarital sexual activity may be worn down quickly as a result of the following:

- *A general sense that "everyone is doing it except me."* Movies, TV, and popular music nurture this idea. Conversations with friends or even offhanded comments overheard between strangers may bring the idea closer to home. A school health-education presentation will confirm this suspicion if it emphasizes contraception and condom use but barely mentions abstinence. As a result, a young person may conclude, *These professionals know more about this than I do. I must be the only seventeen-year-old in town who hasn't had sex.*
- *Personal comments from friends and acquaintances:* "You've been with him for six months and haven't slept together yet? What's wrong?" "Hey, guys, check out Jason, the last American virgin!" "Did you get lucky last night?"
- *Direct pressure from another person who wants a sexual experience or an invitation from a willing potential partner.* Come-ons, smooth talk, whining, haggling, and outright coercion by men who want sex with a woman are timeworn negative behaviors. A woman's resistance may be lowered by a need for closeness and acceptance and by the mistaken belief that physical intimacy will secure a man's love.

  In recent years a turnabout has become more common: A young man is informed by his girlfriend (or new acquaintance) that she wants to have sex with him. Any personal convictions that sex is intended for marriage will be put to the ultimate test in a situation like this, especially if some physical contact is already under way. All the admonitions he has heard and the moral code he embraces may suddenly seem terribly abstract, while the intense pleasure that is his for the taking is very real. Which will prevail?

Lack of reasons (and desire) to wait, or to maintain sex within marriage. Some adolescents and adults are determined to have sex as often as possible with any willing partner, regardless of the risks. Others are unshakably committed to the goal that their only sex partner will be their spouse. In between these opposite poles live a large number of people—mostly single, but not always—who keep an informal mental tally of reasons for and against nonmarital sex. Inner longings and external enticements (or pressure) pull them toward it, while their spiritual and moral values, medical warnings, and commonsense restraints put on the brakes. For many people, decisions about sex tend to be based on an internal vote count. When the moment of truth arrives, the tally may be close—or a landslide in the wrong direction. It may even result in an approach—which some call **serial monogamy**—that attempts to reconcile what are in fact incompatible positions: "I'll be careful with my health and emotions by having sex with only one person at any given time."

The remainder of this section will explore the physical, emotional, and spiritual reasons to preserve the gift of sex for marriage. Many of these involve very real dangers—indeed, some that are potentially lethal—of sexual activity outside of this safety zone. But a number of powerful benefits also result when sex is enjoyed in the context for which it was designed.

Why should sex be reserved for marriage?

Reason No. 1: To take the moral high ground

Despite the rising tide of sexual anarchy in our society, a great many people still believe the words *right* and *wrong* apply to sexual behavior. Even someone with a casual exposure to traditional Judeo-Christian values should pick up an important message: The Designer of sex cares a lot about when it's done and with whom. Sex outside of marriage can be dangerous to one's physical, emotional, and spiritual health. Even for those who do not follow specific religious precepts, basic decency and concern for the well-being of others should curtail the vast majority of sexual adventures, which so often are driven by a selfish agenda.

Unfortunately, even those who have been exposed to explicit teaching about sexual morality at church and home may still become involved with nonmarital sex, which does nothing for spiritual growth. Intimacy with God on Sunday morning (or any other day) may be seriously impaired when physical intimacy the night before has clearly violated the boundaries set forth in the Scriptures.

We need to issue an important reminder at this point: Biblical teachings on sex extend far beyond the words *no* and *don't*. Indeed, there is much more to be gained from adhering to God's prescription for sex beyond avoiding disease, emotional pain, and spiritual derailment (although these are certainly good reasons). Like everything else in life, sexuality is most enjoyable and satisfying when one follows the "Owner's manual."

Reason No. 2: To prevent unplanned pregnancies

For a woman in a stable marriage where husband and wife desire to start or add to a family, the discovery of a pregnancy can create one of the greatest joys life has to offer. For a woman—especially a teenager—who has been involved in nonmarital sex, the same discovery can generate tremendous uncertainty, anxiety, and even panic, and for good reason. Whatever the circumstances of the sexual encounter that began it, a pregnancy cannot be ignored, and whatever is done about it will have a permanent impact on the woman's life. Only two outcomes are possible: The baby will be born, or the baby will die before birth, whether through abortion or miscarriage. There's no quick fix where human life is concerned, no way to rewind the tape and start over as though nothing happened.

Each year more than 800,000 American teenagers become pregnant, and approximately three in ten of these pregnancies end in abortion. (Approximately 10 to 15 percent of teen pregnancies end in miscarriage.) The vast majority of these pregnancies are unplanned, and a sizable percentage begin even though a contraceptive is used. Eight out of ten teenage mothers are unmarried (as opposed to about three in ten in 1970). Altogether, one out of three adolescent girls will become pregnant at least once before the age of twenty.[1]

When an unmarried woman bears a child, her life (and probably the lives of other family members) will be affected for years to come. She must deal with the many challenges that all new mothers face, but nearly always with some additional difficulties. Educational plans may need to be postponed or significantly rearranged, as will any current or future employment. Among teenagers, the impact of a pregnancy is likely to be particularly profound. Only three out of ten adolescents seventeen and under who bear a child will earn a high school diploma. Seven out of ten adolescent mothers drop out of high school, and more than 80 percent of young single mothers eventually become dependent on welfare.[2] Unless she has considerable help and support, a teenage mother is likely to experience struggles with parenting, difficulties in a future marriage relationship, and more unplanned pregnancies.

In some cases, one or both of the mother's parents choose to take on primary care of their grandchild, or other family members participate in the baby's care. This situation can serve to forge new bonds in the extended family, allowing the baby to grow up loved and nurtured in his family of origin while his mother manages part of his care and continues her schooling or vocation. But the added strain of such arrangements can take a significant toll on a family, especially if it is too dysfunctional or lacking in resources to provide adequate care for a new baby.

If a young mother gives up her child for adoption—an act of considerable courage—she will help bring about what is often a relatively positive combination of outcomes. Her baby will be reared by people who are usually better prepared to provide the necessary time, attention, and resources. She in turn can move on with her education, vocation, and social life. But even this solution will not exempt her from pain. She will never forget her baby, and she may experience a sense of loss, sometimes profound, for the rest of her life.

In recent decades **open adoption**, in which there is some degree of interaction between the birth mother (or both birth parents) and the adoptive family, has become more common. In many cases, the birth mother actually selects who will rear her child from a number of potential candidates presented by an adoption agency. That couple may then become involved with the birth mother through an extended period of her pregnancy, and one or both adoptive parents might even attend the birth of the baby. Such a relationship can be fulfilling for all concerned, but it is not without potential pitfalls. It is critical that the relationship between the adoptive parents and the birth mother, and everyone's expectations regarding the amount of contact between mother and adoptive family once the baby is born, be carefully discussed and clarified before the birth.

A woman with an unplanned pregnancy often feels a burning need to find a solution as quickly as possible. As she ponders bringing up a baby or giving one up for adoption, she may find each of these prospects highly uncomfortable, at least at first. This and other strong emotional currents (especially when accompanied by pressure from a boyfriend, parents, or others in her life) may lead to the conclusion that abortion is the only viable alternative. It appears to offer a quick resolution, fewer personal complications, far less financial cost compared to having a baby, and usually confidentiality as well.

But abortion is neither a completely risk-free procedure nor an easy escape from all of the potential fallout from an unintended pregnancy. Damage to the uterus that could jeopardize future pregnancies (or even require major surgical repair), infection, bleeding, future infertility, and even more serious events (including death) are possible, though rare, complications. Furthermore, even if an abortion is performed without any apparent medical hitch, a different type of pain may develop months or years later. Because they want so desperately for the crisis to go away, many women undergo an abortion even though they are knowingly violating their own moral standards. Many come to realize later in life that a human being—a son or a daughter, not a shapeless wad of tissue—was destroyed through abortion. For these and other reasons, many women live with significant, long-term regrets after an abortion, especially if they have difficulty becoming pregnant later in life.

Reason No. 3: To avoid sexually transmitted infections

A few decades ago the typical high school health-education class discussed two sexually transmitted infections (STIs): syphilis and gonorrhea. They were described as potentially hazardous but nothing a little penicillin couldn't handle. But the sexual playground that opened during the late 1960s has resulted in an STI epidemic populated by exotic, dangerous, and often incurable infections.

More than twenty different kinds of infections can be transmitted skin to skin or by exchange of body fluids during sexual activity.[3] Some are fatal, a few are relatively harmless, and many have long-term physical and emotional consequences. A few can be successfully treated with antibiotics—but without creating any long-term immunity. As a result, bacterial infections such as gonorrhea and chlamydia can be acquired over and over by the same individual.

If you are interested in more detailed information about specific infections, you may wish to consult the excellent "Medical Updates" section at the Web site of the Medical Institute for Sexual Health (http://www.medinstitute.org) or call the institute at (512) 328-6268. We will, however, note some important general observations:

"Safe" and *really safe* sex. Despite decades of talk about "safe sex" and "safer sex" (see "'Safe(r)' sex isn't safe," starting on page 583), as far as STIs are concerned the only truly safe sex occurs within the confines of a mutually exclusive relationship in which neither person is or has been infected with any STI. By definition, these diseases are spread through skin-to-skin or mucous membrane contact, or through transmission of infected secretions, involving one or both people's genitalia. If neither individual has ever experienced this type of intimate contact outside of his or her marriage relationship, there is essentially no risk of getting any of these infections, with the unusual exception of medical or occupational exposure (such as a health-care worker acquiring HIV or hepatitis B from an accidental stick with a needle that had been in an infected patient).

Any infection acquired as a result of sexual contact was once called **venereal disease (VD).** The term was eclipsed a few decades ago by the more clinically precise term **sexually transmitted disease (STD).** The recognition that an individual can be infected with a sexually transmitted organism without manifesting disease has recently led to the use of the more encompassing term **sexually transmitted infection (STI)**, which we use throughout this book. STD now specifically refers to disease that manifests as a consequence of a sexually transmitted infection.

Astronomical numbers. A number of important infectious diseases are **reportable**—in other words, the physician or laboratory making the diagnosis is required by law to notify the local county public-health department to help limit the spread of infection and help maintain statistical records. Of the twelve most common reportable infections (of *all* kinds) in the United States, five STIs—chlamydia, gonorrhea, HIV, syphilis, and hepatitis B—account for more than *90 percent* of the total. Furthermore, herpes simplex virus, human papillomavirus (HPV), and trichomonad infections, which are not reportable, are actually far more common. Currently it is estimated that among the United States adolescent and adult population, there are 70 million infections involving sexually transmitted viruses—herpes simplex virus (45 million), human papillomavirus (20 million), hepatitis C (2.7 million), hepatitis B (1.25 million), and HIV (900,000).[4] (Note that a number of individuals have been infected by more than one of these viruses. Also, not all cases of hepatitis B and C infections are sexually transmitted.)

One in five sexually active Americans over the age of twelve has been infected by the genital herpes virus (herpes simplex virus type 2, or HSV2).[5]

Women take the brunt of many common STIs—with an important exception. Gonorrhea and chlamydia may cause some urinary burning and discharge in a male, but in women they can cause a more serious infection known as **pelvic inflammatory disease**, as well as damage to the reproductive organs that can lead to infertility. Some strains of human papillomavirus (HPV) can cause annoying genital warts in both men and women, but in women certain high-risk strains are also directly responsible for all cases of cancer of the cervix (the opening of the uterus), a disease that kills more than four thousand American women every year—and more than two hundred thousand worldwide.

In the United States an estimated 10 to 15 percent of couples (about 6.1 million people) have difficulty conceiving, and more than a million couples seek treatment for infertility each year. Statistics cannot begin to reflect the intense distress this problem creates.

The women at highest risk for developing cervical cancer are those who become sexually active during midadolescence and who have multiple partners.[6]

The exception to this general tendency for women to take the brunt of STIs is the disease burden borne by homosexual men. The propensity for promiscuity in this population, combined with the greater likelihood that they will transmit infectious organisms during oral and anal sex (as well as during oral-anal contact), has resulted in an epidemic of life-threatening and, sadly, life-shortening illnesses.

Homosexual men are likely to have many more sexual partners than heterosexual men. Surveys have found that significant percentages of homosexual males report having hundreds of partners over the course of their adult life. (One study found that fewer than 3 percent report having only one sexual partner.) Not surprisingly, sexual contact with so many individuals results in a marked increase in risk for numerous STIs, including syphilis, gonorrhea, HPV, herpes simplex virus, hepatitis B and C, and the most consistently lethal infection, HIV/AIDS. Centers for Disease Control and Prevention statistics indicate that a sexually active homosexual male is one thousand times more likely to contract HIV than a heterosexual male in the general U.S. population. Currently, 46 percent of AIDS cases in the United States involve men who acquired the infection through sexual contact with other men, while 13 percent of cases involve men who acquired it through heterosexual contact.[7]

The young take the brunt of *most* STIs. Teenagers are disproportionately affected by STIs, including HIV. Statistics published in spring 2004 reveal that there were an estimated 18.9 million *new* STI cases in the United States in the year 2000, of which nearly half (48 percent, or about 9.1 million) occurred among persons aged fifteen to twenty-four. This young population represents only one quarter of the sexually active individuals between the ages of fifteen and forty-four, but it accounts for nearly half of the STIs. Three infections—chlamydia, HPV, and trichomoniasis—account for approximately 88 percent of new cases in this age group.[8] One study of sexually active teenage girls from an inner-city population found that *90 percent* had HPV on the cervix.[9] Another study of sexually active college women found that more than 40 percent became infected with HPV over a three-year period.[10] The immune system's response will eventually clear this infection in most of these women, but about 10 percent will continue to harbor the virus on the skin of the genital area for many years, if not for life.[11] Many develop cellular abnormalities of the cervix, including cancer, as a result of their HPV infection.

Frequently silent, sometimes deadly. Three of the most common STIs—chlamydia, genital herpes, and human papillomavirus—often do not cause noticeable symptoms or visible signs of disease, and thus those who are infected with one or more of them may not know they are contagious. This scenario is also common and particularly worrisome in the case of human immunodeficiency virus (HIV), the virus that causes AIDS. HIV infection may go undetected for years, during which time an infected individual can transmit the virus to dozens or even hundreds of other people.

Oral sex *is* sex. While oral sex—contact between one person's mouth or tongue and another person's genitals—isn't typically a topic of polite conversation, it became a frequent subject for newscasters and talk-show hosts during some high-profile political scandals of the 1990s. These discussions revealed a surprising perception among many people that oral sex really isn't sex, often accompanied by a dangerous—and wrongheaded—belief that it isn't particularly risky. This belief is especially common among teenagers. In a study of twelve- to fifteen-year-olds, one in six reported having tried oral sex, and many of these denied ever having vaginal intercourse.[12] Not surprisingly, alcohol and drug use increase the likelihood that a teenager will try oral sex.[13]

Some adolescent girls who practice oral sex consider themselves to be maintaining their virginity or remaining sexually abstinent. Health-care providers or counselors who are attempting to obtain an accurate sexual history from teenagers must routinely ask not only "Are you sexually active?" but also "Are you giving or receiving oral sex?" It is not uncommon for a teenager or young adult to answer no to the first question and yes to the second. Even significant numbers of college students—as many as one in three in one study—consider practicing oral sex to be compatible with a sexually abstinent lifestyle.[14] This idea is both emotionally and morally naive, and it may be medically misinformed as well if it assumes that oral sex is risk free. True, pregnancy will not result from oral sex, but a number of STIs can be transmitted through oral-genital contact, including syphilis, gonorrhea, herpes simplex virus, HPV, chlamydia, and even HIV. The potential consequences can range from a sore throat (from gonorrhea) or hoarseness (from HPV) to serious systemic illness (syphilis) and even death (HIV/AIDS). Estimates of the number of HIV cases that result from oral sex range from one to 7 percent.[15]

"Safe(r)" sex isn't safe. In spite of a relentless worldwide epidemic of sexually transmitted infections (not to mention unplanned pregnancies), many people—among them, health-care professionals, government agencies, and educators—have been unwilling to give serious consideration to a self-evident truth: These problems and the heartaches accompanying STIs could be eliminated if adolescents and single adults would postpone sex, find and marry one partner, and remain mutually faithful for life. This idea has been widely downplayed as unrealistic by an influential cadre of individuals and institutions that, in response to the AIDS epidemic, began promulgating the notion of "safe sex." When it became clear that only mutually exclusive sex within marriage was truly safe, the concept was redubbed "safer sex."

Presentations that promote safer sex (including those geared to adolescents) typically give a brief nod to abstinence from nonmarital sex before presenting three faulty propositions:

- *If you limit the number of partners with whom you have sex, you'll be safe.*

It is true that having fewer partners means fewer chances for exposure to disease. But it takes only one sexual contact to become pregnant or to acquire a significant or lethal infection.

- *If you know something about a potential partner's sexual history and you avoid having sex with someone who has had many partners, you'll be safe.* This sounds reasonable, but in fact taking a sexual history is tricky, even in a doctor's office. A prospective partner is often not willing to tell the truth if it means a pleasurable evening might be called off. It is virtually impossible to discover the sexual history of the prospective partner's previous partners, or those partners' partners, and so on. From an infectious-disease standpoint, one has sex not just with one person but with all that individual's previous sexual contacts, all of their contacts' contacts, and so on. Furthermore, a significant number of people who are infected with STIs have no symptoms and do not know they are infected.
- *If you use a condom every time, you'll be safe.* True, using a condom correctly (a multistep procedure) during each act of intercourse will reduce the risk of pregnancy and some STIs. But condoms are not a terribly effective form of birth control, with failure rates commonly estimated at 15 percent during the first year of typical use.[16] This means that out of one hundred women who are sexually active, fifteen will be pregnant within a year if condoms are the only form of contraception used. Among adolescents, these failure rates are generally higher, for a variety of reasons. Not only are teens more likely to forget or mismanage some of the fine points of proper condom use during the heat of the moment (including having one available in the first place), many teenagers, and older men as well, simply resist wearing them.

Even if used correctly and consistently, condoms can break, leak, or fall off during intercourse. And while the risk for condom breakage and slippage during a single sexual act may be quite small (one to 4 percent in most studies), the cumulative risk when condoms are used as a long-term prevention strategy is significant.[17] These failure rates are even more alarming since intercourse can lead to pregnancy only a few days each month, while STIs can be transmitted every day of every month.

Scientific evidence shows that condoms are far from 100 percent protective, but rather reduce the transmission of STIs to a variable degree—and with some infections, not well at all. Consistent condom use—that is, use with *every* sexual encounter—has been shown to reduce the risk of transmitting HIV about 85 percent.[18] For gonorrhea, herpes, syphilis, and chlamydia, consistent use reduces the risk of transmission by about 50 percent at best.[19]

One reason for this incomplete protection is that a number of infections such as syphilis, herpes, and especially human papillomavirus (HPV) are often spread through contact between skin surfaces that a condom does not cover. The level of protection provided by condoms against HPV transmission and its potential complications (genital warts and cervical cancer) has been widely acknowledged to be modest.[20]

"Safe" and "safer" sex presentations send a paradoxical message. We tell kids and adults alike that there is no such thing as safe smoking, and no one would say that using filtered cigarettes constitutes "safer smoking." Our messages about the hazards of drinking and driving or riding with an intoxicated driver are unequivocal, and we don't give lessons in "safer driving while under the influence." We don't explain how to survive an auto accident when you haven't buckled up. But when it comes to sex, we essentially tell kids and young adults, "We know you can't control yourself, so be sure to put on a condom and hope for the best. And, by the way, we won't mention that for many STIs condoms aren't terribly effective, because full disclosure would erode your confidence in them, and then you wouldn't bother to use them."

Reason No. 4: To prevent the devaluation of sex

Advocating that sex be kept within the boundaries of marriage is not based on notions that intercourse is dirty or unholy but on a true appreciation for sex as God's fine art. If the original *Mona Lisa* were entrusted to you for a month, you wouldn't leave it in your backyard, use it as a TV tray, or line a birdcage with it. Similarly, sex deserves more respect than our culture gives it.

- What truly devalues sex is the idea that intercourse is no more meaningful than a good meal or a drive in a sleek automobile.
- What stifles sexual satisfaction is casual copulation with little or no emotional involvement.
- What people miss in nonmarital sex is the opportunity for enjoyment far greater than the immediate sensual experience.

While movies and television often portray casual sex as the epitome of sensual excitement, a healthy, long-term marital relationship is actually the best setting for satisfying sexual experiences. Not surprisingly, the landmark 1992 National Health and Social Life Survey (NHSLS), summarized in the book *Sex in America: A Definitive Survey,* found that those who reported the most physical and emotional satisfaction with sex were the married couples.[21] It isn't difficult to understand why this should be the case. The security of commitment can free both husband and wife to relax rather than "perform," and their familiarity over a period of years allows them to please and excite one another with ever-increasing expertise and finesse. In a growing and deepening marriage relationship, sexuality can encompass far more than the superficial, bumper-sticker mentality of merely "doing it." Sex becomes a comfort, a natural stimulant (or relaxant), a playground, a special means of communication, and a bridge that can connect individuals to one another after a difficult day or season. Short-term relationships provide few, if any, of these benefits, and people involved in casual sex cannot approach them—or in some cases even comprehend them.

Reason No. 5: To prevent distorted relationships

Adding sex to a nonmarital relationship is like throwing a thousand-pound weight into a rowboat. The center of gravity drastically shifts, forward motion becomes difficult, and the whole thing may eventually sink. Sex has a particularly toxic effect on teenage romances, generating arguments, secrecy, stress, and guilt that replace laughter, discovery, and meaningful conversation.

Indeed, sex has a way of wrecking good relationships and keeping bad ones going long after they should have ended. After a sexual relationship is broken off, there is likely to be a sense of loss (sometimes severe), abandonment, guilt, regret, and depression, not to mention awkwardness whenever the other person is encountered. Condoms can't prevent a broken heart, and antibiotics can't cure one.

When one or both partners have had prior sexual experience, what's to guarantee that tonight's coupling isn't just another notch on the belt? Trust has become so foreign to the sexual playground that the phrase "trust me" has become the caricature come-on, the phrase uttered by the predator who hopes the intended prey is too dumb not to burst out laughing. Compare this with the experience of two people who have waited until marriage to initiate their sexual experience. For them the wedding night can be a time of discovery and bonding, and whatever they might lack in technique can be learned pleasantly enough at their own pace. Additionally, as we will see next, prior sexual experiences create memories and response patterns that may interfere with bonding and sexual intimacy in a future marital relationship.

Reason No. 6: To avoid devaluing one's sexuality and identity

We have already noted two important ways in which women have borne—and continue to bear—the brunt of the fallout from the sexual revolution that erupted during the 1960s: The woman virtually always pays a far bigger price than her partner when an unwanted pregnancy occurs, and with the exception of syphilis and AIDS, many sexually transmitted infections have more serious consequences in women than in men. But there is another critical arena in which far too many women have reaped a bitter harvest from seeds sown during the sexual revolution: the devaluation of their sexuality and their very identity.

For a woman, the ability to enjoy an uninhibited and healthy sexual response requires that her sexual experiences begin in a setting of complete trust, respect, and love. But if her sexual debut—a medical, not theatrical, term for a woman's initiation of sexual activity—occurs in a nonmarital relationship, it is unlikely that she will experience this nurturing context, even if sex occurs while she is feeling desperately "in love" with someone. All too often, in fact, the context is that of an immature, predatory, or even abusive relationship, especially when sexual experiences begin during adolescence and *inevitably* when they occur during childhood.

While the human race has never been free of sexual predators who seduce and victimize others, never has there been greater opportunity for humans to exploit sexuality than exists today. The resulting emotional and relational damage is incalculable, but it is particularly catastrophic when sexual exposure is both early and casual. When a child or adolescent (or, for that matter, an adult) becomes the object of another's selfish need for sexual release, the lessons are usually devastating. One of these is a strong sense of having been used, violated, and devalued. Instead of learning from experience and resolving not to be burned again, a sexually experienced adolescent—especially one for whom sex has not been entirely voluntary—is likely to think, *What does it matter now? I might as well just go ahead the next time.* Without specific counseling to counteract this damaged-goods mentality, resistance to continuing sexual activity may be seriously weakened. (This devaluation of both sexuality and self, while generally more common and profound in girls, certainly occurs in boys too.)

Another take-home lesson of nonmarital sexual experiences (especially early ones) is that a girl's or woman's sense of self-worth may become closely linked to her sexual usefulness to others. This conclusion is almost certain to have a destructive impact for both sexes, but it is especially significant for women, who more than men are positioned culturally to use sexuality as their power base. Once a woman is experienced or old enough to know how to be in control of sexual situations, her sexuality may become a tool—or even a weapon—that she can wield to get what she needs, especially if she has "learned" that no one else is looking out after her best interests. Sex often becomes a form of barter, both before and after marriage.

Ironically, even though she may look and act sexually sophisticated, this young woman's ability to *respond* sexually is almost certain to be compromised. Rather than something to be enjoyed in an uncomplicated way, sex is more likely to be experienced as a complex—and often contradictory—mixture of functions: as currency and power in a relationship or as a source of anxiety over a partner's approval. The latter can be a major source of conflict if a man is pressuring her into sexual acts that are uncomfortable or even degrading. Indeed, a woman may become so discouraged and embittered by such experiences that she may turn from relationships with men altogether and seek emotional and sexual fulfillment with other women.

We have focused on women in this segment, but we should not ignore the fact that men can develop significant issues regarding sex and their sexual identity as a result of childhood victimization. Men also can be emotionally devastated by the breakup of one or more relationships that involve sexual intimacy. Furthermore, men who have voluntarily and enthusiastically engaged in sex with numerous partners before deciding to settle down may bring a lot of emotional and physical baggage of their own into a marriage. They may have experienced sex repeatedly with partners who have had a variety of agendas and lovemaking techniques, and they may bring expectations for nonstop sexual novelty and excitement that have been shaped by viewing the shallow groping portrayed in pornography. But truly meaningful sex is built on a stable and more mature relationship, one in which sex is freely given and accepted by both individuals. What if a wife doesn't perform in the same way as his other partners? What happens when he wants sex and she isn't feeling well or their communication hasn't been particularly solid during the previous week?

Part Two: Maximizing and Sustaining the Gift of Sex for a Lifetime

God has created our sexuality as a wonderful gift. In this second section, we'll offer some basic principles and general directions for developing a healthy outlook on sex. Depending on the circumstances of your life at this time, you may well want to look deeper into one or more of these topics, perhaps using some of the resources we will recommend.

Understand that God created sex as a gift to enhance our lives

The Bible teaches that God cares about our sexuality and that He has identified the appropriate setting for physical intimacy as between one man and one woman within a marriage commitment. Furthermore, the Scriptures also clearly describe God's disapproval of sexual activity between people who are unmarried, married to someone else, or of the same gender, as well as between humans and animals. Jesus elaborated on Old Testament teachings on sexuality by pointing out to men that harboring lust for a woman is equivalent to having sex with her, a teaching that has rocked more than a few boats over the past two thousand years. (He also brilliantly and calmly rebuked those who might claim moral purity in this area when He invited anyone who was without sin to cast the first stone at a woman caught in adultery. Needless to say, He found no takers.) These teachings and stories have led more than one hormonally driven human to conclude that God must be the front-runner in the "Sexual Killjoy of the Universe" competition. Yet we can find plenty of evidence that the opposite is true.

In creating humankind, God chose to display His image through two very distinct but similar forms: *male* and *female*. The very first chapter of the Bible lays it out for us: "So God created man in his own image, in the image of God he created him; male and female he created them" (Genesis 1:27). Humans are the only part of creation that bears God's image, and He creates each of us in His image *at the level of our gender*. Richard Foster, author of the classic work *Celebration of Discipline*, beautifully summarizes the significance of this fact in his book *The Challenge of the Disciplined Life: Christian Reflections on Money, Sex and Power:*

> Our human sexuality, our maleness and femaleness, is not just an accidental arrangement of the human species, not just a convenient way to keep the human race going. No, it is at the center of our true humanity. We exist as male and female in relationship. Our sexualness, our capacity to love and be loved, is intimately related to our creation in the image of God. What a high view of human sexuality! [22]

Sexual intercourse is the means by which we have the privilege of participating in the creation of new life, something that as both Creator and lover of life God highly esteems. The fact that sex can generate such intense pleasure between a man and a woman is no accident but is in fact celebrated in the Bible, as amply demonstrated in the extended sensual poetry of the Song of Solomon in the Old Testament. Beyond procreation and pleasure, which are wondrous enough in themselves, sex and sexuality are key ingredients in the relationship of a man and a woman in marriage, epitomized by the biblical pronouncement that they become both figuratively and literally "one flesh": "For this reason a man will leave his father and mother and be united to his wife, and they will become one flesh" (Genesis 2:24). Richard Foster writes

> Sexual intercourse involves something far more than just the physical, more than even the emotions and psyche. It touches deep into the spirit of each person and produces a profound union that the biblical writers call "one flesh." Remember, we do not *have* a body, we *are* a body; we do not *have* a spirit, we *are* a spirit. What touches the body deeply touches the spirit as well.
>
> Sexual intercourse is a "life-uniting act," as Lewis Smedes calls it. And Derrick Baily has added, "Sexual intercourse is an act of the whole self which affects the whole self; it is a personal encounter between man and woman in which each does something to the other, for good or for ill, which can never be obliterated.
>
> Thus the reasoning behind the biblical prohibition of sexual intercourse for the unmarried goes beyond the common practical concerns of pregnancy or venereal disease or whatever. Genital sex outside of marriage is wrong [says Smedes] "because it violates the inner reality of the act; it is wrong because unmarried people thereby engage in a life-uniting act without a life-uniting intent."[23]

When viewed from this perspective, the idea that God disapproves of sex or somehow thinks of it as dirty or shameful is revealed to be patently absurd.

His prohibitions on sex outside of marriage arise from an exalted view of human sexuality that sees it as essential to our identity as beings created in His image and likeness, as well as the means by which we create life and as the literal unity of a man and a woman that establishes a new family. The so-called sexual freedom that was set loose in the 1960s—which in fact is an old set of attitudes and behaviors that has recycled through the human race for centuries—debases rather than celebrates the beauty, artistry, and power of sex.

Why belabor this point? Because in today's culture, where opportunities and pressure to be sexually active outside of marriage are so abundant, a spiritual commitment may be the last barrier standing between an individual (or a couple) and a damaging or disastrous sexual encounter. For those who care about God's opinion on this subject, it is important that not only His standards but also the *reasons* for the standards be clearly understood and regularly reflected upon. Otherwise, what was convicting and compelling last Sunday morning may seem theoretical and outdated on Friday night.

Take practical steps to maintain sexual experiences within the boundary of marriage

In theory, understanding the benefits of experiencing sexual activity only within marriage ought to be enough to create a fail-safe defense against sexual misadventures. In reality, even those with strong convictions may find themselves wondering how they wound up with an unexpected pregnancy, a sexually transmitted infection, or a relationship unraveled by one or more sexual encounters. Indeed, these missteps fuel the arguments of those who believe it is unrealistic for teenagers and single adults to remain sexually abstinent until marriage and insist that a detailed understanding of condoms and contraceptives is the only way to prevent the consequences of (inevitable) sexual activity among young and old alike.

Successfully managing internal and external sexual pressure involves a lot more than reciting "just say no" slogans, just as maintaining optimal health in any arena requires some practical and deliberate steps. Here are several to think about:

Guard the most important part of your sexuality: your mind. What movies and TV shows do you watch? What DVDs do you buy and rent? Does your cable carry "premium channels" that bring unedited sexual content into your living room? Do you browse the "adult" channels in your hotel room? What books and magazines do you read? What are your favorite Web sites? Sexual imagery, prose, and music lyrics readily take up residence in the mind and are difficult to dislodge. Furthermore, an abundance of "Do it! Everyone's doing it!" messages eventually wear down even well-fortified resistance to sexual misadventures. In chapter 8 we included a section called "Guarding the mind" (see page 368), which contains a number of practical suggestions to limit your family's exposure to provocative and destructive material. An important question to ponder: If something isn't appropriate for your teenager to watch, is it appropriate for you?

Don't tempt fate. Even when strongly committed to preserving sex until marriage, adolescents and adults alike are often surprisingly naive (or overconfident) regarding the seemingly irresistible urges that build once physical contact begins. Physical touch has powerful effects on us—after all, we're designed to be aroused by it—and a person should decide how much, for how long, and under what circumstances touch should be a part of a budding relationship. Remember, the person you find interesting or attractive—even one you meet in your church's youth or singles group—may have very different expectations and standards about what's appropriate when the two of you are by yourselves. Here are some guidelines to consider (and to teach to your adolescents, if you have any at home):

- *Establish clear and unequivocal respect for your body, your life, and your future.* Decide *before* the conversation, *before* the date, *before* the relationship gets more serious that physical intimacy is reserved for the wedding night.
- *Respecting yourself (and the person you're with) means setting your own limits for physical contact.* Stick to them, and be ready to defend them if necessary. Sexual pressure can become a major problem for a person who is unclear about boundaries, afraid of rejection, or worried about being called a prude.
- *Physical contact—even something as simple as holding hands—may be interpreted in ways you don't intend.* What to you means "I like you" or "I think you're okay" might be interpreted as "I'm madly in love with you" or "I want to go further." It's better to express how you feel in words, rather than through unclear and potentially powerful physical messages.
- *Remember that the events that lead to sex are progressive.* Think of a car gaining momentum as it coasts down a steep hill. Once a given level of intimacy has been reached, it is hard to back up to a more conservative one. Also, it is more difficult to defend a boundary in the heat of the moment.
- *You are much better off setting very conservative limits for expressing affection (holding hands and perhaps a brief embrace or kiss) and progressing slowly, both emotionally and physically, in a relationship.* This isn't old-fashioned but smart and realistic. More intense kissing, lying down together, touching personal areas, and increasing the amount of skin-to-skin contact sets off increasingly intense responses that are designed to lead to sexual intercourse—even if neither person intended this conclusion.
- *If you're not sure whether what you're doing physically is appropriate, ask yourself if you would be comfortable doing it in front of your family*

continued on page 594

THE SCOURGE OF PORNOGRAPHY

The pornography industry, and Internet pornography in particular, is so prolific that the statistics we quote here will almost certainly underestimate the scope of its reach and income by the time you read this book. Pornography is big business, and it does not promote the public welfare. A few disturbing numbers:

- The estimated total revenue of the pornography industry is $57 billion worldwide, of which $12 billion comes from the United States. This is more than the combined revenues of all professional baseball, football, and basketball franchises.
- The biggest component of the pornography business is adult videos ($20 billion), followed by "escort services" ($11 billion), magazines ($7.5 billion), sex clubs ($5 billion), phone sex ($4.5 billion), cable/pay-per-view television ($2.5 billion), and Internet ($2.5 billion).
- Child pornography generates an estimated $3 billion per year worldwide. More than 100,000 Web sites offer illegal child pornography.
- Some 11,000 pornographic movies are produced in the United States every year, more than twenty times the output of mainstream film companies.
- The estimated number of pornographic Web sites is 4.2 million (or 12 percent of the total), containing more than 370 million pages. Fewer than 15 million pages of Internet pornography existed in 1998; the number has increased more than twentyfold since that year.
- Twelve- to seventeen-year-olds are the largest consumer group for Internet pornography.
- Nine out of ten children and teenagers between the ages of eight and sixteen have viewed Internet pornography, most often accidentally while doing homework online. (A common scenario is that a neutral word entered into an Internet search engine links to a pornography site.)[24]

While defenders of uninhibited access to pornography may characterize it as harmless (if mindless) entertainment, this material in fact has profound effects on attitudes and behavior. Research has revealed the following trends among those with ongoing exposure to pornography:

- The emotional discomfort or disgust on first exposures disappears and eventually gives way to overt enjoyment.
- Habituation—like that seen with an addicting drug, where increased doses are required to have an effect—and boredom with depictions of "routine" male-female sex lead to an increased preference for material showing group sex, sadomasochistic practices, and sex with animals.
- Pornography fosters beliefs that premarital and nonmarital promiscuity is normal and healthy, and that "repression" of unrestrained sexual activity is unhealthy.

- Among men, prolonged exposure to pornography tends to promote callousness (sexual and otherwise) toward women, erode attitudes toward marriage, and decrease satisfaction with a spouse's appearance and sexual performance.
- Ongoing exposure to pornography is associated with an increased likelihood of antisocial and criminal behaviors, including sex with prostitutes, date and stranger rape, domestic violence, and incest.[25]

In testimony before a U.S. Senate Committee, Dr. Mary Anne Layden, co-director of the Sexual Trauma and Psychopathology Program at the University of Pennsylvania's Center for Cognitive Therapy, said

> Pornography Distortion is a set of beliefs based in pornographic imagery, sent to the viewer while they are aroused and reinforced by the orgasm. An example of Pornography Distortion would include beliefs such as, "Sex is not about intimacy, procreation or marriage. Sex is about predatory self-gratification, casual recreation, body parts, violence, feces, strangers, children, animals and using women as entertainment."[26]

Some books offering sexual advice to couples have made the misguided suggestion that watching pornography will add some spice to activities in the bedroom. Ironically, ongoing exposure to pornography is associated with impaired sexual performance in men, including premature ejaculation and erectile dysfunction, and mood disturbances in their wives.

As we noted in chapter 10 (dealing with tobacco, alcohol, and destructive drugs), entrenched behavior that has strong reinforcement rarely disappears easily. Confronting the problem, becoming educated about it, accepting responsibility for one's actions, beginning counseling, taking practical steps to limit exposure to provocative material, and maintaining accountability with others who are willing to exercise tough love are all part of the recovery process. Some recommended resources:

- *Every Man's Battle* and *Every Young Man's Battle* by Steve Arterburn and Fred Stoeker with Mike Yorkey (Colorado Springs, Colo.: WaterBrook Press, 2000 and 2002).
- *An Affair of the Mind: One Woman's Courageous Battle to Salvage Her Family from the Devastation of Pornography* by Laurie Hall (Colorado Springs, Colo.: Focus on the Family, 1998).
- "Breaking Free" at the Focus on the Family Web site contains practical information and a number of useful links for those seeking to overcome sexual addiction. See http://www.family.org/married/howtos/A0030352.cfm.
- A number of sexually related topics, including pornography, sexual addiction, and raising children with healthy attitudes toward sexuality, are discussed at http://www.pureintimacy.org. ■

continued from page 591

members or your pastor. Until you both say "I do" on your wedding day, you can't be certain that the person you are with now will be the one you will marry. Would you feel comfortable telling your future spouse you have done this?

- *Stay sober.* Alcohol and drugs cloud judgment and lower inhibitions. They also weaken your resolve against accepting (or offering) sexual overtures, not to mention undermining your ability to resist the pressure of a potential sexual predator.
- *If resisting physical intimacy is becoming more difficult, don't tempt fate.* Stay away from situations where the two of you are alone together. Deliberately plan to be around other people or in places where nothing can happen. Don't lie down on the sofa together to watch a video, and don't watch movies or videos with overt sexual content. Don't banter sexually provocative comments back and forth on the assumption that talk is safer than sex. Remember that your most important sexual organ is your mind, and where it goes your body will follow. (In some school sex-education programs, erotic conversations are actually recommended as an alternative to intercourse.)[27]

Beware of unhealthy relationships that carry an increased risk for sexual involvement

These include

- Relationships that ride a roller coaster of emotions—in which two people are madly in love one day, fighting like cats and dogs the next, crying and then making up after that—distract and drain a couple's time and energy. If "make-up sex" becomes part of the cycle, the drama and perpetual emotion of this type of relationship may make the process of terminating it even more difficult. These relationships routinely turn into difficult and toxic marriages.
- Relationships in which one person intensely needs, clings to, and smothers the other are not only draining, they are also more likely to be the setting for sexual pressure or overtures from the person who feels insecure.
- Relationships in which one person has a position of authority or leverage over some part of the other person's life—as an employer, work supervisor, teacher, family friend, or someone to whom a debt is owed—are inherently unhealthy and a setup for inappropriate contact or even date rape.

Precautions for women

Take prudent measures to protect yourself from date rape. Unless a woman lives a sheltered life, sooner or later she's almost certain to encounter some sort of sexual pressure. Sadly, the odds are at least one in ten (some researchers say one in six) that a woman will experience unwanted sex at some point in her life.[28] Obviously most socializing does not end in rape, and paranoia is an unpleasant mind-set to adopt during every outing with the opposite sex. But a little street wisdom can go a long way toward preventing a devastating or even life-threatening experience. Consider these basic precautions:

- You are much better off dating someone you know fairly well rather than someone who is a casual or chance acquaintance.
- In general, multicouple or group activities are less risky (and can be more fun) than one-on-one dates.
- Single dates—especially the first time with someone—should happen in a public place. An invitation to a play or a sporting event is far preferable to one to watch a DVD at his house by yourselves. Be especially leery of a suggestion to go someplace private to talk. Enjoyable and meaningful conversation can happen anyplace where two people can hear each other's voices.
- Consider accepting a blind date only if the person carries a strong endorsement from someone you trust. Even then, this should not be a single date.
- Bring your own money. Paying your own way in the early stages of a relationship can help establish your independence. Even if your date picks up the tab, you might need cash for transportation home if things get out of hand.
- Stay sober. Alcohol and drugs cloud judgment and put you off guard and off balance.
- Never leave a restaurant, party, or other get-together with someone you've just met.
- Trust your instincts. If you don't feel right about the way the date is progressing, bail out. A little awkwardness is far better than a sexual assault. Teenagers should have a clear understanding that they can call home at any time (no matter how late) and that a parent will come immediately to provide safe transportation, no questions asked.
- Avoid situations in which you do not feel on equal footing with your companion. If you feel intimidated, awestruck, or indebted to your date in some way, your willingness to speak up for yourself may be weakened or delayed. For a teenager, a date with someone more than two or three years older is a risky situation.
- Beware of expensive gifts and lavish dates. Too many men still carry the Neanderthal notion that picking up the tab for an expensive evening entitles them to a sexual thank you. If your date presents that message, don't hesitate to straighten him out. Declining a present that appears to have strings attached is a healthy way to set boundaries.
- Look out for the control freak, someone who insists on his way and ignores your likes and dislikes. If he shows contempt for your taste in

restaurants, movies, and music, he may also have little regard for your physical boundaries.

- Beware of the person who tries to isolate you from your other friends and family or who constantly bad-mouths them. If he is extremely possessive and wants you all to himself, chances are he will eventually want all of you sexually as well.
- Steer clear of men who tell raunchy jokes, listen to sexually explicit music, enjoy pornography, or make degrading comments about women. These behaviors arise from a distorted attitude about women and sexuality, and those who manifest them don't belong in your life.
- Don't waste your time with anyone who won't accept your limits; who begs, pleads, and haggles for physical contact; or who trots out worn and pathetic lines such as "If you loved me, you'd do it" or "Trust me." Anyone who pressures you for sexual favors is a loser and an abuser, and most certainly doesn't love you.

Don't go out of your way to arouse every male who sees you. Most women are well aware of what turns male heads, and many subscribe to the fashion philosophy, "If you've got it, flaunt it!" Because men are rapidly aroused by what they see, if you've "got it" and you wear clothes that reveal a lot of it, you'll certainly get attention—but probably not the type you want. What lies behind the double takes, friendly looks, or outright stares from men who appear to be admiring you is nearly always a mental undressing and some fantasy sex, all of which can occur within a few seconds. Some of those men will have violated their own moral and spiritual commitments in that short span of time, and you will have helped provoke an internal struggle that they will need to resolve with themselves, God, and perhaps another person to whom they are accountable. Other men who lack such restraint may try to figure out how to make their fantasies come true. While there is never an excuse for sexual pressure or rape, regardless of the woman's dress or demeanor, there is no need to tempt fate and risk a devastating experience.

Obviously, women shouldn't have to adopt the fashions of the 1890s when they go out in public, but it's also possible to look terrific without dressing provocatively. If you have any question about the potential impact of your apparel on masculine sensitivities, you might ask the opinion of a trusted and conservative male—an older brother or even your father, for example—before you take it out on the street. Similarly, think twice before you appear in public in the bathing suit that leaves little to the imagination, because men will use their imagination to fill in the details of what they can't see.

Precautions for men

Treat members of the opposite sex respectfully and responsibly. It is impossible to calculate the damage done every day by men who entice, pressure, or force women of all ages into sexual activity. These experiences affect women physically, emotionally, relationally, and spiritually. They may lower her resistance to other destructive sexual encounters in the future. They will almost certainly have a detrimental effect on her emotional and sexual bonding with her future husband. Some of these experiences create wounds that leave permanent scars that never quite heal, even with ongoing counseling. Bottom line: Girls and women are not playthings to be used for whatever sexual gratification they might provide before being shoved aside like leftovers. Each one is someone's daughter and probably someone's future (if not present) wife. Each is of inestimable value to God and is to be cherished, valued, respected, and protected. To that end, men should plant the following messages deeply in their minds and emotions, and teach them fervently to their sons:

- *Never become a sexual predator.* A male who specifically sets out to maneuver women into sexual encounters might be called a playboy, red-hot lover, or Don Juan, but he's basically a jerk. Remember that this type of manipulation isn't only physical. Deploying emotionally charged statements ("I love you, I need you") as a tactic to lower a woman's sexual resistance is as dishonorable as using alcohol, drugs, or even physical intimidation. This is no way to treat any woman.
- *Never push a woman's physical boundaries.* If she says no to anything, even holding hands, that statement is final and not to be questioned.
- *Respect and maintain a woman's body, integrity, and future, even if she is inviting intimacy.* Without question, one of the most difficult challenges for a healthy male is to hold your ground when a desirable female (to whom you're not married) flashes a bright and explicit green light. It is important neither to go full speed ahead nor to be flustered or embarrassed, but rather to decline the invitation in a way that expresses a desire to protect your and her future. Obviously, this requires a prior commitment to this course of action and some forethought about what you might say—or how to walk away—should such a situation arise.
- *Approach any activity or relationship with a person of the opposite sex with the intention of enhancing that person's life and not leaving a wake of regrets.* Thinking in terms of protecting the other person's long-term well-being rather than merely satisfying immediate needs or desires is a sign of maturity.

Within marriage, take deliberate steps that will allow sex to bloom and flourish

The fact that the words "I now pronounce you man and wife" have been uttered does not mean that unbridled sexual bliss is now a certainty. In addition to their suitcases, a husband and wife may bring all kinds of baggage on their honeymoon—such as their past sexual history, guilt about sex, or even expectations that sex will be ecstatic the first time and every time thereafter. The reality is that sex, like the relationship in which it occurs, is a living, growing, blooming, maturing entity. It is likely to involve false starts, misfires, mistakes, pleasant interludes, playfulness, passion, and, yes, some fireworks of the good kind. Overall it needs to be planted in good, rich soil—a relationship that is not only fueled by physical and emotional attraction but also is stable, mutually respectful, deeply committed to each other's well-being, and firmly grounded in each person's devotion to God. Once planted, it needs to be nurtured, studied, and most of all handled with care. Like all other aspects of good health, this is a deliberate process.

Here are some basic principles to keep in mind:

Learn how things work. Many otherwise well-educated adults are surprisingly ignorant about the anatomy and physiology of their own and their spouse's reproductive system, even if they have had a number of sexual experiences before marriage. Unfortunately, what they *have* learned may be a piecemeal mixture of facts and misinformation that has arrived from a variety of sources of variable reliability: a sweaty-palmed "birds and bees" lecture from Mom and Dad years ago; an older sibling or "experienced" friend; a health-education class; or perhaps some steamy scenes in movies, romance novels, or even pornography.

Obviously, when dealing with a subject as emotionally charged as sexuality—especially yours and your spouse's—it is important to consult sources that are not only factually accurate but also morally and spiritually sound. There is no shortage of books that provide lots of explicit details in a context that advocates an anything-goes mentality, whether inside or outside of a marital relationship. Fortunately, other resources provide myth-busting, reliable information about this subject in a way that honors sexuality, marriage, and the Creator of both. The classic books of this genre are *The Gift of Sex: A Guide to Sexual Fulfillment* by Dr. Clifford and Joyce Penner (W Publishing Group, revised edition 2003) and *Intended for Pleasure* by Dr. Ed and Gaye Wheat (Revell, third edition 1997).

Open and maintain lines of communication regarding sex with your spouse. Even couples who enjoy talking about everything under the sun may not communicate at all about what goes on between the sheets. Perhaps they're afraid of hurting the other person's feelings, sounding naive, or "talking dirty." They may mistakenly believe that their bodies, or whatever sounds they make during lovemaking, are saying it all. Many problems arise in marriage because couples don't know how to approach topics that are emotionally sensitive or a potential source of conflict. Few parents deliberately model for their children the process of respectfully resolving an issue—especially one involving their sex life—although far too many foolishly hurl insults at one another while their wide-eyed and terrified kids watch. In other words, talking candidly and carefully about what is and isn't working in the bedroom is an interpersonal skill most of us lack, but one that is worth cultivating. Not surprisingly, most of the basic ground rules of good communication in marriage also apply when sex is the topic:

- When you like something your spouse does before, during, or after sex, feel free to say so—right away, later, or both. (To make things interesting, put one or more of these thoughts in a romantic card, but be sure your beloved will be the only one who reads it.) Nothing builds confidence in this area like positive feedback. Don't hesitate to be specific: "That really feels good" or "I enjoy it when you . . ."
- When you *don't* like something your spouse does before, during, or after sex, you should say something—but pick the time, place, and words carefully. A critique offered immediately after the fact is likely to be discouraging and may set up an unhealthy performance mode for the other person. Likewise, a disparaging comment about last night's sexual encounter that is tossed into an argument about a different subject is like a verbal hand grenade that will injure rather than inform. In chapter 16, we discuss some ground rules for resolving conflicts respectfully and without inflicting damage to the other person. (If this is troubled territory in your marriage, you may want to review this section, which begins on page 802.) All the dos and don'ts for discussing an issue are particularly applicable to conversations about sex. "Why . . ." questions and "You always . . ." statements are likely to be inflammatory. In contrast, mentioning something you *do* like will start things on a constructive note, and then specific suggestions ("Why don't we try . . . " or "I think I would enjoy sex more if . . .") are more likely to yield a positive response. If sex really isn't going well and you can't figure out how to talk through the issues, don't hesitate to go to a counselor for help.
- Think carefully about how much you should disclose to your spouse (or your future spouse, if you are engaged) about any prior sexual experiences. The person with whom you share (or will share) your bed deserves to know something about any sexual partners you have been with, *especially* if you are or might be carrying a long-term infection such as herpes simplex, HPV, or HIV that the other might acquire. (The fact that any of these might be present isn't necessarily a reason to call off an engagement, by the way. But a careful medical review and appropriate diagnostic testing, if necessary, can help clarify whether an uninfected partner-to-be is at risk for an infection in the future.) On the other hand, a detailed account of your prior sexual activities may plant images in your spouse's mind that are likely to be both painful and permanent.

  If you have a complex sexual history—especially one marked by sexual abuse or trauma early in life—you should seriously consider reviewing it with a counselor who is well versed in this subject, because your experiences are almost certain to affect your sexual response to your spouse. The counselor can guide you not only in the healing process but also in determining how much you should disclose.

- Under no circumstances should you ever compare your spouse's sexual performance unfavorably with that of a previous partner. To do so is cruel, disrespectful, and a surefire way to decrease the likelihood of enthusiastic sex in the future. Even a *favorable* comparison with a previous partner is unwise, because it is likely to bring to his or her mind troubling images of your physical intimacy with another person.

Seek to understand the differences between men and women in sexual needs and responses

This is arguably the area in which couples make the most avoidable blunders and in which attention to a few basic principles can make a world of difference in the bedroom. At the risk of greatly oversimplifying concepts about which many books have been written, here are some basic observations about each gender, written for the benefit of the other.

What women need to understand about men

In general, the male libido tends to be a rather straightforward—some might argue primitive—entity throughout the teen and adult years. This is manifested in a number of ways:

Men are strongly visually oriented. When the image of an attractive woman—whether in person, on a page, or on a screen—arrives at the male retina and transmits to his brain, there is immediate interest and potential arousal, even when he is strongly committed to sexual morality and loyalty to his spouse. This immediate interest has nothing to do with the woman's identity, intelligence, personality, accomplishments, or moral character. It is literally hardwired into the male brain, and attempts to prevent it from occurring when the female stimulus is present are futile. Men, especially younger men trying to maintain moral purity, may beat themselves into the ground because they have this response, not realizing that it is normal. *What they do about it* is what counts from the moral and spiritual perspective. (See sidebar: "Looking or Lusting?" on page 603.)

It is the responsibility of the husband to love, honor, and cherish his wife, regardless of the impact that years of living, childbearing, and other forms of wear and tear have had on her physical appearance. Period. It doesn't hurt, however, when wives do what they can to make themselves more physically attractive. But the reason and context for doing so are critical. Is it merely a tactic to keep up with the competition? In the 1960s, women were given the following advice in the popular but not exactly sensitive song "Wives and Lovers": "Day after day, there are girls at the office, and men will always be men. Don't send him off with your hair still in curlers. You may not see him again."[29]

While these rather inane lyrics contain a kernel of truth about the potential for women at the workplace to draw a man's visual attention, they also send an unhealthy message to wives: "Your relationship isn't secure unless you remain more attractive and sexy than the other women who might cross your husband's path." Obviously, a young mother who is exhausted after sleepless nights and busy days caring for infants and toddlers may not feel inspired, as this song suggests, to "wear something pretty . . . and . . . start the music—time to get ready for love."[30]

A healthier reason for making an effort to maintain one's physical appearance (and perhaps to start the music now and then) is that it is one of many expressions of love for the other person and one of many responses to feeling respected and cared for. If you care about your home, you spend time and energy on its upkeep. You could do this because you want to feel superior to your neighbors, but a better reason is to create a place that is inviting and pleasant, where relationships grow and memories are made. Maintaining their physical appearance is not just an agenda item for women, by the way. Wives are not likely to be turned on when their husbands allow themselves to develop a sizeable "spare tire" or pay attention to grooming, clothing, or bodily aromas only when it's time to go to work.

A man's desire for sex not only remains active and constant throughout his adult life, but it also is typically ready for action at a moment's notice. A not-so-old adage says that in sexual matters men tend to be like microwaves—heating up fast and sounding off in a few minutes when they're done—while women are more like Crock-Pots—offering a delicious payoff after some careful preparation and a day of simmering. A couple may have had a difficult week, a long and tiring day, and little communication (or even an ongoing argument) through the evening. For the wife, nothing in the last seventy-two hours has remotely inspired any interest in sex. But before bedtime her husband sees her walk by in a clingy nightgown, and he's ready for sex *right now,* regardless of what has happened over the past several hours.

Unlike most women, men generally do not need a period of feeling loved and cared for before they want to engage in sex. In fact, a man may crave sex even in the midst of conflict or during a "dry spell," because if his wife is willing to have sex it must mean that hostilities are ending. This, of course, is likely to create a negative reaction from an astonished woman who cannot fathom having sex until harmony is restored. If a husband talks, cajoles, pleads with, or threatens her into sex when she truly doesn't want it, when he's done she may feel like a prostitute with a wedding ring. If she refuses, he may feel rejected and deflated. There are, fortunately, alternatives that are far better than either of these outcomes, but they require some understanding and effort. Read on.

Believe it or not, men don't "just want sex." Men desire love and connectedness as much as women. Many wives have a difficult time grasping the fact that a husband hears "I love you" when his partner is sexually responsive. A wife may honestly feel that she is saying "I love you" in countless other ways—bearing and mothering his children, for example—and may be perplexed and frustrated that this seems to pale in comparison with the importance of sex on a frequent basis. A husband, meanwhile, can become extremely confused and frustrated when his wife's libido seems to evaporate within a year or two of the wedding. Because spirited sex is perceived as a declaration of love, a man may feel rejected (or even punished) when his wife displays a lack of enthusiasm in the bedroom and a seemingly endless list of excuses why sex must be put off . . . again.

What men need to understand about women

There are normal variations in a woman's libido. While most men experience relatively little fluctuation in sexual drive throughout their life span, a woman's libido can wax and wane depending on the season of her life and other circumstances. But a host of powerful messages and images throughout our culture propagate a myth that healthy women, like men, are continuously interested in sex once puberty arrives. Consequently, women who experience normal variations in sexual interest may feel inadequate or even defective, and they may be reluctant to discuss their sexual needs with their husband. At the start of a relationship, sex is the by-product of great passion shared between two people. (Indeed, a woman's libido is likely to be at its highest level when seeking a mate or desiring to become pregnant.) But as the relationship deepens and matures, a woman's physiological need for sex decreases and her psychological need for emotional connectedness becomes requisite for a sexual interlude.

Unlike a man's typical willingness to have sex at a moment's notice, a woman's interest in sex directly correlates with how well loved and respected she feels in the relationship *overall*. For a man, sex is an important barometer of the status of the relationship: If sex is happening regularly and is satisfying (at least for him), things must be going okay. By contrast, after (or even during) the honeymoon, his wife's desire for sexual contact will be a *result* of her general satisfaction in the relationship.

Women don't lose interest in sex itself as much as they lose their desire for sex when certain conditions are not being met. Far too many men don't understand that paying attention to the quality of the relationship *prior* to sex stimulates a woman's sexual responsiveness. A woman needs to know that she is supported and respected in the relationship within the day(s) preceding a sexual encounter, and she is likely to be hurt, angry, or at best unenthusiastic when she is asked for sex after days of being ignored. Unlike men, arousal doesn't happen quickly for most women. It happens long before there is physical desire, as she feels sensuous and attractive in response to a man's focused attention—not just in the form of traditional romantic gestures, but (more importantly) in his ongoing willingness both to listen and to perform everyday acts of caring.

LOOKING OR LUSTING?

When does the normal male response to the sight of a female body become lust, an attitude of the mind that is objectionable to God? For thousands of years, men highly concerned about God's standards have agonized over their vulnerability to the female form, sometimes taking extreme measures in a futile effort to suppress it. (One particularly foolish approach in some cultures involves harsh measures against women, who are supposedly to blame for the male response to them.)

A more sensible approach is to consider both the *object of interest* and the *intention of the one who is interested.* As we noted earlier, in the Song of Solomon the Bible offers a vivid account of a couple's enjoyment of emotional and physical intimacy. There is nothing in Scripture to suggest that a man can't or shouldn't relish the sight of his wife's body or contemplate past, present, and future sexual experiences with her. But entertaining the same thoughts about another man's wife or an unmarried woman is another matter, one that involves separating sex from its proper context and mentally violating someone whom God—not to mention a present or future husband—cherishes.

While the question of who should or shouldn't be an object of male sexual interest is relatively straightforward, determining the boundary between normal responses and outright lust can be more difficult. Some might argue that the initial male response to an unintentional viewing of an attractive female form constitutes lust, but to meet this standard of purity a man would somehow have to prevent any woman with a recognizable shape from coming within range of his eyes. Unless one lives in utter seclusion or resides in a culture where women dress in robes and cover their faces, this is impossible—but controlling what happens next isn't. As the old saying goes, you can't keep the birds from flying over your head, but you can keep them from building a nest in your hair.

If a response to an unintentional sighting is unavoidable, a man *can* resist the stare, the second (or third) look, or the deliberate effort to see more. The three-second rule is one guideline—it only takes three seconds (or less) to register the fact that a woman or a visual image is sexually stimulating, so any lingering beyond that time crosses the lust line. So does deliberately thumbing through a provocative magazine (or even swimsuit and lingerie catalogs that arrive in the mailbox), surfing through cable channels and pausing where there's some skin showing, or going out of one's way to get another look at the scantily clad woman who just crossed the street or is lying on the beach. And, of course, so does mentally undressing and fantasizing about sex with whomever one sees on a screen or magazine cover or while strolling through the mall. For many men these behaviors are literally second nature. However, avoiding them is not beyond the reach of a commitment that a man makes to God and to his present or future wife. ■

Author Kevin Leman summarized this reality in the title of one of his books: *Sex Begins in the Kitchen*. While a man is quickly aroused by the sight of his wife's body, she is far more interested in sex when she has heard "I love you" in a variety of ways over the course of the day or the week. The smart husband understands the many ways his wife hears these words. These may include:

- Kind words and compliments on a regular basis. A phone call in the middle of the day to say, "Hi, I was just thinking about you," speaks volumes.
- Kind acts of service: doing the dishes, helping put the kids to bed, filling up her gas tank, pulling out her chair at the dining table or in a restaurant, opening and closing her car door, and so on.
- Specific romantic gestures: giving her flowers and cards (especially when unexpected); making the arrangements for a nice dinner out or a weekend away (including child care); remembering special occasions (not just her birthday and your anniversary, but others, such as the anniversary of your first date or the day you got engaged).
- Physical affection that isn't necessarily sexual or foreplay: hand holding, cuddling, hugging, or giving a foot massage, for example.

HOT TIP

These loving acts are more effective if they are part of the flow of everyday life, rather than appearing to be a contrivance designed to elicit a sexual thank you.

Women don't have to achieve an orgasm in order to feel intimate and connected during sex. Many men mistakenly believe that unless their wife reaches orgasm, they are inconsiderate or inept lovers. The truth is that many if not most normal sexually healthy women have orgasms only some of the time, and it is not necessarily a reflection of the prowess of their partner. But because of a lack of some basic communication, a wife can get into the bad habit of pretending to have an orgasm because (1) she knows her husband's feelings will be hurt if it doesn't appear that the earth moved during sex or (2) she's checked her watch and knows she has to be up in six hours to get the kids up for school and thus needs to hasten the process.

Believe it or not, many wives, assuming their marital relationship is basically healthy, would be willing to have sex more often if they knew it could be "short and sweet." If a man is willing to lower his expectations for how high his wife's Richter scale will register during a given encounter, she may well be agreeable to sex more often—a definite win-win situation.

This doesn't mean that a man shouldn't be invested in his wife's enjoyment of sex. Indeed, making a conscious effort to understand what enhances her sexual experience, and putting that understanding into consistent action, will bear some very rich fruit over the course of a marriage. Here's one idea to think about: If a husband hopes to have a special sexual interlude that will rock his wife's world, he will need to plan ahead to be sure that a few key elements are in place:

- She feels well loved in the days prior to the encounter.
- She doesn't have to get up early the next morning.
- There is plenty of time for as much foreplay (massaging, kissing, etc.) as she needs to become physically aroused.
- He devotes enough time and energy to ensure her complete sexual satisfaction.

Don't ignore trouble spots in your sexual relationship

Be willing to seek counseling for sexual issues. Sex is such a sensitive subject that people often enter the counseling room with fear and trembling if a sexual problem is on the agenda. But far too often this important dimension of life and love remains a source of great personal pain or of turbulence within marriage because it is considered off-limits for discussion with anyone. Obviously this isn't a matter for casual conversation over a quick lunch. Working through one or more sexual issues takes time and careful conversation with an experienced and sensitive counselor. Subjects of particular importance include:

- Healing from the effects of previous sexual experiences, especially any involving abuse or rape and, even more critically, any that occurred during childhood
- Healing from a past pregnancy loss (whether abortion, miscarriage, or stillbirth)
- Dealing with sexual problems within a marriage, including differences in expectations, communication issues, current and past events that are affecting sexual interest and satisfaction, and so on
- Dealing with the fallout from emotional or sexual infidelity, which can have a profound effect on all dimensions of the marriage relationship, including sexuality

Take deliberate measures to affair-proof your marriage. Very often a violation of marriage vows doesn't occur in a sudden act of careless passion, but rather it is the result of a gradual progression of seemingly innocent activities with someone of the opposite sex, such as:

- Increasingly personal conversations at work, online, or even at church, especially when marital problems are discussed
- One or more meals with a coworker that last a little longer than needed to conduct business
- A touch or even a meeting of the eyes that is prolonged just enough to potentially communicate more than innocent friendship

These and similar interactions are more likely to lead to inappropriate behaviors (emotional, sexual, or both) when a marriage is dry or turbulent and when either the husband or wife feels stressed, unappreciated, and worn-out by the daily demands of living. Indeed, affairs of the emotions and body very often arise when another person seems to offer a listening ear, understanding, and compliments that seem scarce at home.

Aside from affirming your commitment to maintain the integrity of your marriage and taking ongoing measures to enhance that relationship, some practical decisions can help prevent a potentially disastrous indiscretion. Most of these involve following a simple but profound advisory from the New Testament: "But among you there must not be even a hint of sexual immorality" (Ephesians 5:3). You can stay out of trouble by asking yourself a simple but important question: *Could what I'm doing [or considering doing] even remotely be construed as inappropriate, even if it is perfectly innocent?* By being careful to avoid what might *appear* out of line or raise questions, you will also avoid situations that are risky or could catch you off guard.

Obvious safeguards include avoiding traveling or dining alone with a

HOW OFTEN IS "NORMAL"?

One question that many husbands and wives wonder about is whether their sex life is "normal." Is there a certain frequency of intercourse that is typical or healthy, too much or not enough? As with many themes related to sexuality, this isn't a typical topic for the family dinner table or casual conversation with friends. Research has provided some idea of the range of sexual frequency among married couples, but this should not necessarily be used as a yardstick by which one person decides "I'm not getting enough" or "We're doing it too often." The 1992 National Health and Social Life Survey (NHSLS), mentioned earlier in this chapter, found that about 45 percent of eighteen- to fifty-nine-year-old married couples reported having sex "a few times a month" while 35 percent said "two to three times a week." Smaller percentages reported less or more frequent sex: 12 percent reported having sex only "a few times a year," while 7 percent said they have sex four or more times a week.[31]

What matters more than these numbers is whether both husband and wife find the frequency and overall experience satisfying. If a husband and wife have a definite and persistent difference of opinion regarding how often each would like to have sex, and how pleasurable (or not) it tends to be, some communication is definitely in order. If the couple can't agree on a course of action that is truly satisfactory to each person, some counseling would be a wise investment. Remember: when dealing with sex, there is no such thing as winning an argument. If one person browbeats or outflanks the other in a verbal duel over their sex life, he or she shouldn't expect an enthusiastic physical or emotional response in the near future. ■

coworker of the opposite sex, as well as maintaining friendships with one or more people (of your own gender) with whom you have absolute accountability in this area and who have your permission to ask tough and penetrating questions.

Be willing to seek medical or counseling help regarding specific sexual dysfunctions. Healthy sexuality is a complex process that is affected both by physical factors—such as the stage of life; the state of neurological, vascular, and endocrine systems; and the effects of medications and alcohol use—and by psychological, emotional, and spiritual factors, such as family upbringing, interpersonal relationships, faith commitment, and history of sexual experiences. Issues arising in any of these areas may lead to what are called **sexual dysfunctions**. The most common of these in men are erectile dysfunction, decreased desire, and ejaculatory disorders. Among women, decreased desire, painful intercourse (called **dyspareunia**), as well as arousal and orgasmic disorders are the most common sexual dysfunctions. We provide an overview in the appendix titled "Common Sexual Dysfunctions" beginning on page 945.

Don't let your sex life become stale. Many married couples leave their imagination at the bedroom door and get into a routine that settles for the "same old, same old" every time they have sex. This may of course be a reflection of many other dimensions of their marriage that perhaps need some attention, but even couples with solid relationships and communication might want to consider exploring some ways to enhance their sexual experiences. This does *not* mean that they should venture into areas of sexuality that are uncomfortable, degrading, or dangerous. Remember that while some sexual self-help books recommend viewing pornography as a way for a couple to spice up their sex life, this is in fact a terrible idea. (See sidebar "The Scourge of Pornography," which begins on page 592.)

The good news is that intimacy can be enhanced with fun, gentleness, respect, and joy. A number of helpful resources, including those listed below, can help you and your spouse explore new and intriguing territory.

FOR MEN:

What Wives Wish Their Husbands Knew about Women
Dr. James Dobson (Tyndale, 1988)

FOR WOMEN:

Intimate Issues: 21 Questions Christian Women Ask about Sex
Linda Dillow and Lorraine Pintus (WaterBrook Press, 1999)

FOR EVERYONE:

The Five Love Languages
Gary Chapman (Moody, 1996)

The Gift of Sex: A Guide to Sexual Fulfillment
Dr. Clifford and Joyce Penner (W Publishing Group, revised edition 2003)

Hedges: Loving Your Marriage Enough to Protect it
Jerry B. Jenkins (Crossway Books, 2005)

The Language of Love
Gary Smalley and John Trent (Focus on the Family, 1999)

Sexual Intimacy in Marriage
Dr. William Cutrer and Sandra Glahn (Kregel Publications, 2001)

Simply Romantic Nights
(FamilyLife, 2001)
Simply Romantic Secrets
(FamilyLife, 2003)
These activity kits to help couples plan meaningful encounters are available from FamilyLife (http://www.familylife.com) or Focus on the Family (http://www.family.org).

QUESTIONS TO PONDER

1. What makes human sexuality one of God's greatest gifts to people?
2. How would you summarize the physical, emotional, and spiritual reasons for preserving sexual activity for marriage?
3. If you are married, how would you rate the level of sexual intimacy between you and your spouse?
4. If you are single, what are your greatest struggles in the area of sexuality? Which suggestions on pages 590–597 might help you keep your head in sexually charged situations?

Action items: If you are married, make a date to sit down and talk openly with your spouse about your sexual relationship. What might you and your spouse do to enhance and protect it? See pages 597–608 for some ideas.

If you or your spouse is dissatisfied with your sexual relationship, talk about some of the possible causes. Consider seeking help from a Christian counselor if the problems seem insurmountable.

Talk about the differences between the sexual response of men and women (see pages 600–605). How might knowing about these differences change your response to your spouse?

If you have teenagers living in your home, do you think they have picked up any of society's misconceptions about sexuality? If so, how might you begin to present them with the truth?

Whether you are married or single, the resources listed on pages 607–608 can help you appreciate your sexuality and better understand its place within marriage. Which one might address any questions you might have about this part of your life? Pick it up at your local Christian bookstore or library, or order online from http://www.family.org.

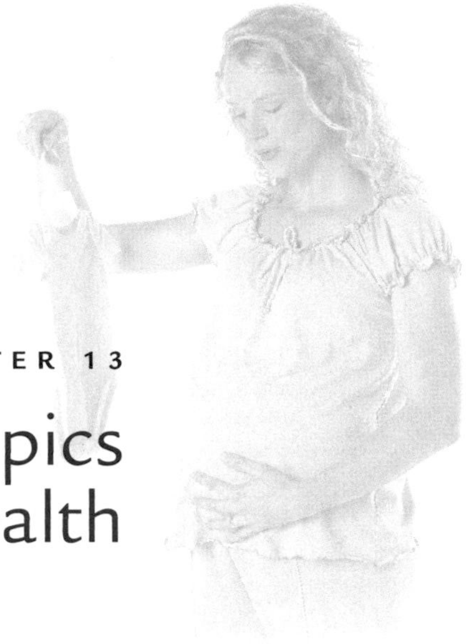

CHAPTER 13

Selected Topics in Women's Health

Most of the information and advice in this book applies equally to men and women (and their children). Regardless of gender, we all need nourishing food, regular exercise, restorative sleep, meaningful work, and time to relax. We all need to monitor the status of our body and take reasonable precautions against threats to life and health. We all need to free ourselves from harmful addictions. We all need to nurture our emotions. We all need to grow in our relationship with God. None of these priorities are unique to men or to women.

There are, however, some health concerns that affect women and not men (at least directly). As you might have guessed, most of these are related to a woman's unique and wondrous ability to reproduce. The hormonal environment that brings a woman to sexual maturity, the monthly cycles that prepare her for the possibility of starting a new life, the dramatic changes of pregnancy and childbirth, and the conclusion of her monthly cycles at menopause—all of these can have a profound impact on her health.

You will notice that this chapter title includes the word *Selected*. Entire books have been written about women's health and, for that matter, about each of the concerns we are covering in this chapter. What follows is a look at some specific subjects involving a woman's reproductive cycle that are not only important but also at times controversial.

Before we begin, it's important to remember that some specific topics of concern to women are covered elsewhere in this book:

- **Cardiovascular disease.** You might think that heart attacks and strokes are a "guy thing," but these are in fact equal-opportunity conditions, and they kill more women than all forms of cancer *combined*.

Chapter 3 discusses this problem in detail, and chapter 4 explains how your risk factors are assessed.

- **Exercise.** Aerobic conditioning and strength training aren't just for athletes, and certainly not just for men. Women of all ages need to make exercise a priority, as we discuss in detail in chapter 7.
- **Breast cancer.** Risk factors, screening options (including self-examination and mammography), and prevention are discussed in detail in chapter 4, beginning on page 88.
- **Ovarian cancer.** Risk factors, screening options, and prevention are also discussed in chapter 4, beginning on page 105.
- **Cervical cancer.** Risk factors (in particular the role of the sexually transmitted HPV virus), screening (including a detailed look at the Pap smear), and prevention are discussed in chapter 4, beginning on page 107.
- **Sexuality.** In the previous chapter, we advocated the medical, emotional, and spiritual wisdom of enjoying sex within the bounds of an exclusive marriage relationship. While this advice flies in the face of the messages broadcast far and wide by popular culture, it is particularly important for women to ponder, since they bear the brunt of the consequences of sexual (mis)adventures. Not only does unintended pregnancy force millions of women to make agonizing—indeed, literal life-and-death—decisions every year, but many (though not all) sexually transmitted diseases are much harder on women than men.
- **Depression and chronic fatigue.** These common problems affect both sexes, but they tend to occur more often among women. We have already looked at depression in chapter 8 and will offer some help for chronic fatigue in chapter 16.

The Cycle of Life

In case your memories of your high school health-education classes and perhaps your childbirth classes are a little fuzzy, the following is a primer on the menstrual cycle, followed by some recommendations to help you deal with any discomfort it might bring.[1]

Under normal circumstances, each month a woman's body performs a three-act play entitled "Preparing for a Baby." What you are about to read is a summary of the essential characters and plot. (As with many other aspects of human physiology, there are thousands of other details that will not be spelled out here and thousands more yet to be discovered. The design of this process is indeed exquisite.)

The main characters in the play are:

- The **hypothalamus**: a multifaceted structure at the base of the brain that regulates basic bodily functions such as temperature and appetite. It also serves as the prime mover in the reproductive cycle.

- The **pituitary**: a small, punching-bag-shaped structure that appears to dangle from the brain directly below the hypothalamus. It has been called the "master gland" because it gives orders to many other organs. But it also takes important cues from the hypothalamus.
- The **ovaries**: a matched pair of organs in the female pelvis that serve two critical functions—releasing one or more eggs (or ova) each month and secreting the hormones **estrogen** and **progesterone**. At birth the ovaries contain about 2 million eggs, a woman's lifetime supply. During childhood, the vast majority of these gradually disappear, and by the time a girl reaches puberty only about three hundred thousand will be left. During her reproductive years, she will release between three hundred and five hundred eggs; the rest will die and disappear.
- The **uterus**: a pear-shaped organ consisting primarily of muscle and containing a cavity where a baby grows during pregnancy. This cavity is lined with delicate tissue called **endometrium**, which changes remarkably in response to estrogen and progesterone produced by the ovaries. The uterus, also called the womb, is located at the top of the vagina and positioned in the middle of the pelvis between the bladder and the rectum.
- The **fallopian tubes**: a pair of tubes, about four to five inches long, attached to the upper corners of the uterus and extending toward each ovary. Their job is to serve as a meeting place for egg and sperm and then to transport a fertilized egg to the uterus.

Act I: Preparing an egg for launch (the follicular phase)

The hypothalamus begins the monthly reproductive cycle by sending a message called **gonadotropin-releasing hormone (GnRH)** to the pituitary gland, which lies directly below it. The pituitary responds by secreting into the bloodstream another biochemical message known as **follicle-stimulating hormone** (or **FSH**), which prepares an egg to be released by the ovary. Each egg within an ovary is covered with a thin sheet of cells, and the term **follicle** (which literally means "little bag") refers to the entire package of egg and cells together. Under the influence of FSH, eight to ten follicles begin to grow and "ripen." Usually only one becomes dominant and progresses to full maturity.

This **follicular phase** of the cycle lasts about two weeks, during which the dominant follicle fills with fluid and enlarges to about three-quarters of an inch. The egg contained within it will soon be released from the ovary. At the same time, this follicle secretes increasing amounts of estrogen, which (among other things) stimulates the lining of the uterus to proliferate and thicken. This is the first stage of preparation of the uterus for the arrival of a fertilized egg.

Act II: The egg is released (ovulation)

As in Act I, this part of the story begins in the hypothalamus. In response to rising levels of estrogen, the hypothalamus signals the pituitary to release a brief but intense surge of **luteinizing hormone** (or **LH**) into the bloodstream. This hormone sets off a chain reaction in the ovary. The dominant follicle enlarges, its outer wall becomes thin, and finally it ruptures, releasing egg and fluid. This mini-eruption called **ovulation** takes only a few minutes and occurs between twenty-four and forty hours after the peak of the LH surge. Sometimes a tiny amount of blood oozes from the ovary as well. This may irritate the lining of the abdomen, producing a discomfort known as **mittelschmerz** (German for "middle pain," because it occurs about halfway through the cycle).

Act III: The egg's voyage and preparation of the uterus (the luteal phase)

The egg is not left to its own devices once it is set free from the ovary. At the end of each fallopian tube are structures called **fimbriae** (Latin for "fingers"), whose delicate tentacles move over the area of the ovary. As soon as ovulation takes place, the fimbriae gently escort the egg into the tube, where it begins a journey toward the uterus. The cells that line the fallopian tube have microscopic, hair-like projections called **cilia**, which move in a synchronized pattern and set up a one-way current through the tube. If sperm are present in the outer portion of the tube and one of them is successful in penetrating the egg, fertilization takes place and a new life begins. The fertilized egg will incubate in the tube for about three days before arriving at its destination, the cavity of the uterus, where it floats for about three more days before implanting. Around the seventh day it "rests," so to speak, implanting in the cavity of the uterus. If the egg is not fertilized, it will live only twelve to twenty-four hours and then disintegrate. (Since sperm live for forty-eight to seventy-two hours, there are three or four days in each cycle during which intercourse could lead to conception.)

Much activity takes place in the ovary after ovulation. The newly vacated follicle has another job to do: prepare the uterus to accept and nourish a fertilized egg, should one arrive. The follicle turns into a gland called the **corpus luteum** (literally "yellow body," because cells lining the inside of the follicle develop a yellowish color), which secretes estrogen and, more important, progesterone. This hormone, which dominates this **luteal phase** of the cycle, promotes growth and maturation of the uterine lining and increases its blood flow. This layer of tissue eventually doubles in thickness and becomes stocked with nutrients. Progesterone not only prepares the uterine "nursery" for a new arrival but also relaxes the muscles of the uterus, decreasing the chance of contractions that might accidentally expel its guest. Progesterone also temporarily stops the preparation of any other eggs within the ovaries.

If a fertilized egg successfully implants and continues its growth within the uterus, it secretes a hormone called **human chorionic gonadotropin** (or

hCG), which sends an important message to the corpus luteum: "Keep the hormones flowing!" The corpus luteum obliges and for ten to twelve weeks continues to provide the hormone support that allows the uterus to nourish the baby growing inside. After ten weeks, the **placenta** (the complex organ that connects the baby to the inner lining of the uterus) takes over the job of manufacturing progesterone, and the corpus luteum retires from active duty.

If there is no fertilization, no pregnancy, and no hCG, the corpus luteum degenerates. Progesterone and estrogen levels fall, resulting in a spasm of the blood vessels that supply the lining of the uterus. Deprived of the nutrients it needs to survive, the lining dies and passes from the uterus, along with blood and mucus, in what is called the **menstrual flow** (also referred to as the **period** or **menses**).

While the menstrual period might seem to be the end of the story, the first day of flow is actually counted as day one of a woman's reproductive cycle. For while the flow is taking place, the three-act play is starting over again as a new set of follicles begins to ripen in the ovaries. This cycle of life will thus normally continue month after month throughout a woman's reproductive years until menopause, unless it is interrupted by pregnancy or a medical condition that interferes with it.

What's normal during menstrual periods?

The words *menstrual* and *menses* are derived from the Latin word for "month," which refers to the approximate frequency of this event. A typical cycle lasts from twenty-eight to thirty-five days, although for some women normal menses occur as frequently as every twenty-one days or as infrequently as every forty-five days. Most of the variability arises during the first (follicular) phase leading up to ovulation. Assuming that a pregnancy does not begin, the luteal phase (from ovulation to menses) is nearly always fourteen days, with little variation.

For a year or two after her first menstrual period, an adolescent's cycles may be irregular because of **anovulatory cycles**, meaning an egg is not released. If ovulation does not take place, the cycle will remain stuck in the first (follicular) phase. Estrogen will continue to stimulate the lining of the uterus until some of it becomes so thick that it outgrows its blood supply. The shedding of this tissue resembles a menstrual period, but it is unpredictable and usually occurs with very little cramping. When ovulation finally takes place, the lining of the uterus will mature and then be shed all at once if a pregnancy has not started. Anovulatory cycles are most common both at the beginning and toward the end of a woman's reproductive years, but they may occur at any time in between as well.

After a girl's first menstrual period, several months may pass before her endocrine system matures to the point of producing regular ovulation. During this time it is not unusual for her to skip two or three months between cycles.

Since cramping doesn't normally occur unless ovulation has taken place, menstrual pains may not be noticed for months (or even one or two years) after the first cycle.

Menstrual flow normally lasts three to six days, although very short (one-day) or longer (seven- or eight-day) periods are normal for some women. One to three ounces of blood is usually lost during each cycle, although more or less than this amount may be a regular occurrence without any ill effects.

Virtually all normal activities can be continued during a menstrual period. Bathing or showering is not only safe but also advisable in order to minimize any unpleasant odor. Feminine hygiene sprays and deodorant pads and tampons may irritate delicate tissue, and douching is unnecessary and should be avoided. Any persistent drainage that is discolored, itchy, painful, or foul smelling should be evaluated by a physician.

What can go wrong with menstrual periods?

Menstrual cramps (the medical term is **dysmenorrhea**) most often are a by-product of the normal breakdown of the lining of the uterus (endometrium) at the end of a cycle. Chemicals called **prostaglandins** are released into the bloodstream by the endometrium, often with unpleasant effects. The most obvious response is a series of contractions of the muscles of the uterus, which may actually be as forceful as contractions during labor. During a strong contraction, blood may be inhibited from circulating through all of the uterine muscle, which like any other muscle temporarily deprived of oxygen, will sound off with genuine pain. (Contractions during menses occur in the fallopian tubes as well.) Prostaglandins may affect other parts of the body during a menstrual period, causing diarrhea, nausea, headaches, and difficulty with concentration. One bit of good news in connection with menstrual cramps is that they do *not* predict what level of pain a woman will feel later in life during childbirth. In other words, a teenager with severe menstrual cramps is not necessarily going to have equally severe labor pains.

Menstrual cramps can be relieved in a variety of ways. Heating pads or warm baths are often helpful, for reasons that are unclear. (It's thought that they may increase blood flow within the pelvis, improving the supply of oxygen to uterine muscle.) Exercise and good general physical condition are often helpful in reducing cramps. Walking is a good exercise during this (or, for that matter, any) time of the month.

Specific prostaglandin-inhibiting medications work well for many adolescents and older women alike. These were formulated to reduce the pain and inflammation of arthritis but were found also to have a significant effect on menstrual cramps. Three are available without prescription: ibuprofen (Advil, Motrin, and other brands), naproxen (Aleve), and ketoprofen (Orudis and others). These anti-inflammatory drugs should be taken with food to decrease the chance of stomach irritation, and they should not be taken with aspirin. They are most effective if they are taken at the first sign of cramping and then continued on a regular basis (rather than "here and there" in response to pain) until the cramps stop. Your physician may recommend one of these medications (sometimes with a dosage schedule different from what is written on the package) or prescribe one of several anti-inflammatory medications. Individual responses vary. If one type doesn't work well, another may seem like a miracle.

Other pain-relief medications that may be helpful include:

- Acetaminophen (Tylenol and others), which does not inhibit prostaglandins but can be quite effective nonetheless. Some women have found that alternating medications is helpful—for example, starting with ibuprofen, using acetaminophen for the next dose a few hours later, then switching back, and so on.
- Midol, which combines acetaminophen with the antihistamine pyrilamine (and thus may be mildly sedating). Depending on the particular formulation, Midol may include ibuprofen or a mild diuretic (to decrease fluid retention).
- Stronger pain relievers may be prescribed by a physician if the discomfort of menstrual cramps cannot be controlled by other measures.

If menstrual cramps are disruptive and are unresponsive to home remedies and nonprescription medications, it is important that they be evaluated medically. Abnormalities of the cervix (the opening of the uterus) or the uterus itself, or a condition called **endometriosis** (in which tissue that normally lines the uterus grows in other parts of the body, usually in the pelvis) can on rare occasions be the cause of significant menstrual pain.

The most significant cause of endometriosis is actually a problem known as **retrograde menstruation**, in which blood flows literally in the wrong direction: from the uterus upward through the fallopian tubes and then into the abdominal cavity.

If the medical examination is normal, a physician may prescribe a diuretic, an oral contraceptive, or both.

Diuretics decrease fluid retention but do not directly relieve cramps; however, discomfort may be less annoying if any fluid retention is relieved (see "PMS and PMDD" later in this chapter).

Oral contraceptives (birth control pills) may be helpful in reducing or eliminating significant cramps that are not adequately controlled by other means. In fact, for many women this may be the only type of medication that is helpful in reducing severe cramps that regularly interfere with normal activity. Each four-week cycle of pills provides three weeks of estrogen and progesterone in a specified amount. This prevents the LH surge and ovulation and also usually results in less proliferation of the lining of the uterus than occurs during a normal cycle. During the fourth week, no hormones are present in the pills, so during this time the lining is shed as in a normal cycle. However, the smaller amount of tissue involved usually generates less cramping. A variation on this approach, known as **continuous oral contraception**, extends the length of each cycle beyond twenty-eight days in order to reduce the number of menstrual periods. For example, with the formulation called Seasonale, a woman takes estrogen and progesterone from twenty-one to eighty-four days, followed by a week of pills containing no hormones. The result: only four menstrual periods per year, which can significantly reduce not only the severity of cramps but also the amount of time a woman must deal with them every year.

If severe menstrual cramps continue while a woman is taking oral contraceptives, she should be reevaluated by her physician, since endometriosis is a definite possibility.

A decision to use birth control pills for this (or any other) purpose should not be made casually. A medical evaluation to rule out other causes of pain may be necessary. Nausea, headaches, bloating, and/or worsening of acne are unpleasant side effects experienced by some users. The pills must be taken consistently each day to be effective.

F.Y.I.

In addition, the use of birth control pills to control menstrual cramps in an adolescent may raise another concern: Could taking them for menstrual cramps (or any other therapeutic purpose) indirectly lower your daughter's resistance to sexual activity? If you don't know the answer to this question, now is the time for candid conversation about sexuality. It would be unfortunate to withhold a treatment that might reduce debilitating pain because of a parent's vague mistrust of an adolescent who is actually fervently committed to remaining abstinent. Furthermore, the decision to postpone sex until marriage should be built on a strong, multilayered foundation. If the absence of contraceptives is the only reason a teen is avoiding intercourse, she needs to hear and understand many more reasons.

Irregular menstrual periods may be a cause for concern if they are (1) too rare, occurring every three or four months after more than a year has passed since the first period; (2) too frequent, with bleeding or spotting occurring throughout the month; (3) too long, lasting more than seven or eight consecutive days; or (4) too heavy, soaking through more than six to eight pads or tampons per day.

For any of these problems, a medical evaluation is usually necessary to discover the underlying cause. A number of physical or even emotional events can also interfere with the complex interaction of hormones that brings about the monthly cycle, including:

- *Medical disorders.* These could include malfunctions of the endocrine system (including pituitary, adrenal, or thyroid glands) or abnormalities of the ovaries, uterus, or vagina.
- *Significant changes in weight.* Women who are significantly overweight can generate enough estrogen in their fat cells to impact the lining of the uterus. At the opposite extreme, stringent diets or the severe reduction of food intake seen with anorexia will effectively shut down the menstrual cycle.
- *Extreme levels of exercise.* Female athletes with demanding training programs may have infrequent periods or their cycles may stop altogether.
- *Stress.* Stormy emotional weather may cause a woman to miss one or more periods, especially during the adolescent years.
- *Pregnancy.* In some cases an unexpected absence of menstrual cycles indicates that an unplanned pregnancy has begun.

It is important that extremes in menstrual flow (whether too much or too little) be evaluated. Not only may the underlying cause have great significance, but the menstrual irregularity could also have damaging consequences of its own.

For example, very frequent or heavy bleeding may outstrip a woman's ability to replenish red blood cells. Often there is an inadequate amount of iron in the diet to keep up with what is being lost each month. This may lead to **iron-deficiency anemia**, which can cause ongoing fatigue, poor concentration, light-headedness, or even fainting episodes.

Absence of menstrual periods related to a continual failure to ovulate may result in months or years of nonstop estrogen stimulation of the uterus. Without the maturing effect of progesterone, the lining of the uterus may be at increased risk for developing precancerous abnormalities or overt cancer. This scenario is one of the concerns for women with **polycystic ovary syndrome**, a metabolic disturbance usually characterized by infrequent menstrual periods as well as excessive weight and body hair.

Women (especially high school or college students) whose cycles stop because of weight loss or intense physical training (or both) may suffer an irreversible loss of bone density, known as osteoporosis. Normally a problem faced by women much later in life (typically well after menopause), osteoporosis can lead to disabling fractures of the spine, hips, wrists, and other bones.

It is impossible to state a single course of action that will resolve all the various forms of menstrual irregularity. However, if there appears to be no underlying disturbance that needs specific treatment and the problem is determined to be irregular ovulation, a doctor may recommend hormonal treatment to regulate the cycle. This may take the form of progesterone, which can be given at a defined time each month to bring on a menstrual period. Or birth control pills may be recommended to restore some order by overriding a woman's own cycle and establishing one that is more predictable.

PMS and PMDD

Most women experience some degree of discomfort that may occur for a day or two prior to menstruation or may extend over the entire two-week period following ovulation. Mild physical or emotional distress during this time, sometimes called premenstrual tension, is very common. But 20 to 40 percent of women experience symptoms severe enough to disrupt normal activities. This is commonly called **premenstrual syndrome**, or **PMS**.

A specific cause for PMS has not been identified, but the effects are all too familiar for many women. Physical symptoms can include bloating and fullness in the abdomen, fluid retention (with tightness of rings and shoes), headaches, breast tenderness, backache, fatigue, and dizziness. More dramatic are the emotional symptoms: irritability, anxiety, depression, poor concentration, insomnia, difficulty making decisions, and unusual food cravings. These can occur in various combinations and levels of severity. The most striking feature is usually the instability and intensity of negative emotions, which can send other family members running for cover. Some women feel literally like Dr. Jekyll and Ms. Hyde—calm and rational for the first two weeks of the cycle and out of control for the second two weeks, with dramatic improvement once the menstrual flow is under way. Between 3 and 5 percent of women have premenstrual emotional storms severe enough to cause significant disturbances at home, school, or work, a condition designated in recent years as **premenstrual dysphoric disorder**, or **PMDD**.

A few decades ago PMS was considered primarily a psychological event, an "adjustment reaction" to reproductive issues or life in general. This is no longer the case. PMS should be taken as seriously as any other physical issue. While no quick-fix remedies or lifetime cures exist for PMS, a number of measures can help you reduce its impact:

- **Make sure the emotional and physical symptoms are, in fact, PMS.** Other life issues or even depression may be at the heart of the problem. If there is any question, symptoms can be charted on a calendar, along with menstrual periods, for two or three months. You should see an improvement for at least a week following menses. Symptoms that continue well after a period is over or throughout the cycle involve something other than (or in addition to) PMS, including depression. Keep in mind that PMS or PMDD may be superimposed on an ongoing depression, and symptoms take a marked turn for the worse—even including suicidal thoughts—during the week or two prior to menses. Anyone whose thinking turns to self-harm, even if it occurs only during certain times of the month, should be evaluated and treated immediately.
- **Keep the lines of communication open with other family members, and plan ahead.** Women with regular menstrual cycles are often able to predict when the more troublesome days are coming. This may give others at home a little advance "storm warning," and hopefully they will respond with an extra measure of TLC—or at least a little slack. This is particularly important if more than one person at home has difficulty with PMS, since the collision of two unstable moods can be quite unpleasant. Needless to say, if you (or your teenage daughter) are irritable because of the time of the month and a change for the better is likely in the immediate future, you would be wise to postpone any conversations about emotionally charged issues for a few days, if at all possible. It is important to acknowledge the reality of PMS and its symptoms without allowing them to become a blanket excuse for any and all forms of unreasonable behavior.
- **Encourage sensible eating and exercise.** Frequent, smaller meals and avoidance of overtly sugary foods may help keep blood glucose

levels (and mood) a little more stable. Avoiding salt can reduce fluid retention. Caffeine may increase irritability, so decaffeinated drinks (and medications) are more appropriate. All-around physical conditioning through the entire month can improve general well-being and help you navigate more smoothly to the end of a cycle.

In addition, a variety of remedies, nutritional supplements, and medications have been recommended at one time or another for this problem. Some have a more consistent track record (and better scientific support) than others, and you should consider getting advice from your physician before trying any of these. Ultimately, the bottom line for any PMS treatment is an honest assessment of the effectiveness, safety, and side effects for the individual taking it.

- *Nonprescription medications* such as acetaminophen or ibuprofen to reduce aches and pains may be of some help.
- *Calcium* (1,200 mg per day) and *magnesium* (200 mg per day) supplementation have both been shown to reduce symptoms of PMS (especially physical discomforts) by 40 to 50 percent. Improvements may not be noticed, however, until two or three cycles have passed while taking supplementation.
- *Vitamin E* supplementation (usually at 400 international units, or IU, per day, but no more than that) has shown mixed results in research studies on PMS.
- *Vitamin* B_6, which has long been advocated as a remedy for PMS symptoms, has performed poorly in controlled studies and probably has limited usefulness at best. If numbness or tingling of the hands or feet occur while taking this vitamin, it should be discontinued. Megadoses of any vitamin or mineral that exceed RDAs (recommended daily allowances) are not recommended for this condition.
- *A number of herbal preparations,* such as evening primrose oil, have been advocated for one or more symptoms of PMS, but research studies investigating such claims have yielded mixed results. While the scientific jury is out, keep in mind that the Food and Drug Administration (FDA) does not certify herbal preparations for safety and effectiveness.
- *Prescription medications* that are most widely used for PMS fall into three basic categories. Obviously, the use of any of these will require evaluation and follow-up by a physician.
    1. *Diuretics.* For many women, much of the discomfort of PMS arises from bloating and fluid retention, so the use of a mild diuretic (or "water pill") to maintain normal fluid levels during the second half of each cycle can be effective.
    2. *Antidepressants.* Many PMS symptoms, and certainly those of PMDD, essentially duplicate those seen in depression. Some women with severe PMS fight milder forms of the same emotional symptoms throughout the entire month. It now appears

For more details about what vitamins do (and don't do), see the appendix "Vitamins and Minerals: What Each One Does and How Much We Need" starting on page 869.

that the fundamental physiological problem in PMS/PMDD involves changes in the levels of biological messengers in the brain known as **neurotransmitters**. New research has shown significant reduction in both physical and emotional premenstrual distress symptoms with a specific family of antidepressants called **selective serotonin reuptake inhibitors** (or SSRIs), such as fluoxetine (Prozac or Sarafem), sertraline (Zoloft), paroxetine (Paxil), and others. These drugs are safe and are not habit-forming, but individual responses and side effects vary considerably. Often doses lower than those needed to treat depression are effective in reducing PMS/PMDD symptoms, and many women obtain satisfactory results by taking one of these medications on an intermittent basis, typically seven to ten days each month. (See chapter 8 for more information about SSRIs in the treatment of depression.)

3. *Hormonal manipulations* have been utilized with variable success. Women who take supplemental progesterone during the second half of the menstrual cycle may report marked improvement, a worsening of symptoms (especially depression), or no effect at all.

Caring for Yourself—and Your Baby—during Pregnancy

As described in the previous pages, the female body is marvelously designed to bring a new life into the world, and the hormonal cycles that a woman experiences from puberty to menopause prepare her body on a monthly basis for the start of that new life. The impact of pregnancy on a woman's health (not to mention the sheer wonder of the phenomenon of developing life) requires that we touch briefly on what happens developmentally during pregnancy and explore how a woman can protect and enhance both her own health and that of her unborn child during these eventful months.[2]

This section is not intended to be a comprehensive resource on pregnancy and is intentionally focused on matters that specifically affect the health of the baby to be born. The length, breadth, and depth of pregnancy care are beyond the scope of this book. If you are pregnant (or may be soon), it is very important that you not only choose a physician who will provide care for you throughout pregnancy but also find books and other materials from which you can learn more about this miraculous process.

Fearfully and wonderfully made: how a baby develops

Many authors and poets, after hearing the cry and seeing the first flailing movements of tiny arms and legs at the moment of birth, have declared that the process of coming into the world is a miracle.

But while childbirth is truly awe inspiring, the real miracles begin long before this transition of the baby from one environment to another. Be assured that many wondrous and marvelous events take place in the warm sanctuary of the womb. Just six days after a new human life begins with the meeting of egg and sperm, a tiny cluster of 64 to 128 cells is embedded in the thickened lining of the uterus. Within seventy-two hours of establishing a temporary residence, he or she sends a powerful hormonal signal to override the mother's monthly cycle, preventing the shedding of her uterine lining.

Then begins the astonishing process of differentiation, as new cells take on particular shapes, sizes, and functions, aligning themselves into tissues and organs, eyes and ears, arms and legs. Each of these cells contains all the information needed to make any of the multitudes of cell types in the body. Yet during the process of constructing and organizing, integrating and communicating with one another, individual cells begin to express unique qualities very quickly and in a seamless and orderly pattern. The intricacy and timing of these events are nothing less than masterpieces of planning and engineering.

Before the end of the first six weeks of life, the child's heart has started to beat, eyes are developing, the central nervous system is under construction, most internal organs are forming, and small buds representing future arms and legs have sprouted. One cell created by the union of egg and sperm has now become millions, and this new child is now one-quarter of an inch long.

By the end of eight weeks, the fingers and toes have been formed. Heart, lungs, and major blood vessels have become well developed. Taste buds and the apparatus needed for the sense of smell have appeared. Tiny muscles have begun generating body movements, which at this point a mother cannot feel.

After twelve weeks of growth, the baby has reached a length of three inches. The heartbeat can be heard using an electronic listening device. All the organs and tissues—including heart, lungs, brain, digestive system, kidneys, and reproductive organs—have been formed and are in place. The only remaining ingredient necessary is time: six more months for growth and maturation.

Sixteen weeks after conception, eyebrows and hair are growing. The baby, now measuring six to seven inches and weighing nearly as many ounces, kicks, swallows, hiccups, wakes, and sleeps. Between sixteen and twenty weeks the mother can begin feeling movement inside, an important milestone still referred to as quickening.

At twenty weeks, with weight now approaching one pound, the baby can hear and react to sounds, including Mom's heartbeat and stomach rumblings, as well as noise, music, and conversations outside the uterus. (Whether any of these sounds are recognized or become part of early memories is uncertain.)

At twenty-six weeks of life, breathing movements are present, although there is no air to be inhaled. Depending on their weight, babies born prematurely at this time have a 65 to 75 percent chance of survival with expert care, although complications are common. With each additional week that passes within the mother's womb, the baby's likelihood of surviving a premature delivery improves, the risk of long-term complications declines, and the medical care needed after birth usually becomes less complex.

The final fourteen weeks are the homestretch, during which the baby grows and gains weight very rapidly. By the end of thirty-two weeks, the bones are hardening, the eyes are opening and closing, the thumb has found its way into the mouth, and the arms and legs are stretching and kicking regularly. The baby is twelve to sixteen inches long and weighs about three pounds. Over the next four weeks, the weight nearly doubles, and Mom feels all sorts of kicks, prods, and pokes much more strongly. A baby born at this age will need some assistance with feeding and keeping warm and could still develop more complicated medical problems as well. However, the vast majority of those born a month or so ahead of schedule do very well.

Finally, after a few more weeks of rapid weight gain (about half a pound per week during the last six weeks of gestation), the baby is fully developed and ready to meet the world outside the womb.

Lifestyle and health questions for mothers-to-be

In a very real and practical sense, parenting begins well before a couple learns that a new family member is on the way. The state of the union of the parents-to-be and the mother's health before pregnancy strongly affect her health during pregnancy, which in turn plays a vital role in the baby's well-being both before and after delivery.

If you are planning to begin a family, or even if your pregnancy is well under way, you would be wise to review the following list of self-assessment questions. Much of what follows is directed toward the mother, but the ongoing health and habits of both parents are very important. (By the way, if you have read chapter 2, many of these will sound familiar.)

In chapter 1 we asked a hypothetical question: What would you do if you were given the car of your dreams tomorrow, but it would be the only car you could ever drive—or ride in? (In other words, if it crashed or wore out, you would be forever stuck without transportation.) How would you treat it? If you liken your one-and-only body to that imaginary car, you get the point: If you mistreat the body you live in, you might be able to make some repairs, but you'll never get another one. For women who are or might become pregnant, there's an additional consideration: Your habits and behaviors don't affect just you. Poor nutrition, smoking, and the use of alcohol and drugs can have a serious impact on your baby's development, especially during the first eight weeks when the vital organs are under construction. But your pregnancy may not even be confirmed until this period has already passed. Therefore, the habits you develop well before you even think about having a child are very important.

So how well are you taking care of your one (and only) body?

How's your nutrition?

Contrary to what talk shows and tabloids say, good nutrition does not involve magic formulas, rigid restrictions, or tackle boxes full of vitamins and supplements. If you read chapter 5, you are already familiar with the basic principles of healthful eating that continue to be reinforced by research and consensus:

- Go easy on the added sugars.
- Gravitate toward whole-grain foods rather than those made from refined or processed grains.
- Eat lots of vegetables and fruits—five to nine servings per day.
- Get an adequate amount of dietary fiber.
- Limit the saturated fat to 10 percent or less of your total daily calories.
- Watch out for the trans fats.
- Get enough of the "good" fats. In particular, become a regular user of olive oil, add seeds and nuts to your diet, and eat at least two servings of fish per week. (As we discussed in chapter 5, this should represent a maximum of about twelve ounces of fish, avoiding shark, swordfish, king mackerel, and tilefish—golden bass or golden snapper—that may carry higher levels of mercury. Tuna should be limited to six ounces per week.)
- Take a vitamin (regular or prenatal) containing folic acid if you are trying to become pregnant. You can also take folic acid by itself. Nonprescription tablets typically contain 0.4 mg (400 mcg), the daily amount recommended for a woman of childbearing age. Once you know you are pregnant, you can increase the amount you take to one-and-a-half or two tablets (0.6 mg or 0.8 mg) daily until your physician prescribes a prenatal vitamin.

The goal is not to become obsessed with meticulous counts of servings or calories but to emphasize higher quality foods on an ongoing basis. If the four food groups in your current diet are burgers, soft drinks, doughnuts, and chips, you need to do some serious revision—primarily shifting to the lower-fat, higher-quality grain, vegetable, and fruit groups.

If you are a vegetarian, you should be able to continue through an entire pregnancy without difficulty, provided that you include a wide variety of foods. If you eat absolutely no animal products, such as milk, eggs, or cheese, you may become shortchanged on protein and calories, as well as iron, calcium, vitamin $B_{12,}$ and zinc. Vitamin and mineral supplementation would be advisable, as would some consultation with a dietitian.

Theoretically, a woman who eats a variety of fresh, high-quality foods should not need to take supplemental vitamins and minerals. But certain substances are so critical to a healthy pregnancy that most physicians will prescribe prenatal vitamins to make up for any deficiencies in the mother's diet. Remember, however, that supplements do not make up for careless eating habits.

There is evidence that taking supplemental **folic acid** will reduce the likelihood that the newborn will have one of several types of major problems known as **neural tube defects**. Within the first month after conception, a tubelike structure forms from which the brain and spinal cord develop. If the tube does not close properly, serious abnormalities of these vital structures can result. Unfortunately, neural tube defects may occur before you know you are pregnant. Therefore, the U.S. Public Health Service now recommends that all women of childbearing age take 0.4 mg of folic acid daily to reduce the risk of a neural tube defect occurring in an unexpected pregnancy.

Once a woman knows she is pregnant, she should be taking 0.6 mg (600 mcg) of folic acid daily. (Prenatal multivitamins typically contain 1.0 mg of folic acid, which allows some breathing room.) If you have already had a child with a neural tube defect, a higher dose of folic acid—4 mg per day—is recommended for three months prior to the time you plan to become pregnant and should be continued through the first three months. (This amount of folic acid requires a doctor's prescription.) You can, of course, obtain folic acid through foods such as dark leafy vegetables, cereals, whole-grain breads, citrus fruits, bananas, and tomatoes. However, in light of the research favoring supplementation, you should check with your physician about the amount of folic acid recommended for your pregnancy.

A pregnant woman needs additional **iron**, both for her increased blood volume as well as for the growing tissues and iron stores within her baby. Iron is necessary for the formation of **hemoglobin**, the protein within red blood cells that binds to oxygen, thus allowing red cells to deliver oxygen to every cell in the body. If the supply of iron in a mother's food is inadequate to meet this increased need, iron-deficiency anemia will eventually result. This can cause her to feel extremely tired—more so than she would normally expect from the pregnancy itself.

An intake of about 30 mg of elemental iron per day will meet the need of most pregnant women. (Those who are already iron deficient may require 60 mg or more to correct this problem.) Since a typical diet provides only 5 or 6 mg of elemental iron per one thousand calories of food, and because consuming five thousand calories per day would be both unwise and impractical, iron should be included in your prenatal vitamin regimen. Absorption of iron is improved when foods containing vitamin C are eaten at the same time.

Folic acid, iron, and other vitamins and minerals are reviewed in detail in appendix B starting on page 869.

A woman's daily **calcium** intake normally should be 1,000 mg per day during the childbearing years, but should increase to 1,200 to 1,500 mg per day during pregnancy because of the new skeleton under construction inside her uterus. Dairy products are a rich source of calcium—300 mg are available in a cup of milk and 450 mg in a cup of nonfat yogurt—so this added requirement is usually readily obtained from foods. If you can't tolerate dairy products, your doctor may recommend that you take calcium supplements, since prenatal vitamins alone typically do not include the full amount. Calcium carbonate or calcium citrate is the most easily absorbed. Natural forms of calcium—oyster shell, dolomite, or bonemeal, for example—may contain heavy metal (such as lead, arsenic, or mercury) and should be avoided.

Do you weigh enough . . . or too much?

Obesity is a health hazard for many reasons, all of which are heightened during pregnancy. Excessive weight during pregnancy is a risk factor for high blood pressure and diabetes, both of which can lead to significant problems for mother and baby. The aches and pains (especially in the lower back) that are so common during the later stages of pregnancy can become intolerable when there is already a burden of excess weight on muscles and joints. Recent evidence suggests that overweight pregnant women are more likely to have babies with neural tube defects, regardless of folic acid intake.

Being underweight before or during pregnancy is no great advantage either, because the nutritional needs of the baby may be compromised. This can result in a baby of low birth weight who is at risk for a variety of problems, including difficulty maintaining normal temperature or blood sugar level after birth.

Is your current weight okay? If you haven't already done so, you can check your body mass index (BMI) and learn how to lose excess weight in chapter 6. Eating disorders, specifically anorexia and bulimia, are reviewed in chapter 8, beginning on page 331.

If you have had a history of erratic nutrition habits or even a full-blown eating disorder (such as anorexia or bulimia), you and your baby will benefit greatly from ongoing counseling and coaching from a dietitian before, during, and after pregnancy. Similarly, if you are struggling with excessive weight, a gradual process of reduction (ideally under the guidance of a dietitian) prior to becoming pregnant would be wise. Attaining a stable weight prior to pregnancy will help prevent rapid regaining of weight after pregnancy begins. If you are already pregnant, however, a weight-loss program is not a good idea, because the nutritional needs of both you and your baby could be jeopardized. Pregnancy would be a good time, however, to modify eating habits toward healthy patterns that will serve you well for the rest of your life.

Are you exercising your muscles, heart, and lungs?

A sedentary lifestyle—that is, one without deliberate exercise—has been specifically identified as a health risk for both women and men. Unfortunately, despite the numerous and well-publicized benefits of regular exercise, a majority of Americans still do not take part in any form of planned physical activity. But a regular habit of exercise established now will serve as an investment in long-term health and also improve the way you feel throughout pregnancy.

Several normal changes during pregnancy put new physical demands on your body. Aside from a normal weight gain of twenty-five to thirty-five pounds, your heart will be dealing with about a 50 percent increase in blood volume. Muscles and ligaments in the back and pelvis will be stretched and subjected to new tensions and strains. Unless you have a scheduled cesarean section, you will also go through the rigors of labor—which is aptly named—

and the birth itself. These are physically challenging events, and those who are well-conditioned usually fare better. In fact, their labor may even be shortened.

The increased stamina and muscle tone resulting from regular exercise will also increase your energy level, improve sleep, reduce swelling of the legs, and probably reduce aches and pains in the lower back. If you are on your feet all day, it may seem ridiculous to spend precious time on additional muscle motion. But unless you are a professional athlete, it is unlikely that your daily activities, no matter how exhausting, will specifically condition your heart and lungs. The good news is that you don't need to become a marathon runner to see some benefit in your health.

If you are not used to exercising, a goal of thirty minutes three or four times per week is reasonable. It is always better to do light or moderate exercise on a regular basis than heavy exercise intermittently. While stretching and muscle strengthening are worthwhile, aerobic conditioning—in which increased oxygen is consumed continuously for a prolonged period of time—has the greatest overall benefit.

The most straightforward and least costly aerobic activity is walking. No fancy equipment, health-club membership, or special gear (other than a pair of comfortable, supportive shoes) is needed. Pleasant and safe surroundings, a flat surface, agreeable weather, and a walking companion are advisable, however. Another person (whether your husband, an older child, a relative, a friend, or another pregnant woman) will add accountability to the process, and the conversation can be enjoyable and help the time pass quickly. Gentle stretching for a few minutes before and after is a good idea, in order to warm up and then cool down leg and back muscles.

Of course, there are many alternatives to walking. First, using a home treadmill ends any concerns about weather, aggressive dogs, or finding someone to watch your children. You can be flexible about the time of day to use it. Its disadvantages include cost, size, and noise.

Many women choose to use an exercise video or book geared to pregnant women, although the constant repetition could become boring. Expectant women may prefer to take a prenatal fitness class at a local hospital or health club where they can interact with an instructor and other women. Of course, the cost, as well as trying to schedule child care for other children, can be drawbacks. Two final possibilities are swimming and stationary cycling, both of which offer good aerobic conditioning without lower back strain. One potential downside to cycling is that many women become increasingly uncomfortable on this equipment as pregnancy progresses.

If you are already well conditioned, you should be able to continue using your specific exercise routine. If you are a confirmed jogger or an accomplished tennis player, you can probably continue these activities through the early months of pregnancy. Snow-skiing, surfing, water-skiing, and horseback riding all pose specific risks during pregnancy because of the possibility of falls—

especially as the uterus enlarges, which shifts your center of gravity and may throw off your balance. All of these activities should be reviewed with your physician throughout the course of your pregnancy. Note: Scuba diving is not recommended at any time during pregnancy.

A few special precautions about exercise during pregnancy:

- Pregnancy is not a good time to take on a new, intense form of exercise, especially if it involves jumping, jerking, high-impact motion, or sudden changes in direction.
- Exercise should not be so vigorous or prolonged as to cause exhaustion, overheating, or dehydration. During pregnancy your heart rate should stay below 140, regardless of the type of exercise you are doing.
- You should avoid significant lifting—and consult with your physician—if you experience any bleeding during pregnancy.
- After the twentieth week of pregnancy, you should avoid exercises that require you to lie on your back.
- Exercise should not continue if any of the following pregnancy-related problems develop: preterm rupture of membranes; poor growth of the baby (intrauterine growth restriction); vaginal bleeding; high blood pressure; preterm labor; or cervical incompetence, a condition in which the cervix or "neck" of the uterus isn't strong enough to prevent a premature delivery. Exercise may also be limited if you are pregnant with more than one baby.
- If you have specific health problems such as heart disease, high blood pressure, irregular heart rate, epilepsy, fainting episodes, asthma, arthritis, or anemia, review any exercise plans with your physician, whether or not you are pregnant.

In addition to aerobic activity, a variety of gentle stretching and muscle-conditioning activities can help prepare your body for the changes of late pregnancy and labor. Your doctor or childbirth-class instructor will have a number of suggestions for such exercises.

Are you taking or inhaling any substances that might harm you or your baby?

In chapter 10 we discussed in detail the destructive effects of smoking cigarettes, drinking excessive amounts of alcohol, and using illicit drugs. As a result of widespread public-health announcements, most people are aware that these are risky and destructive, especially during pregnancy. Yet it's often difficult to believe that "this could happen to me"—that we might actually suffer the bad effects we hear about. Furthermore, even if one is convinced of the dangers of these substances, gaining freedom from their grip can be a real uphill battle. If you need any additional reasons to separate yourself from cigarettes, alcohol, or illegal drugs, or some extra resolve to remain free of these unhealthy habits, consider carefully the following facts:

Cigarettes. This is a form of legalized drug addiction that is harmful to the smoker, those around the smoker, and especially the baby growing inside the smoker. Thousands of chemicals in cigarette smoke flow directly from the mother's lungs into her bloodstream and then directly into the baby. Nicotine specifically causes constriction of blood vessels in both the placenta and the baby, thus reducing the baby's supply of vital blood and oxygen. Carbon monoxide in smoke binds tightly to red blood cells and displaces oxygen. The overall effect is a recurrent choking of the baby's oxygen supply, resulting in smaller (by an average of half a pound) and shorter babies. Unfortunately, these infants (whom doctors refer to as "small-for-dates") are more likely than their normal counterparts to have a variety of medical problems after birth.

The smoker's baby is more likely to be born prematurely or to be stillborn. The tragedy of **sudden infant death syndrome (SIDS)** occurs twice as frequently when the child's mother smoked throughout pregnancy, and the risk increases drastically if there is continuing exposure to secondhand smoke after birth. According to a study published by researchers at the University of California, infants exposed to smoke from ten or fewer cigarettes per day are more than twice as likely to die of SIDS as babies in smoke-free environments. When the exposure involves more than twenty cigarettes per day, the risk soars to more than twenty times that of infants not exposed.[3]

Exposure to cigarette smoke after birth is linked to colds, ear infections, and asthma. And the child who sees Mom and Dad smoke is also much more likely to pick up the habit than are his peers who live in homes where there are no smokers.

Let's not forget smoking's effect on the mother. Aside from the long-term risks of chronic lung disease, heart disease, ulcers, and diseased blood vessels, she is more likely to have unexpected vaginal bleeding during her pregnancy.

The only good news about smoking is that quitting early in pregnancy reduces the baby's risk of problems to the level of a child born to a nonsmoker. For many women, the emotional impact of learning about a threat to their baby is powerful enough to override the compulsion to light up, and a pregnancy usually lasts long enough to help temporary abstainers remain smoke free for life.

But cigarettes are so powerfully addictive that additional support may be necessary to kick the habit. If you are a smoker, it's never too late—or too early—to stop. While we looked at the process of quitting smoking in chapter 10, it is worth recapping within the context of pregnancy. A successful decision to quit usually requires:

- A well-defined list of reasons that have some emotional power. ("I don't want to starve my baby of oxygen" or "I want to live long enough to see my kids grow up.") Since resistance to quitting often hinges on an emotional attachment to cigarettes, your reasons for giving up smoking should likewise motivate you on an emotional level.

- A specified quitting date that is announced to family, friends, and co-workers. Some gentle peer pressure can be a powerful motivator.
- Participation in a stop-smoking class. These are available in most communities through nearby hospitals or local chapters of national organizations (American Lung Association, American Heart Association, American Cancer Society).
- Quitlines, which are free counseling services available by phone in more than thirty states. Counselors are trained to help individuals map out their own quitting strategy and can provide ongoing support, which may be more convenient to access than a meeting. Information about accessing a quitline can be obtained from the American Cancer Society at (800) 227-2345 or the North American Quitline Consortium Web site at http://www.naquitline.org.
- A firm declaration that your home, car, and workplace are smoke-free zones. Nobody, but nobody—spouse, in-laws, guests, visiting heads of state—lights up in your airspace.
- Using prescription or over-the-counter nicotine patches or chewing gum to assist you through the withdrawal process if you are not yet pregnant. If you have any questions or concerns about their proper use, you may want to discuss them with your physician. You should not smoke while using nicotine patches or gum, and you cannot use them during pregnancy.

Alcoholic beverages. Daily consumption of alcohol during pregnancy, with or without binge drinking, may lead to a complex of problems in the baby known as **fetal alcohol syndrome**. Babies with this disorder may have a variety of abnormalities of the head, face, heart, joints, and limbs. In addition, the central nervous system can be affected, causing mental retardation, hyperactivity, and behavioral problems. The damage appears to be directly related to the amount of alcohol consumed, especially during the early months of pregnancy.

A woman who enjoys an occasional drink may wonder how much alcohol might be safe during pregnancy. Some studies suggest that even two drinks a week can lead to a mild withdrawal syndrome in the newborn, with increased irritability and stomach disturbances. The simplest and safest course is to abstain from alcohol altogether during pregnancy. You would be wise to abstain or consume no more than two alcoholic drinks per week if you are not yet pregnant but might become so in the near future. If drinking is not an ingrained habit, this should not be difficult. But if you find it hard to stay away from alcohol or control how much you drink at any given time, total avoidance is even more important. It is likely that you will need outside help, whether in a group setting such as a church support group or Alcoholics Anonymous, or individually with a professional counselor.

Illegal drugs. The use of illegal drugs continues to be a fearsome epidemic in our culture. The popular phrase *recreational drug use* is a contradiction because the word *recreation* implies an activity that has a positive, restoring, re-creating effect on mind and body. These substances, however, have just the opposite effect, draining away the resources, health, and ultimately life of their users. When the user is a pregnant woman, two lives (at least) are being damaged.

Regular marijuana users may deliver prematurely and, even when they go full-term, are more likely to have smaller babies. Cocaine use during pregnancy can cause not only a miscarriage or premature labor but also the eventual delivery of a small, irritable baby who may have serious, lifelong problems. Aside from any difficulties that might arise from premature delivery, cocaine itself can damage the infant's central nervous system, urinary tract, and limbs by constricting their blood supply. Increased irritability during the newborn period, developmental delays, and difficulty with learning and interacting with others have also been associated with cocaine use by the mother. (Frequently these mothers have used other substances such as alcohol and tobacco as well, complicating the question of identifying specific consequences of cocaine.)

A mother's use of narcotics such as heroin or methadone throughout her pregnancy may subject the baby to a difficult withdrawal after birth. Symptoms, which usually begin during the first day or two after birth, can include increased irritability, tremors, a high-pitched cry, constant hunger, sweating, and sneezing. In severe cases, seizures, vomiting, diarrhea, and difficulty with breathing can occur. Furthermore, if these drugs are taken intravenously (that is, injected into the veins), there is an additional risk of acquiring HIV, which without treatment almost always leads to AIDS. This will not only shorten the mother's life drastically but could infect her baby as well.

As serious as all these health concerns are, they do not encompass the vast waste of resources and the chaotic lifestyle that so often accompany the use of illegal drugs. Chronic drug abusers are usually unable to deal consistently with the daily demands of child care. Food preparation, safety in the home, and basic health practices are likely to be compromised. Run-ins with the law and difficulty maintaining steady employment are also common. Healthy relationships with friends and family members may be in short supply. The disturbances and distractions of chronic drug use seriously compromise a parent's ability to bring up healthy children. Whether or not you are pregnant, the time to stop using any of these toxic substances is *now,* and seeking help to do so should be an immediate priority.

Caffeine. This stimulant abounds in everyday beverages such as coffee, tea, and soft drinks, as well as in some headache remedies and pain relievers. A daily intake of up to 200 mg (about the amount in one or two eight-ounce cups of coffee) is widely considered safe during pregnancy. Larger amounts (over 500 mg per day) will keep both you and your baby awake, and his or her increased activity levels before birth may lead to a lower birth weight. If you consume coffee by the potful or sodas by the six-pack, you should begin cutting back to the 200 mg limit (see the table on the next page) before you become pregnant. If you're already expecting, you'll want to reduce your intake immediately. Decreasing the brewing time for coffee or tea will also cut caffeine content.

CAFFEINE CONTENT OF FOODS AND BEVERAGES

FOOD SOURCE	AMOUNT	CAFFEINE CONTENT
Regular coffee	8 oz	100–300 mg
Instant coffee	8 oz.	80–100 mg
Decaf coffee.	8 oz.	3–5 mg
Tea	8 oz	60–65 mg
*Regular cola	12 oz	36 mg
Diet cola	12 oz.	36–47 mg
Chocolate bar.	1 oz	20 mg

*Read labels to determine the presence of caffeine in specific soft drinks, such as Mountain Dew and Dr. Pepper.

Prescription and over-the-counter drugs. In general, you should try to avoid using any type of medication that isn't specifically prescribed or approved by your physician. Always be sure to inform any physician who treats you that you are or might be pregnant, since this could have a significant impact on the medication(s) he or she might recommend.

The fact that you can buy a drug at the supermarket doesn't necessarily mean that it is wise to use it during pregnancy. Pain relievers, cold tablets, laxatives, and other medications, as well as vitamin, herb, and food supplements, may seem harmless merely because they are easily accessible or advertised as "natural." A number of these are, in fact, quite safe during pregnancy, but you should consult your physician, who is familiar with your medical history and the details of your pregnancy, before using any of them. Common examples of nonprescription medications include the following:

- **Pain relievers.** Acetaminophen (Tylenol and various others) is generally recognized as safe for both mother and baby during pregnancy when used in the recommended dosage, but it can be toxic to the liver in an overdose. This drug reduces aches, pains, headaches, and fever. Both aspirin and the various brands of the anti-inflammatory drugs ibuprofen (Advil, Motrin, and others) and naproxen (Aleve) may increase the risk of bleeding in both mother and baby, especially around the time of birth. Anti-inflammatory medications taken late in pregnancy also may inhibit the onset of labor. Furthermore, they can cause a structure in the infant's heart known as the **ductus arteriosus** to close, resulting in potential circulatory problems after birth. While such complications are very unusual, you should avoid these medications during pregnancy (especially during the final weeks) unless they are recommended for a specific purpose by your physician.

- **Cold tablets.** Decongestants, antihistamines, cough syrups, and nasal sprays are sold in a bewildering array of combinations and preparations. All are intended to relieve symptoms, but these drugs rarely have a direct effect on the course of an upper-respiratory illness. Some of the ingredients in cold remedies are considered safe during a normal pregnancy, but you should check with your physician and pharmacist before using any of them. Rest, fluids, and time will take care of the vast majority of these infections. However, you should also contact your doctor if your runny nose, sore throat, or cough continues for more than a week or if you are running a fever over 100°F. If the doctor you speak with is not the one who is caring for your pregnancy, be sure that he or she knows you are pregnant.
- **Antacids.** Many pregnant women develop heartburn and indigestion because of changes in the intestinal tract produced by the growing uterus. Antacids are generally considered safe during pregnancy when used in recommended doses, but they may provoke diarrhea and can interfere with the absorption of prescription drugs.
- **Laxatives.** Constipation is common during pregnancy, but chemical laxatives are not the preferred method of treatment. Lots of fluids and juices, additional fiber in the diet (whether directly from food sources or supplements such as Metamucil or Citrucel), and regular exercise are the best first-line remedies. If you are not able to have a bowel movement for a few days at a time, you should review additional options with your physician.

Are you exposed to any environmental hazards?

During the course of your pregnancy, and especially during the first three months, you should minimize your exposure to **X rays** (also called **ionizing radiation**). Exposure to very large doses during the early weeks when the baby's tissues and organs are under construction could lead to birth defects. Fortunately, the X-ray exposure involved in common medical examinations is a tiny fraction of the amount generally considered risky. If you had one or more diagnostic X rays before discovering you were pregnant, it is extremely unlikely that your baby will be affected. Nevertheless, if this has occurred, you should review what procedures were done with your physician.

You can take a number of precautions to minimize your (and your baby's) exposure to X rays. If X rays (including those in the dentist's office) have been recommended, be sure to tell both your physician and the X-ray technician if you are or might be pregnant.

If at all possible, postpone X rays until after the baby is born, or at least wait until the first three months of pregnancy have passed. Procedures that do not utilize ionizing radiation, such as **ultrasound** or **magnetic resonance imaging (MRI)**, may be alternative options that can supply the necessary diagnostic information. (It is currently assumed but not proven that an MRI study is safe in early pregnancy.) If X rays are needed in an emergency situation, techniques that limit exposure (such as shielding the abdomen with a lead apron or limiting the number of films taken) may be utilized. In fact, it is generally recommended that a woman of reproductive age have her abdomen shielded when she has any type of X ray.

Depending upon location, dose, and timing during pregnancy, radiation therapy for cancer may—or may not—pose a significant hazard to a developing baby. The difficult problem of managing a cancer arises only in about one in one thousand pregnancies. Should this occur, however, the benefits and risks of any proposed treatment—as well as the consequences of postponing treatment—must be reviewed in detail, and decisions should be made after careful deliberation and prayer.

If you work around sources of ionizing radiation (for example, in an office or hospital area where X rays are taken), be sure to follow carefully the occupational guidelines in your facility for minimizing and measuring any ongoing exposure.

Over the past several years, concerns have been raised about the effect of exposure of pregnant women to **nonionizing radiation**—microwaves, radio waves, electromagnetic fields (such as those associated with power lines), and infrared light. Thus far, problems arising from these forms of radiation have not been clearly demonstrated. Specifically, research has not shown an increased risk of birth defects among pregnant women who work full- or part-time at video display terminals (VDTs) such as cathode-ray tube (CRT) computer monitors. (Flat-screen monitors, which are rapidly replacing their bulky CRT counterparts in homes and offices, are for all practical purposes radiation free.) Similarly, adverse effects of living near power lines have not been established.

Some concerns have been raised about prolonged exposure to high temperatures in hot tubs, whirlpools, and saunas. A body temperature elevation to 104°F or beyond during the first three months of pregnancy may increase the risk of a baby having a neural tube defect. Because a maximum safe amount of exposure to high temperatures cannot be established with complete certainty, it is best to avoid hot tubs or extremely hot baths altogether during the course of your pregnancy (and especially during the first three months).

Do you have any medical problems that need to be addressed?

Before 1900, a pregnant woman typically had only one prenatal visit with a physician prior to her delivery, during which her due date was determined—and little else. When next seen, she might be near term and in perfect health—or severely ill with an infection or a complication of her pregnancy. One of the major advances in public health in the early twentieth century was the recognition that a number of health problems that affect both mother and child can be detected, and in many cases corrected, through screening during pregnancy.

Many experts now not only advocate starting prenatal care as soon as possible after a pregnancy is confirmed, but even recommend a preconception visit for those who are thinking about starting a family. Whether before or during pregnancy, a thorough history and physical examination, including a review of important areas such as family background, habits, lifestyle, and general health, are wise. Some basic laboratory tests may also be done. Since all these areas can affect the health of a pregnancy and thus the quality of a baby's start in life, an ounce or two of prevention and protection can save several pounds of costly cure. Areas to consider include:

Family background. If there is a history of any diseases that are passed by inheritance (such as cystic fibrosis, sickle cell disease, blood-clotting disorders, or Tay-Sachs disease) within the family of either parent-to-be, genetic counseling can help to determine the potential risk of having a baby with a similar problem. This information can in turn guide decisions about having certain tests done during pregnancy to detect possible problems in the child.

Previous pregnancies. If you have had a prior pregnancy loss, a complication during labor or delivery, or a child born with a congenital problem of any type, specific tests and preparations may be in order before or during another pregnancy.

General health. Pregnancy is not a disease, of course, but it does have a significant impact on the way a woman's body functions. Furthermore, a number of medical problems can have a profound effect on her pregnancy and the health of her baby. The most important of these are diabetes, high blood pressure (hypertension), epilepsy, heart disease, asthma, kidney disease, and the so-called autoimmune disorders such as rheumatoid arthritis or systemic lupus erythematosus. Any of these problems should be addressed and controlled, if at all possible, before a woman becomes pregnant or as soon as possible after pregnancy is confirmed.

Infections and immunity. Most acute illnesses (such as colds) that might occur during a pregnancy are weathered without difficulty by both mother and baby. However, some types of infection in a pregnant woman can have adverse effects on her unborn child. When one of these occurs, the ultimate outcome will depend on (among other things) the type of organism causing it, the severity of the infection, and the stage of pregnancy during which it occurs. While the more troublesome infections are uncommon, it is well worth taking some basic precautions in order to avoid them.

- **Rubella.** Also known as German or three-day measles, this viral infection causes fever, aches, and a rash for a few days. If a woman becomes infected with rubella during the first month of pregnancy, her baby will have a 50 percent risk of developing one or more serious defects, which together are known as **congenital rubella syndrome**. These can include delayed growth, mental retardation, eye disorders, deafness, and heart disease. If the infection occurs in the third month or later, the risk drops to 10 percent.

Any woman who might become pregnant should have a blood test to see if she is immune to this disease. A vaccine against the rubella virus has been available since 1969, so most young women have had one or two MMR (measles/mumps/rubella) injections during childhood (two is the current recommendation). This does not guarantee that they are protected, although the vaccine is 95 percent effective at preventing rubella. If the blood test does not detect antibodies to rubella, women should have an immunization before they become pregnant. Most experts recommend waiting three months after the injection before becoming pregnant, although congenital rubella syndrome has not been reported even when the injection has been accidentally given during pregnancy. (If a woman is breastfeeding, the rubella vaccine can be administered without any apparent risk to the nursing child.)

- **Chickenpox.** This viral infection, also known as varicella, usually occurs during childhood, although susceptible adults (including pregnant women) can also develop this illness—often with a more difficult course than their younger counterparts experience. If a pregnant woman (or, for that matter, any adult) with chickenpox develops a cough or shortness of breath, it is very important that she be checked for pneumonia—a potentially serious complication—and treated appropriately (usually with intravenous acyclovir).

A small percentage of women who receive the rubella or MMR vaccine will not show immunity on a subsequent blood testing, but they will still be at decreased risk for developing rubella.

A developing baby can be infected with a mother's chickenpox, and the consequences will depend on the timing of the illness. According to the Centers for Disease Control and Prevention, during the first twelve weeks of pregnancy there is a 0.4 percent risk, and between thirteen and twenty weeks a 2 percent risk, of a baby developing **congenital varicella syndrome**, which may include eye, heart, and limb defects. There is no way to determine whether the baby has been affected by the mother's infection. Unfortunately, women who are infected with chickenpox during the first half of pregnancy may be told they should have an abortion without being told that the risk of a congenital problem is in fact quite low.

After twenty weeks of pregnancy, chickenpox in the mother does not result in harm to her baby unless the infection occurs from five days before to two days after delivery. (Before birth, the baby can be infected through the mother's blood via the umbilical cord. If the mother is infected shortly after giving birth, the baby can contract the illness by direct exposure.) When this occurs, a severe infection can result, because the baby may acquire the virus without also receiving any of the mother's protective antibodies. If this occurs, the baby should receive an injection called varicella-zoster immune globulin (or VZIG), which provides a temporary protective dose of "borrowed" antibody.

If you are pregnant and do not believe you have had this disease, you should be careful to avoid any child who has or might have chickenpox, as well as any child who has been given the chickenpox vaccine within the past six weeks. (Of course, this isn't the time for your other children to be given the chickenpox vaccine either.) Finally, avoid contact with any adult who develops shingles, which can spread the same virus.

If you are uncertain whether or not you have had chickenpox in the past and wish to find out prior to or during pregnancy, your doctor can order a blood test that detects antibodies to the virus.

- **Group B streptococci.** These bacteria are present in the vagina or rectum of approximately 20 to 25 percent of pregnant women, and can infect the baby during birth, especially if labor is premature or if the woman's membranes (the "bag of waters") are ruptured for more than eighteen hours prior to delivery. Overall, about one of every one thousand infants is infected during birth, often with severe consequences, including pneumonia and meningitis. The Centers for Disease Control and Prevention now recommends routine screening for group B streptococci at thirty-five to thirty-seven weeks into your pregnancy. A baby born to a woman who is a carrier of group B streptococci has a one in two hundred chance of being infected if the mother is not treated with antibiotics at the time of delivery. If she is treated, however, the risk of group B strep infection drops twentyfold to one in four thousand.
- **Toxoplasmosis.** This infection is caused by a parasite that may contaminate undercooked meat or dead animals and thus can appear in the feces of cats that eat rodents and decaying meat. If a woman develops toxoplasmosis during pregnancy, her baby has about a one in three chance of becoming infected, and of those, about one-third will show some signs of the disease. Significant problems in these infants can include premature delivery, a small head (microcephaly), encephalitis (inflammation of brain tissue), weak muscles, an enlarged liver and spleen, and inflammation of the retina. If recognized in mother or infant, toxoplasmosis can be treated with antibiotics. Unfortunately, this infection can be difficult to diagnose, and treatment doesn't usually change the outcome.

  The most important take-home lesson about toxoplasmosis is that prevention is possible through two simple measures. First, any meat you consume should be well cooked. Second, you should avoid any contact with cat droppings if you are pregnant or might be in the near future. This means staying away from the litter box and avoiding close contact with cats, especially if they spend much time outdoors.

- **Parvovirus.** This virus causes an infection, seen commonly in schoolchildren but also in other age-groups, called **erythema infectiosum**, or fifth disease. Typically seen in winter and spring months, fifth disease is most well known for producing a so-called slapped-cheek rash on the face, although a lacy eruption may be seen on the arms, legs, and upper body as well. Adults who are infected may develop the rash as well as aching joints. However, both children and adults can become infected without any symptoms at all. Unfortunately, this disease is contagious for up to three weeks before the rash breaks out, so it is virtually impossible to prevent exposure of other family members.

  If a woman becomes infected with parvovirus during pregnancy, it's very likely (better than an 80 percent chance) that there will be no adverse effects on her baby. However, sometimes the mother's infection results in a severe anemia in the baby, which in turn can cause congestive heart failure. Therefore, a pregnant woman who is exposed to this infection should have a blood test to determine whether she is immune to it. If she is, there should be no cause for concern. If not, testing may be recommended later in the pregnancy to determine whether she has become infected. Another type of test, called a **polymerase chain reaction** (or **PCR**) **amplification** of parvovirus DNA, can also be used to diagnose this infection if suspicious symptoms occur.

  If infection with parvovirus appears to have taken place during pregnancy—with or without symptoms—the baby should be monitored with ultrasound exams prior to birth for signs of heart failure resulting from anemia. (The PCR test noted above can also be carried out on a sample of amniotic fluid to help determine whether the infant has become infected.) If infection is suspected, the baby may require medication, early delivery, or even a transfusion prior to birth (one of the many forms of medical intervention now available for the preborn).

- **Cytomegalovirus (CMV).** With the dubious distinction of causing the most common congenital infection in the United States, this virus is also both untreatable and rarely (if ever) preventable. Fortunately, significant CMV disease in newborns is very uncommon. Approximately one to three percent of pregnant women experience a primary (first-time) infection with CMV, but the vast majority have no symptoms. About 30 to 40 percent of infected mothers transmit the virus to their babies, but only about 10 to 15 percent of infected infants will have some form of noticeable disease at birth. The overall risk of any infant having serious disease related to CMV (that may involve the central nervous system, vision, hearing, pneumonia, or liver disease) is between one in ten thousand and one in twenty thousand.

At the present time, pregnant women are not screened for susceptibility to CMV because there is no effective treatment for this infection. However, if a woman develops an illness during pregnancy that resembles mononucleosis—with fever, sore throat, enlarged lymph nodes in the neck, and marked fatigue—her physician may at some point request blood tests or even cultures to help determine if CMV might be involved. A polymerase chain reaction (PCR) test for CMV can also be carried out on amniotic fluid to help determine whether the infant has been infected. If this diagnosis is made, she will need careful and accurate counseling regarding the risk of the baby having congenital disease.

- **Sexually transmitted infections (STIs).** Approximately twenty different STIs pose significant risks to both mother and baby, and many begin during intimate contact between people who look perfectly well and have no signs of illness. Unfortunately, the first indication that an infection has taken place may be the birth of a very sick baby, a miscarriage or stillbirth, or even a woman's inability to become pregnant. Chapter 12 in this book contains a more detailed look at STIs, and you would be wise to review that information if you haven't already, even if you consider yourself at low risk for having a sexually transmitted infection.

Family Planning and Birth Control

Contrary to some modern opinions, the family is not a human invention. It is not a societal construct or an arbitrary combination of people who profess love for one another or connect in some other way. The family is in fact an institution designed by God for specific purposes. It is within this context of commitment and security that God intends mankind to reproduce. It also provides a nurturing environment in which children can grow and mature, as well as a framework of relationships in which parents (and grandparents) can pass on a legacy of faith and values to the next generation.

It is of no little significance that God repeatedly declares children to be a blessing, not a burden. They are highly valued in His sight and are to be treasured rather than merely tolerated.

Sons are a heritage from the Lord;
children a reward from him.
Like arrows in the hands of a warrior
are sons born in one's youth.
(PSALM 127:3-4)

Children's children are a crown to the aged.
(PROVERBS 17:6)

Little children were brought to Jesus for him to place his hands on them and pray for them. But the disciples rebuked those who brought them. Jesus said, "Let the little children come to me, and do not hinder them, for the kingdom of heaven belongs to such as these."
(MATTHEW 19:13-14)

Family planning can be defined as a way of regulating the number and spacing of children through contraception or other means of birth control. While it has been widely practiced and considered "standard operating procedure" in the United States and most Western nations for decades, it is not without its controversies and complications. Contraceptive advocates past and present have been passionate about the easing of personal and financial burdens when couples are able to decide when to have children and how large or small their family will be. Some see access to contraception as crucial to ending poverty and privation in many parts of the world. Critics, including some members of Christian, Jewish, and Islamic communities, have raised concerns that availability of contraception to any and all who desire it—young or old, married or single—contributes to a devaluation not only of reproduction but also of sexuality itself.

Throughout the length and breadth of the Christian community, opinions and beliefs about family planning within marriage (and, in some cases, outside of marriage) vary widely. Some hold that no form of family planning is morally acceptable and that a couple acting in obedience to God will be blessed with whatever number of children He chooses, whenever He chooses. Other teachings, including those of the Roman Catholic Church, hold that family planning is acceptable only when artificial contraceptive methods are not used and when the spacing or delaying of children is not pursued for selfish reasons. Still other Christian teachings allow the use of most birth control forms for a number of reasons. These reasons may include but are not limited to:

- **Illness or physical problems associated with childbearing.** Many women delay pregnancy because they are dealing with serious medical problems or are undergoing medical treatment (such as chemotherapy) that can be dangerous to a child developing in the womb. Other women, having experienced health problems in previous pregnancies, delay pregnancy or decide against having another child because a future pregnancy would entail considerable risk.

- **Emotional or psychological reasons.** Some people feel that they are emotionally or psychologically unprepared or ill-equipped to nurture a new life. Some fear that they would be poor parents or perhaps do serious harm to a child because of their own abusive childhood.
- **Financial reasons.** For some couples, the decision to delay pregnancy or avoid it altogether may be based on fears that raising a child might result in a lower standard of living. For poorer women, having another child might actually create crushing financial problems.
- **Career or educational reasons.** Some women choose to delay pregnancy so that they can pursue career goals or obtain a college degree.

Christians of good conscience can and do disagree on the acceptability of using birth control, sometimes strongly. Given this state of affairs, and considering the worth that God invests in children, many Christians who marry or are considering marriage may find family planning to be a complicated subject. If a couple is considering one or several family-planning strategies, it is crucial that they seek guidance through prayer and the Scriptures and obtain wise, godly counsel from a trustworthy source, be it a pastor, counselor, or a physician who is sensitive to matters of faith as well as knowledgeable about reproductive biology.

Some principles to bear in mind when considering birth control

Even if you have no religious or philosophical objections to the use of birth control, it is important to understand some principles that should govern their use. First, however, we need to clarify a distinction between the terms *birth control* and *contraception*. **Contraception** usually refers to specific artificial measures (such as drugs, barriers, or surgery) that prevent the joining of sperm and egg. **Birth control** is a broader term that could refer to any means used to prevent pregnancy or childbirth, including not only contraception but also any approach ranging from abstinence and natural family planning at one end of the spectrum to induced abortion at the other. (Needless to say, abortion is a malignant and uncivilized method of birth control, although it has been utilized for that purpose in some cultures.) In our discussion here, we will use the term *contraception* in the strictest sense of the word: the prevention of the joining of egg and sperm, not interference with the implanting of a fertilized egg in the uterus.

There are a number of family-planning options for women and two for men (wearing a condom or having a vasectomy). With so many alternatives available, understanding (let alone remembering) the various mechanisms, benefits, risks, and various other pros and cons can be a daunting task. There are, however, several principles that should guide men and women as they make decisions about this important subject:

1. **Life begins at conception.** The Bible speaks clearly about the personhood of the unborn child.

> *You created my inmost being;*
> *you knit me together in my mother's womb.*
> *I praise you because I am fearfully and wonderfully made;*
> *your works are wonderful,*
> *I know that full well.*
> *My frame was not hidden from you*
> *when I was made in the secret place.*
> *When I was woven together in the depths of the earth,*
> *your eyes saw my unformed body.*
> (PSALM 139:13-16)

To God, human life does not attain value at a certain stage of pregnancy or at birth. Life is sacred from the moment of conception.

For this reason, elective abortion, whether by chemical (such as the drug mifepristone, formerly known as RU-486) or by surgical means, is unacceptable as birth control. Women should also avoid devices or drugs that prevent an embryo from implanting in the uterine wall, since this results in the loss of a new life.

2. **Sex is designed for, safest, and most fulfilling within the confines of a mutually monogamous marital relationship.** We went to some lengths to explain this proposition in the previous chapter. Why do we belabor this point? Because contraceptives are often prescribed or purchased to prevent pregnancy resulting from nonmarital sex, whether within a long-term "committed" relationship or in a procession of casual couplings. While birth control techniques can reduce the chances of an unplanned pregnancy, they cannot protect either partner from other consequences—emotional, spiritual, and physical—of sexual activity outside of marriage.

3. **Most birth control methods provide no protection from sexually transmitted infections.** Hormonal contraceptives (whether oral, injected, applied to the skin, or inserted into the vagina), intrauterine devices (IUDs), diaphragms, or natural family planning methods do not reduce the risk of acquiring an STI. (Indeed, an IUD may facilitate the spread of certain infective bacteria into the pelvis.) Condoms have been widely promoted as part of a "safer sex" strategy, not only because they reduce pregnancy risk but also because they offer variable protection against many (but not all) STIs. (With human papillomavirus, the virus responsible for the vast majority of cases of cancer of the cervix, condoms have been shown to offer little or no protection against transmission.) Unfortunately, it only takes one sexual encounter

with the wrong person at the wrong time to acquire an infection that can literally change your life—and not for the better.

4. **The method being considered should not violate your religious convictions.** Wholehearted, relaxed, unencumbered—indeed, joyous—sexuality is God's gift to a healthy marriage. If one or both of you feel that whatever you're doing to postpone pregnancy is violating God's intentions for you as a couple, your intimacy with Him and each other will be affected. Any issues in this area need to be addressed—especially if there is a difference of opinion between husband and wife on this subject. If you are questioning whether a particular method is appropriate or acceptable, it is important not to sweep the issue under the bed, so to speak, but rather to obtain godly counsel and to seek God's guidance through prayer and Scripture.

A brief look at family planning methods

Family planning methods can be divided into five basic categories: barrier methods, intrauterine devices, hormonal approaches, surgical interventions, and natural family planning. It should be noted that no birth control method is 100 percent effective in preventing pregnancy, although some are more reliable than others. The effectiveness of a method is usually expressed in terms of a percentage failure rate, based on the number of sexually active women who become pregnant while using the method over the course of a year. For example, a 5 percent failure rate would mean that out of one hundred women relying on that method alone for twelve months, five would become pregnant.

Estimating effectiveness is complicated by the fact that there can be a major difference between a method's theoretical or "perfect use" effectiveness—that is, how well it works if a couple uses it perfectly, month in and month out—and what is called typical use effectiveness, or what happens in the real world. The latter may be affected not only by characteristics of the method itself—how easy or complicated it is to use—but also by factors such as age and marital status. For example, mature, committed married couples using condoms will have a lower failure rate for pregnancy than single teenagers using the same method. The table on page 645 shows both perfect and typical use statistics for a number of methods that we will discuss.

Barrier methods are true contraceptives—that is, they prevent the union of sperm and egg—by physically or chemically preventing sperm from entering the uterus. Of the physical barriers available, the male condom is the most familiar, although there is also a female condom that is placed within the vagina. Both are designed to prevent sperm from entering the vagina. Chemical barriers are spermicidal (sperm killing) compounds, such as nonoxynol-9, which are applied in a variety of ways. For example, contraceptive foam, suppositories, or sponges contain a spermicide that is released after insertion into the vagina. Other barrier methods include the diaphragm, which is inserted into the vagina and covers the cervix, and the cervical cap, which fits more tightly over the cer-

BIRTH CONTROL EFFECTIVENESS
(Number of Pregnancies per 100 Women within the First Year of Use)

TYPE OF METHOD	TYPICAL USE	PERFECT USE
Continuous abstinence	0	0
No method	85	85
Male condom	15	2
Female condom	21	5
Diaphragm	16	6
Cervical cap	16 (32) *	9 (26)*
Sponge	16 (32) *	9 (20)*
Spermicide	29	18
IUD (copper)	0.8	0.6
IUD (hormonal)	0.1	0.1
Oral contraceptive pills/ progestin-only pills**	8	0.3
Ortho Evra (patch)	8	0.3
NuvaRing (vaginal ring)	8	0.3
Depo-Provera (injection)	3	0.3
Surgical methods (tubal ligation)	0.5	0.5
Surgical methods (vasectomy)	0.15	0.1
Natural family planning (rhythm/calendar method)	25	9
Natural family planning (ovulation method)	25	3
Natural family planning (symptothermal method)	25	2

*First number represents effectiveness for women who have never given birth. The number in parentheses represents effectiveness for women who have given birth.

**Progestin-only pills are generally acknowledged to have a higher failure rate than combination oral contraceptives.

Typical Use = effectiveness for couples whose use is not consistent or always correct

Perfect Use = effectiveness for couples whose use is consistent and always correct

Source: Adapted from James Trussell, "Contraceptive Efficacy" in *Contraceptive Technology*, 18th ed. by Robert Hatcher et al., (New York: Ardent Media, 2004), 792. Used with permission.

In 1994 the contraceptive sponge was taken off the market because of problems related to its production. In April 2005, the Food and Drug Administration approved reintroduction of the Today sponge, and it is now available in the United States and Canada.

vix. These do not provide a physical barrier as do condoms, but rather serve as vehicles for spermicidal jellies or creams. Barrier methods can be combined for greater contraceptive effectiveness.

Barrier methods have the advantage of being the most accessible and least hazardous of all forms of contraception. No pills, injections, or procedures (with their potential side effects) are involved. While a diaphragm or cervical cap requires a doctor's visit so that the proper size can be determined, condoms and vaginal spermicidal products (such as foam, cream, suppositories, and other products) can be obtained without a prescription. However, they are also the most user-intensive. Failure rates tend to be higher because they must be used correctly and consistently (in other words, *every* time) to obtain best results, a requirement that can dampen spontaneity—or that may be overlooked in the heat of the moment. Furthermore, condoms may slip off or break, and diaphragms and cervical caps may become dislodged during intercourse.

An **intrauterine device (IUD)** is a small T-shaped object that is inserted through the cervix into the cavity of the uterus to prevent pregnancy. There are two types of IUDs: copper and hormonal. Copper IUDs release small amounts of copper into the uterus, which immobilizes sperm so they cannot swim to the fallopian tubes. Hormonal IUDs slowly release a small amount of hormone into the uterus, causing a thickening of the cervical mucus that can prevent sperm from entering the uterus.

Once inserted, an IUD offers the advantage of long-term birth control—it can be left in place from five to ten years and generally does not affect fertility once removed—but not without some important downsides. It must be inserted or removed in a doctor's office, and in very rare cases it may puncture the uterine wall. Women who are infected with gonorrhea or chlamydia at the time an IUD is inserted, or who become infected while it is still in place, may develop pelvic inflammatory disease (PID). Women who have never been pregnant are at particular risk for this complication, which sadly can result in infertility. (Indeed, even a woman who has had one or more children should understand that there is some risk of future infertility if she uses an IUD for contraception.)

Another important concern is that IUDs (copper and hormonal) can bring about changes in the lining of the uterus that may make it inhospitable to an implanting embryo. This is called a **postfertilization** (rather than a true conception-preventing) effect, and it would terminate a human life in its earliest stages. While IUDs work primarily by preventing sperm from gaining access to eggs, evidence suggests that IUDs prevent pregnancy, at least some of the time, by this other **abortifacient** mechanism. For this reason, IUDs should be avoided as a form of birth control.

Hormonal methods work primarily by preventing ovulation (so that an egg is not available for sperm to fertilize) and secondarily by thickening the cervical mucus so that sperm are prevented from entering the uterus. These include combinations of estrogen and progestin (a synthetic form of progesterone) or progestin-only preparations, and they come in a variety of delivery methods.

Although "the pill" (more technically known as the **combined oral contraceptive pill**, or **OCP**) has been around for over forty years and its formulation has changed many times, the basic idea has remained the same: Each four-week course includes twenty-one pills containing estrogen and progestin that are taken, one per day, starting on the first day of a woman's period (or on the first Sunday following the beginning of a menstrual cycle). Seven additional pills, taken during the fourth week, contain no hormone. (These serve simply to "mark time" for a week, during which a woman normally will have a menstrual flow.) Combined estrogen-progestin contraceptives are also available in a patch that delivers the hormone directly through the skin and in a ring that is inserted into the vagina and releases hormones that are absorbed through the vaginal wall.

Progestin-only preparations are also available and come both in a pill (sometimes known as the minipill) and an injection (Depo-Provera). Progestin-only pills are not as widely used as OCPs and are often prescribed to women who cannot take estrogen or who are breast-feeding. Norplant, a subcutaneous implant consisting of six small, thin silicone rubber capsules that slowly release progestin over five years, was approved by the FDA in 1990 but was taken off the market by its manufacturer in 2002.

Hormonal methods of birth control have the advantage of being highly effective in preventing pregnancy and offering a variety of options with different levels of convenience. One injection of Depo-Provera, for example, will provide three months of birth control. The contraceptive patch can be left on for a week at a time, while the vaginal ring provides coverage for three weeks.

Hormonal contraception is not without side effects and risks. These can include erratic bleeding patterns, nausea, headache, and bloating, as well as a slight risk for developing a blood clot (or **thrombosis**) in the deep veins of the leg or pelvis. (This is now seen far less frequently than in the early days of oral contraceptives, when doses were considerably higher than those used now.) If OCPs are taken inconsistently, or if a dose is missed for two or three consecutive days, their contraceptive effectiveness is significantly diminished. A number of women have become pregnant after missing only one dose. At the opposite extreme, for some women suppression of ovulation may continue for months after the medication is stopped, which may cause some concern when a couple wants to begin a pregnancy. Usually, however, ovulation starts one to three months after an oral contraceptive is discontinued.

A concern about progestin-only pills (and Norplant implants as well) is the fact that they do not reliably prevent ovulation. Five percent of women using progestin-only pills will become pregnant during the first year of use, a higher number than typically occurs with other hormonal contraceptives. Furthermore, they alter the lining of the uterus in a way that appears to increase the likelihood that an embryo might not implant if conception should occur. Another issue with progestin-only pills is that any pregnancies that do occur have a greater chance of being ectopic—that is, outside the uterus (and usually in the fallopian tube)—rather than progressing normally. This may occur because progestins tend to slow the movement of an egg through the fallopian tube. If an egg that has been fertilized becomes "stuck" there, before long the continued growth of the embryo will cause pain, and if not diagnosed and treated, the tube will rupture. The embryo cannot survive, and an ectopic pregnancy ultimately must be treated, usually on an urgent (or emergency) basis with medication or surgery.

Because of the higher likelihood of ovulation, the possibility of interference with implantation in the uterus if conception occurs, and the increased risk of ectopic pregnancy that both terminates a new human life and threatens the mother's life and health, the use of progestin-only pills as a contraceptive method should be avoided.

Similar questions have been raised about the mechanism of action of the Depo-Provera injection, as well as combined oral contraceptive pills, which are used much more widely than progestin-only preparations. While it is known that these medications work by suppressing ovulation and to a lesser extent by thickening the cervical mucus to prevent sperm from reaching the egg, some experts have suggested that they might work, in a very small number of in-

WHAT ABOUT THE "MORNING AFTER" PILL?

You may have heard of emergency contraception, better known as the "morning after" pill, for a woman who has had unintended, unprotected, or forced sex and is concerned about the possibility of pregnancy. What exactly is this medication, and how does it work?

"Morning after" pills contain the same types of hormones found in oral contraceptives, but they are specially packaged and intended to be used within the first seventy-two hours after intercourse. The first brand approved by the Food and Drug Administration (FDA) for this purpose was Preven, which is no longer being manufactured. It contained both estrogen and progestin packaged in a kit with four pills and a pregnancy test (to ensure that a woman wasn't already pregnant from a previous sexual contact, in which case the pills would not be used). Two of the pills were to be taken within seventy-two hours after intercourse; the remaining two twelve hours later. Preven reduced the likelihood of becoming pregnant by 75 percent. About half of the women who took this combination became nauseated, and one in five experienced vomiting. While Preven is no longer available, some health-care providers will recommend multitablet doses of other combination oral contraceptives, although they are not approved by the FDA for this purpose.

The only brand now approved in the United States specifically for emergency contraception is marketed under the name Plan B. It consists only of progestin and is reported to have a higher rate of effectiveness in preventing pregnancy while provoking less nausea and vomiting. (Preven, Plan B, or any other combination of oral contraceptive pills that might be used as emergency contraception does not protect against sexually transmitted infections.)

stances, not by preventing conception but by provoking changes in the endometrium that prevent an embryo from implanting.

However, there is disagreement among pro-life physicians regarding the likelihood, and even the possibility, that OCPs and Depo-Provera might contribute to the loss of human life after fertilization. While the majority of experts believe that these medications do *not* work by an abortifacient mechanism, a minority feel that when conception occurs during their use, there is enough of a possibility for an abortifacient effect, however remote, to warrant informing women about it. Couples who are concerned about the potential implications of OCPs or Depo-Provera should consider reviewing the issue in more detail, consulting with their doctor (though he or she may or may not be familiar with the details of the controversy) and prayerfully considering the facts as they make decisions about this important question.

One additional caution regarding Depo-Provera: Use of this medication

How do these medications work? That depends on the time in a woman's cycle when they are taken. They may prevent ovulation—the release of the egg from the ovary—or they may delay ovulation until sperm are no longer capable of fertilizing an egg. (Sperm cells survive about five days.) They may also interfere with the movement of egg and sperm within the fallopian tube or with the actual union of egg and sperm. All of these mechanisms are truly contraceptive—that is, they prevent fertilization, the union of egg and sperm that starts a new human life.

It is also possible that "morning after" pills have their effect *after* fertilization, by changing the lining of the uterus so that the fertilized egg—a new human in the first few days of life—cannot implant within it. This mechanism is not truly contraceptive, because conception has already occurred, but rather represents a very early abortion. Promoters of emergency contraception pills state that these medications do not cause abortion, but this claim is based on their definition of pregnancy as beginning with the implanting of the fertilized egg within the uterus. For those who hold that human life begins at conception, however, any medication or device that prevents a new life from continuing in its normal development would be considered abortifacient, or abortion inducing.

Because a new human life deserves to be protected at its earliest stages—even in the most difficult circumstances—the various mechanisms by which these pills might work create a real dilemma, because it is impossible to know which of them might be acting in any particular case. This is particularly difficult if a woman has been the victim of a sexual assault. Obviously, this type of medication is not intended to be used on a regular basis or as a primary form of birth control. When deciding whether or not to use this type of medication in a crisis situation, a woman should seek and prayerfully consider counsel from her family, her physician, and her pastor. ■

has been associated with loss of bone density, probably because it tends to lower estrogen levels. Women younger than nineteen (when bone density should be increasing) and those at risk for osteoporosis should consider carefully whether this is an appropriate form of contraception.

Two differing perspectives on whether OCPs and Depo-Provera might have an abortifacient effect may be found at the Web site of the American Association of Pro Life Obstetricians and Gynecologists (http://www.aaplog.org/oral.htm) or in the book *The Reproductive Revolution: A Christian Appraisal of Sexuality, Reproductive Technologies, and the Family,* edited by John Kilner, Paige Cunningham, and W. David Hager (Grand Rapids, Mich.: Eerdmans, 2000).

Surgical methods of birth control are available for both men (specifically, vasectomy) and women. For women the usual surgical means of birth control is **tubal ligation** (sometimes called tubal sterilization), although other procedures such as hysterectomy (removal of the uterus) will also preclude the possibility of pregnancy. Tubal ligation physically prevents the meeting of sperm and egg by altering the fallopian tubes, through which an egg normally travels from ovary to uterus, by severing, cauterizing, or constricting them with bands or clips. This is usually accomplished using **laparoscopic** techniques in which instruments are inserted and the surgery performed through very small incisions in the abdomen (under an anesthetic, of course). Tubal ligation procedures allow women to ovulate normally, and eggs released by the ovaries are absorbed by the woman's body.

In addition to being highly effective, one feature of tubal ligation that makes it attractive to many women is also a potential drawback—it may be permanent. While tubal ligation is surgically reversible in most cases (although some procedures are more reversible than others), after reversal a pregnancy may not occur as readily for most women as it would have before the ligation. Young women who may want to become pregnant at a later date and those who are considering tubal ligation for reasons that might be temporary (such as financial worries or marital problems) should weigh their options very carefully before committing to tubal ligation as a means of birth control.

A newer method involves **hysteroscopy** in which a doctor inserts an optical instrument through the vagina into the uterine cavity and then uses this "scope" to place a small device (called a micro-insert) into the opening of the fallopian tubes. Within twelve weeks the fallopian tubes form a tissue barrier around the micro-insert, blocking sperm from traveling through them. It is important to note that, at the present time, this type of sterilization is *not* reversible.

A **vasectomy** is quite a bit simpler for a man than a tubal ligation is for a woman. A vasectomy is an office procedure, requiring only some local anesthetic, in which the **vas deferens**, a small tube that transports sperm from each testicle, is surgically interrupted. The sperm constitute only a small proportion of the semen released during intercourse, so the procedure has no effect on a man's interest in or enjoyment of sex (other than reducing anxiety over a possible pregnancy). Like tubal ligation for women, it should be considered a permanent event. While surgical reversal is possible, it is much more involved than the original procedure, with variable rates of success.

Any couple considering tubal ligation or vasectomy should assume that they will not be able to have children together after one of these procedures is carried out, and as a result *they should be unified in their decision.* If either husband or wife has reservations about the ultimate outcome, they should postpone—perhaps indefinitely—any such procedure. Needless to say, this is an important question to address with the physician who will perform the surgery, and perhaps even with a counselor or pastor if a couple has a significant difference of opinion about this subject.

Natural family planning (NFP) methods are approaches to birth control that require no drugs, special devices, or surgical procedures, and that rarely if ever pose moral or ethical issues. NFP has had an unwarranted reputation as an ineffective method of postponing pregnancy and is often incorrectly equated with the so-called rhythm method. (An old joke goes, "What do you call a couple that uses the rhythm method? Parents.") Contemporary approaches to NFP are in fact grounded on scientifically based observations of a woman's fertility cycle that indicate more precisely when a woman is least likely to become pregnant. For couples seeking to become pregnant, this method has the added benefit of indicating when a woman is *most* likely to conceive, making it a family-planning tool in the most complete sense of the term.

Natural family planning is a broad term that includes several approaches, but the basic strategy for pregnancy avoidance involves couples engaging in sexual intercourse only on days during a woman's cycle when she is least likely to become pregnant. As mentioned on page 614 of this chapter, there are about three or four days around the time of ovulation during which intercourse could lead to conception. Furthermore, ovulation nearly always occurs exactly fourteen days before the onset of bleeding (assuming there is no pregnancy). For a woman with a twenty-eight-day cycle, ovulation would be expected to occur about fourteen days after the beginning of the cycle (identified as the day on which menstrual bleeding begins).

The older rhythm method for postponing pregnancy involves using a fertility log to keep track of the wife's menstrual periods and then avoiding intercourse for several days before and after the likely time of ovulation. But all too often there is a significant problem with this approach: Most women do not have a predictable, twenty-eight-day cycle, and the variable part of the cycle occurs *before* ovulation. If it were the other way around—that is, if ovulation always occurred exactly two weeks after the first day of the previous menstrual period—the rhythm method would be a snap. But for many couples, using the rhythm method is like asking directions from a passenger on a bus who says, "All you have to do is get off one stop before I do!" What they need, but can never know for certain, is the date of the *next* period. Since a woman's cycle can be as short as twenty-one days or as long as forty-five days, and because the time from day one to ovulation may be variable, women with periods of atypical duration might have difficulty avoiding pregnancy if they schedule their sexual activities according to a twenty-eight-day cycle. In fact, with typical use, couples using the rhythm method have about a 25 percent chance of starting a pregnancy over the course of a year.

Other forms of NFP rely not only on the calendar but also on observing and interpreting physical signs that indicate a woman is entering a fertile time of her cycle. One method takes advantage of the interesting phenomenon that a woman's body temperature rises upon ovulation. With the **basal body temperature method** of birth control, a woman takes her resting temperature when she first awakens and records it on a temperature chart. Although body temperature varies from woman to woman, a normal temperature before ovulation ranges from 96°F to 98°F. When a woman ovulates, her temperature rises between 0.4 and 0.8 degrees, to a range of about 97°F to 99°F. A woman is most fertile (and thus most likely to become pregnant) during the two or three days before the temperature reaches its highest level and for about twenty-four hours afterward. In order to track very small changes in temperature accurately, one should use a basal body temperature thermometer that allows you to read 0.1 degree increments. By charting her basal body temperature carefully, a woman can become familiar with her own temperature patterns and use them to predict the days on which she is most likely to become pregnant.

A third form of NFP takes advantage of another physical sign of fertility. The **Billings ovulation method** (after Drs. John and Evelyn Billings, who discovered and developed this NFP method) is also known generically as the **ovulation method** or the **cervical mucus method**. It is based on the observation that the properties of the mucus produced by a woman's cervix change over the course of her cycle. To monitor her fertility, a woman examines her cervical mucus using her fingers or toilet tissue. As eggs within a woman's ovaries begin to mature, she will be able to observe a vaginal discharge of cervical mucus that is cloudy and white or yellow in color, with a sticky or tacky consistency. As a woman approaches ovulation, her cervical mucus will become more slippery and clear like an egg white, with perhaps a "stringy" texture that allows it to stretch between her fingers or toilet tissue. Within a few days her cervical mucus will again become sticky, and then will eventually cease to be produced as she approaches the beginning of her menstrual period. A woman is most fertile when her cervical mucus is slippery and clear—and especially during the last day in which it demonstrates this consistency.

According to a study by the World Health Organization, the Billings ovulation method, when properly and consistently used, is about 97 percent effective in preventing pregnancy.[4] (This compares favorably with oral contraceptives and other hormonal forms of birth control.) Additional advantages of this method are that it is inexpensive and immediately reversible for couples who want to become pregnant—indeed, it helps them plan sexual activity for times at which they are most likely to succeed in becoming pregnant. Another NFP method, the **symptothermal method** (sometimes known as the **fertility awareness method**), utilizes both the observation of cervical mucus characteristics and the changes in a woman's basal body temperature. Some proponents of the symptothermal method suggest observing an additional

NATURAL PLANNING METHODS

Natural family planning methods are often taught in classes or through printed and video materials. To obtain further information, contact the following organizations:

BILLINGS OVULATION METHOD ASSOCIATION—USA
P.O. Box 16206
St. Paul, MN 55116
(651) 699-8139
www.boma-usa.org

For more about the symptothermal method:

COUPLE TO COUPLE LEAGUE
P.O. Box 111184
Cincinnati, Ohio 45211
(513) 471-2000
www.ccli.org

characteristic: the changes in a woman's cervix during fertile phases of her cycle. Immediately before and during ovulation, the cervix rises, becomes softer, and opens slightly. After ovulation it drops, becomes more firm, and closes.

When the Cycles End: Menopause and Its Aftermath

Strictly speaking, the term **menopause** does not refer to a process but simply to the very last menstrual cycle of a woman's reproductive life. **Perimenopause** refers specifically to the transitional period between normal reproductive cycles and the final menstrual flow. **Postmenopause** refers to the years following the last period. For the sake of simplicity, however, we will use the word *menopause* to refer to the entire transitional time surrounding the end of a woman's reproductive cycles.

When a woman approaches her fifties (and sometimes earlier), the ovaries' supply of eggs (or ova) becomes depleted. At the same time, they begin to reduce their production of estrogen and progesterone, the hormones that prepare the uterus for implantation of a fertilized egg. Essentially, the ovaries "retire" from their thirty- to forty-year career of supplying eggs and hormones, although lesser amounts of various hormones are still manufactured. This may occur rapidly or over several years, during which time a number of important physical and emotional changes occur in a woman—not the least of which is the loss of her fertility.

The cessation of menstrual cycles is usually gradual, marked by increasing length of cycles: 70 percent of all women will experience such irregularity, with thirty-six to ninety days between periods. In contrast, about 10 percent will experience an abrupt end to their periods without warning. Nearly twice that number report *more* bleeding than usual. This may reflect a problem with the lining of the uterus, however, and should be evaluated by a physician.

It's important to remember that menopause is not a disease. It is a universal event in the human female (assuming she lives to the appropriate age), and there is no getting around it, for good reason: Given the physical and physiological rigors of childbirth and the length of time required to raise a newborn to near-adulthood, it would be unwise for a woman to become pregnant after she is well into her fifties. While menopause is unavoidable, its impact on individual women varies greatly. It may occur without notice, or it may produce disruptive symptoms. It may generate little in the way of long-term consequences, or its ultimate effect on quality of life may be profound.

Climacteric is a less commonly used term for menopause.

The vast majority of women experience menopause between the ages of forty-five and fifty-five, with the average age being fifty-one. However, some women enter this stage of life before age forty and some as late as sixty. There doesn't seem to be any relationship between the age at which a woman begins her periods and the timing of menopause. Nor does the age of onset appear to be affected by race, marital status, or geography. Smokers, however, typically experience menopause nearly two years earlier than nonsmokers. And women who have had ovaries removed surgically during their reproductive years have, by definition, an abrupt menopause (referred to as **surgical menopause**). Many women make this important transition with little or no turbulence. Most have one or more symptoms, including hot flashes, night sweats, skin and hair changes, sudden irritability, tingling sensations, sleep disturbances, vaginal dryness, and a decline in sexual desire. (Indeed, it is not uncommon to have to deal with symptoms for two to four years *before* the menstrual cycles actually stop.) And whether or not you experience these acute symptoms, you will need to think about, plan for, and deal with long-term issues: maintaining your overall health, screening for unsuspected disease, preserving the bones, and making decisions about hormone therapy (HT). There are some equally important concerns—personal, emotional, vocational, and spiritual issues—that are affected by menopause. The mental and spiritual attitudes with which you enter this process can greatly influence the direction of the entire experience.

F.Y.I.

Professional organizations now use the term **hormone therapy (HT)** rather than **hormone replacement therapy (HRT)** because the hormones a woman may receive to treat menopausal symptoms are actually supplemental, rather than a replacement for something that is completely absent. (Low levels of estrogen continue to be produced in the ovaries, as well as in fatty tissues throughout the body.) Specific types of hormone therapy are now designated **estrogen therapy (ET)** or **estrogen-progesterone therapy (EPT)**. Unless stated otherwise, throughout this section we will use the umbrella term *hormone therapy* (HT) to refer to any preparation a woman might use to supplement waning hormone levels.

What happens during menopause?

To fully appreciate (if that's the right word) what happens during menopause, make sure you're clear on what happens during a woman's normal reproductive cycle—a wondrous process we described at the beginning of this chapter.

Remember that at puberty a woman's ovaries contain a total of about three hundred thousand eggs, and that over the course of her reproductive years she will release between three hundred and five hundred of them, usually one at a time on a monthly basis. Most of the rest gradually disappear over that thirty- to forty-year period, until about ten thousand are left at the time of menopause. In addition, follicles become less sensitive over time to the follicle-stimulating hormone (FSH) that is released by the pituitary. (Remember that a follicle consists of one egg and a thin sheet of cells that surround it.) After menopause follicles produce some estrogen, but eventually none complete the process of ovulation. As a result, there is no corpus luteum—the gland that forms from the follicle that has released an egg and that secretes progesterone. Thus the uterus receives some stimulation, but its lining (the endometrium) doesn't progress through its usual maturation process because of decreased availability of progesterone. Menstrual bleeding may thus become erratic. Furthermore, if the endometrium becomes overly stimulated, the thicker lining cannot be sustained and bleeding may be much heavier.

As the follicles become unresponsive to FSH, estrogen and progesterone levels decline but don't completely disappear. A low level of hormones continues to exit the ovaries even after the monthly cycles end. Furthermore, some estrogen is created in the adrenal glands and in fatty tissue all over the body. In fact, women with an ample supply of fat may generate enough estrogen to minimize the symptoms that thinner women typically experience when their estrogen levels fall. This is no great benefit, however, because of the many other drawbacks of obesity—one of which, ironically, is increased risk of cancer of the uterus, arising from the increased stimulation of the endometrium by the higher estrogen levels from fat.

Meanwhile, up in the brain, the hypothalamus and the pituitary gland detect lower levels of estrogen and progesterone, and they try to "correct" the situation. In what would appear to be a futile effort to get the ovaries' attention, the hypothalamus secretes high levels of gonadotropin-releasing hormone (GnRH), and the pituitary in turn produces high levels of FSH and LH, but to no avail. Indeed, measuring FSH in the bloodstream serves as a useful confirmation that menopause has occurred. Interestingly, the hypothalamus and pituitary never give up; even the most aged woman will be found to have very high FSH levels (which is not harmful).

What happens when the estrogen levels drop?

Several changes in the peri- and postmenopausal woman can be attributed to the decline of this important hormone.

1. **Irregular menses.** One of the most important signals that the perimenopausal years may have arrived is the onset of irregular menstrual cycles, which may vary considerably depending on the amount of estrogen produced by the ovaries and whether or not an egg was produced that month. As a result, there's no surefire way to tell from the flow pattern whether or not menopause is imminent. For example, a low output of estrogen causes little stimulation for the lining of the uterus to grow, so the menstrual flow may be scant. On the other hand, if ovulation doesn't occur, the progesterone "ripening" of the uterus won't either. This may lead to a steady buildup of endometrial lining in the uterus, which can slough off in bits and pieces (producing spotting) or be released in a veritable flood of tissue all at once.

   In general, a shift toward heavier menstrual flows—whether prolonged in length or very heavy for the usual number of days or both longer and heavier—deserves some attention. While it may reflect a perimenopausal change, it might also be caused by **hyperplasia**, a worrisome buildup of the uterine lining that might progress to cancer. Even worse, the bleeding could be caused by an overt cancer of this tissue. Fibroids, which are benign mus-

Some women develop a pronounced premenstrual irritability during perimenopause, often to their dismay—and their family's as well. This late-onset PMS is not a sign that a woman is falling apart at the seams, but a genuine (if intense) response to hormonal variations.

cular growths in the uterus, can also cause heavy bleeding. Less common, but no less important, are assorted problems such as clotting disorders or thyroid disease. In addition, the ongoing blood loss can outstrip the body's capacity to replace red cells, depleting iron stores and leading to iron-deficiency anemia—which, fortunately, is readily correctable.

If you notice that your menstrual flow is getting longer and/or heavier, for two or three cycles keep track of the number of days you bleed, how heavy the flow appears to be (gauged by the number of pads or tampons you need to use to stay ahead of it), and how many days elapse between cycles. Then review the situation with your primary-care physician or gynecologist. When all is said and done, you may need an ultrasound, an endometrial biopsy (an office procedure), or other diagnostic procedures such as a **dilatation and curettage (D and C)** to make sure nothing serious is happening.

Dilatation and curettage is a procedure performed in the operating room under anesthesia during which the endometrial lining is scraped out and sent to the pathologist for evaluation.

What if you skip one or more periods? This is a common pattern for perimenopausal women, with the time between cycles increasing until they finally stop altogether. The most significant alternative explanation to rule out, believe it or not, is pregnancy. As long as eggs are traveling down the fallopian tubes and sperm are there to meet them, a pregnancy can begin. If there's any such possibility, don't hesitate to bring it up with your doctor, who may not be thinking along these lines.

2. **Hot flashes**. These occur in at least 75 percent of menopausal women. They produce a sensation of heat rising from the chest toward the face and arms, accompanied by flushing of the skin, and less often by an increased heart rate and overt sweating. Hot flashes may occur once in a while or several times a day and last anywhere from a few minutes to half an hour.

   Hot flashes appear to be associated with changes in estrogen levels, which in turn trigger an overzealous response from the hypothalamus. Remember that this area of the brain starts the monthly cycle and tries in vain to get things going after the ovaries sign off. The hypothalamus also regulates body temperature and other primal functions, partly through changes in blood-vessel diameter, and during menopause it seems to send an overabundance of messages to the circulatory system in response to the fluctuation of estrogen. Fortunately, the hypothalamus eventually adjusts to the change in the hormonal level and calms down, although the process may take three to five years or even longer. For those who take supplemental estrogen, disruptive flashes and flushes usually come to an end relatively quickly. For those who opt not to use hormone therapy, there are a number of other ways to deal with them (see sidebar on page 658).

3. **Vaginal atrophy.** The vagina is extremely sensitive to estrogen stimulation, and without it the vagina undergoes a number of changes. The mucous membranes that line it become thinner, and its secretions become less abundant

and less acidic. The vagina also becomes shorter and narrower. Irritation, itching, and burning may result, a condition known as **atrophic vaginitis**. These changes may make sexual intercourse more uncomfortable.

4. **Urinary tract problems.** The cells that line the bladder and urethra (the short tube connecting the bladder to the outside world) and the muscular layers of these structures become thinner after estrogen levels decline. This may lead to difficulty controlling the release of urine (**incontinence**), a sensation of needing to void more often (known as frequency), and burning with the passage of urine (called **dysuria**). These changes also reduce the normal defenses against bacteria, sometimes causing repeated bladder infections.

   Furthermore, loss of muscle tone in the pelvis may lead to **stress incontinence**, an annoying loss of urine with anything that causes pressure on the abdomen (such as coughing, sneezing, or laughing). Stress incontinence is less a hormonal problem than a mechanical one, and it may be improved by a type of exercise that strengthens the "hammock" of muscles (called **pubococcygeals**) that support the pelvic organs and vaginal tissue. You may have been taught this (known as a **Kegel exercise**) during pregnancy: The next time you urinate, try to stop the flow of urine before the stream ends. Hold it for a count of three, then let go. This tightening of muscles constitutes a Kegel exercise, and to strengthen the pelvic floor you need to repeat this process several dozen times per day. Fortunately, you don't have to pass urine every time. Simply tighten and relax these muscles five or ten times when you stop at a red light, or during a commercial break on the radio or TV. If conservative measures don't correct the disruptive symptoms of stress incontinence, surgery may be an appropriate option.

Bladder symptoms arising from lack of estrogen are so similar to those caused by infection that, if and when they show up, the urine should be checked and possibly cultured to clarify the nature of the problem.

Kegel exercises were named for Dr. Arnold Kegel, a Los Angeles obstetrician-gynecologist who during the 1940s carried out pioneering work in the use of pelvic-muscle exercises to cure urinary incontinence.

5. **Skin changes.** Both layers of skin—the epidermis and dermis—are sensitive to estrogen support. At the surface, estrogen promotes lubrication and water retention. In the deeper dermis, estrogen stimulates production of collagen, a protein that maintains thickness and elasticity of skin. As a result, declining estrogen levels accelerate the thinning, drying, and wrinkling of skin. But so do sun exposure and cigarette smoking. With or without depletion of the ozone layer, ultraviolet (UV) light not only destroys elasticity and promotes wrinkling, but it also provokes anarchy at the cellular level, leading to various forms of skin cancer. It is important to take appropriate measures to protect your skin from the sun, as well as to avoid deliberate exposure to UV rays, whether from the sun or in a tanning booth.

6. **Formication.** That's for*m*ication, with an *m*. Derived from the Latin word for *ant* (formica), it is a sensation that insects are crawling on the skin, experienced at least once by 15 to 20 percent of postmenopausal women. Oddly

continued on page 660

AIDS TO COPING WITH HOT FLASHES IF YOU'RE NOT TAKING ESTROGEN (OR EVEN IF YOU ARE)

Hot flashes can be maddening, but there are a few strategies that any woman can implement to reduce the frequency and severity of hot flashes.

- An effort to identify and avoid hot-flash triggers can pay off. These triggers might include certain foods, especially spicy dishes, caffeine, alcohol, and even sugar; rapid changes in temperature, such as entering a chilled office building on a hot summer day; and stressful situations that provoke the autonomic nervous system into action.
- Along with all of its other benefits, regular aerobic exercise (see chapter 7) may help reduce hot flashes.
- Likewise, along with all of its other hazards and hassles (see chapter 10), cigarette smoking tends to worsen hot flashes and should be avoided.

In addition to these avoidance mechanisms, a number of medical therapies can help reduce hot flashes. For many women, the favored approach over the past several decades has been estrogen therapy. However, estrogen can stimulate the growth of breast tissue, which may be problematic for women who have (or have had) breast cancer. Women who are at risk for developing breast cancer may also be wary of estrogen supplementation.

As we will see later, some recent medical research has raised other concerns about the safety of short- and long-term estrogen or estrogen-progesterone use. Whatever your reason for wanting to avoid hormone therapy, a number of medical treatments may be effective in reducing the frequency or severity of hot flashes.

- Doctors sometimes prescribe progesterone or **progestins** (progesterone-like drugs) as a treatment for hot flashes, for which they may be at least somewhat effective.
- Several **antidepressant medications** are effective in reducing hot flashes. This is not an indication that hot flashes are "all in your head." Rather, it appears that some of the same neurotransmitters (namely serotonin and norepinephrine) whose imbalance in the brain can result in depression also transmit hot-flash signals. The antidepressant venlafaxine (Effexor) is thought to work by inhibiting the reuptake of both serotonin and norepinephrine. Several selective serotonin reuptake inhibitors (SSRIs), a class of antidepressants mentioned in chapter 8, have also been found to reduce hot flashes. These drugs include fluoxetine (Prozac), sertraline (Zoloft), citalopram (Celexa), and paroxetine (Paxil). Common side effects of antidepressant medications include dizziness, nausea, sexual dysfunction, and mood changes.

- **Gabapentin (Neurontin)** is a drug used to control seizures and to treat postherpetic neuralgia (an intense nerve pain that persists after a shingles outbreak in some people). Researchers have found that the drug can reduce hot flashes. Side effects include drowsiness, dizziness, mood changes, and swelling.
- **Clonidine (Catapres)**, a drug normally used to treat hypertension, can reduce the frequency of hot flashes in some women. Side effects include dizziness, drowsiness, constipation, and dry mouth.

While some women will not have any problems using medical treatments to relieve hot flashes, other women may not be able to tolerate them because of side effects. Still others may simply wish to avoid prescription-drug options as much as possible. For these women, the following alternatives may be helpful.

Among the herbal preparations promoted to treat menopausal symptoms, the most popular is **black cohosh**, which has been used extensively in Europe to reduce hot flashes. While several studies have found that black cohosh offers some relief from hot flashes, others show little or no benefit. Side effects can include an upset stomach and headaches.

Because black cohosh is considered a dietary supplement rather than a pharmaceutical, it is not regulated by the Food and Drug Administration as a drug. Therefore manufacturers do not have to prove the safety or effectiveness of black cohosh, and the purity of preparations supplied by different manufacturers can vary widely. Women who wish to try black cohosh for relief of hot flashes may be interested to know that a standardized formulation of black cohosh, called Remifemin, is available.

Based on the limited research available, the American College of Obstetrics and Gynecology (ACOG) suggests that black cohosh may be helpful for short-term (less than six months) treatment of hot flashes, although it states that data demonstrating the safety and efficacy of black cohosh beyond six months is lacking.

Another popular nonprescription treatment that some women find helpful is **soy**. Soybeans contain phytoestrogens, a type of estrogen found in plants that can weakly mimic the effects of estrogen in a woman's body. Women—especially women from Asian countries—whose diets contain high amounts of soy are less likely to suffer from hot flashes and other symptoms of menopause, and it was suspected that soy isoflavones (a type of phytoestrogens abundant in soy) might be the reason. Unfortunately, studies examining the effects of soy on hot flashes have shown mixed results. Further research is needed to determine the full benefits of soy in relieving menopausal discomforts. ■

continued from page 657

enough, it tends to occur one or two years after the last menstrual cycle. This condition may be related to sudden changes in small blood vessels.

7. **Night sweats and disturbed sleep.** Night sweats related to estrogen withdrawal are similar to hot flashes but with the added attraction of soaking nightgowns and sheets. Obviously, such an event isn't conducive to uninterrupted sleep. In addition, some women have difficulty falling asleep or staying asleep, even without the nocturnal soak.

   Unfortunately, you can't automatically assume that these events are caused by estrogen changes. Night sweats on their own may also be caused by infections or more serious illnesses, including certain malignancies. If these are occurring in the midst of hot flashes and other menopausal events and are relieved decisively by estrogen, then the diagnosis is straightforward. But if you have any doubt, talk to your health-care provider.

   Similarly, sleep disturbances may be caused by a variety of problems, especially depression. Again, if a trial of supplemental estrogen brings on a dramatic improvement, the cause is probably hormonal.

8. **Emotional disturbances.** There is no doubt that many women experience irritability, mood swings, anxiety, and overt depression during the years surrounding menopause. There has also been no shortage of controversy surrounding the relationship between hormone fluctuations and these emotions. Medical research has not established a consistent link between them nor has it uncovered evidence that hormone therapy routinely solves this problem. Some women have found, however, that supplemental estrogen seems to help calm emotional storms. For many more, however, there are a host of other factors that may need to be addressed: changes in overall health, losses of friends and family members, conflicts at home, and imbalances in chemical messengers in the brain (called neurotransmitters) that play a pivotal role in many cases of depression. (We have reviewed this problem, known as endogenous depression, in detail in chapter 8, starting on page 323.) It is very important that mood problems during this period of life not be ignored or trivialized and that they be addressed using any and all appropriate investigations and treatments.

This list of symptoms experienced by many women during the menopause and postmenopausal years might sound discouraging. The good news is that, while some of the structural changes (such as thinning of the vagina) are essentially universal, many women sail past menopause as if nothing much has happened. And others who are having a lot of the problems we just listed can get some impressive relief with lifestyle adjustments and medical treatment (including, for some, hormone therapy).

Like so many other physical characteristics, much of the response to the events of menopause is determined by genetics. Some women have a gradual decline in estrogen, for example, which tends to generate fewer symptoms than an abrupt drop or wild fluctuations in hormone levels. Others make enough estrogen away from the ovaries that the symptoms they experience are limited. Also, the hypothalamus and other estrogen-responsive structures may vary in their sensitivity to hormone levels. On the other hand, the quality of prudent self-care can make a major difference as well. Someone who is in poor condition to begin with—whether physically, emotionally, or spiritually—may find any added hormonal hassles of menopause to be intolerable.

There is one other important physical problem that many women must address before and after menopause. Unlike the others we have described, it is typically silent over many years until announcing its presence in a most unpleasant manner. That problem is osteoporosis, or thinning of bone.

Dealing with thinning bones

Osteoporosis, which means "porous bone," is a condition in which bone mass is gradually lost, resulting in decreased strength and thus an increased risk of fractures. Thin, porous bones break easily, often with very slight or even no trauma. Simply shifting position or bending over can provoke a fracture. Osteoporosis affects some 10 million Americans and is responsible for about 1.5 million fractures every year in the United States. Of these, more than three hundred thousand involve the hip, generating an $18 billion bill annually for acute and long-term care.[5] But more ominous is the fact that more than 20 percent of those who suffer a broken hip will die within a year after the fracture. Hundreds of thousands of other people suffer painful fractures of the vertebra and forearm every year. And gradual compressing of the weight-bearing segments of the spine eventually leads to the deforming curvatures—especially the impolitely named dowager's hump—that bother so many elderly women. As our population continues to age, the annual number of fractures will double within forty years unless perimenopausal women begin to take some meaningful preventive measures.

Contrary to a common perception that the skeleton is lifeless, bone is living tissue. At any given time, various areas are undergoing turnover and remodeling, which blends microscopic tearing down and rebuilding processes. These normally are tightly coupled to one another, but any imbalance between them will lead to a net gain or loss of bone. Unfortunately, after reaching a peak at about age thirty, the bone mass of both men and women begins a steady and relentless decline with age. The speed of loss and its impact are determined by several factors:

- **Gender.** The peak bone mass reached in early adulthood is about 30 percent more in men than in women.
- **Race.** African American women tend to have a greater bone density than white or Asian women and are less commonly affected by osteoporosis.

- **Age.** Between the ages of fifty and eighty, a woman loses *30 percent* of her bone density. During the first five years after menopause, the loss is fastest—about 2 percent per year, after which the rate drops to one percent per year. It stands to reason that the oldest women have the thinnest bones and thus the most fractures. Half of all hip fractures occur after age eighty.
- **Early menopause.** As soon as the ovaries retire, or if they are surgically removed, the accelerated bone loss begins. Some research suggests that it is the *total number of reproductive years* (that is, the age at menopause minus the age of the first menstrual period) that makes the difference. Women with thirty or fewer reproductive years tend to have significantly lower bone density than their counterparts with forty or more reproductive years. Thus a late start and early end of cycles do not bode well for strong bones. When estrogen levels drop, the balance in bone remodeling is lost: The cells that rebuild bone (called **osteoblasts**) slow down, while those that tear it down (called **osteoclasts**) pick up steam. And the longer estrogen levels are low, the more bone a woman loses.
- **Thin body build.** Osteoporosis is about the only health problem for which being heavy is a theoretical advantage. Higher weight leads to a greater peak in bone mass when young, more production of estrogen (in fatty tissue) after menopause, and increased bone formation stimulated by weight-bearing forces throughout life. These advantages, of course, are greatly offset by other risks when the scale reads too high.
- **Sedentary lifestyle.** As just mentioned, bones that support weight are stimulated to preserve their density by muscles pulling and moving them. Prolonged immobility (while recuperating from chronic illness or injury) or a lifestyle devoid of exercise (or decreasing activity with increasing age) can contribute to thinning bones.
- **Smoking.** Cigarettes contribute to osteoporosis both before and after menopause. This is probably caused by an anti-estrogen effect of nicotine.
- **Alcohol.** Medical truism: The relationship between alcohol consumption and bone mass before menopause is both inverse and dose dependent. English translation: The more alcohol you drink and the longer you drink it, the thinner your bones will be.
- **Low calcium intake.** Of all the dietary factors studied by osteoporosis researchers, calcium (in food or supplement) has been found to make the most important contribution to bone strength throughout life.
- **Certain medications.** Oral cortisone preparations, such as might be used to treat chronic bronchitis, asthma, or severe arthritis, definitely accelerate bone loss. For most long-term lung problems that need cortisone, the medication can be inhaled (with far less absorption into the rest of the body). But some people with rheumatoid ar-

thritis, lupus, and related disorders may need oral cortisone to control their symptoms, although physicians invariably try to use alternative approaches. Anyone on long-term oral cortisone should take special precautions to protect against excessive bone loss.

Other medications that can contribute to bone loss when used on a frequent basis include the antiseizure medication phenytoin (Dilantin), as well as antacids that contain aluminum. In addition, high levels of thyroid hormone, whether coming from the thyroid gland itself or from an ongoing dose of a thyroid supplement that is too high, can reduce bone density. (The proper dose can be determined using routine blood tests.)

You can't change your age, sex, race, body build, or (usually) the time of menopause, but if you are at higher risk, you need to pay close attention to the risk factors that you *can* change. If chapter 10 didn't give you enough reasons to quit smoking and limit (or eliminate) alcohol use, perhaps some additional concern about the fate of your bones might help you make these important changes. In addition, you can also take the following bone-preserving measures:

Regular exercise. Of the many benefits of moving your muscles on a regular basis, preserving bone density is one of the most important for women. Both weight-bearing aerobic exercise (in which feet are making contact with the ground and bones are supporting the body) and strength-training exercise cause very slight distortion of bone, which in turn stimulates the bone to build more supportive tissue.

Calcium and vitamin D. For some time the National Institutes of Health and various professional organizations have recommended that women routinely consume 1,000 mg of calcium per day before menopause. The Food and Nutrition Board of the Institute of Medicine recommends that older women get at least 1,200 mg per day, but some nutrition experts consider 1,500 mg a more advisable calcium intake for older women. Much of this can come from dietary sources, especially dairy products. A one-cup (eight-ounce) glass of *any* form of milk (anything between whole and skim) contains about 300 mg of calcium, so consuming a quart per day (or four of these servings) approaches 1,200 mg and thus provides nearly the entire recommended daily allowance for a postmenopausal woman. An eight-ounce serving of low-fat plain yogurt contains more than 400 mg of calcium.

In this section when we mention amounts of calcium, we are referring to *elemental* calcium. When checking the content of a calcium supplement (or a food containing calcium), look for the amount of elemental calcium that it contains.

One concern with any of these dairy items might be the fat and calorie content, but the numbers actually aren't too bad. Skim milk, for example, contains 90 calories per eight ounces, or 360 per quart. One percent milk, which many find much more palatable, contains only 15 more calories per eight ounces than nonfat (105 vs. 90 calories), or 420 per quart.

Nondairy sources of calcium include salmon and sardines: Three ounces of these provides about 160 mg and 370 mg respectively. Leafy green vegetables such as collards, kale, and turnip greens are also respectable calcium sources.

The more common greens in a small salad provide about 100 mg, an orange or a half cup of raisins about 50 mg, and a half dozen figs about 150 mg. Some vegetables such as spinach and Swiss chard contain oxalic acid, which may decrease absorption of the calcium that they contain. This should not present a problem if you obtain an adequate amount of calcium from other sources.

For many women, a typical daily intake of calcium from diet provides about 400 to 500 mg, and thus some sort of supplementation is usually a good idea. If you check your typical all-purpose daily multivitamin, you'll notice that it probably contains much less than 1,000 mg of calcium, because this amount of calcium would make the tablet too bulky. Instead, various preparations (many of which are quite inexpensive) can be purchased at your local supermarket or pharmacy.

Calcium is always attached to another compound, the character of which may affect absorption and overall cost. The most commonly used and most cost-effective preparations use calcium carbonate, the active ingredient in many chewable antacids. (Tums E-X, for example, contains 300 mg of elemental calcium per tablet, so four of these per day provide a very respectable supplement for less than 25 cents.) Absorption is usually enhanced by taking these with food, and the total amount should not be consumed in one sitting but should be divided into two or three doses. Obviously, if you are already consuming a pint or more of milk per day, your intake should be adjusted accordingly.

Some people who feel bloated or otherwise distressed with calcium carbonate may want to consider alternatives such as calcium gluconate, lactate, or citrate. Of these, calcium citrate is considered to be particularly well absorbed, but women may still need to consume several tablets per day to reach recommended doses.

Loading up on higher-than-recommended doses of *anything* is rarely a good idea, and calcium is no exception. Doses that far exceed the 1,500 mg level may increase your risk for kidney stones or actually raise your blood concentration of calcium, which is normally tightly regulated.

In addition to dietary and supplemental calcium, an adequate supply of vitamin D is also critical for bone health. This vitamin is manufactured in the body in response to sun exposure and is also added to many foods (such as milk and vitamin-fortified cereals) as well as multivitamin and calcium supplements. The amount most commonly recommended for a person between the ages of fifty and seventy who gets no sun exposure is 400 international units (IU) per day. (For someone over seventy, the amount is 600 IU.) Deliberately taking large doses of vitamin D (more than 2,000 IU per day), unless under supervision for a specific medical reason, is unwise and may cause other medical problems. (For more detailed information about vitamin D, check appendix B entitled "Vitamins and Minerals: What Each One Does and How Much We Need.")

Estrogen. For decades physicians have prescribed hormone therapy (HT) as a preventive measure to preserve bone mass, a decision that was well supported in the medical literature. It was noted that the most protective benefit occurred when HT was started soon after menopause (within the first few years, and preferably right away) and when it continued as long as a woman took hormone supplementation. Furthermore, hormone therapy has long been a therapeutic option for women with thinning bones (whether full-blown osteoporosis or its less severe stage known as osteopenia). However, recent research has caused many women to be concerned about the safety of long-term HT, and today most physicians do not prescribe estrogen specifically to treat osteoporosis. We will discuss this momentarily.

Bisphosphonates. These drugs work to prevent or reverse bone loss by inhibiting bone resorption by osteoclasts. By reducing the rate at which osteoclasts break down bone, bisphosphonates restore the balance between resorption and bone formation and can actually skew it toward the net formation of bone mass. In women with a high risk of fractures, bisphosphonates have been shown to reduce the risk of breaks. Drugs in this class include alendronate (Fosamax), risedronate (Actonel), and ibandronate (Boniva).

Calcitonin. Naturally produced by the thyroid gland, calcitonin is a hormone that inhibits bone resorption by osteoclasts and appears to promote bone formation by osteoblasts, leading to a net increase in bone mass. It reduces the likelihood of fractures of the spine, although it does not appear to reduce the risk of hip fractures. Calcitonin is often given to women who cannot take estrogen or bisphosphonates. It is available in a nasal spray (Miacalcin).

Selective estrogen receptor modulators (SERMs). These drugs bind to estrogen receptors, producing estrogen-like effects in some tissues while blocking those effects in others. One of the estrogen-simulating effects of these medications is the reduction of bone resorption. Subsequently, bone mass density increases and fracture rates decrease in menopausal women taking SERMs. The first SERM approved by the FDA to treat osteoporosis was raloxifene (Evista), although others are being studied. While raloxifene reduces bone loss through an estrogen pathway, it does not appear to have estrogen's effects on the uterus or breasts. An added benefit of the drug is that it lowers LDL (the "bad cholesterol") and total cholesterol while leaving the level of "good cholesterol," HDL, unchanged. It may also reduce a woman's risk of developing breast cancer. However, like supplemental estrogen, it can also increase a woman's risk of developing blood clots in the veins, and anyone who has had this problem in the past should avoid using this drug.

Human parathyroid hormone. A form of this hormone, produced using recombinant DNA technology, is one of the newer therapies used to fight osteoporosis.

F.Y.I.

The **parathyroids** are four small glands situated beside (actually within, though not part of) the thyroid gland. These help regulate calcium levels in the blood by releasing **parathyroid hormone,** a compound that mobilizes calcium from bone.

Available as teriparatide (Forteo), this drug must be injected daily. Unlike other prescription medications that treat osteoporosis by reducing the activity of osteoclasts (the cells involved in bone resorption), teriparatide actually increases the formation of new bone by stimulating the activity of osteoblasts, the cells that build bone. Because the drug has been shown to increase the incidence of bone tumors in rats, the long-term safety of teriparatide is uncertain, and it should not be used longer than two years. It is also very expensive, about five hundred dollars per month. Teriparatide is recommended only for patients with severe osteoporosis who are at high risk for fractures.

Should I use hormone therapy?

Over the past few decades, the status of hormone therapy (HT) has swung wildly, both in the general public and among medical professionals. In the 1950s the successes of estrogen in relieving acute symptoms such as hot flashes, vaginal atrophy, and (for some) mood swings led to a naive "wonder drug" mentality. Estrogen seemed to be good for "whatever ails ya" if you were female and over forty, and by the early 1960s it was the fifth most commonly written prescription in the United States.

Then in the mid-1970s, a new series of studies showed that long-term estrogen users were at a higher risk for developing cancer of the uterus. As other concerns were raised about links between estrogen and breast cancer, blood clots, and other problems, the general perception of HT changed from that of a panacea to a rather drastic and risky intervention to be used only for those with severe menopausal difficulties.

Over the next twenty years clinical experience and research refined HT and demonstrated what appeared to be some important long-range benefits. These included not only relief of many of the symptoms described earlier in this chapter, but also prevention of osteoporosis and cardiovascular disease. A number of studies suggested that starting estrogen supplementation at menopause and continuing indefinitely would not only drastically reduce the risk of fractures but also cut the number of heart attacks experienced by postmenopausal women *in half*. Given the significant burden of both fractures (especially those involving the hip) and cardiovascular disease among women, physicians routinely advised long-term HT to women as soon as menopause arrived (and often before), unless there was a compelling reason not to. That situation has again changed considerably with two recent well-publicized studies that have raised questions about the usefulness and safety of long-term hormone therapy.

The **Heart and Estrogen/Progestin Replacement Study** (or **HERS**) attempted to assess whether hormone therapy might protect women with known coronary heart disease (CHD) from further heart attacks or lethal heart events. The study not only demonstrated no protective effect, but those taking a combination estrogen/progestin pill were two to three times more likely to develop blood clots in the deep veins of the leg or pelvis than those who did not take hormones. (Remember that a progestin is a synthetic form of the hormone progesterone.)

The massive **Women's Health Initiative** (or **WHI**)—a fifteen-year study designed to identify strategies to prevent heart disease, cancer of the breast and colon, and osteoporosis in postmenopausal women—enrolled more than

27,000 women in a study of the effects of either an estrogen/progestin combination or estrogen alone on several health outcomes. Women taking the combination were found to have a higher risk of developing breast cancer, heart attack, stroke, and pulmonary embolism (a blood clot traveling from the legs or pelvis to an artery supplying a lung), but also a lower risk of developing colorectal cancer or suffering fractures of the hip or vertebra. Those taking only the estrogen were also found to have a higher risk of stroke, along with a lower risk of fracture and also a slightly reduced risk of breast cancer. Despite the benefits that were documented, both components of this study were stopped ahead of schedule because the benefits that were observed appeared to be outweighed by the potential dangers of continuing hormone therapy.

These results sent shock waves through the medical community, and they were widely interpreted by the media and general public as compelling evidence that women should avoid hormone therapy altogether or stop using it as soon as possible. However, a number of issues have been raised regarding the design of these studies, the validity of their conclusions, and especially the interpretation of the risks of hormone therapy that have been publicized in popular media. For those interested in more information about these studies, their conclusions, and some of the issues surrounding them, we have included a more detailed analysis in an appendix entitled "Hormone Therapy Controversies: A Closer Look at the HERS and WHI Studies" beginning on page 953.

The HERS and WHI studies, and the intense media coverage they generated, have restructured the conversations between menopausal women and their health-care providers about hormone supplementation. In some ways this has been useful, in that there is no longer a "one size fits all" approach to this subject. Many women and their physicians who have been renewing hormone prescriptions for decades now have had some overdue conversations about the pros and cons of continuing on the current course. However, there has also been some unfortunate fallout. Many women for whom hormones might offer a significant improvement in troubling menopausal symptoms have been so frightened that they refuse even to consider their use. Some have wasted money on inferior or worthless concoctions offered on the Internet and elsewhere as a treatment for these symptoms.

The need to individualize treatment for each woman should be the true take-home message from the HERS and WHI studies. At this time hormone supplementation is prescribed specifically for relief of postmenopausal symptoms—hot flashes, sweats, and atrophic changes in the vagina. For women whose symptoms are very disturbing and disruptive, alternatives to HT may not be effective, and the small risks posed by taking hormones might be acceptable in light of the relief they provide. For other women, the passage through menopause might be accompanied by few if any uncomfortable symptoms, and these women might opt against HT, especially if they have a family history of breast cancer or other risk factors that would raise concerns about hormone use. While HT is known to help maintain bone density and appears to reduce the risk of colon cancer, these are now considered incidental benefits. At this time hormones are not prescribed specifically for these purposes. Furthermore, based on current research findings, HT should not be used as a strategy to prevent cardiovascular disease or dementia.

There are a few more cautions to be aware of when considering HT, and most of the following apply to the various forms of both estrogen and progesterone/progestin that are currently available.

- **HT should not be used if you are pregnant.** Remember what we mentioned earlier about irregular or skipped periods during the perimenopausal years: As long as eggs are traveling down the fallopian tubes and sperm are there to meet them, a pregnancy can begin. If there is any possibility that you could be pregnant, you should discuss this with your doctor and certainly not use hormone therapy, which poses potential risks to the developing fetus, especially during the first three months.
- **HT should not be used if you have an undiagnosed breast lump.** Because estrogen can stimulate the growth of certain breast tumors, it is imperative that you determine the identity of any breast mass before considering using HT.
- **HT should not be used if you have abnormal vaginal bleeding that has not been evaluated.** As with breast lumps, you must know what is happening in this part of your body before adding hormones to the mix. If you have definitely completed the passage into menopause (that is, a year has passed since your last cycle, or the diagnosis has been confirmed by a doctor's exam and lab studies) and you start bleeding again, check with your physician so he or she can evaluate the lining of the uterus for any abnormalities.
- **HT should be used with extreme caution if you have a history of problems with abnormal blood clotting.** If you have ever been treated for a blood clot in the veins of the leg or a pulmonary embolism (in which a clot travels from a vein in the leg or pelvis into an artery supplying the lung), HT might increase your risk of another incident of this type.
- **HT should be used with caution if you have liver disease.** Because in very rare cases estrogen provokes jaundice, those who already are dealing with an ongoing liver problem should review this situation with an internist or gastroenterologist before beginning HT. Estrogen also may slightly increase the risk of developing gallstones.
- **Some form of progesterone/progestin should be taken with estrogen in women who have a uterus.** If the uterus has not been removed surgically, a woman who takes estrogen by itself has an increased risk of developing cancer in the endometrium (the tissue that lines the inner cavity of the uterus). The overall risk for a woman developing this cancer is about one in one thousand, and this number increases four- to eightfold when estrogen is added by itself. This, indeed, is the reason why a progesterone/

progestin preparation is included in nearly every woman's hormone regime if she still has a uterus. Progesterone rounds out the development of this lining every month during the reproductive years. After menopause, it prevents ongoing stimulation of the lining that might induce precancerous changes. In fact, women who use appropriate progesterone doses every month appear to have *less* risk of endometrial cancer than those who don't take anything at all.

A few more notes and considerations regarding HT

As stated earlier, over time there appears to be a small but real increase in the risk of breast cancer for those using estrogen plus progestin. (The WHI hormone study did not find this to be the case in women taking estrogen alone, for whom there was a slightly lower risk of breast cancer.) Interestingly, studies show that women who develop breast cancer while on HT have a better life expectancy than those who develop it without hormone supplementation. This advantage may result from earlier detection. Women receiving HT will usually be required to have annual Pap smears, breast checks, and mammograms in order to continue their refills. Those without a specific reason to show up regularly for these examinations might be inclined to let them go or carry them out with less consistency.

Some women experience side effects from one or both hormones. The severity of these annoyances (compared to the relief HT might provide) will have to be taken into account when women consult their health-care provider about individualized treatment. These are the most common side effects:

- *Fluid retention*, manifested as swelling in the hands, feet, or breasts, may be provoked by either hormone.
- *Headaches* may develop or established patterns may worsen.
- Women who dealt with *tender lumps* in their breasts every month during their reproductive years may not be thrilled with a series of encores. This may be treated by adjusting the type or dosage of hormone, or in rare instances using a mild diuretic for all or part of the month. Breast tenderness may also be reduced by avoiding caffeine and chocolate.
- *Elevated blood pressure*, perhaps related to fluid retention, may occur.
- *Irritability* (specifically PMS-like symptoms) from the progesterone/progestin preparation may arise.
- *Spotting* or outright vaginal bleeding will depend greatly on the pattern of HT used.

Before considering whether or not to use HT, you will need to go over your history and have an appropriate physical exam. Your physician will need to confirm that you are postmenopausal, review risk factors for various problems, screen for breast and cervical cancer, and arrange follow-up. You should take time to discuss the pros and cons of HT for you as an individual (not just as a statistic) and have any questions answered.

You'll also want to consider the costs of medications and physician consultations. Keep in mind, however, that nearly all the screening done in connection with using HT should be done routinely anyway. Remember also that it is quite all right to use HT on a trial basis, observing how it affects you (for better or worse) and then regularly reviewing your progress (or lack thereof) with your health-care provider. A decision to try a form of hormone is not a lifetime commitment.

Assuming you decide to proceed, you may use one of several options. Most women who have a uterus will take some form of estrogen and progesterone every day of the month. This may result in some unpredictable spotting, but this usually disappears after a few months. Most women without a uterus will take only the estrogen, since the primary function of the progesterone in HT (at least thus far) is to protect the uterine lining from overstimulation and reduce the risk of cancer. Obviously, that risk is nonexistent if the uterus is gone. Some researchers have suggested that progesterone may confer some added protection against osteoporosis, but this has not yet translated into widespread use in women who have had a hysterectomy.

The vast majority of women using HT take their hormones orally. Some women, however, do not absorb estrogen through the digestive tract as well as others and find a **transdermal** patch, in which the hormone is absorbed through the skin, more effective. Examples of these are Estraderm and Vivelle (which contain only estrogen) and Climara Pro (which contains both estrogen and progesterone). Since transdermal hormones also bypass the liver, they may hold an advantage for women with liver disease. The patch can be applied to any area of the skin and is changed at an interval (typically every three-and-a-half days) determined by the release pattern of the patch. If progesterone is needed and not included in the patch, it is normally taken separately. One common annoyance is the development of a skin sensitivity, which leaves a rash whenever the patch is removed.

Some women need only to be relieved of vaginal itching and burning, and they may wish to use one of the vaginal applications instead of an oral form. While these exert an effect locally on the vagina, some of the hormone may be absorbed and taken up into the bloodstream as well. Hormone therapy can be applied locally via a vaginal cream (Estrace and Premarin creams, for example), or through a vaginal ring. The latter is a small, pliable device that is placed within the vagina and releases estrogen into the surrounding tissues. Estring is one type of vaginal ring that provides relief of local symptoms. Another type, Femring, provides a higher dose of estrogen that can be absorbed by the vagina and may also provide relief of other symptoms such as hot flashes. However, this could be a concern for a woman who has other medical issues (such as a significant risk for breast cancer) for which estrogen supplementation may not be advisable. Vaginal tablets containing estrogen are also available. One preparation called Vagifem is typically inserted into the vagina once daily for two weeks and then twice a week, providing local benefits with very little absorption into the bloodstream and thus little risk of significant side effects.

Over the years some women have received their HT in the form of monthly injections. Because these result in unpredictable blood levels of estrogen over the course of a month, these have fallen out of favor, except in those very rare circumstances when a woman cannot tolerate oral or transdermal forms or when vaginal applications are not sufficient.

All of the estrogens in common use for postmenopausal HT in the United States are referred to as "natural," because they duplicate those forms of estrogen manufactured in the human body. (Synthetic estrogens, on the other hand, are much more potent and utilized in oral contraceptives, whose purpose is to prevent ovulation.) The most familiar and widely used of these is Premarin, a mix of what are called conjugated estrogens derived (believe it or not) from the urine of pregnant mares. (Thus the name: *Pre* for pregnant, *mar* for mare, and *in* for urine.) Despite its equine origin, this preparation has held its own for years and has served as the supplement in the majority of studies on the benefits and risks of HT. The typical starting dose is 0.625 mg, although higher doses may be needed to control symptoms.

Other commonly used forms of estrogen are estrone (the weaker estrogen produced by the ovaries and peripheral fat cells), which is marketed as Ogen, and estradiol, a more potent form found in Estrace cream, the Estraderm patch, the Vagifem vaginal tablet, and many other preparations. At present there is no consensus in the medical literature that one of these variations is more effective or safe than the others. Individual variations in effectiveness and side effects largely determine which of these a woman will use over the long haul.

In contrast to the estrogens, the forms of progesterone used in HT very often are synthetic compounds called progestins. Medroxyprogesterone (Provera, Amen, and Cycrin) is the most commonly utilized of these. (The widely used preparation Prempro combines the estrogen mix in Premarin with various doses of Provera—hence the name.) Some women and their physicians are more comfortable using natural progesterone, which for years was available only in the form of a vaginal suppository. An oral form of natural progesterone—many physicians prefer the term **bioidentical**, since *natural* is more of a marketing word than a scientific one—is available as Prometrium.

What about hormones for the woman who is not yet at menopause?

Remember that perimenopause may last for many months prior to the actual end of menstrual cycles, and during this time fluctuations in estrogen levels can cause not only irregular cycles, but also hot flashes, flushing, and sweats. Women in this situation have traditionally been in a bind because physicians were reluctant to give any hormone supplementation to someone who was still having cycles.

Now, however, it is not uncommon to use very low-dose oral contraceptives in this situation. As long as the woman is not a smoker and the appropriate screening has been done, this form of hormone supplementation not only relieves symptoms of estrogen withdrawal but also regulates erratic cycles.

QUESTIONS TO PONDER:

(Note: These questions are addressed to women, but men are welcome to think about these as well.)

1. Do you have a clear understanding of what happens during the monthly cycle and what is changing as you transition into menopause? Would you be able to explain it to an adolescent in your family or your husband?
2. Do you know when your next Pap smear is due? What about your next mammogram? Are you avoiding either of these because you find them unpleasant? (You are aware, we assume, that *everyone* finds these unpleasant.)
3. If you experience painful cramps or other discomfort during menstruation, what are some ways you might be able to better manage those symptoms?
4. If you are pregnant or might become pregnant, what aspects of your health or lifestyle might you need to improve or change *now* in order to give your baby the best possible start in life?
5. If you are married and physically capable of having your first child, or one or more additional children, have you decided on the number you might ultimately have? What factors did you evaluate as you considered this decision?
6. If you and your spouse are using a method of family planning, how did you select it? Did you take into consideration the factors covered in the section "Some principles to bear in mind when considering birth control" on page 642?
7. If you are in perimenopause, menopause, or postmenopause, what physical changes are you experiencing, if any? Do you think you could take any steps to better control the symptoms?
8. If you have been using hormone therapy for many years, have you considered whether or not you need to continue doing so?
9. What can you do now to prevent developing osteoporosis later in life? Are there any habits such as tobacco use or lack of exercise that you need to address?

Action items: If you're not sure you understand the basics of the monthly cycle, take some time to review the material at the beginning of this chapter.

If you haven't done so already, read the material in chapter 4 about breast, cervical, uterine, and ovarian cancer. Check with your health-care provider to be sure you're up-to-date on appropriate screening tests.

If you are experiencing disruptive symptoms of PMS or PMDD, talk to your health-care provider about treatment options.

If you are using one or more methods of family planning, set aside some time once a year to discuss with your spouse your current approach and your understanding regarding the ultimate size of your family. Are you both in complete agreement on these important topics? If not, or if either of you is uncomfortable with what you are doing now—especially if you are concerned that the family planning methods you are using do not appropriately safeguard life from the moment of conception—you should strongly consider having a discussion with your physician, pastor, or a counselor.

If you are bothered by menopausal symptoms, talk to your health-care provider about methods of treatment that might be helpful. If hormone therapy is an option but you have concerns about its safety, take time to review the material in this chapter, as well as the appendix entitled "Hormone Therapy Controversies: A Closer Look at the HERS and WHI Studies" starting on page 953.

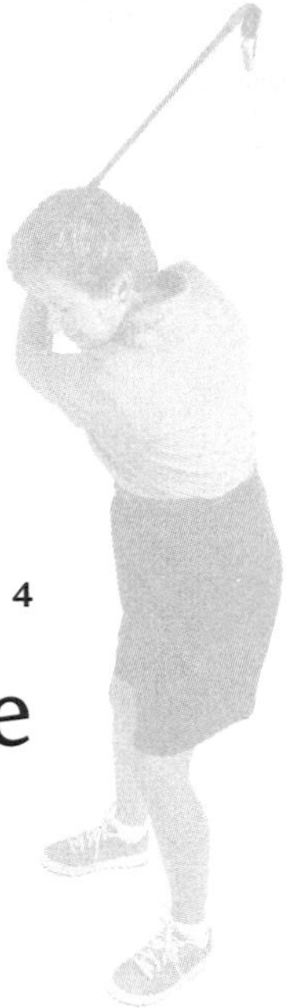

CHAPTER 14

Senior Maintenance

If you have passed the big 4–0, 5–0, or another birthday milestone with bigger numbers, you have probably thought about your future. How do you envision your senior years?

Here are some scenarios that most of us would welcome:

- Having time—more than we could afford while raising children and pursuing a career—to do projects, read, fix up the house, tend to a garden . . .
- Traveling to places near and far, and spending as much time as we'd like once we got there . . .
- Serving God in our church, neighborhood, and faraway places . . .
- Enjoying and spoiling grandchildren, and perhaps great-grandchildren, and providing them with experiences for which their parents might not have the time or money . . .
- Hosting everyone at our home for the holidays, and lots of other days as well . . .
- Offering our experience, wisdom, and values to younger generations, and seeing them profit from it . . .
- Enjoying clear vision, keen hearing, a taste for well-prepared food, a strong heart, mobile joints, energy during the day, and restful sleep at night . . .
- Transitioning from this life, "full of years," to the next with peace and expectancy . . .

On the other hand, other scenarios of the future provoke some uneasiness—or flat-out anxiety:

- Experiencing a relentless progression of infirmities: forgetfulness, clouded vision, loss of hearing, sleepless nights, lousy appetite, shortness of breath, frail muscles, and creaky joints . . .

- Submitting to the orders of multiple physicians (who may or may not be aware of what the others are doing) . . .
- Enduring and recovering from a series of operations to repair things broken, worn out, obstructed, or out of place . . .
- Facing a squadron of prescription bottles that have been deployed like overpriced toy soldiers, with names we can't recall, functions we don't understand, and side effects we don't appreciate . . .
- Attending a progression of funerals for family members and friends who were our age—or younger—when they passed on . . .
- Seeing a lifetime of possessions, and the memories they hold, dispersed far and wide, save for whatever will fit into a room or two at the assisted-living facility or the spare bedroom of an accommodating child . . .
- Losing the ability to balance the checkbook, drive to the store, use the stove, remember what happened ten minutes ago, carry on a conversation, recognize our own child or spouse . . .
- Spending months or years living, and then dying, lonely, unnoticed, unheeded, and uncomforted . . .

Few of us will spend our senior years in nonstop bliss or abject misery. We can anticipate that a number of things in our future will go our way, while others will not. Some aspects of aging may prove unpleasant or difficult for reasons that are largely beyond our control: unexpected reversals in health, relationships, or material welfare. But we may also enjoy the benefits of a lifetime spent cultivating our physical, emotional, and spiritual health, as well as our relationships with those around us.

In 1900, the average life span for someone living in the United States was forty-seven years. At the beginning of the twenty-first century, that number has increased dramatically to seventy-seven years. The primary reasons for this increase in longevity—public-health measures, innovations in prevention such as vaccines, and improved medical care—have also changed the causes of mortality. Whereas most deaths in 1900 were due to infectious disease (influenza, pneumonia, and tuberculosis) or acute illness (particularly diseases of the digestive tract), today's main killers are chronic diseases like cardiovascular disease, cancer, and complications of diabetes.[1] As we have described at length elsewhere in this book, much can be done to prevent or forestall today's leading causes of death and disability. But much of the responsibility (or opportunity) to do so rests on our own shoulders.

The baby boomers are becoming increasingly interested in anything with the word *anti-aging* attached to it. As with every other phase of their life, they do not intend to accept the status quo for their final laps or to "go gentle into that good night," to quote the poet Dylan Thomas. In some ways, they have a point. Is it really inevitable that the quality of our health should be inversely related to the number of candles on our birthday cake? Is there anything we can do to stay alert, active, and independent in our seventies, eighties, and nineties? Can we fulfill the promise of the August 30, 2004, *Time* magazine cover story, "How to Live to Be 100 (and Not Regret It)"? And if things really are unraveling, is there any way to turn the tide?

This chapter is not a comprehensive look at the ills and ailments that become more common as we gain our seniority. (For a guided tour, you can consult some relevant chapters in the Focus on the Family *Complete Guide to Caring for Aging Loved Ones.* That book also provides invaluable information regarding self-care for those who have become primary caretakers of a senior.) Instead, we will focus on how seniors can stay healthy and prevent problems as much as reasonably possible.

Note that while this chapter is dedicated to the health maintenance of older adults, *age* and *aging* are concepts that may not be perceived or experienced in the same way by everyone. For example, someone in his fifties who has spent years neglecting and mistreating his body may feel (and look) much older than someone twenty years his senior. Similarly, a woman well into her seventies or eighties may enjoy the vitality of someone much younger and may feel a bit indignant when categorized as an "older adult" or a "senior citizen." How many birthdays make one a senior? In an attempt to avoid oversimplifying (or offending someone), we've defined our target audience for this chapter as men and women who are sixty-five and older—and anyone else who anticipates being sixty-five and older.

Before we start, however, we need to issue a major reality check for young and old alike: Whatever you do as a younger adult to promote—or damage—your health will most likely bear all kinds of good—or rotten—fruit as you get older. The principle is obvious, but millions of people seem oblivious to it.

By the year 2030, one in five people in the United States will be older than sixty-five.[2]

Two analogies are worth noting. Remember in chapter 1, where we told the story of the free car of your dreams? We asked what you would do if you could have any car you wanted with the catch that it would be the only one you could ever own (see page 8). If you mistreat your one and only car (i.e., your body) for years, how will it run as the dents accumulate and the tires wear thin? Take good care of it, and your ride will be a lot smoother as it becomes a vintage model. Drive it fast and hard for years or never take it out of the driveway, and you can expect a breakdown sooner than you would like.

On a broader and more profound scale, consider Jesus' timeless illustration comparing the results of building on different foundations (Luke 6:47-49). This is a story about everyone's life, in all of its dimensions. Note that Jesus did not say *if* the storms come and the waves crash, but rather *when.* Here's a big news flash: Those storms are inevitable. If we live long enough, we will all face setbacks and heartaches of every shape, size, and severity. No one gets every wish granted, every desire fulfilled, every goal achieved. How will we respond when things don't turn out the way we want—or for that matter, when they do? Here's a second big news flash: The emotional and spiritual attitudes you have cultivated through the seasons of your life will usually intensify as you age. If the themes of your life have been defined by an ongoing, vibrant relationship with God and the fruits of living under His control—love, joy, peace, patience, kindness, goodness, faithfulness, gentleness, and self-control—it is likely that the fruit will ripen and sweeten, even during years of physical frailty. If the themes of your life have been dominated by self-centeredness, envy, hostility, anxiety, bitterness, and outbursts both physical and verbal, then you should be prepared for an even more unpleasant ride when the body you inhabit begins to wear out.

Put another way, the best time to optimize your health for the golden years is *not* at the time you arrive at them (whenever that might be). To be the healthiest older adult tomorrow, you need to start making healthy choices *today*. That being said, you or your loved ones may already be older adults. You may be concerned that the damage has already been done, that too much time has passed for you to make any meaningful progress at this point.

Wrong. Many people get a wake-up call at midlife or later—perhaps from an alarming lab report or a stay in the coronary-care unit—that results in a health makeover, after which they are in much better shape and feel much better than they did years before. The good news is that it's never too late to take steps (however faltering) that contribute to better health.

"Old age isn't so bad when you consider the alternatives."
—MAURICE CHEVALIER

One more thing before we begin. You will notice that many of these recommendations will seem to cross-reference others. For instance, exercise has been demonstrated to provide not only physical benefits, but also cognitive and emotional ones. Similarly, the state of our emotions, thought processes, and relationships (especially the one with our Creator) affects our physical well-being. We are more than an aggregate of separate mental, emotional, or spiritual components, and these are not independent of one another. We are fully integrated creatures, and research consistently shows that what promotes good health in one area of our life usually promotes good health in others. This is true throughout our life—but it becomes more obvious as we age.

In the following pages, we'll review the top ten ways to protect, preserve, and promote health during the senior years.

1. KEEP MOVING

In chapter 7, we described at length how a regular investment in physical activity pays off in overall health, both over the long and short run (no pun intended). Unfortunately, older adults have the dubious honor of leading the pack of those who do not get adequate amounts of exercise. While one in four American adults does not intentionally participate in even moderately intense recreational activities, that number climbs to one in three among older adults. A sedentary lifestyle is perhaps the most notable behavioral health risk for which prevalence increases with age.[3] For many, a career of inactivity begins in young adulthood or midlife and then carries into the senior years, where it is reinforced by the aches and ailments that can accompany aging—especially when physical activity has long been avoided. While a consistent pattern of exercise that begins early in life and continues into older adulthood is likely to have the most far-reaching benefit, it's never too late to start: Regular exercise and activity initiated late in life will also have significant benefits.

The abundant physical benefits of exercise include:

- Reduced risk of cardiovascular diseases such as heart disease and stroke
- Reduced risk of diabetes
- Reduced risk of osteoporosis
- Reduced risk of certain cancers, such as colon and possibly breast cancer
- Improved balance and coordination
- Increased strength, endurance, and mobility
- Reduced risk of obesity
- Reduced pain and disability from chronic diseases such as osteoarthritis
- Reduced risk of dying

That last point doesn't mean that regular exercise leads to physical immortality. We will all cross the Great Divide at some point, of course, but exercise decreases one's overall likelihood of dying in a given year from any cause. (Medical researchers refer to this as "a reduction in all-cause mortality.")

The physical benefits of exercise also overflow into other areas of life. Fewer health problems mean lower medical expenses—and perhaps even avoiding a financial crisis arising from a medical one. Furthermore, older adults with chronic illness and physical frailty often need daily living assistance, including nursing-home care. Physical activity can help many older adults delay or avoid the need for such assistance and thus prolong their independence, an increasingly valuable possession as the years pass.

Older adults should regularly engage in exercise that increases aerobic capacity, strength, and flexibility. Moderately intense aerobic activity (such as a brisk walk) is recommended at least three to five times per week for at least thirty minutes each session, although some research indicates that many health benefits still can be obtained if the activity is broken down into shorter segments. For example, three 10-minute workouts of moderate intensity may yield some of the benefits of a thirty-minute workout. Carrying a light weight in each hand while walking can help to build stamina and muscle strength. If you are concerned about contending with weather, local terrain, stray dogs, and other elements of the great outdoors, consider walking inside a climate-controlled mall. For those with significant problems of the back, hips, knees, or feet, exercising in a pool (also called **water aerobics**) can be a pleasant alternative to walking, as well as a good way to keep joints moving without generating aches and pains. Check with your local YMCA, senior center, community recreation center, or health club for information about water aerobics classes for seniors.

The purpose of strength training in older adults—indeed for the vast majority of younger ones—is not to build huge, rippling muscles, but to prevent the decrease in muscle mass that naturally accompanies aging. (This process actually begins much earlier, at about age thirty.) Two to three strength-training sessions every week (exercising every second or third day) can prevent or even reverse much of that muscle loss. (In other words, use it or lose it.) As in younger adults, increased muscle mass also makes it easier to control weight, since lean muscle tissue burns calories at a faster rate than fatty tissue. Strength training is also effective in countering age-related bone loss that can lead to osteoporosis.

While osteoporosis is often perceived as a woman's health issue, about 20 percent of osteoporosis cases occur in older men. For more on osteoporosis in men, see the sidebar on page 722.

Flexibility exercises become increasingly important as we age because our joints, tendons, and ligaments tend to stiffen with time and disuse. By stretching on a daily basis, many everyday range-of-motion problems that become more annoying as the years pass—such as difficulty reaching a cup in the pantry or even tying one's shoelaces—can be avoided. Senior centers, YMCAs, private health clubs, and many churches schedule stretching classes specifically for seniors.

What If I Can't Do Intense (or Even Moderate) Exercises?

Your current physical condition may make it impossible to exercise even with moderate intensity. Although current recommendations call for a person to do at least three sessions per week of moderate-intensity exercise lasting thirty minutes per session, this does not mean that you won't benefit if you cannot meet this level of activity. The point of physical activity is not to become a star athlete but to extend life as you preserve and maintain your health. While the greatest health advantages are gained with more vigorous levels of aerobic activity, research also clearly indicates that graduating from a sedentary lifestyle to modest levels of physical activity such as brisk walking can reduce one's risks for heart disease.[4]

Exercising with care

In chapter 7 we included a number of precautions regarding exercise. These are particularly important for older adults with medical problems that could be aggravated by exercise that is too vigorous, too long, or simply too much for someone who has been out of shape for a number of years.

Older adults should consult a physician if they are interested in starting an exercise program after a long period of inactivity, or if they are already active but desire to increase the intensity of their exercise. This is especially important for:

- Anyone with a history of heart disease, including coronary artery disease, congestive heart failure, an irregular rhythm, an abnormal valve, or a congenital abnormality (one present from birth).
- Anyone with symptoms that might suggest something is wrong with the heart, including episodes of chest pain or pressure, pounding or fluttering sensations in the chest (called **palpitations**), or shortness of breath from mild exertion, such as climbing a flight of stairs or walking a short distance. Remember that chest discomfort caused by a shortage of blood supply to the heart may not even be felt in the chest; sometimes it's noticed in the left arm, jaw(s), or even upper abdomen.

In addition, some types of exercise may not be appropriate for people with certain medical conditions. For example, a high-impact aerobic activity such as jogging would not be wise for someone with severe osteoporosis. If you have a chronic medical condition such as heart or lung disease, diabetes, or arthritis, be sure to discuss any new exercise program with your health-care provider. Likewise, if you experience chest, arm, neck, or jaw discomfort during exercise, discontinue it and seek medical attention before trying it again. If a particular exercise repeatedly causes pain elsewhere (for example, in your back, hips, knees, or feet), you should also talk to your doctor or an appropriate specialist before deciding whether to press on and endure it.

Remember that in these situations, pain is your ally, signaling that something is wrong and helping you to prevent more serious injury.

Old and young adults alike with type 1 diabetes—the type that requires insulin injections for survival—will need to track glucose (blood sugar) levels carefully using a glucose monitor so that they can balance activity with food intake and insulin use. Failure to do so could result in a dangerous drop in blood sugar level. For older adults with the more common type 2 diabetes, exercise is an extremely important part of an overall strategy to manage this disease. Physical activity usually does not lead to hypoglycemia (low blood sugar) in type 2 diabetics, although this could occur if a person is using medications (including insulin) that directly lower glucose levels. It is imperative that diabetics of either type discuss exercise options with their physician before starting a new program, since they are at higher risk for cardiovascular disease. In addition, diabetics should be careful to wear comfortable, properly fitting footwear, since their disease can lead to both poor circulation and decreased (or absent) pain sensation in the feet, which in turn is a setup for injuries, sores, and serious infections.

2. KEEP INVOLVED

In preindustrial society, there was no such thing as a mandatory or even typical retirement age. Men (and women) worked until they were no longer physically able, at which point they turned over the family farm or business to the oldest son or, in the absence of an heir, sold it. Older people who were not financially independent usually moved in with their grown children, making whatever contributions to the household their health would allow. In the United States, this scenario continued to be the norm well into the twentieth century, until Congress passed the Social Security Act (SSA) in 1935. While imperfect in many ways, this law provided older Americans with a modest safety net when they reached a point at which they could no longer work. The architects of the SSA settled upon sixty-five as the minimum age at which older adults could receive retirement benefits. While it was necessary for the government to designate an age for Social Security entitlements, the implications of choosing age sixty-five as that milestone had unintended consequences. Before long, societal norms and expectations began to converge around this milestone, and eventually it was assumed by employers and workers alike that upon reaching the "ripe old age" of sixty-five, an individual would retire from his or her chosen field of occupation.

This was not particularly problematic in 1935, when the average life span in the United States was about sixty-two. The SSA's age for retirement was chosen at a time when the effects of the aging process, combined with the rigors of labor in the 1930s, would force most workers to consider seriously giving up work by their midsixties. But as life expectancy (and the quality of health enjoyed by older adults) improved through the years, senior citizens began to face a new dilemma: They were arriving at "retirement age" without the physical promptings to retire. Instead of retiring because they no longer felt able to meet the demands of the job, older adults found themselves hanging up their spurs simply because they had reached society's designated age, with considerably better health than their forebears, and today they have an average of twelve years of life ahead of them.

The combination of increased longevity (a blessing by all accounts) and a customary retirement age of sixty-five produced several predicaments, including the prospect of outliving one's retirement savings or facing a Social Security system destabilized by a shrinking worker-to-retiree ratio. Even if finances aren't an issue, another question arises sooner or later: *What will I do with my remaining years now that I'm no longer spending my days (and nights) working for a paycheck?* Perhaps the more important question is this: *How will I use the time I have left in a purposeful manner?*

That word *purposeful* is crucial. To live purposefully means to live a life of useful endeavor, personal growth, and service to others. The need to have and fulfill a purpose is deeply ingrained in each of us. Unfortunately, many adults arrive at their later years with portfolios in order but without any sense of purpose.

They may hit sixty-five intending to spend the rest of their days on the golf course, but they quickly find an emptiness of spirit that the links just don't fill.

Please don't misunderstand: We don't mean even to hint that enjoying golf or any other recreational activity is somehow selfish or wrong. After decades of hard work, many people reasonably look forward to their retirement years as a time to devote a little attention to simple pleasures that they may have sacrificed or delayed most of their life. However, people tend to find very quickly that a life in which leisure is the main course, not just a side dish, is devoid of much of the zest that makes it seem worthwhile.

One reflection on the importance of purpose in the twenty-first century: By the end of 2004, Rick Warren's book *The Purpose-Driven Life* had spent one hundred consecutive weeks on the *New York Times* best-seller list. With more than 20 million copies sold (an average of 833,000 per month), it is the best-selling hardcover nonfiction book in U.S. history, according to *Publishers Weekly*.

Deciding When to Retire

Assuming that you or your loved one is approaching or has reached the nominal age of retirement and is still working, you may wish to consider whether or not this is the time to call it quits at the workplace. As we just noted, some people retire at age sixty-five primarily because doing so is what is expected—but this may not be the best option for everyone. Of course, the decision may be out of your hands if your employer has a mandatory retirement policy. But besides continuing to work because you need the income, you may wish to consider whether your work continues to provide enough fulfillment and purpose to continue for a few more years—or longer. Are you making a difference in someone's life? Does your job provide enriching experiences or contacts with others that you might not enjoy otherwise? Does it give you access to others' lives in ways that allow you to make a positive impact? Do you simply like what you do? If you answered yes to any of these questions and you are not hampered by any health concerns (and, of course, if your employer is amenable to the idea), you may wish to consider extending your occupational lifetime. In addition, you could look into working part-time if doing so would be practical and acceptable in your workplace.

Obviously, if your job has been a nonstop source of aggravation for years and you can't wait for the door to close behind you for the last time, you needn't bother asking that question. (What you should be asking is why you are spending so much of your life doing what you don't like.) At the other extreme, workaholism isn't just a young person's disease, and some older adults find themselves reluctant to relinquish a career or turn over the reins of a business to someone else. If work has been your emotional center of gravity, you may need to consider carefully what that orientation may be costing you in neglected relationships and other missed opportunities that cannot be recovered "someday when I have more time." Men in particular may have a more difficult time retiring because their occupation is so often the centerpiece of male identity. Even after quitting for good, a man is more likely to introduce himself as a "retired ________ [engineer, lawyer, contractor]" than as "the father of three and grandfather of eight." Because women—even those with careers outside of the home—tend to identify with relational roles (mom, wife, daughter), retirement from the workplace may not be as significant an event in terms of their sense of identity.

Making a Difference after You Retire

For most older adults, there does, indeed, come a time when retirement is the best option. Whether because of failing health, a need to slow down into a more relaxed lifestyle, or a desire to move on to different endeavors, the majority of seniors will spend their final years in retirement. The great news—indeed, the important news—is that retirement isn't the end of a useful life. Some people, in fact, find that their pursuits during the postoccupational years provide a greater sense of purpose than anything they did on the job. What often makes a crucial difference is that they aren't merely vegetating, rocking on the front porch (or in front of the TV), or focusing on maintaining their own "stuff." (Most male retirees find that after about six months they have run out of fix-its and honey-dos around the house.) Instead, *they are exploring avenues of service to others.*

There are virtually an unlimited number of ways you can make positive contributions to the lives of other human beings in your own home, your neighborhood, or in faraway places. Living a life of purpose later in life is, in fact, a lot like enjoying good health during those years: For the best results, you should begin doing the right thing (in this case, cultivating your avenues of service) early in life, rather than waiting until you arrive at your retirement age, whatever that might be. But even if you're a late bloomer, you can make a difference for others and for your community, regardless of your age or situation. In so doing, you'll avoid being overtaken by boredom, restlessness, and frustration.

Investing in your own family is a great way to pursue purpose during retirement. A few decades ago, the interactions between older adults and their children followed a traditional pattern. Children grew up, left home, and started their own families, and perhaps Grandmother or Grandfather would eventually move in with a grown son or daughter. Today, interactions between older adults and their families have entered new territories. Many grown children move back in with their parents, sometimes with grandchildren in tow. An increasing number of seniors find themselves in the role of primary caregiver for their grandchildren, years after they raised their own kids. Divorce, remarriage, and blended families complicate the landscape even further. But regardless of the "plot developments" that occur in your unique family story as the decades pass, one thing is certain: At *any* stage of life, the best investment you can make is in your own family.

As a grandparent you can have a profound impact on the lives and outlook of your children and grandchildren. Your ability to appreciate and enjoy grandchildren is likely to be much greater than what you experienced with your own children, for several reasons. Without the relentless, 24-7, "the buck stops here" duty required during early parenthood, you have the luxury of greeting grandchildren with fresh delight each time they walk through the door. The errands and chores of life can be suspended while you are with them because (unlike their own mom and dad) you know you will have time later on, when the house is quiet once again, to tend to those details. Also, hopefully by this time of your life, most of your striving to "be somebody" will have been resolved (see chapter 8), and (even more important) you will now have allotted more time in your life for cultivating relationships.

The value of the perspective gained *after* raising children cannot be overstated. Even those who are happy about how their grown children turned out will often reflect on their parenting careers and wish they had put a little more emphasis on *enjoying* the relationship instead of worrying so much about messy rooms or crayon marks on the walls. Having gained that understanding and without the responsibility for daily guidance and correction (although they can certainly make a contribution), grandparents are wonderfully positioned for a unique and highly enjoyable relationship with their grandchildren.

It is an incredible gift to help grown children see their offspring through the eyes of a hopelessly love-struck grandparent. When Grandma's face lights up the instant Jenna toddles through the front door, it helps Mom remember why she became a mommy in the first place. When Grandpa values playing with Travis more than watching a football game, it helps Dad renew his commitment to being a good father. When grandparents regard these little ones with perpetual awe and wonder rather than seeing them as a source of nonstop responsibility, they are blessing two generations at once.

Speaking of blessing, older adults have an opportunity to make (or continue making) a spiritual investment in their children and grandchildren. Perhaps when your children were younger, your faith was nonexistent or not sufficiently mature for you to provide much spiritual guidance as your kids were growing up. It is not too late for you to have some heart-to-heart conversations with grown children about your faith and its importance to you. You might even surprise them by having a candid conversation in which you attempt to make amends for your own shortcomings as a parent.

By the way, here's an important piece of advice about *giving* advice: If you are not in complete agreement with the way your grown children are raising your grandchildren, spiritually or otherwise, be *very* careful about the way you broach that subject, especially with a daughter-in-law or son-in-law. Remember: as parents they have the final say and responsibility for the way their children are reared, and your duty in nearly every situation is to abide by their decisions. (As one seasoned grandparent put it, "Your job is to keep your wallet open and your mouth shut. . . . ")

The exception to this guideline, of course, is when an irresponsible parent's behavior or neglect is exposing your grandchildren to harm. Otherwise, you can offer advice if asked and work at building a relationship in which you can compare notes and share the benefits of your parenting experience. Suggestions that are presented simply as "take it or leave it" opinions or observations are more likely to be welcomed than grand pronouncements.

You also have the opportunity to communicate a legacy of faith to a new generation both by word and (more important) example. Whether your spiritual roots and those of your family are old and deep or newly planted, you can pray for your children and their children daily. The impact of that time logged in conversation with God on their behalf may ultimately be more profound than any advice or gift you'll ever bestow.

Involvement in ministry opportunities will also give you a sense of purpose. While activities such as teaching Sunday school or participating in a choir or worship team at church can easily be categorized as ministry, there are a number of other ministry opportunities for which time might not be available until later in life. If you knew you had ten to fifteen healthy years after retirement, what might you accomplish? Does your church partner with a sister church in another country? You may be able to lend a hand to that congregation for several weeks or longer, now that you don't need to report for work every Monday. Could you raise some money, pound some nails, or serve some meals as part of an outreach project? Now that you finally have some time, what vision that has been percolating in your mind and heart might now come to fruition?

Giving back to the community and helping others are important ways that many older adults find or express purpose, and the opportunities are practically limitless. You can participate in an adult literacy program and give another person the gift of reading. You can teach English as a second language to immigrant adults or their children. You can provide living assistance to people in your community with physical or mental disabilities. You can donate your time to nonprofit or community organizations, most of which are grateful for any volunteer service they can get. Such organizations might include the Red Cross or Salvation Army, or your local homeless shelter, soup kitchen, or food pantry. If you love animals, your local animal shelter may need your help. If you're handy with tools, or you want to help in other ways to provide housing for needy families, consider Habitat for Humanity. For more information, go to http://www.habitat.org or call (229) 924-6935. If you have a heart for women with crisis pregnancies and their unborn children, consider volunteering at a pregnancy resource center.

An organization that provides this type of service to women may also be called a crisis pregnancy center, pregnancy care center, or women's resource center. Your church may already be involved with a center, or you can check with umbrella organizations such as Care Net at (703) 478-5661 or http://www.care-net.org, or Heartbeat International at (888) 550-7577 or www.heartbeatinternational.org.

If you'd like to enhance the lives of other older adults, call a local church to inquire about nursing-home ministries or in-home visitation programs. The Senior Companion Program is sponsored by the Senior Corps, a national service organization that helps older Americans find ways to use their experience to benefit their communities. You can find more information about Senior Corps at http://www.seniorcorps.org. And you can get a list of other volunteer opportunities in your region by calling your local Area Agency on Aging or by visiting http://www.volunteerfriends.org.

F.Y.I.

There are more than 650 Area Agencies on Aging (AAAs) and more than 230 programs for aging Native Americans in the United States, for which the National Association of Area Agencies on Aging (N4A) serves as the umbrella organization. These agencies coordinate and support a variety of services for seniors, encompassing meals, transportation, employment, adult day care, and others. To find and contact these resources, you can use the Eldercare Locator, a national toll-free number funded by the United States Administration on Aging. The number is (800) 677-1116, at which specialists are available to take calls Monday through Friday, 9 A.M. to 8 P.M., eastern standard time. (Voice messages are recorded twenty-four hours a day.) The Eldercare Locator can also be accessed on the Internet at http://www.eldercare.gov.

You may assume that young people don't want older people around. If they're struggling at all with their parents and other adults of the "older" generation—a timeless phenomenon, by the way—why would they want to spend time with someone who is *really* older? Won't the gap be just too wide and deep? *What have I got that they might want or need?* If this is your mind-set about engaging with teenagers and young adults, you need to take another look. Perhaps now more than ever, young people need the wisdom, experience, or even just the attention that older people can offer. Giving your time to one or more of them may change lives—theirs *and* yours.

There are many arenas in which you can work with young people. Organizations such as 4-H and Junior Achievement provide an environment in which you can share life skills and knowledge. Your local school district may have tutoring opportunities available. Many communities have mentoring programs that partner older adults with young people in need of guidance. One program, foster grandparenting, puts seniors in contact with children or teens who have emotional needs or physical disabilities and could benefit from the love of a surrogate grandmother or grandfather. Contact your Area Agency on Aging for more opportunities. And don't forget your local church. Getting involved in a youth group or teaching Sunday school is an excellent way to make a positive impact on children and young people.

3. KEEP CONNECTED

Many of us know people who shun the company of others because of past unpleasant interpersonal experiences. They may minimize contact with other people, fearing that interaction might be too painful. Others become socially isolated not by choice, but because of physical illness, lack of transportation, or the loss of friends or a spouse. For whatever reason, isolation is hazardous on many levels, and one of the best ways to maintain good health is to stay connected with others.

Humans are social creatures, and we function optimally when we enjoy healthy relationships. This isn't just touchy-feely pop psychology. Study after study shows that people who experience healthy social interactions live longer and fare better—physically, cognitively, and emotionally—than loners.

When it comes to maintaining social connectedness, some of us are naturals. We tend to think of extroverts as having an advantage in this area, and it might even seem unfair that an aspect of aging as important as the ability to socialize can come so easily to some and be such a challenge to others. Fortunately, having a core of solid relationships does not mean that one must become the life of the party or gather an army of friends. It's not the quantity but rather the quality of our relationships that is most likely to yield the greatest benefits. However, cultivating these connections requires more intentional effort for some than it does for others.

There are a number of ways to keep socially connected as we age. First, we can go to church. We can pray, study the Bible, and even worship on our own—indeed, these are important spiritual disciplines, as we discussed in chapter 9. But we are also designed to experience our journey with God in community with others, and we are explicitly instructed to do so in the New Testament: "Let us not give up meeting together, as some are in the habit of doing, but let us encourage one another" (Hebrews 10:25).

This exhortation and others like it throughout Scripture remind us that our faith is not intended to be experienced in a social vacuum. It's important not only to attend regular worship services but also to gather in smaller groups that allow individuals to support, encourage, and care for one another.

Rev. Michael Green of the Church of England once said in a sermon: "If you want only good teaching and worship, come only on Sunday morning, but if you want someone to remember your birthday, you'll have to join a small group."

Another way to become involved with people whose interests are similar to yours is by joining a club. Are you civic-minded and interested in bettering your community? You may wish to investigate the local Lions Club or Rotary Club. Do you have a green thumb? Try the local garden club. If you like to read or discuss good books, contact your local library to investigate area book clubs. If you like woodworking, a supply store or home-improvement retailer may be able to put you in touch with others who share your enthusiasm. The great thing about clubs like these is that they allow you to delve deeper into your area of interest while providing enriching social involvement at the same time.

We talked about the importance of volunteering in our second step toward keeping healthy as we age. While volunteering our time has the primary effect of helping others, it also has the additional and delightful benefit of connecting us with others. This may include interaction with other volunteers, or it may mean meeting and forming bonds with the people we serve.

While making new friends through new activities will bring great satisfaction, maintaining healthy relationships with grown children and their families can also play an important role in staying connected. While this may seem more challenging if the children have moved away, you can still use the phone or e-mail to keep in touch. By the way, if you don't hear from your family as often as you'd like, you would be wise to limit your complaining about it. Guilt is never a good motivator. Remember that your children (and even your grandchildren as they get older) probably have plenty of concerns of their own. If they have to listen to a litany of complaints every time they speak with you—especially if some involve your disappointment with *them*—you can expect fewer calls and visits. If you're normally a source of encouragement and conversations with you are bright spots in their week, you'll be more likely to hear from them.

While it may be discouraging if calls from the kids are a rare event, don't let that stop *you* from picking up the phone. Also, a letter (especially a handwritten note) in the mailbox, as antiquated as it may seem in this era of electronic communication, remains unmatched as a means of expressing your affection or thoughts, and it may provide a keepsake for years to come.

4. KEEP YOUR BRAIN HEALTHY

A decline in cognitive abilities—the complex mental processes of thinking, learning, and remembering—is arguably the change associated with aging that people fear most—even more than cancer. Some seniors do indeed experience dementia, a permanent deterioration of cognitive function, but a noticeable or severe decline is not inevitable with the passage of years. Most of us know men and women who have lived to a very old age while remaining sharp as the proverbial tack. Unfortunately, most of us also know people—perhaps within our own families—who have suffered serious or even catastrophic deterioration in mental function, sometimes at a surprisingly early age.

The good news is that cognitive decline is not a necessary consequence of aging. While some mental changes appear to be linked to factors that are not easily controlled or that may be out of our hands altogether, there are steps we can take now to reduce the likelihood of mental decline later. Before we examine the types of cognitive problems that can occur as we grow older, let's look at the changes in the brain that normally accompany the aging process.

What Happens to the Brain as We Age?

The physical transformations that accompany aging become readily apparent sooner or later: wrinkles, gait, hairline, stature, and many other features speak

"By the time you're eighty years old, you've learned everything. You only have to remember it."
—GEORGE BURNS, who lived to be 100

eloquently before the person utters a word, so that a quick glance can distinguish an eighty-year-old from a man in his twenties. However, we can't see physical changes to the brain directly, although CT scans, MRIs, and other modern technologies have revealed much over the past few decades.

During normal aging, few if any of the roughly 100 billion neurons in the brain die, but the brain's volume decreases, and 5 to 10 percent of its weight is lost between the ages of twenty and ninety.[5] The grooves on the surface of the brain tend to widen, and the raised convoluted structures on the surface of the brain shrink. The activity of neurotransmitters—the chemical messengers that transmit signals between neurons—slows somewhat. In spite of these changes, most people experience little actual loss of cognitive ability. Many older adults complain that they can remember vividly events that happened fifty years ago, but not what they had for breakfast. Nevertheless, most individuals do not experience appreciable memory loss, although *accessing* some items stored in memory may take longer. Similarly, unless some debilitating disease is at work, mental operations such as problem solving and verbal memory remain intact, though these processes tend to slow down as people grow older.

Dementia, Delirium, and Cognitive Decline

Dementia is a chronic and usually progressive loss of cognitive functions, including memory and reasoning ability. People with dementia may experience confusion, disorientation, emotional instability, depression, and personality changes. **Delirium** is a mental state marked by confusion, disorientation, difficulty thinking, hallucinations, and agitation. It can be caused by toxic substances, acute illness, or a metabolic disorder. Dementia and delirium may have similar outward manifestations, but delirium is generally short-term and usually reversible, while dementia generally progresses more slowly and is essentially irreversible. The brain of a person with dementia is likely to demonstrate physical changes of neurodegenerative disease, while the brain of a person with delirium may be essentially normal for its age.

Most of us have lost track of where we parked the car at the mall, misplaced our keys, searched high and low for a pair of glasses (that embarrassingly showed up in our shirt pocket), or racked our brain for the name, often on the tip of the tongue, that goes with a familiar face. If we have had enough birthdays, we usually laugh off these episodes as "senior moments"—although a series of them may generate an anxious visit to the doctor. (*Is there a test for Alzheimer's? I think I may have it!*) Yet these are common experiences, not necessarily signs of dementia or delirium. Indeed, many of these forgetful moments seem to arise from an overabundance of details (such as phone numbers, passwords, schedules, and procedures) that can accumulate and clutter our life and brain. More significant memory lapses, however, may indicate a true health problem. Here are a few symptoms of memory loss and cognitive impairment that should prompt a discussion with a health-care provider:

- Forgetting the way home from a familiar place
- Misplacing items on an increasingly frequent basis
- Forgetting names with greater regularity
- Having difficulty calculating simple arithmetic problems
- Confusion carrying out simple everyday tasks such as brushing teeth, combing hair, or using the telephone
- Putting clothes on backward or inside out
- Having difficulty completing sentences or recognizing the meaning of common words
- Having difficulty reading or writing
- Forgetting conversations or events that just took place, often manifested by asking for the same information over and over again

Often these cognitive glitches are reversible and result from adverse drug interactions or reactions, thyroid disorders, inadequate oxygen levels caused by lung or heart disease, infections, malnutrition, vitamin deficiency, dehydration, depression, or head injury. Serious cognitive problems occur very commonly with depression in the elderly, and such cases are called **pseudodementia**. In cases of delirium, the onset of symptoms is usually relatively rapid—another clue that a reversible medical problem may be the culprit.

Symptoms such as those listed above deserve a careful medical evaluation. To get the most out of the visit, be ready to give the doctor a clear idea of the time frame involved, along with some specific examples of episodes you have experienced or observed. Complaints such as "I think I'm losing it" or "Mom just isn't right" are too vague. However, explaining that "I can't seem to remember what day of the week it is" or "Yesterday, Mom got lost driving home from the store" is much more likely to be useful to the physician as he or she determines whether or not dementia is present. Also be sure to bring a current list of medications, including nonprescription drugs, vitamins, supplements, and herbal preparations. Something as simple as an antihistamine taken for a cold can set off a frightening episode of altered thinking or behavior in an elderly individual. While it's normal to desire a quick and certain answer, the diagnosis may not be clear, and you may need to exercise some patience while the doctor (or a consultant) goes through the necessary detective work. Unfortunately, sometimes even the most diligent diagnostic efforts don't yield a definite conclusion.

Many cases of dementia in older adults are not caused by reversible factors but by progressive diseases. You may hear these referred to as **senile dementias**, because they occur primarily in older adults. The two most common types of irreversible dementias are **vascular dementia** (sometimes called **multi-infarct dementia**) and **Alzheimer's disease**.

The word *senile* comes to us from the Latin word *senex*, meaning "old."

Vascular dementia

When a blood vessel hemorrhages or becomes blocked, the tissue that receives oxygen through that vessel can die quickly. This area of dead tissue caused by insufficient blood supply is called an **infarct**. When there is an infarction of brain tissue, the functions carried out by the damaged area of the brain will be affected to varying degrees. If this occurs on a large scale, as in a stroke involving a sizable artery, a person will experience sudden and dramatic symptoms: numbness or paralysis on one side of the face or body, confusion, or the inability to speak or understand speech. In vascular dementia, interruption of blood flow to one or more areas of the brain results in cognitive impairment. The most common form of this disorder is called multi-infarct dementia, in which a series of small strokes affects multiple locations in the brain. Sometimes the impairments are slight and difficult to notice, becoming more obvious only after a succession of these so-called **ministrokes** has occurred. Symptoms may include confusion, short-term memory impairment, emotional swings, laughing or crying inappropriately, depression, garbled speech, and loss of bowel or bladder control. A variation on this theme involves a single stroke to a critical area of the brain that results in cognitive disturbances without the loss of sensory or movement functions.

A noticeable change in cognitive function occurs in some seniors who undergo coronary bypass surgery—an unfortunate instance in which a procedure designed to prevent one problem (in this case, a heart attack) causes another.

Because neurons in the brain do not regenerate, the damage involved in vascular dementia is irreversible, and the prognosis for significant improvement may be poor unless other reversible problems can be addressed. Some individuals have a genetic risk for developing vascular dementia, but other risk factors can be reduced by behavior modification, medication, or both. These modifiable risk factors are the same as those for heart attack and stroke: the "usual suspects," including hypertension (high blood pressure), diabetes, elevated cholesterol, and smoking.

We discuss the various types of strokes, their risk factors, and strategies to prevent them in chapter 3.

Alzheimer's disease

The most common form of senile dementia is Alzheimer's disease (AD), which accounts for as much as 60 to 70 percent of this problem among seniors. Approximately 4.5 million people in the United States live with AD, and since symptoms are typically noticed after age sixty, that number is expected to rise as more baby boomers move into their sixties and beyond.[6] It is estimated, based on current projections, that by the year 2050 more than 13 million Americans will have this disease.[7]

Alzheimer's disease is a progressive neurodegenerative illness for which there is currently no cure. People live, on average, between eight and ten years after the diagnosis of AD is first made, although some may live with this disease for more than twenty years.[8]

Because of its prevalence and the level of disability that it creates, AD has a tremendous impact on society. The total cost of caring for people afflicted with this disease is estimated to be as much as $100 billion per year in the

United States. But more significant than the national economic impact of Alzheimer's are its devastating effects on its sufferers and their families. People with AD experience sadness, frustration, and anger at their progressive loss of memory and inability to communicate and think clearly. They may also be fearful because of their uncertain future and the potential pain the disease will cause family and loved ones. It is important to note, however, that individual experiences with AD (and with other chronic dementias) vary considerably. Not everyone progresses relentlessly to a full-blown, incapacitating condition. Taking the process one step at a time, while planning for potential developments, is wise and reasonable. Worrying incessantly about the future is not.

The impact on loved ones is no less significant. It is one thing to watch a grandparent, parent, spouse, or other loved one weaken and die because of heart disease, cancer, or another disorder that leaves the basic identity intact. But with AD (and the other dementias as well), physical death is but the final loss after a seemingly endless series of losses, a literal death by inches over years or even decades. The person you know gradually seems to fade into someone else whose thoughts, behavior, and personality are usually anything but pleasant. Since more than half of people with AD receive in-home care (as opposed to residing in a nursing home), spouses, children, and friends of the Alzheimer's victim experience not only the heartbreak of watching this relentless decline, but they may also become exhausted—physically, emotionally, and perhaps financially as well—as they deal with the realities of full-time care for this person.

A classic book written for those who care for individuals with Alzheimer's disease is aptly titled *The 36-Hour Day: A Family Guide to Caring for Persons with Alzheimer Disease, Related Dementing Illnesses, and Memory Loss in Later Life* by Nancy L. Mace and Peter V. Rabins (New York: The Johns Hopkins University Press, 1999).

As a young adult, raising a baby or toddler is also a demanding job, but at least the parent is bigger and stronger, and can confine the child to a crib at night and (if needed) a playpen during the day. (It is also relatively easy to arrange for a babysitter.) This is not the case with a full-sized, confused adult who may wander through the house (or outside) day or night, turn on the stove, undress at inopportune moments, urinate in the closet, and so forth. Well before this type of disruptive behavior develops, you may find yourself answering the same question about some seemingly minor event—going to the bank or visiting the doctor—twenty times a day, and then doing so again the next day. A combination of faltering memory, anxiety, and agitation may lead an impaired loved one to suspect and accuse you of all sorts of vile deeds—stealing his money, plotting against him, even trying to kill him. The caregiver's frustration and hurt are indescribable and must be countered by constant self-reminders that these acccusations are the direct result of a physical disease.

Needless to say, caregivers need all the help they can get and should feel comfortable asking for help as well. Conversely, the community, and especially the church, needs to step up and support those who bear the primary responsibility for the care of ailing seniors, with or without dementia. If you know someone who is in this situation, call and make a specific offer to help (for example, "What would be a good morning or afternoon for me to stay with your mom for a few hours?"). If you are facing this situation yourself, don't try to do it alone. Admit when you need help and don't be afraid to ask for it or accept it.

Symptoms and stages of Alzheimer's disease

Alzheimer's disease manifests itself in three stages. The progression of the disease is different in each person, and some stages may appear shorter or more prolonged in certain individuals.

A person in the early stage of AD will likely be able to carry out a range of normal activities but may need guidance with various tasks that require multiple steps, such as balancing a checkbook. She may have difficulty remembering people's names, as well as recent events and conversations. Finding the right word when speaking becomes a challenge, and she might misplace items with increasing regularity. Mood swings, depression, or anxiety may develop.

In the intermediate stage, a person with Alzheimer's is still able to carry out many daily activities but begins to have greater difficulty caring for herself. She may need assistance bathing, dressing, and using the toilet. She will need help cooking (for her own and everyone else's safety) and may need to be reminded to eat. Sleep patterns can become reversed, so that she sleeps during the day and stays awake at night, often with a tendency to wander around rather than simply rest in bed. These nocturnal adventures can be doubly unsettling because confusion may increase after the sun goes down. Communicating with and understanding others becomes difficult. The emotional weather may grow more turbulent, with anxiety, anger, and agitation dominating the landscape. When combined with impaired memory and confusion, these feelings can also generate suspicion or outright paranoia. As the condition worsens, she may no longer recognize family members.

In the late, severe stage of AD, she becomes dependent on others for assistance with the most basic functions of life: walking, standing, dressing, eating, and using the toilet. If she hasn't done so already, she may begin to lose bowel and bladder control. Her verbalizations will usually dwindle to a few words (or to syllables repeated endlessly), and she may appear not to remember or recognize anyone. Eventually, she may lose her interest in food and finally the ability to swallow. Unfortunately, as the person reaches the very end stage of this disease, interventions such as feeding tubes will only prolong the dying process. Unless she dies from an acute illness (usually an infection such as pneumonia) or the consequences of some other disease, AD will eventually take her to a state of increasing unresponsiveness, coma, and death.

As bleak as this picture might look, it is crucial to remember that the person with Alzheimer's—or any other form of dementia, even in its most advanced stages—is still a human being who must not be devalued or disrespected. He or she needs love and gentle care, as do the caregivers, through the full course of the illness. We must resist any campaign that would push our culture toward allowing deliberate measures to terminate the life of those with dementia because they'd be "better off dead."

Managing and treating Alzheimer's disease

The brain of a person with AD, if examined under a microscope, would reveal tangled nerve fibers (called **neurofibrillary tangles**) and abnormal, sticky clumps of protein (known as **amyloid plaques**). While these hallmarks of the disease are well defined, the precise physiological steps that lead to AD are poorly understood, and thus there is currently no cure for the disease. However, there are some medical treatments that can slow its progression or at least decrease the severity of some of the symptoms. The currently approved classes of treatment include:

Cholinesterase inhibitors. Drugs in this class include donepezil (Aricept), rivastigmine (Exelon), tacrine (Cognex), and galantamine (Razadyne). Reduced levels of the neurotransmitter **acetylcholine** are believed to be responsible for some of the symptoms of AD, such as declines in memory, attention, and reasoning. These drugs inhibit the activity of **acetylcholinesterase**, the enzyme that breaks down acetylcholine. While cholinesterase inhibitors can help Alzheimer's patients maintain their current level of ability, these medications do not address the underlying causes of decline. As a result, the evidence indicates that they will not prevent the dementia from progressing, but they may temporarily *slow* that progression. This treatment can thus stabilize the individual for several months and potentially make a major difference in the lives of the patient and his family members for that time. Unfortunately, these drugs are very expensive. Also, patients taking cholinesterase inhibitors often experience an ongoing loss of appetite or overt nausea.

NMDA receptor antagonists. This class includes the drug memantine (Namenda). The amino acid glutamate is a neurotransmitter (chemical messenger) in the brain that plays an important role in learning and memory through its effects on a nerve cell structure known as the N-methyl-D-aspartate (or NMDA) receptor, which alters the chemical environment within the cell.

Researchers believe that some of the symptoms of Alzheimer's disease may be due to improper regulation of glutamate levels, which, if too high, can lead to disruption and death of nerve cells. Memantine is believed to work by limiting access of glutamate to NMDA receptors, thus helping to protect these cells. While memantine has been approved by the FDA for use in treating moderate to severe Alzheimer's disease, like the cholinesterase inhibitors, it has not been shown to alter any of the underlying processes that cause dementia. It has the same advantages as cholinesterase inhibitors. When combined with one of them, the stabilizing effect may be even more significant, and the appetite and nausea problems may be diminished. However, it also is expensive, especially when taken with one of the cholinesterase inhibitors.

NMDA receptors are so named because they are selectively activated by N-methyl-D-aspartate (NMDA), an artificial molecule that is structurally similar to glutamate.

Risk factors for Alzheimer's disease

The best way to deal with any disease is to avoid it, but with diseases like AD, whose causes are poorly understood, it can be difficult to make strong recommendations for prevention. Of the known risk factors for this disease, two are unalterable.

Age. The average age of onset for AD is in the mid to late sixties, and the risk of developing the disease increases as one ages. The incidence of AD—that is, the number of people who develop it in a given year—is about one percent at age sixty, but that number doubles every five years.[9]

Genetics. Alzheimer's disease can be classified as either familial or sporadic. The familial, or hereditary, form of the disease occurs in only a small percentage of cases but can result in the horrific scenario of a person developing the disease well in advance of the average age of onset. The sporadic form of Alzheimer's does not show any evident inheritance pattern, but it does appear to be affected by a gene for apolipoprotein E (apoE). Apolipoproteins are proteins that combine with lipids to form lipoproteins, large molecules such as low-density lipoprotein (LDL) and high-density lipoprotein (HDL), which help transport cholesterol through the bloodstream.

For a closer look at lipoproteins, especially HDL and LDL, which play an important role in the risk for developing cardiovascular disease, see "Cholesterol Basics" in chapter 3, beginning on page 56.

There are multiple forms of the gene that codes for the apoE protein, and one form, the APOE e4 gene, appears much more frequently in individuals with sporadic AD. The exact link between APOE e4 and the disease is uncertain at this time, although it is known that the apoE protein is involved in the repair of neuronal membranes.

The encouraging news about Alzheimer's disease is that biology is not destiny. Even if a person has risk factors of age and genetics going against him, it is not certain that he will develop AD. Other factors that *are* within our control may make us less likely to experience Alzheimer's, or may at least delay onset of the disease. These include:

Smoking. Here is yet one more reason to quit (or never start) smoking. The research is not definitive, but some studies (and a basic understanding of the effects of smoking on blood vessels) indicate that smokers are more likely than nonsmokers to develop vascular dementia and AD. Do your brain a favor and don't light up.

Nutrition. Some reports claim that vitamin E may reduce the risk of developing Alzheimer's disease. One study published in 2004 suggests that a daily combination of 500 mg of vitamin C and 400 IU (international units) of vitamin E may reduce the risk of developing AD.[10] (This amount of vitamin E cannot be obtained from diet alone and requires a vitamin supplement. Some experts question whether long-term use of high doses of vitamin E is safe, and they suggest limiting daily intake to no more than 400 IU. Some research indicates that doses of vitamin E supplements should be kept below even that level.) Curiously, other research indicates that vitamin E intake from food—but not from vitamin supplements—offers a protective benefit against AD.[11] In addition, studies suggest that people with elevated blood levels of homocysteine are at greater risk for AD. Elevated homocysteine levels may be tied to low levels of folic acid and vitamin B_{12}, and supplementing these nutrients may lower blood homocysteine. It is important to note, however, that it has yet to be proven that lowering homocysteine levels in this way will reduce a person's risk of AD.

For more information about homocysteine and its possible connection with coronary artery disease, see "Other Screening Tests for Cardiovascular Disease" in chapter 4 on page 83. For more information about vitamin E, see appendix B, "Vitamins and Minerals: What Each One Does and How Much We Need" starting on page 869.

Physical activity. Remember earlier in the chapter when we mentioned how our top ten ways to promote health during the senior years would seem to cross-reference each other? This is definitely one of those instances. In addition to the physical benefits it brings, exercise offers a protective effect against cognitive decline. Studies suggest that physical activity can enhance cognitive performance, stimulate formation of new connections between neurons (synapses), and promote resistance to neurodegenerative disease and injury within the brain. To keep your brain healthy, stay active.

Cardiovascular health. A number of studies suggest that several of the factors that increase the risk of heart disease and stroke (such as elevated blood pressure and unfavorable cholesterol levels) may also increase the risk of AD. Bringing these under control may thus reduce the risk of developing AD. (Doing so will certainly reduce the risk of developing vascular dementia.) You'll find detailed and practical information about these factors in chapters 3 and 4 of this book.

Mental activity. It has been hypothesized that regular mental stimulation and activity (such as reading, solving puzzles, and doing math problems) help the brain form more synapses. And while damaged neurons in the brain do not appear to regenerate, there is evidence that learning and mental stimulation may cause new neurons to be generated in certain parts of the brain. This may reduce the likelihood of developing dementia or cognitive decline, since the creation of new neurons and synapses could compensate for the loss of others due to injury or disease. Interestingly, level of education has also been identified as a factor that may affect the risk of developing Alzheimer's disease. Researchers hypothesize that the learning process increases the number of synapses that are generated in the brain, which could help prevent cognitive decline. This research is far from definitive, however, and it is likely that overall mental activity is more important as a protective factor than the number of academic degrees hanging on the wall.

There are many things you can do to keep your mind alert. (These include activities that connect you with other people—another of those cross-references we keep mentioning.)

- Shut off the TV and start reading. Become a regular at the library or your favorite bookstore. For even more stimulation, gather some friends together to create an informal book club where you can discuss interesting and worthwhile reading material.
- Become a lifelong learner. Take a class at your local community college

on a subject that interests you, or perhaps go back and complete that degree you never quite finished.

- Look into Elderhostel, a nonprofit organization that provides exceptional travel and learning opportunities for older adults all over the world (and at far less cost than commercial tour groups). Check http://www.elderhostel.org or call (877) 426-8056 for more information and a catalog.
- Keep a journal. Do more than just list the day's events; pour out your feelings in a diary. One day your children will treasure being able to gain a deeper understanding of what made you tick.
- Write your memoirs. Your experiences, insights, and descriptions of past events and family traditions will be a treasure for future generations.
- Write letters. Keep your family and friends updated not only on what you're doing, but also what you're thinking about. Write to your elected representatives (city, state, or federal) about matters that concern you. (Believe it or not, your opinion does make a difference.)

HOT TIP

Want to have an impact on someone's life with your letters? Contact Prison Fellowship, an organization that is changing the lives of prisoners all over the world, about becoming a pen pal with someone who is incarcerated. (Prison Fellowship, The Pen Pal Program, P.O. Box 2205, Ashburn, VA 20146-2205; phone: (800) 497-0122; Internet: http://www.pfm.org.) A less time-consuming (but no less meaningful) form of letter writing can take place when you support a little one through World Vision, which provides the opportunity to have an ongoing written communication with the child. You can begin this process by calling (888) 511-6592 or visiting http://www.worldvision.org on the Internet.

- Become computer literate. Many older adults see the world of computers and the Internet as foreign or even hostile territory. Wrong! These are powerful tools, and you're never too old to learn how to use them for all sorts of worthwhile purposes (including e-mailing friends and family—especially grandchildren who may be more at home with a computer than paper and pen).

HOT TIP

Take a basic computer course at your local community college or senior center. Better yet, ask a teenage computer whiz in your family (or even outside of your family) to teach you. (You might offer to pay for this tutoring, either in cash, gift certificates, or treats from your oven.)

- Do the daily crossword puzzle.
- Tutor a student.
- Learn to play a musical instrument.
- Learn to paint.
- Learn a foreign language.

Get the idea? The list is nearly endless!

5. KEEP EATING RIGHT

As men and women grow older, they are at greater risk for nutritional problems for several reasons. Nutritional needs can change if the capacity for digesting certain foods or absorbing nutrients becomes impaired, and people often do not adjust their eating habits—or even know that they need to—in order to accommodate these new needs. Furthermore, many older people simply do not eat adequate amounts of nutritious foods, for reasons we will explore shortly. A recent federal survey concluded that the quality of diet for two out of three older Americans "needs improvements," while for 14 percent, diet quality is considered poor.[12] This is a sad state of affairs in a nation so blessed with an ample and stable supply of food.

Let's take a closer look at the nutritional problems faced by older adults.

Changes in Digestion and Nutritional Needs

As we age, many processes in our body slow down, including metabolism and the movement of food through our digestive system. Absorption of nutrients is often affected as well. Most changes in digestive capacity are natural, but certain prescription medications can interfere with digestion and cause nutritional deficiencies.

Seniors often don't utilize dietary proteins as efficiently as younger adults and thus may need greater amounts of high quality proteins to preserve lean muscle tissue.

One important disorder related to nutrient malabsorption is **pernicious anemia**. With advancing years, the tissue that lines the stomach can begin to atrophy. When healthy, this tissue produces a substance called **intrinsic factor**, which is essential for the absorption of vitamin B_{12} in the small intestine. Vitamin B_{12} is necessary for the normal production and maturation of red blood cells. A decrease in production of intrinsic factor or certain diseases involving the small intestine can lead to inadequate levels of B_{12}, which in turn results in anemia (a shortage of red blood cells). This condition is called pernicious (i.e., exceedingly harmful) because it can also cause serious and permanent nerve damage. On rare occasions, pernicious anemia arises from an inadequate intake of foods containing vitamin B_{12} (specifically meat and dairy products) over an extended period of time, and eating foods rich in this vitamin (or taking a vitamin supplement) will correct it. In most cases, however, the problem is an inability to absorb vitamin B_{12}, and treatment consists of monthly B_{12} injections.

Inadequate Nutritional Intake

Many older adults face nutritional deficits for reasons that have nothing to do with malabsorption or changing physiological needs.

- Economics. Many seniors live on fixed (or shrinking) incomes that often limit the types and amounts of foods they can buy. For some, buying nutritious food on a regular basis requires financial juggling. Nowadays, it is not uncommon for older adults to accrue a list of medications that cost hundreds of dollars every month, and sadly there may be occasions when one has to choose between picking up a prescription or buying groceries.
- Diminished appetite. A gradual decline in the senses of taste and smell, which is not uncommon during the aging process, makes food less appealing. Also, a number of medications can reduce appetite or cause nausea, but the connection between drugs and symptoms may not be obvious. If you have any concern that this might be happening, you should discuss it with your physician.
- Social factors. Loneliness, isolation, and depression can also contribute to a poor appetite. For some widowed women (and men) who have cooked for years for a large family, cooking for one may not seem worth the effort.
- Restricted mobility. Seniors who no longer drive or who need other assistance obtaining groceries have more limited access to food and less variety in the refrigerator and cupboard. Furthermore, reductions in stamina and mobility within the home can make it difficult for many older adults to prepare food.
- Difficulty chewing and swallowing. Seniors with dental problems or ill-fitting dentures have limited food choices. Strokes and other neurological problems that affect the ability to swallow slow the eating process or even make mealtime hazardous if solids or liquids are repeatedly aspirated into the airway.

Loss of taste or smell in older adults can present a health hazard, as they may find it more difficult to determine whether foods have started to go rancid. To prevent food poisoning, older adults should be sure to cook all meats fully and refrigerate any leftovers promptly. Refrigerated foods should be dated. And as always, when in doubt, throw it out. For more information on food safety, see pages 553–555 in chapter 11.

Fortunately, there are many ways to address these problems and improve nutritional intake. The appeal of foods for older people with diminished taste or smell can be increased by experimenting with different flavors, spices, and textures. Varying colors of foods and even temperatures can make them more appetizing.

Because many causes and consequences of a poor appetite are medical, a thorough and thoughtful medical evaluation is important. This should include a review of medications, as well as careful evaluation for depression. To deal with appetite loss related to isolation and loneliness, consider the advice in the second and third segments of our top ten list ("Keep Involved" and "Keep Connected"). Obviously, gathering with others—family members, friends, and neighbors—at church or at a senior center can help solve this problem, although the logistics, challenges, and opportunities to do so will vary substantially with individual circumstances.

A number of community-based, government-funded programs provide meals to seniors at reduced or no cost. Meals On Wheels is an excellent program that provides nutritious meals to housebound older adults, and volunteers who deliver meals often spend some time socializing with them, thus helping relieve their feelings of isolation. Also, many grocery stores will deliver free to seniors who can call, fax, or e-mail their orders. Sometimes, the delivery person will even assist in putting away the food. For older people who are mobile, many local senior centers provide not only meals but also companionship.

If you or an aging loved one is not eating enough because of financial limitations, you can call your local Area Agency on Aging to find out if assistance is available. (See page 687 for information about Area Agencies on Aging.)

Contact information for Meals On Wheels: Meals On Wheels Association of America, 203 S. Union Street, Alexandria, VA 22314; phone: (703) 548-5558. Check the Web site (http://www.mowaa.org) to locate the program nearest you.

Vitamin and Mineral Needs in Older Adults

According to guidelines established by the Food and Nutrition Board of the Institute of Medicine, most of the Recommended Daily Allowances (RDAs) and Adequate Intakes (AIs) for vitamins and minerals are the same, or very similar, for both older and younger adults. We have listed these in appendix B, entitled "Vitamins and Minerals: What Each One Does and How Much We Need"—a question that is addressed there at some length.

The following details, however, are important for seniors:

- While the RDA for vitamin C is 90 mg per day for adult men who do not smoke (and 125 mg per day for those who do), experts at the National Institutes of Health recommend a daily intake of 100 mg to 200 mg, to be obtained from fruits and vegetables whenever possible. And as referenced in our discussion of Alzheimer's disease, research suggests that 500 mg a day of vitamin C, along with 400 IU a day of vitamin E, may offer some protection against AD.
- Calcium, as mentioned in chapter 13, is essential to maintaining bone health—for both men and women. The Food and Nutrition Board of the Institute of Medicine recommends that older men and women get at least 1,200 mg of calcium per day, but some nutrition experts consider 1,500 mg of calcium per day to be a more advisable intake for both older men and women. Since this amount may be difficult for some older adults to obtain from dietary sources alone, a calcium supplement is a good investment (see chapter 13, page 664).
- Vitamin D is necessary for proper calcium absorption. Adults fifty to seventy should receive 400 IU per day, while those over seventy should be getting 600 IU per day. Milk produced in the United States is fortified with 400 IU of vitamin D per quart, as are many breakfast cereals. Many calcium supplements include vitamin D as well in order to help maintain bone density.

Older adults are frequent users of supplements, many of which are marketed to them with extravagant claims and impossible promises. To avoid wasting money on products of dubious value, review the nutritional basics presented in chapter 5 and the vitamin and mineral appendix. Chapter 17 also addresses the challenge of separating the wheat from the chaff in the world of health information.

Because vitamin D is produced in the skin upon exposure to sun, some experts believe that 1,000 IU of vitamin D per day is more appropriate for adults who have no sun exposure.

Concern about getting adequate amounts of vitamins and minerals leads many people to consider taking a nutritional supplement. *Remember that the best source of nutrients is from food,* and like everyone else, older adults should try to get as much of the recommended amounts of vitamins and minerals as they can from their plate rather than a pill bottle. Follow the general recommendations in chapter 5 (summarized at the end of that chapter) to reach that goal. However, this may be difficult for individuals dealing with appetite loss, certain chronic illnesses, or other problems that impair their dietary intake. Even for younger adults who are able to eat three square meals a day, many reputable authorities consider a daily multivitamin and mineral supplement a good investment. For seniors who may have a number of problems obtaining, preparing, and digesting adequate amounts of quality food, this recommendation is even more compelling.

A good multivitamin should provide 100 percent of the daily value (DV) of most of the vitamins and minerals listed in appendix B. In particular, it should supply 100 percent of the B vitamins (including folic acid), C, D, E, iron, iodine, zinc, selenium, copper, manganese, chromium, and molybdenum. Typically, multivitamins do not supply the higher doses of vitamin C or E noted above nor do they include the amounts of calcium normally recommended for seniors, but all of these can be purchased separately. A good multivitamin does not need to be a senior formulation, which is more of a marketing term than a nutritional one. (What distinguishes most of these formulations from other adult multivitamins are minute variations in nutrients and bigger variations in price.) Most important, *it should not be expensive.* The total supplement package for adults, young or old, shouldn't cost more than ten to twenty cents *per day*. If you're dropping twenty or fifty dollars every month on supplements, you are spending money that would be much better used to buy good-quality food (especially fresh fruits and vegetables). There are several other useful guidelines for buying and taking vitamin and mineral supplements at the end of appendix B beginning on page 918.

Weight Gain and Loss during the Senior Years

As we age, our metabolism slows down for a variety of reasons, including a decreased amount of lean muscle mass and a decline in physical activity. As a result, older adults generally need fewer calories to maintain necessary body functions and overall weight. However, it is not always easy to balance decreasing metabolic needs with established eating habits. In other words, it isn't unusual for a person with a senior citizen's metabolism to still have the appetite of a much younger adult. As a result, many enter their senior years with a significant number of excess pounds. Combine this with a body that isn't all that willing to burn extra fat, a generous food supply (and many opportunities to enjoy it), and one or more physical limitations that may interfere with vigorous or sustained exercise, and it shouldn't be surprising that about 70 percent of Americans age sixty-five and older are overweight or obese.[13] As with all other age groups, the statistics regarding excessive weight and obesity have worsened over the past few decades for older adults. In the early 1960s, 55 percent of men and women sixty-five to seventy-four were overweight, and 18 percent were obese. At the turn of the twenty-first century, 73 percent of men and women in this age group are overweight, and 36 percent are obese.[14] Unfortunately, this aggravates nearly all of the common health problems facing seniors: cardiovascular disease, decreased lung capacity, diabetes, osteoarthritis, sleep disorders, even some cancers.

The issue of excess weight (including criteria for being overweight or obese) is addressed in detail in chapter 6, and the general principles of weight loss given there apply to all adults, young and old. Because getting an adequate supply of nutrients can be challenging for many older adults, the smaller portions that are needed to shed some pounds must consist of nutritious foods, such as fruits, vegetables, and whole grains. Overweight seniors should seek medical input about the impact of their weight on their health and strategies to deal with it. And like younger adults, they should beware of "quick fix" diets (that may be inappropriately restrictive) and "miracle" weight-loss supplements that waste money and may compromise health.

Other Nutritional Matters

Dehydration occurs far more often in older people than in younger people, especially among those living in institutional settings. It may develop so gradually as to go unnoticed until it is relatively severe. Contributing factors can include a diminished sensation of thirst, difficulty communicating a desire for liquids, and certain medications—specifically diuretics—that increase water loss from the body. (Diuretics, also known as water pills, are used to treat elevated blood pressure and congestive heart failure, two problems that are common among seniors.)

Changes in bowel function in the elderly leave many prone to constipation, a problem aggravated by insufficient water intake. This can eventually lead to fecal impaction, a condition in which dry, hard stool accumulates in the colon or rectum and cannot be evacuated with normal bowel movements. More dramatic consequences of dehydration include cognitive decline and even death. Dehydration accounts for a significant number of hospitalizations among older adults. Unless a doctor specifically recommends restricting the amount of fluid a person is to consume, older adults should aim for eight 8-ounce glasses of water every day (or more on hot days or in drier climates).

Speaking of constipation, other nutritional factors can also contribute to it. Certain prescription or over-the-counter medications are known to cause difficulty in passing stools, as can a diet low in insoluble fiber and high in fat or dairy products. The Institute of Medicine recommends that men fifty-one and older consume 30 grams of fiber daily, and women fifty-one and older should get 21 grams of fiber per day. If you feel you are getting the recommended amount of fiber but still struggle with constipation, ask your doctor if ramping up your fiber intake would be appropriate. If you are not accustomed to eating a lot of fiber, you should increase your consumption gradually. (A sudden increase in insoluble fiber may lead to cramping, gas, and other uncomfortable events in the digestive tract.) If water and fiber intake are adequate but constipation is still a problem, a laxative may be in order, but only as a short-term solution. Your doctor can offer further help and rule out other possible causes (including side effects from medications).

If constipation or other bowel symptoms are new to you, your doctor may recommend a colonoscopy. This may seem like an overzealous response, but you would be wise to comply. See page 708 later in this chapter.

6. KEEP UP ON HEALTH SCREENINGS

In chapter 3 we presented three health problems to be avoided (cardiovascular disease, cancer, and diabetes), and in chapter 4 we looked at a number of screening tests for these and other disorders for which early detection could be life- and health-preserving. Often the importance of these tests is emphasized for those in their midlife years: More health problems are likely to be detected at age forty or fifty than at twenty or thirty, and there is still enough potential "mileage" for a timely intervention to make a difference in life expectancy.

Yet health screening is important for older adults as well. There is no reason for a person at age sixty-five, seventy, or even much older to assume that "I made it this far, so there isn't much point in doing a bunch of tests (that are likely to be uncomfortable and expensive) just to help me add a few more years to my life span." Some believe that no one will care or do anything about the problems that are discovered in a senior citizen. This is not true. Life and health are gifts from God, and they deserve to be preserved and protected for His continued use at any age. That being said, we should note that experts do not always agree on how frequently (or whether) certain common screening tests should be performed on people over sixty or seventy. This is not because older seniors have less value. Rather, it is simply not clear whether carrying out these tests will extend the quantity and quality of life for the oldest among us.

At the beginning of chapter 4, we described nine characteristics that make a screening test useful—or a questionable use of time and money. We won't repeat them here, but you might want to take a few minutes to review them. In addition, the American Geriatrics Society has developed some helpful guidelines for screening seniors:

- If a person has a very short life expectancy because of one or more serious medical conditions, screening tests should be focused on discovering whatever might be causing symptoms and problems *now*, rather than at some point in the distant future.

- Screening decisions should be based on how burdensome the test(s) will be in *all* respects for the senior adult, not to mention how burdensome additional tests and treatments might be if something wrong is discovered. Someone with dementia, for example, might not understand the reason for the test and could perceive certain procedures not only as frightening and uncomfortable, but also as a literal assault. And what if the initial screening test uncovers a problem that might need further evaluation and treatment? Is the person a candidate for whatever the next steps might be? In other words, given the person's current health condition and personal preferences, *what can be done with the results of the tests?*
- Screening should be individualized rather than determined strictly by age. Someone who is a "young" eighty-five—healthy, alert, and active—may benefit from tests that would be inappropriate for another person who is an "old" seventy—chronically ill, with an uncertain or short life expectancy.
- Screening decisions for seniors should take into account the desires and expectations of the individual. For example, if someone has made it abundantly clear that he isn't going to change his diet or take medication to lower his cholesterol, there's little reason to keep checking it every year. On the other hand, an elderly woman may desire a mammogram even if she wouldn't undergo treatment for breast cancer, because the results of the test could affect personal planning decisions for the remaining years of her life, not to mention providing reassurance that she does not have breast cancer if the test is negative.[15]

These important guidelines could be boiled down to a simple question: Will the test provide information that is truly useful to the individual being screened in light of his or her current health, life expectancy, willingness to undergo further tests and treatments, and need for life planning? Keep that question firmly in mind as we look at several screening tests that are of particular relevance to older adults. We have included page numbers that will refer you back to the more detailed explanations of tests that were provided in chapter 4.

An important note: Over the past several years Medicare, the federally funded health-care program for seniors sixty-five and over, has expanded its coverage to include a number of screening procedures. This has helped alleviate some of the financial burden of health screening for seniors.

Medicare is also available for some younger individuals who have long-term disabilities, as well as for those with permanent kidney failure.

We will make note of the tests that are covered (at the time of this book's publication), although the extent of coverage will depend on the specific test and a patient's deductible. Medicare still does not cover physician charges for annual physical exams, with one exception: In 2005 Medicare began covering a one-time "Welcome to Medicare" physical exam during the first six months after a person enrolls.

To obtain current information about Medicare coverage, check http://www.medicare.gov or call (800) MEDICARE. For more information about Medicare, see chapter 17, beginning on page 860.

Screening for Major Diseases

Cardiovascular screening (see pages 80–86). Blood pressure should be checked every time you see a doctor. If you have hypertension (elevated blood pressure) or other heart-related problems, your doctor will make specific recommendations as to how often it should be checked. A screening lipid profile, including total cholesterol, HDL, LDL, and triglycerides, should be carried out at least every five years. (If your blood pressure is abnormal or under treatment, your lipids will be checked more often.) Some experts do not recommend routine screening of adults older than age seventy-five, but this should be discussed with your doctor.

Fasting blood glucose (see page 81). This blood test is an essential screening test for type 2 diabetes. The American Diabetes Association recommends that glucose (blood sugar) be checked every three years if your blood glucose levels are in the normal range, but your doctor may request it more frequently if you are at risk for developing diabetes. Risk factors include (but are not limited to) having a parent or sibling with type 2 diabetes, excess weight, physical inactivity, and hypertension.

Thyroid screening (see page 117). A blood test for thyroid stimulating hormone (or TSH for short), a hormone secreted by the pituitary gland at the base of your brain, can signal the presence of too high or too low a level of thyroid hormone. (Physicians commonly measure thyroid hormone at the same time, and the two tests provide a useful snapshot of this important function.) The American Thyroid Association recommends that adults thirty-five and over have thyroid screening every five years unless they are already taking thyroid hormone, in which case it will be measured more often. Testing every five years is particularly important for postmenopausal women.

Mammography and breast exams (see pages 90–93). Seventy-five percent of breast cancers are diagnosed among women over the age of fifty, but more than 20 percent of women sixty-five and older have not had a mammogram in the past two years.[16] Women over forty should have a mammogram done every year, and Medicare covers this annual procedure for seniors who are enrolled. Breast self-examination (see page 91) should be performed monthly, and a clinical breast exam should be carried out by a health-care provider annually. (Medicare covers 80 percent of the physician charge for a clinical breast exam every twenty-four months.)

Cervical cancer screening (see pages 108–109). As we discussed in chapter 4, the familiar Pap smear is a simple and important routine test that can detect and intercept this cancer. If you're sixty-five or older, you may feel that you're ready to retire from regular Pap smears and pelvic exams. You're not alone: More than half of women in this age group have not had a Pap smear in the past three years. But you also need to know that nearly 25 percent of the more than ten thousand new cases of cervical cancer annually, and more than 40 percent of the deaths from this disease, occur in women sixty-five and older. Bottom line: Don't forgo this important screening test if you are still a candidate for it.

Generally speaking, unless your uterus has been completely removed, the Pap smear should be an annual event, with the following exceptions:

- If the newer, liquid-based tests are used, testing every other year may be considered.
- Women over thirty who have had three consecutive normal tests and are not at increased risk for cervical cancer may consider having a Pap smear every two or three years. However, less frequent testing should *not* be considered unless a woman has had no new sexual partners—and her partner has not had any new partners—since the last Pap smear.
- Another option for women over thirty is to be tested every three years with either the regular or liquid-based Pap test, along with a test for human papillomavirus DNA (which detects infection of the cervix with HPV strains that can cause cervical cancer).
- A woman over seventy who has had at least three consecutive normal Pap smears and no abnormal results over the previous ten years may elect to discontinue this test.

Women with certain risk factors, including diethylstilbestrol (DES) exposure before birth, HIV infection, or a weakened immune system due to organ transplant, chemotherapy, or chronic steroid use, should be tested annually.

Medicare covers a pelvic exam and Pap smear every twenty-four months—or every twelve months if you have had an abnormal smear within the past three years. (Medicare also covers annual Pap smears for women who are at increased risk for cervical or vaginal cancer—for example, if you have had a sexually transmitted infection, or if your mother took the hormone diethylstilbestrol [DES] during pregnancy.)

Prostate cancer screening (see pages 94–97). Of the more than 230,000 men diagnosed with prostate cancer each year, 70 percent are over age sixty-five. Because benefits have not been clearly shown to outweigh risks (including the consequences of false positive tests), there is not a clear consensus among experts and professional organizations regarding prostate cancer screening (specifically, whether a digital rectal exam or a blood test for prostate specific antigen [PSA]—or both—should be done). This is particularly problematic for elderly men, among whom prostate cancer is both common and frequently slow-growing and for whom the treatment may be much worse than the disease. (It is often said that men in their eighties and beyond are more likely to die with prostate cancer than because of it.) Nonetheless, men fifty and older should at least discuss the pros and cons of these tests with their doctor. Medicare provides coverage for both a screening digital rectal exam and PSA blood test every year for men over fifty who are enrolled, and more often if necessary for diagnostic purposes.

Diethylstilbestrol (DES) was used between 1940 and 1971 to prevent miscarriage and has been linked to unusual forms of vaginal and cervical cancers among women whose mothers took this medication.

Colon cancer screening (pages 100–104). Most colon cancers occur in men and women older than sixty-five, and risk factors include smoking, obesity, a diet high in animal fats, excessive alcohol consumption, physical inactivity, diabetes, inflammatory bowel disease, and a family history of colon cancer. To screen for colon cancer, the American Cancer Society recommends the following for men and women beginning at age fifty:

- fecal occult blood testing or fecal immunochemical test every year, *or*
- sigmoidoscopy every five years, *or*
- fecal occult blood testing or fecal immunochemical test every year *plus* sigmoidoscopy every five years, *or*
- double-contrast barium enema every five years, *or*
- colonoscopy every ten years.

As we explain in detail in chapter 4, there are pros and cons for each of these five approaches, but the colonoscopy is the gold standard. It is also the most expensive, but Medicare now pays for a screening colonoscopy once every ten years (though not within four years of a screening sigmoidoscopy). It also covers yearly fecal occult blood testing, as well as a screening sigmoidoscopy every four years. For those who can't or won't undergo a sigmoidoscopy or colonoscopy, Medicare will cover a screening barium enema every four years. For seniors at higher risk (for example, with a history of colon polyps or a parent or sibling with colon cancer), Medicare will cover a colonoscopy or barium enema every two years.

Ovarian cancer screening (page 106). In the United States, half of the new cases of ovarian cancer are diagnosed among women who are older than sixty-three. Risk factors include a family history of ovarian cancer, use of fertility drugs, early age of first menses, late onset of menopause, delayed pregnancy or having never been pregnant, long-term menopausal estrogen therapy, and breast cancer. While routine screening is not recommended for women at low risk, you should talk with your doctor about having a pelvic ultrasound or CA-125 performed if you are at high risk.

Skin cancer screening (starting on page 112). This is the most common type of cancer in the United States, with more than one million new cases every year, nearly as many as all other forms of cancer combined. Fortunately only a small percentage of these spread to other parts of the body, and less than one in one hundred cases lead to death. But seniors need to be aware that once they reach the age of sixty-five, they have a *40 to 50 percent chance* of developing one of the three main types of skin cancer (squamous cell carcinoma, basal cell carcinoma, or malignant melanoma). Older adults should regularly examine their skin and consult with a physician if they find anything unusual or are uncertain about the significance of a lump, bump, mole, or scaly area.

For more information about what to look for on the skin, see the sidebar "Inspecting the Skin" on page 113 in chapter 4.

Sun-exposed areas of the skin—especially the back of the hands and forearms, the top surfaces of the ears, the nose, forehead, and scalp (especially in men who are bald)—are most vulnerable. (These areas should be carefully protected with sunscreen.) One of the most common abnormalities in these regions is a mildly scaly patch, known as an **actinic keratosis**, that results from sun damage. One or more of these may appear in sun-exposed areas, and while often subtle in appearance, they have the potential to evolve into squamous cell carcinoma, one of the more aggressive types of skin cancers. Fortunately, actinic keratoses (that's the plural—often there are many of them) are treatable. If you notice any irregularity of the skin surface that persists over time, especially in one of these areas, have your physician or a dermatologist check it.

Eye Exams

Like slowing metabolism, some deterioration of vision is virtually inevitable as we grow older. There are a number of reasons why we may not be able to demonstrate our eagle eyes or read the fine print as the years pass, and many of these are related to normal changes in the aging eye, including:

- **Stiffer lenses (presbyopia).** This is the most common vision problem associated with aging, noted to some degree (with some chagrin) by nearly everyone as they pass through their forties or fifties. The lenses of the eyes are clear, flexible structures. Lenses focus light entering the eye on the retina, the membrane that lines the inner surface of the eye and detects light, sending electrical impulses to the brain, which then interprets them as images. Muscles attached to the lens can deform the lens slightly, allowing us to focus on objects nearer or farther away. As we grow older, the lenses lose some of their flexibility, affecting our ability to focus on objects closer than about two feet away. We begin to notice that we can't read the fine print or decipher a road map. We may compensate by holding objects at arm's length, but sooner or later we yield to this annoyance and buy a pair of reading glasses—or a half-dozen pairs to leave in strategic places around the house. Those who also need correction for distant vision will usually find bifocals or variable-focus lenses more convenient than switching from one pair of glasses to another.
- **Denser lenses.** With aging, the lenses become more dense, allowing less light to pass to the retina. This can be aggravated by the development of cataracts (see next page).
- **Less sensitive retinas.** With aging, the retina becomes less sensitive to light. Combine this with a denser lense, and you'll understand why you need more light in order to read as you get older.
- **Slower adjustment to changes in light.** A number of factors, including smaller and less reactive pupils, reduced speed of metabolism in the retina, and other retinal disease, conspire together to reduce our adaptation to changing light conditions. As we age, it becomes more difficult to see when we walk into a dark room or exit a building into the sunshine. This can be a momentary nuisance—or a

potential hazard if you trip over an object you can't see in a dark room or if you can't adjust to sudden changes in light while driving a car through a tunnel.

Unfortunately, there are a number of other eye problems that can rob us of our vision as the years pass. The most common of these are:

Cataracts

A **cataract** is a clouding of the eye's lens. Usually cataracts form very gradually or affect only a portion of the lens, so that vision does not seem impaired for months or even years. Over time, however, the clouding becomes more dense or widespread, resulting in blurred vision. Cataracts cause light coming into the lens to scatter, making bright light (such as oncoming headlights) seem glaring and uncomfortable. Colors often do not appear as sharp.

The word *cataract* comes from the Latin word for the grated gate in a castle wall that would be dropped suddenly to bar entrance to invaders. Cataracts usually don't appear suddenly, but they can certainly "bar the entrance" of the eye to incoming images.

Risk factors for cataracts include long-term sun exposure, smoking, diabetes, injury, heredity, and perhaps low vitamin C intake. Once a relentless thief of vision in the elderly, today cataracts are easily treated by surgically replacing the clouded lens with an artificial one.

Age-related macular degeneration (AMD)

Visual images sent from the eye to the brain originate from a thin but intricate layer of tissue at the back of the eyeball called the retina. Near the center of the retina is a small area known as the **macula** that is responsible for central vision—the part of your visual image that is straight ahead and critical for seeing fine detail, as when you read or drive. In **macular degeneration**, cells in the macula that generate visual signals become damaged, leading to distortion or loss of the image in the center of the field of vision.

AMD is often described as **wet** or **dry**. All cases of AMD begin as the the dry type, in which cells of the macula gradually break down, typically affecting both eyes and accounting for 90 percent of AMD cases. People with dry AMD become aware of gradual blurring and the need for more light to read. These changes may be less obvious if the problem develops only in one eye. Dry AMD often gradually progresses from an early to an intermediate or advanced stage—or at any of these stages it can suddenly turn to the wet form.

Wet AMD is the feared complication of dry AMD, in which a new blood vessel grows under the retina. This develops in only 10 percent of cases and typically affects only one eye at a time, but it is responsible for 90 percent of blindness caused by AMD. (A person who develops wet AMD in one eye is at significant risk of developing it in the other.) These new and abnormal blood vessels leak blood and other fluid that distort and quickly damage the normal retinal cells. One of the first symptoms can be a wavy appearance to lines that should appear straight. *A person who notices this should see an ophthalmologist as soon as possible for an evaluation.*

Age is the greatest risk factor for AMD; most cases occur in people over fifty (although it has been known to arise during the forties), and it is the leading cause of vision loss among those sixty and older. Heredity appears to play a role, and AMD is more common among Caucasians, women, and those with fair skin. Smoking is also a risk factor, while zinc and antioxidants in the diet may offer some protection. Some research suggests that frequent and prolonged exposure to ultraviolet light is also a contributing factor.

Sadly, vision loss caused by either form of AMD is permanent, and this disease is the leading cause of legal blindness in North America. However, the risk of progression of dry AMD with certain high-risk characteristics to the wet form is reduced by taking a specific high-dose combination of zinc and antioxidants known as the **AREDS formulation**. It is not yet known whether this supplement mixture is helpful for other stages of the disease, although those with AMD are often advised to take it since it appears to pose little, if any, risk.

The progress of wet AMD can be slowed with laser surgery or a treatment called photodynamic therapy, both of which destroy abnormal blood vessels. Neither treatment can restore vision loss, however, nor is either of these considered a cure.

WHAT IS THE AREDS FORMULATION?

AREDS stands for **Age-Related Eye Disease Study**, a research project conducted by the National Eye Institute (one of the National Institutes of Health) that demonstrated the potential benefits of the following formulation in dry AMD:

- Zinc—80 mg as zinc oxide
- Vitamin C—500 mg
- Vitamin E—400 international units
- Beta-carotene—15 mg (equivalent to 25,000 international units of vitamin A)
- Copper—2 mg, in a form called cupric oxide, to prevent a form of anemia caused by copper deficiency associated with high doses of zinc. The amount of zinc in the AREDS formulation is more than five times the amount found in the typical multivitamin—most contain 15 mg, or 100 percent of the daily value.

While it is possible to concoct the AREDS ingredients from individual supplements, the eye-care company Bausch & Lomb markets the exact formulation used in the study under the brand name Ocuvite PreserVision. This preparation can be purchased without a prescription, but it would be prudent to consult with an ophthalmologist as well as your primary-care physician before taking this or any similar high-dose antioxidant combination—*especially* if you are taking a number of medications or other supplements. ■

Glaucoma

Inside the front portion of the eye is a space called the **anterior chamber**, through which a clear fluid circulates at a constant pressure. Glaucoma develops when, for unknown reasons, the passages that allow fluid to drain from the chamber become clogged and pressure builds up within the eye. The increased pressure can damage the optic nerve, resulting in loss of vision. In the most common form of the disease, known as **open angle glaucoma**, pressure increases gradually, and changes in vision may not be noticed until the optic nerve has been significantly damaged. If allowed to progress, blindness can result. In the rarer form called **closed angle glaucoma**, pressure within the eye increases suddenly, causing severe pain in the eye, headache, blurred vision, halos around lights, and nausea and vomiting. This is a true emergency, and a person with these symptoms must be seen immediately by an ophthalmologist, both to preserve vision and relieve the symptoms.

Risk factors for glaucoma include a family history of the disease, diabetes, long-term corticosteroid use, prior injury to the eye, and a variety of structural abnormalities of the eye. African-Americans and Hispanics are also at an increased risk for glaucoma.

Vision lost to glaucoma cannot be restored, but if diagnosed early it can be controlled. Treatment usually involves daily, lifelong use of eye drops that reduce the pressure within the eye. Occasionally, oral medication may be prescribed as well. In addition, a variety of laser and surgical techniques are available to correct abnormalities within the eye that lead to increased pressure. People who have glaucoma must be sure to inform (or remind) their primary-care physician of the diagnosis whenever a new drug is prescribed, because certain medications aggravate this problem.

The good news is that many common eye problems can be corrected, or their progress slowed, *if caught early*. The American Academy of Ophthalmology recommends that adults over sixty-five have an eye exam every one to two years. People with a history of eye disease or diabetes should see an eye specialist more often.

Dental Exams

While dental health among older adults in the United States has improved substantially over the past half century, almost one in four Americans sixty-five and older does not have any of his or her natural teeth. Almost a third of older adults have untreated cavities, and about one-fourth have lost tooth-supporting structure in the gum and jaw because of advanced gum disease.[17]

Some older adults may consider poor oral health nothing more than a matter of inconvenience or discomfort, but it can represent a true health hazard. Seniors with painful dental problems or ill-fitting dentures are likely to eat less and thus are at greater risk for malnutrition. Ninety-five percent of oral cancers occur in people older than forty.[18] In addition, research suggests a link between poor oral health and an increased risk for coronary artery disease, although the exact reasons for this connection remain unclear.

Adults age sixty-five and older should get a routine dental exam every six months. Medicare does not pay for routine dental care, but even if you have to pay out of pocket, routine dental checkups are a worthwhile investment. If you cannot afford private dental care, consider other options. For example, many dentistry and dental hygiene schools offer low-cost examinations and cleanings. Neighborhood health clinics may also offer dental services. Your local Area Agency on Aging or your state dental association should be able to provide information about other resources in your community.

7. KEEP SAFE

We review safety and injury-avoidance strategies in chapter 11. There are, however, several safety concerns that are especially important for older adults. Because of decreased muscle and bone strength, as well as deterioration of eyesight and balance, everyday circumstances that would represent little or no threat to younger adults can pose special hazards to seniors. When cognitive decline enters the picture, the dangers become even greater.

Managing Medications in Older Adults

The average adult over age seventy-five has three chronic illnesses and uses five prescription medications along with two or more over-the-counter (OTC) preparations.[19] While these may play a vital role in relieving symptoms, preventing the progress of disease, and even prolonging life, they can also create trouble in a variety of ways:

- **Enhanced drug effects.** Because of age-related changes in metabolism, liver and kidney function, circulation, and a host of other functions, seniors may be more vulnerable to side effects than younger adults. For example, diphenhydramine (Benadryl and other brands), a common antihistamine also found in many "PM" products, can cause marked sedation in the elderly. It has also been found to inhibit or temporarily block the flow of urine in a man with an enlarged prostate.
- **Drug-drug interactions.** Most older adults see more than one doctor, and each may prescribe one or more medications. As the medication list lengthens, the possibility for unexpected consequences from drug inter-

actions rises dramatically. Indeed, the prescribing physician(s) may not be aware of all of the potential interactions, and the situation becomes even more perilous if one physician is not aware of what others are doing. Drugs can inhibit or enhance the metabolism of other drugs (thus increasing or nullifying each other's actions). Nonprescription drugs can interact with prescription medications as well. Furthermore, the side effects of one medication can amplify similar side effects of another. OTC nighttime sleep aids, for example, may intensify the effects of a sedating prescription drug—possibly to a dangerous degree—if both are taken during the same time frame.

- **Drug-food interactions.** Drug absorption can be altered dramatically by the presence of food in the digestive tract. Less commonly, some drugs may affect the absorption of nutrients in the intestines. In some cases, substances within specific foods alter drug metabolism. Grapefruit juice, for example, contains compounds that can interact with enzymes involved in the metabolism of certain drugs. As a consequence, concentrations of these drugs in the blood rise to unexpected and potentially unsafe levels. Drugs affected by grapefruit juice include the antidepressant sertraline (Zoloft), the sedative diazepam (Valium), certain cardiovascular drugs such as nifedipine (Procardia), and the cholesterol-lowering drugs simvastatin (Zocor), lovastatin (Mevacor), and atorvastatin (Lipitor). If you are a regular grapefruit-juice drinker and you are taking (or starting) one or more prescriptions, you should inform your doctor or pharmacist and discuss any possible interactions.
- **Drug-alcohol interactions.** Alcohol consumption can enhance the sedative effects of a number of common drugs in the family called benzodiazepines, which are used to relieve anxiety or induce sleep—such as alprazolam (Xanax), clonazepam (Klonopin), or diazepam (Valium). Dizziness, drowsiness, or even an increased risk of overdose may result from combining alcohol with these medications. Alcohol can also alter the metabolism or effects of other drugs.
- **Drug-supplement interactions.** They may be advertised as "all natural," but dietary supplements often have a variety of distinctive medical effects and can also interact with prescription drugs. For example, the herb Ginkgo biloba, promoted for improving cognitive function, contains substances that inhibit aggregation of platelets, the microscopic structures in the blood that initiate clotting. Episodes of spontaneous bleeding have been reported in people taking Ginkgo biloba along with aspirin or the anticoagulant drug warfarin (Coumadin). Similarly, the herb kava, used to relieve insomnia and anxiety, may significantly intensify the effects of sedating drugs (including alcohol).[20]

Remember that while dietary supplements are not regulated as drugs by the FDA, their potential effects and interactions should not be underestimated. It is very important that you *inform your physician(s) about any supplements and herbs you are taking,* especially when you are discussing prescriptions.

- **Dose and timing errors.** Aside from the dangers of multiple drugs interacting with one another or other substances, older adults also are at higher risk for taking medications in the wrong amounts, at the wrong time, too often, too infrequently, or not at all. The odds of one or more medication errors can be increased by poor eyesight, impaired coordination, memory lapses, or mental illness, not to mention the sheer number of medicines an elderly person may be taking.
- **Noncompliance.** As a person's medication list lengthens, the monthly price tag may become unmanageable. Seniors who have to choose between prescriptions and necessities (like food) may decide to cut pills in half, skip doses, or simply not fill one or more prescriptions, increasing their risk for other health problems.[21] Sometimes a news report, a random symptom, or a side effect will scare a person into stopping a medication—without informing his or her physician. If you feel that you can't or shouldn't take a prescription for *any* reason, review the problem with your physician first. Solutions may include medication changes, less expensive alternatives (including generics), simplified drug regimes, samples from the office, assistance programs offered by many drug companies for patients on a fixed income, one of the Medicare-approved drug discount cards, or public programs such as Medicaid for those who qualify. You may want to contact a Medicare representative or your local Area Agency on Aging (see page 687) for additional assistance. Information about Medicare-approved drug discount cards is available on the Internet at http://www.medicare.gov.

The symptoms that might occur as a result of drug interactions, side effects, or overdosing in older adults are, as you might imagine, extremely variable. But you should think about a problem with medications if you or your elderly loved one experiences any of the following, especially after starting a new drug:

- Dizziness
- Upset stomach
- Blurred vision
- Headache
- Sleep changes (e.g., difficulty falling or staying asleep, or excessive drowsiness during the day)
- Constipation
- Diarrhea
- Incontinence

- Mood changes
- Rash

If you experience any symptoms after embarking on a new prescription, supplement, or herbal remedy, you should review the situation with your doctor. Remember also that medication issues might have nothing to do with the new problem.

Safety and the Older Driver

To paraphrase Mr. Shakespeare, "To drive or not to drive—that is the extremely delicate but nonetheless important question," one that inevitably confronts older adults (and their families or caregivers) if they live long enough.

TIPS FOR SAFE USE OF MEDICATIONS

By following these simple tips, you can decrease the likelihood of experiencing problems with your prescription and nonprescription medications:

- To reduce the risk of an adverse (or disastrous) drug event, it is crucial that *every* doctor you see knows *all* of the prescription medicines you are taking, as well as any nonprescription drugs, vitamins, or herbal supplements you may be using. Don't forget eyedrops or medications you apply to your skin.
- Maintain a current list of all your medications and bring it to *every* doctor's visit—especially if something has been added by another physician since your last visit. If you can't keep a list, put all of your pill bottles in a plastic bag and take them with you to your next appointment.
- Work with your doctor to try to keep your medication list as short as possible.
- Ask your doctor to give you written instructions that you can read and understand, especially for new medications. It is also important to receive clear information about proper dosing *in writing* if the doctor gives you samples from the office.
- If you aren't sure why you're taking one or more medications, don't be shy about asking.
- Be sure to find out whether you are supposed to take a medication every day or whether it is to be taken as needed for a particular symptom.
- If you regularly (or even occasionally) eat grapefruit or drink grapefruit juice, or if you drink alcohol (even if it's only a little or just once in a while), be sure your doctor knows this.

The subject is fraught with emotion because driving represents much more than a way to get from point A to point B. For young and old alike, it embodies independence like few other privileges in life. Just as teenagers look forward to driving as a means of gaining a new measure of autonomy, many older adults see losing driving privileges as the death knell to their independence. Beyond this emotional response lie some very practical concerns that will arise as soon as the keys are turned in.

Operating a motor vehicle is serious business, one that can have a profound impact on the safety of older adults and the public at large. We should state up front, however, that no particular number of birthday candles automatically signals that driving must come to an end. In fact, older adults often get a bad rap when it comes to driving and are frequently and unfairly stereotyped as

- If you have any questions about the possibility of alcohol interacting with any drug you are currently taking—especially one that might be sedating—consult your doctor or pharmacist.
- Try to fill all of your prescriptions at one pharmacy. The pharmacist will be more likely to identify potential drug interactions, including some that your physician might not anticipate.
- Ask your pharmacist to use labels with large print.
- The information sheets that now come with most prescriptions can be informative, but often they list literally dozens of warnings, cautions, and potential side effects. If these raise concerns, be sure to ask your doctor or pharmacist to clarify which of these are common and which are less likely.
- Don't be a prescription collector. Each year it's a good idea to comb through your medicine cabinet and get rid of old or expired medications. These should *not* be flushed down the toilet or dumped in the trash, by the way. Contact your pharmacist, who can either take them back for proper disposal or advise you regarding where this can be done.
- If your medication regimen is so complex that it is difficult to remember what should be taken and when, buy a pill box with compartments for each day of the week. You may need a separate box for nighttime dosages.
- If you are caring for an aging loved one, you may need to assist him with some of these safety measures, respectfully making sure that he not only takes his medications but also that he takes them at the right dose and time. You may want to dispense a week's worth of medications into the correct compartments of a multiday pill box and provide a checklist for medications taken at various times of the day (e.g., breakfast, lunch, dinner, and bedtime). If your elder is mentally impaired, you or someone else should dispense the medications directly to him rather than risk a potentially serious accident. ■

unsafe drivers. Much of the negative image of older drivers is reinforced by news stories that sensationalize tragic accidents in which seniors are at fault. Obviously, some seniors should never get behind the wheel, but there are also many young and middle-aged drivers who ought to be riding the bus. Age alone does not determine whether or not a person is a safe driver.

As a group, older drivers actually display several traits that contribute to safe and responsible driving. Seniors wear seat belts more often than any other age group except for infants and preschoolers. They are much less likely to drive under the influence of alcohol than younger adults. Seniors are more likely to restrict their driving to the safest road conditions. They tend to avoid nighttime driving and stay off the roads when the weather is bad. They also drive fewer miles than younger drivers.[22] The net result is that drivers ages seventy and older, who represented 10 percent of the driving-age population in 2003, were involved in only 10 percent of fatal accidents that year.[23]

That's the good news. The bad news is that, on a per-mile-driven basis, older adults have a greater chance of dying in a crash than all other groups except teenage drivers. There are several reasons for this. As they age, most adults experience a decline in central or peripheral vision, loss of hearing, as well as a slowing of their reflexes. Impairments in cognitive function can also affect judgment or reaction time. Increased frailty makes older adults more vulnerable to injuries—especially involving the chest—in an accident, or from complications in its aftermath.[24]

Because people age differently, the assessment of someone's fitness to drive must be made on an individual basis, and it should not be based solely on age. If you are concerned about the impact of your age on your driving skills (or if you're wondering whether an aging loved one is becoming a potential threat to self or others when behind the wheel), the following questions are worth considering:

How's my vision? Is it difficult to read street signs? Can I clearly see pedestrians, other cars, or obstacles in the road? Can I see these people and objects only during the daytime, or can I see them clearly at dusk, dawn, on overcast days, and at nighttime as well? Am I bothered by the glare of oncoming headlights?

Am I up to the physical demands of driving? Do I have trouble turning my head to look over my shoulder before changing lanes or turning my head to look for oncoming cars before making a turn? Do I have difficulty moving my foot rapidly from the gas pedal to the brake? Can I turn the steering wheel quickly to avoid an accident? Can I hear the siren of an oncoming emergency vehicle in time to pull over and get out of the way?

Do I have the cognitive skills to drive safely? Do I get confused or anxious in heavy traffic or when merging onto busy roadways? Do I have difficulty judging when it is safe to make turns or merge into traffic? Is it difficult for me to pay attention to several things at once (such as pedestrians, street signs, stoplights, and other vehicles), as a driver must do at times? Do any of the medications I take make me drowsy or reduce my alertness? Do I often get lost? Do I slow down or even stop at intersections when the light is green or accidentally roll through red lights?

What are other people or circumstances telling me? Do other drivers frequently honk at me? Have I had any moving violations, near misses, or accidents in recent years? Have I been pulled over by a police officer because of erratic driving, even though I might not have received a ticket? Have friends or relatives expressed concern about the safety of my driving? Has my doctor suggested I stop driving or restrict my driving?

Maintaining automotive safety and independence

Fortunately, answering yes to one or more of these questions does not mean that you need to turn in your driver's license and hand over the keys, but it does mean you should consider taking measures to help you maintain safe driving skills. If your vision has been declining in recent years, by all means visit an eye-care professional to identify the problem. If you need corrective lenses, make sure that your glasses have the right prescription—and that you wear them. Keep your windows, headlights, and glasses clean. If glare from oncoming headlights is uncomfortable, do not try to compensate by wearing sunglasses at night. It is better to avoid driving at night or at other times (such as sunrise or sunset) when glare might be a problem.

If the physical aspects of driving are too demanding, pinpoint specific problems and talk with your doctor about them. He may recommend stretching and exercise programs to increase your mobility and ability to react quickly. An occupational therapist may be able to suggest vehicle modifications that can make it easier to steer or use the brake or gas pedals.

When the mental tasks of driving are a concern, ask your physician or pharmacist whether any medications (or combination of medications) you take might be having detrimental side effects. Try to avoid heavy traffic and consider taking routes to your destination that might be less congested. Give yourself more time to react to potential hazards by keeping a greater distance between your car and the one in front of you. Consider limiting your driving to short distances for essential errands—to and from the grocery store, the bank, the doctor's office, and your church, for example. For a trip across town, see if you can arrange for a friend or relative to take you (offer to buy lunch!), or see if public transportation is available and accessible for your destination.

Sometimes it is difficult for even the most objective person to make an accurate judgment about the safety of his or her own driving habits. In such cases, it can be helpful to consult with an occupational therapist who is specially trained to perform a driving evaluation. This evaluation assesses an individual's visual, physical, and cognitive skills in areas that affect driving safety, including visual acuity, reaction time, and decision making. The evaluation includes tests administered in an office setting, as well as a behind-the-wheel driving test.

Based on the results, the occupational therapist can recommend actions (such as restricting driving to daylight hours) or may suggest training that can help a person maintain his or her driving skills. To find an occupational therapist trained in driving evaluation, look in the yellow pages under occupational therapists or rehabilitation centers. You can find more information on the Internet at http://www.aota.org/olderdriver/driving-evals.html, a Web site of the American Occupational Therapy Association.

Another option for those who wish to maintain safe driving skills is a refresher driving course designed specifically for older adults. These are offered by the AARP, some affiliates of the AAA, and some chapters of the National Safety Council. Not only will these courses help you keep your safety skills up to date, but they can sometimes even help you get a lower rate on your auto insurance.

When it's time to quit . . .

Many older adults are able to drive safely throughout their entire life. Others, however, eventually begin to pose a risk to themselves and others whenever they back out of the driveway. If you suspect—or if others are telling you—that your presence on the road is creating a safety risk, you need to make an honest assessment of your driving abilities. If you have taken remedial steps to improve your driving safety—such as restricting your driving to daytime hours, taking a refresher driving course, or seeking the help of an occupational therapist—and this has not resolved the concerns, you owe it to yourself and others to perform a brave and unselfish act: turning in your keys.

Relinquishing the right to drive is a difficult choice for practical as well as emotional reasons. Without a car, it is more difficult to go shopping, run errands, go to medical appointments, attend church, and visit family and friends. While these are all compelling reasons to keep driving, you need to ask yourself if any of them are worth risking your (or another person's) life. The answer, of course, is a resounding no.

Talking to your loved one

Confronting an older friend or family member who is demonstrating unsafe behaviors on the road is extremely difficult. It can be traumatic to the adult who has been self-reliant for years to be faced with the prospect of losing or having restrictions placed on her automotive independence. If you are convinced that your loved one's driving represents a danger, you need to broach the subject candidly but respectfully. While expressing your concern for her well-being, you should be very specific about the driving problems you have noticed. If she denies the problem—which, in fact, is very likely—you may need to ask a physician, pastor, family member, or trusted friend to speak with her. You should be aware that if a doctor has concerns about a patient's driving safety, he or she may be obligated to notify the Department of Motor Vehicles (DMV), which will then evaluate the situation. (In extreme circumstances, a physician may intervene by sending a report to state authorities specifically recommending that a driver not be allowed to drive for medical reasons.) Indeed, one way to force the issue is to ask your aging family member or friend to be retested for driving skills by the DMV, which then shifts the responsibility for the decision to a more objective party.

Exploring transportation alternatives

Going without a car can create inconvenience and hardship, but there are alternatives available. Walking, carpooling with friends and family, and using public transportation, taxicabs, and shuttle buses or vans are all options. Many local senior centers, churches, and agencies on aging offer special bus services. Contact a representative from your local agency on aging to find out what services are available in your area.

Preventing Falls

About one in five emergency department visits involving accidental injuries is the result of a fall, the leading cause of unintentional injury among people sixty-five and over in the United States.[25] While not exclusive to any particular age group, falls are all too common—and too often devastating—among aging adults. One in three adults aged sixty-five and over suffers at least one fall each year. More than 1.8 million seniors are treated each year in emergency rooms, and 421,000 require hospitalization because of falls. Not surprisingly, the likelihood of a long-term complication resulting from a fall is greater in this age group. A person seventy-five or older who suffers a fall has a four- to fivefold greater risk of needing placement in a long-term nursing facility for at least a year.[26]

Fractures from falls are a leading cause of disability among older adults. While bones of the hands, arms, and legs can all break during a fall, perhaps the most ominous location for a fracture is the hip. Only about a third of hip-fracture victims regain the level of independence they enjoyed before their fracture, and *an astounding 24 percent of hip-fracture victims age fifty and older die within a year following their injury.*[27] Hip fractures, as well as other breaks in older adults, are often intimately linked to osteoporosis.

Here are some suggestions for helping older adults avoid or prevent falls:

- **Start exercising.** Diminished lower-body strength and poor balance and physical coordination contribute to many falls. Exercise can help increase strength and promote improved coordination.
- **Stand carefully.** When rising from a sitting position, be sure that you are fully balanced before you start moving. If you feel light-headed, pause before you walk.
- **Make your home safe.** Check your stairs and other places where you walk, removing obstacles (such as shoes or electrical cords that

might trip you, especially in the dark. Remove throw rugs or secure them firmly to the floor. Avoid floor finishes that are slippery, and wipe up wet spots. Install bars next to the toilet or in the shower to give you greater stability. Install brighter lighting in your home if needed, and install night-lights in bathrooms and hallways.

- **Talk with your doctor about medications.** Some medications or combinations of medications can make you drowsy, affect your balance, or cause you to feel light-headed momentarily when you stand up. Let your doctor know if you experience any of these problems.
- **Check your vision.** Many household tumbles result from obstacles that are difficult to see because of impaired vision.
- **Consider an emergency-response device.** A nightmare scenario for an older adult living alone is falling, sustaining a major injury (such as a hip fracture), and then lying helplessly on the floor for hours—or days—because the phone is out of reach. While it won't prevent a fall, an emergency-response device worn around the wrist or neck may save untold pain, or even a life, by enabling a person to call for help after an accident in the home.[28]

OSTEOPOROSIS IN MEN

Osteoporosis is commonly regarded as a disease of older women, and indeed it affects fewer older men than women, in part because of the protective effects of testosterone and the tendency of men to arrive at adulthood with stronger, thicker bones. Nevertheless, 2 million men in the United States have osteoporosis, and another 12 million are at risk for it.

The major risk factors for osteoporosis in men, aside from age, include long-term use of steroid medications, smoking, excessive alcohol consumption, low calcium intake, physical inactivity, and low levels of testosterone. A family history of osteoporosis may also put some men at risk.

As in women, osteoporosis in men can be slowed or prevented by quitting smoking, cutting out excess alcohol consumption, and receiving adequate daily amounts of calcium and vitamin D. Physical activity, especially weight-bearing exercise, helps prevent this disease. If you already have osteoporosis, your doctor may advise against high-impact exercise.

The drugs alendronate (Fosamax) and risedronate (Actonel) have been approved for use in men with steroid-induced osteoporosis. A doctor may also prescribe supplementary testosterone for men who have both osteoporosis and low levels of the hormone. However, because testosterone stimulates the prostate gland, physicians typically monitor PSA on a regular basis when prescribing this hormone as a supplement. ■

Immunizations: Not Just for Kids

Most immunizations are given during the first few years of life, but a few must be repeated later in adulthood, perhaps many times.

Tetanus is caused by a type of bacteria that can be introduced to the body through contaminated wounds. A toxin produced by the bacteria causes painful muscle spasms and can be fatal. Because these spasms and contractions are particularly severe in the neck and jaw, you may remember warnings about how "lockjaw" might result from stepping on a rusty nail. Immunity to the tetanus toxin does not last for life, and thus most authorities recommend that adults (including seniors) receive a booster shot for tetanus every ten years. This is usually combined with the vaccine for diphtheria in a form called adult Td. (Diphtheria can cause severe sore throat, heart problems, and sometimes death.)

An adult who has *never* been immunized against tetanus should receive three doses of tetanus/diphtheria vaccine—the first two at least four weeks apart, and the third dose six to twelve months after the second. If an adult sustains a contaminated wound and the last update was more than five years ago, he may be advised to receive another update. If an adult has a contaminated wound and has never been immunized against tetanus, he should receive tetanus antibody (immunoglobulin) as soon as possible, along with an initial dose of the tetanus/diphtheria vaccine, followed at least four weeks later by a second dose of the vaccine, and a third dose six to twelve months after the second.

The **influenza** vaccine must be given on an annual basis because of the influenza virus's exceptional ability to mutate, or alter itself, just enough to escape recognition by the immune system. Since the immune system may not identify the mutated form of the virus as a familiar foe, by the time the body's defenses are rallied, the new strain will have already provoked an unpleasant or even dangerous illness. In an effort to reduce the number of cases of influenza, every year health officials try to predict which strains are most likely to make the rounds during the upcoming flu season and then create a specific formulation that can be produced for widespread distribution.

The Centers for Disease Control and Prevention occasionally alters its age guidelines for the influenza vaccine, depending on the availability of vaccine supplies. Anticipating a shortage in the 2004–2005 flu season, for instance, the CDC recommended that those sixty-five and older, along with other especially high-risk groups, receive the vaccine. Later in the flu season, the CDC expanded the guidelines to include all adults fifty and over in those regions with an adequate vaccine supply.

Influenza can be dangerous for older adults, especially for those with chronic respiratory or cardiovascular illnesses, and thus routine annual vaccination is recommended for everyone fifty and over. (Exceptions are those who are severely allergic to eggs and egg products or who have had a significant adverse reaction to the vaccine in the past.) Seniors living in long-term care facilities are also at risk and should be routinely immunized. Influenza can be particularly hazardous for men and women eighty-five and older, as people in this age group are sixteen times more likely to die from influenza-related complications than individuals sixty-five to sixty-nine years old.[29]

Flu season usually runs from December through March, and flu shots typically become available in October or November in a variety of venues, including private medical offices, local or county health departments, senior centers, pharmacies, and even supermarkets. Medicare normally covers the cost of yearly influenza vaccination.

Pneumococcal pneumonia is not only the most common form of bacterial pneumonia, but it is also frequently associated with more severe illness. It is responsible for the deaths of thousands of older adults each year. The pneumococcal pneumonia vaccine prevents or reduces the severity of this infection, as well as other types of infections (such as **septicemia**, in which bacteria enter the bloodstream) caused by strains of bacteria known as pneumococci. This vaccination is recommended for all adults ages sixty-five and older, yet only 56 percent of older adults have ever received it.[30] Individuals who have had the vaccine at an earlier age are advised to get a one-time booster at age sixty-five if their initial immunization was more than five years before.

8. KEEP CLEAR OF BAD HABITS

The problems associated with tobacco use, as well as alcohol and drug abuse, have been presented in detail in chapter 10, but it is worth revisiting a few points (and making a few fresh ones) with regard to aging.

Tobacco. Smoking makes a major contribution to the most common causes of death among older adults: heart disease, stroke, cancer, and chronic respiratory diseases. It also plays a role in important age-related problems such as Alzheimer's disease, vascular dementia, osteoporosis, eye diseases, and oral-health problems. The combination of smoking and diabetes—especially type 2 (adult-onset) diabetes, which usually emerges during the fifties and later—is a time bomb. Indeed, there is hardly a health problem faced by seniors (including accidental fires) that *isn't* aggravated by tobacco use.

In 1965, approximately 29 percent of men age sixty-five and older and 10 percent of older women smoked. Today, 10 percent of older men and 9 percent of older women smoke.[31] That's a significant positive trend (at least for men), but still far more people are smoking than should be. Seniors who have been long-term smokers or tobacco chewers may believe that quitting won't make any difference at their age, but that is absolutely not true. It is never too late to benefit from reducing or abandoning the use of tobacco products.

Alcohol. Roughly half of older adults in the United States drink alcohol, and as many as 15 percent of seniors are at risk for health problems directly related to the amount of alcohol they consume, or from the interaction of alcohol and medications or ongoing medical conditions. Approximately 2 to 4 percent of older adults abuse or are addicted to alcohol.[32]

Alcohol's intoxicating effects are more profound among seniors than in younger drinkers because older adults generally have a lower concentration of the enzyme that metabolizes alcohol so that it can be cleared from the body. Furthermore, the aging brain may be more sensitive to alcohol's effects. Needless to say, the impact of alcohol on driving skills is a serious concern at any age, but it is likely to be more profound for seniors than for younger people.

Alcohol also interacts with a number of medications commonly taken by older adults. Additionally, excess alcohol consumption is a risk factor for several disorders common to seniors, including osteoporosis and diabetes. Many alcohol abusers and addicts are late-onset drinkers. They may not have had an alcohol problem earlier in life but started drinking later, often during crises or difficult transitions such as the death of a spouse, a health problem, or retirement.

Drug abuse. Illegal drug use is far less common among seniors than the abuse of tobacco or alcohol. Government research indicates that less than one half of one percent of adults sixty-five or older use illicit drugs. This figure may rise, however, as more baby boomers—whose attitudes about taking drugs have been notably more relaxed than those of prior generations—reach seniority: In the year 2000, more than 2 percent of adults aged fifty-five to fifty-nine reported using illicit drugs in the past month.[33]

Seniors are more likely to get into trouble with prescription painkillers and sedatives. These are usually prescribed in good faith—often by more than one physician—to relieve pain, anxiety, or insomnia. Usually older adults are not involved in overt drug-seeking behavior (for example, deliberately exaggerating pain symptoms for the specific purpose of obtaining narcotics). But sometimes physicians, faced with a variety of discomforts, difficult diagnoses, short appointments, and a desire to bring about relief as quickly as possible, prescribe a number of habituating drugs that cannot be discontinued without an uncomfortable withdrawal. It should be noted, however, that older and younger adults alike may develop chronic problems (especially pain) that, after careful evaluation, cannot be adequately managed without long-term use of medications that are potentially habit-forming. When this occurs, it is critical that *every* physician involved in the person's care know *all* of the medications being taken. Also, multiple doctors should not prescribe the same drug (unless they are part of the same practice and use the same medical record).

Breaking the Addiction (or Better Yet, Not Starting One)

If tobacco use or unsafe alcohol consumption—which current medical wisdom places at more than two drinks per day for men, and more than one per day for women—are established habits in your life and you're having trouble stopping, *get help*. If you're not interested in stopping, you should get an honest opinion from your physician, or at least read chapter 10 in this book. We've all heard anecdotes about someone's distant aunt or uncle who smoked two packs a day, drank copious quantities of alcohol for decades, and died at ninety-five while skydiving. But here's the truth: People like that (and there are a *very* small number of them) are definitely exceptions to the rule. What is much more common among those who chronically indulge in tobacco, alcohol, or illicit drug use is a turbulent entry into older adulthood with an abundance of habit-related health problems—assuming that they actually make it to their senior years. If you've arrived at sixty-five or beyond and find yourself caught up in substance addictions, you can still improve and extend your life by breaking these habits. You may have tried a thousand times already, but the fact remains that you *can* quit—though you'll find the task much more manageable once you acknowledge that you don't have to do it on your own. Take a close look at chapter 10, especially the segments dealing with breaking free of these habits.

9. KEEP YOUR "SUNNY SIDE UP"

We discussed the importance of mental and emotional health, as well as their effects on the entire body, in chapter 8. For older adults, the interconnection and interaction between mind and body are often even more apparent. Disturbances in mental, emotional, and social well-being can have a profound effect on the overall health of seniors, in part because their tools for coping with loss and change may be more limited. Furthermore, chronic conditions that become more prevalent as we age, including the fallout from heart disease, stroke, and cancer, may cause biochemical changes in the brain that bring on depression (even in someone who has not had emotional problems in the past), provoking a downward spiral in overall health.

When It's More Than Just the Blues

Anxiety and depression are serious health hazards for seniors. Seniors with depression and anxiety may experience diminished functional capacity, reduced appetite and energy, unexplained aches and pains, and memory loss. Clinical depression affects 15 to 20 percent of adults sixty-five and older, and it is more common among adults who are socially isolated, housebound, functionally impaired, or chronically ill.[34] Depression has been found to be a major risk factor for death in older patients who have experienced a heart attack, and not surprisingly, older adults in nursing homes are at a higher risk for mortality if they suffer from major depression.[35] It should come as no surprise that depression is also a risk factor for suicide among the elderly. Sadly, the number of suicide deaths among older adults is disproportionately large compared to the number of seniors in the population.[36] Anxiety disorders appear to be as common in older people as in young people and at least as debilitating, if not more so. Anxiety and depression frequently appear together in older people; a fourth of seniors diagnosed with anxiety show signs of major depression, and almost half of adults with major depression exhibit the criteria for anxiety.[37]

As we explained in chapter 8, depression and anxiety are not defined as simply the lack of a pleasant outlook or sunny disposition, nor are they, contrary to popular opinion, a normal part of aging. As with younger people, these disorders are frequently caused by chemical imbalances in the brain. Dementias and cognitive decline are often accompanied by depression and anxiety. Mood shifts or other signs of depression may also be caused by a specific illness, the side effects of one or more medications, or by drug interactions. Needless to say, if you are experiencing symptoms of depression, you should be evaluated by your physician, who should (among other things) review the medications or supplements you are taking. In many cases, depression and anxiety are triggered by stresses common to old age, and especially by the *losses:* loss of loved ones, loss of health, loss of financial status and security, loss of home and possessions, loss of independence. In depression and anxiety brought on by accumulated stress, the critical factor is not just the stressors themselves, but also the capacity—or lack thereof—to cope with them effectively.

As in younger adults, depression and anxiety in the elderly can often be successfully treated using one or more approaches, including psychotherapy, antidepressant medications, and, in more severe cases that do not respond to other treatments, electroconvulsive therapy. Note that in some older seniors, antidepressants can have side effects that are more dangerous than those seen in younger people, including increased risk of falls.[38] It is worth noting that there are psychiatrists who specialize in the care of emotional and behavioral problems of seniors. They are known as **geropsychiatrists**, and their input may be extremely valuable, especially when an elderly person is manifesting more severe and disruptive agitation, disorientation, or depression.

Unfortunately, one other important factor that can profoundly affect the mood of seniors is not always treatable. Some adults enter their seventies, eighties, and beyond with long-entrenched negativity, pessimism, and bitterness. As general health and cognitive abilities deteriorate, so does the capacity to contain these attitudes and maintain basic civility. The end result—nonstop complaining, insults, even physical assaults—can be harrowing for family members and friends alike, often alienating all but the most gracious, patient, and thick-skinned caregivers. Sadly, these deep-seated attitudes are often extremely resistant to treatment by talk, medication, or even loving care. They represent a cautionary tale, illustrating the practical importance of an admonition from the New Testament: "Get rid of all bitterness, rage and anger, brawling and slander, along with every form of malice. Be kind and compassionate to one another, forgiving each other, just as in Christ God forgave you" (Ephesians 4:31-32).

Staying Positive in Older Adulthood

At the beginning of this chapter, we emphasized that the way you treat your body, mind, and spirit as a young adult will have a profound effect on your life as an older adult. We looked at several ways to protect and promote your emotional and spiritual health in chapters 8 and 9, and we will not repeat them all here. But it's worth noting once again that changes—including many that are unplanned and unwelcome—are inevitable as you take the final laps of your life. Do you cope with change graciously or grudgingly? Do you accentuate the positive or obsess over the negative? Do you light candles or curse the darkness? Even if you haven't been proactive about grooming your attitude over the years, it's never too late to take stock of your emotional weather and start making changes. But no one can do it for you.

Here are a few practices and habits that can help you remain positive, even if it's late in your life. You will note that the first six suggestions may sound familiar, but they are worth repeating.

- **Stay physically active.** Regular exercise has been strongly correlated with positive emotions and a reduced risk for depression. Keep moving!
- **Get involved.** Engaging in meaningful, helpful activities will engender a sense of purpose and reduce listlessness. If you are retired, volunteering in your church and community is a great way to start.
- **Nurture relationships and recruit social support.** Social isolation is a major contributor to depression and emotional difficulties. By cultivating new friendships and nurturing old ones, you can build a network of support that can help you through hard times.
- **Keep mentally active.** Read any good books lately? Have you learned anything new? engaged in any lively conversations? listened to some stimulating audio recordings? Learning, reading, and discussion not only keep a person mentally active but emotionally fit as well.
- **Eat right.** Proper nutrition is as essential for mental and emotional well-being as for physical health. Even if you have moved into a facility or a relative's home where the menu isn't what you're used to, you can still make healthy choices from the food that is provided or supplement your diet with nutritious snacks.
- **Clear out bad habits.** Tobacco use and alcohol and drug abuse can be as detrimental to emotional health as to physical health. Remember that tobacco use is a risk factor for developing Alzheimer's disease, which is often accompanied by depression and anxiety. Alcohol intoxication and illicit drug use may seem to provide a temporary escape from life's challenges, but repercussions, both physical and emotional, are inevitable in their wake.
- **Re-create through recreation.** Listening to music, gardening, fish-

ing, and enjoying a stroll in the park or along a beach are some of the inexpensive pleasures of life that can refresh the body and the mind. When enjoyed with friends and family, these activities can also build and bond relationships. You may have more time to enjoy these simple pastimes with grandchildren than their parents can afford, and the memories you create for them (and you) will be priceless.

- **Get the focus off yourself and onto others.** Instead of waiting or demanding to be served, consider ways you can become a servant, especially to someone who is more disadvantaged than you. Helping to ease someone else's discomfort is a reliable way to lift your spirits and provide perspective on your own circumstances.
- **Attend to your spiritual life.** We will talk more about the overall importance of this in the next section, but it is worth stating here that a healthy relationship with God and daily study of His Word are perhaps the most important ingredients in maintaining a positive outlook. By growing closer to Him, we can come to more fully realize that the problems we face in this world are but "light and momentary troubles" (2 Corinthians 4:17) that will quickly be eclipsed by the joy we will experience when we are reunited with our loved ones in His presence.

10. KEEP THE FAITH

For those who have had the benefit of a vibrant spiritual life spanning many decades, older adulthood offers a time of reflection and refocusing on what is truly important from an eternal perspective. For those who have become acquainted with Christ only recently, the senior years can be a time of spiritual discovery and a chance to make positive changes. For those who have yet to begin a walk of faith, the golden years can truly be golden, a time of rebirth and a season of renewal even as this earthly life draws to its conclusion. No matter which group you may be in, the comforting truth is that the limitations that age places on the physical body do not hamper the spirit.

On the other hand, many seniors whose faith has been strong for decades are now bewildered by feelings of barrenness in their relationship with God. The losses have piled up, and instead of sensing His close comfort, older people may feel distant from or even abandoned by the God they have loved and served for so long. Confusion and bitterness can eclipse clarity and contentment. Such people may even question whether their faith ever was genuine, because it doesn't seem to be bearing fruit at this point in life.

There is no greater test of one's faith than loss. Your faith is tested when you feel overwhelmed by all you have had to surrender—not merely possessions, but health, independence, even loved ones. Rather than feeling shame and guilt for not pulling through these tough transitions with utter tranquillity and joy, this is the time to remember God's compassion for the brokenhearted. The first words of Jesus' Sermon on the Mount address this: "Blessed are the poor in spirit, for theirs is the kingdom of heaven" (Matthew 5:3). Like no other time in your long life, this is when head knowledge must become heart knowledge. The very definition of faith is believing that God is still in charge of your life and has not withdrawn from it, even when current events don't make sense. This is not the time for *you* to withdraw from others but rather it's the time to draw strength from fellow believers in your family and church (or better yet, in a small group) with whom you can share these burdens.

God indeed loves you so much that He made arrangements (at an extremely costly price) for you to survive physical death and to join Him in a setting where faith will never again be tested—or needed. You will soon be unshackled from the limitations of an aging body in a broken world, and He will never leave you as you approach that inescapable transition.

Spiritual health, as discussed in chapter 9, is a vital topic. Indeed, from an eternal viewpoint it is the most important subject in this book, and it pertains to each and every person, regardless of age. How one stands with God is a concern that everyone must consider eventually, but for our discussion of aging we need to look now at a few aspects of faith and spiritual health that are especially relevant to older adults. These include thoughts on our own mortality and questions of how we plan to make the best use of our time in service to God.

Are You Ready to Meet Your Maker?

If you're not sure of the answer to that question, there is no better time than the present to get some certainty. Perhaps religion is something you have always thought would best be attended to later . . . perhaps *much* later. You might even be planning to hold out for a deathbed conversion, a last-minute settling of accounts with God before you actually meet Him. Here is some sound advice: Few people have the luxury of knowing the time and place at which they will make that final passage.

One of the great advantages of living many decades is that a person can reach a point where the illusion of life's permanence, which colors the judgments of most younger people, no longer has as strong a hold. And yet, even when staring their own mortality in the face, many continue to look the other way and imagine that spiritual issues can be addressed another day.

Sometimes the first steps in beginning a spiritual life are the hardest for older adults. For those who have ignored God for years, rebelled against religious teachings, or flatly denied His existence, it may be difficult to believe that

God could be interested in starting a conversation, let alone a loving relationship. Older people may assume that they are beyond God's reach and redemption because of past (or present) sins or that they are too entrenched in their habits to make any meaningful change. But Jesus' story of the Prodigal Son speaks volumes to this situation. In this story—which can be found in Luke 15:11-32—a young man squanders his inheritance but eventually comes to his senses and returns home, where he is embraced by his father even before repenting of his misdeeds. No matter when or under what conditions a person comes to his senses and turns toward his eternal home, God is waiting with open arms to welcome and celebrate that the dead is alive again, and the lost is found (see Luke 15:32). If you are sure of nothing else, you can be sure of one thing: God knows everything about you, and yet He has been pursuing you all your life. Don't let your final years slip away without responding to Him.

How do you take that first, all-important step? If you're not sure, go back to page 399 in chapter 9.

Finishing Strong

Perhaps the best thing about older adulthood is that it offers a chance to "major in the majors," to concentrate on the things that are most important: faith and service to God and others. Unlike the vocational world, where a final departure from the office or workplace is customary (or mandated) at a certain age, there is no retirement from ministry. God never intended for His people to settle permanently into an easy chair after a long life and say, "Well, I guess it's time to let someone else pick up the slack." There is no point at which we should assume that God can't use us or declines our service. Indeed, older adults can make some unique contributions to His Kingdom by virtue of their age and experience. Older adulthood provides a multitude of opportunities for ministry. Even if you have no formal training or you think you are inadequate for the task, God can and will use you. Consider the following arenas where you might become involved:

- **Missions.** Many seniors can help expand God's Kingdom and demonstrate His love by serving on short-term mission projects lasting from a few days to several months. Missionaries and national workers often need the help of people with experience and skill in a number of fields, from construction to computers, from accounting to health care. Whatever you did to earn a paycheck for decades—and what may not have seemed particularly inspiring at the time—might make a world (and an eternity) of difference serving God and people in a distant country. Indeed, in this setting you may find your work far more enjoyable, energizing, and fulfilling than it ever was during your nine-to-five years. Information about short-term missions options can be obtained through your denomination or local church.

- **Sharing your faith.** Many older people want to share their faith with others but feel ill equipped to do so. Perhaps you have never learned how to explain clearly and genuinely to others how they can enter into a relationship with God.

  If you would like to gain greater confidence in expressing your faith publicly, find out if your church offers an evangelism training program. You may want to read books such as *Evangelism Explosion* by D. James Kennedy or *Going Public with Your Faith* by William Carr Peel and Walt Larimore. The Web site http://www.evangelism.com, sponsored by Campus Crusade for Christ, can also provide encouragement and practical help with the important assignment of sharing the Good News about Jesus Christ with those who have not yet heard or embraced it.
- **Encouragement.** No one is beyond the need for encouragement, but too often we forget that even the most competent, capable, and independent individuals need to be affirmed. During years filled with career and commitments, we may feel too pushed to spare any time expressing our appreciation for what others have done in our life. After retirement, we have more opportunities to do so.

  Purchase a journal and begin filling its pages with all the things, people, and events for which you have felt grateful during your life. From those entries, start sending out written communications. A thoughtful letter, card, or e-mail could have a major impact on a family member, friend, pastor, or even a public figure who has made a difference in your life.
- **Prayer.** It is always a great encouragement to find out that someone is praying for us—especially when we know that this person's prayer is more than a cheerful "thinking of you" spiritual greeting card. We describe in chapter 9 a number of purposes and benefits of prayer, but one worth repeating is the fact that God responds to our conversations with Him, as the Bible teaches clearly and repeatedly. When God's people spend time in thoughtful intercession and prayer, good things indeed happen, though not always in ways we anticipate. Prayer is an especially powerful, though often unseen, ministry.

  If disabilities limit your participation in more physically demanding forms of ministry, seek God's guidance and ask if prayer might be your special area of service. Whether first thing in the morning, when you lie down at night, or any time in between, think about every member of your extended family and pray for them individually, remembering to thank God for what He has already accomplished in their life. If you are able to let others know that you are praying for them, this can be a profound source of encouragement to them.

- **Service.** God equips so many people in so many ways that you can always do something to help someone else, whatever your gifts or abilities. If you're handy around the house or garage, you can put your abilities to work for others who are in financial straits or other difficult situations by changing the oil in their car, doing small household repairs, or using your carpentry skills. Cooking, house-cleaning, or taking other older adults to medical appointments or church are other practical ways of serving others and sharing Christ's love. You can multiply your efforts by starting a ministry in your local church to recruit help for those in need.
- **Teaching and mentoring.** Your knowledge and experience are valuable. Consider passing them on by teaching and mentoring others. Don't fall into the trap of feeling that you must reach spiritual perfection before you are qualified to teach. The process of preparation and sharing actually strengthens your faith.

  You might feel called to teach a Sunday school class, or you may prefer spending time one-on-one with others, encouraging and assisting them in their faith and the issues of their life. Either way, you can make a lasting impression and a valuable investment in the life of someone else.

QUESTIONS TO PONDER:

1. How do you envision life during your golden years? Do you think it is a realistic picture in light of your current physical, emotional, and spiritual health, as well as your financial situation?
2. What type of physical exercise would you be most likely and most able to engage in (or continue in) as your body ages?
3. Do you plan to retire when you reach retirement age or continue working at your current job until you are no longer able? If you do retire, what purposeful activities are you interested in pursuing?
4. What personal relationships might you be able to spend more time on as life "slows down"?
5. What are some activities you might enjoy that would provide mental stimulation and keep your brain healthy and active?
6. According to the information in this chapter (and elsewhere in this book), and perhaps according to your health-care provider, which health screening tests should you consider having done?
7. Which issues of safety (medications and supplements, driving, falls, contagious disease) are most likely to concern you, and how can you prevent or manage such problems?
8. Are you content with your spiritual condition and relationship with God as you approach the end of your life on this earth?

Action items: If you are not physically active, talk to your health-care provider to help you devise an appropriate and appealing plan for getting regular exercise. Remember, it's never too late to benefit from physical activity.

Be aware of how your nutritional needs may change as you age. Ask your health-care provider to help you determine what changes you should make to your diet.

Look again at the symptoms of anxiety and depression on pages 317–318 and 324–325 in chapter 8. If you are experiencing one or more of these symptoms, schedule appointments with both your physician and your pastor to discuss them.

If you are not sure where you stand with God, turn back to page 392 in chapter 9 and read the sections entitled "Our terminal condition" and "The cure." Don't wait another day before taking the all-important step of accepting God's gift of forgiveness and making your eternal relationship with Him a certainty.

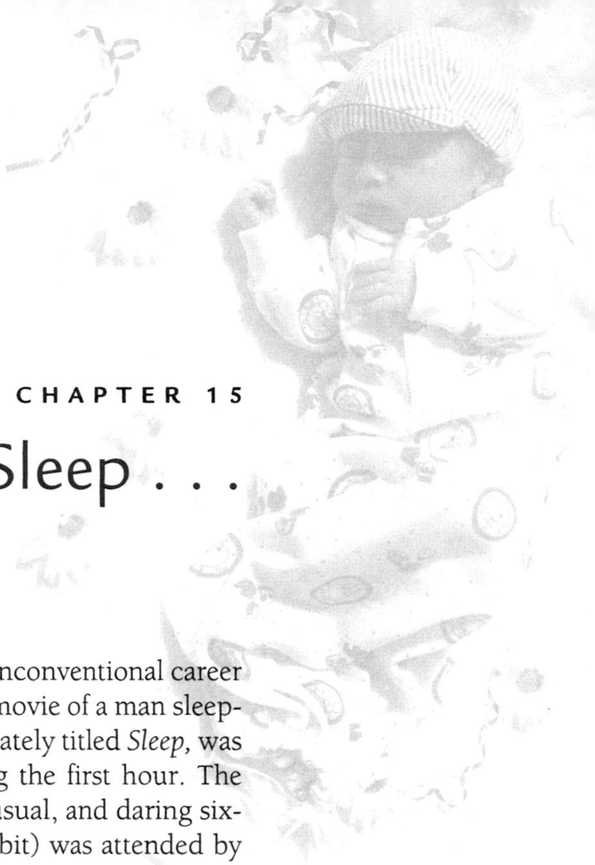

CHAPTER 15

To Sleep . . .

In 1963, pop artist Andy Warhol embarked on a highly unconventional career as a filmmaker with his first feature, an eight-hour silent movie of a man sleeping. The New York premiere of this masterpiece, appropriately titled *Sleep,* was attended by nine people, two of whom departed during the first hour. The film's Los Angeles premiere, advertised as a "strange, unusual, and daring six-hour film about sleep" (apparently it had been edited a bit) was attended by some five hundred unwary art-house filmgoers. After the first forty-five minutes, consisting entirely of a close-up of the sleeping man's abdomen, the audience became decidedly restless. Later, during a shot of his snoozing face, a viewer ran up to the screen and shouted, "Wake up!" to the delight of the increasingly agitated crowd. Fearing that a riot would erupt, the manager handed out free passes to the two hundred remaining patrons. Fifty diehards (not counting the projectionist, who fell asleep) made it to the bitter end.

Obviously, watching someone sleep is not the world's most popular spectator sport, for the obvious reason that there doesn't appear to be much to see. (There are exceptions, of course: loving parents or grandparents watching a new baby slumber, or a new husband gazing at his bride on the first daybreak of their honeymoon. In these situations, the interest is definitely in the eye of the beholder.) But if it were possible to create a window into the brain or a video screen showing what was happening inside a sleeper's head, the Sleep Channel would be one of the most popular destinations on cable TV.

"I lie down and sleep; I wake again, because the Lord sustains me."
Psalm 3:5

As it turns out, sleep—and not merely the dreams that inhabit it—is one of the most interesting phases of our life. The term *phase* is quite appropriate, by the way, because most of us will spend about one-third of our life asleep (depending on how many hours we average per night). While we may take this daily dose of altered consciousness for granted, it is mind-boggling to ponder that a person celebrating his ninetieth birthday will have spent three decades snoozing. For those who claim not to need a lot of sleep, or those who are drawn like an excited moth to the bright lights in a bustling city, dozing for a few hours every day may seem like an incredible (but unavoidable) waste of time. But in fact, sleep is a crucial daily event, designed for specific and important purposes. Researchers are only now beginning to explore the physiology of sleep and to understand the intricate events going on inside the brain and body during those many hours when so little appears to be happening. In this chapter we'll take an eye-opening look, so to speak, at this fascinating part of our life.

> *My help comes from the Lord, the Maker of heaven and earth. He will not let your foot slip—he who watches over you will not slumber; indeed, he who watches over Israel will neither slumber nor sleep.*
>
> (PSALM 121:2-4)

While far too many people make the grave mistake of trying to play God, one characteristic of the Almighty that no human can duplicate is His eternal wakefulness. For all of us, sleep is a physiological necessity, as vital as oxygen, water, and food. Why is this? The answer is not entirely clear, but we do know that sleep is definitely more than a temporary time-out from a stressful day. Sleep researchers generally propose that these times of physical rest and altered brain function are needed for restoration and repair—not just within the central nervous system, but throughout the body.

Whatever the reasons may be (and there are no doubt many more to be discovered), we all know how poor we feel during—and especially after—the times we've been up for an all-nighter brought on by an overdue school assignment, medical emergency, colicky baby, red-eye flight, or some other compelling event. If we don't make up the lost sleep the next day (or night), our thought processes and emotions will become increasingly frayed as the hours pass. Sleep loss has been found to impair memory, learning, and logical reasoning. During prolonged sleep deprivation, poor concentration will eventually deteriorate into hallucinations, and irritability into overt mood swings. Rats, which normally live for two to three years, will survive only about five weeks if deprived of rapid eye movement (REM) sleep (see page 739) and will not survive a month if not allowed to sleep at all.

F.Y.I.

Mammals, birds, reptiles, amphibians, and at least some fish are known to sleep, though often in patterns very different from humans. Among animals (not counting those that hibernate), the champion sleeper is the brown bat, which logs nearly twenty hours of sleep every day. Cats (with their famous naps) spend about twelve hours per day snoozing; dogs, about ten and a half. At the short end of the sleep spectrum are elephants and horses, averaging about three hours per day. Among mammals, giraffes—which never lie down—sleep the least: less than two hours per day. Dolphins, some species of seals, and probably whales and manatees have the amazing capacity to allow half (or one **hemisphere**) of their brain to sleep while the other remains awake. (Talk about sleeping with one eye open!)

Sleeplessness is both a significant predictor of absenteeism and a cause of lost productivity. In the United States alone, sleep loss is estimated to cost employers more than $18 billion every year in lost productivity. The total cost of sleeplessness, which also includes absenteeism, accidents, hospitalization, and medical fees, is about $100 billion annually.[1] The National Highway Traffic Safety Administration has estimated that fatigued or sleepy drivers (especially those age twenty-five or younger) are responsible for more than 100,000 car crashes per year, resulting in 1,500 deaths and more than 70,000 injuries and disabilities. Contrary to popular belief, someone who is severely sleep deprived cannot successfully maintain wakefulness, even with the help of caffeine or other stimulants. Anyone fighting sleep while driving—repeatedly yawning, struggling to keep his or her eyes open, or forgetting the scenery passed in the last few miles—shouldn't be behind the wheel.

How Much Sleep Do You Need?

The answer: Probably more than you are getting.

Sleep research has consistently shown that most adults actually *do* need the proverbial eight hours of sleep a night in order to perform at their best and avoid general tiredness, daytime drowsiness, and even fatigue-related illnesses. There are, of course, some who actually have a physiological need for as many as nine or ten hours and some who are fine on a routine of six or seven.

The need for sleep varies as we age. Newborns often sleep twenty hours per day, while children may need anywhere from eight to thirteen hours, depending on their age. Teenagers, who are notorious for gravitating toward a "late to bed and late to rise" schedule, also generally need nine hours. While most adults need eight hours of sleep per night, this amount may be altered by genetics, sleep habits (or sleep hygiene, a topic we will discuss later), and certain problems that can interfere with the quality of sleep. As we age, it's harder to fall asleep and stay asleep. Our sleep also tends to become less restful and more easily disrupted, and we spend less time in deeper phases of sleep.

F.Y.I.

While many parents may be exasperated by their teenagers' propensity to stay up late and then sleep until noon, this behavior actually has a formal name among sleep researchers: delayed sleep phase syndrome, or DSPS. We will look at it later in this chapter.

For more information about children and sleep, see "Sleep Concerns during Infancy and Childhood" beginning on page 761.

How much sleep *you* need is best judged by how well you feel and perform during your waking hours. If you feel refreshed shortly after getting up and are generally alert throughout the day, you're probably getting enough sleep. But if you are sleep-deprived, you may identify with one or more of these situations:

- Your hand "dive-bombs" the snooze button on your alarm several times every morning.
- You have come to hate whatever program is playing when your clock radio goes off.

- The first word out of your mouth upon arising is "Coffee. . . ."
- You often feel sleepy and fatigued during the day.
- You have difficulty staying awake when you have to sit still, such as during a class or meeting or while driving.
- You struggle with irritability, poor concentration, or remembering facts.
- You find yourself relishing the chance to catch up on sleep on weekends or your day off.
- You fall asleep almost immediately when your head hits the pillow.

It is estimated that in the 1850s the average American slept eight to nine hours each night. Today, an American adult typically sleeps seven hours or less a night during the workweek and then crashes on the weekends. Unlike our forebears, who relied on candles and lanterns to participate in a limited number of activities after it got dark outside, we keep our nights alive with lights, entertainment, and activities long after the sun has gone down. The busyness of our life and an endless list of diversions seduce us into sacrificing sleep on the altar of extended work hours, evening meetings, and late-night entertainment. Sleep is a gift from God, but we live in a culture that does not give it much value. Indeed, so many of us have become accustomed to a harried, sleep-deprived existence that we may have come to accept its consequences of fatigue, irritability, and daytime drowsiness as normal.

A National Sleep Foundation "Sleep in America" poll showed that about 75 percent of adult Americans report having one or more symptoms of a sleep problem at least a few nights each week.[2] When a person fails to get the sleep that he or she needs for more than two or three days, whether due to an overextended lifestyle or a sleep disorder, that person begins to build what doctors call a **sleep debt**. Unfortunately, even with a steady flow of caffeine and a lot of activity, it's not really possible to adjust to sleeping fewer hours than are needed. As our sleep debt builds over several days, fatigue increases and mental and physical performance begin to suffer. The need for sleep will continue to grow until we sleep in on a weekend or a day off, become ill, or start napping during normal waking hours. In order to feel (and be) properly rested, the sleep debt will at some point need to be repaid. Sleep debt has been blamed for many major industrial and aviation accidents, and it is now implicated in overall poor health as well. The only way to repay a sleep debt is to get an hour or two more sleep than we typically need for several nights in a row—an assignment that can be surprisingly difficult. Once the debt has been dealt with, the brain reverts to seeking whatever amount of sleep it normally needs.

Fatigue and sleep debt also affect **sleep latency**, the actual amount of time it takes to fall asleep. If you're not fatigued or short on sleep, it can take twenty minutes or more to fall asleep. At the end of a long, demanding day, or with a buildup of sleep debt, sleep latency can shorten to a few minutes or less. If you experience a very short sleep latency night after night, this is usually an indication that the amount or quality of your sleep is inadequate. A short sleep latency should be noted as a warning sign, especially by anyone (such as a long-distance driver) whose life and safety depend upon staying awake.

If you have a restful vacation planned in the near future, try this experiment in order to help determine how much sleep you need on an ongoing basis. Once you are unpacked and settled in, go to bed each night when you feel tired and then sleep until you wake up spontaneously. Keep the room dark, set no alarms, and don't let other people awaken you. You may be paying back a sleep debt for several days, but after that you should start sleeping for about the length of time you actually need. If you don't have a vacation planned soon or will be following a busy itinerary on your next trip, you can try a similar experiment at home. Try to go to bed about fifteen minutes earlier each night (fifteen minutes the first night, thirty minutes the second night, and so on) until you discover the amount of sleep that leaves you feeling completely restored the next day.

How Do We Sleep?

This sounds like a silly question with a simple answer: We lie down and close our eyes when we get tired and then wake up several hours later.

But in fact, the brain is undergoing all kinds of activity while asleep, cycling repeatedly through phases of sleep known as stages 1, 2, 3, 4, and **REM (rapid eye movement)**. The first four stages, together called **non-REM sleep**, make up about 75 percent of our sleep time.

MAKING THE MOST OF A NAP

Most toddlers or preschoolers are not enthused about lying down for a nap during a busy day. Years later, a nap may feel like a luxury, a wonderful way to spend a good chunk of a quiet afternoon. But you may be surprised to learn that a brief "power nap" may be as refreshing as a two-hour snoozefest.

Napping can be particularly helpful when you are fatigued during the day or when you know you will need to stay up late at night. Napping is usually easier during the period of normal sleepiness that occurs from about two to five in the afternoon. An effective short nap should typically last no longer than twenty minutes. If you sleep longer, you are likely to enter the deeper phases of sleep from which it is much more difficult to awaken and stay alert. Sleep research suggests that a short (fifteen- to twenty-minute) nap can improve performance and alertness, sharpen memory, and delay the need for sleep later in the day.

If you have a significant sleep debt, then napping as long as one and a half to two hours will allow you to pass through a complete REM cycle, providing more rest and making it easier to wake up. Remember, however, that napping during the day should not take the place of a full night's sleep. ■

The first and lighter phases of non-REM sleep are stages 1 and 2. When we struggle to stay awake and keep nodding off, we may drift in and out of stage 1 sleep, from which it is easiest to awaken. During this stage, our eyes often move and muscles twitch, and we may even remember some images ("I got so drowsy that I was starting to dream. . . ."), but this in fact is not the stage in which we do our dreaming. We spend about 50 percent of our total sleep time in stage 2, when eye movements and brain waves slow down. From there we progress to stages 3 and 4, known as **deep sleep**, which is the most restorative. Blood pressure, pulse, and breathing rates all decrease, and eye movements and muscle activity essentially stop. It is more difficult to awaken from deep sleep, and when it is interrupted, we may feel groggy or even disoriented for several minutes. Bed-wetting, sleepwalking, and night terrors in children occur during stages 3 and 4.

Rapid eye movement sleep—so named because our eyes move actively under the eyelids during this phase—is the stage during which we dream. Breathing becomes more rapid and less regular, and arms and legs become temporarily paralyzed as the brain electrically disconnects from the spinal cord and stops sending messages to the muscles. This is an important safeguard, because when it fails people literally act out their dreams, often with disastrous results. (We will look at this phenomenon, called REM movement disorder, in more detail later in this chapter.)

REM sleep makes up about 20 to 25 percent (up to two hours) of total sleep time in adults and children older than two. Newborns spend about 50 percent of their sleep time in the REM phase. This amount drops to about 40 percent REM sleep after the first few weeks of life and then decreases to about 30 percent between the ages of about six months and two years. This high percentage of REM sleep time may be important for brain development because this phase stimulates areas of the brain that are utilized in learning. Several studies have shown that individuals deprived of REM sleep have more difficulty with cognitive (thinking-related) learning and motor skills than those who are not REM-deprived.

F.Y.I.

Most mammals and birds display signs of REM sleep, while reptiles and other cold-blooded animals do not. We can only guess whether Rover's occasional kicks and moans while asleep on the floor represent an exciting dream chase in progress.

When we first fall asleep, we generally pass through stages 1 through 4 in sequence, then return to the lighter phases of sleep, from which we enter the first REM phase about sixty to ninety minutes after dozing off. Brain waves—the electrical activity that can be measured on an **electroencephalogram (EEG)**—slow down more and more as we pass from stage 1 through stage 4. But during REM sleep, brain-wave activity is very similar to what occurs when we're awake. We continue cycling through the non-REM stages during the night, interrupted by periods of REM, each complete cycle lasting around 90 to 110 minutes. During the first of these, the deeper stages of sleep last longer with a relatively short period (fifteen to twenty minutes) of REM sleep. As we

WHY DO WE DREAM?

Because dreams can be sweet, ecstatic, irritating, terrifying, and often bizarre, they have always fascinated people. Many have tried to understand, interpret, or even predict the future based on images in the dreams. The Bible documents a number of occasions in which dreams and their interpretations played a key role in the lives of people in the Old Testament, including Abraham, Jacob, Joseph, and Daniel. In the New Testament, both Joseph and the magi who visited Mary's young son, Jesus, received guidance and warnings from God in dreams.

But while relating these stories and describing communications from God to prophets in dreams (as in Numbers 12:6, for example), the Scriptures also sternly caution about the dreams and interpretations of false prophets (see Jeremiah 27:9 and 29:8). What shows up in a dream should not automatically be accepted as "gospel truth." Psychics and seers of all stripes have offered their fanciful interpretations of dreams to paying customers for thousands of years, and their contemporary counterparts are thriving on the Internet. Sigmund Freud and his followers went to great and convoluted lengths to interpret their patients' dreams through the grid of their elaborate theories of the human psyche that are now widely discredited.

Indeed, legitimate sleep investigators today virtually ignore the content of dreams, which, incidentally, reflects what the brain usually does as well. While REM sleep—and thus dreaming—is universal, we routinely remember very little (if any) of our nocturnal adventures. Since we spend up to two hours in this phase of sleep and thus presumably have all sorts of images and stories playing in our heads for a significant amount of time every night, it is a blessing that our brain's default setting is to *forget* dreams. (Imagine the mental clutter and confusion that would accrue if we actually remembered the entire contents of one or two hours of dream material, much of which is highly illogical, every single day.) Even if we awaken with a dream in progress, it will fade away within moments unless we immediately and deliberately "replay" it. This mental process will usually store some or all of the dream more permanently in our memory banks.

One contemporary theory holds that dreams are primarily an effort by the frontal cortex (the part of the brain that does our learning, thinking, and organizing) to interpret the assorted signals arriving from the **pons**, an area at the base of the brain that initiates REM sleep. Does the content of a given night's dreams have any greater significance? Are we blowing off psychological steam or expressing our deepest concerns and desires in our dreams? Perhaps. Can God communicate with us in a dream? No doubt He can, but whether a specific dream truly is a message from Him, as opposed to a creation of our own brain, may take some time and counsel to sort out. To seek other messages in our dreams, presuming that they communicate hidden wisdom about ourselves and others or contain all sorts of obscure symbolic meaning, is to embark on a pursuit based on pure conjecture at best and misleading fantasy at worst. ■

continue through the night, REM becomes more predominant and deep sleep less so, such that sleep cycles closer to morning consist almost entirely of stages 1 and 2 and REM sleep. This is an important observation, because those of us who are getting only five or six hours of sleep per night may be unintentionally eliminating a significant amount of our much-needed REM sleep.

Researchers refer to the particular pattern of REM and non-REM sleep stages that occur throughout the night as our **sleep architecture**. The quality of our sleep architecture—the correct amount, proportion, and patterns of REM and non-REM sleep—is as important as the total amount of sleep. Unfortunately, many environmental factors, medications, jet lag, tobacco and alcohol use, and a number of specific sleep disorders can disrupt it. Therefore, if a person's sleep architecture is disturbed, he or she can actually sleep for what seems to be a reasonable amount of time but still feel exhausted and drowsy the next day.

Imagine (or remember) being awakened every thirty minutes during the night by a barking dog or a crying child. Even if you fell asleep fairly quickly after each interruption, you would need to reenter sleep through stage 1, then cycle into the other stages. Since it usually takes at least thirty to forty minutes to enter the deeper, restorative phases of sleep and REM, you would have difficulty reaching them. In the morning you would probably feel pretty miserable, even if you managed to cobble together seven or eight hours of sleep, because the quality of your sleep architecture would have been disrupted.

Taming Sleep Disrupters

We've already noted that many of us are routinely shorting ourselves of sleep because of overcrowded schedules and late-night activities. There are several other ways in which our circumstances and habits can cheat us of restorative sleep.

Before we look at these sleep disrupters, however, we need to introduce another important factor that impacts our patterns of sleeping and waking: our **circadian rhythm**. Derived from Latin words meaning "around the day," this term refers to changes in the physiology of our body that occur in roughly twenty-four-hour cycles. The internal clock that drives the circadian rhythm is a pair of tiny structures (called the **suprachiasmatic nuclei**, or **SCN**) located in the hypothalamus, an important area of the brain designed to regulate hundreds of functions throughout the body. The SCN direct some two hundred circadian fluctuations, including variations in our blood pressure, body temperature, and hormone levels. In addition, their location in the brain—just above the area at which the optic nerves cross—is strategic in that they receive input from the eyes as to the presence of light and darkness.

During the day the SCN signal a structure called the **pineal gland** to reduce the production of melatonin, a hormone that increases drowsiness. Rising levels of melatonin after dark help induce sleepiness. For most people, circadian-driven sleep-wake patterns linked to darkness and light cause a marked increase in the desire to sleep between midnight and 6 A.M. (no great surprise) and bring about another drowsy period during the midafternoon. The tradition of an afternoon nap or siesta in some cultures undoubtedly arises from a combination of this normal fluctuation in sleepiness and the burden of laboring or conducting business during the heat of the day.

F.Y.I.

Research has determined that if deprived of external cues such as clocks or the presence of light and darkness, the human circadian cycle gravitates to about twenty-five hours. Everyday stimuli repeatedly "reset" our circadian rhythm to line up with a twenty-four-hour day.

Jet lag is a common sleep disruption brought about by flying long distances. After a flight across several time zones, a person's circadian rhythm suddenly becomes out of sync with the local time. Jet lag is an entirely modern phenomenon. Prior to the introduction of commercial jetliner travel in the late 1950s, people didn't travel far enough east or west in one day to experience circadian disruptions. The pioneers never had to deal with "covered wagon lag" and sailors never have "ship lag," because these forms of travel don't cross time zones fast enough to demand a rapid readjustment of circadian rhythms.

Depending on the number of time zones changed, the length of travel, and the level of sleep deprivation associated with the trip, jet lag can significantly affect a person's mental performance, sleep-wake cycle, and general well-being for several days after arrival. Symptoms of jet lag include irritability, fatigue, daytime drowsiness, poor concentration, intestinal disturbances (including diarrhea), and nighttime awakening. Most people find that jet lag is more troublesome when traveling eastward than westward. Generally it takes about one day to adjust for each time zone traveled east or west. (When a person travels north or south along a time zone, there is generally no disruption to the circadian rhythm, though the traveler may still be tired from making the trip.)

An estimated 15 million Americans perform **shift work**, which is another common cause of significant sleep disruption. A person who works an 11 P.M. to 7 A.M. shift is completely out of phase with the environmental daylight/nighttime cycle and is therefore "fighting circadian city hall," so to speak. Studies of night-shift workers almost always reveal significant disruptions of circadian rhythms, including **circadian dysynchrony**, in which the various cycles of blood pressure, temperature, alertness, and hormone secretion are out of sync not only with the clock but with each other as well.

Shift workers can have particular trouble if they don't avoid sunlight, because the pattern of outside light and darkness is a powerful cue to the internal clock. As we just mentioned, normal circadian physiology causes most people to gravitate to a pattern of wakefulness during the day and sleep at night—the opposite of the night-shift work schedule. When they get a day or two off, many who have worked several consecutive night shifts may try to stay awake

BEATING AND TREATING JET LAG

Seasoned travelers—especially those who have suffered through the discomforts of jet lag on one or more trips and don't care to repeat the experience—have learned several techniques that speed the alignment of their circadian rhythm with the local time zone. These include:

- If you have a few days to prepare for a west-to-east cross-country flight, try to synchronize your inner clock with your destination's time zone over three or more successive nights. If your normal bedtime is midnight, go to bed at 11 P.M. one night, 10 P.M. the next, and then 9 P.M. for a night or two. If you can get up earlier as well, even better. When the time comes to fly to the east coast, you'll be less likely to lie awake at midnight (9 P.M. Pacific time) and then wonder what hit you when the alarm goes off at 7 A.M. (4 A.M. Pacific).
- Trans-Atlantic west-to-east flights cover even more time zones, so resynchronizing can be challenging. If you can travel on an overnight flight and sleep for a few hours on the plane, the transition will be much easier. (This may require a little help from your doctor in the form of a short-acting sleeping medication, assuming that its use is appropriate for your current health status.) An alternative is to arrange your flight(s) so that you arrive in the evening, and then go to bed at 10 or 11 P.M. If you arrive earlier and need to nap, avoid sleeping more than two hours.
- As soon as you depart, set your watch for the time zone of your destination.
- Avoid common sleep disrupters for a few hours prior to bedtime at your destination. These include alcohol, caffeine, nicotine, or intense exercise.
- Once you have arrived, get outside during the day as much as possible in order to cue your brain to the current timing of day and night.
- Melatonin supplementation has been widely promoted as a treatment for jet lag and appears to be helpful at least for some long-distance travelers. It is typically taken for a few days after arrival, in doses of 1 to 3 mg about a half hour before going to bed. Melatonin's safety during pregnancy or while nursing has not been established, and it is not recommended for long-term use. ■

More information about melatonin can be found later in this chapter on page 752.

during the day in order to spend time with family and friends. Then it's back to the night shift.

Not surprisingly, attempting to adjust the circadian rhythm so quickly usually results in drowsiness at work and insomnia at home. As many as 10 to 20 percent of night-shift workers report falling asleep on the job, especially toward the end of the shift. Overall they tend to get five to seven fewer hours of sleep each week compared to their counterparts on day or evening shifts. As a result, night-shift workers are at an increased risk not only for health problems (including heart disease, digestive disorders, and emotional disturbances), but also for more frequent and serious accidents. The Three Mile Island and Chernobyl nuclear-power-plant accidents, the *Exxon Valdez* oil spill, and the Bhopal, India, chemical gas leak that killed 3,800 people all occurred during the night shift and have been attributed, at least in part, to errors made by fatigued workers.

Environmental factors are notorious for disturbing sleep. A barking dog, catfight, crying baby, noisy neighbors, thunderstorm, police siren, or other unpredictable racket can cause one or more awakenings. More constant types of noise—city traffic, crickets, soft rain, even a train that passes so regularly that one can tune it out—are less disruptive. One type of noise that few people become accustomed to is the snoring of a bedmate, especially if it comes in fits and starts throughout the night. Aside from driving a spouse into another room, snoring could have more ominous significance, as we will discuss shortly. Someone whose sleep is particularly sensitive to noise might have to take measures to block unwanted sounds (such as using earplugs) or to mask them using a device that generates neutral sound (white noise) or simulates a pleasant sonic environment, such as a mountain stream or breeze in a forest.

Too much light in a room can interfere with sleep, especially for a shift worker trying to sleep during the day. A room that is too hot, too cold, or too stuffy will also keep slumber at bay. High altitude can interfere with the quality and quantity of sleep for a few nights until a person becomes accustomed to it. Many people who have adapted to a particular set of surroundings (especially their own mattress) might also have considerable difficulty falling asleep or staying asleep in a hotel or guest room.

Perhaps the most notorious combination of sleep disrupters occurs during hospitalization. In addition to whatever illness or medical problem led to the admission, a patient is usually confined to a less-than-comfortable bed, perhaps with a few tubes and wires attached to his or her body. Those who have experienced a hospital stay are well aware of the many disruptions: staff members who come in and out at all hours (including the proverbial nurse who awakens the patient to deliver a sleeping pill), roommates who are sick or noisy (not to mention *their* caregivers and visitors coming and going), noise in the hallways, blood draws at 5 A.M., and the discomfort of a hospital gown that is notoriously thin and missing a back side. If it doesn't interfere with the treatment plan or worsen a patient's condition, this is one time when he or she may want to ask the doctor to order a sleep aid.

A number of popular habits can disrupt sleep. Caffeine is well-known for its mild stimulant effects, but for some a cup of coffee or a caffeinated soft drink can promote wakefulness for up to twelve hours. Tobacco use can interfere with sleep because of nicotine's stimulant effects. Alcohol has a temporary sedating effect, depending upon the amount consumed, but it can lead to frequent waking later in the night. A large meal eaten shortly before retiring can lead to reflux—a backflow of stomach acid into the esophagus—and heartburn during the night.

Many health problems, arising from virtually any organ system, can interfere with sleep, including:

- An acute illness such as a cold or flu that brings on aches, pains, coughing, or an intestinal upheaval.

HELP FOR THE NIGHT CREW

If we have an emergency in the middle of the night, we certainly appreciate the hardy souls who run the emergency department or arrive in the police car in response to our distress call. Indeed, we owe a lot not only to those who help with crises, but also to the millions who serve meals, monitor vital resources such as water and power, guide air traffic, and provide hundreds of other services that keep the country running when most of us are sound asleep. What steps can these workers take to help them do these important jobs without suffering unreasonable health consequences?

First and foremost, become familiar with the principles of good sleep hygiene, which apply to everyone, regardless of work or sleep schedules. These can be found later in this chapter, beginning on page 749. One important recommendation that can be particularly tough to follow is going to bed at the same time every day—even on days off or weekends, when you want to get other things done during the day. This can help prevent seesawing circadian rhythm disruptions.

If you are a shift worker who must sleep during the day, you have two major challenges: limiting the daylight cues that tell your circadian clock to stay awake and minimizing the interruptions to your sleep when others are up and about. These mean:

- If you're going to sleep in the morning after a night shift, wear dark glasses on the way home and keep your exposure to the morning daylight to a minimum.
- Keep your bedroom dark, quiet, and at a comfortable temperature.
- Turn the phone off in your bedroom.
- Ask family members to do their best to keep noise levels down. Wear earplugs if necessary.

- Chronic pain from arthritis, injury, cancer, surgery, or other conditions.
- Breathing problems, such as those that occur with chronic lung disease, asthma, and congestive heart failure.
- Ongoing digestive upsets, such as heartburn, nausea, cramps, and diarrhea.
- The need to get up several times at night to urinate, whether arising from fluid shifts in the body that generate more urine or from actual bladder or prostate disorders.
- Anxiety and depression, as well as more severe mental disturbances such as schizophrenia, are notorious for disrupting sleep. Many people with chronic insomnia have a treatable depression or anxiety disorder.

Your other major concern is staying awake and safe on the job. To the degree that your job, workplace, and employer permit, the following can help you:

- Keep your work area as well lit as possible.
- Talk with coworkers to help keep you alert.
- Move around briefly and stretch as often as possible, especially if you start to feel drowsy.
- If your routine is to sleep soon after your shift is over, and if you use coffee or other caffeinated beverages, try to avoid drinking them late in the shift. (A mug of coffee at 6 A.M. may make it difficult to fall asleep at home a couple of hours later.)
- If possible, walk briskly or do some other light exercise during your breaks.
- If your job involves tasks that are particularly boring, try to do them when you are most alert (which is usually early in the shift).
- To state the obvious: If your work involves any tasks that are potentially hazardous to yourself or others and you are fighting drowsiness (yawning, blinking, or even nodding off), stop what you are doing as quickly as possible. Talk with a coworker or supervisor, move around, get some fresh air, and drink a caffeinated beverage. If possible, you might even try to arrange for a brief nap. A twenty-minute sleep may provide a surprising improvement in alertness and performance.

Don't forget about safety on the way home. If you carpool, let the person who feels (and acts) the most alert do the driving, and help to keep that person engaged in conversation. If you have a lengthy solo drive and repeatedly fight drowsiness behind the wheel, consider a short nap before leaving work, look into carpooling, or even consider public transportation. ■

Many medications, including some prescribed or recommended for the problems just listed, can interfere with sleep:

- Decongestants—especially pseudoephedrine—in common cold remedies can be very effective in keeping people awake for hours. They are often added to cold and sinus preparations or combined with antihistamines (often with the suffix *-D* attached to their name).
- Caffeine is added to some pain relievers, especially those geared for treating headaches.
- Many diet pills (prescription and otherwise) have a stimulant effect that can interfere with sleep.

Other medications disrupt sleep in some—but by no means all—people. These include oral cortisone (steroid) preparations, including birth control pills; certain types of blood pressure medications (diuretics, nifedipine, and a class known as beta-blockers); aminophylline and a class of drugs called beta-agonists, which are used to treat asthma; and antibiotics in the family called **fluoroquinolones** (such as Cipro, Levaquin, and Avelox).

F.Y.I.

Aminophylline is no longer widely prescribed for treating asthma. But beta-agonists are frequently used in inhalers such as **albuterol** (Ventolin, Proventil), which relieve wheezing for several hours. While this medication is intended to work only in the airways, some may be absorbed through the lining of the mouth or throat and cause a mild stimulant effect. This can be minimized by rinsing the mouth out with water after using one of these inhalers.

Aging is frequently associated with disturbed sleep: More than 50 percent of people over age sixty-five report some type of sleep problem. As we mentioned earlier in this chapter, seniors are more likely to have difficulty falling asleep, spend less time in the deeper stages of sleep, experience early morning awakening, and accrue less total time asleep. Contrary to a commonly held notion, the elderly do not need less sleep. Instead, they more frequently experience decreased sleep efficiency and are vulnerable to more factors that can impair sleep. These include:

- Poor sleep habits, including irregular sleep-wake times and daytime napping, that interfere with falling asleep at night.
- Acute and chronic illnesses, and the medications that treat them.
- Significant social changes, usually involving profound personal losses, such as leaving a familiar home/community, the death of a loved one, separation from loved ones and friends, a move to a long-term care facility, and so on.
- Emotional upheavals, including anxiety and depression, as well as changes in overall mental function. Dementia (deteriorating cognitive abilities stemming from Alzheimer's disease, stroke, and other illnesses) often is accompanied by agitation, disorientation, and disruptive behaviors at night that wreak havoc on sleep, not only for the individual but also for his or her live-in caregivers.

- Sleep disorders, including sleep apnea, restless legs syndrome, and periodic limb movement disorder, are more common later in life. We will look at these problems later in this chapter.

Getting a Good Night's Sleep

Sleep hygiene refers to the conditions, practices, and habits that assist and promote effective and continuous sleep. These recommendations are the ABC's of a good night's rest and the first steps to review when insomnia becomes an issue.

- Establish consistent sleep and wake-up times that provide enough sleep *every* day—and thus don't change radically on weekends or days off.
- Develop a "winding down" routine that serves as a cue for your mind and body to get ready for sleep. This might include a warm bath, some diverting or inspirational reading, or pleasant music—and *not* the evening news. In case you hadn't noticed, bedtime newscasts are routinely jammed with the most lurid, disturbing, and unpleasant events of the day. (This strategy grabs and holds the viewers' attention but does nothing for their sleep.) An uplifting psalm or other Scripture passage containing some spiritual good news will provide better raw material for your sleeping brain to process.
- Exercising regularly is helpful for a good night's sleep, but try to avoid vigorous activity within three hours of bedtime. This raises body temperature and tends to stimulate the brain rather than sedate it—which is why morning is a better time for your workout. Your body cools down (a condition more favorable to sleep) about five to six hours after exercise, so a late-afternoon or even early evening workout can be conducive to sleep.
- If at all possible, avoid personal turbulence prior to bedtime. If you have an important issue to discuss with someone (especially your spouse), don't start the conversation at bedtime. Fatigue at the end of the day (and the irritability, frustration, and short tempers that accompany it) will not only lead to a full-blown argument but also generate enough agitation to interfere with sleep. Schedule the conversation for a time and place when you are both rested and calm.
- Avoid going to bed hungry, but also avoid going to bed shortly after a large meal. A feast before bedtime may provoke heartburn or bloating, and the liquids that typically accompany it may fill up the bladder during the night. Some people, however, find that a light snack at bedtime helps them fall asleep more easily.
- Make your sleeping area as quiet, dark, and comfortable as possible, avoiding extremes in temperature. Most sleep experts recommend sleeping in a cooler room rather than a warm one, because a hot envi-

ronment tends to cause lighter sleep and more awakenings during the night.

- Avoid caffeine (not only in coffee, but also in tea, soft drinks, and even chocolate), nicotine (from smoking or patches/gum), or alcohol late in the day. Caffeine and nicotine are stimulants that tend to keep you awake, and alcohol, while initially sedating, interferes with sleep architecture.
- Don't use your bed for anything other than sexual relations or sleep. Your bed isn't meant to be your office, your primary TV viewing area, or the place in which you unravel the mysteries of your life. Attempting to deal with work tasks and other issues in your bed can definitely interfere with relaxing and falling asleep.
- If you can't sleep after thirty or forty minutes, don't continue to lie awake in bed. Get up and do some sort of relaxing activity, such as reading (something rather boring might be helpful) or listening to calming music, until you get sleepy. Try not to solve the world's problems, or your own, in the middle of the night. If some issue has you pacing the floor when everyone else is asleep, write a short list of specific "action items" that will help you deal with it the next day, and then go to bed. When you are tempted to revisit the problem instead of sleeping, remember that you now have a to-do list . . . for tomorrow . . . in another room. Now it's time to rest. If you truly cannot stop the flow of thoughts racing through your head during the night, you may need some help from your physician.
- Napping can be a useful short-term strategy when you know you won't be getting much sleep that night or when you have an accumulating sleep debt. But if you have trouble falling asleep night after night, avoid daytime napping, which can delay the onset of sleep later.

When Sleep Will Not Come

In Shakespeare's historical play *Henry IV,* King Henry's troubles are robbing him of sleep. The king laments his miserable wakefulness amidst royal comforts while his subjects in meager surroundings enjoy sweet slumber:

> *How many thousand of my poorest subjects*
> *Are at this hour asleep! O sleep, O gentle sleep,*
> *Nature's soft nurse, how have I frighted thee,*
> *That thou no more wilt weigh my eyelids down*
> *And steep my senses in forgetfulness?*[3]

Indeed, few experiences in life are as frustrating as lying awake at night unable to sleep, periodically glancing at a bedroom clock that delivers nothing but bad news. It's 3:15? *I'm supposed to be up in less than four hours! This is going to be one rotten day!* **Insomnia** is generally defined as the awareness of having trouble getting to sleep or staying asleep, or the perception of not sleeping well and not waking up refreshed. It is, needless to say, commonly associated with daytime sleepiness or fatigue.

Insomnia is often categorized by its duration: transient, short-term, or chronic. *Transient* insomnia lasts a few nights and is generally caused by stress, jet lag, changes in sleep timing, or an alteration of the sleep environment. Many people, especially as they get older, become so accustomed to the feel of their own bed that an overnight stay anywhere else—whether in a hotel, guest room, campground, or hospital—becomes an ordeal until they become acclimated to the new surroundings. *Short-term* insomnia is poor sleep lasting two to three weeks, often caused by stress, medical issues, or psychological problems. Addressing the cause will usually bring sleep back to normal. *Chronic* insomnia involves difficulty falling or staying asleep that continues for a month or longer—sometimes *much* longer. This is usually related to an underlying medical, behavioral, or psychological problem such as depression.

"As goods increase,
so do those who consume them.
And what benefit are they to the owner
except to feast his eyes on them?
The sleep of a laborer is sweet,
whether he eats little or much,
but the abundance of a rich man
permits him no sleep."
Ecclesiastes 5:11-12

It is important to note that insomnia is a symptom, like headache or fatigue, that can have many different characteristics, causes, and possible treatments. If the cause is readily identifiable and self-limited, no specific evaluation or treatment may be necessary. But if insomnia is a recurrent or chronic event, it should not—and usually cannot—be ignored. Very often the solution lies in addressing a basic area of sleep hygiene that needs adjustment: taming a caffeine habit, for example, or acquiring a pair of earplugs to reduce the impact of a spouse's snoring, which itself may need to be evaluated. If you or a loved one is struggling with insomnia, *a review of sleep habits should be the first order of business.*

A common response among people who are dealing with insomnia is to try some form of self-medication. One of the most common methods (and definitely a bad one) is a nightcap, an alcoholic beverage at bedtime. Needless to say, alcohol is definitely not a good choice for a sleep aid. While it may induce a little drowsiness, alcohol actually keeps some people awake. It suppresses REM sleep until it is metabolized, delaying this phase until later at night. It can also cause more frequent waking (including an additional trip or two to the bathroom), thus reducing the overall quality of sleep.

One Gallup poll found that almost 60 percent of adults with sleeping difficulties had tried at least one nonprescription medication to promote sleep.[4] The most common of these is the antihistamine **diphenhydramine**, sold as Benadryl (and other brands) and commonly found in "PM" forms of cold and pain relievers. A dose of 25 to 50 mg of diphenhydramine commonly brings on drowsiness, which makes it a poor choice for treating allergies during the day. (Some people, however, do not become sleepy on this medication.) Another sedating antihistamine is **doxylamine**, which is usually found in nonprescription cold remedies such as NyQuil. Either of these antihistamines can help induce sleep, and they're particularly useful if a person has both allergic symptoms and insomnia. However, they can also have an effect lasting beyond the sleep period and may cause daytime drowsiness the next day. They may also interfere with sleep architecture, resulting in a poorer quality of sleep. People with asthma or chronic lung disease should avoid these medications because they can thicken respiratory secretions, and men with symptoms arising from an enlarged prostate may have difficulty passing urine when taking one.

Many people who struggle with insomnia have tried taking **melatonin**, which can be purchased at any supermarket or pharmacy without a prescription. As we mentioned earlier, melatonin is a hormone that is known to induce drowsiness. Produced by the pineal gland within the brain, it normally increases during the night and falls to very low, almost undetectable levels during the day. Taken about thirty minutes before bedtime in doses from 1 to 3 mg (although the optimal dose is unknown), melatonin induces drowsiness in many individuals. It is also used by travelers as a treatment for jet lag, and it may help synchronize a person's circadian rhythm to the local time zone. But very few studies have examined melatonin's side effects, its interactions with other drugs, or the consequences of taking it on a long-term basis. Also, because there is very little regulation of the manufacture of herbal and food supplements, the amount and quality of melatonin may vary among the many formulations currently on the market.

Valerian, an extract of the root of the valerian plant, has a mildly relaxing effect and has been utilized widely in Europe as a treatment for insomnia. Its effects may not be noticeable for several days or even a few weeks, and thus it would not likely prove useful for transient or short-term insomnia. Because valerian may boost the effects of other sedating medications or alcohol, you should not take it with these drugs. Many preparations are available, and as with melatonin, quality and exact quantity may vary among them. A typical dose is 400 to 500 mg taken one or two hours before bedtime. (One major U.S. pharmaceutical company has entered this herbal arena with a valerian preparation called Alluna.)

Several types of prescription medications have been used to promote and maintain sleep. One class of drugs, the barbiturates (such as Nembutal, or pentobarbital), was widely used a few decades ago but is prescribed far less frequently today. Barbiturates adversely affect the quality of sleep, have significant side effects, tend to be addictive (both psychologically and physically), and can be extremely dangerous when taken in an overdose.

A class of drugs called **benzodiazepines** is well known for its members that reduce anxiety: diazepam (Valium), alprazolam (Xanax), lorazepam (Ativan), and clonazepam (Klonopin). All of these are sedating to some degree, and many people who take them for anxiety also use a bedtime dose to help with sleep. Other benzodiazepines that produce overt drowsiness have been widely prescribed as sleeping medications. The most common of these are triazolam (Halcion), temazepam (Restoril), and flurazepam (Dalmane). Estazolam (ProSom) and quazepam (Doral) are used less often. These medications vary dramatically in the duration of their activity:

- Triazolam takes effect relatively quickly and then wears off in about four hours, making it an ideal drug for inducing sleep on an overnight cross-country or transoceanic flight. Typical doses are 0.125 or 0.25 mg. Taking more than 0.25 mg is not recommended: When the drug was first introduced, a 0.5 mg dose was available, but its use was found to be associated with amnesia and erratic behavior.
- The effects of temazepam extend over about eight hours, which makes it more useful for people who have trouble both falling and staying asleep.
- Flurazepam stays in the bloodstream for so long that a person taking it for the first time may be groggy for much of the next day. Even if that doesn't occur, flurazepam tends to accumulate in the body if taken over several successive nights, which can lead to persistent daytime sedation. The elderly are particularly vulnerable to this consequence.

While no sleeping medication is recommended for long-term use, the sedating benzodiazepines are particularly ill suited for this role because they tend to interfere with sleep architecture, thus affecting the overall quality of sleep. Ongoing use can also lead to **rebound insomnia**, an unpleasant worsening of sleeplessness when the drug is discontinued. These medications should never be taken with alcohol because the combination can cause excessive sedation (including suppression of respiration), and they can be hazardous when taken in an overdose.

These problems with benzodiazepines have fueled interest in a new class of sleeping medications that are much safer and do not seem to affect sleep architecture. The three forms currently available, zolpidem (Ambien), zaleplon (Sonata), and eszopiclone (Lunesta), are effective for most people and do not appear to be physically addictive. Like any sleeping medication, however, ongoing use can lead to psychological dependence: *I've run out of my pills. . . . I won't be able to sleep tonight!* Also, until they become available in generic forms, they will be much more expensive than the benzodiazepines.

Sleep experts routinely counsel against using any sleeping medication regularly for more than a few weeks, if that long. There are a number of reasons for this. Long-term use may result in psychological and even physical dependence, disruption of sleep architecture (though not with zolpidem, zaleplon, and eszopiclone), daytime sedation (with longer-acting drugs), and adverse interactions with other medications. More importantly, treating chronic insomnia with sleeping medications is not appropriate if the reason for the problem has not been explored. If someone has wakeful nights because of depression, for example, a prescription for sleeping pills will treat only one symptom and not the underlying problem.

If a significant sleep problem lasts more than a week, you should see a health-care provider for an evaluation. Keeping a sleep-wake diary (see sidebar on the next page, "Helping Your Doctor Track Down Your Sleep Problem") may be useful in determining what is wrong and what can be done about it. In some situations your doctor might refer you to a physician with special training in managing sleep problems, if one is available in your area.

A Brief Look at a Few Sleep Disorders

Sleep specialists frequently distinguish between insomnia, the general feeling of not getting enough (or good quality) sleep, and **sleep disorders**, which are specific abnormalities in the physiology of sleep that can affect its duration and quality. An estimated 40 million Americans suffer from one of more than eighty identified sleep disorders. These are responsible for many cases of chronic insomnia, but few of the millions of people who have transient or short-term insomnia have an identifiable or diagnosable sleep disorder.

One of the most widely used (but by no means simplest) steps in diagnosing a sleep disorder is a **sleep study** (called **polysomnography**). This usually involves an overnight stay in a **sleep laboratory**, which may be set up in a specialist's office or in a center utilized by many physicians. During such a study, a person sleeps in a private room that is monitored by closed-circuit television and microphones. Sensors attached to the head and face using nonallergic tape record brain waves (EEG) and eye movements. Other skin sensors detect muscle activity. Elastic bands around the chest and abdomen track respirations. A special clip on one finger measures oxygen levels and heart rate.

F.Y.I. It is best to use an American Academy of Sleep Medicine accredited center or laboratory if you are going to have a sleep study. A list of these can be found at the academy's Web site, http://www.aasmnet.org.

It takes about an hour to make all these preparations, and while none of the attachments are painful, falling asleep under such unfamiliar circumstances would seem to be challenging. One might envision trying to sleep in a brightly lit laboratory, surrounded by beeping electronic equipment and technicians circulating in lab coats. But the technologist(s) and equipment are in another room, the sleeping rooms are comfortably furnished, and once everything has been set up, lights are dimmed to a low level. The vast majority of people who need a sleep study don't usually lie awake all night in the lab.

Some organizations offer sleep studies in the home, which sound appealing in many respects but may or may not provide the quantity and quality of information that can be obtained in a fully equipped lab. Before having a home study done, a person should confirm that both the provider and the physician interpreting the study are properly credentialed. Because a sleep study can be expensive (five hundred to one thousand dollars or more), it is also important to check with one's medical insurance provider before having it done, because many plans have restrictions or may require prior authorization.

Sleep apnea

It is estimated that as many as 18 million Americans have **sleep apnea**, which is characterized by interruptions of breathing lasting ten seconds or longer (in

HELPING YOUR DOCTOR TRACK DOWN YOUR SLEEP PROBLEM

Like any health concern that you bring to a health-care provider, a good history is extremely important as the first step toward finding causes and solutions. A complaint such as "I can't sleep" is a starting place, but your doctor needs much more information than that. Before the appointment, be prepared to offer some basic facts. (You may want to write them down.)

- How long have you had the problem?
- Do you have trouble falling asleep, staying asleep, or both?
- How long does it take you to fall asleep?
- How many times do you wake up during the night? Do you go right back to sleep, or do you stay awake (and if so, for how long)?
- Does anything specific awaken you during the night?
- What time do you normally go to bed? What time do you normally get up? Are these times different on weekends or days off?
- Do you feel refreshed in the morning?
- Do you become drowsy during the day if you have to sit still (as in a meeting) or while driving?
- Do you know if you snore?
- Has anyone (spouse or roommate) noticed any pauses in your breathing while asleep?
- Do you use caffeine, tobacco products, or alcohol? How much, and when?
- Are you taking any medications (prescription or nonprescription) or supplements?
- Are there any major stresses or changes in your life at this time?

It may be helpful to keep a simple diary for a few days. In the morning, write down when you went to bed, when you got up, and estimates of how long it took to fall asleep, how many times you were awake (and for how long), and how many hours of sleep you got. In the evening, note how you felt during the day and the time and length of any naps you took. ■

some cases, up to two minutes). By far the most common form is called **obstructive sleep apnea (OSA)**, which occurs when soft tissues at the back of the nose, mouth, and throat relax during sleep, gradually obstructing the passage of air flowing into the upper airway. People with this disorder often snore loudly, and as their airways become more obstructed during sleep, the snoring becomes even more pronounced, until breathing stops. The short lapse in breathing causes the level of oxygen in the blood to drop precipitously. This provokes an arousal from sleep, during which the person gasps, coughs, chokes, or snorts as the obstruction clears and breathing resumes. It is possible for breathing to slow down without stopping, which is called **hypopnea**. The severity of sleep apnea is determined by the number of episodes of apnea or hypopnea per hour (five to fifteen is mild, sixteen to thirty is moderate, and more than thirty episodes per hour is severe), as well as by the level to which blood oxygen levels drop during the episodes.

F.Y.I. The words *apnea* and *hypopnea* are derived from the Greek *pneuma,* meaning "breath" or "spirit," a word used frequently in the New Testament. Since the prefix *a-* means "no" or "not," the word *apnea* literally means "no breath." *Hypo-* means "below," so hypopnea literally means "low (or decreased) breath."

A person may slow or stop breathing hundreds of times during the night without awakening and will rarely if ever remember any of these episodes (although he or she may drive a spouse seeking some peace and quiet into another room). Remembered or not, such episodes repeatedly disrupt the normal transitions between sleep stages and the amount of time spent in each sleep phase, so that a person with OSA is usually sleep-deprived even if logging eight or more hours in bed. The obvious consequence is fatigue and drowsiness during the day, especially when sitting still. People with OSA are at increased risk for having an accident at work or while driving, and those with severe cases may actually fall asleep while eating or talking.

Other medical problems linked to sleep apnea are equally important. As many as 50 percent of people with this disorder have high blood pressure (hypertension). Oxygen levels sag whenever breathing stops, which can provoke potentially dangerous irregular heart rhythms, as well as an increased risk for heart attack in people with coronary artery disease. Stroke is also linked to sleep apnea.

Hypertension, heart attack, and stroke are discussed in detail in chapter 3, starting on page 41.

A person who thinks he or she may have sleep apnea should undergo a thorough medical evaluation, not only to assess the primary complaints but also because other health problems (such as high blood pressure, heart disease, and obesity) will usually need to be addressed as well. A sleep study can provide both the diagnosis and an opportunity to try, if appropriate, a widely used treatment option called **continuous positive airway pressure**, or **CPAP**, which can be very helpful for those with moderate to severe sleep apnea. CPAP involves wearing a face mask, with straps extending around the head, that is connected to a machine that increases air pressure in the mouth and throat.

YOU MIGHT HAVE SLEEP APNEA IF . . .

Several factors put people at risk for having sleep apnea, including:

- **Age.** Most people with this condition are over thirty (although children can have this problem as well).
- **Gender.** Men are three times more likely to have this problem than women.
- **Ethnicity.** Sleep apnea is more common among African-Americans, Hispanics, and Pacific Islanders.
- **Obesity.** Most people with this problem are overweight.
- **Neck size.** The presence of extra tissue in obese people can obstruct air flow. The risk for sleep apnea is higher for men whose neck circumference is greater than seventeen inches (for women, greater than sixteen inches).
- **Excessive soft tissue in the mouth and throat.** Enlarged tonsils and adenoids (especially in children), a prominent uvula (the "punching bag" that hangs from the back of the palate), or a large tongue increases the risk.
- **Sleep position.** Sleeping on one's back and using multiple pillows aggravate the collapse of soft tissues that obstruct airflow.
- **Use of alcohol or other sedatives before bedtime.**
- **Smoking.**

The above risk factors do not guarantee that sleep apnea is present, but the following symptoms should definitely raise one's suspicions:

- **Loud snoring during the night and drowsiness during the day.** Not everyone who snores has sleep apnea, nor does everyone who is sleepy during the day. But when these two symptoms occur together, sleep apnea is a very strong possibility.
- **Episodes in which breathing stops for ten seconds or more,** whether a few or many times per hour, especially if they end with gasping or other distressing sounds. Obviously, these must be heard by someone else.

Several other symptoms are common with sleep apnea, but these can have other causes:

- Rarely, if ever, feeling refreshed after sleeping
- Poor concentration, irritability, and fatigue during the day
- Morning headaches
- Tossing and turning during the night

In children, symptoms may be less obvious. Snoring may be present but daytime drowsiness may not. Parents may also notice restless sleep, frequent waking, and poor school performance. ■

This helps keep air passages open and thus reduces or prevents the episodes of obstruction. While using such a contraption during the night may sound unpleasant, most people with sleep apnea do become accustomed to it. More importantly, they nearly always notice an immediate and dramatic improvement the next day: a sense of feeling refreshed, alert, and energetic, and often relieved of morning headaches as well.

Other approaches to treating sleep apnea include:

- **Losing excess weight.** While easier said than done (see chapter 6), this can make a definite difference in both sleep and a number of other health problems.
- **Sleeping on one's side.** One low-tech approach involves attaching a tennis ball to the back of a person's pajama top, either by creating a pocket for it or (for those lacking sewing skills) using duct tape. This simple but effective annoyance prevents one from sleeping on his or her back and therefore keeps the airways unobstructed.
- **Avoiding alcohol and other sedatives, especially before bedtime.**
- **Relieving chronic nasal congestion** with decongestants, cortisone, antihistamine nasal spray, or even surgery when there is a significant but correctable obstruction (such as a deviated septum or nasal polyps).
- **Using certain dental appliances** that sometimes help position the jaw in a way to relieve the obstruction.
- **Surgery to shrink or remove excessive soft tissue in the mouth and throat.** Occasionally other types of surgery, such as removal of large nasal polyps or correction of a congenital facial deformity, may be appropriate. For most people with sleep apnea, it is wise to try other approaches before resorting to a surgical solution. In children, on the other hand, removal of large tonsils and/or adenoids that are interfering with breathing at night may be more appropriate as a first step.

Restless legs syndrome

Restless legs syndrome (RLS) is a disorder affecting 2 to 5 percent of the population. It is often difficult to describe, but for those who have experienced it, the sensation is unmistakable. While sitting quietly at the end of the day or trying to fall asleep, a person with RLS will feel an overwhelming need to move his or her legs in order to relieve an odd crawling, tingling, or prickling sensation, but not pain. (The arms are involved occasionally, but much less often.) Moving, rubbing, or massaging the legs, getting up and walking around, or even taking a hot shower may offer some relief, but usually only temporarily. For many, RLS is little more than a temporary annoyance during a late movie or airline flight, but for some it can prove to be very disruptive to sleep.

Many people with RLS also have what is called **periodic limb movement disorder (PLMD)**, which is characterized by jerking or twitching of arms or legs that can occur as often as every twenty to forty seconds during sleep. These cause interruptions of sleep that can interfere with the quality and cycling of the sleep stages.

RLS is not considered a health risk in itself, except for its tendency to disrupt sleep. Pregnancy, stress, or hormonal changes can cause worsening of symptoms in some people. This disorder can start at any age but tends to worsen in middle-aged and older adults. RLS and PLMD may be the cause of as many as one out of three cases of insomnia in people over sixty. Certain medications can offer relief and may be prescribed after an appropriate evaluation has been carried out.

Narcolepsy

Narcolepsy is a disorder involving almost irresistible "sleep attacks" that can last from a few seconds to more than thirty minutes at a time. Narcolepsy seems to affect the part of the brain that regulates sleep and wakefulness, resulting in the sudden onset of REM sleep during the day, even when a person has had a normal amount of sleep the night before. The sleep attack may be preceded by hallucinations and can be embarrassing—when a person suddenly falls asleep during a social occasion or a class at school, for example—or dangerous, should it occur while one is driving or operating power equipment. Symptoms of narcolepsy commonly begin between puberty and the midtwenties and may be difficult to diagnose. Narcolepsy is associated with a phenomenon called **cataplexy**, in which a person suddenly loses muscle control and falls to the ground. Cataplexy can be brought on by strong emotions such as anger, laughter, or surprise. If all of these weren't irritating enough, people with narcolepsy may also experience **sleep paralysis**, brief periods of inability to move or speak while falling asleep or awakening.

People with narcolepsy should generally avoid night-shift work, irregular bedtimes, heavy meals, or alcohol intake. Once narcolepsy is diagnosed, a number of medications are available to manage these episodes, including stimulants to increase alertness, antidepressants (which help control the other phenomena associated with sleep attacks), and a newer drug called Provigil, which also improves alertness but without the other effects of stimulants.

F.Y.I.

The word *narcolepsy* was coined by combining the prefix *narco,* meaning "numbing" (as in *narcotic*), with the suffix *-lepsy,* meaning "seizure" (as in *epilepsy*). The word *cataplexy* comes from a Greek word meaning "to startle or terrify," suggesting the action of someone suddenly paralyzed by fear.

Parasomnia

A simple definition of **parasomnia** is an unusual (even bizarre) or disturbing behavior occurring during sleep. The more formal definition is a disorder of sleep characterized by unwanted motor, verbal, or experiential phenomena associated with certain sleep stages or transitions. The major categories of parasomnia are nightmares, sleep terrors, REM movement disorder, sleepwalking, and sleep talking.

At one time or another we have all experienced **nightmares**—frightening or unpleasant dreams that disrupt sleep. They are more common among the young than among adults, occurring in 35 to 45 percent of children between the ages of two and eighteen. Nightmares occur during REM sleep and are more common later in the sleep period. The dreams usually involve some sort of danger or threat. Upon awakening, a child having the nightmare is usually alert and aware of the present surroundings. Nightmares can be brought on by fever, illness, or certain medications but may also be related to stress or some other physically or psychologically traumatic event. For a child, some calm reassurance from Mom or Dad that the particular subject of the nightmare (the monster in the closet, the space alien, or whatever) isn't a true threat is very important, especially for a younger child who is still learning what is real and what isn't. We will look at nightmares in small children in more detail later in this chapter.

Night terrors (or **sleep terrors**) involve the sudden awakening from an early phase of deep sleep with physical behavior associated with fright and intense fear, including screaming, thrashing, jabbering, and even fighting with whomever enters the room. Night terrors occur in 2 to 4 percent of young children (the first episode usually between the ages of two and four) and typically last ten to thirty minutes, after which the child usually goes back to sleep. Because night terrors occur during deep sleep (stage 3 or 4), the child will have no memory of his outburst, unlike his parents, who may lie awake for quite a while trying to calm down after the uproar is over. Fortunately, night terrors do not commonly continue into adulthood. (When they occur in adults, they may be difficult to distinguish from agitated sleepwalking.) We will take a closer look at night terrors (and the best way to manage them) later in this chapter.

Sleepwalking, like night terrors, is probably a malfunction of the deeper phases of non-REM sleep. It occurs more commonly in childhood—the peak age is between four and eight—although if it persists into adolescence or adulthood, sleepwalking can be more dangerous. Episodes tend to occur earlier rather than later in the night. A glassy-eyed sleepwalker may wander aimlessly, carry objects around the house, get something to eat, urinate in an unusual location, go outside, and (when older) even attempt to drive. In children, no intervention is really needed other than to protect the sleepwalker from injury. A frequent sleepwalker may need additional safeguards, such as locking windows and doors and placing an alarm on the bedroom door. Sleepwalking adults who have had an injury (or a narrow escape) may be candidates for a bedtime medication that can effectively limit the number of episodes or stop them altogether.

Sleep talking is a vocalization at night, which may range from a few words of nonsense to entire speeches. It is a harmless and usually temporary phenomenon, although it may startle or even frighten others within earshot. Sleep talking is sometimes associated with stress or an illness but does not need specific treatment.

Episodes of **REM movement disorder** (or **REM sleep behavior disorder**) resemble sleepwalking run amok. These are, in fact, very different events. Remember that during REM sleep the brain is very active generating dreams, but paradoxically (and for our safety) the body is virtually paralyzed. (REM sleep is, in fact, also called **active sleep** because so much is going on in the brain and **paradoxical sleep** because muscles are so quiet at the same time.) REM movement disorder demonstrates why this is so important. A person with this problem literally acts out his dreams, which unfortunately are not usually peaceful. Instead, the typical dreams involved in REM movement disorder seem to have been dialed in by a hyped-up video-game programmer. They are intense, full of action, often violent, and their dreamer may respond not merely with walking and talking, but with yelling, punching, kicking, jumping out of bed, running around, and at times even injuring himself or others.

While REM movement disorder may affect men or women at any age, more than 85 percent of people with this problem are men over fifty. Usually the person's temperament while awake in no way resembles the wild behavior that occurs during these episodes. Unfortunately, at least half of the people with this problem have other neurological disorders, such as Parkinson's disease, narcolepsy, or stroke. In fact, REM movement disorder may be the first manifestation of a different neurological disease that may not become apparent for months or even years. However, once the correct diagnosis has been made, both the sleep disturbance and its unruly manifestations can usually be controlled effectively with bedtime medications.

Sleep Concerns during Infancy and Childhood

Up to this point, this chapter has emphasized sleep patterns and problems in adults. But good sleep is obviously critical to the health and welfare of infants and young children, who may present some unique challenges for their parents at bedtime or nap time. If you have a young child, the following section will help you understand how your son or daughter sleeps—and what you can do to help you both get the sleep you need.

The first three months of life

Whenever we watch a young infant in deep, relaxed slumber, the phrase "sleeping like a baby" is likely to come to mind. Wouldn't it be nice if we could sleep like that?

Well, not exactly.

During the first three months of life, a baby's sleeping patterns are quite different from those she will experience over the rest of her life. A newborn sleeps anywhere from twelve to eighteen hours every day, but this is not unbroken slumber. Her small stomach capacity and her round-the-clock need for nutrients to fuel her rapid growth essentially guarantee that her life will consist of ongoing three- or four-hour cycles of feeding, wakefulness, and sleep. Like it or not, two or three feedings will be on the nighttime agenda at least for the first several weeks.

Furthermore, a newborn's patterns of brain activity during sleep are unique. We have already discussed the cycles of two different types of sleep—rapid eye movement, or REM, and non-REM—throughout the night and noted that adults spend about one-fourth of their sleep in REM sleep and the rest in non-REM. Babies also manifest these types of sleep but spend equal time in each, alternating about every thirty minutes. During non-REM sleep, they appear very relaxed, breathing regularly and moving very little. During REM or active sleep, they seem to come to life, moving arms and legs, changing facial expressions, breathing less regularly, and perhaps making a variety of sounds. They may be experiencing their first dreams during these periods.

Adults and children older than about three months pass through the increasing depths of non-REM sleep before they enter a REM phase. *But newborns reverse this pattern,* starting with a period of REM sleep before moving into non-REM stages. As a result, the new baby who has just fallen asleep can easily be awakened for twenty minutes or more until she moves into her non-REM phases.

This accounts for those character-building situations in which some parents feel they are dealing with a little time bomb with a short fuse. A fed, dry, and apparently tired baby fusses and resists before finally succumbing to sleep after prolonged cuddling and rocking. But when placed ever so gently into the cradle or crib, she suddenly startles and sounds off like a fire alarm. The cycle is repeated over and over until everyone, baby included, is thoroughly exhausted and frustrated. This baby isn't getting past her initial REM phase and therefore is easily aroused. The problem usually resolves itself by the time the baby is three months old; at that time, she begins to shift gears and enter non-REM sleep first.

Helping a new baby enter the slumber zone

If you have a newborn and don't want to wait twelve weeks for a good night's sleep, there are two basic but quite different approaches to helping your baby fall asleep. Each approach has advocates who tend to view their ideas as vital to a happy, stable life for both parent and child while seeing the other as producing troubled, insecure babies. In reality, both have something to offer, and neither will work for every baby-parent combination.

One method calls for you to be intimately and directly involved in all phases of your baby's sleep. Proponents of this approach recommend that he be nursed, cuddled, rocked, and held continuously until he has fallen asleep for at least twenty minutes. He can then be put down in his customary sleeping place, which may even be your bed.

The primary advantage of this approach is that it can help a baby navigate through drowsiness and REM sleep in the comfort and security of closeness to one or both parents. Those who favor it claim that a baby does best when he has more or less continuous contact with a warm body, having just exited from inside one.

Those who challenge this approach argue that a baby may become so accustomed to being "manipulated" into sleep that he will not be able to fall asleep on his own for months or even years. Every bedtime or nap time will thus turn into a major project, and parents (or whoever is taking care of the baby) will be hostage to a prolonged routine of feeding and rocking well into the toddler years.

A second approach suggests that a baby can and should learn to "self-calm" and fall asleep on his own. Rather than nursing him to sleep, you should feed the baby thirty to sixty minutes before a nap or bedtime and then put him down before he is asleep. He may seem restless for fifteen or twenty minutes and may even begin crying. But he'll likely settle and fall asleep if left alone.

Proponents of self-calming feel this approach frees Mom and Dad from hours of effort and allows the baby to become more flexible and independent.

Critics argue that leaving a baby alone in a bassinet or crib represents cruel and unusual treatment at such a young age. Some even suggest that this repeated separation from parental closeness leads to sleep disorders (or worse) later in life.

You'll be relieved to know that neither of these methods was carved in stone on Mount Sinai along with the Ten Commandments. Parents need to tailor their approach to each baby's unique temperament and style and to their (and their family's) needs. When dealing with newborns and very young infants, a fair amount of adjusting and pragmatism is not only wise but also necessary. "Let's see if this works" is a much more useful approach than "We *have* to do it this way." Most babies give clues when they are ready to sleep—yawning, droopy eyelids, fussiness—and you will want to become familiar with your child's particular signals. If he is giving you these cues, lay him down in a quiet, dimly lit setting and see if he will fall asleep. If he is clearly unhappy after fifteen or twenty minutes, check on him. Assuming that he is fed and dry, comfort him for a while and try again. If your baby is having problems settling himself, especially during the first few weeks of life, do not attempt to "train" him to calm himself by letting him cry for long periods of time. *During the first few months of life, it is unwise to let a baby cry indefinitely without tending to him. Babies at this stage of life cannot be spoiled by adults who are very attentive to their needs.*

If you need to help your new baby transition into quiet sleep, any of these time-honored methods may help:

- **Feeding.** Nursing (or a bottle, if using formula) may help induce sleep, especially at the end of the day. However, don't overfeed with formula or, worse, introduce solids such as cereal at this age in hopes of inducing a long snooze. A stomach that is too full will interfere with sleep as much as an empty one. Solids are inappropriate at this age and will not lengthen sleep. Also, never put a baby to bed with a bottle propped in her mouth. Not only can this lead to a choking accident, but it also allows milk to flow into the eustachian tubes (which lead into the middle ears), increasing the risk of ear infections.
- **A rocking chair.** Rocking gently while you cuddle your baby can calm both of you. If this works for your baby, relax and enjoy it. (You may find that a contemporary "glider" rocker is smoother, quieter,

and more comfortable—especially if it has a matching, gliding ottoman for your feet—than Grandma's time-honored oak rocking chair, which might become a little creakier with each passing generation. If you have a baby-supply store near you, sit in a few models to see what suits you and your budget.)

- **A cradle.** This is an alternative to the rocking chair—again, it should be rocked smoothly and gently. A baby swing is also a good option, but it must be one that is appropriately designed for this age group.
- **Swaddling.** Many new babies settle more easily if they are swaddled—wrapped snugly in a light blanket.
- **Quiet sounds.** The whirring of a small fan (not aimed toward the baby), a tape or CD recording of the ocean, or even small devices that generate monotonous white noise may help settle your baby and screen out other sounds in the home. If you are musically inclined, you might choose to play a lovely anthology of lullabies, quiet classical music, or gospel songs and hymns that might soothe your fussy baby.
- **A gentle touch.** Sometimes a simple touch, pat, or massage will help settle a baby who is drowsy in your arms but squirmy in bed.
- **A car ride.** Many babies routinely fall asleep when they are gently and continuously jostled during a car ride. Occasionally, a frustrated parent who is dealing with a wakeful baby during the night may take her out for a 3 A.M. automobile trip—although this does not guarantee that she will stay asleep once the ride is over. Since staggering out into the night isn't much fun, especially in the dead of winter, this measure should be considered a last resort for a very difficult sleeper.

All of the above, except for the white noise and the swaddling, involve ongoing parental activity to help settle a baby. Occasionally, however, prolonged rocking, jostling, patting, and singing may be counterproductive, keeping a baby awake when she needs *less* stimulation in order to settle down. If a few weeks of heroic efforts to induce sleep don't seem to be working, it may be time to take another look at self-calming. Steps that may help the self-calming process when a baby has been put down but is not yet asleep include the following:

- Guide a baby's flailing hand toward her mouth. Many infants settle effectively by sucking on their hand or fingers.
- Identify a simple visual target for the baby's gaze, such as a single-colored surface; a small, nonbreakable mirror in her crib; or a nearby window or night-light. Then place her in a position where she can see it. (Complex visual targets such as moving mobiles or busy patterns are not as useful for settling during the earliest weeks, especially when a baby is very tired.)

What about sleeping through the night?

Newborns do not typically sleep in long stretches during the first several weeks of life, nor do they know the difference between day and night. By two months, however, they are capable of lasting for longer periods without a feeding. You may go through the pulse-quickening experience of awakening at dawn and realizing that your baby didn't sound off in the middle of the night. "Is he okay?" is the first breathless concern, followed by both relief and quiet exultation: "He slept through the night!"

By three months, much to their parents' relief, a majority of babies have established a regular pattern of uninterrupted sleep for seven or eight hours each night. However, some will take longer to reach this milestone. A few actually drift in the wrong direction, sleeping peacefully through most of the day and then suddenly snapping awake—often fidgeting and fussing—just when bleary-eyed parents are longing for some rest. If you have a baby who favors the wee hours, you will want to give him some gentle but definite nudges to use the night for sleeping:

- Make a specific effort to increase his time awake during the day. Don't let him fall asleep during or right after eating, but instead provide some gentle stimulation. Talk or sing to him, lock eyes, change his clothes, play with his hands and feet, rub his back, or let Grandma or Grandpa coo over him. Don't make loud noises to startle him, and do not—under any circumstances—shake him. (Sudden movements of a baby's head can cause physical damage to the brain.) Let him nap only after he has been awake for a while after feeding. This can also help prevent a baby from becoming dependent on a feeding to fall asleep.
- If your baby is sleeping for long periods during the day and fitfully at night, consider gently awakening him while he is in one of his active sleep phases when a nap has lasted more than three or four hours.
- By contrast, make nighttime interactions, especially those middle-of-the-night feedings—incredibly boring. Keep the lights low, the conversation minimal, and the diaper change (if needed) routine. This is not the time to play.
- Remember that babies frequently squirm, grunt, and even seem to awaken briefly during their REM sleep phases. Try to avoid intervening and interacting with him during these times, because you may unknowingly awaken your baby when he was just shifting gears into the next phase of sleep.
- If your baby tends to awaken by the dawn's early light and you don't care to do likewise, try installing shades or blinds to block out the first rays of sunlight. Don't assume that his rustling around in bed necessarily means he is waking up for good. Wait awhile before tending to him, because he may go back to sleep. Sometimes, however, he will wake up with the local roosters no matter what you do, at which point you may

want to consider adjusting your schedule to follow the famous "early to bed, early to rise" proverb until a few more months pass.

Where should your baby sleep?

By the time your baby arrives home for the first night, you will have had to address a basic question: Will she sleep in your bed right next to you, in a cradle or bassinet next to your bed, or in her own room? There are advocates for each of these arrangements.

Those who espouse sleeping with a baby (a practice often called "co-sleeping" or "shared sleep") point out that this is widely practiced throughout the

IF YOU'RE GOING TO SHARE YOUR BED WITH AN INFANT

Later in this chapter we outline several measures to reduce the risk of sudden infant death syndrome (SIDS). One of the key points is that an infant needs a safe sleep environment in which suffocation or disrupted breathing is unlikely to occur. Critics of "shared sleep" argue that the parents' bed is more likely to be unsafe than a properly equipped crib. Proponents of this practice claim otherwise, provided that a number of important safeguards are followed.

In one sense, the critics are right: Many common sleeping environments for older children or adults are not appropriate for infants. *If you are thinking about "co-sleeping" with your baby, you must be willing and able to abide strictly with all of the following:*

- You must use a wide bed with a firm mattress. Do not sleep with your baby on a water bed, sofa, or beanbag chair.
- Do not use fluffy bedding or cover your baby with your comforter.
- Your baby must sleep on her back.
- There must not be any gaps between the mattress and a wall or bed frame in which your baby might become trapped.
- The baby should sleep next to her mother, not between her mother and father.
- Don't let your baby fall out of bed. If the baby is going to be positioned on the side of a mattress from which she could potentially fall, use a mesh guardrail that fits flush against the mattress.
- Do not sleep with your baby if you are using alcohol, sedatives, sleeping pills, or any medication that might affect your ability to awaken.
- Don't sleep with your baby if you are a smoker. The risk of sudden infant death syndrome associated with co-sleeping is significantly higher among smokers. Important: Exposure to cigarette smoke increases *any* baby's risk of dying of SIDS.
- Older siblings or babysitters should not sleep with the baby.
- Don't leave a baby sleeping unattended in an adult bed. ■

world. These proponents claim that it enhances parent-infant bonding, facilitates breast-feeding, and gives the newborn a sense of security and comfort she won't feel in a crib.

Shared sleep advocates also argue that this practice reduces the risk of sudden infant death syndrome (SIDS), although the National Institute of Child Health and Human Development states that there is no scientific proof to support this claim.[5]

In fact, some researchers believe that adult bedding can—in rare instances—contribute to SIDS. A newborn should sleep on his back on a fitted sheet, not on soft bedding materials (such as down mattresses or feather beds) or on a water bed.

Sleeping in an adult bed can pose other dangers to infants and toddlers as well. In 2002, the U.S. Consumer Product Safety Commission (CPSC) issued a warning about the potential hazards of infants sleeping in adult beds, citing reports of more than 100 deaths of children under the age of two during a three-year period that appeared to be specifically associated with physical features of adult beds.[6]

If you are thinking about sharing your bed with a newborn or young infant, be sure that your bedding and sleeping arrangements meet specific safety criteria, such as those outlined in the sidebar on pages 770–771 "Preventing Sudden Infant Death Syndrome," and that pillows, blankets, quilts, and other coverings are kept away from your baby's face.

One of the tricky issues for parents who share their bed with one or more children is deciding when and how to reclaim their bed for themselves. Most children are more than happy to sleep with Mom and Dad well into or beyond their toddler years, and making the transition to their own bed may be easier said than done. Parents who routinely allow one or more babies and children in bed with them for months or years should regularly take stock of the effect this custom is having on their marriage. Regaining sexual intimacy after the birth of a child normally requires some time and effort for both parents. It will be far more challenging if there are more than two bodies in the bed.

Many parents prefer to place their newborn in a cradle next to their bed. This arrangement may be useful with a newborn who has a difficult time settling during the night. It prevents one or both parents from having to get in and out of bed in response to repeated bouts of crying or fussing. These infants and their parents may have an easier time if they sleep in close proximity so that Mom and Dad can offer feeding and comfort as often as needed without having to get up several times throughout the night.

Unfortunately, when young children sleep in your room—whether in your bed or a nearby cradle or crib—your sleep, intimacy, and privacy are likely to be disrupted. New babies don't quietly nod off to sleep at 10 P.M. and wake up calmly eight hours later. They also don't typically sleep silently during the few hours between feedings. As they pass through their REM sleep phases, they tend to move around and make all sorts of noises, often sounding as if they're waking up. All of this activity isn't easy to ignore, especially for new parents who tend to be tuned in and concerned, if not downright worried, about how their new arrival is doing. Unless you learn to screen out these distractions and respond to your child only when she is truly awake and in need of your attention, you will find yourself woefully short on sleep and patience within a few days.

Before bringing your baby into your room at bedtime, be sure to consider the potential effect on your relationship with your spouse as well. If Mom and Dad are equally enthused about having a new bedmate, great. But many young couples aren't prepared for the demands a new baby places on them. A father who feels that his wife's attention is already consumed by the baby's needs may begin to feel completely displaced if the baby is in his bed too.

If you prefer to have your baby sleep in another room but wonder whether you will hear her if she needs you, don't worry. An infant who is truly awake, hungry, and crying during the night is difficult to ignore. And new parents are uniquely tuned in to their baby's nighttime vocalizing.

The advantage of having your child sleep in another room is that you will be less likely to be aroused repeatedly through the night by your baby's assorted movements and noises during sleep. You are also less likely to intervene too quickly during a restless period, which can accidentally interrupt a baby's transition from active to quiet sleep. Having your baby sleep in another room can also increase her nighttime adaptability, allowing her to go to sleep in a variety of environments.

If you are truly concerned about hearing your baby when she first begins to cry, you can purchase an inexpensive wireless electronic baby monitor, which will allow you to hear what's happening in the nursery long before crying reaches even a modest intensity. In fact, the monitors can be so sensitive that you may find yourself hearing (and possibly being kept awake by) a lot of false alarms as your baby stirs and makes a variety of sounds without actually awakening, just as if she were in the room with you. And, like the rooming-in arrangement, you will have to train yourself not to respond immediately to every rustle or chirp you hear over the speaker, because you may unintentionally awaken a baby who is simply transitioning from one phase of sleep to another.

F.Y.I.

A note of caution with monitors: It would be unwise to leave your baby in a place where you would be totally unable to hear her and then rely on a monitor to be your electronic ears. If the monitor failed for some reason, your baby might lie uncomfortable, crying and unattended for an extended period of time.

As with the techniques you choose to help your baby settle down to sleep, you will need to determine which sleeping arrangement works best for your family and be flexible about the various possibilities. Moreover, it is important that parents continue to communicate with each other about this subject. If

Mom is the one getting up to nurse a fussy baby and as a result spends more hours in the baby's room than in her own bed, Dad may need to assume a larger share of the nighttime duties. He could, for example, bring the baby to Mom for nursing and then return her to her crib when the feeding is done. Similarly, if Dad is feeling an increasing distance from Mom because of a baby in their bed, Mom may need to be willing to empty the nighttime nest of offspring.

Three to twelve months: establishing a routine

Between the fourth and sixth months, your baby will probably settle into a more predictable sleeping routine. Two naps during the day, one in the morning and one in the afternoon, are a good habit to encourage and maintain. These may last from one to three hours, and at this age you need not awaken your baby from a long nap unless it seems to be interfering with his sleep at night. (Some infants continue to catnap during this period.) Between two and four months or shortly thereafter, your baby should be skipping a night feeding. By six months, he should be able to handle an eight-hour stretch without being fed unless he was premature or is exceptionally small. But whether this translates into uninterrupted sleep will depend both on your baby and your sleeping arrangements.

If he's down for the night by 8 P.M., he may be genuinely hungry at 4 A.M. But at that hour, unless he's sounding off with a sustained howl, you might want to wait a few minutes to see if he might go back to sleep. Delaying his bedtime may help extend his and your uninterrupted sleep in the morning, but a decision to allow him to stay up later must be weighed against other family needs. Ideally, before he is put to bed he should be given some time to wind down with quiet activities: a feeding, some cuddling, some singing, and perhaps a bath. With a routine, he will begin to associate these particular activities with bedtime and a surrender to sleep. If at all possible, have different people work through this process with him so he won't come to expect that Mom or Dad is the only person in the world who can bring the day to a close.

Now is a good time to let him learn to fall asleep on his own if he hasn't been doing so already. When he is drowsy but not yet asleep, lay him down, pat him gently, and leave the room. Make sure there's a night-light on so he can see familiar surroundings. If he fusses for more than a few minutes, you can come back for a brief reassurance (perhaps offering some gentle patting)—but not a full-blown recap of the nighttime routine. If he persists, let a little more time go by before you return. If he will not stop crying and you can't stand to let it continue, do whatever it takes to get him to sleep and then try again at a later date, perhaps on a weekend night when you have some flexibility in your evening and morning schedules.

If he isn't able to fall asleep by himself by six months of age, the window of opportunity for learning this skill may not be open again for several months. After six months, he is likely to begin a normal phase known as **separation anxiety**, in which a nightly howl may erupt when you or his closest caregivers are out of his sight, especially at bedtime. As a result, if after six months he's still used to being nursed, held, and rocked through several rounds of "Hey Diddle Diddle" until he's sound asleep, you can plan on repeating this ritual for months on end unless you are prepared to endure a vigorous and prolonged protest.

Remember that your baby's nighttime activity may include one or more awakenings that do not necessarily need your attention. If you rush into your baby's room to feed, cuddle, and rock him with every sound he produces, he will become quite accustomed to this first-class room service, and you may find that he is rather reluctant to give it up. Obviously, if he sounds truly miserable and is keeping everyone awake, do whatever is necessary to comfort him and calm things down. At this age it is still better to err on the side of too much attention than too little.

PREVENTING SUDDEN INFANT DEATH SYNDROME

For many years, **sudden infant death syndrome (SIDS)**, also called crib death, has been the subject of intense research. While the exact cause is uncertain, SIDS involves a disturbance of breathing regulation during sleep. It is relatively rare, occurring in two or three out of every thousand newborns, most often between the first and sixth months, with a peak incidence between the second and third months. For unknown reasons, it is more common in the winter months.

SIDS is more common in males with low birth weight and in premature infants of both sexes. Breast-fed babies seem to have a reduced risk. In addition, some potential contributing factors to SIDS can be minimized by taking a few basic preventive measures:

- **Stay completely away from cigarettes** during pregnancy, and don't allow anyone to smoke in your home after your baby is born.
- **Lay your baby down on his back.** For decades, child-care guidebooks recommended that new babies sleep on their stomachs, based on the assumption that this would prevent them from choking on any material they might unexpectedly spit up. However, recent evidence suggests that this position might be a risk factor for SIDS. *Therefore, it is now recommended that a newborn be positioned on his back to sleep.* Exceptions to this guideline are made for premature infants, as well as for some infants with deformities of the face that might cause difficulty breathing when lying faceup. In addition, your doctor may advise you against laying your baby on his back if he spits up excessively. If you have any questions about sleeping position, check with your baby's doctor. Sometime after four months of age, your baby will begin

After a few months pass, however, you can become more hard-nosed if he seems intent on having a social hour several times a night. By the time he reaches the six-month mark, he shouldn't need any middle-of-the-night feedings. If you continue offering them, you'll be providing bleary-eyed calories and companionship but not meeting any nutritional needs. It's certainly appropriate to check that he isn't ill, grossly wet or soiled, or tangled in his blanket. But the encounter should be quick and quiet.

If your infant is older than nine months and is still routinely rousing everyone from sleep two or three times a night, you may want to consider more deliberate measures to bring this behavior to a close. This would involve picking a time (usually on a weekend) when you can say good night and then resolve not to return until the next morning—if you can handle it—no matter how often and how long the crying goes on. *Keep in mind that returning to your baby after a*

rolling over on his own, at which point he will determine his own sleeping positions. By this age, fortunately, SIDS is extremely rare.

- **Put your baby to sleep on a safe surface.** Don't place pillows or any soft bedding material other than a fitted sheet under the baby. His head or face might become accidentally buried in the soft folds (especially if he happens to be lying facedown), which could lead to suffocation. Sheepskin, down mattresses, and feather beds pose a similar risk. Don't put your baby to sleep on a wavy water bed or beanbag chair. Even on one of these plastic surfaces, a baby whose face shifts to the wrong position could suffocate.
- **Don't overbundle your baby.** Overcompensating for the cold of winter by turning up the thermostat and wrapping a baby in several layers of clothing should be avoided. If he looks or feels hot and sweaty, start peeling off layers until he appears more comfortable.

A few parents experience the terror of seeing their baby stop breathing, either momentarily or long enough to begin turning blue. It is obviously important in such cases to begin infant CPR and call 911 if he does not start breathing on his own. A careful evaluation by your doctor or at the emergency room is mandatory. It is also likely that this baby will be sent home with an **apnea monitor**, which will sound off if a breath is not taken after a specified number of seconds.

Parents who have suffered the loss of an infant for any reason must work through a profound grieving process. When SIDS is the cause, many parents feel a great sense of guilt as well as intense anxiety over the safety of their other children. It is important that they obtain support from family, church, and, if available, a local support group for families who have dealt with such a devastating loss. ■

prolonged bout of crying may convince him that endurance pays off. Obviously, you would not want to try this "commando" approach with a child who is sick, or on a hot summer night when the windows are open, or when you need to be wide-awake the next day, or (most important) if *both* parents are not wholeheartedly ready for it.

You should greet your baby in the morning with smiles, hugs, and reassurance. Yes, indeed, you love him as much as the day is long, but nighttime is for sleeping. Normally after three or four nights, he will get the picture and sleep through the night thereafter (unless, of course, something else is wrong). Obviously, if interrupted sleep doesn't bother anyone, you may choose to leave things alone. Eventually your child will sleep through the night on his own, but with some children it may take many more months before this occurs spontaneously and (hopefully) routinely.

Toddlers and two-year-olds: dealing with bedtime resistance

By her first birthday, your child should have been sleeping through the night for some time. If not, take note that by now her nocturnal awakenings aren't the result of any nutritional needs. Instead, she has become accustomed to the fact that having company or a snack feels good during the night. Why go back to sleep when there are other pleasantries to enjoy?

If your child is otherwise well, you can usually establish uninterrupted sleep for everyone within a few days as just described, once you decide to take the plunge.

Even a seasoned all-night sleeper, however, may depart from her pattern during an illness, while on a trip, after a move, or because of a bad dream. Under these circumstances, you'll need to provide care and comfort (though not snacks, unless you have been specifically directed by the doctor to push fluids when she is sick) until things settle down and then nudge her back toward her old habits.

For many toddlers the *Good Ship Slumber* may be rocked in other ways. At some point, you're likely to run into bedtime resistance, manifested either by winsome appeals (requests for another kiss, one last drink, and in subsequent months, answers to riddles of the universe) or by outright rebellion against getting or staying in bed. Some of this may arise from separation anxiety, from negativism, or simply from the fact that other people are up doing interesting things, and lying in a crib or bed seems awfully boring by comparison. You may be tempted to take the path of least resistance and let her decide when she's ready to sleep—in other words, when she eventually collapses from sheer exhaustion. This is definitely a bad idea, for a number of reasons:

- You need to spend time with older children (if you have any) without an increasingly tired and irritable toddler wandering around.
- You need to spend time with your mate or by yourself without *any* children wandering around.

- Your toddler needs the sleep—a good ten or eleven hours at night, which probably won't happen if she's staying up until your bedtime.

If not already in place, developing a fixed bedtime and standard bedtime routine will be an important task this year. Even if her vocabulary is limited, you can talk her through the steps you choose: bath, jammies, story, song, prayer—all carried out in a manner that winds her down. A raucous wrestling match or chasing the dog right before bedtime probably won't help set the stage for turning in. Keep in mind that whatever bedtime routine you establish (including one that takes one or two hours to complete) may become entrenched and expected every night for years to come.

As with a blessing before meals, your child can learn the routine of a short bedtime prayer even before she understands the words or the theology. Over the coming months and years, however, this brief but important moment should take on new meaning and not become a singsong patter repeated every night for no apparent reason.

As with infants, your toddler should be placed in her crib or bed sleepy but not asleep. If she becomes accustomed to falling asleep on the sofa, floor, or your bed, she is more likely to resist signing off on her own pillow—both at bedtime *and* during the night.

Parents who have maintained a "family bed" through the first year should take the baby's first birthday as an occasion to review the current sleeping arrangements. Does your child need a parental body next to her to fall or stay asleep? (If one or both parents were to go away on a retreat for a night or two, would there be a problem?) More importantly, how is the presence of a much larger and more mobile baby affecting your sleep and your intimacy? Mom and Dad should be in complete agreement about this situation or seek to resolve any difference of opinion if they are not—even if counseling is needed. Serious and damaging rifts in a marital relationship can develop if one spouse feels displaced physically and emotionally by a child who is taking over an ever-increasing area of bed space. In general, if either Mom or Dad feels that it's time for the baby to sleep elsewhere, the other parent should oblige—not only out of respect for the other's feelings, but also in recognition that the marital relationship needs to be nurtured and preserved.

At their first birthday, most children are still logging three to four hours of daytime sleep, usually in two naps. The amount of daytime sleep will decline to two or three hours over the next year, and as a result, the morning nap will eventually phase out. When your toddler shifts to a one-nap-per-day routine, don't start too late in the afternoon or you may increase her bedtime resistance. (Who wants to go to bed after just getting up?) And, though she may seem intent on playing through the entire afternoon, don't be conned into eliminating nap time altogether, even if she resists it. Without daytime sleep, afternoons will probably be more notable for combat than for companionship.

Two-year-olds generally need nine to thirteen hours of sleep a day, including about eleven hours at night and a two-hour nap at midday. Some will still do best with two shorter naps, while others will regularly fight nap time with a vengeance. How long you continue a daytime sleep routine will depend upon its impact on your child. If she resists but eventually falls asleep for an hour or two, most likely the nap is worth maintaining. Similarly, if she turns into a three-foot-tall tyrant by the end of the day whenever she skips her nap, you should overrule her objections to a siesta. The time to phase out naps, whether this year or later, will arrive when she can regularly make it through the entire day without having a prolonged attitude meltdown.

Your more important assignment will be to maintain a bedtime routine in the face of increasing resistance, which in some children can become impressive. Some of the turbulence can arise from the following issues:

- **It's not her idea.** The recurring cry for many two-year-olds will continue to be a heartfelt rendition of Frank Sinatra's theme song "My Way." If the all-important question "Who's in charge here?" has yet to be settled, bedtime can be one of the great battlegrounds in a contest of wills between you and your child. You will certainly want to make sure that bedtime is a calm, relaxing, reassuring time of day and that other concerns are dealt with. But ultimately someone will have to decide when it's bedtime, and it shouldn't be your two-year-old.
- **Separation anxiety.** As independent as she may want to be, she may not feel she's gotten quite enough time and attention by the end of the day. Or she may be unsettled about being away from you, even in the familiar surroundings of your home. Often this can be resolved by making sure that the bedtime routine isn't rushed; by providing security/comfort objects (a favorite toy or blanket); by playing quiet, soothing music in her room; or by leaving the door to her room open—provided that other sounds in the home won't keep her awake. If she hears the family having noisy fun without her, she will have little interest in lying down and closing her eyes.
- **Other fears.** Your child is reaching an age at which she may become worried about scary sounds she hears, funny shapes in the closet, or darkness itself. A night-light in her room or light from the next room coming through an open doorway is likely to be a necessary fixture at this age and for a number of years to come. Unexpected loud noises, such as a catfight outside her window, a siren passing nearby, or a booming thunderstorm, may frighten a small child and require some hands-on comforting. Your two-year-old may also be unsettled about what went on during the day. Noisy arguments between parents are alarming, even when she can't understand their content. A move to new living quarters, a new baby in the house, the first trip to a preschool or day-care facility, or changes in family routines related

to one or both parents' job schedules may also rock her sense of security. Ongoing overtures for attention at bedtime may signal a need for more (or more reassuring) attention during the daylight hours.

New sleeping quarters

One of the important transitions most two-year-olds must navigate is the move from crib to "real bed." This will become necessary when the side rail of his crib reaches to less than three-quarters of his standing height (usually at about thirty-six inches), since the risk of scaling the rail and falling out increases after this point. The arrival of a younger sibling may also prompt the move.

The move to a bed can be a happy occasion, an indication that he is a "big boy" and no longer a baby. If he is unhappy about leaving the crib, affirming how grown-up he is may help change his opinion. You may help him gain more enthusiasm for moving to a bed if you let him help pick it out (assuming you are shopping for one) or at least choose fun sheets and pillowcases to adorn his new sleeping quarters.

One potential drawback of a bed is that it allows your toddler to get up if he doesn't want to stay put. A more unsettling possibility is that your toddler may decide to wander around the house—or even go outside—when everyone is asleep. You may be able to limit these nighttime explorations (and certainly prevent accidental falls from bed) by installing a simple safety rail. However, a determined toddler can easily climb around the rail and get out of bed. For this reason, if size and circumstances permit, it may be wise to maintain the crib until he is closer to three years of age and possesses a little more wisdom and training. If you aren't already doing so, keep all doors and windows locked.

Night terrors and nightmares

Night terrors are unpleasant events that affect 2 to 4 percent of children (more commonly boys) and scare the daylights out of everyone who sees them. During the middle of the night a confused, wild-eyed child will suddenly begin screaming, kicking, thrashing, sweating, moaning, and jabbering incoherently. His heart will be pounding and his breathing rapid—and so will yours. He may climb out of bed, stumble around and injure himself, and if he is older, try to run out of the house. What is especially unsettling during a night terror is that your child won't respond to you or even seem to know you. When you attempt to calm him, he may thrash more violently and try to push you away.

Despite all of the wild activity, children do not actually awaken during a night terror. They are instead having a disordered arousal from deep (phase 3 or 4 non-REM) sleep. The first episode typically occurs between the ages of two and four years, and other family members may have done the same thing during their toddler years.

Your job during a night terror is to sit tight through the interminable ten to thirty minutes, provide soothing reassurance that you're there and that he's okay. Hold him if he'll let you, and prevent him from hurting himself. You may also need to calm down any older children who have been awakened by the commotion and are witnessing this wild event. *Don't leave him alone,* because there is a very real risk of injury, and *don't try to wake him up.* He is actually in a state of sleep that does not readily progress to wakefulness, and shaking or speaking forcefully to him ("Wake up! Wake up!") will only compound his (and your) agitation. Furthermore, if you succeed in bringing him to full consciousness, he will be unhappy and irritable and may have difficulty going back to sleep. Instead, if you sit tight and stay cool, you will be surprised at how quickly the night terror ends once it has run its course. Your child will suddenly fall back to sleep, and in the morning he will have no memory of the previous night's uproar. You, on the other hand, may stare at the ceiling for a while as your adrenaline surge calms down.

Your child may have only one night terror, or you may have to endure many episodes before he outgrows them. Identifying a cause may be difficult, although it is possible that a sudden pain, such as a cramp in the abdomen, during the wrong phase of sleep may set off a night terror. In rare cases, night terrors may be frequent enough to require preventive medication prescribed by a physician.

Nightmares are different from night terrors in all respects. They are scary dreams, occurring during active (REM) sleep late in the night or very early in the morning. In contrast to the bug-eyed thrashing of the night terror, a child who cries out after a nightmare will be wide-awake, aware, and responsive to your presence and comfort. Instead of the sudden return to sleep that follows a night terror, a nightmare may leave a child unwilling or unable to fall back to sleep.

Whether or not she can tell you about the dream will depend upon her age and vocabulary. Even if she can't fill you in on the details, it's safe to assume that whatever she experienced was frightening and that her need for comfort is genuine. In particular, she will need your reassurance that the dream was not real, a difficult concept to grasp at this age. A few moments of prayer can also help impart the idea that Jesus is truly in charge and looking after your child whether she's asleep or awake. Be sure, however, that you are not contributing to the problem by reciting "Now I Lay Me Down to Sleep." This poem's infamous lines "If I should die before I wake, I pray the Lord my soul to take" are alarming and inappropriate for children.

How you deal with nightmares will depend on your perception of what is going on. A child who suddenly awakens at 4 A.M. crying and frightened will need conversation and cuddling. When she was younger, you may have worked diligently to end routine nighttime awakenings by holding back during the wee hours. But after a real nightmare, your reluctance should be set aside.

Rarely you may find it expedient to let her fall asleep in your bed if she won't calm down any other way. However, if she repeatedly wanders into the family room a half hour after bedtime and calmly announces that she "had a bad dream" or crawls into your bed night after night using *nightmare* as the password, she may be trying to change the bedtime ground rules, and a more businesslike approach will be needed.

Unlike night terrors, nightmares are influenced far more by daytime input. The adage about turning off the scary movie because "it might give you nightmares" is certainly appropriate for small children, who cannot readily distinguish reality from fantasy. Because television, videotapes, and video games can bring hair-raising images before your toddler's undiscerning eyes, you will need to exercise nonstop vigilance in this area. Even films such as *Pinocchio* or *Snow White and the Seven Dwarfs,* widely considered to be childhood classics, contain sequences that could definitely scare a toddler.

Dealing with bedtime confrontations

All the factors just described can add up to bedtime confrontations. If your toddler is no longer in a crib, not feeling the least bit sleepy, unhappy about missing out on grown-up company, worried about bad dreams, or in a challenging mood, he may try to get up several times after he's been tucked in. Another drink of water, another trip to the potty, curiosity, boredom, interesting aromas from someone's snack, a "tummy ache," a claim of a "bad dream" (probably bogus if he just went to bed), or anything else he might think of may all be reasons he feels compelled to exit his bed and his room.

As in every other area in which you are shaping your child's behavior, a consistent response—loving but firm—will be necessary. Once he has been through the bedtime routine, any further interactions should be calm, brief, and businesslike. "It's time for bed" should be your response, and his return to bed should be enforced without any further fun, games, food, or ceremony. The problems come when there's a lot of variation at bedtime, or if one or both parents feel guilty about the kind of interactions they've had with him during the day. But the time to remedy the need for more quality time with your two-year-old shouldn't be at 11 P.M. If you give in and let him fall asleep on the couch or agree to a snack or another story, be prepared for more of the same tomorrow night.

If your two-year-old is a late-night or early-morning explorer, you may need to install a barricade (the same type of folding gate used to keep toddlers off the stairs) across his exit route. Otherwise, you may awaken to find him finger painting on the walls, dumping flour on the floor, or worse—turning on appliances, leaning precariously over the toilet bowl, or perhaps checking out the garage.

You will also need to decide what to do if your toddler occasionally slips into your bed in the middle of the night. If you feel too weary to escort him back to his room or you don't mind the extra sleeper when you're already conked out, you may choose not to make this an issue. But if you decide that your bed is off-limits except by special invitation, enforce your policy consistently, no matter how tired you might feel. One approach to consider is designating some special snuggle times—for example, on weekend mornings.

Preschool sleeping routines . . . and monster patrol

Most three- and four-year-olds will sleep about twelve hours each night. Don't be surprised if your child's daytime nap is phased out during the next several months.

If you are struggling with your child over bedtime, work toward implementing the principles described in the previous section. Remember that bedtime should be *early* because your child needs the sleep and you need time with other children, your spouse, or yourself. During the middle of summer, this can be a challenge. The sun may still be shining, and all sorts of activity may still be going on outside at what is normally bedtime. You will need to decide how much to bend your routines to match the seasons or perhaps invest in heavy window shades if you need to darken your child's room at this time of year. You may also need to exercise sensible flexibility to accommodate family work schedules.

The activities that surround getting tucked in should become a familiar and quieting routine. At this age, bedtime can be a delightful, enlightening experience. You can introduce your child to some wonderful stories, including books with several chapters that can create eager anticipation for the next night's installment ("I wonder what's going to happen to Pooh and Piglet tonight. Better get ready for bed so we can find out!"). Your child's desire to keep the lights on and you in the room as long as possible will usually cause her to be remarkably transparent and receptive.

Expect to hear some of her private thoughts or to tackle some riddles of the universe ("Are there cats in heaven?" "Where did the sun go?"). Without being manipulated *too* much, allow enough slack in your day so you can relax during these wide-eyed sessions. You will probably have many more opportunities at bedtime to talk about God and the values you care about than during family devotions or even at church, Sunday school, or other formal religious teaching sessions.

You will also need to deal with some childhood fears when it's time to tuck in. Monsters in the closet, under the bed, or outside the window may need to be banished. Be sure to ask what your child is actually worried about. Is the creature something from a book or video, or perhaps a tall tale spun by an insensitive adolescent next door? Are we talking about space aliens, Brothers Grimm concoctions, or something from the nightly news that is in fact a reality somewhere in the world or the community? Are there tensions at home creating a need for reassurance?

Very often the beast in question doesn't exist except in someone's imagination. In this case it can be tempting to give a lighthearted, direct inspection ("I don't see any monsters in your closet—just a lot of junk!"), but you may leave the impression that there are monsters or aliens running around *somewhere*—they just don't happen to be here at the moment. For these fears, more decisive reality checks are important ("Bigfoot isn't under your bed or anywhere else").

When the issue is burglars or other villains who actually *do* exist out there, you will need to be more specific about the safeguards in your home: You are present (or if you are going out, someone whom you trust will be there), the doors are locked, and perhaps you have a dog or an alarm system that adds to your home's security. In addition, remind your child that God is keeping watch over her twenty-four hours every day. What your child really wants is reassurance and confidence that things are under control.

If a fearful bedtime resistance persists or escalates, take time to find out if something else is bothering her. Did your child see a disturbing image on TV or a video? Did she hear an argument the other night? Did something else frighten her? Once you have spent time exploring the problem, it's okay to make some minor adjustments to reduce the anxiety level: leaving a light on in the hallway or the door open a little wider, for example.

Healthy Sleep during the Adolescent Years

The teen years are often fast paced and packed with activities. School, sports, part-time jobs, church, and youth group functions all conspire to overload teens' schedules—and this doesn't include socializing (either in person, on the telephone, or online) that may continue long into the night. Add to this active lifestyle the physical changes that occur during adolescence, and it's not hard to understand how teenagers might become shortchanged on sleep.

Because sleep deprivation diminishes one's capacity for processing information, it should come as no surprise that inadequate sleep can impair a student's academic performance. A 1999 National Sleep Foundation survey found that 60 percent of children under the age of eighteen complained of being drowsy in school within the previous year, with 15 percent reporting that they have fallen asleep during the school day.[7] Drowsiness at school is correlated with lower grade performance.[8] Sleepiness can lead to more tragic results when a teenager is behind the wheel. Young drivers (under age twenty-five) are involved in more than half of the one hundred thousand automobile crashes every year directly related to fatigue, lapses in attention, and delayed response time associated with drowsiness.[9]

Just how much sleep does your adolescent need? Each person is different, but research suggests that the average teen needs at least 8.5 to 9.25 hours of sleep each night. Only 15 percent of adolescents get that much; one-fourth of teens get 6.5 hours of sleep or less. Physical changes during adolescence have curious effects on sleep and sleepiness. For many teens, daytime drowsiness increases even when they are able to get an optimal amount of sleep.[10] Likewise, sleep patterns appear to shift later in the day, so that the typical high school student's natural time for falling asleep moves back to 11 P.M.—or much later.[11]

Adolescence is likely to be the time in which **delayed sleep phase syndrome** (or **DSPS**) first occurs. Sometimes known as the "night owl syndrome," DSPS involves a shift in the circadian rhythm such that the affected person has difficulty falling asleep any earlier than from midnight to 3 A.M.

He or she then has great difficulty awakening in the early morning. If allowed to sleep seven or eight hours, the person with DSPS feels perfectly refreshed and ready to work. For many self-employed individuals—especially those who write or do computer work and find evening hours less distracting—this schedule may not pose any problem. Unfortunately, classes or workdays frequently start at 8 or 9 A.M.—well before the night owl is ready to get up. As many as 7 percent of the general population may have DSPS, and some research suggests that it is more than twice as common among college students.[12]

If it is truly disrupting school and work performance, DSPS should not be ignored or written off as simple laziness. Sleeping medications are generally not effective in helping the person with DSPS fall asleep earlier in the evening, although melatonin has been found helpful for some. Exposure to bright light for thirty to sixty minutes after awakening early in the morning (typically between 6 and 8 A.M.) may help reset the internal clock. Light boxes that emit a standardized amount of white light are available commercially for this purpose. Because night owls usually find it easier to stay up later than to go to bed earlier, another approach called **chronotherapy** can help many with DSPS. This involves going to bed three hours later each night over a week's time, essentially resynchronizing a person's circadian rhythm to the schedule necessary for optimal school and work performance. Once a new (earlier) wake-up time is established, it must be maintained in order to avoid a relapse into the old late-night routine. Sleep experts generally recommend consulting with a physician trained in sleep disorders before embarking on a week of chronotherapy.

Helping teenagers establish healthy sleep habits

Even though your teen might feel the need for more sleep, getting it may not always be easy. Here are some tips from the National Sleep Foundation that can help young people obtain the rest they need:

- Help your teen establish regular times for going to bed and getting up. When she departs from her normal schedule (such as on weekends), she should avoid delaying bedtime by more than an hour and waking more than two hours later than her regular schedule. If she is sleepy during the day, she may benefit from taking a nap in the early afternoon or after school. She should try not to take a nap much later in the day, however, since it may interfere with sleeping at night.
- Help your teen determine how much sleep she actually needs in order to feel refreshed and ready to start the day. Even if she gets the recommended amount of sleep, she could still awaken feeling tired. If this happens repeatedly, she may have to adjust her sleep routine (for example, go to bed earlier).

- Getting into bright light as soon as possible in the morning and avoiding it in the evening are wise at any age. Light signals the brain that it's time to be awake.
- Once your teen knows her body's rhythm, she should try to adjust her schedule so that she is engaged in activities that are best suited to her level of alertness. For example, she can try to avoid scheduling lecture classes—or activities that require mental alertness for safety, such as driving—during times when she tends to be sleepy.
- Your teen should stay away from caffeine in the afternoon, as it may interfere with her nighttime sleeping pattern.
- Encourage your teen to relax before going to bed, while avoiding intense studying, exercise, computer games, or other activities that stimulate the brain.

Here are some things that parents can do to help their teenagers obtain the proper amount of rest:

- Educate yourself about the sleep needs of adolescents. Many parents automatically interpret an increased need for sleep as laziness. Don't berate a teen for sleeping later on Saturday mornings.
- Look for signs of sleep deprivation in your teen and talk with him about his level of sleepiness and sleep habits. *Do not allow your teenager to drive if he is drowsy or sleep-deprived.*
- Encourage your adolescent to take ownership of his own sleep schedule. Keeping a sleep diary for seven to fourteen consecutive days can help pinpoint areas of the daily routine that need attention.
- At the end of summer vacation, help your teen adjust his sleep routine to fit his school schedule. A sudden drastic change in the sleep schedule is not likely to work, since the body's internal clock is rather resistant to such changes. Going to bed fifteen minutes earlier each night over several days may be more successful in shifting his sleep schedule. If simple measures are not working, you may wish to consult your adolescent's health-care provider or a sleep-disorder specialist.
- As with so many other areas of parenting teens, set a good example. Examine your own habits. Do you regularly burn the candle at both ends and then fight drowsiness much of the time? If so, make whatever changes are necessary to model healthy sleeping patterns that you would want your teen to imitate.

QUESTIONS TO PONDER:

1. How many hours of sleep do you get on a typical weeknight? Is it the same on weekends? Do you feel refreshed when you get up on most days?
2. If you are getting by on six hours of sleep or less every night, what is preventing you from getting more? Is it overcommitment? Are your projects and deadlines keeping you up late night after night? Are you squandering valuable sleep time watching TV or surfing the Internet late at night? What would you have to change in order to get eight hours of sleep every night?
3. Are you frequently drowsy during the day? Do you have trouble staying awake during meetings or while driving?
4. Are your nighttime habits setting you up for troubled sleep? Are you watching disturbing programs (especially late-night news) before you go to bed? What could you do late in the evening that would relax your body and calm your heart before going to bed?

Action items: If you are allowing yourself less than seven hours of sleep most nights and don't feel refreshed when you get up, take a hard look at your evening habits. As an experiment, try going to bed fifteen minutes earlier every night until you find the amount of sleep that leaves you refreshed and alert the next day.

If you are frequently drowsy during the day despite an apparently adequate amount of sleep time (at least seven hours), discuss this problem with your physician or if possible consult with a sleep specialist. This is particularly important if you snore during the night.

Get into the habit of reading an uplifting, reassuring passage of Scripture (such as a psalm of praise) every night before you fall asleep.

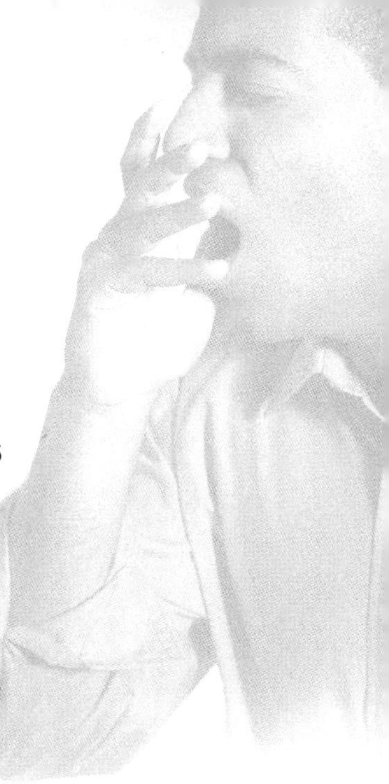

CHAPTER 16

"Why Am I So Tired All the Time?"

The Problem of Fatigue

Why am I so tired all the time?

When I get home after work, all I want to do is crash in front of the TV or go to bed.

I wonder if my doctor could give me something to pep me up.

Say the word *epidemic*, and most people think of infections such as influenza or HIV/AIDS, or perhaps conditions such as cancer, coronary artery disease, or even obesity. But when we think about the most common symptoms adults experience on an ongoing basis, we might consider adding fatigue to the list. As many as one in four patients visiting a primary-care physician is likely to consider fatigue a significant problem, even when something else is the stated complaint.[1] Millions more who feel chronically tired still carry out their daily routines, whether out of habit, necessity, or self-discipline, even if they feel tired while doing it. For some, fatigue is so severe that they have difficulty fulfilling even their most basic responsibilities.

Medically speaking, fatigue is not a diagnosis but rather a symptom, one that may have numerous causes. When we say we're tired, we may in fact be referring to a number of different experiences: a transient feeling arising from a day of physical labor or a sleepless night, a symptom produced by a serious illness, drowsiness at some point in the day (or all day), or a generalized sense of feeling poorly that has lasted for months or years.

When evaluating fatigue, one of the most important characteristics to consider is its duration. Acute fatigue is nearly always related to a specific event or cause, such as a cold or other illness, an unusual amount of physical exertion, or perhaps one or more nights of disrupted sleep. Usually this type of fatigue will be relieved by a good night's sleep or a few days' rest, but if loss of sleep is disruptive or severe, it should be evaluated by a physician. The Centers for Disease Control and Prevention (CDC) defines **prolonged fatigue** as persistent fatigue lasting one month or more, while **chronic fatigue** is defined as persistent or relapsing fatigue of six or more consecutive months. This chapter will focus on prolonged and chronic fatigue, with a particular emphasis on tiredness for which there is no apparent medical diagnosis. Chronic fatigue syndrome (CFS) is a specific, severe form of fatigue that is defined by several specific criteria established by the CDC. We discuss CFS in detail in appendix G beginning on page 959, but for now it is important to note that the vast majority of people who feel chronically tired do not have CFS.

Both acute and chronic fatigue can have a host of physical, emotional, and even spiritual causes. More than one of these may be present in a given individual at the same time, and not all may be recognized by the person who feels tired. We can group them into a few basic categories:

1. **Physical fatigue caused by disease.** This is the type most readily identifiable by a doctor. It may be acute (such as the malaise of a flu) or chronic (such as the draining effects of a widespread cancer). If a medical disease is not readily apparent from a health history and physical exam, only in a small percentage of cases will additional studies (such as X rays and laboratory tests) reveal an unexpected physical disorder. Chronic fatigue syndrome (CFS) appears to fit in this category, although the exact nature of the physical disturbance remains unclear. We will look at some important medical causes for fatigue later in this chapter.

2. **Habits and lifestyle.** Poor physical conditioning, erratic eating patterns, obesity, stress, disrupted sleep, the use (or abuse) of certain prescription and nonprescription drugs, tobacco use, and excessive alcohol intake can all contribute to tiredness. While these issues cannot be resolved overnight, addressing them over time can definitely improve energy. If you are dealing with one or more of these problems (with or without chronic fatigue), we would recommend that you review the chapters in this book that address them in more detail:
    - basic nutritional concepts—chapter 5
    - excessive weight and obesity—chapter 6
    - exercise and fitness—chapter 7
    - tobacco, alcohol, and drug abuse—chapter 10
    - sleep disturbances—chapter 15

3. **Acute mental and emotional fatigue.** This is usually tied to a specific event: working on a difficult homework assignment, preparing tax returns, packing for a long trip, hosting a large family gathering, and so forth. Many of these

situations and the tiredness they create have a limited impact and duration (typically a few days or perhaps weeks). More serious events such as the sudden death of a loved one, a business reversal, or a divorce will have both immediate and long-lasting repercussions that can contribute to fatigue that lasts for months or years.

4. **Chronic mental and emotional fatigue.** Long-term conflict or dissatisfaction with relationships, work, and the circumstances of everyday life can be stressful and draining. Ongoing responsibility for elderly parents or for a spouse or other loved one with failing health, a significant disability, dementia, or other chronic problems can be a setup for fatigue. Very often someone with this type of fatigue is fighting battles on more than one front: Pressure all day on the job may be followed by ongoing conflict at home, for example.

5. **Depression.** Frequently the primary cause of ongoing fatigue, depression may be **reactive** (related to outside circumstances), **endogenous** (related to biochemical processes in the brain), or a mix of both. Depression may be acute, chronic, or recurrent. Very often a person visiting a physician's office to address fatigue may not be aware of a mood problem, although often those who live and work with him or her have noticed it. Needless to say, it is important that depression be considered during an evaluation for fatigue, as many tired people feel considerably better after they are treated appropriately for this problem. Other mood and thought disturbances, such as bipolar disorder, schizophrenia, and eating disorders (anorexia nervosa and bulimia nervosa), may be associated with fatigue as well. For more information on these important subjects, see chapter 8.

6. **Spiritual and moral issues.** These can't be detected through a physical exam or laboratory tests, but they may play a role in causing fatigue. A person who has a vibrant relationship with God and who senses His loving presence on a daily basis has a reason to feel optimistic and energetic even when other factors that might generate fatigue (such as a physical illness) are present. It should be noted, however, that spiritual health does not guarantee freedom from physical or even emotional disturbances—including fatigue. At the same time, one who feels estranged from God, who consciously behaves in ways that violate God's standards, or who believes that there is no God and that life is pointless may eventually experience a melancholy that can be relieved only by establishing or restoring a relationship with his Creator. Spiritual malaise may also be a by-product of other types of fatigue. If we're tired for other reasons—or simply overcommitted—we may not feel we have the energy or time to connect with God on our own or to gather with others for that purpose. God may seem distant, detached, or even ab-

sent. We discuss this very important issue beginning on page 389 in chapter 9, ("More Than Molecules: Spiritual Health").

Some Characteristics of Chronic Fatigue

People who are chronically tired usually spend a fair number of waking hours (or sleepless nights) thinking about possible causes and remedies for their problem. Some come up with reasonable ideas, many more remain perplexed, and a few arrive at far-fetched conclusions. In order to gain some perspective on this problem, it is helpful to understand some basic principles that apply to most cases of chronic fatigue.

Fatigue, like pain, is subjective. Fatigue is a symptom that one can feel and describe. It is not a physical characteristic, such as heart rate or blood sugar, that can be measured. More importantly, fatigue is usually drastically influenced by one's emotional state, and especially by expectations for the immediate future. If you're feeling lethargic at work in the middle of the afternoon, an unexpected call from the president of the company will most likely spring you to life in a matter of seconds. Mild symptoms of fatigue may be ignored when circumstances are enjoyable and interesting, but they become a ball and chain in the face of an unpleasant task. It may take a crowbar to get children out of bed on a typical school morning, but watch the miraculous burst of activity when they suddenly realize that it's snowing and school has been canceled.

Chronic fatigue often has more than one cause. Occasionally a single medical problem (for example, anemia caused by iron deficiency) is the cause of ongoing tiredness. More often, fatigue is like a river fed by several streams. Several years of consuming more calories than needed every day may have created a physical burden of twenty, fifty, or one hundred extra pounds. There may be ongoing frustration at work. The daily round of chores at home may feel like an endless treadmill. A stack of bills may overwhelm the paycheck. A relationship with one's spouse or children may be in constant turmoil. And a medical problem may be lurking behind the scenes. Defining the problems and mapping these various "streams" can be a major challenge. Yet identifying causes is only the beginning.

Chronic fatigue infrequently has a single, "magic bullet" cure. The person who comes to a physician asking for "something to pep me up" will usually walk away disappointed, especially if the practitioner takes a careful and methodical approach to evaluating the cause of fatigue. There is, however, no shortage of supplements, potions, diets, and eccentric therapies that are promoted as surefire energy boosters. Some people find that these approaches seem to improve matters for a while, often for reasons that make little or no sense biologically. This may happen because the tired person feels energized by the belief that someone has found an answer to this problem, no matter how far-fetched the "cure" may be. Unfortunately, this apparent solution may divert attention from more important issues, such as lack of exercise or excessive weight.

Paradoxically, in most cases managing chronic fatigue requires *effort* by the individual who is tired. This is especially true when lifestyle changes, such as exercise and weight loss, are needed. While many who are chronically fatigued may feel too tired to do what is needed to reduce their tiredness, there are in fact few passive cures for this problem. What is done *to* us or *for* us tends to be less effective in raising energy levels on a lasting basis than what is done *by* us.

Raising one's energy level is usually a slow process. This should come as no surprise, given the multitude of factors that may contribute to chronic fatigue, the shortage of effective magic bullets, and the need to expend some effort and make changes if we are to improve how we feel. Most chronically tired people cannot say exactly when their weariness started, and few can identify exactly when things begin to turn around. Managing this problem is like steering an ocean liner. It usually requires a number of small course corrections that result in a change in position some time later.

When Should a Doctor Be Consulted about Fatigue?

In general, it is important to be evaluated medically for significant fatigue lasting more than two or three weeks, unless there is a cause that will eventually resolve on its own (for example, lack of sleep caused by a fussy newborn in the house). In addition, certain symptoms indicate the need for a medical evaluation *sooner* rather than later:

- fever over 100°
- unusual sweating, especially during the night
- significant headache, especially if it is new, persistent, or unusual
- light-headedness or overt fainting episodes
- shortness of breath
- persistent or recurring pain, especially in the chest or abdomen
- nausea and vomiting
- jaundice (a yellow-orange color of skin)
- persistent diarrhea
- dark or bloody bowel movements
- painful, frequent, or difficult passage of urine
- blood in the urine, with or without pain
- painful or swollen joints
- pain or swelling in the legs
- intolerance of heat or cold
- change in menstrual flow, whether increased, decreased, or absent
- unexplained weight loss

Keep in mind that these symptoms may or may not be related to the cause of fatigue—indeed, they may or may not even indicate the presence of a significant medical condition. Shortness of breath, for example, may result from anxiety, congestive heart failure, or a number of other problems. Each of these symptoms may be associated with fatigue, and any of them must be addressed, though in different ways. It is well beyond the scope of this chapter to explore all of the conditions that might cause these symptoms, which if present should be discussed in detail with your physician.

Questions health-care providers routinely ask about fatigue

If you are going to seek help from your physician about fatigue, make an appointment specifically to address that question. Don't ask "Why am I so tired all the time?" at the end of a visit for another problem, because it is impossible to address this concern appropriately in a few minutes. In addition, you will get a lot more accomplished if you are prepared to offer specific details about your fatigue. Your health-care provider may ask the following questions:

How long have you been tired, and did your fatigue problem begin suddenly or gradually? If you feel as if you've been tired for years, these questions may be hard to answer, but the more specific you can be, the better. When the time frame is uncertain, it sometimes helps to consider the last time you truly felt well. If fatigue began recently (within the past several weeks), or you can state specifically when the trouble started ("I felt great until June 15"), an identifiable medical problem is more likely. If the answer is "I can't remember when I really felt well," you should be open to the possibility that ongoing mood and lifestyle issues need to be addressed.

Does the fatigue interfere with any daily activities? Have you canceled any plans because of fatigue? Many people *feel* tired even while they remain very active and productive. (In fact, their fatigue may be related to overcommitment.) Some, however, are so profoundly affected by tiredness that work, recreation, and even the basic functions of life may be disrupted. In this case, certain diagnoses should be ruled out by a careful medical evaluation. Significant depression can cause a person to withdraw from normal activities. By definition, chronic fatigue syndrome (CFS) is tiredness that significantly limits a person's ability to function at work or home.

When your fatigue began, was it accompanied by any other symptoms? Symptoms that occurred at the onset of the fatigue problem (or perhaps preceded it) may provide important clues about the cause. For example, a combination of fever, aches, loss of appetite, and headache followed by prolonged tiredness usually suggests that a virus started the problem and left fatigue in its wake. Another example: The passage of one or more very dark stools followed by ongoing fatigue could signal blood loss in the intestine and a resulting anemia.

Are specific physical symptoms accompanying the fatigue now? Symptoms that accompany fatigue on a long-term basis can suggest directions to explore. Some—fever, unexplained weight loss, and the others listed on page

787—may indicate the presence of a specific disease and require further medical evaluation. Symptoms such as insomnia, poor concentration, dizziness, and numbness or tingling that migrate all over the body may also point to specific illness, but often they are related to mood disturbances such as anxiety and depression. (When physical symptoms and mood problems mix, it can be difficult to determine which is the cause and which is the effect.) As with fatigue, it will help the physician if you can offer specific characteristics of these other symptoms (e.g., How long have they been present? What, if anything, makes them better or worse? Have they ever happened before?). If you have a number of complaints, don't be disappointed if all of them are not addressed fully in one sitting.

Is fatigue relieved by a good night's sleep? Do you have any trouble falling or staying asleep? The relationship of fatigue to sleep is an important one. If tiredness stems from an overabundance of activities and a shortage of hours left for sleeping, an extra couple of hours one night or a weekend of "catch-up" sleep can work wonders. On the other hand, chronically tired people often complain that they feel no better when waking in the morning than they did when crawling under the covers. Disturbed sleep—whether difficulty falling asleep, waking early, a strong desire to sleep both night and day, or a combination of these—is also an important issue for the depressed person, who almost invariably complains of chronic fatigue.

Is the fatigue problem actually chronic drowsiness? Do you fight sleepiness during the day (especially when sitting quietly or while driving)? Do you fall asleep right after dinner or as soon as your head hits the pillow? Has anyone noticed that you snore or have erratic breathing patterns during the night? If the answer to one or more of these is yes, the problem may be a sleep disorder—especially sleep apnea, which is often associated with snoring. Because they interfere with the normal restorative effects of sleep, these disorders can cause a person to feel drowsy even after seven or eight hours of sleep. Also, many of us become fatigued during the afternoon, often immediately after lunch or between 2 and 4 P.M. This is at least partly due to a normal phenomenon known as circadian rhythm, which can cause a dip in energy and increased sleepiness during this time frame. Sleep disorders and the circadian rhythm are reviewed in more detail in chapter 15.

Does fatigue improve on weekends and vacations? If your fatigue disappears at 5 P.M. every Friday or evaporates on the beach at Maui, chances are you have some issues related to the responsibilities of the workweek. On the other hand, if weariness interferes with or aborts an activity you normally relish, a medical problem or a significant depression is more likely.

Are you taking any medications? Sedation and fatigue are common side effects of a number of prescription and over-the-counter drugs, which can contribute to chronic fatigue. Occasionally a medication that normally does not cause fatigue may prove to be a major energy drainer for a particular individual.

In some cases, a medication review may uncover a chain reaction leading to fatigue. For example, the chronic use of an anti-inflammatory drug to treat arthritis might cause ongoing blood loss into the intestine, which in turn could eventually lead to a tiring iron-deficiency anemia.

Even if one or more medications may be contributing to chronic fatigue, it is important *not* to change dosage (or stop taking a drug) before checking with your physician. Furthermore, if possible it's wise not to make more than one change at a time in an established medication regime, because the results can be confusing. If you feel better (or worse) after making multiple changes, it will be hard to tell which is responsible. Finally, be careful not to assume there's a relationship between symptoms (especially fatigue) and medications. Some people assume that if they're not feeling well, whatever was prescribed most recently must be the culprit—especially if they weren't too excited about taking it in the first place.

What types of medications can be associated with chronic fatigue?

Antihistamines. The older (sometimes called first generation) forms of these common remedies for colds and allergies can cause immediate drowsiness or ongoing fatigue when taken on a daily basis. They may be sold as single agents, such as diphenhydramine (Benadryl) or chlorpheniramine (Chlor-Trimeton), or in combination with decongestants, which by themselves rarely produce this effect. (Examples of combination agents are Actifed, Contac, Drixoral, and Dimetapp, among dozens of others.) Newer antihistamines—loratadine (Claritin), fexofenadine (Allegra), cetirizine (Zyrtec), and desloratadine (Clarinex)—are far less likely to cause drowsiness or fatigue.

Drugs that lower blood pressure (antihypertensives). Some medications that reduce blood pressure can cause fatigue. Certain **beta-blockers**, which slow the heart rate and decrease the forcefulness of each contraction, are known for this effect. Propranolol (Inderal) and nadolol (Corgard) are more likely to cause tiredness than atenolol (Tenormin) and metoprolol (Toprol XL and Lopressor). Clonidine (Catapres), which affects the nervous system's control of blood pressure, is often sedating in the oral form, although less so when used as a patch. Neither clonidine nor methyldopa (Aldomet), another older medication that tends to be sedating, is commonly used today.

For more information about high blood pressure (hypertension), see "Blood Pressure Basics" in chapter 3 beginning on page 52.

Fortunately, the blood pressure medications that are most widely used today usually do *not* cause fatigue. These include the **diuretics** (or water pills) that decrease the body's fluid volume, the angiotensin-converting enzyme inhibitors (more commonly called **ACE inhibitors**), the **angiotensin receptor blockers** (or **ARBs**), the **calcium channel blockers**, and the **alpha-blockers**. Nevertheless, even a drug that normally causes no (or minimal) side effects may cause some individuals to feel tired. If this seems to be occurring, some careful trial and error should be carried out under the supervision of one's physician. One important reminder: Some people who have had hypertension for a long time, especially the elderly, may feel fatigued with a lower blood pressure—at least for a while. Therefore, it is not a good idea to give up on a medication until enough time has passed to assess its various effects.

Antidepressants. Ironically, these are often the medications prescribed to treat chronic fatigue caused by depression. The right agent in the right patient can produce a dramatic improvement, but individual responses vary. For some people these drugs can be sedating, particularly during the first few days. As with blood pressure medications, it is wise not to discontinue one of these drugs too quickly, since side effects are often temporary and benefits may not be noticed for a few weeks.

Anxiety-reducing medications (anxiolytics). The drugs most widely used to reduce anxiety are the **benzodiazepines**, which include alprazolam (Xanax), diazepam (Valium), clonazepam (Klonopin), and lorazepam (Ativan), among others. They are by definition sedating and thus can produce fatigue. In some people this occurs because these medications relieve the nervousness that accompanies an underlying depression, but not the depression itself, which may make other symptoms (including fatigue) more apparent. For others, severe anxiety itself drains energy, and so one of these medications can improve both anxiety and fatigue—at least for a while. Unfortunately, long-term use can result in both psychological and physical dependence. (The anxiety-reducing drug buspirone [BuSpar], which is not a benzodiazepine, is both minimally sedating and non-habit-forming. However, it does not relieve symptoms as quickly or reliably as the others and so it is less widely used.) If you take one of these drugs regularly and feel tired, a discussion with your physician is definitely in order.

Antidepressants and anxiety-reducing medications, as well as the mood problems they are intended to treat, are discussed in detail in chapter 8.

Medications used for neurological disorders. Drugs that treat epilepsy, Parkinson's disease, and Alzheimer's disease can produce fatigue, among other symptoms. Treating these illnesses requires careful monitoring of the benefits and side effects of medications, although often these can be alleviated or prevented by using newer agents, tracking blood levels, and adjusting dosing schedules. An important caution: *Under no circumstance should any treatment for epilepsy be changed without consulting the prescribing physician.* The most common cause of an unexpected seizure is reducing or stopping medication.

Pain relievers in the opiate class. These medications are inherently sedating. When they are taken chronically, this effect becomes less noticeable because the body becomes habituated, or accustomed, to the drug. Anyone who takes prescription pain medications—especially codeine and its derivatives hydrocodone (Vicodin) and oxycodone (Percodan, Percocet, OxyContin, and others)—for a prolonged period may feel fatigued for other reasons. Chronic pain syndromes are draining and frequently associated with depression. Addressing the pain problem (and finding the most appropriate medications to help manage it) usually is a multidisciplinary task, which may require help from a primary-care physician, a pain specialist, a counselor, and a psychiatrist, among others. Frequently a team approach, such as is used in pain clinics associated with medical centers and university hospitals, is most appropriate.

Drugs used to treat certain intestinal disorders. These drugs also can cause fatigue, although not many are taken on an ongoing basis. Medications for nausea such as prochlorperazine (Compazine) and promethazine (Phenergan) are inherently sedating, but fortunately these are rarely needed for long periods of time. (Other less sedating options are also available.) The antinausea patch Transderm-Scop is an effective treatment for seasickness, but for some it can be quite sedating. Metoclopramide (Reglan), once prescribed widely for heartburn and still used for certain types of ongoing intestinal problems, can cause fatigue in some people. Antispasmodics used to treat the cramps of irritable bowel syndrome can be sedating. Some of these, including Donnatal and Librax, actually contain small doses of tranquilizers, while pure cramp relievers—hyoscyamine (Levsin) and dicyclomine (Bentyl), for example—can also cause fatigue. The newer agent tegaserod (Zelnorm) is often more effective and better tolerated, but its use is limited to those who are prone to constipation.

What health-care providers may—or may not—do about fatigue

People who seek medical help because of tiredness will probably experience something like the following scenario: Their health-care provider will ask a number of questions about the nature of the fatigue, specific symptoms, current medications, and overall health status, as we have just described. Lifestyle—diet, exercise, sleep, tobacco and alcohol use, work, and recreation—hopefully will be discussed as well, along with any current life events or stresses. An examination of variable length and detail will be done. Blood and urine will probably be checked, and other tests may be ordered.

WHAT MEDICATIONS NORMALLY DON'T CAUSE FATIGUE?

Some medications are *rarely* directly responsible for a chronic fatigue problem. These include antibiotics of all kinds, the nonprescription painkiller acetaminophen (Tylenol and other brands), anti-inflammatory agents used to treat arthritis and other musculoskeletal pain (aspirin, ibuprofen, and naproxen are everyday examples), and medications that reduce stomach acid. The latter include antacids, the older **H_2 blockers**–cimetidine (Tagamet), ranitidine (Zantac), famotidine (Pepcid), and nizatidine (Axid), all of which are sold without prescription–as well as the newer and more effective **proton pump inhibitors (PPIs)** such as omeprazole (Prilosec), lansoprazole (Prevacid), pantoprazole (Protonix), rabeprazole (AcipHex), and esomeprazole (Nexium). Hormones used in birth control pills and as treatment for the symptoms of menopause also rarely cause fatigue. ■

When all has been reviewed and evaluated, the majority of those with chronic fatigue will hear this verdict: "I do not have an explanation for your fatigue." For some, this is good news. (*Whew! What a relief to know that I don't have a serious illness.*) Others feel great frustration and discouragement. (*I've spent all this time and money, and there's still no answer. What do I do now?*)

Occasionally, the medical evaluation will reveal a specific cause for the fatigue. This may be good news—an underactive thyroid, for example, that can be readily treated—or it may be a devastating diagnosis, such as a widespread cancer. (See sidebar, "Important Medical Causes of Fatigue," below.)

Sometimes if the fatigue is severe and prolonged and other tests are normal, the diagnosis of **chronic fatigue syndrome (CFS)** may be considered. CFS usually involves not only disabling tiredness but also a number of other

IMPORTANT MEDICAL CAUSES OF FATIGUE

This list of medical problems that are often associated with prolonged and chronic fatigue is not intended to alarm you, but rather to give you a feel for the breadth of conditions that your physician might consider when addressing this symptom.

- *Chronic failure of one or more vital organs:* heart, lungs, liver, or kidneys
- *Infection,* such as acute infectious mononucleosis, influenza, HIV/AIDS, hepatitis, tuberculosis, Lyme disease, and chronic sinusitis
- *Anemia* (an abnormally low red blood cell count), which may have a number of possible causes
- *Neoplasm,* a benign or malignant (cancerous) growth, including uncontrolled proliferation of certain types of blood cells (such as leukemia) or lymph tissue (lymphoma)
- *Endocrine (hormonal) disturbances,* including abnormally high or low levels of thyroid hormone, diabetes (especially when blood glucose is markedly elevated), abnormalities of adrenal gland function (which are quite rare), menopause, or in men, low testosterone levels
- *Autoimmune (often called rheumatologic) syndromes,* such as rheumatoid arthritis, systemic lupus erythematosus, Sjögren's syndrome, dermatomyositis, and thyroiditis, that occur when the immune system inappropriately inflames and damages the body's own tissues
- *Neurological disorders,* including multiple sclerosis and Parkinson's disease
- *Heavy metal exposure and toxicity,* such as lead poisoning
- *Chronic pain problems* that provoke both physical and emotional fatigue as well as depression, or that are controlled by medications that contribute to fatigue ■

symptoms, including headache, muscle and joint aches, tender lymph nodes, and difficulty concentrating (what some call brain fog). This syndrome is challenging to diagnose, difficult to treat, and thoroughly unpleasant to experience. Furthermore, it is not always accepted as a legitimate diagnosis by medical professionals. CFS is reviewed in detail later in the appendix beginning on page 959.

Those patients who leave their doctors' offices without a specific, treatable diagnosis may or may not be given ideas to help resolve the fatigue, depending

TWO NONDIAGNOSES FOR CHRONIC FATIGUE

The frequent failure to find a clear-cut diagnosis for chronic fatigue has, not surprisingly, led to a number of theories about its cause that have not passed scientific scrutiny. Two that continue to circulate in books, Web sites, and other media are **hypoglycemia** and **chronic candidiasis**.

For decades, hypoglycemia or **low blood glucose** (also referred to as low blood sugar) has been blamed for causing chronic fatigue and numerous other symptoms. We reviewed this phenomenon in chapter 5, and for many reasons it is an unlikely suspect for causing long-term fatigue. The most compelling of these is that our body is engineered to ensure that any drop in blood glucose level will be transient rather than chronic. Even if a person's blood sugar drops far enough to cause fatigue or other symptoms, the body's response (or the next meal, snack, or glass of juice) will raise it relatively quickly. (The exception would be a profound hypoglycemia caused by an excessive dose of insulin or other glucose-lowering medication taken by a person with diabetes. In that case, however, emergency medical care would be necessary to correct the problem.) Bottom line: Even if a person experiences brief periods of hypoglycemia for whatever reason, these would not be expected to cause *chronic* fatigue. If you are concerned that you might have this problem, read "Do I Have Hypoglycemia?" starting on page 128 in chapter 5.

Chronic candidiasis is sometimes blamed for chronic fatigue and many other problems, but this explanation lacks scientific credibility. The yeast species *Candida albicans* is no stranger to the human body, and it is best known for growing in places that are wet and warm: skin folds (especially in those who are overweight and in the diaper area of babies), the vagina, and occasionally the mouth, where the infection is called thrush. It can also be troubling for diabetics and for people who have been on prolonged or intensive courses of antibiotics. These common infections with *Candida* produce local irritation and itching, at times intense, and usually respond to appropriate medications applied directly to the affected area. In a small number of people with immune deficiencies (such as cancer patients receiving chemotherapy or AIDS patients), *Candida* can spread throughout the body, causing a devastating illness.

on the expectations of the patient and the inclinations of the doctor. Everyday medical practice is so demanding that even the most caring physician may be hard-pressed to look very far beyond medical problems into other causes of chronic fatigue, which may involve important conflicts at home or work, mood disturbances such as depression and anxiety, personal habits and lifestyle, and spiritual problems. After a thorough medical evaluation, if a specific cause of fatigue cannot be identified, a patient might consider seeking professional counseling to learn how to cope with persistent fatigue.

The term *candidiasis hypersensitivity syndrome* (sometimes called the "yeast connection" because of a book that popularized this concept[2]) refers to a constellation of symptoms that are said to arise from a disturbance in immune function caused by excessive growth of *Candida albicans* in the body. The list of symptoms encompasses nearly every organ system and includes fatigue, depression, hyperactivity, headaches, abdominal discomfort, respiratory disease, and many more. The diagnosis is not based on any specific test but rather on the individual's history and response to treatment. Commonly recommended approaches include following a special diet designed to limit simple carbohydrates, avoiding refined foods (as well as "all foods containing yeast and mold," which are said to encourage the growth of *Candida*), plus using nutritional supplements and possibly antifungal medications.

Unfortunately, the symptoms of candidiasis hypersensitivity syndrome are so numerous that nearly everyone may experience at least one or two at any given time. There is no specific test that identifies it, only an assumption that the diagnosis is confirmed if a person feels better in response to the proposed therapies. Furthermore, this concept lacks a credible explanation of the mechanism by which *Candida albicans* might produce so many generalized symptoms or how the treatments (other than the antifungal agents) might have any impact on this process. One could just as easily substitute another potential biological offender for *Candida*—for example, one of the many species of bacteria that normally live on the skin—give the syndrome a name ("chronic *Staph. epidermidis* hypersensitivity syndrome," for example), claim that it causes dozens of common symptoms, and devise a combination of dietary advisories and supplements to treat it. The fact that some people feel better as a result would in no way prove the underlying theory correct. The bottom line: The promoters of candidiasis hypersensitivity syndrome have yet to present convincing evidence to support their claim that chronic fatigue (and numerous other everyday ailments) is caused by this common organism. ■

What to Do about Chronic Tiredness

While there is no surefire cure for chronic fatigue, don't lose heart or give up, even if your doctor hasn't come up with a diagnosis. There are a number of steps that you can take to address this problem. All of the suggestions that follow will be helpful, regardless of the cause of your fatigue. We have already mentioned some of these in passing, but they bear repeating.

Get enough restorative sleep. This is both fundamental and critically important, but it's often overlooked because so many of us attempt to do too much on too little sleep. Most adults function best with eight hours or more of sleep every night, but too many of us see that amount as a luxury that we cannot afford. In addition, sleep disorders—especially sleep apnea, which may be related to snoring and excessive weight—are very common. If you feel that you might have a sleep disturbance or if you struggle with chronic insomnia, consult a physician who is trained to deal with these important problems. For more details, see chapter 15 ("To Sleep . . .") beginning on page 735.

Get regular exercise. People who exercise regularly and are fit are less likely to struggle with fatigue. Even if you feel too tired to make the effort, regular physical activity—even a modest amount that you gradually increase every day—is one of the few measures that will reliably improve chronic fatigue. For more information about exercise, see chapter 7, beginning on page 275.

Deal with excess weight. The further your weight climbs above a body mass index (BMI) of 25—and especially as it rises to 30 or above—the more likely you are to develop physical problems that contribute to fatigue. For more information about excess weight and a look at strategies to deal with this important and often stubborn problem, see chapter 6, beginning on page 189.

Take a careful look at your mood. As we mentioned already, ongoing anxiety and depression are among the most common and treatable causes of chronic fatigue. Assessing these conditions may require a visit with your physician, a qualified counselor, or both. This important area of life and health is discussed in detail in chapter 8 ("The Emotional Weather"), beginning on page 315.

Take a careful inventory of the quality of your relationships. Ongoing conflict at home, work, or school can be a major energy drainer in your life. If you experience constant turmoil with your spouse, children, or parents or are having difficulty developing a network of supportive friends, an honest and open discussion with a counselor or your pastor is in order. We will look at the problem of ongoing conflict at home in more detail later in this chapter.

Evaluate your relationship with God and your purpose in life. Do you feel stuck in a routine? What motivates you to get out of bed every morning? Do you have any goals, spiritual or otherwise? Lack of a worthwhile purpose or an ongoing pursuit of possessions and pleasures that ultimately amounts to a "chasing after the wind" (as described by King Solomon in the book of Ecclesiastes) will eventually bring a person to a state of weariness and even despair.

Even a cursory reading of the Bible makes it clear that God does not suffer from chronic fatigue and that those who are empowered by His Spirit to accomplish His purposes manifest remarkable energy. (See the book of Acts in the New Testament for some noteworthy examples.) If your spiritual life is dead in the water or has never been launched in the first place, we encourage you to review chapter 9 ("More Than Molecules: Spiritual Health") in this book, meet with your pastor, or become involved in a church that is manifesting life, love, and growth.

Addressing Nine Potential Lifestyle Energy Drainers

Whether or not you are dealing with medical illness, depression, spiritual dryness, or turbulent relationships, the following nine issues can affect anyone. They are important enough to examine a little more closely.

1. **Overcommitment: too many irons in the fire.** Do you ever attempt to set a date for a night out with your spouse or close friends and find nothing available in your schedule for three weeks? Do you ever look at your calendar for the coming week and ask in exasperation, "Who made up this schedule?" Do you feel like your life consists of an unending series of brushfires, with the hottest and the closest flames getting the most attention? Do you often get the sinking feeling that you're doing a half-baked job on a number of projects rather than an excellent job on a few?

   If you answered yes to one or more of these questions and feel perpetually tired, you should turn to page 362 in chapter 8 and read carefully the section entitled "Create 'margin.'" Then begin the challenging (and often lengthy) task of dealing with your cluttered calendar. Remember that you must do this prayerfully and carefully. You may not be able to disengage from ongoing commitments without giving plenty of advance notice and perhaps assisting in passing the baton to someone else. If you are married, involve your spouse in these discussions. Whether you're married or single, you may want to ask one or more trustworthy friends to hold you accountable to this de-commitment process.

2. **Undercommitment: too few meaningful activities.** In contrast to the overcommitted, some people attend only to the most basic needs of life. They are stifled and usually tired because they lack the energizing purposes and goals that would take them beyond the four walls of home. In chapter 14 we note that this is a particular risk for those who find themselves adrift after retirement. We mentioned earlier the energizing effects of sensing a compelling purpose for your life, and the good news is that there are unlimited opportunities to make a difference in the lives of other people. Consider what might be your purpose beyond attending to everyday routines. There is no shortage

of worthwhile projects in your own church, a local hospital or nursing home, the neighborhood, or even in some distant country. What skills do you have that could assist someone else? Can you teach a disadvantaged person something you know—perhaps how to read or how to balance a checkbook? You may change his or her life. Is there a nursing home in town? Many who are confined there would be overjoyed to have a regular visitor. Does your community have a crisis pregnancy center? These ministries, which provide practical assistance to women, are always in need of volunteers for all sorts of projects.

An organization that provides services to pregnant women in crisis may also be called a pregnancy resource center, pregnancy care center, or women's resource center. Your church may already be involved with a center, or you can check with umbrella organizations such as Care Net, which you can reach at (703) 478-5661 or www.care-net.org, or Heartbeat International, (888) 550-7577 or www.heartbeatinternational.org. Those seeking help with a crisis pregnancy can call (800) 395-HELP.

Is there a prison or jail nearby? Prison Fellowship can put you to work in all sorts of significant activities that make a decisive difference in inmates' lives. For information about local projects, contact Prison Fellowship at (877) 478-0100 or online at http://www.pfm.org. If you help change the world for even one or two people, you'll feel better as well.

3. **Clutter: the accumulated stuff of life.** When we combine our all-too-human urge to acquire things with a reluctance to let go of them, our gradual accumulation of possessions can become an indoor overgrowth of weeds that will suffocate us unless it is periodically pruned. A home or apartment crammed from one end to the other with "treasures" can be a major energy drainer.

   In chapter 8 we note that decluttering can be a step toward tranquillity. It can also be an energizing experience, especially if you turn on some upbeat music while tossing out junk that will never be missed. Limit yourself to one room or closet per session to avoid feeling overwhelmed. Has an article of clothing not been donned for a year or more? Goodwill will find it a nice home. Have you looked at those magazines from last year? You won't this year either. How about those cans of paint with just a little bit left? Toss them (safely, of course, following the disposal protocols in your community). Do you need to keep every piece of artwork Johnny brings home from preschool? Unless you want to be buried alive by the time he reaches junior high, pick the best of the lot, preserve them carefully and faithfully, and toss the rest. What about the old videocassettes of shows you recorded years ago for viewing at some later date? You can probably rent most of them at the video store any day of the week (assuming they're worth watching). And so on. Once some order is restored in your home or workplace, notice how good you feel. To maintain that positive emotion, remember that the "round file" can be one of your best friends.

4. **Debt: the paper chain.** In chapter 8 we discuss financial bondage as a component of an overcommitted and frantic lifestyle—one that we would call "marginless"—and a contributor to emotional distress. Significant debt and pressing financial obligations can also be an enormous energy drain. As we

note in that chapter, getting out from a serious burden of debt requires an approach similar to that needed to lose weight. We need to face the reality that there are more things to buy than we can afford, and we need to get a grip on the flow of our own income and expenses. We then need to develop a plan that we can live with for a long time, and stay with it. More than one financial planner has suggested taking the smallest debt first and paying it off while maintaining the minimum requirements on the others. Each account sent to zero can be the occasion for a "retirement party." In addition, being accountable to someone else will help us maintain the chosen course when temptation is at hand. In chapter 8, we recommend the resources of Crown Financial Ministries, and we will mention them again here. Its ten-week small group study, which many churches offer on an ongoing basis, is particularly useful. For more information check http://www.crown.org on the Internet, call (800) 722-1976, or write to Crown Financial Ministries at P.O. Box 100, Gainesville, GA 30503-0100.

5. **Workaholism: breaking the fourth commandment.** This specific form of overcommitment can occur both in the corporate world and among the self-employed. The common denominator is a compulsion to attend to the job, the business, the clients, the patients, the project, or the store without reasonable boundaries on the number of hours in the day or the number of days in the week.

Hard-driving corporate types are actually not the worst violators of the fourth commandment. The self-employed, especially those with small businesses, are always vulnerable in this area. They frequently don't feel secure enough to forget about their enterprises for a day, so they carry work home in their mind (if not in their briefcase) after business hours and may deprive family members of the precious time and attention that they need. Second on the list for workaholic risk are caregivers: physicians, psychologists, social workers, and pastors. Since the dimensions of human need in any community are virtually limitless, those who meet needs for a living can easily burn out with exhaustion if they are always "on call."

The fourth commandment: "Remember the Sabbath day by keeping it holy. Six days you shall labor and do all your work, but the seventh day is a Sabbath to the Lord your God. On it you shall not do any work, neither you, nor your son or daughter, nor your manservant or maidservant, nor your animals, nor the alien within your gates" (Exodus 20:8-10).

Obviously diligence, responsibility, and excellence are noble goals for corporations and small businesses. Family enterprises can be meaningful for all concerned, and reaching out to those in need is a high calling. But there is always infinitely more work to do than can ever be done, and there are more needs within one city block than any of us can ever meet. Solid lines must be drawn in our life, across which work must not be given a toehold. The line may involve a *place* (such as home, unless the office *is* at home) or more importantly, a *time*. Here's the bottom line and the essence of the fourth commandment: *It is extremely important to have a minimum of one day per week—very often, but not always, Sunday—during which one's primary vocation is off-limits.* Those who fail to set aside this day over an extended period of time can count on being tired. When Jesus noted that the Sabbath was made for man and not man for the Sabbath (see Mark 2:23-28), He was talking about more than religious observances. God commanded a day off every week for the sake of the survival and sanity of the humans He loves.

Ideally, the day off is not the time to clean the garage or check off the first five items on a honey-do list. (Of course, for many people some physical effort exerted on behalf of one's home or garden can actually be diverting or even refreshing.) It should be a time to refresh, reflect, recreate, worship, and spend time with people we care about. Sometimes it is necessary to escape to a park, beach, zoo, movie, museum, or whatever puts distance between us and our vocational brushfires. Unfortunately, cell phones and pagers, as useful as they can be, can tether us to our work. One of life's most courageous and difficult decisions may be declining to answer calls during time that has been set aside for family or personal restoration.

6. **The TGIF syndrome: why work?** Pop quiz—(1) If you suddenly inherited a million dollars, would you keep working at your present job? (2) Does a cloud of gloom hang over your workplace (or your kitchen table) every Monday morning? Does it gradually lift as the week progresses? Obviously, the vast majority of us find it necessary to be gainfully employed. However, if your work generates no greater satisfaction than a paycheck every other week, you may spend five or six days each week fighting fatigue.

   If you're not particularly enthusiastic about your job, reflect on what your work accomplishes. Who benefits from what you do? If the answer is no one in particular and if after careful assessment you decide that your work is essentially meaningless, think creatively about other ways to spend forty or more hours of work per week. On the other hand, before blowing off steam about "this lousy job" and making noises about quitting, some precautionary prayer and wise counsel are in order. Jumping from job to job may be symptomatic of a deeper lack of contentment or a permanently critical and ungrateful attitude. Furthermore, perhaps your workplace is an arena God has provided in which you are to be salt and light. There are usually plenty of needs to be met within a few feet of any desk or workbench. The apostle Paul did not consider his occupation as a tentmaker to be his primary mission in life—but he didn't belittle it either, since it gave him a certain level of independence as he pursued his goals of preaching and teaching.

7. **Raising small children: on call at all times.** Some of the most tired people who pass the portals of doctors' offices are the parents of infants and toddlers. Anyone who has assumed responsibility for young children for more than a few minutes understands that parenting them is one of the most demanding full-time tasks on earth. Bringing a newborn home is challenging even for a married couple who is well prepared, motivated, and supported

by family and friends. The cry of a newborn baby is not a particularly pleasant sound, but it serves a vital purpose—it's a powerful stimulus for parents to feed, change, rock, and provide other necessary care frequently both day and night. When a baby cries on and on, especially during the night, even the most committed parents can begin to feel edgy and put-upon. For those in less favorable circumstances—single moms, young couples with very limited resources, or parents whose feelings about the child-rearing process are mixed—the response to a combination of unending responsibility and chronic fatigue arising from sleepless nights may escalate into frustration, anger, and even child abuse or neglect.

After newborns and infants have graduated to toddler and preschooler status, staying at home with them may feel rewarding, exhausting, stimulating, and mind-numbing—sometimes all in the same day. What do you do when the kids have left the room and you're still watching *Sesame Street*? How many times can you hear the latest Barney CD before you start singing it—when no one else is around? What does it mean when the high point of your day is watching reruns of a twenty-year-old sitcom while the kids lie down for a nap? Why bother to clean up the house when it automatically returns to total disorder within thirty minutes? Is it possible to be attentive to the needs of small children without your brain turning to mush?

Lack of sleep, lack of adult conversation, and lack of any sense of forward motion (except watching the kids get bigger) drain vast amounts of energy from the most talented, motivated, and dedicated stay-at-home parents. In addition, and probably most importantly, lack of recognition for the job being done drives many stay-at-home parents into unnecessary despair, as they picture their friends advancing in what may appear to be glamorous (or at least more interesting) careers and wonder if they're foolish for staying home.

There are many ways to plug (or at least slow) this very important energy drain. If you are a parent who stays home, consider the following ideas.

- Develop some appropriate expectations for this season. This is a surprisingly brief passage, though it may seem like an eternity now. Life is not passing you by. There will be many years ahead to carve your niche in society, if that is what you are called to do.
- Remind yourself of the importance of this job, even if no one else seems to appreciate it. These years are significant for both you and the children, and being an eyewitness to your children's daily changes and growth can be fascinating.
- Keep learning. Who says the mind has to go numb for several years? What books do you want to read besides *Goodnight Moon* and *The Runaway Bunny*? What was your favorite course in high school or your major in college? No one said you couldn't keep exploring those topics or continue taking courses at a local college when the children get a little older.

- Cultivate relationships with other adults (of the same sex). Regularly scheduled times of grown-up conversation are critical, and your spouse may not be able to meet all of your needs in this area. (This is especially important for the single parent, who is bearing all of the responsibility single-handedly.)
- Find the best babysitters in the area, and reward them well (if you can). Doing so will allow you to have some time-outs on a regular basis—not for errands but for brief periods of personal refreshment. Going out with friends or having some time alone is both legitimate and necessary. When cash is short, a resourceful alternative is the babysitting co-op, an arrangement in which several people use a barter system to swap child care. If you are blessed with loving grandparents nearby, let them spoil the kids for a few hours (or even overnight) while you get a break.
- If you are a single parent, take strong measures to maintain your sanity and balance. You have some of the greatest challenges of all, since there may not be another adult in the vicinity to share child-rearing responsibilities with you. Don't be afraid to let your church family know about some of your needs, and be patient if its activities seem geared to couples or childless singles. Most importantly, don't be too proud to accept what help is offered.

If you are the spouse of the stay-at-home caregiver, you have a critical role in maintaining his or her sanity. Stay-at-home parents need to hear that they are important and desirable. They need adult conversation, not more prattle from the television. They need someone to take charge of the kids for a while, even when they're right there in the room. They need to go out for an evening with you, even to be taken away for a weekend if possible. They need to be sent cards and love notes for no particular reason. They need to be encouraged to develop their mind and skills; caring for the kids one night a week while they go to a class is considerate and would also give you an intense appreciation for the magnitude of their daily work.

Above all, those who raise children need to stay on their knees, because no one has all the answers, wisdom, and energy needed for the job—but God does. Don't forget: More than any other experience, this process will teach you about your relationship with God, who is the ultimate loving parent.

8. **Conflict on the home front: verbal (and other) warfare.** One of the most common and highly damaging contributors to chronic fatigue is a state of trench warfare at home. All too often those who have promised to "love, honor, and respect" at the altar find themselves in the midst of searing conflict before the honeymoon is over because they never learned how to address common (and inevitable) life issues while honoring and respecting their spouse's opinions and personhood. If the verbal battles continue un-

checked, children soon learn to imitate this behavior, until the home becomes the most dangerous place in town. The ongoing prodding, accusing, put-downs, sarcasm, arguing, and in some cases physical fighting create an atmosphere that is draining and polluted. Since the patterns are usually ingrained and automatic, the combatants may be aware only of their constant dissatisfaction and fatigue.

Of all the contributors to chronic fatigue, this can be one of the toughest to resolve, because two or more people not only need to recognize the problem but also must learn to communicate without using verbal clubs. (However, one highly motivated person can model some constructive patterns for the others.) An astute counselor can facilitate this process, as can a mature couple or family whom you have observed relating in healthy ways. While it is not possible to detail all the principles involved in settling disagreements within the family in this book, the following basic concepts can serve as a foundation for those who desire to work on this important area.[3]

Mutual respect is an absolute necessity. Without respect on all sides, any relationship will ultimately deteriorate or become destructive. With mutual respect, it is possible to have an intense disagreement with another person without causing damage to the relationship or those who are affected by it. Respect acknowledges the ultimate worth of the other person—because he or she is made in God's image, not because of any other attributes or accomplishments—and affirms that worth in attitudes, words, and actions. If family members do not respect one another or if respect flows only in one direction, attempts to resolve issues are likely to be unsuccessful or hurtful. This fundamental problem must be addressed—usually in a counseling setting—if a marriage is going to survive and thrive through the years of raising children and beyond.

During a disagreement, conversation should focus on the issue and not the person. If Mom feels she needs more help with the kids in the evening, it isn't productive for her to begin the discussion with the statement "You care more about that TV than your own children!" If Dad is getting worried about the family budget, he won't get very far by saying, "All you ever do is spend the money I work so hard to bring home!" Once the issue is defined (How do we care for the kids when we're both tired? or How can we keep better track of our finances?), the focus can shift toward generating and evaluating a potential solution.

When an issue needs to be discussed, pick an appropriate time and place. The right time is not at the end of the day when energy is low and fuses may be short; not right before bed; not when anger is at a fever pitch; not when there isn't time to work through it; not when the TV is on, the phone is ringing, the kids are arguing, and the dog is barking. If it is clear that an issue needs to be addressed later, it's quite all right for either person to call time and say, "This isn't a good time to discuss this" or "I don't feel like talking about it right now"—as long as a specific time is set to talk about it in the very near future. The best time to talk is when both parties are rested, focused, and attentive. It's helpful to work through an issue in a place that is relatively free of distractions and interruptions. This may be a particular room, somewhere out in the yard, or a place away from home. Many couples do their best negotiating at a coffee shop or on a long walk.

Pray together before discussing the issue. Laying the issue before God can help keep it in perspective and reinforce your common ground. Be careful not to use this prayer time unfairly to express your viewpoint or claim God's backing for your side of the conflict. Prayer should be an exercise in humility, not a power play.

Each person must be able to express his or her viewpoint fully, without interruption. A key element of respect is listening carefully to what the other person is saying, without thinking about one's own response. One technique that encourages attentive listening involves picking an object (such as a pen) and stipulating that whoever holds it is entitled to speak without interruption. The other person cannot say a word until the pen is passed, and the pen will not be passed until the person receiving it can summarize what was just said to the speaker's satisfaction—without argument, rebuttal, or editorial comment. If the listener doesn't get it right, the pen doesn't pass. This approach may seem awkward and ritualistic at first, but it is surprisingly effective at improving listening skills. Get in the habit of checking frequently to be sure that you understand what the other person is saying. "I hear you saying . . ."

Avoid "You . . ." statements—especially those containing the word *always, never, should,* or *shouldn't.* Replace them with statements that express your own feelings. "You *never* spend any time at home anymore!" essentially demands a rebuttal ("That's not true!"). In contrast, "It seems as if the kids and I are spending more evenings by ourselves than ever before, and it makes me feel lonely" is a straightforward observation and an expression of a genuine feeling. Similarly, a statement such as "You *shouldn't* make commitments for both of us without talking to me first!" is likely to provoke a defensive response. The one way in which a "you" statement can legitimately enter a conversation is in this form: "When you say (or do) _____, I feel _____ ." (For example, "When you make commitments for both of us without talking to me first, I feel as if my opinion doesn't count.") This type of statement can help one person understand how specific words or actions are affecting the other person.

Avoid "Why . . . ?" questions—especially those containing the word *always* or *never.* "Why do you *always* leave the back door open?" can be answered in only one of two ways: defensively ("I don't either!") or sarcastically ("Because I'm an idiot!") "Why . . . ?" questions automatically turn a discussion into a battle.

Avoid bringing up events from the distant past. Statements like "Here we go again!" or "This is just what you did on our vacation in 2002, when you . . . " are not helpful. If current problems are related to grievances from the past, then those specific concerns need to be discussed and resolved apart from any current problems.

Name-calling and other forms of insults are disrespectful and should be banned from all conversations within a family (or anywhere else). Verbal insults live in everyone's memory long after apologies have been made. One of the most powerful lessons that children can learn from their parents is how to disagree or be angry with a person without resorting to labeling, name-calling, or insults. Remember that body language (such as sighing and rolling the eyes), gestures, and tone of voice can communicate disrespect as powerfully as the most explicit insult.

When discussing an issue, participants should eventually explore possible courses of action. Questions like "What can I do to help you not feel so tired at the end of the day?" or "How can we make Sunday morning less hectic?" can lead to productive solutions. It may help to list a number of possibilities and then talk through the pros and cons of each one.

Realize that sometimes you may have to "agree to disagree," and that in doing so, neither person's viewpoint is to be subject to constant ridicule. This will mean compromising in some cases. There is usually, however, some solution that will allow for each person's needs to be met.

If your discussions of issues frequently deteriorate into shouting matches or glum stalemates, get some help. It takes courage and maturity to go to a counselor (or to a mature couple whom you know to be experienced in conflict resolution) to determine what goes wrong when disagreements arise in your home. Constructive suggestions from an unbiased third party, if acted upon consistently, can drastically improve the quality and outcome of these conversations.

9. **Unmet expectations and desires.** These can cause fatigue at any season of life, and they will never be detected during a medical examination. Generally, a person with unmet expectations thinks: *Things aren't turning out the way I had hoped.* Perhaps deep longings for companionship, children, recognition, or other measures of success have not been met, and there are no prospects on the horizon. Or the desires *have* been met, and they aren't all they were cracked up to be. The degree, the spouse, the home, the kids, the job, the raise, or the title isn't supplying lasting contentment. The restless search for the next source of satisfaction continues—and fatigue may well accompany it.

   This scenario is nothing new. Centuries ago King Solomon surveyed all that he had acquired: unimaginable wealth, political superiority, worthwhile building projects, education, and the sexual satisfaction from one thousand partners. Yet he was still not at all satisfied:

I denied myself nothing my eyes desired;
I refused my heart no pleasure.
My heart took delight in all my work,
and this was the reward for all my labor. . . .
Yet when I surveyed all that my hands had done
and what I had toiled to achieve,
everything was meaningless, a chasing after the wind;
nothing was gained under the sun. . . .

So I hated life, because the work that is done under the sun was grievous to me. All of it is meaningless, a chasing after the wind. . . . What does a man get for all the toil and anxious striving with which he labors under the sun? All his days his work is pain and grief; even at night his mind does not rest. This too is meaningless.

(ECCLESIASTES 2:10-11, 17, 22-23)

This type of fatigue, this world-weariness, will not be resolved by medication, supplements, exercise, or other physical remedies. It is at its core spiritual and involves settling a primary issue that we addressed in chapters 8 and 9: Is true contentment generated internally, or is it the result of how things are going? What dictates mood—circumstances or a forward-looking, others-oriented, stable attitude sustained by God's transforming work at the core of our being?

The Scriptures use vivid imagery to portray the person who has a vibrant, energizing relationship with God:

He is like a tree planted by streams of water,
which yields its fruit in season
and whose leaf does not wither.
Whatever he does prospers.

(PSALM 1:3)

The image of the tree here is powerful, one worth comparing to our own day-to-day experience. It is solid, stable, and productive at the right time, constantly drawing life from the waters nearby. And we can be as secure as that tree as we develop our relationship with God and are transformed by Him. If you are not certain how this happens, turn to "Our terminal condition" on page 392 in chapter 9 and read carefully from that point through the end of the chapter.

Some Final Thoughts on Fatigue

Throughout this book, we describe symptoms and health hazards that arise from the frantic pace of our life. This point bears repeating as we conclude our look at fatigue. Jesus made a compelling offer: "Come to me, all you who are weary and burdened, and I will give you rest. Take my yoke upon you and learn from me, for I am gentle and humble in heart, and you will find rest for your souls. For my yoke is easy and my burden is light" (Matthew 11:28-30). Many who are "weary and burdened" are in fact straining and exhausted under yokes of their own making.

Far too many of us are overcommitted, underrested, and overstressed, and this often results in our feeling *tired*—physically, emotionally, and even spiritually. We fill our life with activities, most of which are good when considered individually. However, as they accumulate, they can lead to overload and then fatigue. Much of what we buy and accumulate is supposed to make our life simpler, easier, and less stressful. But in fact many of these items (including those that are supposed to save time or labor) actually consume more time, attention, resources, and energy than we ever intended.

We are the victims of **hurry sickness** as well, responding to an ongoing push to see and do more in less time. Like the drive to accumulate more possessions, some of this relentless pursuit is fueled by media and marketing. To own more and do more, we need to *make* more as well, so we push the throttle at work and often look for other sources of income while we're at it. Often the reward in the distance isn't financial but rather status and recognition, but these can capture our time and energy as effectively as any quest for a bigger paycheck. We seem unwilling to wait for anything anymore: Buy the big house *now*, get the new car *now*, take the exotic vacation *now*, and don't worry about that inevitable *pay later* part of the equation.

All the while, the most important things in life—relationships with God, family, and friends, not to mention time for exercise, sleep, reading, prayer, and other critical restoratives—are most often pushed to the background or out of the picture entirely. Our kids (who may have developed a frantic schedule of their own) not only suffer directly but may also see a mom and dad who can't say no. They may later mimic this example as adults.

In chapter 8, which deals with emotional health, we note the importance of margin, as discussed so eloquently by Dr. Richard A. Swenson is his books *Margin* and *The Overload Syndrome*. Dr. Swenson describes a process of "pruning the activity tree," which can be a major challenge for many families. But the reality is that we have limited resources of time, money, and energy, and we need to spend each of them wisely, with God as our adviser. We must realize that *no* can be a sacred word and have the courage to say it. We also need at times to ask ourselves why we feel compelled to have, to do, or to be something, to push ourselves and our families to the point of exhaustion.

We each have reserves to "run on empty" for a while, but we don't have an unlimited capacity. To some degree this serves to remind us that we were designed to live within physical, mental, emotional, intellectual, and spiritual boundaries. We are not God, and one of the reminders of this reality is that we have limits. This may seem obvious, but too often our decisions reflect an unconscious assumption that *I can do it all!* Sooner or later, however, the challenges of life will bring us to the end of our intelligence, our knowledge, or our physical and emotional strength. Recognizing this may cause some to feel despair, but in fact this acknowledgment of our limits is the beginning of wisdom. Indeed, doing so *before* we reach the end of ourselves reflects even greater wisdom.

History, literature, and pop culture are abundant with would-be supermen and wonder women, but those who are not fictional or mythological inevitably prove to have feet of clay or chinks in their armor. Real people have been created for a relationship with God that is grounded on a humbling but also comforting reality: We are dependent on Him for every breath we take and every decision we make, and we need *each other* as well. The apostle Paul illustrates this mutual dependence with the analogy of a physical body whose various parts serve the whole:

> *Do not think of yourself more highly than you ought, but rather think of yourself with sober judgment, in accordance with the measure of faith God has given you. Just as each of us has one body with many members, and these members do not all have the same function, so in Christ we who are many form one body, and each member belongs to all the others.*
>
> (ROMANS 12:3-5)

> *God has arranged the parts in the body, every one of them, just as he wanted them to be. If they were all one part, where would the body be? As it is, there are many parts, but one body.*
>
> *The eye cannot say to the hand, "I don't need you!" And the head cannot say to the feet, "I don't need you!" On the contrary, those parts of the body that seem to be weaker are indispensable, and the parts that we think are less honorable we treat with special honor. . . . God has combined the members of the body and has given greater honor to the parts that lacked it, so that there should be no division in the body, but that its parts should have equal concern for each other. If one part suffers, every part suffers with it; if one part is honored, every part rejoices with it.*
>
> (1 CORINTHIANS 12:18-26)

Our family, our friends, and our fellow believers in a community of faith fulfill different (and interdependent) roles in our lives so that all can live more abundantly without feeling overburdened and worn out. Acknowledging our limits—the reality that we can't be and do everything—is not a liability or a sign of weakness. Instead, doing so provides opportunities to experience God's utter sufficiency and to serve one another in love—and in so doing, to avoid wearing ourselves out.

QUESTIONS TO PONDER

1. If you have been experiencing fatigue, do you have another illness or physical problem that may cause or accompany your fatigue? Do you have any of the symptoms listed under "When Should a Doctor Be Consulted about Fatigue?" on page 787? If so, make an appointment with your doctor as soon as you can.
2. Consider your habits and lifestyle (weight; eating patterns; physical condition; sleeping habits; use of any prescription, nonprescription, or illegal drugs, or alcohol or tobacco). Think about stressors in your life, whether temporary (e.g., work or homework projects, events you oversee) or long term (e.g., work, relationships, people in your life who require special attention). If you often feel tired, how might you change any of these patterns or address any causes of stress, in order eventually to feel less tired?
3. If you do not have problems with chronic fatigue now, can you identify any lifestyle choices that may take their toll on you several years down the road?
4. When was the last time you took a day or a weekend to relax or do something just for fun? How did you feel when you returned to your normal routine?

Action items: If you are experiencing chronic fatigue, a medical evaluation is an important initial step toward recovery. Prepare for your visit by answering each of the questions under "Questions health-care providers routinely ask about fatigue," which begins on page 788.

Ironically, reducing fatigue is a fairly active process. Review the steps listed under "What to Do about Chronic Tiredness" on page 796 and begin putting them into practice. If you've been keeping a journal, record any lifestyle changes or progress you make toward overcoming chronic fatigue—no matter how small. Look back over the journal if you ever feel discouraged about your ability to curtail your fatigue. Remember that it may take awhile before you notice some improvement in your energy level.

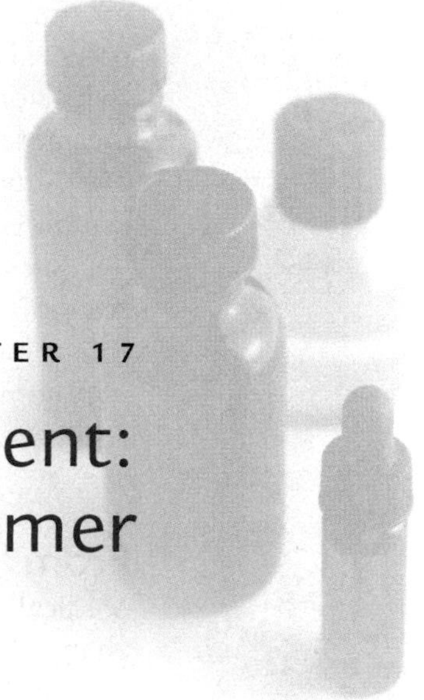

CHAPTER 17

Health-Care Discernment: How to Be a Wise Consumer

A health-care conversation fifty years ago:

Doctor: There are a number of medicines available now that can help your problem. I'd like you to fill this prescription and come back in two weeks so I can see how you're doing.

Patient: Okay. You're the doctor.

A health-care conversation today:

Doctor: There are a number of medicines available now that can help your problem. I'd like you to fill this prescription and come back in two weeks so I can see how you're doing.

Patient: You want me to take *what*? How long do I have to use it? What are the side effects? How long has this been on the market? I've read on the Internet that this type of drug can damage my liver. Are we going to keep an eye on my liver functions? What about my kidneys? Also, I don't know if this particular brand is covered by my insurance. Could you check on that before we get started?

These dialogues are a little exaggerated, of course, but they reflect a definite shift in the relationships between patients and their doctors over the past several decades. A few seasoned physicians still in practice recall and pine for the good old days, when doctors gave orders and everyone followed them without uttering a peep. Today medical decisions are often so complex that the doctor (or other health-care provider) is but one person in the loop, and the patient practically needs a scorecard, if not a full-blown guidebook, just to know "who's on first" and how to navigate the health-care system successfully. Furthermore, there are all kinds of practitioners (both conventional and alternative), hundreds of books, thousands of products, and zillions of Web sites claiming to offer you and your family better health or relief from whatever ails you. How do you distinguish between beneficial, borderline, and bogus information? Whether you're a newcomer to this realm or a seasoned veteran of things medical, this chapter is intended to give you a sense of direction (along with some practical pointers) that can help you make informed and sound decisions about health care.

From "Patient" to "Health-Care Consumer"

Medical science in the United States and other developed countries has changed so drastically over the past century that the tools used today for diagnosing and treating disease would be completely unrecognizable to a physician or a patient of the early 1900s—or for that matter, the early 1950s. Most likely these citizens of the past would also be perplexed by the ways in which we now receive health care, and they would—along with most of us today—no doubt express some bewilderment over the ways in which that care is paid for.

Indeed, dramatic increases in health-care costs, growing disenchantment with health-insurance companies, and increasing numbers of therapeutic options are among the factors that have converged in a single generation to change the way people interact with the health-care system. Instead of passively waiting (and waiting and waiting) for a time-pressured doctor to "make them better," individuals began to explore new ways to maintain or improve health on their own. Instead of enrolling in a single health plan chosen by an employer, they began to pick and choose from a menu of options. Instead of automatically following the advice of their doctor regarding a particular therapy or drug, they began to ask questions about benefits, risks, side effects, and costs. Instead of routinely going to local physicians and the nearest hospital when seeking care for complex problems, they sought second opinions from experts across town and traveled long distances to centers that specialized in treating their ailment. In other words, they started to see themselves as *consumers* of health care rather than as helpless patients, taking more responsibility for decisions and treating health care much like any other commodity on which their hard-earned money was spent.

These trends represent a major shift in attitude and behavior, which has been—for the most part—a positive one. An informed recipient of health care is more likely to make thoughtful choices and then follow through with them, having developed a sense of ownership and responsibility for the process of maintaining or restoring health. But there's a catch: A critical element of any intelligent consumer decision is having accurate, reasonable, and understandable information. What good is an "informed" decision that is actually *misinformed*—based, for example, on inaccurate information, or even propaganda, in the media or on the Internet? How does a health-care consumer sort through all of the claims and counterclaims about various drugs or therapies? And even when people have a clear idea of what they want or need in terms of health care, how do they go about obtaining it?

In this chapter we will look at two important elements of being a wise health-care consumer. First, we will explore how to evaluate health-care claims, introducing the fundamental principles that researchers and health-care professionals apply to diagnostic tests and treatments to determine whether they are helpful, harmful, or merely ineffective. Unfortunately, a good deal of the health information disseminated through the media needs to be taken with a sizable grain of salt. We will offer some ideas to help you weed out the plausible from the implausible. This is particularly important when dealing with the realm of alternative medicine, a broad array of therapies that may be beneficial, dangerous, or have little impact one way or the other. Without going to exhaustive lengths, later in this chapter we will discuss some popular alternative therapies, help you spot questionable claims, and direct you toward more detailed sources of sound information about alternative medicine.

In the second part of this chapter we will explain the importance of finding a primary-care provider for you and your family and will suggest ways to develop a good working relationship with him or her. We will also discuss the various types of insurance or payment options and how they might be best utilized.

How Do We Know What Works?

Bookstores and the Internet are awash with offerings from innumerable experts—some actual, many self-proclaimed—who claim to have the latest and greatest insights into curing health problems, relieving symptoms, or promoting wellness. Many books and Web sites steer readers to therapies, regimens, or dietary supplements that are likely to be quite different from those you might receive from your own physician or another conventional health-care provider. Pharmaceutical manufacturers make their own claims, too, spending billions of dollars each year to induce consumers to "ask your doctor or pharmacist" about their various medications. TV and radio infomercials—including a lineup of programs that fill a great deal of weekend airtime on some Christian radio stations—promote cure-all products that sound too good to be true. (In fact, they are.)

How do you sort out which claims made about a product or treatment are reasonable, whether they come from your own doctor, a best-selling book, a radio broadcast, or the Internet? Just how can you know what works and what doesn't? For example, ponder the following questions:

- Will a cholesterol-lowering drug reduce my chance of having a heart attack?
- Will megadoses of vitamins help me fight off a cold?
- Will certain herbal supplements help my mood or memory?
- Will the product I just heard advertised on the radio get rid of my excess fat?

Answering questions such as these responsibly and then applying those answers appropriately is much easier said than done. For example, to evaluate whether a new drug is a useful treatment for osteoporosis (a thinning of the bones that is commonly seen among women after menopause), researchers might first identify appropriate measures of bone density. They would then design a study to determine what happens to bone density among a number of women who take the drug, compared to a similar number who don't. But how long should women take the drug before researchers test the difference? And what about other factors besides the drug that might affect bone density? Even more important is the question of whether the drug's effects on bone density actually make a difference in the risk of suffering a fracture. (What if the drug makes the bones more dense but not actually stronger?) What about safety and side effects? Do the risks outweigh the benefits? Is the cure worse than the disease? Even if the drug appears to be safe and effective in large-scale studies, is it appropriate for Mrs. Smith, who is sitting in Dr. Jones's exam room?

A Primer on Research and Evidence: How Do We Know What Causes What?

The primary means by which modern conventional medicine tackles this question, whether it concerns medications, supplements, surgical procedures, or diets, is an approach known as **evidence-based medicine**. Evidence-based medicine can be defined as "the conscientious, explicit, and judicious use of current best evidence in making decisions about the care of individual patients. The practice of evidence-based medicine means integrating individual clinical expertise with the best available external clinical evidence from systematic research." Boiling down this fancy verbiage to its essentials leaves us with a great example of both "stating the obvious" and "easier said than done": The overall goal of evidence-based medicine is to take the best available information about what works to keep us healthy (or helps us when we're not) and to apply it intelligently to individual patients.[1]

Evidence of a therapy's efficacy (its capacity to produce a desired effect) and safety comes in many forms, some of which are definitely more reliable than others. Several types of evidence you might see or hear are listed below in order from the least to the most trustworthy.

Advertisements are a familiar source of claims—and occasionally useful information—about medications, supplements, and other types of therapies. Ads for nonprescription drugs and supplements have been a staple of radio, TV, and print media for decades. Prescription drugs have long been marketed intensively to physicians—the ones who recommend and prescribe them—but more recently they have been promoted to nonphysician audiences as well. "Ask your doctor about. . ." ads for prescription-only medications for problems ranging from allergies to sexual dysfunction now routinely appear during network television broadcasts. Because of time limitations (and expense), these may offer little more than the name of the drug and some pleasant images to make it appear user-friendly. (If the ad states what the drug is intended to do, by FDA mandate it must also include a list of possible hazards and side effects.)

A newer form of advertisement is the **infomercial**. Usually encompassing thirty minutes of non-prime-time TV or radio airtime, these hard-sell infomercials pitch a nonprescription product (typically a nutritional supplement), inevitably with a toll-free number for viewers to place their order *right now*. Many of these programs use deceptive titles to imply that they are evenhanded health reports or talk shows, and most make extravagant claims for the effectiveness of the product, often for a host of conditions. Needless to say, advertisements—especially infomercials—are the *least* reliable source of health information because their primary goal is not to educate consumers or present unbiased information. Even if the ads feature a trusted or authoritative spokesman, they are all designed to do just one thing: *convince you to purchase the product.*

Advertisements and infomercials, especially those for dietary supplements, often include **testimonials**, self-reported stories about a product's benefits. (For example, "It helped me lose weight, feel more energetic, improve my sex life . . ." and so on.) In a best-case scenario, testimonials are offered spontaneously by those who truly feel that they benefited from the product. In less honorable situations, they come from someone who is selling the product or who is being paid to give the testimonial. In a worst-case scenario, the claim is made falsely by someone who has never used the product. Unless you personally know the individual and his or her experience with the product, the validity of a testimonial can be difficult to gauge.

Furthermore, even an endorsement from a trustworthy source doesn't guarantee that the product's claims are true or that it will work for you. For example, imagine that a principled and trusted friend tells you that her alertness and energy increased after she started taking a new dietary supplement. Her perception is that these welcome changes resulted from using the product. But it's possible that some other factor—perhaps beginning an exercise program, quitting a sedating medication, resolving a conflict, or even believing that the product would help her—is responsible for her newfound vigor. Testimonials and word of mouth may certainly pique our interest in a product, but they can never substitute for **objective** and **systematic observations** when it comes to determining whether a treatment is truly effective.

Researchers intent on determining the effectiveness and safety of a drug, therapy, or supplement have a variety of research tools at their disposal. One source of information that can yield important evidence is a **case report**. A case report is a description of a single patient's case of a disease, including how the problem was manifested, the therapy undertaken to address it, and the results of that therapy. Case reports are referred to as **anecdotal evidence**, and they are considered more valid than testimonials because the course of the illness and its outcome have been documented by a qualified (and hopefully unbiased) party. The main weakness of case reports is that the human population contains tremendous variability. In other words, what might work wonderfully to treat a disease in one person might be ineffective in another or might cause side effects in the second person that are absent in the first. While case reports are generally considered a weaker form of evidence, they may stimulate or provide direction for more powerful studies.

One of the most important types of health research is the **observational study**, so named because individuals or groups of people are observed in an effort to determine a link between one or more variables—a particular diet, supplement, behavior (such as exercise or smoking), treatment (such as hormone therapy), or an even broader characteristic (such as age or ethnic background)—and a particular outcome. Observational studies not only can explore the efficacy and safety of a drug or other treatment, but they also can be used to determine the effects of a substance when deliberately exposing people to it would be unethical. For example, it would be inappropriate to conduct an experiment in which individuals are told to inhale asbestos fibers for several months or years to see whether they develop various lung diseases. However, one could investigate the association between asbestos and lung disease by performing an observational study of those who are known to have had exposure to asbestos fibers and comparing their health histories with a comparable group (or control group) of individuals who did not have that exposure.

There are two basic types of observational studies. **Retrospective studies** look back in time, comparing a given number of people who have a certain disease with an equal number of similar age (and other characteristics) who do not have it, in order to determine what factors might have played a role in causing that particular disorder. A retrospective study related to estrogen supplementation after menopause, for example, would correlate certain health outcomes (such as hip fractures) with a history of hormone therapy. One problem with retrospective studies, however, is that they rely both on the researchers' ability to collect pertinent and complete data (which can be difficult) and on the patients' memory of long-term habits (which may be faulty). Both of these drawbacks can introduce bias into even well-planned research. **Prospective observational studies**, by contrast, identify several characteristics in a group of people and then follow them over time to see who gets certain health problems and who doesn't. As you might imagine, this can take many years and requires tireless effort to keep track of people and their health status over extended periods of time. If the researchers lose contact with too many people who began the study, for example, the results may not be valid.

Conclusions from both types of observational studies may be open to criticism because people's lives contain so many variables—what they eat, how much they exercise, what risks they take, and so on—that researchers cannot control. Furthermore, these studies may suggest or support a connection between something a person does (or doesn't do) and a particular health problem, but it is difficult for them to establish cause and effect. Observational studies are thus not considered the gold standard of scientific research, but they can build a powerful case. For example, such strong links between smoking and cancer, heart disease, and many other types of health problems have been established that no one seriously questions whether or not smoking contributes to these conditions. In the case of hormone therapy, a convincing body of observational studies suggested that taking supplemental estrogen soon after the onset of menopause and continuing it indefinitely would help prevent osteoporosis and coronary artery disease. Some argued, however, that women who went to the trouble to use estrogen might have been inclined to take better care of themselves, get regular checkups, exercise more regularly, and so on. Perhaps those factors affected their health as much or more than the estrogen. Indeed, experimental studies, which we will describe momentarily, have been unable to prove that estrogen prevents coronary artery disease, although they have supported its role in maintaining bone density.

This brings up an important problem with observational studies: The fact that two factors appear to be associated with one another does not always mean that one causes the other. One way to answer the question of causation is to perform an **experimental study**, in which researchers deliberately adjust one or more variables for some individuals but not others, according to a carefully planned design. Participants who volunteer for such a study are randomly assigned either to the **test group**, which receives the medication or other treatment being studied, or to the **control group**, which receives either a treatment of known efficacy or a placebo (an inert substance that appears identical to the one being tested). Researchers can thus more directly compare the effects of an experimental drug or treatment to the effects of a known drug or placebo.

An application of research to everyday life: We tend to assume a cause-and-effect relationship if one event follows another closely in time. Sometimes our conclusions are reasonable: If you break out in hives shortly after starting a new prescription, chances are you may be allergic to that drug. But we have to be careful with these assumptions. If you borrow a friend's Toyota one day and then come down with the flu the next, it would be illogical to conclude that driving a Toyota impairs your immunity.

To add more insurance against bias, prospective studies can be **blinded**. That is, they can be carried out so that the participants have no idea whether they have been assigned to the experimental group or the control group. To add yet an additional layer of protection against bias, many studies are **double-blinded**: Neither the participants nor the researchers know whether a given subject is in the treatment or control group, although records are kept so that the results of the study can be correctly interpreted later. (This might seem overly cautious, but it is well-known that a physician experimenter who knows what the patient in front of him or her is receiving may unconsciously give off cues that could affect the patient's response.) The gold standard for clinical research is thus the **randomized placebo-controlled double-blind study**, although not all types of medical questions can be studied in this fashion. (Current medical literature often uses a shorter phrase—a **randomized controlled trial**, or **RCT**—to refer to this type of study.)

Unfortunately, even the gold standard is not foolproof. Conclusions that are based on a single study may prove to be erroneous, even if that study is well designed and well executed. Therefore, if a team of researchers obtains a noteworthy result from a well-designed study, it is often appropriate to see whether a different team can perform the same experiment (or one that is very similar) and come up with a comparable outcome. If a study's results cannot be duplicated, its conclusions may not be trustworthy. This is called **reproducibility**, and it is very important in validating experimental results—especially those that are unusual or surprising.

Even a carefully planned study, whether observational or experimental, can suffer from bias or subtle flaws in design or data analysis that escape the notice of researchers and reviewers. Problems can arise, for example, if there are too few people participating in the experiment or if the wrong criteria are used to select participants. Any of these defects can skew results and lead to differing conclusions when similar studies are performed by different researchers. For example, by the early 1990s there were nineteen retrospective observational studies investigating the link between environmental tobacco smoke (secondhand smoke) and lung cancer. Of these, fifteen suggested an increased risk of lung cancer associated with secondhand smoke, three found a decreased risk, and one found no difference between women who were exposed to secondhand smoke and those who were not.

In an effort to make sense of conflicting conclusions from different studies (or to confirm what appears to be an emerging trend in similar studies), researchers may evaluate the results of multiple studies in what is called a **meta-analysis**. A meta-analysis is a quantitative statistical analysis—in simpler terms, a giant number-crunching exercise—encompassing several separate but similar studies. By systematically comparing, combining, and synthesizing the data from several studies, a more complete conclusion can be drawn on a given subject of study. In the example above, researchers performed a meta-analysis of the existing studies on lung cancer and secondhand smoke. They found that exposure to secondhand smoke resulted in a 42 percent increased risk of lung cancer, prompting the Environmental Protection Agency to declare secondhand smoke a carcinogen.

One other important safeguard against erroneous or misleading results is accountability, which occurs when researchers submit their work to others who are qualified to make unbiased judgments on a study's design, execution, and analysis. In scientific circles this system of accountability to colleagues is known as **peer review**, and it is a requirement for publication of a study in all credible scientific journals. While the peer-review process is not perfect, it can provide constructive criticism that in turn can help researchers improve their methods and analyses. On a more basic level, peer review encourages a healthy sense of skepticism. It is not enough for an individual or company simply to announce that a particular treatment is effective or that a new drug is safe. Peer review forces scientists to demonstrate that the methods they used to arrive at their conclusions are valid. This is especially important in medicine, where a person's life and health may depend on the reliability of the research backing a particular therapy or medication.

So why does all this matter? You may not feel inspired at this point to subscribe to the *New England Journal of Medicine* or take a statistics course so that you can analyze the research supporting the next prescription your doctor writes for you. But as we will see later, both reliable and bogus health information abounds in the media, and knowing a little about the way legitimate research is done may help you detect the difference. For now, you should be aware of two basic principles:

1. **Talk is cheap, but solid evidence isn't.** It's easy to make all kinds of claims (especially for a product that could make a profit), but building a reliable body of knowledge about the complexities of health and disease requires extraordinary effort, time, patience, and resources.

2. **When it comes to valid scientific inquiry, there are no lone rangers.** You should quickly head for the exit if any practitioner claims to have a one-of-a-kind device that can diagnose anything or a "unique" product that cures all manner of disease (especially one that no one else knows about). You should also be highly suspicious of any self-appointed expert who claims to have answers to complex health problems (such as cancer or Alzheimer's disease) that have been missed or ignored by researchers all over the world. Furthermore, no one—the pharmaceutical industry, the American Medical Association, the government, or anyone else—is trying to suppress "natural" cures that are supposedly better than conventional treatments. Such allegations are fueled by a dangerous combination of ignorance and arrogance, and they are not worthy of your attention.

Defining Alternative Medicine

Earlier in this chapter we mentioned the term **alternative medicine** without actually defining it. While exact definitions can be elusive, many who examine alternative medicine would agree with what Potter Stewart, a former U.S. Supreme Court justice, once said about obscenity: "I know it when I see it." One common definition isn't much more specific: Alternative medicine is whatever does not come under the heading of conventional therapy. While rather vague, this description is to a large degree true. Generally speaking, alternative therapies are not taught as first-line approaches in conventional medical schools, they are not the primary modes of care offered in most hospitals or health-care professionals' offices, and they are not extensively covered by most health-insurance plans.

But there are some important exceptions and qualifiers to those generalizations. For example, while alternative therapies are not taught in conventional medical schools as standard approaches to treating disease, their popularity has caused many schools to include courses on integrating certain alternative therapies into mainstream treatment modalities. Most primary-care practitioners now routinely ask their patients about any supplements and herbal remedies they may be using and have at least a rudimentary understanding of the more common preparations. Chiropractic is so widely practiced in the United States, Canada, and Europe that the term *alternative* might not seem appropriate to describe it. A number of health-insurance plans now cover therapies such as chiropractic and acupuncture, at least under certain circumstances.

Types of alternative therapies

The number and diversity of alternative therapies are truly staggering, so much so that categorizing them is a daunting task. For more than a decade, the National Center for Complementary and Alternative Medicine (originally called the Office of Alternative Medicine and part of the National Institutes of Health) has refined and revised its lists and categories of these practices, and it now groups them into some domains that have a loose conceptual association. They are as follows:

- **Mind/body medicine** involves techniques intended to enhance the mind's effects on functions and symptoms in the rest of the body. Examples include meditation, yoga, and prayer, as well as pursuits such as art, music, and dance when used as part of the healing process.
- **Biologically based practices** represent the realm of alternative therapy that the average citizen is most likely to use and for which scientific research will arguably yield the most fruit. It encompasses the gamut of **dietary supplements**, including herbal or botanical products; vitamins and minerals taken in unusual doses for specific therapeutic purposes; and **probiotics**, specific strains of bacteria that may have beneficial effects. This category also includes certain dietary regimens, some of which are very strict, that purport to improve health.
- **Manipulative and body-based practices** involve movement or manipulation of certain parts of the body, as exemplified by chiropractic and osteopathic manipulation, as well as massage therapies.
- **Energy medicine** encompasses two extremely diverse realms. One involves the alternative use of verified and widely studied energy

fields, such as magnetism or low-intensity electrical pulses, for therapeutic purposes. The other encompasses techniques claiming to manipulate "human energy fields" (sometimes called biofields) that are said to circulate within and beyond the body. (Think of the Force in the *Star Wars* films, minus the special effects and light sabers.) Examples include therapeutic touch, Reiki, and qi gong, all of which have strong ties to Eastern religious worldviews.

NCCAM previously identified a fifth domain, called **alternative medical systems**, that encompasses complete, self-contained systems of diagnosis and treatment such as traditional Chinese medicine, *ayurveda* (traditional East Indian medicine), homeopathic medicine, and naturopathy. Because these employ elements of all the other domains, to varying degrees, they are now classified separately as **whole medical systems**.

This classification scheme is useful to some degree, but it offers little guidance regarding the plausibility and underpinnings of the various alternative therapies, let alone their efficacy and safety. Some critical questions should be asked of any alternative therapy, and they are as important as the basic questions, "Does it work?" and "Is it safe?" The more penetrating questions are:

- Does the particular therapy or system make sense?
- What are its basic assumptions about the way the body works?
- Are the therapy or system and its assumptions compatible with the long-established and widely validated principles of biology, physiology, chemistry, and physics? Put in more basic terms, if the therapy or system was assumed to be true, would we need to rewrite every science textbook to accommodate it?
- If I receive or practice this therapy, am I accepting—or promulgating—ideas that will compromise my faith or that of someone else? This is a significant issue not addressed by NCCAM or by many of the books and Web sites that promote alternative medicine but one that needs to be seriously considered by those who believe in the truthfulness of Scripture. A number of alternative therapies and systems are built on spiritual foundations that are incompatible with—or overtly hostile to—the basic teachings of the Bible.

One simple but useful classification approach divides alternative therapies into four basic groups according to their underlying assumptions, and more specifically their compatibility with well-established scientific principles, as well as their involvement with supernatural forces or entities.[2] The four classes of therapies are: (1) those that conform to biologically plausible mechanisms; (2) those that stray from these mechanisms to varying degrees; (3) those that are overtly implausible or incompatible with well-established principles of biology, chemistry, and physics; and (4) those that rely to some extent on supernatural powers. A thorough review of the gamut of alternative therapies is available elsewhere. Later in this chapter we will list a number of resources that offer more information on this subject. Nevertheless, as you hear claims for various therapies, you may find it helpful to consider which of these four categories best describe them.

Therapies that are biologically plausible

The principles and practice of these therapies do not strain or violate the laws of physics or established facts of biology and physiology. Most of the biologically based practices noted on page 820 (such as the use of dietary supplements) fall into this category because the efficacy, safety, and mechanism of action of these substances can be determined through straightforward research. Chiropractic manipulation as a form of physical therapy (especially for back pain) does not violate any principles of biology, although its original claims to cure disease by aligning the spine are not plausible (see sidebar "Chiropractic: Alternative or Mainstream?"). Certain uses of acupuncture may serve to relieve pain through

CHIROPRACTIC: ALTERNATIVE OR MAINSTREAM?

Chiropractic, which means "hand work," has been so widely practiced throughout the United States and around the world over the past century that one could reasonably argue that it represents mainstream (as opposed to alternative) health care. There are more than sixty-five thousand chiropractors in the United States, and as of 1997 they carried out an estimated 190 million treatments (including care for one out of three people with low back pain).[3] Chiropractic practitioners are licensed in all fifty states and are reimbursed by most major medical insurance plans, as well as by Medicare Part B coverage.

Widespread public acceptance of chiropractic has not entirely settled the question of whether it represents mainstream or alternative health care. The original premise of chiropractic and the claims of a number of its contemporary practitioners fall well outside of the bounds of biological plausibility. On the other hand, many chiropractors are strongly committed to evidence-based therapy and serve effectively as musculoskeletal consultants within their health-care community.

The founder of chiropractic, D. D. Palmer (1845–1913), proposed that good health requires the unimpaired flow of an invisible energy (which he called "Innate Intelligence," or simply "the Innate") throughout the body, and more specifically through the spinal cord and its branches. He taught that the flow of the Innate was impeded by misalignments (known as **subluxations**) in the spine, and that proper alignment of the spine through "hands-on" adjustments could not only relieve back pain but also treat other illness and disease throughout the body. Palmer's notion that spinal manipulation is the key to overall health generated controversy and conflict with conventional medical practitioners for decades and is not taken seriously by any mainstream scientific body today.

neurological mechanisms; this is entirely different from uses involving invisible energy flow that are taught in traditional Chinese medicine.

Therapies that stray from plausibility

Alternative therapies fall into this category when they use the vocabulary of contemporary science and medicine but make claims for which evidence (or logic) is spurious, scant, or nonexistent. These include diets that are promoted to "detoxify" the liver, colon, or other organs or suggest that food choices should be based on your blood type. They also include "treatments" for a host of symptoms supposedly caused by the common yeast *Candida albicans*, as well as other products marketed through infomercials for cure-all products on radio and television. Other biologically implausible alternative approaches include iridology (in which health problems are supposedly diagnosed or predicted by changes in the iris, the colored area of the eye surrounding the pupil) and can-

Indeed, strict adherence to this idea (sometimes referred to as **straight chiropractic**) has long been debated among chiropractors themselves, along with other issues such as the existence of the Innate, the definition of subluxations, and the scope of illness that can be treated by manipulation.

The dissenters (known as "mixers") who abandoned the doctrine of subluxations as the cause of all disease gradually became the clear majority and also helped chiropractors gain credibility in the mainstream of health care. Most limit the scope of problems treated with manipulation to those involving the musculoskeletal system, often using other treatments as well, including ultrasound, exercise, and postural training. Many are skilled in the assessment of workplace ergonomics (the physical design and arrangements of chair, desk, and other equipment such as computer hardware) that may contribute to chronic pain.

Many chiropractors see themselves as providing a broader scope of care for the "whole person," providing input on topics ranging from nutrition to athletic training. Claims that ongoing chiropractic treatment for months or years is necessary for optimal health maintenance definitely strain credibility—Medicare, for example, will not cover ongoing "preventive" chiropractic treatments—and some practitioners promote manipulative care for conditions that are not clearly related to spine or muscle function, such as asthma and attention deficit hyperactivity disorder (ADHD).[4] There remains a significant burden of proof for claims that chiropractic can play a credible role in treating problems such as these.

The bottom line: Chiropractors function both in the mainstream of health care and in the eccentric fringes, depending on their scope of care and willingness to embrace evidence-based treatments as opposed to more implausible alternatives. ■

cer treatments that involve unproven (and often peculiar) regimens such as coffee or castor oil enemas.

What determines whether an alternative therapy falls into the first or second category? Not the position of a promotional book on the current best-seller list. Not an endorsement by a celebrity. Not the number of satisfied customers, although reports of success can certainly stimulate further study. The answer is *the quality of the evidence supporting it.*

Occasionally an alternative approach that goes against the grain of mainstream medical opinion will migrate from the second category to the first. This can and should occur when enough solid evidence accumulates to suggest not only that the therapy may be beneficial, but also that there exists a reasonable scientific basis to explain how it works. Both of these qualifications are important because it is always possible for people to respond to a highly suspect treatment through the placebo effect (see sidebar "Alternative Therapies and the Placebo Effect") or for reasons other than those given by the treatment's promoters.

The Atkins diet provides one example of a therapy that has gradually gained a modest degree of respect from the medical community. When it was first introduced, it ran counter to the prevailing wisdom that the only way to lose weight was to reduce fat in the diet. Many medical professionals concluded that there was no basis in reality for such a diet, that it absolutely could not work, and that it would lead to disastrous consequences. Then something interesting happened: Controlled studies began to suggest that a diet high in protein and low in carbohydrates, as proposed by Atkins and others, might help some people lose weight without causing a worsening of cardiovascular disease risk factors.[5] While most health professionals still do not believe that a diet high in protein (and generous in fat) is the best way to control weight, many have been willing to acknowledge that this approach might be successful for some patients (at least for a while) and that there is in fact a reasonable physiological explanation for it.

For a detailed look at the conflict between low-fat and low-carb diets, see chapter 6, beginning on page 231.

Therapies that defy plausibility

In this category are alternative therapies whose theory and practice clearly contradict an extensive body of knowledge about the way humans actually work (not to mention animals and plants). Not only do these treatments run counter to widely validated principles of biology, physiology, and physics, but they often cannot be studied using any scientific means. This category includes a number of therapies claiming to restore health by manipulating invisible energy that is said to circulate within and outside of the human body. **Traditional Chinese medicine** (including classical acupuncture and acupressure techniques) purports to adjust the flow of an energy called **Ch'i**, while practitioners of traditional East Indian practices known as **ayurveda** claim to manipulate **prana**—which by the way, is described as flowing in patterns that are completely differ-

ALTERNATIVE THERAPIES AND THE PLACEBO EFFECT

Why do many implausible therapies appear to work, at least for some people? One important factor is the **placebo effect**, which we mentioned in chapter 2 (page 21). This is the mechanism by which a person's condition improves in response to his or her own *expectation* that a treatment or medication will make a difference. It has played a role in medical practice for hundreds of years, but its effects have been largely ignored in today's world of high-tech and often impersonal health care. (The effect *isn't* ignored in clinical research, where an inert substance—the placebo—is an important component of a well-designed study, as we described earlier in this chapter.)

Alternative therapies often provide an ideal arena for the placebo effect to work, for several reasons:

- They are often "kinder and gentler" than conventional therapies. You aren't likely to suffer side effects from the extremely dilute solutions used in homeopathy, for example, because there is no plausible reason for these remedies to have *any* effect on human physiology. It's always easier to feel better when the treatment isn't making you feel worse.
- Many seek alternative care for problems that their conventional physician couldn't solve or for multiple symptoms that have been dismissed or ignored. An alternative therapist may not only take these tough complaints seriously but may also offer explicit solutions. "I've figured out what's wrong with you, and I can help you feel better" is a powerful statement, whether or not the diagnosis and treatment make any sense.
- Alternative therapies are often promoted with enthusiasm, using positive vocabulary and imagery. Phrases such as "all-natural," "gets rid of toxins," "helps the body heal itself," "burns fat," and "boosts immunity" sound encouraging and promising, even if biologically unrealistic.
- Individuals who seek alternative care often see themselves as taking charge of their own health, rather than submitting to the orders of a doctor or the bureaucracy of the health-care system.

Ironically, conventional physicians who take the time to explain carefully the risks and benefits of their treatment plan may be playing against the placebo effect and activating its evil twin, the **nocebo effect**. This involves a worsening of symptoms in response to taking a medication or other treatment that a person perceives as harmful, toxic, or otherwise unpleasant.

Needless to say, whether a practitioner is conventional or alternative, intangible but very important factors—empathy, genuine interest, optimism, and honesty—play a powerful role in the healing process. ■

ent from those taken by Ch'i. Not one of these energies has ever been detected by reputable researchers using even the most sensitive technologies, despite their central role in so many alternative systems.

Two other therapies in this category are worth noting. Therapeutic touch—a misnomer, because there is no touch involved—purports to redirect invisible energies through the movement of the therapist's hands above the surface of the patient's body. It has been taught to thousands of individuals (primarily nurses) around the world, although its validity has been convincingly discredited in relatively simple scientific experiments.[6] **Homeopathy**, which dates from the eighteenth century, claims to treat symptoms by giving infinitesimally small doses of materials that *cause* those symptoms when taken in higher doses. Reviewing the specifics of this system is not possible in this chapter, but suffice it to say that homeopathy, and the use of homeopathic remedies, is burdened with so many profound biological and physiological inconsistencies that it is a thoroughly unreliable approach to restoring health. For those interested in a detailed review of the issues raised by these methods, we recommend the books *Examining Alternative Medicine: An Inside Look at the Benefits & Risks* by Paul C. Reisser, M.D., Dale Mabe, D.O., and Robert Velarde (Downers Grove, Ill.: InterVarsity, 2001) and *Alternative Medicine: The Christian Handbook* by Dónal O'Mathúna, Ph.D., and Walt Larimore, M.D. (Grand Rapids, Mich.: Zondervan, 2001).

When challenged regarding the lack of scientific backing for the precepts of these therapies, proponents invariably fall back on the argument, "We don't completely understand it, but that doesn't matter—it just works." The problem is that people may—or actually may not—respond to these approaches as well as their proponents claim. Careful research often shows that these don't "just work" as advertised. Furthermore, when a person does respond positively to a therapy whose underlying assumptions fly in the face of what we know about the way the body works, the benefits can invariably be explained using far more straightforward mechanisms, such as the body's incredible ability to repair itself or a healthy dose of the placebo effect. In other words, the fact that a person feels better after a particular treatment—whether alternative or conventional—does not necessarily validate that approach. A person who feels better, of course, may not particularly care about whether the explanation makes any sense, but the question is important and must not be ignored. (As an extreme example, would you feel comfortable seeing a practitioner who explained that his treatments were based on astrology, Tarot cards, the lines on your palm, or advice he or she received during a séance—even if you felt better after the visit?)

Integrating these more implausible approaches into the mainstream of medical care requires an awkward compartmentalizing of thinking, because if they accurately reflected how the human body works, then all knowledge of biology, chemistry, and physics accumulated over the past two centuries would have to be declared utterly wrong. Furthermore, with few exceptions the basic assumptions of these approaches are metaphysical rather than scientific. Most are deeply rooted in Eastern religious understandings of reality, God, and humanity that are incompatible with the most basic teachings of the Bible, as we will summarize momentarily. As a result, practitioners of these therapies who also embrace biblical teachings must undergo a sort of spiritual compartmentalizing—in essence, operating from two contradictory worldviews at the same time.

Therapies that court the supernatural

Everyone should be free to practice and promote his or her religious convictions, whether Eastern, Judeo-Christian, or otherwise. But many advocates of alternative therapies that fall in this fourth category (and the previous one as well) are disingenuous about their spiritual underpinnings and agendas. Some link their ideas to quantum physics, for example, or invoke quasiscientific words such as *bioenergy* while downplaying or even denying the overtly religious nature of their approaches. As we describe in some detail in chapter 9, the Scriptures teach clearly that God is God, and we are not. If we are to follow biblical precepts, any philosophy or health-care practice that has the potential to shift one's worldview from "I need God" to "I *am* God" deserves to be scrupulously avoided.

A fundamental component of the biblical worldview is that God created a universe that operates on orderly principles and mechanisms that can be discovered and understood through diligent investigation. At the same time, the Scriptures state that God can intervene supernaturally to bring about healing, and that it is appropriate to petition God on behalf of those who are ill. James 5:14-15 says: "Is any one of you sick? He should call the elders of the church to pray over him and anoint him with oil in the name of the Lord. And the prayer offered in faith will make the sick person well; the Lord will raise him up."

Of course, such intervention is entirely at God's discretion. However, certain alternative practices seek to bring about healing by gaining mastery of supernatural forces or engaging the help of spiritual beings other than God. This category encompasses a diverse collection of approaches that are as old as humankind and its perennial desire to have godlike powers, although they may be presented in language that sounds quasiscientific (and less spooky) to appeal to modern audiences.

Psychic diagnosis and healing falls into this category, although different terms may be used. In the 1970s participants in holistic health conferences marveled at tales of psychic surgeons in the Philippines and elsewhere who, under the direction of spirit guides, supposedly could remove diseased tissue painlessly using rusty knives. Psychic surgeons have been largely debunked by trained illusionists who can duplicate their feats using sleight of hand. Other contemporary claims for psychic abilities have been toned down somewhat, although they never disappear. For example, some practitioners claim to be "medical sensitives" who can diagnose a patient's problem after hearing little more than his or her name. A variation on psychic healing is now given the less exotic title **distant healing** and might be referred to as prayer, although this does not involve petitioning God. Rather, it is an attempt to extend a person's consciousness across space and time to benefit—and hopefully not harm—another. (We discuss this in more detail in chapter 9, beginning on page 386.)

In **shamanism**, a healer (often the traditional medicine man in remote cultures) enters an altered state of consciousness to interact with spirit "helpers" for the purpose of exerting power over the material world. While this might seem exotic for contemporary Western patients, some popular books on healing have promoted the idea of using meditative techniques to identify an "inner guide" who can provide wisdom and insight on health and other matters. These stray dangerously close to or overtly violate what we might call a biblical no-fly zone. The Scriptures clearly teach that the spiritual realm is not all sweetness and light, that some of its inhabitants are cunning and dangerous beings bent on deceiving and ruining us, and that we are not to engage any spiritual entities other than God Himself. (See Deuteronomy 18:10-12 and Isaiah 8:19, for example.) These warnings are issued not merely because God alone is worthy of our attention, but also for our own safety—like swimmers entering shark-infested waters, we are not equipped to plunge into this realm and return unscathed.

A number of alternative-medicine best sellers have taught that healing essentially involves adjusting our core beliefs to align with **monism**, the notion that "all is one" in the universe. According to this worldview, which underlies Hinduism and other Eastern religious traditions, we are spiritual entities indistinct from one another or from God. Monism insists that if we are one with God, then we are inherently divine—another proposition that does not square well with everyday experience. According to monism, our problem is not that we are alienated from God and need to repent of our rebellion against Him but rather that we don't realize we are God and need to be enlightened of our true nature. Our experiences during normal waking consciousness—including the awful things human beings do to one another every day—do not seem to corroborate this idea, but Eastern traditions have provided various techniques designed to alter our consciousness so that we might *experience* our godhood and the unity of all things. As we discussed in chapter 9, meditation that seeks to empty the mind of conscious thought (typically by repeating a word called a **mantra** over and over) is one of the most widely used of these techniques.

Even **yoga**, a familiar fixture in fitness centers (and even some churches), has a spiritual agenda far more profound than learning simple ways to stretch and relax. The word *yoga* comes from the Sanskrit for "union" or "yoke" and points toward the ultimate goal of the various exercise, breathing, and meditative techniques. Yogic stretching and breathing exercises are likewise ultimately intended to lead a person to an *experience*, not merely a belief, that he or she is "one with all things," or God. The degree to which this idea will be expressed will depend on the individual teacher and class setting, but the fact remains that a profound, experiential worldview adjustment is the primary agenda of yogic practices.

For more information about alternative therapies

If you are investigating one or more alternative therapies, be sure to consider not only their scientific credibility but also any underlying (or overt) spiritual implications. One great place to start is *Alternative Medicine: The Christian Handbook*, which provides an insightful look at the spectrum of alternative medicine from both a spiritual and a scientific perspective. It lists and defines numerous therapies, discusses therapeutic claims, reviews research on efficacy, and provides specific cautions or recommendations. The book *Examining Alternative Medicine: An Inside Look at the Benefits & Risks* provides a studied observation of the assumptions and philosophies that underlie many popular alternative therapies. (For publication information on these books, see page 826.)

There are literally thousands of Web sites devoted to alternative therapies, but most promote specific approaches or products and thus may be biased or unreliable sources of information. Some exceptions include:

- The Web site for the National Center for Complementary and Alternative Medicine (NCCAM), http://nccam.nih.gov, offers information about alternative therapies in general, some reviews of specific therapies, and the findings of NCCAM research projects. In attempting to be evenhanded—some would argue favorably inclined—toward complementary and alternative medicine, the site offers little critical assessment of therapies other than reporting the results of research studies. (NCCAM's overall mission has been to disseminate information about alternative therapies that are deemed safe and effective, rather than to protect consumers from those that are not.)
- The section on alternative medicine at Healthfinder, a service of the National Health Information Center of the U.S. Department of Health & Human Services, contains numerous links to other Web sites, including those of professional organizations, academic institutions, and federal agencies. Most of these are informative; however, some links are to groups that advance alternative therapies, where the content is more promotional than analytical. The Healthfinder Web site is http://www.healthfinder.gov, and the alternative medicine links are at http://www.healthfinder.gov/Scripts/SearchContext.asp?topic=35.
- A different approach is taken at Quackwatch, a nonprofit Web site operated by Stephen Barrett, M.D., a longtime critic of alternative therapies. As the title suggests, this site, accessible at http://www.quackwatch.org, is dedicated to critiquing and debunking

therapies that lack scientific credibility. A similar critical approach is taken at http://www.ncahf.org, the Web site of the nonprofit National Council Against Health Fraud. Articles posted at both sites provide information and analysis that is generally unfavorable to alternative therapies but nonetheless informative (and never boring).

Evaluating Drugs and Supplements

The rising popularity of alternative therapies in the United States over the past two decades has been accompanied by a dramatic increase in the use of herbal remedies and other dietary supplements. At the same time, as a nation we remain avid users of prescription drugs and over-the-counter (OTC) medications. Americans filled an estimated 3 billion prescriptions in 2003, generating more than $216 billion in sales of these medications.[7] According to the Consumer Healthcare Products Association, three out of four Americans use one or more OTC drugs to treat common symptoms (such as a headache or runny nose), and their purchases amounted to more than $15 billion in 2004.[8] We are also the world's leading consumers of dietary supplements, with more than 100 million Americans taking daily vitamins and minerals and over 35 million using herbal products on a regular basis. As of 2000, annual sales of these products were approximately $17 billion.[9]

Nearly half (44 percent) of Americans take at least one prescription drug, and more than 15 percent take three or more. More than 60 percent of visits to physicians' offices or outpatient clinics are associated with the writing of at least one prescription medication.[10]

About one thousand active ingredients are used in more than one hundred thousand different nonprescription drug preparations currently on the market.[11]

Many people assume that dietary supplements in general and herbal products in particular have an advantage over OTC and prescription drugs in terms of overall safety, even effectiveness. Supplement marketers routinely reinforce this belief by referring to their products as all-natural, implying that if a product is natural it must be safe (and good for you too). In fact, the only truly natural products are those found in the produce section of your local supermarket or at a local farmers market. Once a compound is extracted and concentrated into a pill or tonic, it is no more natural than a prescription or OTC drug. But even if the word *natural* on the label doesn't necessarily guarantee a dietary supplement's safety or effectiveness, promoters of these products are correct when they point out that a significant number of injuries and fatalities result every year from drug reactions. A widely quoted 1998 study in the *Journal of the American Medical Association* estimated that adverse reactions to prescription and OTC drugs resulted in more than 2.2 million serious events and over 100,000 deaths among hospitalized patients in 1994 in the United States.[12] These were not the result of overdose, abuse, noncompliance, or errors made by health-care personnel in the hospital. While the estimates in this study have been challenged as being significantly inflated, even if only a tenth as many serious or fatal drug reactions occur every year, the number is still highly significant.

Dietary supplements (including herbal preparations) generally are less potent than OTC and prescription drugs and are thus less likely to provoke serious side effects. That being said, there are three potential problem areas with the use of supplements. First, a person might use supplements and herbal remedies to self-medicate a problem for which more effective conventional treatments exist or delay having a medical evaluation that would lead to the correct diagnosis. Of course, self-treatment and procrastination could occur with or without the use of supplements, but some promoters of dietary supplements may contribute to the problem by implying (or claiming outright) that their products are superior to mainstream treatment.

A second problem area is that of potential interactions between supplements and other medications. Unfortunately, supplement users may forget to inform their physicians that they are using these products (mistakenly believing that they won't have any effect on other medical care) or say nothing out of concern that the doctor may not approve. However, it is crucial to inform anyone who is providing health care for you of *everything* you take—prescriptions, OTC drugs, vitamins, minerals, herbs, and any other supplements. This is particularly important if you are taking one or more drugs for blood pressure, diabetes, any heart condition, anxiety, or depression, or if any of your medications affect liver function or inhibit blood clotting, such as warfarin (Coumadin) or aspirin. The popular herb ginkgo biloba, for example, can inhibit blood clotting, which could be hazardous for someone having surgery or using anticoagulant medications.

The third potential problem is the possibility of an allergic or toxic effect of the supplement or one of its ingredients. The burden of evidence for the safety and efficacy of drugs required by U.S. law is very different from that required for dietary supplements. While new medications (prescription and OTC) must go through a stringent approval process to be marketed in the United States (see sidebar "How Medications Are Approved for Sale in the United States"), dietary supplements are *not* subject to the same type of regulation. In 1994, Congress enacted landmark legislation known as the Dietary Supplement Health and Education Act (or DSHEA), which set the tone for marketing supplements in the United States. DSHEA's underlying assumption was that good health can be promoted—and a host of diseases averted—through optimal nutrition and that dietary supplements play a role in improving the nation's nutritional status. Therefore, the government should erect few if any barriers to the sale of safe nutritional or dietary supplements to the public. A broad range of substances falls under DSHEA's definition of a dietary supplement: "a product (other than tobacco) that is intended to supplement the diet that bears or contains one or more of the following dietary ingredients: a vitamin, a mineral, an herb or other botanical, an amino acid, a dietary substance for use by man to supplement the diet by increasing the total daily intake, or a concentrate, metabolite, constituent, extract, or combinations of these ingredients."[13]

DSHEA has two significant features. One is that a supplement manufacturer can make what is called a "structure or function" claim for a product without FDA evaluation or approval of the evidence supporting that claim, as reflected in the familiar disclaimer that you will find on nearly all supplement labels: "This statement has not been evaluated by the Food and Drug Administration. This product is not intended to diagnose, treat, cure, or prevent any disease." The manufacturer need only notify the FDA that the product bearing a given claim is being marketed (within thirty days of its release) and is only supposed to be able to substantiate that the claim is truthful and not misleading. A supplement's label might say the product "promotes cardiovascular health" or "supports immune function" without any explanation to consumers as to what aspect of cardiovascular health is promoted or what specific immune function is supported. What the promoter *cannot* do is claim that the supplement actually treats or prevents a specific disease.

Critics of DSHEA have complained that manufacturers' ability to make claims with-

HOW MEDICATIONS ARE APPROVED FOR SALE IN THE UNITED STATES

When a company wants to bring a new prescription or over-the-counter medication to the market, it must take the product through an involved (and expensive) approval process by the Food and Drug Administration (FDA). The first step is submitting an **investigational new drug application**, along with results from animal testing and proposals for human experimentation. Clinical trials begin only after the FDA reviews the research plan and **institutional review boards** (which approve the protocols of clinical trials) make sure that human subjects are fully informed of any risk, have given full consent, and are appropriately protected from harm during the trials. Clinical trials then take place in three phases.

- **Phase 1 trials** are performed mainly on animals and healthy human subjects to examine drug safety, usually involving twenty to eighty subjects. The most common side effects of the drug—along with the frequency with which they occur—are determined. Researchers also evaluate how the drug is metabolized or excreted.
- **Phase 2 trials** begin if the drug is judged to be adequately safe. Controlled studies are performed to provide preliminary data on the drug's efficacy for patients with a given disease. Safety and side effects continue to be monitored. These studies may involve up to several hundred subjects.
- **Phase 3 trials** are started if phase 2 trials provide evidence of therapeutic benefit. Clinical trials in this phase gather more data, looking at more subjects and at different populations, and examine the medication at different dosages or in combination with other drugs. These studies may include several hundred to several thousand subjects.

The final step toward FDA approval is for the drug's sponsor to submit what is formally known as a **new drug application**, which includes all data from

out FDA evaluation of the evidence supporting them has created an unregulated Dodge City marketing environment, governed only by the phrase *caveat emptor* ("let the buyer beware"). Also, promoters of supplements often push the envelope with the prohibition against claiming their products treat disease. On infomercials, for example, a person offering a testimonial may proclaim that his diabetes, depression, or other malady disappeared when he took the product, and the promoter won't make any effort to qualify those statements. Often outrageous claims are made for months before the Federal Trade Commission (which polices this aspect of DSHEA) actually identifies and cracks down on the perpetrators.

DSHEA's other significant feature is that it inverts the regulatory system for

animal studies and human clinical trials. The FDA scrutinizes data from the clinical trials, along with any other pertinent research or information, to evaluate the drug's effectiveness and safety. Reviewers look for any weaknesses or flaws in the sponsor's studies or data analysis and decide whether they agree with the sponsor's conclusions about the drug's fitness to be released as a product that physicians can prescribe (or that may be purchased without prescription). Needless to say, no drug is 100 percent safe in the sense of having absolutely no side effects. (One could argue that aspirin might have trouble obtaining FDA approval if it were introduced today, given its known risk of causing stomach irritation and bleeding.) Instead, the overriding consideration is whether a drug's benefits are determined to outweigh its risks.

Although the FDA approval process is rigorous, it is not always the last word on a medication's efficacy and safety. Occasionally problems are not discovered until after a drug has been approved by the FDA and used by thousands or even millions of people. These unpleasant discoveries can and do occur after the drug is on the market (in what is called the **postmarketing phase**) because most clinical trials involve, at most, several thousand subjects, and very rare side effects may not be apparent until many more individuals—perhaps millions—take the drug. If the problem is potentially serious, physicians and pharmacists throughout the United States are notified, and the manufacturer may be required to add what is called a "black box" warning to the drug's prescribing information. If a medication's newly discovered hazards are deemed to represent an unacceptable risk to patient safety, the manufacturer may be ordered to take it off the market.

Needless to say, the removal of a drug from the market is a serious setback for the manufacturer. Not only must all the investment in the medication's development and approval be written off, but the manufacturer will also usually find itself facing hundreds or thousands of lawsuits filed on behalf of those who were harmed (or think they were) by the drug. In addition, the FDA's approval process for that medication is likely to be scrutinized and criticized. ■

supplement safety, which, like effectiveness, does not need to be proven before a product enters the marketplace. An unsafe dietary supplement (or a hazardous ingredient present in many supplements) can be sold for months or years, and nothing can be done about it until the FDA *proves* it to be unsafe. This usually happens only after health officials have linked the supplement to a pattern of health problems in many individuals. Such was the case with **ephedra** (also called *ma huang*), which contains compounds known as ephedrine alkaloids that have multiple stimulant effects. Ephedra was added to a host of supplements that were promoted for losing weight, boosting sports performance, and increasing overall energy. As early as 1997 the FDA proposed warnings that products containing ephedra not be taken for more than seven days. Over the next several years, hundreds of case reports associated this compound with incidents of heart attack, stroke, seizure, and even death. Finally in February 2004, the FDA banned it from sale in the United States, although that decision has been subjected to legal challenge.

It is vital to note that the laxity of the laws governing dietary supplements compared with those regulating prescription or OTC drugs does not mean that all supplements are unsafe or ineffective, or that all FDA-approved medications are guaranteed to work without a hitch. A good deal of peer-reviewed research indicates that in the right doses and formulations, certain supplements may be beneficial for treating a variety of conditions. Similarly, as we have already noted, significant side effects from prescription or OTC drugs are far more common than those caused by supplements. What must be stressed, though, is that because the law does not require supplement manufacturers to test their products and provide evidence of safety and effectiveness, it is vital that consumers find quality information about supplements.

Using medications and supplements wisely

Listing all types of medications and supplements, let alone the various preparations themselves, would be impossible. However, some basic principles will help you get the most out of any you take and may prevent some problems as well.

Prescription medications

Make sure that whoever is writing a new prescription for you knows *everything* you are taking at the time, including nonprescription drugs, vitamins, minerals, and supplements. Bring a current list to every appointment with every health-care provider you see. This is particularly important if more than one physician is writing prescriptions for you. For your safety, *everyone must know what everyone else has been giving you and what you're taking on your own.*

If you are receiving one or more new prescriptions, make sure that you understand the purpose for each medication and how each is to be taken: the number of times per day, with or without food, and any other cautions or restrictions. You should also know whether a medication is intended for long-term use (for example, as would be typical for drugs that lower blood pressure or cholesterol) or "as needed" (such as for relief of pain or cough). Get directions *in writing* from your health-care provider for any medications you receive as samples.

If you think you are having an adverse reaction to a medication, contact the prescribing physician for further advice. If it is determined that the problem was an actual allergic response (as opposed to a nonallergic side effect), make

WHAT EXACTLY IS IN THOSE SUPPLEMENTS?

A buyer staring at shelves lined with supplements faces a dilemma: How does he or she know whether the products actually contain what the labels advertise and whether the ingredients in Product A are better or worse than those in Product B? This is particularly important when it comes to herbal preparations because so many variables can affect their quality and effects: the strain of the plant, the soil composition and growing conditions, the time of harvesting, the herb's concentration in the product, and the form of consumption (for example, tablet, capsule, tea, or other solution).

Because no rigorous quality control standards exist for herbal supplements, different preparations of the same supplement may contain variable amounts of the marketed ingredient (or perhaps none at all). In one notable investigative report published in 1998 by the *Los Angeles Times*, an independent testing laboratory was commissioned to evaluate preparations of St. John's wort from ten different companies. The lab found an eye-opening variability among samples, with active ingredients ranging from 20 percent to 140 percent of the values listed on the labels. Half the brands contained less than 80 percent of the stated value.[14] More worrisome have been cases in which certain products, especially Chinese and ayurvedic herbal mixtures, have contained adulterants (such as heavy metals), other drugs (such as diazepam, the generic form of Valium), and substitutions of key ingredients.[15]

How can you find out whether your favorite dietary supplement passes muster? One excellent source of information is http://www.ConsumerLab.com, a Web site that provides information on a variety of supplements as well as results from independent lab tests indicating which preparations contain stated and appropriate amounts of the active ingredient and which have been found to contain contaminants. A number of products that have passed ConsumerLab.com's voluntary certification program are also listed. Some of the information on this site is free, while much more is available for a modest subscription fee. ■

note of that information and be sure it is also marked prominently in the medical chart kept by your physician. (For a more detailed look at the differences between allergic reactions and side effects related to medications, see chapter 2, beginning on page 20.)

F.Y.I. Medical personnel use the shorthand **PRN** to refer to medications that are taken as needed. The letters stand for the Latin phrase *pro re nata*, which means "as needed."

If you have taken medications that have caused problems (or simply haven't worked), keep your own list, including the date and the nature of the problem. This may keep a physician from wasting your time and money—and possibly provoking an adverse reaction—by using a medication that you have already tried unsuccessfully.

F.Y.I. Ever wonder about the lengthy (and alarming) list of potential side effects that you receive from the pharmacist along with your prescription? During clinical trials, *every* symptom and problem that develops while the subjects are taking the drug is dutifully recorded and tabulated. These are all listed as **adverse effects** on what is called the **product information sheet** (or PI), an FDA-mandated summary of what is essentially the fine print on any prescription drug. (The *Physicians' Desk Reference*, a massive volume that is updated annually, contains the PIs for hundreds of medications.) Needless to say, the list of adverse effects found on the PI (or on the patient information sheet from the pharmacist) is invariably so exhaustive that it may not be the most useful source of information about what you might expect from a given drug. Your doctor or pharmacist can usually better answer the question "What should I *really* worry about when I take this medication?"

Never "borrow" someone else's prescription medication to treat yourself, and never offer someone else one of your prescriptions that you think might help. You could be wrong, with serious consequences.

Nonprescription (OTC) medications

Follow the directions for use on the product's label, unless you are given explicit directions for a different dose from your physician.

If you are taking one or more prescription drugs or have chronic medical problems (for example, high blood pressure, a heart condition, diabetes, or ongoing liver or kidney disease), be sure to check with your health-care provider before taking OTC medications.

Dietary supplements, including herbal preparations

As with OTC medications, be sure to check with your physician before taking a dietary supplement—especially an herbal preparation—if you are taking one or more prescription drugs or have chronic medical problems (for example, high blood pressure, a heart condition, diabetes, or ongoing liver or kidney disease).

If you are going to have surgery, be sure that all physicians involved—especially the anesthesiologist—know about any supplements or herbs you are using.

When taking dietary supplements, be careful about your sources of information. Extravagant claims about the benefits of a product—especially from someone who is attempting to sell it to you—are not likely to be accurate, let alone unbiased. More reliable sources of information include:

- **Books** with a balanced view of the benefits and potential risks of using supplements. *Tyler's Honest Herbal: A Sensible Guide to the Use of Herbs and Related Remedies* and *Tyler's Herbs of Choice: The Therapeutic Use of Phytomedicinals* are among the many books written by the late Varro Tyler, Ph.D., that are widely regarded as reliable and evenhanded sources of information from an expert on botanical medicine.[16] (Dr. Tyler wrote many books and well over 250 research articles, and he served for thirty years as a professor of pharmacognosy and dean of the School of Pharmacy at Purdue University.) *Alternative Medicine: The Christian Handbook* by Dónal O'Mathúna, Ph.D., and Walt Larimore, M.D., contains an excellent summary of the evidence supporting (or refuting) the proposed benefits of numerous supplements.
- **Web sites** with balanced and responsible information. In the sidebar "What Exactly Is in Those Supplements?" we introduce http://www.ConsumerLab.com. Another helpful resource is http://www.NaturalDatabase.com, the Web site of the Natural Medicines Comprehensive Database. As its name implies, this database provides comprehensive information about hundreds of ingredients and brand-name products. It has earned high marks from a number of professional organizations. Full access to the database requires an annual subscription fee, which is somewhat more expensive than that of ConsumerLab.com.
- **A pharmacist or a physician** (ideally one who knows your medical history) who is knowledgeable about the use of supplements and herbs and is well-grounded in conventional medicine. Be cautious about accepting advice from someone who is also seeking to sell products (especially an entire product line).

Beware of the tackle-box approach to supplements. Some promoters of vitamins, minerals, and supplements would have you believe that it is impossible to be healthy without taking dozens of products, sometimes costing hundreds of dollars every month. Remember that the best source of nutrition is a wide variety of quality foods, as we described at length in chapter 5 and in our appendix dealing with vitamins (see page 869).

Talk with your pediatrician or family practitioner—and think very carefully—before giving a child any dietary supplement or herbal preparation, other than a vitamin that has been specifically recommended for him. In general, there is little reliable data regarding safety, efficacy, and appropriate dosage for most of these substances in infants and children. Sadly, some are inappropriately promoted as miracle cures for common childhood problems such as recurrent colds and ADHD.[17]

All preparations: prescription, OTC, or dietary supplements

Avoid a "pill for every ill" attitude. One of the potential pitfalls for caregivers and patients alike is a quick-fix mentality that assumes every symptom of a health problem is best solved by taking a medication or supplement. Some problems are better solved with lifestyle changes—food choices, exercise, getting more or better sleep, taking a day off, and so on. The vast majority of colds will resolve on their own with some rest and comfort measures and without antibiotics or other concoctions.

Never assume that because a little of any substance is helpful, more will be better.

If you are pregnant, do not take *anything* without checking with the physician who is caring for your pregnancy. You should also check with your health-care provider before taking any preparation if you *might* be pregnant or will be attempting to conceive in the near future.

Be very careful about the doses of any preparation you give to children—especially infants and toddlers. A physician will normally determine the dose for a prescription medication based on your child's current weight. OTC medications may or may not provide adequate dosing guidance, especially for younger children. If there is any doubt, you should check the dose with your child's physician before giving any to an infant or toddler younger than two.

For more information on preventing accidental ingestion of these and other substances, and what to do should this occur, see "Protecting young children against poisoning" beginning on page 512 in chapter 11.

Never underestimate a child's ability to find and sample any medications or supplements that might be in your home. Make sure that *all* preparations are stored where little ones cannot possibly get their hands on them.

Finding Reliable Health Information

We have a problem today that didn't exist a century (or even a half century) ago: We have access to more information about health and illness than we know what to do with. As noted previously, not all of that information is reliable. Furthermore, applying what you may read or hear to your own unique situation can be challenging. How do you separate the wheat from the chaff in order to make responsible health decisions for you and your family without wasting time and money? First, let's consider some of the unhelpful or misleading types of information:

- **Health information that is geared toward making a sale.** You should be highly suspicious of radio or television health programs that purport to inform you about a certain condition (such as arthritis, diabetes, or excess weight) but in fact are promoting a product for sale. Such programs typically announce that the product is completely unique, available only by calling a toll-free number, and that those who call within the next half hour will receive a special offer. Printed materials with the same commercial objective should also be considered questionable.

- **Claims that seem too good to be true.** The dictum "if it seems too good to be true, it probably is" definitely applies when it comes to therapies and health products. When you hear an infomercial for a product that is supposed to do it all for you—give you energy, help you lose weight, boost your immune system, rev up your sex life, and so on—you can guarantee that any money spent on it will be wasted. Cure-all therapies, potions, and pills have been the stock and trade of health hucksters for centuries, and too many people still fall for their empty promises.
- **Claims that are supported only by anecdotes and testimonials.** As we mentioned earlier in this chapter (see page 815), testimonials are one of the most unreliable forms of evidence for the value of a health product. Even if a trustworthy friend swears by a product, that does not mean it will work for you.
- **Therapies or products presented in "attack mode."** If a therapy or product is presented with a lot of verbiage attacking the health-care system, drug companies, the government, or "other practitioners who don't know what they're doing," beware. At best this is a ploy to distract your attention from the lack of credible evidence supporting the supplement or therapy in question. At worst, the claims are so outrageous that they deserve to be challenged by state or federal regulatory agencies.
- **Appeals to God's pharmacy.** A popular notion among those who are leery of conventional medicine is that it is based on human wisdom, and God has provided all of the remedies we need through herbal or dietary regimens. There is, to be sure, much to be said for avoiding health problems by eating well, exercising regularly, avoiding tobacco use, and so on. Furthermore, evidence consistently shows that fruits and vegetables provide healthful antioxidants and phytochemicals that have never been duplicated in any supplement or medication. (Indeed, this is a compelling argument for obtaining nutrients from food sources rather than from multiple supplements.) Some people, however, promote the idea that God has spelled out remedies for specific diseases—cancer, arthritis, and so on—in the Bible and that other treatments are suspect. However, the Scriptures also do not contain information about electronic devices, automobiles, or hundreds of other products of human invention, but we use them without a second thought. God has provided us with the mental capacity to investigate both the world around us and the body we inhabit, without including many specific details about either in the Scriptures. We gather knowledge—including ways to treat illness and promote health—while the Bible provides direction and wisdom regarding its proper use.

continued on page 842

ONLINE HEALTH INFORMATION

SPONSORING ORGANIZATION	WEB ADDRESS	DESCRIPTION
American Academy of Allergy, Asthma & Immunology	http://www.aaaai.org/patients.stm	Patients and Consumers Center deals with concerns related to allergies and asthma
American Academy of Family Physicians	http://familydoctor.org/	Links to information on dozens of topics related to all age groups
American Academy of Pediatrics	http://www.aap.org/parents.html	Information for parents on a variety of specific conditions and topics
American Cancer Society	http://www.cancer.org	Disease and treatment information
American Dental Association	http://www.ada.org/public/topics/alpha.asp	Information on dozens of topics related to oral health
American Diabetes Association	http://www.diabetes.org	Diabetes news and information
American Dietetic Association	http://www.eatright.org	Links to a variety of nutritional subjects
American Heart Association	http://www.americanheart.org	Covers cardiovascular disease and stroke
American Lung Association	http://www.lungusa.org	Facts on lung disease and health
Arthritis Foundation	http://www.arthritis.org	Covers arthritis and related conditions
Centers for Disease Control and Prevention	http://www.cdc.gov	Useful information on infectious diseases, including prevention and vaccination; updated advisories for travelers to foreign countries
ConsumerLab.com	http://www.ConsumerLab.com	Provides results of independent testing on health, nutrition, and wellness products
Harvard Medical School	http://www.health.harvard.edu	List of online topics, newsletters (by subscription), and books that are well researched and informative
Mayo Clinic	http://www.mayoclinic.com/	Excellent summaries of a variety of health conditions
Medem	http://www.medem.com/pat/pat.cfm	Provides links to health information and offers the option of creating a free, secure, updatable online health record (called iHealthRecord)

SPONSORING ORGANIZATION	WEB ADDRESS	DESCRIPTION
National Center for Complementary and Alternative Medicine	http://nccam.nih.gov	Information about alternative therapies, reviews of specific therapies, and findings of NCCAM research projects (with little other critical assessment of therapies)
National Council Against Health Fraud	http://www.ncahf.org	Like those at Quackwatch, articles posted here provide analysis that is generally unfavorable to alternative therapies, but nonetheless informative (and never boring)
National Health Information Center, U.S. Department of Health & Human Services	http://www.healthfinder.gov	Links to Web sites of professional organizations, academic institutions, and federal agencies
National Institutes of Health (NIH)	http://health.nih.gov/	Includes multiple subdivisions on a variety of health issues; for example, if you click on "Cancers" in the area marked "Browse Categories," you can find extensive information on various types of tumors through the National Cancer Institute
National Library of Medicine	http://www.medlineplus.gov	Type in a topic, and it will bring you several informative articles from a number of reliable sources; also contains information on prescription and OTC drugs
Natural Medicines Comprehensive Database	http://www.naturaldatabase.com	Comprehensive information about hundreds of ingredients and brand-name products; full access requires annual subscription fee
The North American Menopause Society	http://www.menopause.org/	Many educational resources dealing with this important phase of a woman's life
Quackwatch	http://www.quackwatch.org	Founded by Stephen Barrett, M.D., this site critiques and debunks therapies lacking scientific credibility
Virtual Hospital, University of Iowa	http://www.vh.org	Digital library of health information for patients and health-care providers

continued from page 839

What are some characteristics of reliable health information?

- **Evenhanded in tone.** There are a few topics, such as the destructive effects of tobacco use, where research findings are so compelling that you may find solid material with a decisive viewpoint. (For example, "You should quit using tobacco as soon as possible.") Otherwise, well-researched material will present facts in a straightforward manner, offer a variety of viewpoints on a topic when appropriate (which is most of the time), and draw conclusions that are reasonable and balanced.
- **Well referenced and committed to evidence-based medicine.** Solid health information will cite references or other resources. It will state whether a given perspective is widely accepted, speculative, or controversial.
- **Free of any commercial, political, or ideological bias—or willing to state its underlying position or worldview.** If an author or organization has an agenda, it should make that vantage point clear to the reader.
- **Understandable.** You won't get much from material that is loaded with vocabulary you don't understand or that doesn't explain basic concepts.

What are some reliable sources of health information? First, you would be wise to have a trusted primary-care provider serving as your medical "home base." This individual (or clinic) is the resource for applying health information specifically to *you*. Needless to say, not everything you read or hear about health may be scientifically valid, and even if you become aware of important findings arising from a well-designed study, the media's spin on the story may be sensationalized and, more importantly, not relevant to your individual health status. Someone who is both properly trained and directly involved in your medical care should be available to apply health information to you, especially when it involves treatment that you may—or may not—want to pursue. We'll discuss this in more detail later.

In the early twenty-first century, the **Internet** has become a—perhaps *the*—preeminent resource for learning about health topics or investigating new developments in this field. The World Wide Web is truly helpful in its ability to connect us immediately with current information, but at the same time, it is treacherous because of the number of sites containing questionable or overtly unreliable material. If you enter a medical condition into your favorite search engine, it will probably bring up a number of commercial ventures promoting products that supposedly treat the condition, though with dubious evidence to back such a claim. In general, you are better off gathering information from sites that will do some screening for you or whose content you can trust for medical accuracy.

You can nearly always rely on material on Web sites (or in print) from nationally recognized nonprofit organizations that are dedicated to research and education regarding specific health problems. Professional organizations, along with a number of medical schools and nationally recognized health centers, also provide online medical information for the public. See the table on pages 840–841 for some of the most noteworthy.

Internet beginners should be aware that commercial Web sites are usually identified by the letters ".com" (for example, the Web site for the publisher of this book is www.tyndale.com), federal government Web sites by ".gov" (for example, as we just noted, the Centers for Disease Control is www.cdc.gov), and organizations by ".org" (for example, Focus on the Family is www.family.org).

Working with a Primary-Care Provider

Earlier we mentioned the importance of having a primary-care provider to consult about your health-care concerns. This is an individual or a team who serves as the entry point into the health-care system for you and your family, providing preventive and screening health care and also helping you navigate the potentially complicated waters of modern medicine. Primary-care providers should be knowledgeable about the specialists, hospitals, home-health agencies, counselors, social services, and other resources in your community, and they usually will assist in the overall coordination of health care. This becomes particularly important in complex medical situations involving multiple physicians and medications. Ideally, every specialist should know what the others are doing, but in addition it is wise for one person to keep the total picture in view. Thus all consultations, procedures, and diagnostic studies should be sent to the primary-care provider, who in turn can assist in the referral and coordination of further specialty care and testing.

Even when specialists are providing complex interventions that extend well beyond a primary-care provider's training and expertise, the primary provider is often in the best position to explain and interpret what is going on. In addition, because the primary provider may care for the entire family, he or she may be the first to recognize that a particular problem may affect other family members and can institute appropriate diagnostic and treatment measures for them.

Who provides this type of service? Typically it will be either a **physician** (M.D. or D.O.) who has been trained in one of four specialties—family practice, internal medicine, pediatrics, or obstetrics and gynecology—or one of two types of nonphysician providers: a physician assistant or a nurse practitioner.

A **family physician** (also referred to as a **family practitioner**) cares for individuals and families of all ages, from birth through the senior years. During a three-year residency, a family physician is trained to recognize and treat a variety of conditions, encompassing nearly all areas of medicine. Health promotion and disease prevention are emphasized, as is coordinating care among medical specialists and community resources. Family physicians are trained to perform minor surgical procedures (such as vasectomies or suturing wounds), and in many communities they offer prenatal care and deliver babies as well. In some rural or remote areas, they may be called upon to provide care that in larger communities would typically be delivered by specialists.

M.D. OR D.O.: WHAT'S THE DIFFERENCE?

A physician with a doctor of medicine degree typically has earned an undergraduate college degree and then has completed four years of medical school to earn the initials "M.D." after his or her name. Medical school lays the groundwork in anatomy, physiology, pathology, and pharmacology. It also provides training and experience in the basics of taking a medical history, performing a physical examination, and understanding the essentials of hospital and outpatient care. Then comes an intense period of training (known as a **residency**) during which the actual "nuts and bolts" of caring for patients are learned and experienced. Depending on the specialty, residency may last three to seven years, though in some fields (known as subspecialties) it may be even longer, especially when the physician must learn complex procedures. (In some programs, the first year after medical school is called an **internship**.)

A physician with a D.O. (doctor of osteopathic medicine) degree usually has had training very similar to that of an M.D.: four years of medical education at a college of osteopathic medicine after earning an undergraduate degree. Though the curriculum at osteopathic and medical schools is similar in most respects, D.O. physicians receive specialized training in musculoskeletal manipulation techniques in addition to their medical education. The degree to which this will be emphasized in a particular physician's practice may vary considerably. Many if not most D.O.s enter medical residency programs and then function in a manner identical to that of M.D.s in their communities, including prescribing medications and performing surgical procedures for which they have received appropriate training. A small minority gravitate toward practicing unconventional forms of treatment such as cranial therapy, which purports to improve health by manipulating the bones of the skull. (Since the cranial bones fuse with one another during infancy, the premise of such treatment is seriously flawed.) If you are planning to receive care from an osteopathic physician, it would be prudent to confirm that he or she has completed an accredited medical residency program.

After completion of residency training, both M.D.s and D.O.s normally seek **board certification**. Each specialty has its own board certification process, which entails intensive written examinations and, in some specialties, oral exams as well. Some specialty boards require periodic recertification. (A physician who has completed training but has not yet passed the specialty board certification process is said to be **board eligible**.) ■

F.Y.I.

The older designation of a "general practitioner" as someone with an M.D. but limited postdegree training has been phased out over the past few decades. Family practice is now considered a formal specialty in its own right, with residency programs accredited by the Accreditation Council for Graduate Medical Education and periodic board certification requirements established by the American Board of Family Medicine.

An **internist** provides general nonsurgical medical care for adolescents, adults, and the elderly. Internists often care for individuals with multiple long-term medical problems such as diabetes, congestive heart failure, kidney failure, and lung problems, both in the office and in hospital settings. Some internists focus specifically on the health needs and problems of the elderly, a field known as **geriatric medicine**. After completing a residency in internal medicine (typically three years in length), many physicians receive additional training in nonsurgical specialties such as **cardiology** (heart disease), **pulmonology** (lung disease), **gastroenterology** (disorders of the intestinal tract, including the liver and pancreas), **nephrology** (kidney disease), **rheumatology** (diseases involving joints as well as what are called autoimmune disorders, such as rheumatoid arthritis), **allergy/immunology** (allergic disorders and problems with immune function), **endocrinology** (disorders of hormone function), **infectious diseases, oncology** (medical management of cancer), and **hematology** (disorders of blood cells; the vast majority of hematologists are also oncologists). Some who specialize in one of these areas function as primary-care physicians and manage the general care of their adult patients, but most focus exclusively on the area in which they have been trained. (**Neurology**, which deals with disorders of the nervous system, is also a nonsurgical specialty, but one that does not require completion of a residency in internal medicine.)

Pediatricians provide general health care to infants, children, and adolescents. They are specifically trained in the physical, emotional, and behavioral development of children, and they provide routine and preventive health care (including immunizations) and manage most acute illnesses in this age group. After a three-year residency in general pediatrics, some pediatricians, like internists, obtain additional training in specialties such as pediatric cardiology, pediatric neurology, and so forth. (Because they involve specialty care limited to a certain age group, these areas are often called **subspecialties**. Not all of these may be available in a local medical community, and often one must travel to a large city or university medical center to obtain a consultation in one of these areas.) Some pediatricians focus more specifically on older children and teenagers, practicing what is called **adolescent medicine**. As with adult internal medicine specialists, pediatric subspecialists may provide general health care for their patients but usually delegate these concerns to general pediatricians.

An **obstetrician/gynecologist (OB/GYN)** specializes in the medical and surgical care of the female reproductive system. Obstetrics involves care for women during pregnancy, labor, and delivery, while gynecology encompasses the entire female reproductive system, including infertility problems. For many women, routine Pap smears represent the only ongoing contact with a health-care provider, so an OB/GYN may serve as their primary-care physician by default. For that reason, some will treat problems such as colds, urinary tract infections, and even depression, but they will refer more serious or complex problems that are not gynecologic in nature to other specialists. In general, it is advisable for women to have a family practitioner or internist to care for medical concerns involving other body systems.

A **physician assistant (PA)** has completed a two- to three-year training program (usually an extension of an accredited medical school) that includes both classroom and clinical training, comparable to the first and third years of medical school. (All have previously completed two to three years of undergraduate education, and most hold a bachelor's degree.) After graduation, a physician assistant must pass a national board certifying exam to earn the title PA-C (physician assistant–certified). Physician assistants are licensed in their state and must practice under the supervision of a licensed physician, but they may participate in any medical specialty. PAs may receive additional training focused on a specialized area of practice (such as surgery or emergency medicine). Typically these extended PA training programs are one or more years in duration. Physician assistants can perform many of the same duties as their supervising physician, including routine physicals, diagnosis and treatment of illness, and minor surgical procedures (lacerations, mole removals, cyst excisions). They can also assist with surgery and prescribe medication.

A **nurse practitioner (NP)** is a registered nurse (RN) who has completed advanced training in diagnosing and managing common medical conditions and illnesses through graduate nursing school. Nurse practitioners are often trained in a specific area of interest, such as gynecology or pediatrics, and when training is completed, the NP's scope of practice is limited to the chosen specialty. In many states, nurse practitioners do not have to practice under the supervision of a physician (although most do), and NPs and PAs generally play similar roles in health-care settings.

Choosing a primary-care provider

If someone asks you, "Who is your doctor?" what is your answer? If your response is "I don't have one" or "I go to the nearest urgent care center when I get sick," you have a new assignment: Identify and establish a relationship with a physician, medical group, or clinic that will serve as your medical base of operations. This may be easier said than done. Important factors may limit your options, such as a health-insurance policy that requires you to pick from a list of individuals who have signed up to be providers for that particular company. You may have Medicare, Medicaid, or no coverage whatsoever, any of which may hamper or prevent your access to many providers in your community. Perhaps you have just moved and have barely become acquainted with your neighbors, let alone a physician or medical group. If you're not sure how to carry out this task, here are a few ideas that may help.

Identify your available options. If your insurance has provided a list of "preferred providers" (those who have signed on for your particular plan), mark the pages where family physicians, internists, pediatricians (if you have children), and obstetrician/gynecologists are listed. You'll need to refer to these names as you seek out potential caregivers. If you are in an HMO plan that requires you to designate a primary-care physician or group as a gatekeeper—one whom you must contact (and probably see initially) in order to access care—you will need to be particularly attentive to the names on their list.

Ask around. People who have had particularly good (or bad) experiences with a physician or group are usually more than happy to tell you about them. Ask your neighbors, friends, fellow church members, or other people whom you trust in your community for recommendations, and see which names are mentioned most often. Those who work in health care, especially nurses—and *especially* those who care for patients in the hospital or emergency department—can often give you the lowdown on the good, bad, and mediocre in the local medical community.

Check with your local hospital. Most hospitals maintain a referral list of physicians who are members of their medical staff. While the presence of a person's name on such a list does not guarantee that you'll find him or her to your liking, it does at least indicate that the physician has the credentials—education, training, licensure, and possibly certain other factors (such as specialty board certification)—that are required to admit patients to that facility.

In a best-case scenario, you will find a primary-care provider who is supremely competent, compassionate, good at listening, intuitive, flexible, available whenever you need help, always on time but never rushed, aligned with your moral and spiritual convictions, affordable, and able to leap tall buildings with a single bound. In reality, you may have trouble finding a "Superdoctor" in your community (or on our planet) who fulfills all of the items on this wish list. In fact, you may have to decide which characteristics are the most important to you. For example:

Competence. This is critical in a health-care provider. It does not mean that the person is a walking encyclopedia but rather that he or she applies training, experience, and ongoing education intelligently—including knowing when (and whom) to ask for help. Great interpersonal skills are no substitute for knowing which end of the stethoscope is which. Most, if not all, physician groups will verify that their providers have received a degree from an accredited school, completed a residency program in their specialty, passed certifying exams, and are duly licensed to practice medicine. This information can also be obtained by contacting state medical licensing boards or hospitals with which the provider is affiliated. Additionally, one can determine if a physician is certified by calling (866) ASK-ABMS or accessing the Web site of the American

Board of Medical Specialties (a nonprofit organization comprised of twenty-four medical specialty boards) at http://www.abms.org.

Compassion and communication skills. These components of the proverbial bedside manner rank just below competence as important traits to seek in a primary-care provider. If the doctor won't listen to you, doesn't seem interested in or concerned about your symptoms, won't answer questions, and generally treats you disrespectfully, you shouldn't plan on building a long-term relationship. There may be occasions when you require care from someone with unique technical skills—for example, a subspecialist trained to perform an unusual procedure that you need—who has the personality of a brick or the social skills of a porcupine. You can probably put up with his or her behavior for a short time, as long as it isn't overtly disrespectful or inappropriate. But with a primary-care provider, your intent is to be in a long-term relationship, and that may prove difficult with someone you find irritating.

Worldview compatibility. It is extremely helpful if your primary-care provider shares your moral and spiritual outlook, since this can impact many health-care decisions. This is particularly important if this individual is going to provide input to your children or teenagers, especially in matters regarding sexuality. (It is frustrating to teach your adolescent standards of conduct in this arena, only to have those standards undermined behind closed doors in the office or clinic.) Even if you and your health-care provider have differing moral views, it is crucial that he or she respects your commitments. Remember also that, as with bedside manner, there are a number of situations where you may need the technical expertise of a physician who does not share your faith.

Accessibility and availability. Your primary-care provider or medical group is the one you call when you need help. Ideally, making an appointment, refilling a prescription, or asking a question shouldn't feel like running a gauntlet. Some questions to ponder: When you call the office, do you have to wade through a ten-step menu to talk with someone or routinely wait on hold for fifteen minutes? Is there anyone available to talk to after hours or on weekends, or do you get a recording that says, "If you're having a problem, go to the emergency room"? Do you have to wait for several weeks to get an appointment? In some busy practices, a physical exam may have to be scheduled months in advance, and the next nonemergency opening may be a few weeks in the future. But is there a provision for seeing you or your child for an illness *today*?

There are times when it's reasonable for the physician to refer you to another caregiver within his or her practice. Often the person who is designated to see patients for acute problems will be a physician assistant or a nurse practitioner. We encourage you not to be resistant to that option, for reasons we will explain shortly. Also, certain situations—for example, crushing chest pain that started a few minutes ago—do not belong in the doctor's office but rather in an emergency department. If your primary-care provider instructs you to go directly to the emergency room (or call 911), don't ignore that advice.

On time vs. giving you time. A provider may be behind schedule on any given day for many reasons, and most of them arise from the unpredictability of the problems that arise in a medical practice. For example, it takes only one patient with an acute, complicated problem to disrupt the schedule for the rest of the day. Another reason may be that the caregiver takes enough time to evaluate each patient's problems carefully, explain the treatment options, and answer whatever questions arise. Very often a person with a fifteen-minute appointment brings forty-five minutes worth of symptoms into the exam room. If the provider feels that these cannot be reasonably postponed to another time, delays will be inevitable. When a few of these show up on the same day, the person at the end of the schedule may have a long wait. If your primary-care provider resists rushing with patients, he or she may frequently be behind schedule. Ideally, the office staff will inform those arriving in the waiting room when there is a major delay and offer the option of coming back later in the day or making an appointment on a different day. On the other hand, you may want to seek a different provider if your routine experience is a long wait followed by a rushed exam.

Starting and maintaining a good working relationship with a primary-care provider

Ideally, your relationship with a primary-care provider will be a productive one lasting many years. Here are some ideas to get things off to a good start—and to keep them that way over the long haul.

Consider a "get acquainted" visit. If you're seeking more information about a particular provider or office, it isn't unreasonable to set up an introductory visit. Some offices and medical groups have a patient representative or office manager who can answer your questions and even show you around. If you want to meet the physician but are not certain whether you are going to become a patient, make sure this is understood when you call, and clarify whether there is a charge for this visit. If you're not going to be charged, don't expect a half-hour conversation and don't suddenly ask for medical advice. (If you want medical attention, you need to establish a formal relationship with that practice.) During this encounter you can get a sense of how you are treated on the phone, see what the office looks like, learn what services are provided, and determine if the practice seems to be a place you can comfortably call home, medically speaking.

When making an appointment, state your agenda as best you can. You need much more time for a complete physical or an evaluation for chronic fatigue than for a sore throat or a wart. If the visit will focus on issues that you don't feel comfortable explaining to the front-office staff (for example, a problem related to sexuality), let the person know that the concern is of a personal nature. If she presses the issue, ask if you can speak with a nurse in the office to clarify what you need.

Bring pertinent information to your first (and any other) visit. If you have records from another physician, lab results, a summary of your health history, and a list of medications you are taking (including supplements), by all means bring them.

Don't hesitate to ask questions. If you don't understand what the caregiver is saying about your problems or have concerns about the tests and treatments that are being recommended, ask *questions* until you have a reasonable grasp of the information. You might ask if the office has any written information or pertinent handouts.

Take notes if necessary. If your visit results in a to-do list involving several items—diagnostic tests, medications, perhaps a referral—the caregiver should write these down for you. If not, do so yourself. You should not leave the office without a clear idea, in writing, of what you're supposed to do next.

Avoid the fateful phrase "by the way . . ." If you have a list of five concerns for a given visit, let the caregiver know all five topics, and which is most important to you, as you begin. Few events are more frustrating to a provider than spending time discussing a cold or a sore ankle and then hearing, "By the way, I've been having some terrible headaches recently." When this occurs, the caregiver must either give an off-the-cuff answer (not a good idea), delay everyone else in order to evaluate the complaint properly (necessary if it sounds urgent), or schedule a follow-up visit (usually the best solution, but not what most patients want to hear).

Avoid bringing "surprise guests" to your visit. If one child is scheduled for a checkup and another suddenly becomes ill, for example, check with the appointment desk or the nurse *before* the visit to see if it would be possible to have your sick child seen as well (or to take the other child's appointment).

Respect—and better yet, become good friends with—the office staff. A physician depends on his or her staff to help a demanding day go more smoothly. Some patients make the mistake of being all smiles with the doctor but repeatedly being rude or hostile to the office personnel. An angry exchange that rattles or upsets anyone on the office staff can actually disrupt the care of other patients for the rest of the day. On the other hand, if someone who works for a physician has in fact treated you poorly, your doctor will certainly want to know about it. Your best course of action is to send a note marked "personal and confidential" to the caregiver and explain in a straightforward way what happened.

HOT TIP

If the doctor has a nurse who works with him or her on a regular basis, do your best to be friendly and cheerful toward that person. Most often she (or he) is the physician's right arm and "control tower," and can help you deal with a variety of questions and concerns.

Respect the caregiver's boundaries. Believe it or not, the vast majority of physicians do not like to be on call 24-7 to answer medical questions, and few are excited about being accosted in the store or at church for an informal "consultation." Don't be offended if you get what is, in fact, the most appropriate response, both medically and legally (assuming the situation isn't an emergency):

"Why don't you give the office a call on Monday so we can set a time to talk about this?" This is definitely better than "Why don't you take off your clothes and lie down on the pew so that I can examine you right now?" Similarly, even if you are a friend and have your doctor's home phone number, don't use it to do an end run around office hours and staff. If you have a medical question after hours, have the courtesy to check with the exchange to find out who is actually on call, and contact that person. The off-call doctor/friend whom you call at home will probably feel obliged to deal with your problem and may have to abandon some much-needed family time or other respite from the demands of practice to do so.

Don't hesitate to be seen by a physician assistant or nurse practitioner. We have already mentioned that these allied health professionals may be an integral part of your physician's medical office; indeed, they may become your primary-care providers. In many practices, these individuals are able to address acute problems on short notice, and you may find that they give you more time than the physician. If you have a problem that is indeed beyond their scope of care, they can still perform an initial assessment and then bring the doctor into the room to continue the evaluation.

Paying the Bills: Dealing with Health Insurance

A century ago most people who were ill received treatment (including surgery) and recuperated under their own roof. Most babies were delivered at home. Medicine was considered a vocation, and professional training was inconsistent in content and quality. In many cases a doctor would visit the patient, hold his hand, offer words of encouragement or advice, provide some form of rudimentary medicine by today's standards (if any was available), and leave the healing entirely up to God. Today the diagnostic and therapeutic tools are much more sophisticated—and expensive. (Some have lamented that we now may often miss out on the therapeutic benefits of kind words and gentle touches that were the primary tools of many physicians of bygone days. In addition, all of our modern advances notwithstanding, healing remains in God's hands.)

For generations people paid for doctor visits and medicines out of their own pocket, or perhaps bartered for these services. Given the rudimentary state of medical technology, for most of our history medical expenses usually represented a very modest portion of the family budget. Indeed, before 1920 the main cost associated with sickness or injury in the United States wasn't medical care but rather loss of income from being unable to work. As a result, few households bought health insurance, but many purchased "sickness" insurance, somewhat like today's disability insurance, to cover lost wages in the event of illness. In addition, insurance companies were reluctant to offer health insurance out of concern that they couldn't accurately estimate a person's risks in order to calculate appropriate premiums. (What if someone claimed to be in good health when buying a policy but really wasn't?)

During the 1920s and 1930s, four emerging trends began to increase the cost of health care: advances in medical knowledge and technology; more stringent requirements for physician training and licensure; increasing use of the hospital (rather than the home) as the place in which people would receive treatment for acute illness and injury; and rising income (at least until the Great Depression), which increased the demand for medical services. In 1929, hospital costs accounted for less than 15 percent of the average American family's annual medical bills; by 1934, that number had increased to 40 percent.[18] As health-care costs began to rise, so did the need to make medical care affordable for average citizens. Organizations began offering health insurance, pooling the risks and resources of individuals and promising to pay a part of necessary health-care expenditures in exchange for a premium. Blue Cross plans were first organized in the 1930s as nonprofit programs to provide prepaid hospital care, and Blue Shield soon emerged as a nonprofit counterpart to cover physi-

SIGNS THAT YOU MAY NEED A DIFFERENT PRACTITIONER

When you establish a relationship with someone who is going to provide care that will affect your health—and perhaps your life as well—several characteristics indicate that you will be in good hands, and a few suggest otherwise. Here are some red flags that should serve as warnings to proceed with caution—or even turn around and head in a different direction.

- **"Hi/Good-bye."** Some physicians habitually rush in and out of the room like the White Rabbit in *Alice in Wonderland*, as if in a big hurry because of a "very important date"—somewhere else. While you can't expect every visit to be an extended conversation about multiple subjects, if a practitioner is always in a rush and seems impatient when you ask a question or two, you may want to look elsewhere.
- **"My way or the highway."** You deserve to have legitimate questions answered and to have mutually respectful dialogue about treatment options. Beware if a practitioner refuses to discuss alternatives to his diagnostic and treatment plan or appears offended by the idea of getting a second opinion (especially for a complex problem). While those practicing conventional medicine are more often accused of authoritarianism, alternative therapists occasionally manifest a similar attitude by urging their patients to abandon mainstream care. For example, advocates of unconventional cancer therapy may appeal to normal apprehensions about surgery, radiation, and chemotherapy by insisting that their all-natural treatments can avoid the "cutting, burning, and poisoning" of mainstream medicine. Beware of such

cian expenses. Observing the success of these plans, commercial insurance companies entered the arena, and the number of Americans with health-care coverage exploded from about 20 million in 1940 to more than 140 million in 1950.

The basic type of health insurance first offered was **indemnity coverage**, the traditional fee-for-service plan in which the insurance company paid a portion of medical expenses and the patient paid the rest. In 1965, Congress passed legislation creating the Medicare program, which provides coverage for hospital expenses (known as Part A) for all Americans sixty-five and over, as well as optional supplemental coverage for physician services (known as Part B). The 1970s saw the development of a new health-insurance structure called **managed care**, which ostensibly placed greater emphasis on health maintenance and illness prevention with the professed goal of reducing the need for expensive medical treatments over the long haul.

We will look at these various forms of coverage in more detail momentarily, but for now we should note that, for a variety of reasons, many people

advice, whether regarding cancer or any other condition, not only because it is almost certainly poorly informed but also because it may lead to a delay in treatment that could be potentially hazardous.

- **"I'm the only one who knows about this treatment."** Legitimate advances in health care represent the joint effort of many investigators and rely on accountability to peers who can evaluate the validity of research findings. It is never a lone-ranger enterprise. A practitioner who claims to have a unique, one-of-a-kind treatment that no one else knows about is either fraudulent or delusional, either of which disqualifies him from providing health care for you and your family. Furthermore, a practitioner's claim that he or his unique approach to health care is being smeared by the "medical establishment" or persecuted by the government is a sure sign that something is wrong—with him.
- **"I've got some products that you need."** Offices and clinics may supply medications and other services at an appropriate price as a convenience for their patients. However, some practitioners, both conventional and alternative, may lean on you to buy a dietary supplement or other type of product—or even a whole line of products. In a worst-case scenario, a practitioner claims to have "diagnosed" several exotic deficiencies (often using tests of dubious reliability, such as hair analysis, muscle-pulling techniques, or electronic "black boxes" that magically reveal what's wrong with you) and insists that you need to take a unique (and pricey) collection of supplements that happen to be for sale in the office. If this occurs, head immediately for the exit. ■

have become frustrated or disillusioned with the world of health insurance. Every year it seems as though higher premiums cover fewer benefits. Many have a jaundiced view of the term *managed care* as a euphemism for "limiting my options and refusing to pay for care my physician thinks is necessary." That is not always or even routinely true, of course, but the reality is that those who pay the bills—insurance companies and government programs (federal and state)—

WHAT MAKES HEALTH CARE SO EXPENSIVE?

Most of us experience sticker shock when we receive a hospital bill or when the pharmacist tells us how much that new prescription will cost. Over the past few decades the costs associated with health care have increased steadily, outpacing the rate of inflation by large margins. While it's easy to play the blame game (labeling whomever you don't like as greedy, wasteful, or incompetent), it's more productive to understand some of the factors that keep costs rising. In no particular order, they include:

More high-tech diagnostic options. CT scanners and MRIs are available everywhere, and PET scanners, which are sometimes used to scan the heart and brain, as well as to detect cancer, are becoming more widely used as well. An office sigmoidoscopy, costing a few hundred dollars at most, used to be considered adequate for routine screening of colon cancer. Colonoscopy, which can cost ten times that much (because of the time, expertise, sedation, and vital-sign monitoring involved), is now the gold standard. The more these expensive tests become the standard of care for evaluating common complaints or for screening, the more they are ordered. While they may be more effective, they aren't cheap.

More high-tech therapeutic options. New and exotic surgical techniques, transplants, immunotherapy, chemotherapy, and other technological advances make their debut every year. None are inexpensive for a variety of reasons, including research and development costs, and complex manufacturing processes. In addition, many are used for a relatively small number of patients so that they cannot be mass-produced.

Lack of awareness of costs. One of the effects of the widespread availability of health insurance (particularly managed-care insurance) and Medicare is that many people are not aware of the actual costs of health-care decisions, especially those involving sophisticated technologies and hospital care. This is frequently true of physicians as well, who for generations have been trained to carry out whatever tests or treatments appear necessary without regard for the price tag.

"Do whatever it takes. . . ." When confronting a serious medical problem, few of us are willing to cut corners when our life, or that of a loved one, is on the line. Because many more treatment options are available now than even ten years ago, costs can escalate quickly.

have literally become the third person in the exam room, along with the physician and the patient, making health-care decisions.

For the person who does *not* have health coverage, instead of a third person in the exam room, there is an eight-hundred-pound gorilla blocking the entrance to the doctor's office and the local hospital. That creature is the cost of care, and he gets more gigantic and unruly every year. (See sidebar: "What

The pharmaceutical business. Pharmaceutical manufacturers spend hundreds of millions of dollars in research, development, and clinical trials to get a single drug approved and onto a pharmacy shelf. They also spend huge sums marketing those drugs to physicians and the general public. A by-product of this process is a wide-scale diversion of attention and money to costly brand-name drugs and away from inexpensive generics.

People are living longer. As people age, they tend to develop more medical problems and may find themselves taking multiple medications to treat ongoing problems, prevent new ones, or alleviate symptoms.

Defensive medicine. Health-care professionals want to offer the best available care to their patients—but they also are well aware of an increasingly litigious climate in which a physician who fails to diagnose a serious problem may face a malpractice suit, an extraordinarily stressful event. The legal assault may be unavoidable, but the defense may hinge on the lengths to which the caregiver went to prevent or diagnose the problem.

Bill payers. Many health-care providers (both caregivers and facilities) are aware that insurance companies pay only a fraction of the amount charged for a given service, and they are often contractually bound to accept that lesser amount. As a result, providers may charge more than they expect to get so that the amount they actually receive is within a reasonable range. An unfortunate consequence is that the uninsured (cash-paying) patient may be presented with charges that are much higher than the amounts a well-funded insurance company would pay for the same services.

Overhead. The costs of doing business—salaries, supplies, insurance, and many other expenses—can be impressive for any health-related business, and they never decrease over time.

Fraud and abuse. According to the National Health Care Anti-Fraud Association, at least 3 percent of America's health-care bill, or $51 billion for the calendar year 2003, was lost to overt fraud. Other government and law-enforcement agencies estimate the amount lost to fraud to be as much as 10 percent, or $170 billion.[19] This arises both from dishonest providers (who might, for example, bill for services that were never provided) and patients (who might file a claim for reimbursement for services or medications that were never obtained). ■

Are generics as good as brand-name drugs? The answer depends on the specific medication, the particular problem, and the response of the individual patient being treated. The decision to use a brand-name drug or a generic should be made on a case-by-case basis with the prescribing physician.

Makes Health Care So Expensive?") One illness or accident for the uninsured or underinsured individual or family can result in financial ruin. Currently about half of personal bankruptcies in the United States are the result of a costly illness.[20] The purpose of health insurance is to help pay the costs associated with health care and hopefully avoid financial disaster. Understanding medical coverage is a feat in its own right, and having some knowledge of the system can empower you to obtain appropriate health insurance and navigate its complex terrain.

Most people obtain health insurance as an employment benefit through private insurance organizations. Some publicly funded government plans such as Medicare and Medicaid are available only to specific individuals such as the poor, elderly, or handicapped. Those for whom health insurance is not available through employment or the government can purchase a private plan. The expense of obtaining insurance privately is prohibitive for many, and as medical costs continue to escalate, more Americans are finding themselves uninsured or underinsured. Similarly, many who may be able to afford insurance are denied coverage because of health conditions that render them "high risk." (Most physicians are familiar with patients who were denied coverage because of relatively minor problems that have been inappropriately deemed high risk for future claims.) Unlike many countries, the United States does not have universal national health coverage, although Medicare is in fact this type of program for citizens sixty-five and over. Needless to say, this continues to be a hotly contested issue, especially near Election Day.

Private health-insurance plans

Private insurance comes in two basic varieties: indemnity and managed care.

Indemnity

Also known as **fee for service**, these plans allow the subscriber to go to any physician, specialist, or hospital without obtaining preauthorization or approval from the insurance company. Typically, the subscriber pays an annual **deductible** and a percentage of the cost of their care—usually 20 percent, with the insurance plan covering the other 80 percent. After a certain predetermined out-of-pocket expense has been paid by the subscriber, the plan typically covers 100 percent of other medical expenses. Indemnity plans tend to be the most costly, but they also provide the most flexibility for the subscriber. Some indemnity plans may offer incentives to subscribers who choose certain medical providers, an approach taken by most managed care plans.

Managed care

These plans place certain restrictions on patient choice in exchange for lower coverage rates and (at least in theory) more comprehensive care. Typically physicians, hospitals, laboratories, X-ray/imaging facilities, and other types of health-care providers (for example, physical therapists) sign contracts to serve as providers, usually agreeing to take less than their "usual and customary" fees. In exchange they are listed as providers for patients in their community and are usually paid relatively promptly for services rendered. Most managed-care plans also encourage health promotion and disease prevention, based on the assumption that preventing illness and injury is less costly than treating it. They may provide incentives for subscribers to obtain preventive health care such as routine physicals and immunizations, and they encourage consumers to maintain good health in a variety of ways. For example, a smoker will usually be able to seek reimbursement for a smoking-cessation program. Managed care plans, which became widespread in the 1990s, fall into three basic categories:

1. **Health maintenance organizations (HMOs)** provide all-inclusive medical care (preventive exams, treatment of illness or disease, immunizations, specialist referral, hospital services, allied care or social services, and medications) to participants but in a manner very different from that of indemnity plans. Instead of paying for each separate visit or service, HMOs pay participating primary-care providers a flat amount every month (known as a **capitation fee**) for each patient assigned to them, regardless of the amount of care obtained by the participant. (This is also called **prepaid care**.) In order to contain costs and prevent abuse of the system, consumers typically have a **co-pay** with each visit that usually ranges from five to twenty dollars.

   The primary-care physician or group chosen by the patient approves and coordinates any specialty or referred care. Therefore, tests or specialist visits cannot be covered unless they are authorized by the primary-care provider, who is thus referred to as the gatekeeper. Furthermore, the specialists, hospitals, and providers of other services are designated by the HMO or the gatekeeper. However, once a referral is approved, the HMO typically assumes the entire cost of care.

   If a participant chooses to seek care outside of this framework, the costs are generally not covered or caregivers are paid at a significantly reduced rate (with the patient responsible for the difference). Exceptions are made for emergencies requiring care in the closest available facility. Also, if the HMO has not contracted with a specific type of specialist needed to treat a certain condition, the primary physician can request authorization for that patient to be seen by an out-of-network physician. Typically, approval is granted, but it may take considerable time and effort to coordinate referrals.

   Similarly, HMOs have strict pharmaceutical formularies (a listing of all the medications that the HMO agrees to cover). If a health-care provider writes a prescription for a drug that is listed on the formulary, then the patient gets the full drug benefit offered by the plan. If, however, a prescription is written for a drug not listed on the formulary, the patient will have to assume most, if not all, the cost of that medication. To help control costs, generic drugs make up the vast majority of the formulary, and drugs new to the market or those used for cosmetic purposes (e.g., for treating toenail fungus) are typically not covered.

Capitation-based HMOs have been criticized because a potential conflict of interest exists for the primary-care provider. In many plans the individual physician or group must pay for services and specialty referrals out of its capitation income, which can create an incentive to provide as little care as possible. Some plans have restructured financial arrangements to remove much of this pressure from primary-care providers, but in many HMOs patients still feel as though they must deal with challenging and time-consuming protocols in order to obtain the care they need. Certain HMOs, such as Kaiser Permanente, hire their own full-time physicians (including specialists) and operate their own hospitals and clinics, thus providing all services within a self-contained medical system.

2. **Preferred provider organizations (PPOs)** are much more like indemnity plans than HMOs. A group or several groups of physicians (called network providers) contract with the PPO and agree to provide services at a reduced fee for plan participants. Members are provided with a list of these primary-care physicians and specialists from which they can choose their caregivers. As with HMOs, patients will pay more if they go out of network. They may also have access to prescriptions at a reduced rate, though formulary restrictions often apply. Furthermore, preauthorization from the company is usually required before certain costly tests (such as MRI scans) or elective surgeries will be covered.

3. **Point of service plans (POS)** combine elements of PPO and HMO plans. Like a PPO, a group of providers contracts with the insurance company to provide care to subscribers, who must choose a primary-care provider. Where a member of a PPO can choose any specialist within the network, a POS member must first see the primary-care provider about the problem and then obtain a referral (or some other form of approval) to see a specialist. Unlike an HMO, however, the primary-care gatekeeper is paid for each visit and has no incentive (financial or otherwise) to limit referrals that he or she feels are appropriate. POS plans may be less costly because straightforward problems are usually managed less expensively by primary-care providers than by specialists.

Whatever type of plan you have, you can maximize your health-care benefits and avoid a tremendous amount of frustration simply by *reading and under-*

standing your policy. When you sign up for a health-insurance plan, you agree to a set of rules. Similarly, the health-care providers who accept your insurance agree to a set of rules. In order to successfully navigate the system, you must know what your plan offers and what it doesn't. Specifically:

- How big is the deductible? (A deductible is the amount you must pay at the beginning of a new year before the policy begins to cover expenses.)
- After the deductible is met, how much are you responsible for? Is there an upper limit to the amount you might have to pay in a given year?
- Can you see any doctor you want, or must you pick one from a list of preferred (or network) providers?
- Do you need a referral to see a specialist?
- What services are covered if you are in the hospital? What about emergency visits and ambulance fees?
- When you go to an office, is there a co-pay, and how much is it? Are any routine or preventive exams covered? What about checkups and immunizations for children?
- Is obstetrical care covered?
- What about dental and eye exams?
- Are blood tests and X rays covered? Are these expenses covered only at certain facilities?
- Is there coverage for prescriptions? Is there a formulary list of medications that are covered?
- Are nonphysician services such as physical therapy and chiropractic care covered?

Though most health-care providers attempt to stay abreast of insurance plans, it is unlikely that your physician keeps track of the various (and constantly changing) provisions of the insurance plans that he or she has agreed to accept. You must know the terms, conditions, and definitions of your policy. If you don't know what something means, call the administrator of the plan and educate yourself. The more you know about your specific policy, the more likely you are to obtain the maximum benefit, and the more comprehensive your coverage will be.

HOT TIP

If you receive a formulary list for medications covered (or preferred) by your insurance plan, give it to your physician to place in your chart. You'll save yourself and your doctor a great deal of hassle if new prescriptions are chosen (when appropriate) from the current list.

Think proactively. It is much easier to obtain authorization ahead of time for treatment that otherwise might not be covered than to request payment after the fact. When you communicate with the administrator of the insurance plan, keep records. Document the date, time, and name of the individual you spoke to, including the question asked and the answer received. If possible, channel all future inquiries through the same individual. If you get an answer that does not make sense or satisfy you, request to speak to someone in a superior position, such as a manager. The goal is not to manipulate the system to get the answer you want but rather to have a clear understanding of how you can maximize your benefit and avoid pitfalls.

Government plans

Established in 1965, these plans are funded by the Department of Health and Human Services and provide services to people sixty-five years or older, individuals with certain disabilities, and some low-income individuals.

Medicare

Medicare consists of two parts: Part A is compulsory for individuals sixty-five years and older (and others with certain disabilities) and covers hospital expenses. Part B is an optional supplemental medical insurance to cover physician services. Funding for Medicare comes from federal payroll taxes, income taxes, government trust-fund interest, and premiums paid by individuals. Medicare is not an all-inclusive insurance plan, and there are gaps in coverage and services. However, it does offer a relatively solid foundation of care.

Most people with Medicare obtain a supplemental private policy, either provided to them by an employer or purchased individually, to provide more comprehensive coverage. Supplemental insurance policies are regulated by states and can vary from state to state. In addition, a variety of Medicare-approved drug discount programs (now referred to as "Part D") have recently been initiated. The extent (or limits) of Medicare coverage evolves from year to year, and current and comprehensive information can be found at the official Web site: http://www.medicare.gov.

Medicaid

Medicaid is a program funded by both the federal government and individual states that provides medical coverage for individuals with certain disabilities and people with low income, especially pregnant women and children. Acting under broad federal guidelines, each state is responsible for determining eligibility and benefits for its residents. The initial intention of Medicaid was to provide health coverage for those who fall below the poverty level. However, the excessive cost of the program and budget shortfalls have forced states to vary the qualifications and coverage for Medicaid insurance, since individual states bear much of the responsibility for caring for their residents. To obtain current information about coverage in your state, go to http://www.cms.hhs.gov/medicaid, a gateway site that will link you to a specific Medicaid Web site for your state.

Other health-coverage options

Health savings accounts (HSAs), sometimes known as medical savings accounts, operate somewhat like IRAs (individual retirement accounts) in that pretax dollars—that is, money not subject to income taxes—can fund an account that is used to pay for qualified medical expenses. (Money in the account can grow tax free.) At the same time, an individual purchases high-deductible, lower-premium health-insurance plans (also known as **major medical** or **catastrophic plans**) that will cover major medical events. (HSAs are not used in conjunction with a regular health plan such as a PPO.) Then, if an individual incurs medical expenses that are not covered under the major medical plan, he may draw money from the account to pay for them. A variety of health-related expenses usually can be covered, including co-payments, deductibles, medications (over-the-counter and prescription), eye or dental care, mileage (to appointments), and even counseling. Money remaining in the account at the end of the year rolls over and is available the next year (and beyond) to pay for expenses.

Flexible spending accounts (FSAs) are employer-sponsored accounts in which individuals may deposit pretax earnings. When medical expenses are accrued, the individual submits a claim to the account manager, and the out-of-pocket costs are reimbursed to the individual. As with HSAs, a variety of health expenses may qualify for payment from an FSA, but unlike HSAs, an FSA may be used in conjunction with regular health insurance (such a PPO plan). Also, FSA accounts return to zero every twelve months; if you have not incurred enough qualified expenses, any money remaining in your account at the end of the year is forfeited. A person with an FSA should attempt to predict with some accuracy what the year's medical expenses might be. If uncertain, it may be best to err on the side of undercontributing.

If I don't have insurance, what can I do?

There are a multitude of reasons why people may not have health insurance. Some simply cannot afford it. Others believe that they should save their money and trust God to care for them, and still others believe insurance is a waste of money. While no system is perfect, we believe that health insurance is a wise investment, and we would encourage people to purchase at least some protection. Remember that one accident or illness can incur jaw-dropping expenses—one night of room and board alone at a hospital can cost a thousand dollars or more—and we question the wisdom (and the stewardship) of taking an enormous financial risk if there are reasonable provisions available to prevent it. It may not be feasible to have a top-of-the-line health plan that covers every conceivable expense, but there are many major medical plans that have high deductibles but reasonably low premiums and will cover major medical expenses and prevent a catastrophe.

If you truly cannot afford health-insurance coverage and do not qualify for

Medicaid or Medicare, this does not mean that you cannot or should not obtain appropriate care. Here are some options to consider.

Seek to establish a relationship with a primary-care provider (such as a family physician) who will serve as your guide to the local medical community. If you cannot afford the entire fee at the time of the visit, see if payments may be made over time. Generally speaking, the cost of a visit to a primary-care physician is the least expensive component of medical care—less than any X ray, most lab fees (unless heavily discounted), an emergency-room visit, and a visit to almost any type of specialist. Often medication costs can be reduced by the use of samples from the office, and many drug companies offer free or discounted prescriptions for individuals with a limited income—but these are all initiated from a physician's office.

Some other possibilities:

- Most communities have hospitals and clinics (typically funded at the county level) that take everyone, regardless of insurance. In addition, there may be clinics in your community run by volunteers, including some that are church based, where you can obtain some basic medical advice and care.
- Some local hospitals run annual or semiannual health fairs, where a number of simple screening tests may be carried out for a nominal fee. They may also provide low-cost immunizations, especially during flu season. If you use these types of services, keep a basic medical record of your own—when and where you were seen, what medications you received, and what advice you were given.
- Your church may have an emergency fund for medical expenses or may have contacts with medical professionals who, as a form of ministry, would be willing to see you for a nominal (or no) fee.

If you have a true emergency—crushing chest discomfort, severe abdominal pain, a significant injury that may involve a fracture, and so forth—you should go to the nearest emergency department, even if you are uninsured. All emergency departments are required to render appropriate care without regard to insurance status, and you must not risk a medical catastrophe because of concerns over finances.

QUESTIONS TO PONDER

1. After reading this chapter, where do you think you would go to evaluate a health claim you hear on radio or TV or read about on the Internet or in a magazine?
2. Have you or a family member tried any alternative therapies? If so, which ones? In which of the four categories of alternative medicine (see pages 820–821) do you think it falls?
3. If you or a family member takes any supplements, how can you evaluate their safety and effectiveness?
4. How satisfied are you with your family's primary-care providers? What might you do to strengthen your relationship?
5. If you or a family member doesn't have a primary-care provider, what steps might you take to find one?
6. What type of health-insurance plan do you have? How familiar are you with its benefits and procedures?
7. If your family is not currently covered by a health-insurance plan, how can you best prepare yourselves for upcoming medical expenses? See pages 861–862 for some ideas.

Action items: If you have not yet compiled a complete list of all the prescription and over-the-counter medications, along with all dietary supplements, you currently take, do so now. Do the same for each member of your family, and be sure to pass along this information to your primary-care provider, especially if another physician (for example, a specialist) has added or changed a medication.

Whenever you have a new health-related question, refer to the table providing reliable online sources of health information on pages 840–841.

If you have a primary-care provider, evaluate your satisfaction with his or her services, and consider what steps you might take to improve your relationship. If you are unsatisfied or have no primary-care provider, follow the steps beginning on page 846 and come up with a plan for selecting a primary-care provider.

If you have a private insurance plan but are unsure what type it is or how it works, pull out your benefits booklet and familiarize yourself with it. If you have a plan provided by your employer, don't hesitate to contact your human resources department for additional information.

If you have Medicare or Medicaid, consider visiting http://www.medicare.gov or http://www.cms.hhs.gov/medicaid to be sure you have all the appropriate coverage for which you qualify.

If you do not have health insurance, don't assume there is nothing you can do to deal with the costs of a health problem. See pages 861–862 for some ideas on preparing for future medical expenses.

APPENDIX A

Abortion: A Risk for Breast Cancer?

A Working Paper from Focus on the Family's Physicians Resource Council

Is there support for the claim that abortion is a risk factor for breast cancer?

Epidemiological evidence of an association between elective (induced) abortion and an increased risk of developing breast cancer first appeared in the Japanese medical literature in 1957.[1] (**Epidemiology** is the branch of medicine that studies not only specific epidemics but also the presence, distribution, causes, and control of all types of disease in populations.) Since that study was first published, more than fifty research papers in peer-reviewed medical journals and several others included in reviews or presented at scientific conferences have addressed this issue.

Among the many factors that impact a woman's likelihood for developing breast cancer are some that are related to her reproductive history. Specifically, the American Cancer Society notes that:

> Women who have not had children, or who had their first child after age 30, have a slightly higher risk of breast cancer. Being pregnant more than once and at an early age reduces breast cancer risk.[2]

One or more abortions might play a role in a woman never having a child, having only one child, or delaying her childbearing (especially until after age thirty). In these situations, abortion is but one of many types of decisions that affect the number and timing of a woman's childbearing, and thus her risk of developing breast cancer. But some have raised a concern that abortion is an *independent* risk factor for breast cancer.

Consider this question: A childless woman who never became pregnant and a childless woman who aborted one or more pregnancies would both be considered to have a slight increase in breast cancer risk based on the fact that neither bore a child. But does the childless woman who had one or more abortions carry a greater risk for developing breast cancer than she would have if she had never become pregnant?

In 1996, Dr. Joel Brind published an extensive review of the available research dealing with the possibility of an independent link between abortion and breast cancer. He reviewed thirty-eight epidemiological studies of this link published worldwide, including fifteen studies on women in the United States. Twenty-nine of the studies, including thirteen in the United States, showed an increased risk of breast cancer among women who had undergone an abortion. From this review Brind concluded that the average lifetime risk for developing breast cancer is increased 30 percent among women who have had an abortion.[3]

Other prominent scientists and professional organizations disagreed with this conclusion, leading the National Cancer Institute (NCI), the federal government's principal agency in cancer research, to hold a conference on the abortion–breast cancer issue in 2003. While the conference's stated purpose was to review the evidence in the world's literature on the subject, it was in fact strongly weighted in favor of those who reject an association between abortion and breast cancer. While recognizing that full-term pregnancy provides an element of protection against the development of breast cancer, the NCI panel concluded that "induced abortion is not associated with an increase in breast cancer risk."[4] This conclusion was reached without the benefit of testimony from any scientist who supported the abortion–breast cancer link.

Most of the studies dealing with this issue have been observational "case-control" studies, meaning that the medical histories of women who were diagnosed with breast cancer were compared with those of a similar group of women who did not have breast cancer. (These types of studies are also referred to as "retrospective," because they "look back" at the histories of women in an effort to see what might have affected the disease in question—in this case, breast cancer.) However, a potential bias of many of these retrospective studies is that they are based on patients' self-reporting of their medical histories, rather than their actual medical records or exams. Some researchers claim that this approach can lead to inaccurate information, especially when a woman is questioned about a procedure such as abortion that may have emotional repercussions and social stigmata. Other researchers believe that the data from these retrospective studies are, on the whole, trustworthy, but they have pointed out design flaws in certain studies that they believe invalidate their conclusions.[5] One comprehensive review of fifty-three studies in sixteen countries found that the prospective studies that were reviewed did not reveal an independent association linking breast cancer with abortion, but the retrospective studies did show an increased risk.[6] Needless to say, the debate is far from settled.

Why Might Breast Cancer Be More Likely after an Elective Abortion?

Prolonged exposure to estrogens, especially at increased levels, is known to be a risk factor for developing breast cancer. During early pregnancy there is a significant increase in estrogen levels, which in turn stimulates the proliferation of primitive, immature cells within the breast. These are called **undifferentiated** cells, which are more easily stimulated to becoming malignant. During the last eight weeks of pregnancy, these mature into **differentiated** cells that form the milk-producing glands of the breast. They are also more resistant to becoming cancerous. The theoretical explanation for the association between elective abortion and breast cancer is as follows: When a pregnancy ends in spontaneous abortion (miscarriage), estrogen levels are often abnormally low before the pregnancy loss, and the undifferentiated cells are not stimulated to grow. However, in a pregnancy terminated by an induced abortion, the sudden termination of the pregnancy allows the estrogen levels to remain elevated afterward for a longer period, and large numbers of breast cells are left in an undifferentiated state where they are more vulnerable to becoming malignant.[7]

The Physicians Resource Council (PRC) of Focus on the Family recognizes the biological fact and affirms the biblical teaching that human life begins at conception/fertilization. The PRC holds that abortion not only destroys an innocent human life but also is harmful to women who undergo this procedure. Before any woman decides to have an abortion, we believe that she has the right to be adequately informed not only about all the physical, emotional, and spiritual consequences of abortion, but also that abortion may increase her risk for developing breast cancer later in life.

APPENDIX B

Vitamins and Minerals: What Each One Does and How Much We Need

Did you chew (or gag) on a vitamin pill every day when you were growing up, cheered on by Mom's pronouncements that it would "help you grow big and strong"? Do you become glassy-eyed in the aisle at the supermarket where battalions of vitamins, minerals, and other supplements line the shelves? Do you wonder whether you can get all the vitamins you need from a bowl of fortified cereal, or if you need to spend a small fortune every month on a tackle box of supplements?

You've probably gotten an earful of advice on this subject from just about every direction—except one. If you haven't heard much from your doctor about vitamin and mineral supplements, you're not alone. Professional organizations and physicians have generally taken the "food is enough" approach: If you're a healthy individual consistently eating three square meals a day, all of the vitamins and minerals necessary for good health should be available on your plate. Taking a lot of supplements wastes money and may even risk toxicity.

Other voices argue that our food isn't as good as it used to be in the good old days: Modern technology, processing, and pollutants, the stresses of life, and fast-food eating habits have all conspired to downgrade what's on our daily table, so every day we need to take a comprehensive vitamin/mineral tablet or elixir, and perhaps a whole assortment of supplements, to stay healthy.

Which of these positions is right?

If sales figures mean anything, Americans are buying into the second approach. According to the American Dietetic Association, estimated U.S. sales of dietary supplements of all types increased from $8.6 billion in 1994 to $18.7 billion in 2002. Of this amount, 40 percent was spent on vitamins, 8 percent on minerals, and the rest on herbal and botanical products, sports supplements, and various specialty items—altogether some 29,000 different products.[1] An estimated 40 percent of Americans take at least one vitamin or mineral supplement regularly.[2]

But sales figures and cultural trends don't always reflect sound judgment. Are vitamin and mineral supplements a wise investment or a waste of money? To get a handle on this question, we'll need a little background information about these substances. What do they do? How much do we need? Can we get enough from our food, or do we need to supplement at least some of them?

What Exactly Are Vitamins?

Vitamins are nutrients with the following characteristics:

- They are **essential**, in that they are vital to health, even life itself. In addition, the term *essential* in nutritional vocabulary means that *they cannot be created within the body from other nutrients* but must be obtained from food (or supplements). An exception to the second meaning of *essential* is vitamin D, which for its synthesis requires a modest amount of sun exposure. (Without adequate sun exposure, vitamin D must be supplied from food or supplements.)
- They are **organic**—that is, they contain carbon (as opposed to minerals, which are *inorganic*).
- They are *needed only in tiny amounts*, and thus are **micronutrients**. Daily requirements for vitamins are measured in milligrams (mg) or micrograms (mcg), as opposed to grams or ounces, which are used for **macronutrients**—carbohydrates, fats, and proteins.
- Unlike macronutrients, vitamins *do not serve as fuel* (they are not broken down to create energy), nor do they form any structures. Instead, most of them participate in important biochemical reactions.

Early in the twentieth century, when researchers began to uncover the connection between nutritional deficits and certain diseases, it was believed that there were only two vitamins, one water soluble and one fat soluble.

During the first half of the twentieth century, thirteen compounds were identified as vitamins. Since 1948, when vitamin B_{12} was isolated, no new vitamins have been discovered. (Several compounds have been proposed as vitamins, but none have incontrovertibly met the scientific criteria to be designated as one.) The thirteen well-identified vitamins are divided into two groups:

- The **water-soluble vitamins**—eight **B vitamins** (also called the **B complex**) and **vitamin C**
- The **fat-soluble vitamins—vitamins A**, **D**, **E**, and **K**

What's the Difference between Water- and Fat-Soluble Vitamins?

Carbohydrates and proteins are water soluble and thus disperse freely throughout the bloodstream and tissues, while fat molecules must be "escorted" by special proteins because they do not dissolve and disperse in blood.

Similarly, the water-soluble vitamins enter the bloodstream directly. They disperse freely throughout tissues and are excreted by the kidneys, which are capable of removing some (but not all) of these substances when more is available than we need. (Critics of high-dose vitamin supplementation are fond of pointing out that this tends to create "expensive urine.") Vitamin C and most of the B complex are not stored for long periods of time, so regular replenishment from food or supplements every few days (if not more often) is necessary to maintain health. Vitamin B_{12} is a notable exception.

As might be expected, the fat-soluble vitamins tend to be found in the fats and oils of foods. They enter the bloodstream by way of the lymphatic system and usually require a protein carrier to circulate in the blood. Excess amounts are stored in fat and the liver rather than being excreted by the kidneys—a useful process if there is an extended dietary shortage, because these vitamins may then be available even if none are taken in food for weeks or even months. But if very large doses are taken on a regular basis, toxicity is more likely to occur with fat-soluble than with water-soluble vitamins. (As with any nutrient, there is always the possibility of too much of a good thing.)

All of the B vitamins serve as **coenzymes** in vast numbers of biochemical reactions throughout the body. You may recall from chapter 5 that **enzymes** are complex proteins that serve as catalysts—compounds that allow chemical reactions to occur rapidly at body temperature. (See page 155.) A coenzyme is a substance that attaches to a particular enzyme and allows it to function properly. The B vitamins are necessary for the proper function of enzymes that are involved in the release of energy from carbohydrate, fat, and protein, as well as the creation of DNA, the genetic blueprint needed for the construction of new cells.

Ladies and Gentlemen, May We Introduce the Vitamins . . .

Water-soluble vitamins

Vitamin B_1 (Thiamin)

What does it do? Thiamin serves as a coenzyme in a key reaction in energy metabolism in all cells. It also plays a significant role in normal nerve function.

F.Y.I.

Unless otherwise stated, the amounts of vitamins and minerals listed in this chapter are either **recommended daily allowances (RDAs)** or **adequate intakes (AIs)** from the 1997–2001 Dietary Reference Intakes published by the Food and Nutrition Board, a component of the Institute of Medicine which in turn is one of the four National Academies. (We introduced these influential advisory organizations in chapter 5, starting on page 160.) The RDA represents the amount of the vitamin or mineral that is considered appropriate for most healthy people in the age and gender groups listed. When there isn't enough data to determine an RDA, the Food and Nutrition Board provides adequate intakes (AIs) based on surveys of nutrient contents in foods consumed by Americans. For some vitamins and minerals, the recommended amounts during pregnancy and lactation (breast-feeding) are slightly different for women younger than nineteen.

How much do we need?

AIs:

Infants, birth to six months	0.2 mg/day
Infants, seven months to one year	0.3 mg/day

RDAs:

Children, one to three years	0.5 mg/day
Children, four to eight years	0.6 mg/day
Children, nine to thirteen years	0.9 mg/day

Teenage boys and men, fourteen and older	1.2 mg/day
Teenage girls, fourteen to eighteen	1.0 mg/day
Women, nineteen and older	1.1 mg/day
Women, pregnant or breast-feeding	1.4 mg/day

Where do we get it? Good dietary sources of thiamin include whole-grain or enriched breads and cereals, legumes and nuts, and pork products.

What happens if we don't get enough? Two significant syndromes related to inadequate intake of thiamin are **beriberi** and **Wernicke-Korsakoff syndrome.**

The word *beriberi* literally means "I can't, I can't" in the Sinhalese language of Sri Lanka. It is an apropos and poignant tribute to the profound weakness of the legs and arms that is the hallmark of this disease. Beriberi can also result in severe heart failure that in turn causes edema (fluid retention) in the legs and elsewhere. When this occurs, beriberi is called "wet," as opposed to "dry" beriberi in which there is only muscle wasting. The disease normally is a consequence of malnourishment, but it became particularly common in the early 1900s among Asian laborers who lived primarily on milled (polished) rice. Some detective work by a number of researchers determined that a dietary deficiency was the culprit, but it was not until 1912 that Polish-born biochemist Casimir Funk determined that substances in rice husks—the part removed in milling—would prevent beriberi. Funk coined the term *vitamines*, short for *vital amines*, for these compounds, but the word was later changed to "vitamins" when it was determined that a number of them were not amines (that is, nitrogen-containing compounds derived from ammonia). He determined that serious diseases such as scurvy, rickets, and pellagra were also caused by vitamin deficiencies, although other scientists would eventually figure out which substances would prevent them.

In Western nations today overt thiamin deficiency is relatively uncommon, occurring primarily among individuals who are severely malnourished—for example, a homeless person who cannot obtain food for an extended period—as well as among alcoholics whose primary source of calories is the bottle. (Needless to say, alcoholic beverages provide little nutritional value.) Alcohol also interferes with the absorption of thiamin and increases its excretion in the urine, such that as many as four out of five alcoholics may be deficient in this vitamin.[3] When the deficiency is severe, a neurological disorder called Wernicke-Korsakoff syndrome may occur, notable for disorientation, staggering gait, and memory loss. (Indeed, long-term alcohol abusers with memory loss are notorious for making up information to fill in the gaps, a symptom called **confabulation**.) An alcoholic admitted to the hospital for treatment will routinely receive an injection of thiamin, along with ongoing vitamin supplementation.

Need help with an alcohol problem? Check out chapter 10, starting on page 447.

People who might not get enough: Those who abuse alcohol, especially if they fail to eat while drinking, may be deficient in thiamin. People with **malabsorption** syndromes that cause inadequate absorption of nutrients may also be deficient. Otherwise, a person eating enough food of reasonable quality to meet basic energy needs will nearly always get enough thiamin.

Too much of a good thing? No specific toxicity has been observed among people taking high amounts of thiamin in supplements. However, as we will discuss later, there are good reasons to avoid taking massive quantities of any vitamin.

Interesting tidbits: Thiamin was the first vitamin identified. Prolonged cooking (especially in water) destroys thiamin, but it is preserved when foods are steamed or microwaved with little added water.

Vitamin B_2 (Riboflavin)

What does it do? Like thiamin, riboflavin serves as a coenzyme in reactions where energy is released in all cells throughout the body.

How much do we need? The amounts are very similar to those for thiamin.

AIs:

Infants, birth to six months	0.3 mg/day
Infants, seven months to one year	0.4 mg/day

RDAs:

Children, one to three years	0.5 mg/day
Children, four to eight years	0.6 mg/day
Children, nine to thirteen years	0.9 mg/day
Men, fourteen and older	1.3 mg/day
Teenage girls, fourteen to eighteen years	1.0 mg/day
Women, nineteen and older	1.1 mg/day
Women, pregnant	1.4 mg/day
Women, breast-feeding.	1.6 mg/day

Where do we get it? Milk and milk products, whole grains and enriched cereals, fish, poultry, eggs, and liver. Dark leafy green vegetables such as spinach, asparagus, and broccoli are also excellent sources of riboflavin.

What happens if we don't get enough? No specific disease is associated with riboflavin deficiency, but inadequate intake may lead to cracked and scaling skin, especially around the nose, ears, and corners of the mouth. Inflamed lips and a sore tongue may also occur.

People who might not get enough: Those who avoid all dairy and meat products and don't eat plenty of leafy greens and whole or enriched grains may not get enough riboflavin.

Too much of a good thing? No specific toxicity has been observed among people taking high amounts of riboflavin in supplements. However, as we will discuss later, there are good reasons to avoid taking massive quantities of any vitamin.

Interesting tidbits: Riboflavin has also been called vitamin G, as well as lactoflavin, ovoflavin, and hepatoflavin, in honor of its presence in milk, eggs, and liver. (The prefix *lacto* refers to milk, as in "lactate"; *ovo* to eggs, as in "ovulate"; and *hepato* to liver, as in "hepatitis."

Riboflavin in milk may be destroyed by exposure to direct sunlight.

Vitamin B_3 (Niacin)

What does it do? Niacin serves as a coenzyme in many energy metabolism reactions, especially those involving glucose, fat, and alcohol. (The term **niacin** actually refers to two compounds called nicotinic acid and nicotinamide, which is also called niacinamide.)

How much do we need?

AIs:

Infants, birth to six months	2 mg/day
Infants, seven months to one year	4 mg/day

RDAs:

Children, one to three years	6 mg/day
Children, four to eight years	8 mg/day
Children, nine to thirteen years	12 mg/day
Teenage boys and men, fourteen and older	16 mg/day
Teenage girls and women, fourteen and older	14 mg/day
Women, pregnant	18 mg/day
Women, breast-feeding	17 mg/day

Where do we get it? Niacin is unique among the vitamins in that our body can make it from **tryptophan**, an amino acid found in protein-rich foods such as meat, fish, poultry, eggs, and nuts. It takes about 60 mg of tryptophan to make 1 mg of niacin, so this amount of tryptophan is called a **niacin equivalent**. There is about 1 mg of tryptophan in 100 mg of protein, so to get one niacin equivalent's worth of tryptophan you need about 6 grams of protein that aren't being used for other body functions. (Most tables showing the amount of niacin present in a given food indicate only *preformed* niacin and don't include what might be obtained from any protein present.) Needless to say, high-protein diets are not short on this vitamin. Niacin can also be readily obtained from whole- and enriched-grain foods as well as leafy green vegetables.

What happens if we don't get enough? A person who is chronically deprived of niacin develops **pellagra**, a disease known for "four Ds"—dermatitis (inflammation of the skin), diarrhea, dementia, and death. For centuries pellagra has been seen in parts of southern Europe and the Middle East, and during the early twentieth century, tens of thousands died of this disease in the southern United States. Like beriberi, pellagra occurs among people living on a subsistence diet who are dependent on an inadequate staple crop—in this case, corn or maize. While corn contains tryptophan, it is present in a form that isn't easily absorbed. Furthermore, corn is abundant in another amino acid, **leucine**, that inhibits the conversion of tryptophan to niacin. The first researchers who studied pellagra believed that it was caused by an infection transmitted in corn, and considerable effort was put into searching for the responsible bacteria, fungus, or toxin before the true culprit—the *lack* of a critical dietary factor—was discovered.

The dry, crusty, scabby skin seen with pellagra gave the disease its name, from the Italian words *pelle* ("skin") and *agra* ("rough").

People who might not be getting enough: Without supplementation, those whose diet is extremely restricted in protein, grains, and vegetables may be deficient in niacin.

Too much of a good thing? Niacin has a property unique among the B vitamins. In very high doses—typically 1,000 mg to 1,500 mg or more per day, or about 100 times the RDA—the nicotinic acid (but not the nicotinamide) form can have a beneficial effect on lipid levels, lowering total and LDL (bad) cholesterol, reducing triglycerides, and raising HDL (good) cholesterol. Before the arrival of the more effective statin drugs, high-dose niacin was widely used to treat high cholesterol. It is still used for this purpose, though less commonly. High doses of niacin can dilate small blood vessels, causing a colorful and annoying flush, though this is less common with time-release forms. (The flush is also reduced when niacin is taken with food or with a dose of aspirin.)

We introduced the various components of cholesterol, as well as the statin drugs, in chapter 3, beginning on page 48. Statins currently on the market include atorvastatin (Lipitor), lovastatin (Mevacor and Altoprev), fluvastatin (Lescol), pravastatin (Pravachol), rosuvastatin (Crestor), and simvastatin (Zocor). The preparation Advicor combines lovastatin and niacin in the same tablet.

More importantly, even though niacin is a vitamin, at high doses (which can be purchased without a prescription) it should be considered a drug—complete with benefits and risks, just like any other product from the pharmacy. As a result, you should not attempt to use high-dose niacin (nicotinic acid) to treat cholesterol without consulting a physician. It may provoke intestinal symptoms such as nausea, vomiting, and diarrhea, and even aggravate peptic ulcer disease. It can raise uric acid levels (which could provoke an attack of gout in a susceptible individual) and may also raise blood glucose levels, making it a less attractive option for diabetics. It can also irritate the liver, so people taking high doses of niacin should have blood tests on a periodic basis not only to check cholesterol and triglycerides but also to confirm that all appears to be well with the liver. (Needless to say, high-dose niacin should be avoided by people with known liver disease.)

Interesting tidbit: For decades, high-dose niacin was prescribed or recommended as a treatment for vertigo and ringing in the ears (tinnitus), apparently based on the assumption that if it increased blood flow in the face (manifested by the annoying flush), it would do likewise in the inner ear. Perhaps this medication-induced hot flash distracted people from their other symptoms, but this use of niacin is no longer recommended in mainstream medical practice.

Biotin

What does it do? Biotin is yet another coenzyme involved in energy production, as well as in the creation of glucose from noncarbohydrate sources, the synthesis of fatty acids, and the metabolism of fat and protein.

How much do we need? Biotin is needed in such tiny quantities that the Institute of Medicine's Food and Nutrition Board has determined adequate intake (AI) levels rather than recommended daily allowances (RDAs). Note that these are measured in **micrograms** (abbreviated **mcg**), so the amounts are nearly a thousand times smaller than those recommended for the previous B vitamins.

AIs:

Infants, birth to six months	5 mcg/day
Infants, seven months to one year	6 mcg/day
Children, one to three years	8 mcg/day
Children, four to eight years	12 mcg/day
Children, nine to thirteen years	20 mcg/day
Teenage boys, fourteen to eighteen years	25 mcg/day
Men, nineteen and older	30 mcg/day
Teenage girls, fourteen to eighteen years	25 mcg/day
Women, nineteen and older	30 mcg/day
Women, pregnant	30 mcg/day
Women, breast-feeding	35 mcg/day

Where do we get it? A wide variety of foods contain biotin, especially egg yolks, soybeans, fish, and whole-grain foods.

What happens if we don't get enough? Skin rash and hair loss have been reported, along with a variety of neurological symptoms including depression, lethargy, and tingling sensations in the arms and legs. Because so little is needed, an isolated biotin deficiency is very uncommon.

People who might not get enough: Those who adhere to the Super-Duper Raw Egg White Diet. Raw egg white contains avidin, a protein that interferes with the absorption of biotin. (Cooking the egg destroys the protein, and egg yolks contain plenty of biotin.) A person would need to eat two dozen raw egg whites every day for several months to demonstrate biotin deficiency.

Too much of a good thing? No specific toxicity has been observed from high intakes of biotin in supplements. However, as we will discuss later, there are good reasons to avoid taking massive quantities of any vitamin.

Interesting tidbit: At one time biotin was called vitamin H.

Pantothenic acid

What does it do? Pantothenic acid is a component of a compound called coenzyme A, which itself is part of another compound called acetyl CoA, a key structure in a vast number of biochemical reactions.

How much do we need? As with biotin, only AIs have been established for pantothenic acid.

AIs:

Infants, birth to six months	1.7 mg/day
Infants, seven months to one year	1.8 mg/day
Children, one to three years	2 mg/day
Children, four to eight years	3 mg/day
Children, nine to thirteen years	4 mg/day
Teenage boys and men, fourteen and older	5 mg/day
Teenage girls and women, fourteen and older	5 mg/day
Women, pregnant	6 mg/day
Women, breast-feeding	7 mg/day

Where do we get it? Just about everywhere. (*Pantothenic* comes from a Greek word meaning "from every side.") Meats, whole grains, potatoes, tomatoes, and broccoli are excellent sources, although this vitamin can be destroyed during freezing, canning, and refining processes.

What happens if we don't get enough? Fatigue, abdominal discomfort, and a burning sensation of the feet were among the symptoms observed in adult volunteers fed a diet deficient in this substance.

People who might not get enough: It is difficult for people to become deficient in this vitamin if they eat even modest amounts of food from one or two major groups.

I THINK I HAVE A BIOTIN DEFICIENCY!

You may notice throughout this chapter that many of the vitamin deficiency syndromes *(a)* sound very similar and *(b)* involve a lot of common symptoms, such as fatigue, aching, unusual sensations, and so on. Symptoms such as these can have dozens of possible causes, and unless you have an extremely restricted diet, it's very unlikely that an overt vitamin deficiency is the cause.

Unfortunately, millions of people spend billions of dollars every year hoping that a supplement (or several of them) will relieve ongoing discomforts. Those who market these items will be quick to describe the miraculous improvements that their products will provide, and they may throw in a testimonial or two to prove it.

You should beware of such age-old selling tactics for two reasons. First, while the supplements probably won't hurt you, you will probably pay more than you need to for something you actually *don't* need. Second, those symptoms may have one or more important causes that need to be identified. Make sure you have them checked out by a competent physician before you hit the supplement aisle or the Internet. ■

Too much of a good thing? No specific toxicity has been observed with high intakes of pantothenic acid in supplements. However, as we will discuss later, there are good reasons to avoid taking massive quantities of any vitamin.

Interesting tidbit: Pantothenic acid deficiency may have accounted for a "burning feet" syndrome seen among prisoners of war in Asia during World War II.

Vitamin B_6 (Pyridoxine)

What does it do? Vitamin B_6 is a family of compounds, the major forms of which are pyridoxine, pyridoxal, and pryridoxamine. All three of these are converted to a coenzyme called PLP, which plays an important role in more than one hundred reactions related to protein metabolism. Two of these reactions involve the conversion of the amino acid tryptophan into two different but important compounds: the vitamin niacin (which we discussed earlier in this chapter) and **serotonin**. Serotonin is one of several neurotransmitters, chemical messengers within the brain and central nervous system whose activity influences mood, sleep, and many other functions. PLP is also needed for the synthesis of **heme**, a component of hemoglobin, the molecule that carries oxygen within red blood cells.

Vitamin B_6 has become a hot item over the past several years because of ongoing research suggesting its importance in the proper function of the nervous and immune systems, as well as its possible role in reducing the risk of coronary artery disease.

How much do we need?

AIs:	
Infants, birth to six months	0.1 mg/day
Infants, seven months to one year	0.3 mg/day
RDAs	
Children, one to three years	0.5 mg/day
Children, four to eight years	0.6 mg/day
Children, nine to thirteen years	1.0 mg/day
Teenage boys and men, fourteen to fifty years	1.3 mg/day
Men, over fifty	1.7 mg/day
Teenage girls, fourteen to eighteen years	1.2 mg/day
Women, nineteen to fifty years	1.3 mg/day
Women, over fifty	1.5 mg/day
Women, pregnant	1.9 mg/day
Women, breast-feeding	2.0 mg/day

Where do we get it? A wide variety of foods contain vitamin B_6, including meat, poultry, fish, whole and fortified grains, potatoes, beans, and noncitrus fruits.

What happens if we don't get enough? A full-blown deficiency in vitamin B_6 is uncommon but can cause serious problems, including anemia, dermatitis (skin inflammation), depression, confusion, and even seizures. There has been ongoing discussion and debate as to whether a mild deficiency of B_6, which may occur more commonly in the elderly (especially among those with a limited variety of available foods), could increase the risk of coronary artery disease.

People who might not get enough: Alcoholics may lack sufficient B_6, since abusing alcohol accelerates the loss of this vitamin from the body. Also, the drug INH (isoniazid), which is used to treat tuberculosis (or prevent its spread if one has become infected), inactivates this vitamin and can cause symptoms of deficiency. Those who take INH are commonly given a B_6 supplement. The drug theophylline, once widely used to treat asthma, can deplete stores of this vitamin, and a supplement may be appropriate for someone using this medication. A full-blown deficiency in vitamin B_6 from poor eating habits is rare because the vitamin is found in so many foods. However, low levels have been observed in the elderly.

Too much of a good thing? Unlike many of the other B vitamins, you can overdose on B_6, a fact that was not fully appreciated until the early 1980s. Impaired nerve function—specifically altered sensations in the arms and legs, which can be very aggravating—may result from daily doses of 500 mg per day or less. The symptoms are usually reversible when this oversupplementation stops. However, at extremely high doses—2 to 6 *grams* per day, well above 1,000 times the recommended daily dose—symptoms tend to be more severe and may reverse more slowly once the excessive dose is stopped. The National Academy of Sciences has set an upper limit (UL) of 100 mg per day for vitamin B_6 in adults and well below that for children.

Interesting tidbit: Sales of high-dose vitamin B_6 supplements have been fueled both by traditional usage and by enthusiastic claims that they are effective in treating depression, premenstrual syndrome, insomnia, and carpal tunnel syndrome, among other ailments. Unfortunately, confirmation of these uses in well-controlled research studies has not been impressive, and overdose symptoms have often occurred among those trying to relieve other problems with high doses of this vitamin.

Folic acid

What does it do? Like most of the B vitamins, folic acid—also known as **folate**—is a coenzyme. It plays an important role in the synthesis of DNA, the complex compound in the nucleus of cells that transmits genetic information. It is particularly critical in tissues where cells are rapidly multiplying and growing, such as the lining of the intestine and the bone marrow (where blood cells are produced). Folic acid has a unique relationship with vitamin B_{12}—each requires the presence of the other to be activated and function properly.

How much do we need? Note that, just as with biotin, these quantities are given in *micrograms*, which is equal to one millionth of a gram.

AIs:

Infants, birth to six months	65 mcg/day
Infants, seven months to one year	80 mcg/day

RDAs:

Children, one to three years	150 mcg/day
Children, four to eight years	200 mcg/day
Children, nine to thirteen years	300 mcg/day
Teenage boys, fourteen to eighteen years	400 mcg/day
Men, nineteen and older	400 mcg/day
Teenage girls, fourteen to eighteen years	400 mcg/day
Women, nineteen and older	400 mcg/day
Women, pregnant	600 mcg/day
Women, breast-feeding	500 mcg/day

Where do we get it? The name says it all: *folic*, as in "foliage." Folic acid is abundant in legumes and vegetables, especially the leafy green variety, although cooking can destroy a significant percentage of it. Because of its role in preventing birth defects, by federal mandate folic acid is routinely added to products such as flour, bread, rice, pasta, and cereals. A large number of breakfast cereals now contain 100 percent of the adult RDA for folic acid per serving.

What happens if we don't get enough? Folic acid deficiency is most notable for causing a form of anemia (a shortage of red blood cells) characterized by **macrocytosis**, a fancy word meaning "big cells." As red blood cells progress from their earliest, just-created state to full maturity within the bone marrow where they are manufactured, they actually become smaller. Without an adequate supply of folic acid, red blood cells cannot mature properly, and those that begin circulating are deficient in their ability to carry oxygen or travel through tiny capillaries where the cells are supposed to deliver it.

In addition, adequate folic acid taken by a woman before and during early pregnancy plays an important role in preventing a type of birth defect called a neural tube defect. (See sidebar: "Preventing Birth Defects with Folic Acid" on page 882.) Some research also suggests that it can help prevent heart disease and cancer. In chapter 4 (beginning on page 83) we described how an elevated level of homocysteine in the blood is associated with a higher risk for coronary artery disease and that this level can be reduced by taking a folic acid supplement, along with vitamins B_6 and B_{12}. Some have suggested adjusting the amount of folic acid depending on the level of homocysteine and its response to the supplement, but the most effective doses of folic acid and the two other B vitamins—and whether they will truly prevent coronary disease—remain to be determined. Recent research suggests that folic acid, whether obtained through supplements or leafy greens, may help prevent both colon and breast cancer. This appears to be particularly beneficial for women who consume more than one alcoholic drink per day.

People who might not get enough: Certain intestinal problems that cause malabsorption, as well as conditions in which cells multiply at an increased rate, incuding cancer, blood loss, a major burn, or a multiple-gestation pregnancy—that is, involving more than one baby—can lead to a deficiency. Also, certain medications, including a number of anticancer (chemotherapy) drugs, as well as aspirin and antacids when taken multiple times per day on an ongoing basis, can interfere with the function of folic acid. Alcohol also interferes with both absorption and utilization of folic acid, and daily users should be particularly careful about getting enough folic acid through food or supplements.

Too much of a good thing? Supplementing folic acid beyond 1000 mcg (1 mg) per day is generally not recommended, with one exception: Women who have had a child born with a neural tube defect should take 4 mg of folic acid per day if they are planning to become pregnant again. In general, higher doses of folic acid aren't likely to be toxic, but they might mask the neurologic consequences of vitamin B_{12} deficiency. (Remember that their functions are interrelated.) This in turn could lead to a delayed diagnosis of a serious condition called pernicious anemia, which is discussed in the next section.

Interesting tidbit: The number of cases of neural tube defects in newborn infants dropped 25 percent in the United States within five years of the 1998 FDA mandate that all enriched cereal grains be fortified with folic acid.

Getting enough folic acid every day is one of the most compelling reasons to consider taking a multivitamin supplement. (However, don't forget the many benefits of five to nine servings of fruits and vegetables every day—especially those leafy greens.)

Vitamin B_{12} (Cobalamin)

What does it do? Vitamin B_{12} is a coenzyme, which, with folic acid, participates in the synthesis of DNA necessary for the multiplication of cells. In addition, this vitamin helps maintain the insulating sheath that surrounds nerve cells.

How much do we need? As with folic acid, quantities are in micrograms (mcg), but notice how much smaller the recommended amounts are:

AIs:

Infants, birth to six months	0.4 mcg/day
Infants, seven months to one year	0.5 mcg/day

RDAs:

Children, one to three years	0.9 mcg/day
Children, four to eight years	1.2 mcg/day
Children, nine to thirteen years	1.8 mcg/day
Teenage boys and men, fourteen and older	2.4 mcg/day
Teenage girls and women, fourteen and older	2.4 mcg/day
Women, pregnant	2.6 mcg/day
Women, breast-feeding	2.8 mcg/day

Where do we get it? Unlike its B vitamin counterparts, vitamin B_{12} is obtained almost entirely from animal products: meat, poultry, fish, eggs, dairy products, and cheese. It is also commonly added to cereals.

PREVENTING BIRTH DEFECTS WITH FOLIC ACID

One of the most important developments affecting prenatal care and prevention of birth defects was the discovery that adequate daily doses of folic acid during the first month of pregnancy can reduce the risk of a **neural tube defect** in the newborn. Beginning at the seventeenth day after conception, a structure called the neural tube forms within the growing baby. Normally this will develop into the brain, skull, spinal cord, and spine, and by the thirtieth day the neural tube should be closed. If it is not, the brain or spinal cord will not form properly, causing what can prove to be a major or even lethal defect.

The most common neural tube defect is **spina bifida**, a condition affecting the lower end of the spine and spinal cord. A fluid-filled sac, which may contain part of the spinal cord, may protrude from an opening in the back. While spina bifida isn't commonly fatal, it can be associated with a number of neurological problems, including paralysis of the legs, difficulties with bladder and bowel control, and learning disabilities. Less common but far more severe is **anencephaly**, in which the upper end of the neural tube fails to close, resulting in lack of development or complete absence of the brain. Anencephaly commonly results in miscarriage, but if the baby is born he or she usually will die within a few days of birth.

Current research indicates that taking folic acid during the first month of pregnancy can reduce the likelihood of having an infant with a neural tube defect by 50 to 70 percent. Unfortunately, this critical period of pregnancy usually has come and gone before a woman realizes she is pregnant. Therefore, any woman of childbearing age who plans to become pregnant or *might* become pregnant should take 400 mcg (0.4 mg) of folic acid daily. Once a woman knows she is pregnant, she should take 600 mcg (0.6 mg) daily. (Prenatal multivitamins typically contain 1.0 mg of folic acid, which allows some breathing room.) For a woman who has already had a child with a neural tube defect, the amount should be ten times greater—4 mg of folic acid daily, an amount that is usually obtained by prescription. ■

What happens if we don't get enough? The primary calling card of vitamin B_{12} deficiency is **pernicious anemia**, a name rightly indicating that more is wrong than a shortage of red blood cells. The anemia is much like that seen with folic acid deficiency, involving the presence of immature, large red blood cells in circulation. But B_{12} deficiency also causes insidious, progressive, and ultimately permanent nerve damage. Symptoms include altered sensation, weakness, and, if not corrected in time, paralysis. Folic acid supplements will cure the anemia of B_{12} deficiency, but if the vitamin is not also replenished, the nerve damage will continue.

The word *pernicious*, a nonmedical term meaning "exceedingly harmful or destructive," comes from a Latin word meaning "to slay outright."

People who might not get enough: Strict vegetarians (or **vegans**) who shun all animal products, including eggs and dairy products, may become deficient in vitamin B_{12}. They should consider taking a supplement that contains this vitamin. But because so little of this vitamin is needed each day and because the body's supply is continuously and efficiently recycled through a clever mechanism called the **enterohepatic circulation**, it is actually hard to become deficient in this vitamin merely by failing to consume enough of it.

The term *enterohepatic* (literally "intestinal-liver") *circulation* refers to a process in which substances such as vitamin B_{12} are recycled. In a nutshell, a substance that has been used by some process within the liver is secreted into bile, which flows via a system of tubes called **bile ducts** into what is called the **common duct**. This in turn opens into the **duodenum**, the first segment of the small intestine. Downstream in the small intestine, the substance is reabsorbed and sent back to the liver, where it is used again.

Most cases of vitamin B_{12} deficiency actually involve a problem with absorption. Stomach acid and a digestive enzyme called **pepsin** separate B_{12} from the proteins in food to which it is attached. Then a compound called **intrinsic factor**, which is secreted by the stomach, must be attached to B_{12} for it to be absorbed in the small intestine. If the stomach has been seriously damaged such that it no longer makes adequate amounts of acid and intrinsic factor (especially the latter), B_{12} deficiency will eventually occur. Also, most of this vitamin is absorbed in the segment of the small intestine that is farthest from the stomach and closest to the colon (large intestine). If this segment is damaged or removed, B_{12} deficiency may occur.

Too much of a good thing? There is no known toxicity syndrome for vitamin B_{12}, other than money wasted on unnecessary megadoses (especially injections). In the past, some physicians provided their patients a zingy placebo and supplemented their own incomes handsomely by routinely giving a shot of vitamin B_{12} or B complex for a wide variety of complaints (especially fatigue). Today the only well validated role for B_{12} injections is the treatment of pernicious anemia, for which a monthly dose is normally adequate for long-term maintenance.

Interesting tidbit: Most of the B vitamins are heat sensitive and may be lost when foods containing them (usually vegetables and fruits) are cooked in water. Cooking these foods in a microwave oven usually preserves the B vitamins. However, vitamin B_{12} in meat and dairy products is destroyed during microwave cooking, so these foods should be prepared in an oven or on a stovetop.

Time Out—A Brief Introduction to Free Radicals, Antioxidants, and Oxidative Stress

We need to take a brief intermission in our vitamin survey to introduce some important concepts. Over the past several years, attaching the word *antioxidant* to any product has become a buzzword meaning "It's good for you, no matter what the problem," much like the words *natural* or *organic* in previous decades. What exactly are antioxidants, and what do they do for us? To answer that question, we have to understand a little basic biochemistry.

Earlier in this book we noted that the Old Testament proclaimed quite accurately that "the life of a creature is in the blood" (Leviticus 17:11). Blood, of course, carries oxygen, and any tissue that doesn't get it for more than a few minutes is doomed. But while a steady supply of oxygen is necessary for basic metabolic operations in every cell, oxygen's reactions with a variety of compounds generate **free radicals**: highly unstable molecules containing one or more **unpaired electrons**, which are definitely *not* content to live a biochemical "single life." Instead, free radicals actively seek out other molecules from which they can swipe an electron and regain their stability. Those molecules may in turn become free radicals, stealing electrons from their neighbors and turning *them* into free radicals, and so on, in a literal chain reaction reminiscent of some horror-movie scenario.

There are a number of different types of free radicals, but those derived from oxygen are the most abundant in humans.

Unfortunately, molecules that have lost an electron to a free radical may be altered or even damaged in ways that can affect their function. Free radicals inflict their electron thievery on all kinds of important compounds: fatty acids; proteins; and even DNA, the complex blueprint containing the genetic information needed to make proteins and new cells. (It is estimated that within each cell the genetic material alone sustains as many as ten thousand oxidative "hits" every day.[4]) Free radicals not only arise from ongoing reactions involving oxygen within our body, but from other sources as well: polluted air, cigarette smoke, even the food we eat and water we drink.

Not all free radicals are bad for us. Some are harnessed by the immune system and used as weapons against invading organisms.

The totality of this nonstop biochemical onslaught by free radicals is often called **oxidative stress**, and fortunately our bodies are designed to carry out ongoing repair operations to counter it. Furthermore, a number of enzymes inactivate free radicals. With the passage of time, however, these wondrous mechanisms may become less effective or may simply be overwhelmed. Current research has implicated free radical damage in many of our modern plagues: cardiovascular disease (heart attack and stroke), cancer, eye disorders (specifically cataracts and macular degeneration), and arthritis, not to mention the aging process itself.

Coming to the aid of our cells and biochemical repair mechanisms are the **antioxidants** in our foods (and, for some, in supplements). These include the **antioxidant vitamins C** and **E** and a host of **phytochemicals** (compounds found in plants, some of which we introduced in chapter 5), including the **carotenoid compounds** (of which the best known are **beta-carotene** and

lycopene), **phytoestrogens**, **flavonoids**, **phenols**, and **polyphenols**. Some of these, such as vitamins C and E, work by sacrificially donating an electron to a free radical, thus stabilizing it and preventing it from grabbing an electron from another molecule. What makes these types of antioxidants particularly virtuous is that they remain stable after giving away the coveted electron. Other compounds join in the battle by stimulating the body's own enzymes that are antioxidant or that repair free radical damage. In addition, certain minerals—notably **selenium**, **manganese**, **copper**, and **zinc**—while not antioxidants themselves, are necessary for the proper function of antioxidant enzymes.

A growing body of research suggests or demonstrates the benefits of foods containing various antioxidants:

- Laboratory experiments show that various antioxidants can prevent the oxidation of LDL (bad) cholesterol by free radicals, an event widely considered to be a critical step in the development of diseased arteries.
- Large population studies indicate that those whose diets are rich in antioxidants, and to some degree those taking vitamin E supplements, have lower rates of coronary artery disease.
- Similarly, research suggests a link between diets abundant in fruits and vegetables in general, and vitamin C in particular, and lower rates of a number of cancers, including those in the mouth, larynx, esophagus, stomach, pancreas, colon and rectum, lungs, breast, and cervix.
- A number of studies suggest that antioxidants in the diet—especially vitamin C, as well as the carotenoids **lutein** and **zeaxanthin**—may reduce the risk of both cataracts and macular degeneration, the leading causes of visual problems among the elderly.

If a number of antioxidants in food have been identified and associated with health benefits, then taking generous amounts of them in supplements should seriously improve one's health and well-being—right? For years a multi-billion-dollar supplement industry has been shouting "Amen!" all the way to the bank, but hard data to back its enthusiastic claims has been difficult to come by. One notorious example: Beta-carotene, an antioxidant found in deeply pigmented fruits and vegetables, appeared to be a prime candidate for supplement superstardom. But in four large randomized controlled studies comparing the health of people who were given a beta-carotene supplement with that of an equal number of people given an identical-appearing placebo (with no biological effect), the supplement group struck out. Only one study, involving a concoction of antioxidants given to a poorly nourished population in rural China, showed some benefit. One study of U.S. physicians found no difference between those who took the supplement and those who didn't. And two large studies involving smokers showed an *increased* risk of lung cancer among those taking the beta-carotene supplement.

Indeed, this type of discouraging scenario—where a concentrated supplement of a specific nutrient in a controlled experiment doesn't seem to work as well as expected—has been rather common. There are several important reasons why this should not come as a big surprise:

- Diseases such as cancer and cardiovascular disease aren't like scurvy, where a single missing ingredient added to the diet will produce dramatic results. (See the next section, which deals with vitamin C.) Their causes and prevention involve complex interactions of many variables.
- Similarly, hundreds of antioxidants and antioxidant-enhancing substances work in a variety of ways in different environments within the body, and in turn they interact with one another in complex ways. Attempting to isolate one substance that would prove to be the key antioxidant may prove to be a lost cause.
- Even in well-designed experiments involving supplements, it can be difficult to control the effects of individual dietary choices on a long-term basis. Furthermore, even an experiment lasting for several years may not last long enough to pick up a very subtle effect from a supplement.
- Even with antioxidants, it is possible to take too much. As we saw with niacin, at doses found in foods this compound acts as a vitamin; but when a large amount is packed into a pill, it acts as a drug, with very different effects. Some antioxidants perform their appointed tasks when consumed in food, but when they are taken at the much larger dose found in a supplement, they may have the opposite effect, acting as **pro-oxidants**—substances that induce oxidative stress rather than protect against it.

There's an important take-home lesson here, one that we cannot state often enough: While vitamins and other supplements can be beneficial (and for some, even lifesaving), *they are not a substitute for wise food choices*. As clever as we might become through research and development of nutritional products, no one can duplicate the rich and complex blend of nutrients and phytochemicals in food, especially fruits and vegetables. Remember, the only truly natural products are found in the produce section of the supermarket. An important corollary: Supplements cannot compensate for a lifetime of poor lifestyle choices (smoking, overeating, abusing drugs and alcohol, refusing to exercise, and so forth). You can't fill your gas tank with turpentine and then expect the fancy additive to take care of your engine.

And now, back to our vitamins.

Vitamin C (Ascorbic acid)

When European adventurers began to launch long voyages of exploration and conquest across the world's oceans in the fifteenth century, little did they know that for the next three hundred years the greatest threat to life and limb would *not* be storms or hostile inhabitants of faraway lands. Instead, it would be the disease hailed by scales and scabs, known as scurf, on rough, dry skin. What came with scurf would be worse: swollen and bleeding gums, loosening teeth, massive bruises, wounds that refused to heal, bones that softened and broke, depression, heart failure, and severe fatigue.[5] If death didn't draw near during one or more of these torments, it would eventually be summoned by internal bleeding and would arrive quickly.

The disease was **scurvy**, whose name was originally an adjective meaning "covered with scurf." On a long seagoing voyage it would routinely claim the lives of at least half the sailors on board, none of whom knew that the cook held the power of life and death. During the first weeks, the fruits and vegetables on board would be served. Once they were gone, scurvy would begin to accompany the rancid food that remained. It is estimated that between the years 1500 and 1800, scurvy took the lives of more than 2 million sailors worldwide.[6]

In 1747, a Scottish naval surgeon named James Lind conducted a pivotal experiment in nutrition at sea on the HMS *Salisbury*. Twelve sailors with scurvy were selected to receive a daily dose of one of six potential remedies: a quart of cider; sulfuric acid ("oil of vitriol"); vinegar; seawater; a mixture of garlic, myrrh, radish, and resin from a central American tree ("balsam of Peru"); or oranges and lemons. The two sailors who ate the citrus fruits recovered within a week and ultimately cared for the other ten, who remained ill. Taking a cue from Lind while also instituting some additional hygienic measures, the legendary explorer Captain James Cook lost only one sailor on his second round-the-world voyage, which lasted from 1772–1775. It would take the British Royal Navy another twenty-five years to routinely issue lemon juice to every sailor in the fleet, thus eliminating scurvy altogether. The curative fruits and juice were referred to as antiscorbutic in honor of their scurvy-curing power, but it would not be until the 1930s that **ascorbic acid** would be identified as the sailor-saving compound in citrus fruits.

What does it do? Vitamin C does plenty, and probably more than we currently recognize.

1. It serves as a powerful antioxidant, helping to protect cells and tissues against ongoing damage from free radicals, especially those found in cigarette smoke and polluted air. Needless to say, this property of vitamin C has given it star billing as a likely risk reducer for cardiovascular disease, cancer, two common eye disorders—cataracts and macular degeneration—and possibly disorders of aging such as Alzheimer's disease.

   Vitamin C's antioxidant effects have inspired a faithful following among many who are convinced that very large doses can prevent (or even treat) cancer and heart disease. Perhaps the most famous mega-C advocate was Linus Pauling, Ph.D., winner of two Nobel Prizes (for chemistry and for peace) and author of numerous books and articles extolling the benefits of this vitamin. He advocated routine doses of 2 grams per day for adults, and much larger doses—10 grams per day, more than 100 times the current RDA for adult men and roughly the amount present in 120 oranges—as beneficial for cancer patients. (Pauling routinely took 12 grams per day and increased that amount to 40 grams per day when he felt a cold coming on.) In spite of his credentials, Pauling's advisories were not widely accepted in the scientific community for a variety of reasons. There is, however, general agreement that *foods* rich in vitamin C and other antioxidants offer a protective effect against heart disease and cancer.

We already mentioned that the B vitamins serve as coenzymes, compounds that attach to enzymes in a way that allows them to function properly in a particular reaction. A cofactor is a compound that is required for an enzyme to function but that does not attach to an enzyme as a coenzyme does.

2. It serves as a **cofactor** in several important biochemical reactions. Vitamin C is critical for the proper formation of **collagen**, a fibrous protein that serves as the body's "glue." Collagen provides the foundation upon which bones and teeth are built. It is involved in forming scar tissue when an injury occurs. It helps keep cells attached to one another, a particularly important role in the tiny arterioles and capillaries through which blood flows. This particular function of vitamin C explains many of the disastrous symptoms of scurvy.

3. It participates in the conversion of the amino acid tryptophan into the neurotransmitter serotonin—the one that also depends on vitamin B_6—which plays an important role in mood, sleep, and many other functions.

4. It appears to play a role in the body's response to stress, based on its presence in the adrenal glands and its release by the adrenals in response to events such as infection or fever.

5. Large doses (a gram or much more—many times the RDA) of vitamin C have long been touted as useful for preventing or treating the common cold. Many people swear by this approach, but controlled studies have shown marginal (if any) differences between those who do and those who don't take large quantities every day or at the first sign of a sniffle. On average, doing so may trim a day off the illness, but even this effect may result from an antihistamine effect much like that seen with cold tablets. However, some new research indicates that vitamin C at a dose of a gram per day may in fact provoke a brief boost in at least one group of virus-fighting substances (called cytokines).[7]

How much do we need? As the last paragraph suggests, there are differences of opinion on this subject. As little as 10 mg of vitamin C per day will prevent scurvy. Until recently, the adult RDA for vitamin C was 60 mg per day. In 2000, however, the Food and Nutrition Board of the Institute of Medicine increased the RDAs to those shown below, and experts at the National Cancer Institute have recommended doses of 100 to 200 mg per day. Some recent research suggests that a combination of 500 mg of vitamin C and 400 IU of vitamin E may reduce the risk of developing Alzheimer's disease. Note that smoking increases one's need for vitamin C.

AIs:

Infants, birth to six months	40 mg/day
Infants, seven months to one year	50 mg/day

RDAs:

Children, one to three years	15 mg/day
Children, four to eight years	25 mg/day
Children, nine to thirteen years	45 mg/day
Teenage boys, fourteen to eighteen years	75 mg/day
Men, nineteen and older	90 mg/day
Men who smoke	125 mg/day
Teenage girls, fourteen to eighteen years	65 mg/day
Women, nineteen and older	75 mg/day
Women who smoke	110 mg/day
Women, pregnant	85 mg/day
Women, breast-feeding	120 mg/day

Where do we get it? Citrus fruits—oranges, grapefruit, and lemons among others—and their juices are the most familiar sources of vitamin C, but berries and green vegetables such as broccoli, Brussels sprouts, and spinach are also excellent sources. Potatoes, kiwi, and mango contain generous amounts, and red bell peppers are particularly rich in vitamin C. An eight-ounce glass of orange juice contains about 100 mg of this vitamin.

People who might not get enough: Tobacco users may be deficient in this vitamin, since the oxidants in tobacco products deplete it. Also, those who shun fruits and vegetables and don't get a regular dose of vitamin C from a supplement or a fortified food (such as a cereal with added vitamins) may not be getting enough.

Too much of a good thing? While some people advocate massive doses of vitamin C, most professional organizations recommend taking no more than 2 grams per day. Higher doses taken on an ongoing basis may increase the risk for a mixed bag of health problems:

- Kidney stones among people with impaired kidney function, gout, or a certain genetic abnormality that affects the metabolism of vitamin C
- Interference with the action of anticoagulant medications
- Potentially harmful elevations of iron levels in people with iron overload syndromes
- Interference with screening tests for glucose in urine or occult (hidden) blood in stool, which could affect medical decisions

- Intestinal symptoms such as nausea, cramps, and diarrhea

Interesting tidbit: It has been suggested that "lemons perhaps did as much as Nelson to defeat Napoleon,"[8] referring to the outnumbered but no doubt healthier British seamen who destroyed the French fleet near Cape Trafalgar under Admiral Horatio Nelson in 1805. Later, when British sailors began routinely drinking lime juice to prevent scurvy, they would be called "lime juicers" or "limeys"—as an insult.

Fat-soluble vitamins: A, D, E, and K

Vitamin A

Vitamin A exists in three distinct forms—retinol, retinal, and retinoic acid—each of which has a distinct and important function. (These compounds, along with some relatives with similar activity, are as a group called retinoids. In order to avoid getting too technical, we will refer to all of them as vitamin A.) No doubt you have noticed the similarity of these names to the word *retina*, the pigmented inner surface of the eye that converts light to nerve impulses. These compounds are appropriately named because of retinal's critical function in the retina, not to mention the disastrous effects on vision for those who are deficient in vitamin A.

The word *retina* comes from the Latin word for "net," reflecting the delicate netlike structure of that tissue.

What does it do?

- Vitamin A is a vital component of a pigment molecule called **rhodopsin** found in the cells of the retina. There are approximately 100 million cells in each retina, and each cell contains about 30 million molecules of rhodopsin. When light strikes rhodopsin, it undergoes a structural change and creates a tiny electrical impulse within the cell. This in turn leads to the generation of a nerve impulse that travels to the brain, where in a split second millions of incoming signals are organized into recognizable images. On an ongoing basis, a small amount of the vitamin A in the eye is irreversibly converted to a form that cannot function in the retina, and this drain must be continuously replenished.
- Vitamin A is necessary for the formation and function of the cells (called **epithelial cells**) that line every surface of the body, both inside and out. On the outside, epithelial cells form the skin. Surfaces on the inside of the body, most of which have contact with substances from the outside world, are also lined with epithelial cells, and these tissues are called **mucous membranes**. These include the inside of the nose, mouth, throat, intestine, airways, bladder, urethra (through which urine flows out of the body), vagina, and uterus.
- Vitamin A helps regulate the processes by which cells divide and assume their proper function. This role suggests that vitamin A may also help inhibit the growth of cancer cells.
- Vitamin A participates in a process called **remodeling**, which is nec-

essary for the growth of bone. As a child grows, his bones don't merely enlarge, but rather are continuously sculpted toward their mature size and shape. This requires that cells be removed from some surfaces of bone while cells are added to others. This intricate process will not proceed properly without adequate amounts of vitamin A.

How much do we need? Describing quantities of vitamin A is confusing because there are different forms in which it occurs, not to mention various precursors of vitamin A (especially beta-carotene) found in plants. (See "Where do we get it?" below.) The basic unit of measurement for vitamin A is a microgram of retinol, and the amount of any other form (or precursor) that provides the same vitamin A activity as a microgram of retinol is called a retinol activity equivalent (RAE). Researchers and nutritionists now describe vitamin A quantities in RAEs, but your vitamin bottle and the Nutrition Facts label on your box of cereal still use the older and more familiar measure, international units (IUs). In the table below we have included both, and we'll use IUs for the rest of this chapter so that you can interpret labels without a calculator.

AIs:

Infants, birth to six months	400 mcg/day (1,333 IU)
Infants, seven months to one year	500 mcg/day (1,667 IU)

RDAs:

Children, one to three years	300 mcg/day (1,000 IU)
Children, four to eight years	400 mcg/day (1,333 IU)
Children, nine to thirteen years	600 mcg/day (2,000 IU)
Men, fourteen and older	900 mcg/day (3,000 IU)
Women, fourteen and older	700 mcg/day (2,333 IU)
Women, pregnant	770 mcg/day (2,567 IU)
Women, breast-feeding	1,300 mcg/day (4,333 IU)

Where do we get it? Vitamin A that is preformed (that is, ready to be used in the body) is abundant in the fat or oil of certain animal products: milk and dairy products, butter, eggs, liver, and fish-liver oils. Removing the fat from milk takes out the vitamin A as well, so commercial nonfat milk is fortified with vitamin A (about 40 percent of the adult RDA per quart).

Plants do not contain any preformed vitamin A. However, the family of compounds called **carotenoids**, which provide the red and yellow colors of plants, contains precursors. The body can convert certain carotenoids (called **provitamin A carotenoids**) into vitamin A, with the vast majority coming from beta-carotene. Yellow and orange vegetables and fruits such as carrots, yellow squash, sweet potatoes, pumpkin, and cantaloupe—but not corn or bananas—are among the richest sources of provitamin A. Spinach, broccoli, and kale are among the dark leafy greens that also contain respectable amounts of provitamin A.

What happens if we don't get enough? Unlike water-soluble vitamins that aren't stored by the body for long periods, we can store a substantial amount of vitamin A that we don't immediately need. (The vast majority is stored in the liver.) A healthy adult has enough on board to meet daily requirements without taking any vitamin A or precursors from food or supplements for many months. This time may be shortened if a body is deficient in calories, protein, or zinc, because these are necessary to make the protein that transports vitamin A from the liver to destinations throughout the body. (Remember: Fat-soluble vitamins are like cholesterol and triglycerides—they can't float freely in blood, which is water-based, but must instead be "escorted" by specific carrier proteins.)

The first visual disturbance that occurs in vitamin A deficiency is a diminished capacity to see in dim light called **night blindness**, as the retina cannot replenish the pigments that are altered by light. For those with night blindness in parts of the world where electric or other light sources are scarce, life comes to a screeching halt after the sun goes down. If the deficiency isn't corrected, the cornea—the clear "dome" through which light first enters the eye—becomes affected as well, first by increasingly severe dryness (a condition called **xerophthalmia**) and then eventually by irreversible damage that leads to blindness.

Unfortunately, compared with adults, children are able to tolerate a much shorter amount of time without vitamin A. When their body stores run out, as occurs all too frequently in impoverished areas, the results can be devastating. According to the World Health Organization (WHO), between 100 and 140 million children worldwide (especially in Africa and Southeast Asia) are deficient in vitamin A, and of these between 250,000 and 500,000 will go blind each year. They lose more than their sight: Within twelve months, half will die.[9] Vitamin A deficiency is the leading preventable cause of blindness in children, but this shortage also impairs the immune system. Children who lack sufficient vitamin A are vulnerable to pneumonia, infectious diarrhea, and especially measles, which infects 30 million children annually and kills more than 750,000.[10] This susceptibility to infection is aggravated by a less than healthy status of the mucous membranes, which normally serve as the first line of defense against invading organisms. For vitamin A–deficient children, supplementation cuts the death rate from measles in half. Both measles vaccination and low-cost vitamin A supplementation among children in developing nations are major priorities for a number of relief organizations.

People who might not get enough: Full-blown vitamin A deficiency is rare in the United States, although certain situations may lead to what is called subclinical deficiency, especially among young children who then become more susceptible to infection. These situations include:

- Ongoing lack of basic nutrients, either in an extreme form (such as in areas of famine or severe poverty) or arising from long-standing, unwise choices (such as a diet consisting mainly of hamburgers, fries, and soft drinks)
- Diseases of the pancreas or intestine that impair digestion and absorption of nutrients
- Iron deficiency
- Inadequate intake of protein and zinc, which are needed to create the protein that transports vitamin A
- A strict vegetarian diet—one that does not include dairy products or eggs and that does not include regular intake of orange and yellow vegetables and fruits
- Excessive alcohol intake, which depletes stores of vitamin A

Too much of a good thing? Unlike the B vitamins, for which high doses are unlikely to produce actual illness, too much vitamin A can cause a host of problems. This can occur in one of two ways. Preformed vitamin A is abundant in the liver of animals, and frequent servings of liver can cause an overload. Beta-carotene from fruits and vegetables is converted to vitamin A too slowly to cause toxicity, but it may be stored under the skin, resulting in a slight orange-yellow hue in an eager consumer of these foods (especially during childhood). More common is the "more must be better" syndrome of the supplement taker who goes overboard on vitamin A or beta-carotene.

How much is too much? To provide some guidance, the Institute of Medicine has established tolerable upper intake levels (ULs) for vitamin A for healthy children and adults:

Infants, birth to twelve months	600 mcg/day (2,000 IU)
Children, one to three years	600 mcg/day (2,000 IU)
Children, four to eight years	900 mcg/day (3,000 IU)
Children, nine to thirteen years	1,700 mcg/day (5,667 IU)
Teenagers, fourteen to eighteen years	2,800 mcg/day (9,333 IU)
Adults, nineteen years and older	3,000 mcg/day (10,000 IU)

(These guidelines do not apply to malnourished people who are receiving intermittent large doses of vitamin A as part of treatment or prevention programs.)

In general, the more one takes above the ULs, the worse the toxicity may be. Someone who takes large amounts of vitamin A over a short period of time may develop headaches, blurred vision, nausea, vomiting, dizziness, and poor coordination. Women who take 10,000 IU or more of vitamin A during the first three months of pregnancy (especially before the seventh week) significantly increase their risk of having a baby with a birth defect. Unless necessary to correct a known deficiency, *a woman should not take a vitamin A supplement during early pregnancy*, other than what is present in the comprehensive prenatal multivitamin recommended by her physician. Indeed, women of childbearing age shouldn't take separate vitamin A supplements, and men and women alike would be wise to avoid multivitamins that supply more than 5,000 IU of vitamin A per day. Possible long-term effects of excessive doses of vitamin A include thinning of bone (osteoporosis), dryness and peeling of skin, fatigue, and insomnia, as well as the symptoms of acute toxicity listed above.

The Institute of Medicine has not established ULs for beta-carotene. However, based on the results of controlled studies involving beta-carotene supplements (see page 885), it has also recommended against the general population taking beta-carotene supplements.

Interesting tidbit: While many useful acne medications are derived from vitamin A, taking large doses of vitamin A does not help this common condition.

Vitamin D (Calciferol)

Vitamin D is unique among the vitamins in many ways:

- It is the only vitamin that is actually a hormone—a compound manufactured in one part of the body that affects one or more functions in others. (Insulin, estrogen, testosterone, and thyroxine, or thyroid hormone, are examples of other well-known hormones.)
- It is a steroid molecule, derived from cholesterol and chemically related to other steroid molecules such as cortisol, estrogen, and testosterone.
- Given enough exposure to sunlight, a healthy individual can make an adequate amount of vitamin D without getting any from food. A molecule similar to cholesterol that is made by the liver is converted to a previtamin called cholecalciferol (or D_3 for short) in the skin in the presence of ultraviolet light—more specifically, the high energy form called UVB—from the sun. Foods that serve as sources of vitamin D also contain D_3. Once the body ingests previtamin D_3, it must undergo two separate reactions, one in the liver and one in the kidney, to be converted to the final form of vitamin D (called calciferol) that the body actually uses.

What does it do? Vitamin D plays profound roles in bone metabolism. It helps maintain blood levels of calcium and phosphorus, which are essential for bone growth and maintenance, by enhancing their absorption from the intestine and slowing their loss from the kidney. Vitamin D also regulates the deposition of these minerals in bone.

How much do we need? Because we generate vitamin D in response to sun exposure, it is difficult to determine a recommended daily allowance (RDA) for this vitamin, so current recommendations are based on an estimate known as the adequate intake (AI). Note that the AI is the same for everyone (including pregnant and breast-feeding women) from birth to age fifty, and then it increases for those who are older. Also, *these recommendations assume that a person has no sun exposure.* As with vitamin A, there is an old but familiar measure for vitamin D—the international units, or IU—and a newer measure, micrograms (mcg) of the previtamin cholecalciferol (D_3), which for convenience we will refer to as vitamin D through the rest of this section.

AIs:

Infants, birth to one year	5 mcg/day (200 IU)
Children, one to thirteen years	5 mcg/day (200 IU)
Teens and adults, fourteen to forty-nine years	5 mcg/day (200 IU)
Adults, fifty to seventy years	10 mcg/day (400 IU)
Adults, over seventy years	15 mcg/day (600 IU)
Women, pregnant	5 mcg/day (200 IU)
Women, breast-feeding	5 mcg/day (200 IU)

Remember the definition of adequate intake (AI) from earlier in the appendix: an educated guess of the necessary amount of a specific nutrient based on observations and scientific findings. It is given when the available evidence is not conclusive enough to arrive at an RDA. Some experts believe that 1,000 IU of vitamin D per day is more appropriate for adults who have no sun exposure.

Where do we get it? First, from the sun: In light-skinned individuals, as little as fifteen minutes of sun exposure to face, hands, and arms every week will typically generate an adequate amount of vitamin D. (This could occur in one sitting, or in five- to ten-minute exposures two or three times per week.) In areas closer to the equator, only a few minutes every week may be adequate. Pigments in the skin that protect against ultraviolet damage from the sun also inhibit the synthesis of vitamin D, so darker-skinned people must spend much more time in the sun to bring about the same effect (up to six times more than those who are light skinned). While you can get too much vitamin D from supplements (see page 897), you can't get too much from sun exposure. (Obviously, however, prolonged sun exposure can damage your skin and increase your risk for skin cancer, as we discuss in chapter 4.) On the other hand, several other factors can reduce or block the effects of the sun on the creation of vitamin D:

- Sunscreen with a sun protection factor (SPF) of 8 or more, which decreases the ability of the skin to produce vitamin D by more than 90 percent.
- Smog, smoke, fog, and clouds.
- Time of day. More of the sun's UVB rays reach us between 11 A.M. and 2 P.M. than earlier or later in the day.
- Geography and seasons. People who live in latitudes above 35° north—the geographical line roughly connecting Los Angeles and Atlanta—obtain little or no vitamin D from the sun from November through February. Above 50° north—roughly the level of the northern border of the western United States, the straight line between Canada and the states of Washington, Idaho, Montana, and North

Dakota—that period lasts from September through March. (The same is true for those who live in the southern hemisphere below 35° south.)

- Staying indoors. To state the obvious, someone who rarely if ever goes outside will need to obtain vitamin D entirely from food or supplements.
- Age. At age seventy a person makes much less vitamin D than he or she did at age twenty with the same amount of sun exposure.

Why do geography and time of day make such a major difference? Even under a blazing noonday sun at the equator, 99.9 percent of the UVB energy—which our bodies need to produce vitamin D—is absorbed by the earth's ozone layer and doesn't reach the surface. If you travel to higher or lower latitudes or if you go outside earlier or later in the day, the sun's rays arrive at an angle and pass through more ozone, which filters out more (or all) of the UVB light before it ever reaches your skin.

We can also get vitamin D from food, although there are very few foods that naturally contain substantial amounts of vitamin D. Perhaps the most well-known are the fatty fish—salmon, tuna, mackerel, and sardines in particular—and the notoriously foul-tasting fish liver oils. Cod liver oil, which previous generations of disgruntled children choked down at the insistence of their parents, contains a whopping 1,300 IU of vitamin D per tablespoon, along with a generous amount of vitamin A.

Children now obtain vitamin D primarily from milk, which has been routinely fortified with this vitamin since the 1930s. By law, in the United States milk contains 400 IU of vitamin D per quart, so a pint per day supplies the entire recommended intake for a child or adult up to the age of fifty. Note that other dairy products such as yogurt, ice cream, and cheese are generally *not* fortified with vitamin D. However, it may be added to other foods, such as fortified breakfast cereals. (Check the label.)

Remember that these foods actually contain the previtamin D_3 rather than vitamin D itself. For convenience, we refer to this compound in food and supplements as vitamin D.

What happens if we don't get enough? It's all about the health of your bones. A shortage of vitamin D leads to inadequate absorption of calcium and phosphorus from food (and losses from the kidneys) that can cause low levels in the blood. Serious and even life-threatening consequences may arise if calcium is not maintained within precise limits in the blood, and a low level will provoke a hormonal response that draws calcium out of bone.

Children who receive inadequate amounts of vitamin D develop **rickets**, a disorder in which bones contain an inadequate amount of calcium, fail to grow properly, and actually bend when they have to support the weight of a growing body. (A classic finding in an older child with rickets is bowed legs.) Deformities of the spine, pelvis, skull, and chest may occur, as well as impaired growth and vulnerability to fractures.

F.Y.I. If you are deficient in vitamin D, you typically absorb only 10 to 15 percent of the calcium in your food or any supplement you might take.

The adult version of rickets is called **osteomalacia**, which also can cause softening, bowing, aching, and breaking of bones. The person at highest risk for this disturbance is a woman who has poor calcium intake, little or no sun exposure, and multiple pregnancies in succession.

A more widespread consequence of vitamin D deficiency is **osteoporosis** (thinning of bones) among senior citizens, a serious problem that we address in more detail in chapter 14 ("Senior Maintenance"). Several factors contribute to osteoporosis, and vitamin D intake isn't the only factor to be concerned about, but inadequate levels definitely increase the risk for fractures in the elderly. Unfortunately, the elderly are less likely than others to spend time outdoors, may not drink milk on a regular basis, and may have declining skin, liver, and kidney functions that are necessary for vitamin D synthesis. Age does *not* affect how much vitamin D a person absorbs from food or supplements—but remember that food and supplements actually contain the previtamin cholecalciferol (D_3), and its conversion to the active molecule may be hampered if liver or kidney function is abnormal. (As we already noted, the recommended amounts for vitamin D supplementation are higher in the elderly.)

Some research indicates that vitamin D deficiency may increase the risk for developing type 1 diabetes (the less common form that usually occurs early in life and requires insulin injections) and hypertension (high blood pressure). Animal research suggests that vitamin D deficiency also may play a role in the development of multiple sclerosis—a disease that is known to be more common the farther one lives from the equator. There is some preliminary evidence that vitamin D may have a protective effect against cancer. The active form of vitamin D is known to inhibit proliferation of cells, and vitamin D receptors are found throughout the body. Compounds similar to vitamin D are being investigated as possible treatments for certain types of cancer. However, it is unclear whether vitamin D deficiency is a risk factor for cancer and whether taking extra vitamin D would help protect against it.

People who might not get enough: Those who have little or no sun exposure, don't drink milk, avoid eating fish, and don't take a supplement may be deficient. Because vitamin D is fat soluble, any disorder that results in poor fat absorption may lead to vitamin D deficiency. Chronic liver or kidney disease also can cause vitamin D deficiency, because as we noted earlier, these organs must each carry out a reaction that converts the previtamin D_3 into the functional vitamin D. Prolonged use of oral corticosteroids, which are prescribed for certain medical problems such as severe asthma or arthritis, may contribute to osteoporosis. One mechanism for this side effect may be interference with vitamin D metabolism.

Too much of a good thing? Like the other fat-soluble vitamins, vitamin D toxicity is a risk for those who overuse supplements (or who override their taste buds and take large amounts of cod liver oil). A variety of symptoms, including nausea, constipation, weakness, and weight loss, may result. Of greater concern is the tendency for high doses of vitamin D to raise calcium levels in the blood, which can cause a number of medical problems, depending on the severity and duration of the elevated level. The Food and Nutrition Board of the Institute of Medicine has established a tolerable upper limit (or UL) of 1,000 international units (IU) of vitamin D per day for infants up to one year of age and 2,000 IU per day for all other age groups. A number of experts believe that intakes as high as 5,000 IU per day are safe for adults, but there is no reason to take this much, even when a deficiency in vitamin D has been diagnosed.

Interesting tidbit: It may be appropriate to check your vitamin D level in the fall—especially if you are over fifty and have limited sun exposure. The test to request is 25-hydroxyvitamin D (not 1,25 dihydroxyvitamin D, which can yield misleading results).

Vitamin E

Vitamin E has become a hot item over the past several years because of conflicting reports that it might—or might not—protect us from heart disease, cancer, and a host of other chronic ailments.

What does it do? Vitamin E is a potent antioxidant, protecting cells and tissues by donating an electron to unstable free radicals. (See page 884.) Specifically, it is known to prevent the oxidation of low-density lipoprotein (LDL) cholesterol, which is generally considered to be an important step in the development of atherosclerosis, the clogging of arteries that can lead to heart attack and stroke. (We reviewed this process in chapter 3.) However, this benefit of vitamin E occurs only with doses far greater than any that can be obtained from food. There are actually eight forms of vitamin E, but the form called **alpha-tocopherol** is the most active in the human body.

How much do we need? The recommended daily allowances (RDAs) for vitamin E are relatively small compared to the amount typically found in supplements. Note that as with the other fat-soluble vitamins, the RDA is expressed in milligrams (of alpha-tocopherol) as well as the older but more familiar international units (IU), which is the measure you are likely to see on food and supplement labels.

AIs:

Infants, birth to six months	4 mg/day (6 IU)
Infants, seven months to one year	5 mg/day (7.5 IU)

RDAs:

Children, one to three years	6 mg/day (9 IU)
Children, four to eight years	7 mg/day (10.5 IU)
Children, nine to thirteen years	11 mg/day (16.5 IU)
Men and women, fourteen and older	15 mg/day (22.5 IU)
Women, pregnant	15 mg/day (22.5 IU)
Women, breast-feeding	19 mg/day (28.5 IU)

Most adults typically obtain about 5 to 15 IU per day in food. But studies of the effects of vitamin E on heart disease or cancer involve doses of 400 to 800 IU per day, at which antioxidant effects are likely to be seen—and which can only be obtained with supplements. To complicate matters, some research has observed that adults who take 100 IU or more per day are less likely to develop heart disease. But attempts to duplicate this finding in controlled studies have led to inconsistent results, as have studies of the effects of vitamin E supplementation on cancer.

Where do we get it? Vegetable oils, nuts, whole grains, and leafy green vegetables are considered good sources of vitamin E, but the quantities they contain are relatively small. An ounce of dry roasted almonds, for example, contains 7.5 units, while other nuts contain considerably less—2.4 units of vitamin E in an ounce of peanuts, for example.

What happens if we don't get enough? True vitamin E deficiency is very rare. People who have unusual disorders of fat metabolism or who can't absorb fat may develop disturbances in muscular coordination, vision, and speech that can be corrected by vitamin E supplementation. Premature, very low birth rate infants (less than 3½ pounds) may develop a form of anemia that will respond to vitamin E. (Normally vitamin E is transferred from mother to infant during the last weeks of pregnancy.)

Too much of a good thing? Vitamin E is less likely than other fat-soluble vitamins to cause toxicity at doses far beyond the recommended daily allowance. Individual studies of older adults taking 800 IU of vitamin E for at least four months have not detected any adverse effects, although the consequences of long-term use at this level have not been determined. The Institute of Medicine has established a tolerable upper limit of 1,000 mg (1,500 IU) of vitamin E per day for adults—more than 65 times the RDA. (At doses beyond this level, the vitamin may interfere with blood clotting.)

Recently some controversy has been raised by an evaluation (known as a meta-analysis) of nineteen studies that included more than 135,000 patients. The analysis found death rates from all causes *increased* among those taking 400 IU or more of vitamin E daily.[11] Though it's unclear at this point whether taking a vitamin E supplement is beneficial, you may want to consider taking supplements of both vitamins C and E, as we will discuss at the end of this chapter. (See "Getting Back to the Original Question: Should I Take a Vitamin/Mineral Supplement?" beginning on page 917.)

Interesting tidbit: Vitamin E was originally identified as a component of vegetable oil that was necessary for reproduction in rats, and it was given the name **tocopherol** in honor of that function. The word *tocopherol* is derived from Greek roots meaning "to bring forth birth."

Vitamin K

What does it do? Vitamin K plays a vital role in activating several proteins that are necessary for blood clotting. Some of the same proteins appear to be involved in the building of healthy bones, and inadequate intake of vitamin K may increase the risk of fracture, especially in the elderly.

How much do we need? As with vitamin E, it is difficult to determine a recommended daily allowance (RDA) for vitamin K, because the amount produced in and absorbed from the intestine will vary from person to person. Thus the Institute of Medicine has established only adequate intakes (AIs) to serve as guidelines.

AIs:

Infants, birth to six months	2 mcg/day
Infants, seven months to one year	2.5 mcg/day
Children, one to three years	30 mcg/day
Children, four to eight years	55 mcg/day
Children, nine to thirteen years	60 mcg/day
Teenage boys, fourteen to eighteen years	75 mcg/day
Men, nineteen and over	120 mcg/day
Teenage girls, fourteen to eighteen years	75 mcg/day
Women, nineteen and over	90 mcg/day
Women, pregnant	90 mcg/day
Women, breast-feeding	90 mcg/day

Where do we get it? Some of the vitamin K that we need is produced by the bacteria that live within our intestine and is then absorbed. The rest comes from a variety of foods, especially leafy green vegetables, cabbage, and liver. Some can also be obtained from milk, meat, eggs, and cereals.

What happens if we don't get enough? The immediate and most serious problem brought on by vitamin K deficiency is the threat of hemorrhage: uncontrolled bleeding from an injury, an ulcer, or any other damaged tissue.

People who might not get enough: Those with a rare digestive disorder that prevents absorption of fat (remember that vitamin K is the last of our four fat-soluble vitamins) may be deficient. Antibiotics may temporarily depopulate the bacteria in the intestine that make vitamin K, but under normal circumstances this is unlikely to result in hemorrhage. Vitamin K is stored in the liver, and those stores can be mobilized if the normal intake falls.

The newborn infant has a temporary shortage of vitamin K until her bowel becomes colonized with bacteria, a process which may take a few weeks. (None are present at birth.) In order to prevent potentially harmful bleeding during the first weeks of life, newborns in the United States are routinely given a dose of vitamin K, a standard practice since the early 1960s.

Too much of a good thing? Toxicity from vitamin K is rare and would only be expected if someone took an excessive amount of this vitamin as a supplement. Of more concern is the reaction that may occur when people who are taking the anticoagulant warfarin (Coumadin) consume foods or supplements containing vitamin K. This medicine is prescribed to prevent the formation of blood clots in a number of medical conditions, and monitoring its effect requires regular blood tests. Because vitamin K reverses warfarin's effect on clotting, those who take this medicine should avoid dramatic alterations in their diet that might change the amount of this vitamin (such as suddenly increasing their intake of leafy green vegetables, as health promoting as that might be).

Interesting tidbit: The K in vitamin K stands for *koagulation,* the Danish word for clotting—similar to our word *coagulation*.

And Now a Look at the Minerals

While the vast majority of our diet consists of organic compounds—that is, molecules both simple and complex that contain carbon—we also need a steady supply of certain minerals to stay healthy. In the realm of nutrition, minerals are distinct from vitamins in some important ways:

They are **elements**—the basic building blocks of chemistry—which means they cannot be broken down into simpler components. For example, table salt is sodium chloride: one atom of sodium combined with one atom of chloride. Salt is a **compound**, while the minerals sodium and chloride are chemical elements: they cannot be broken down further.

Not only are minerals elements, they are also elements other than carbon. By definition, then, they are **inorganic** (so don't let anyone try to sell you "organic" minerals). Unlike vitamins, minerals cannot be broken down or destroyed by exposure to light or heat.

While an element cannot be broken down into simpler components or lose its basic identity, it can exist in different forms, depending in large part on how it is combined with other elements. In its pure form, the element chlorine is a poisonous gas. Chloride, on the other hand, is the form of chlorine that is present (and very necessary) in our body, found in combination with sodium, hydrogen, and other elements.

All vitamins are micronutrients—present and needed in the body in very small amounts—but minerals are divided into two categories based on the quantities we need. **Major minerals** are present in the body in amounts totaling more than 5 grams. These include **calcium**, **phosphorus**, **potassium**, **sulfur**, **sodium**, **chloride**, and **magnesium**. **Trace** or **micro minerals**, on the other hand, weigh in at well under 5 grams in a normal adult, and they are needed in quantities measured in milligrams or even micrograms. They are no less important, however. Trace minerals include **iron**, **zinc**, **copper**, **manganese**, **iodine**, **selenium**, **fluoride**, **chromium**, and **molybdenum**.

Unlike many of the vitamins (especially the B complex and C), with trace minerals and magnesium *there is a narrow margin between amounts that are needed for normal function and amounts that are toxic*. Therefore, it is especially desirable to obtain these substances from foods if at all possible. If you use supplements for trace minerals, you should avoid taking more than 100 percent of the RDA on an ongoing basis.

In this section we're going to look specifically at the trace minerals and at magnesium (the least abundant of the major minerals in our bodies), because they are most commonly found in supplements. Of the other major minerals, calcium may need to be supplemented to promote bone health, which we discuss in chapter 13 ("Selected Topics in Women's Health").

Magnesium

What does it do? Despite the relatively small quantity of magnesium in the body—most adults have little more than 25 to 30 grams (about an ounce)—magnesium is crucial for hundreds of reactions involving energy metabolism as well as the synthesis of proteins and DNA. It also plays vital roles in muscle, nerve, and immune function. Like calcium, a very small amount of magnesium (less than one percent of your total) circulates in your blood at levels that are precisely regulated. A much larger amount (about half of the magnesium in your body) is stored in bone, and most of the rest is present in muscle and other soft tissues.

How much do we need?

AIs:

Infants, birth to six months	30 mg/day
Infants, seven months to one year	75 mg/day

RDAs:

Children, one to three years	80 mg/day
Children, four to eight years	130 mg/day
Children, nine to thirteen years	240 mg/day
Teenage boys, fourteen to eighteen years	410 mg/day
Men, nineteen to thirty	400 mg/day
Men, thirty-one and over	420 mg/day
Teenage girls, fourteen to eighteen years	360 mg/day
Women, nineteen to thirty years	310 mg/day
Women, thirty-one and over	320 mg/day
Women, pregnant	360 mg/day
Women, breast-feeding	320 mg/day

Where do we get it? Green leafy vegetables, fruits, nuts, seeds, whole (but not refined) grains, and fortified breakfast cereals contain magnesium, although only a few foods (notably spinach and avocados) are particularly rich sources. (Once again, this is a good reason to sample a wide variety of foods—especially fruits and vegetables.) In some areas, magnesium found in the water supply contributes to daily intake as well. Hard water is actually a better source of magnesium than the more desirable soft water.

What happens if we don't get enough? A true magnesium deficiency is rarely a dietary problem but more often is related to specific diseases or medications. When present, a variety of symptoms may occur. These usually involve nerves and muscles (confusion, disorientation, numbness, tingling, cramps, even seizures) or the heart (rhythm disturbances).

Some evidence suggests that ongoing shortfalls of magnesium may be associated with an increased risk of high blood pressure, stroke, and coronary artery disease, as well as diabetes, although this is not conclusive. Nevertheless, maintaining an adequate dietary intake of magnesium is one recommendation of the Joint National Committee on Prevention, Detection, Evaluation, and Treatment of High Blood Pressure as a lifestyle measure that may help prevent or manage high blood pressure.

The Joint National Committee on Prevention, Detection, Evaluation, and Treatment of High Blood Pressure (or JNC for short) is a component of the National High Blood Pressure Education Program (NHBPEP), a coalition of thirty-eight major professional, public, and voluntary organizations and seven federal agencies. The NHBPEP is coordinated by the National Heart, Lung, and Blood Institute (NHLBI), one of the National Institutes of Health (NIH). Those are a lot of acronyms, but they add up to an important set of guidelines that are updated every few years. The periodic unveiling of a new set of JNC guidelines is an important event in U.S. health-care circles.

People who might not get enough: Those who have a medical problem or take medications that cause them to lose magnesium or prevent their body from absorbing it may have a magnesium deficiency. These conditions include:

- Chronic diarrhea, recurrent vomiting, or both
- Malabsorption—difficulty absorbing nutrients because of chronic intestinal disease, surgery, or infection
- Alcoholism—30 to 60 percent of alcoholics have low levels of magnesium in their blood, as do 90 percent of those going through withdrawal
- Poorly controlled diabetes, which leads to loss of magnesium in the urine
- Use of certain drugs: diuretics (water pills), which are relatively common, as well as the cancer chemotherapy drug cisplatin and certain potent antibiotics, which are less common

Too much of a good thing? Magnesium toxicity can occur, though not from food or hard water. As with many vitamins and minerals, overzealous use of magnesium supplements or products containing magnesium (see below) could lead to trouble. (Claims abound on the Internet for the healing powers of magnesium supplements for virtually every ailment.) At particular risk are the elderly, who might be taking extra magnesium in the form of a multivitamin, a calcium ("cal-mag") supplement, and laxatives. Normal kidney function is needed to clear excessive magnesium, and seniors often live with diminished kidney function. Interestingly, the symptoms of magnesium toxicity are similar to those arising from very low levels of this mineral.

The Institute of Medicine has established a tolerable upper limit (UL) for adults for magnesium at 350 mg per day from *nonfood sources* (i.e., supplements). A typical multivitamin contains 100 mg.

Interesting tidbit: Two compounds containing magnesium have served as common household remedies for generations. **Magnesium hydroxide** is a common ingredient in antacids (for example, Maalox). In larger doses, under the alias **milk of magnesia**, it draws fluid into the bowel, resulting in a well-known laxative effect. **Magnesium sulfate** is an even more potent laxative, but in its crystal form, widely known as **Epsom salts**, it has been tossed into hot water and used for hundreds of years as a remedy for sore feet. (Epsom salts are named for the town of Epsom, which became England's first spa in the seventeenth century when the purgative effects of its well water, rich in magnesium sulfate, became famous.)

Iron

What does it do? Iron is an essential nutrient, but we cannot synthesize it; we must obtain it from food. Iron's major claim to fame is its starring role in the function of hemoglobin, the protein that carries oxygen in red blood cells, and in the function of myoglobin, a protein that plays a similar role in muscle. Iron also participates in a number of other reactions throughout the body. About two-thirds of your body's total iron supply is present in hemoglobin. Another 15 percent is in storage, where it can be mobilized if dietary intake isn't adequate or if an unusual amount is needed, as might occur during pregnancy or after blood loss.

How much do we need?

AIs:

Infants, birth to six months	0.27 mg/day

RDAs:

Infants, seven months to one year	11 mg/day
Children, one to three years	7 mg/day
Children, four to eight years	10 mg/day
Children, nine to thirteen years	8 mg/day
Teenage boys, fourteen to eighteen years	11 mg/day
Men, nineteen and older	8 mg/day
Teenage girls, fourteen to eighteen years	15 mg/day
Women, nineteen to fifty years	18 mg/day
Women, fifty-one and older	8 mg/day
Women, pregnant	27 mg/day
Women, breast-feeding	9 mg/day

Where do we get it? Iron comes to us in food in two forms. **Heme iron** is found only in meat, fish, and poultry, while **nonheme iron** is found in meats and in green vegetables, legumes, and lentils, as well as in flours, cereals, and other grain products to which iron has been added. Only about 10 percent of the iron in a typical Western diet is heme iron, but about 25 percent of that is absorbed. A much smaller percentage of nonheme iron is absorbed, but that percentage is increased when food containing heme iron (that is, meat) is eaten at the same meal. Vitamin C also increases iron absorption. The body regulates how much iron is absorbed based on how much is available in storage. When there's plenty of iron on board, absorption from food—especially from the nonheme sources—drops significantly. When we need more, we absorb more.

What happens if we don't get enough? Some people become iron deficient simply because they do not consume enough foods containing iron. Others may experience iron deficiency because of blood loss that depletes iron stores faster than they can be replenished. When iron stores are depleted, a person will develop **iron-deficiency anemia**. Over time not only are there fewer red blood cells in circulation, but those that are present are both smaller and contain less hemoglobin. Immune function is compromised as well. As this problem evolves, a person is likely to become pale, chronically tired, irritable, apathetic, and more prone to infection. A person with heart or lung disease may also become short of breath because there is less hemoglobin—and thus less oxygen—available in the blood.

Vegetarians who eat no animal products must obtain all their iron from nonheme sources, so they should be sure to include foods that are good sources of vitamin C (such as citrus fruits) or consider taking a vitamin C supplement to enhance the absorption of iron.

More recently it has become apparent that iron deficiency can cause decreased energy and interest in work—whether at home, on the job, or at school—*long before anemia develops*. Learning and behavior problems that might suggest a child has attention deficit hyperactivity disorder (ADHD) may in fact be due, at least in part, to low iron levels. Sadly, infants with severe chronic iron deficiency may have learning and behavioral problems later in childhood or adolescence, even after the iron deficiency has been corrected.

People who might not get enough:

- Women during the reproductive years, because of the monthly losses of blood during menstruation.
- Pregnant women, who need additional iron to support not only their baby's growth but also their own increased blood volume.
- Infants over six months, since they may have used up the stores provided by their mother while in utero. The normal newborn has enough iron stored at birth to last four to six months, and a breast-fed baby can absorb about half of the iron present in her mother's milk. In contrast, an infant can use less than 12 percent of the iron in formula and very little from cow's milk (which doesn't have much to begin with). Cow's milk can also provoke blood loss, and thus loss of iron as well, when fed to babies younger than twelve months old. An infant who isn't getting all of her milk from Mom should be fed iron-fortified formula and should not drink cow's milk before her first birthday.
- Teenagers, because of a combination of the nutritional demands brought on by rapid growth (especially in boys), menstrual blood loss in girls, and erratic eating habits that may occur in this age group.

In addition, people who have ongoing blood loss can develop iron deficiency. In a man, or in a woman who is no longer having menstrual cycles, the discovery of iron deficiency with or without anemia should prompt a visit with a doctor to discuss a search for possible blood loss in the intestinal tract. Such blood loss could occur anywhere from the esophagus, which carries food from mouth to stomach, to the colon (large intestine), and might involve inflammation, an ulcer, a polyp, or even cancer. Unfortunately, very often the leak of red blood cells is so gradual it goes unnoticed.

Iron deficiency is the world's most common nutritional disorder. The World Health Organization (WHO) estimates that as many as 4 to 5 billion people, or 66 to 80 percent of the world's population, may be iron deficient. Ninety percent of these live in developing countries. Roughly 2 billion people (more than 30 percent of the world's population) are anemic, most commonly from iron deficiency, which may be aggravated by parasite infections such as malaria and intestinal worms. The worldwide loss of productivity, learning capacity, and even life is staggering. Iron deficiency increases the risk of death among pregnant women and young children, and WHO estimates that eliminating iron deficiency in a number of countries would result in a 20 percent increase in national productivity.[12]

Too much of a good thing? Though it can rid itself of many substances (such as vitamins) taken in excess, the body has no way of disposing of excessive amounts of iron. Therefore, **iron overload** is a potentially serious medical problem. This can result from unnecessary use of iron supplements (especially among adult men and postmenopausal women), repeated blood transfusions, or **hemochromatosis**, a genetic disorder in which iron is absorbed too efficiently. Excessive iron may accumulate in organs such as the liver or heart, where it can cause tissue damage and lead to problems such as cirrhosis or heart failure. Common symptoms of iron overload are fatigue and apathy—the same symptoms seen in iron deficiency.

Acute iron poisoning is the leading cause of poisoning death among children under six in the United States. As few as a half-dozen adult iron tablets can be lethal for a small child, and thus *any vitamin or supplement containing iron—including children's formulas—must always be tightly capped and kept completely out of reach of any children in your home.* If you suspect that your child may have taken iron supplements by mistake, immediately contact his physician or your local poison control center, or take him to the nearest emergency department for evaluation.

Interesting tidbit: Iron deficiency provokes an unusual craving for eating ice, clay, or paste. This behavior is called **pica**, from the Latin word for "magpie," a bird notorious for picking up random objects with its beak.

Zinc

What does it do? Zinc is an essential mineral found in nearly every cell. It promotes the activity of about a hundred enzymes involved in basic metabolism. It also plays a role in the proper function of the immune system, the senses of taste and smell, wound healing, and growth and development during pregnancy, childhood, and adolescence.

How much do we need?

AIs:

Infants, birth to six months	2 mg/day

RDAs:

Infants, seven months to one year	3 mg/day
Children, one to three years	3 mg/day
Children, four to eight years	5 mg/day
Children, nine to thirteen years	8 mg/day
Teenage boys and men, fourteen and older	11 mg/day
Teenage girls, fourteen to eighteen years	9 mg/day
Women, nineteen and older	8 mg/day
Women, pregnant	11 mg/day
Women, breast-feeding	12 mg/day

Where do we get it? We can obtain zinc from a variety of foods, including meat and poultry, as well as beans, nuts, whole grains, and fortified cereals.

What happens if we don't get enough? Zinc deficiency can cause or contribute to a host of disturbances, especially among people who are chronically malnourished. Among other problems, it can cause diarrhea and poor absorption of food. It hampers the immune response, including the body's defense against infections in the intestine, which can in turn cause more diarrhea. All of these can lead to a downward spiral of worsening malnutrition. Among children, severe zinc deficiency can lead to slow growth, poor development of motor (movement) and cognitive (thinking) skills, and delayed sexual maturation. Delayed wound healing, lethargy, and altered taste may be other manifestations.

People who might not get enough: Certain groups of people are particularly vulnerable to zinc deficiency: pregnant women, growing children, the elderly, the poor, and chronic alcohol abusers. Diets (such as are common in some Middle Eastern regions) in which meat is scarce and legumes and grains are abundant may predispose some individuals (especially children) to zinc deficiency. This occurs because fiber and compounds called phytates that are present in these foods may inhibit the absorption of zinc. (Note, however, that zinc deficiency is uncommon in developed countries.)

In the elderly, several factors may contribute to potential zinc deficiency: poor food intake, decreased absorption of zinc from food, interference with absorption from calcium and fiber supplements, and increased loss of zinc in the urine among those taking diuretics. As many as 50 percent of alcoholics may be zinc deficient because of poor food intake, as well as alcohol's tendency to interfere with zinc absorption and increase its loss in urine. People with intestinal disturbances that cause poor absorption or long-term diarrhea are also at risk for zinc deficiency.

What about zinc supplements for treating colds? During the winter months, zinc lozenges and nasal sprays fly off store shelves because of their reputation for shortening the length and severity of colds. Do they really work? Research studies have provided mixed results: Some have suggested that zinc preparations might reduce the number of days you spend feeling ill, while others show no particular benefit. On the downside, zinc lozenges aren't known for their pleasant taste. Also, concerns have been raised about reports of long-term loss of smell among a small number of users of zinc gluconate nasal sprays.

Too much of a good thing? As with most minerals, there is a very small gap between the amount of zinc we need and the amount that will harm us. And as is common with minerals, you won't develop zinc toxicity from food, but rather from overzealous use of supplements. The tolerable upper intake levels for zinc—the highest intake not associated with ill effects—have been established as follows:

Infants, birth to six months	4 mg/day
Infants, seven to twelve months	5 mg/day
Children, one to three years	7 mg/day
Children, four to eight years	12 mg/day
Children, nine to thirteen years	23 mg/day
Teenagers, fourteen to eighteen years	34 mg/day
Adults, nineteen and older	40 mg/day

Chronic intake of zinc above these levels can interfere with the absorption of copper, another essential mineral, and provoke many of the same symptoms of zinc deficiency, including decreased immune function, loss of taste and smell, and poor wound healing.

Interesting tidbit: By far, the food richest in zinc is oysters.

Selenium

What does it do? Selenium is an essential mineral that has gained some notoriety as an antioxidant and potential anticancer agent. Its antioxidant role in the body is actually indirect, as a component of enzymes that break down oxidizing agents (called peroxides) and thus limit free-radical formation. (For more information about free radicals and antioxidants, see page 884 earlier in this appendix.) Selenium is also a component of another enzyme involved in the formation of thyroid hormone.

Because of selenium's role in supporting antioxidant enzymes, one might assume that it would help prevent cancer, heart disease, and other common diseases in which free radicals participate. Those who sell selenium supplements enthusiastically advertise these benefits and many others, although the evidence supporting these claims isn't quite so conclusive. Some research links increased selenium intake or blood levels with lower death rates from cancer (especially lung, colon, and prostate). People with rheumatoid arthritis have been found to have lower selenium levels. Adults and children with HIV/AIDS who are selenium deficient have been found to have higher death rates. These findings are intriguing, but they don't automatically mean that taking this mineral as a supplement will protect against or treat these diseases. Thus far, no professional health organization has recommended selenium supplements for disease prevention, but several ongoing research projects may clarify whether or not this might be helpful. (Remember some of the paradoxical findings about beta-carotene that we noted earlier; a substance that appears to provide benefits in our food doesn't always do the same in a supplement.)

How much do we need?

AIs:

Infants, birth to six months	15 mcg/day
Infants, seven months to one year	20 mcg/day

RDAs:

Children, one to three years	20 mcg/day
Children, four to eight years	30 mcg/day
Children, nine to thirteen years	40 mcg/day
Men and women, fourteen and older	55 mcg/day
Women, pregnant	60 mcg/day
Women, breast-feeding	70 mcg/day

Where do we get it? Plant foods are the primary source of selenium, although the amount they contain will vary depending on the amount of this mineral found in the soil. The soil of the high plains of Nebraska and the Dakotas is particularly rich in selenium. (Meat from animals that have eaten plants grown in this soil can also be a source of dietary selenium.) Selenium deficiency has been reported in some areas of Russia and China where the soil lacks this mineral.

What happens if we don't get enough: Selenium deficiency is associated with an uncommon heart disorder called Keshan disease, named for a province in China where the soil lacks selenium. In Keshan disease, fibrous tissue replaces normal heart muscle, resulting in enlargement and failure to pump adequate amounts of blood.

People who might not get enough: Those who have had a serious intestinal disorder or who have had surgery that prevents adequate absorption of nutrients (for example, removal of more than half of the small intestine) may not get enough. In such cases, there are usually a host of nutritional deficits beyond selenium deficiency that need attention and treatment. Some people with serious medical problems must be sustained with specially prepared nutrients that are infused directly into the bloodstream by vein. This treatment is called total parenteral nutrition, or TPN for short, and requires medical expertise to set up and maintain. Selenium deficiency was at one time seen among some patients receiving TPN, but this mineral is now routinely included in TPN solutions. Unless you have one of these extreme nutritional problems or live in one of the selenium-poor areas of China or Russia, it is extremely unlikely that you will become deficient in selenium.

Too much of a good thing? As with the other minerals, there is a relatively small gap between the amount of selenium we need and the amount that can cause trouble. The Institute of Medicine has set the tolerable upper intake level (UL) for selenium at 400 mcg per day for adults. Taking 1,000 mcg or more can lead to symptoms of toxicity, including intestinal disturbances, hair loss, and nerve damage.

Interesting tidbit: The champion food source of selenium is the Brazil nut. One ounce of dried Brazil nuts can contain over 800 mcg of selenium—more than ten times the adult RDA for this mineral.

Iodine

What does it do? Iodine is an indispensable micronutrient that the body converts to an ion form called **iodide**, which has one very crucial function: It is trapped by the thyroid gland (a butterfly-shaped structure located at the base of the neck, below the Adam's apple) and incorporated into thyroid hormone. This compound regulates your body's "idle speed," impacting metabolic rate, body temperature, growth, reproduction, nerve and muscle function, and other vital roles.

How much do we need?

AIs:

Infants, birth to six months	110 mcg/day
Infants, seven months to one year	130 mcg/day

RDAs:

Children, one to three years	90 mcg/day
Children, four to eight years	90 mcg/day
Children, nine to thirteen years	120 mcg/day
Men and women, fourteen and older	150 mcg/day
Women, pregnant	220 mcg/day
Women, breast-feeding	290 mcg/day

Where do we get it? The ocean is the world's great iodine repository, and land that is near or was once under the ocean usually has iodine-rich soil. Plants grown in these regions, and animals that eat those plants, are food sources of iodine, as is seafood. In places where the land has been exposed to the elements and erosion for millennia—for example, mountainous areas, or regions where repeated flooding leaches iodine from the soil—inadequate amounts of iodine may be available in food. In the United States and Canada, the widespread use of iodized salt has virtually eliminated iodine deficiency.

What happens if we don't get enough? Without an adequate supply of iodine, the thyroid gland cannot make an adequate amount of thyroid hormone. The pituitary gland, located at the base of the brain, detects this problem and secretes a hormone called thyroid stimulating hormone (or TSH), a wake-up call designed to prod the thyroid gland into action. Among other responses, the thyroid cells will enlarge in an effort to capture as much iodine as possible. If the deficiency isn't corrected, the gland itself will enlarge, forming a bulge in the neck called a **goiter**.

The word *goiter* comes from the Latin word for "throat." A goiter can have a number of causes, but in the United States and Canada it is rarely the result of iodine deficiency.

Inadequate levels of thyroid hormone, a condition called **hypothyroidism**, can eventually cause a number of symptoms, including fatigue, intolerance to cold, puffy skin (especially of the face), hoarseness, heavy menstrual periods, and weight gain. The most devastating effects of hypothyroidism, whether caused by iodine deficiency or other problems, impact infants and children. During pregnancy, hypothyroidism in the mother can affect her baby before the child's own thyroid gland is functional, resulting in severe and irreversible mental and physical retardation. (This severe congenital deficit is called **cretinism**, a clinical term that has been cruelly modified to form the slang insult "cretin.") During infancy and childhood, thyroid hormone is essential for normal brain development, and inadequate levels can result in variable degrees of impaired intellectual development or learning disabilities.

F.Y.I.

Many overweight people are convinced (or hope) that their problem is caused by an underactive thyroid gland. Unfortunately, this is the case in only a small number of cases, as a simple lab test will usually demonstrate. Even when it is present, hypothyroidism will only account for about ten to twenty pounds of excess weight. Some overzealous physicians and weight-loss clinics have inappropriately given thyroid hormone to patients who in fact don't need it, in a misguided effort to "rev up" their metabolism.

Iodine deficiency is the world's most common and preventable cause of brain damage. The World Health Organization (WHO) estimates that 740 million people worldwide are affected by some form of iodine deficiency disorder and that 50 million of these have some degree of brain damage related to iodine deficiency.[13] Significant progress has been made over the past decade through programs designed to provide iodized salt on a permanent basis within countries (primarily in Asia and Africa) where there are iodine-deficient regions.

People who might not get enough: Because of the widespread use of iodized salt in the United States and Canada, iodine deficiency is rare in these countries. Only those on a very restricted diet that includes scrupulous avoidance of salt, seafood, meat, and other animal products such as milk and eggs may be deficient.

Too much of a good thing? At very high daily doses—more than ten times the RDA—iodine actually interferes with thyroid function and can cause a goiter to develop. While iodine is critical for the normal development of a baby before birth, excessive amounts taken by a pregnant mother can also be harmful. The Institute of Medicine has established the tolerable upper limit (UL) for iodine at 1,100 mcg for adults.

Interesting tidbit: The champion food source of iodine is seaweed. An ounce of dried seaweed may contain as much as 18,000 mcg of iodine—more than one hundred times the adult RDA. In some coastal areas of Japan, the local diet includes enough seaweed to push the iodine intake to more than 50,000 mcg per day.

Copper

What does it do? The dime in your pocket contains more than twenty times the amount of copper in your entire body (only about 100 mg), but this essential mineral plays a role in a number of enzymes with diverse and important tasks. These include energy production, iron metabolism, the formation of collagen (a key component of connective tissue and scars), and antioxidant functions, among others.

How much do we need?

AIs:	
Infants, birth to six months	200 mcg/day
Infants, seven months to one year	220 mcg/day

RDAs:	
Children, one to three years	340 mcg/day
Children, four to eight years	440 mcg/day
Children, nine to thirteen years	700 mcg/day
Teenagers, fourteen to eighteen years	890 mcg/day
Adults, nineteen and older	900 mcg/day
Women, pregnant	1,000 mcg/day
Women, breast-feeding	1,300 mcg/day

Where do we get it? Copper is found in a variety of foods, including seafood, nuts, legumes, whole grains, and seeds.

What happens if we don't get enough? Anemia (a low number of red blood cells) and **neutropenia** (a shortage of an important type of white blood cell) may arise from copper deficiency, as can osteoporosis and abnormalities in bone development. However, copper deficiency is by no means a common cause of these problems.

People who might not get enough: Copper deficiency severe enough to cause overt health problems is very uncommon, but it may occur in certain groups of vulnerable infants and children. These include premature and low birth-weight infants, as well as babies and children with chronic diarrhea or malnourishment, especially if they are fed only cow's milk.

Too much of a good thing? Copper toxicity is extremely uncommon, occurring only as a result of environmental exposures (such as a contaminated water supply) or rare genetic disorders that affect copper metabolism. Symptoms of acute copper toxicity can include abdominal pain, nausea, and vomiting, and in severe cases coma and death. The Food and Nutrition Board of the Institute of Medicine has set the tolerable upper limit (UL) for copper in food and supplements at 10 mg per day for adults, or about five times the amount found in a typical multivitamin/mineral supplement.

Interesting tidbits: As of 1982, our copper-looking pennies are actually made of zinc, with a copper coating that is only 2.5 percent of the total weight. All of the rest of our coins are made almost entirely of copper, with a small amount of nickel added.

Coins are one of the most common objects accidentally swallowed by children, and as long as they don't obstruct the airway or the esophagus (the tube between the throat and the stomach), they should pass uneventfully in a bowel movement after a day or two. The copper or nickel present in these coins will not be absorbed into the bloodstream.

However, if a child accidentally swallows a penny and it remains in the stomach rather than passing into the intestine, the *zinc* it contains can react with stomach acid, forming a corrosive compound that can cause significant damage to the stomach lining. For that reason, if a penny doesn't pass within a couple of days, and especially if abdominal pain develops after one or more pennies have been swallowed, the child should be evaluated by a physician.

Chromium

What does it do? Chromium is an essential mineral that has appeared on the supplement radar because of its apparent effect on glucose metabolism. Specifically, it appears to enhance the action of insulin, the hormone essential for the transport of glucose into the cells that use it as their basic fuel. As we described in detail in chapter 3, lack of sensitivity to insulin (called **insulin resistance**) plays a central role in the development of type 2 diabetes, a disorder that impacts the health of millions of Americans. A compound containing chromium appears to increase the sensitivity of cells to insulin.

Because of chromium's apparent ability to enhance the body's processing of glucose, it has been marketed as a supplement (usually in a form called **chromium picolinate**) to help increase muscle mass, decrease body fat, and lose weight—all without any additional effort, of course. As with so many extravagant promises that are made for dietary supplements, controlled studies have not supported these claims. However, some research supports the notion that chromium supplementation may improve blood glucose control in people with type 2 (adult-onset) diabetes. Some physicians give chromium picolinate to their patients with type 2 diabetes or metabolic syndrome, typically in doses up to 200 mcg, but at this time no professional organization recommends doing so. Future research may clarify whether chromium should be a routine part of the treatment of these disorders.

How much do we need? It is difficult to determine precisely how much chromium we need each day, and therefore the Institute of Medicine has provided adequate intake (AI) estimates rather than recommended daily allowances (RDAs):

AIs:

Infants, birth to six months	0.2 mcg/day
Infants, seven months to one year	5.5 mcg/day
Children, one to three years	11 mcg/day
Children, four to eight years	15 mcg/day
Boys, nine to thirteen years	25 mcg/day
Girls, nine to thirteen years	21 mcg/day
Teenage boys and men, fourteen and older	35 mcg/day
Teenage girls, fourteen to eighteen years	24 mcg/day
Women, nineteen to fifty years	25 mcg/day
Men, over fifty	30 mcg/day
Women, over fifty	20 mcg/day
Women, pregnant	30 mcg/day
Women, breast-feeding	45 mcg/day

Where do we get it? Chromium content has not been determined for many foods, although many familiar foods—whole grains, bran cereals, broccoli, and processed meats, among others—are known to contain it.

What happens if we don't get enough? This is a difficult question to answer because there are no accurate and reliable tests to determine whether one is deficient in this mineral. Some limited and indirect evidence (involving people receiving fluids by vein on a long-term basis) supports the idea that chromium might indeed improve the body's ability to use glucose.

People who might not get enough: As with many of the other essential minerals, chromium deficiency is unlikely unless one is severely malnourished.

Too much of a good thing? Doses of 1,000 mcg of chromium per day for an extended period have been taken without apparent harm in some studies, but there have been isolated reports of both kidney failure and altered liver function with doses ranging from 600 to 2,400 mcg per day. People with known kidney or liver disease should limit their intake of chromium supplements.

Interesting tidbit: Foods high in simple sugars not only tend to be low in chromium but may promote its loss as well.

Manganese

What does it do? Like many trace minerals, manganese is a cofactor in enzyme reactions required for a variety of functions, including the metabolism of carbohydrates, amino acids, and cholesterol; the synthesis of glucose from noncarbohydrate sources; as well as the healing of wounds and formation of bone. Manganese is also present in the primary antioxidant enzyme in mitochondria, important structures within cells that provide energy in a form that the cell can use. Mitochondria consume the vast majority of oxygen within cells, and they are potentially vulnerable to oxidative stress.

How much do we need? Only adequate intakes (AIs) have been established for manganese:

AIs:

Infants, birth to six months	0.003 mg/day
Infants, seven months to one year	0.6 mg/day
Children, one to three years	1.2 mg/day
Children, four to eight years	1.5 mg/day
Boys, nine to thirteen years	1.9 mg/day
Girls, nine to thirteen years	1.6 mg/day
Teenage boys, fourteen to eighteen years	2.2 mg/day
Teenage girls, fourteen to eighteen years	1.6 mg/day
Men, nineteen and older	2.3 mg/day
Women, nineteen and older	1.8 mg/day
Women, pregnant	2.0 mg/day
Women, breast-feeding	2.6 mg/day

Where do we get it? A variety of foods, including leafy vegetables, pineapple, whole grains, beans, and nuts, supply manganese.

What happens if we don't get enough? No specific human deficiency syndrome has been described, although in animals manganese deficiency has been associated with growth, reproductive, and central nervous system abnormalities.

People who might not get enough: Those who take daily iron supplements, which can interfere with manganese absorption, may have a manganese deficiency.

Too much of a good thing? Environmental exposures—inhaling manganese dust, or drinking water contaminated with high levels of manganese—have been associated with the development of neurological symptoms similar to Parkinson's disease. Comparable results have not been observed in studies of people taking oral supplements containing 30 to 40 mg (up to twenty times the AI), but because of concern over potential damage to the nervous system, the Food and Nutrition Board of the Institute of Medicine has established upper levels of intake (UL) for manganese that are only two to five times greater than the AI. (Manganese supplements containing a whopping and excessive 50 mg per tablet can be purchased on the Internet.)

People with chronic liver disease are more vulnerable to manganese toxicity because this mineral is removed from the body in the bile (fluid that drains from the liver). They should avoid supplements containing more than the adequate intake.

Interesting tidbit: Be careful not to confuse *magnesium* (discussed earlier in this chapter) with *manganese* if you are shopping for supplements. The amount of magnesium you need is well over 100 times greater than the amount of manganese.

Molybdenum

What does it do? Aside from having a tongue-twisting name, molybdenum is an essential trace element that serves as a cofactor for a few important enzymes, including one that is vital for the metabolism of certain amino acids (the building blocks of proteins).

Where do we get it? Legumes (beans, peas, lentils); nuts; and grains are good dietary sources of this mineral, but amounts may vary depending on soil conditions.

How much do we need? Though we need little of this mineral, recommended daily allowances (RDAs) have been established for it:

AIs:	
Infants, birth to six months	2 mcg/day
Infants, seven months to one year	3 mcg/day
RDAs:	
Children, one to three years	17 mcg/day
Children, four to eight years	22 mcg/day
Children, nine to thirteen years	34 mcg/day
Teenagers, fourteen to eighteen years	43 mcg/day
Men and women, nineteen and older	45 mcg/day
Women, pregnant	50 mcg/day
Women, breast-feeding	50 mcg/day

What happens if we don't get enough? It's hard to say because we need so little. A specific molybdenum deficiency syndrome has not been observed in anyone eating even a modest amount of food, and someone who is severely malnourished will have so many health problems that identifying the role of molybdenum in the total picture would be virtually impossible.

Too much of a good thing? Unlike most of the trace minerals, there appears to be a wide margin between RDA and toxicity for molybdenum. Based on animal studies, the Institute of Medicine has set tolerable upper levels for molybdenum that are quite high—2,000 mcg for adults, or roughly fifty times the RDA. Very high intakes of molybdenum may increase the level of uric acid in the bloodstream, which could lead to an episode of **gout**—painful, acute inflammation of one or more joints (usually involving one of the big toes) that occurs when uric acid crystals form within a joint space.

Interesting tidbit: *Molybdenum* comes from the Greek for "piece of lead" and is used in industry to strengthen steel.

Getting Back to the Original Question: Should I Take a Vitamin/Mineral Supplement?

We mentioned at the outset that the traditional viewpoint of physicians and dietitians (and their professional organizations) has been that a well-balanced diet and a little sun exposure should supply all the vitamins we need. This view makes sense. Remember that whole foods contain not only macronutrients, vitamins, and minerals, but also complex compounds that no supplement can duplicate—especially the fiber and disease-preventing phytochemicals found in fruits and vegetables. A supplement may wear the label all-natural, but the *real* natural substances are in the produce aisle.

Nevertheless, as we took our tour of the thirteen vitamins and the important trace minerals, you may have noticed that, even in our well-fed society, certain groups of people may be vulnerable to one or more shortfalls in these substances. These include people who are unable to obtain, prepare, swallow, or absorb an adequate supply of basic nutrients because of

- Chronic illness, especially when it affects appetite or the absorption of food
- Poverty
- Alcoholism or other drug addiction
- Major psychological or emotional problems—especially schizophrenia, significant depression, or certain behavioral problems, including eating disorders

Along with these more extreme situations, a number of people do not consume a balanced or adequate diet every day. Others might need an extra supply of one or more nutrients because of a special situation:

- The elderly, who may have to cope with chronic illness, multiple medications, depression, memory problems, and loss of mobility. Seniors who are living alone may develop erratic eating habits, and some may battle alcoholism.
- Dieters, especially those on weight-loss plans that banish entire groups of foods (such as very strict low-carbohydrate or low-fat ap-

"I do not like broccoli. And I haven't liked it since I was a little kid and my mother made me eat it. And I'm president of the United States and I'm not going to eat any more broccoli."
—GEORGE H. W. BUSH

proaches). A variation on this theme is the picky eater, young or old, who sticks to a narrow repertoire of foods.

- Fast-food addicts, especially those whose primary source of fruits and vegetables is whatever is found between the burger and the bun.
- Adolescents, who not only may frequently eat fast-food meals but also may have erratic eating habits (such as skipping breakfast before running off to school). Furthermore, their rapid growth and development requires a steady supply of high-quality nutrients.
- Smokers whose habit depletes the body of vitamin C.
- Strict vegetarians (vegans) who consume no animal products of any kind.
- People recovering from surgery, a major injury, or a burn.
- Women who are pregnant or breast-feeding (or who may become pregnant).
- Women with heavy, lengthy, or more frequent menstrual periods, who are at risk for iron deficiency.

Despite the dire warnings of many would-be nutritional experts (who more often than not have some expensive products to sell), it is not necessary to take handfuls of supplements to remain healthy. Nevertheless, a number of reputable, conservative researchers and organizations consider a daily multivitamin and mineral supplement to be a good investment—especially for someone who falls into one of the categories listed above.

But how do you choose from the hundreds of products that line the shelves of your supermarket or drug store, not to mention all of the preparations on the Internet? Here are ten basic guidelines that can help you:

1. **Think of a supplement as a safety net.** It should serve as nutritional insurance—not as a quick way to get around making good food choices. Putting an additive in your gas tank can't substitute for poor-quality fuel or no fuel at all.

2. **Look for a comprehensive supplement.** It should supply 100 percent of the daily value (DV) for most of the thirteen vitamins and the trace minerals we have reviewed in this chapter. (See sidebar: "What Exactly Does *DV* on the Supplement Label Mean?" on page 920.) In particular, look for 100 percent daily value for the B vitamins (including folic acid), C, D, E, iron, iodine, zinc, selenium, copper, manganese, chromium, and molybdenum.

3. **Beware of inflated prices.** Your comprehensive supplement should be inexpensive—no more than ten to twenty cents per day. If you're shelling out thirty dollars or more every month for vitamins and minerals, you're spending too much. Pick a less expensive brand and spend the difference at the produce section or a local vegetable stand.

4. **Beware of inflated doses.** Taking up to 200 percent of the daily value for the B vitamins won't hurt you, but unless you have specific directions from a

physician to use high doses of other vitamins and minerals, think carefully before buying a megadose preparation. (Two exceptions are vitamins C and E, which we will discuss momentarily.) As we have already described, vitamin A and many of the minerals can be toxic in large doses.

5. **Beware of inflated claims.** Many advertisements and infomercials claim that a concoction has special, unique, all-natural, superpotent, stress-reducing, life-extending, youth-restoring, energy-boosting, cosmic, good-for-what-ails-ya ingredients and additives. They want $29.99 or more per month, usually with a special offer if you call right now ("Operators are waiting!"). If you suspect that it sounds too good to be true, you'll be correct 99.9 percent of the time.

6. **Look for the letters "USP" on the label.** This indicates that the product meets the standards of the United States Pharmacopeia (USP), a nonprofit, nongovernmental organization that sets manufacturing standards for drugs, supplements, and other health-care products.

7. **Better yet, look for a logo that says "USP-Verified Dietary Supplement."** This indicates that the product has undergone more rigorous voluntary testing for verification of ingredients, good manufacturing procedures, absence of contaminants, and dissolving characteristics (to ensure that it can be absorbed effectively once swallowed). Products that have passed this muster are also checked over time using random samples from store shelves. A current list of verified supplements can be found at http://www.usp.org/USPVerified.

8. **Don't worry about getting 100 percent of the daily value for phosphorus, potassium, chloride, biotin, or vitamin K from your multivitamin.** These typically appear as low percent DVs on multivitamins because you get the vast majority from your food. (Also remember that the current RDA for biotin, 30 mcg, is now 10 percent of the amount used in estimating the DV.) If you are low in potassium, your doctor will prescribe an appropriate preparation and follow your progress with blood tests.

9. **You don't need to use a liquid supplement unless you can't swallow tablets.** Some liquid supplements are marketed with the claim that vitamins and minerals are better absorbed in liquid form than from tablets. This may indeed be true—if the tablet doesn't disintegrate. USP recommends that a vitamin tablet disintegrate completely thirty to forty-five minutes after being swallowed, another reason to seek brands that meet USP standards. Unfortunately, claims that liquid vitamins are uniformly superior to tablets originate from marketers and not from professional organizations. Similarly, some

continued on page 922

WHAT EXACTLY DOES *DV* ON THE SUPPLEMENT LABEL MEAN?

Throughout this chapter we have listed adequate intakes (AIs) and recommended daily allowances (RDAs) for each vitamin and trace mineral. These usually vary quite a bit depending on age, gender, and pregnancy or nursing status. But when you pick up a bottle of vitamins and minerals and look at the label, you'll notice that it includes not only the amounts of the various nutrients but also the percent of something called the **daily value (DV)**. We encountered the daily value in chapter 5 when we looked at food labels, where the percent DV is listed not only for vitamins and minerals but also for nutrients such as carbohydrates, fats, saturated fats, and cholesterol.

Here is a list of the quantities of vitamins and trace minerals that constitute 100 percent of the daily value.

Nutrient	**Daily Value**
Thiamin (B_1)	1.5 mg
Riboflavin (B_2)	1.7 mg
Niacin	20 mg
Biotin	300 mcg
Pantothenic acid	10 mg
Vitamin B_6	2 mg
Folic acid	400 mcg
Vitamin B_{12}	6 mcg
Vitamin C	60 mg
Vitamin A	5,000 IU
Vitamin D	400 IU
Vitamin E	30 IU
Vitamin K	80 mcg
Iron	18 mg
Iodine	150 mcg
Magnesium	400 mg
Zinc	15 mg
Selenium	70 mcg
Copper	2 mg
Chromium	120 mcg
Manganese	2 mg
Molybdenum	75 mcg

Remember: A milligram (mg) is 1/1,000 of a gram. A microgram (mcg) is 1/1,000 of a milligram.

Notice that the daily value is a "one size fits all" number that isn't broken down by age or gender but is meant to apply to adults. Also, there are some notable differences between the DV and the RDA for several nutrients, including these:

Nutrient	**Daily Value**	**RDA for adults**
Biotin	300 mcg	30 mcg
Pantothenic acid	10 mg	5 mg
Vitamin B_{12}	6 mcg	2.4 mcg
Vitamin C	60 mg	75 mg (women); 90 mg (men)
Vitamin A	5,000 IU	2,330 IU (women); 3,000 IU (men)
Copper	2 mg	0.9 mg

Why the differences? The daily value is based on the recommended daily allowances (RDAs) set by the National Academies (specifically, the Food and Nutrition Board of the Institute of Medicine) in *1968*, not the current RDAs we have listed in this chapter. For any given vitamin or mineral, the daily value is based on the highest 1968 RDA for anyone, regardless of age or gender. (Usually this was the level for adult males.)

In a nutshell, the daily value is a reasonable guideline for gauging the quantities in a supplement, although it is not based on the most current recommendations from the Food and Nutrition Board. Indeed, many comprehensive supplements are more in line with the newer RDAs than the daily values. You'll typically find less biotin (30 or 40 mcg, or about 10 percent of the DV), more vitamin C (90 to 120 mg, or 150 to 200 percent of the DV), and less vitamin A (3500 IU, or 70 percent of the DV) in a good, all-around supplement. ■

continued from page 919

notoriously misleading advertisements for "colloidal" liquid mineral preparations have been in circulation on cassette tapes and the Internet for years. Assuming you can swallow a good-quality tablet, there is no reason to pay inflated prices for a liquid formulation.

10. **Keep all vitamin and mineral preparations in a safe place where children cannot find and accidentally swallow them.** Remember that the amount of iron in a few adult multivitamin/mineral tablets can be lethal to a small child.

In addition to using a single comprehensive supplement as a nutritional safety net, you may want to consider some additional vitamins and minerals for your daily routine:

- **Additional vitamin C (250 to 500 mg) and vitamin E (200 IU).** These are doses at which you may obtain antioxidant benefits from these two vitamins. Recent research suggests that daily doses of 500 mg of vitamin C and 400 IU of vitamin E on an ongoing basis may reduce the risk of developing Alzheimer's disease.[14] But, as we noted earlier in this chapter, analysis of multiple studies has raised concern that ongoing vitamin E doses of 400 IU or more may be associated with higher rates of death from all causes. The jury is still out, but you may obtain some overall benefit and are probably safe in taking 250 to 500 mg of vitamins C and 200 IU of vitamin E daily. These quantities are not found in typical multivitamin tablets, and while it's possible to take in this much vitamin C from food sources, there is no way to obtain this much vitamin E from food. Remember that if you are a smoker, you need more vitamin C.
- **Additional calcium.** Because calcium is so bulky, most multivitamins contain only 100 to 200 mg. The recommended daily allowance for adults ranges from 1,000 to 1,300 mg, with many experts suggesting 1,500 mg for women after menopause. Because calcium intake from food may vary, many adults should add a calcium supplement, with or without vitamin D. Because of its importance in bone health and the vulnerability of many women to osteoporosis (thinning of the bones), we examine calcium in food and supplements in chapter 13 ("Selected Topics in Women's Health").
- **Additional iron and folic acid if you are pregnant.** The RDA for iron during pregnancy is 27 mg, while a typical multivitamin contains 18 mg. Similarly, the RDA for folic acid during pregnancy is 600 mcg, while most multivitamins contain 400 mcg. Rather than looking for additional iron and folic acid tablets, however, your best bet would be to use prenatal vitamins prescribed by your physician, which usually contain 1,000 mcg of folic acid and 25 to 30 mg of iron.

APPENDIX C

Body Mass Index: Tables for Adults and Children

A simple but meaningful way to assess whether or not your weight may pose a health risk is by determining your body mass index (BMI), which is explained in chapter 6. The BMI figures correlate closely enough with body fat to serve as a general indicator of the health risk associated with your weight.

To determine whether or not your weight is in the normal range, refer to the BMI table on the next two pages. Find your height in the vertical column on the left, and then look across the row until you find the column that is closest to your weight. The number at the top of the column where your height and weight intersect is your BMI.

Remember, however, that the BMI calculation for an adult is based solely on height and weight. Age or gender is not a consideration. This makes the table easy to use; however, when classifying someone as normal, overweight, or obese, it can't take into account variables such as the higher percentage of body fat in most women and older adults.

These differences are much more significant in children and adolescents, which is why separate tables that consider age and gender have been created for them. (The normal amount of body fat not only differs between boys and girls but also changes as children grow and mature.)

The tables for children and adolescents from two to twenty years of age show a series of curved lines, each of which represents a certain **percentile** rank. Given a child's height and weight, a BMI can be calculated using the same formula as for adults (see page 193). By looking at the appropriate chart, one must then determine the percentile rank for that BMI, depending on age. If the child's BMI falls on the 50th percentile curve, it means that half of the children at his or her age have a higher BMI, while half have a lower one. For example, a five-year-old boy with a BMI of 18 would fall on the 95th percentile curve, and this would raise concerns about his weight. But the same BMI for a twelve-year-old boy falls on the 50th percentile curve, indicating a normal combination of height and weight.

Measuring a child's height and weight is an important component of every checkup, and a child's physician is likely to track a child's growth using this tool.

BODY MASS INDEX TABLE FOR ADULTS

	NORMAL						OVERWEIGHT					OBESE	
BMI	19	20	21	22	23	24	25	26	27	28	29	30	31
Height (inches)	Body Weight (pounds)												
58	91	96	100	105	110	115	119	124	129	134	138	143	148
59	94	99	104	109	114	119	124	128	133	138	143	148	153
60	97	102	107	112	118	123	128	133	138	143	148	153	158
61	100	106	111	116	122	127	132	137	143	148	153	158	164
62	104	109	115	120	126	131	136	142	147	153	158	164	169
63	107	113	118	124	130	135	141	146	152	158	163	169	175
64	110	116	122	128	134	140	145	151	157	163	169	174	180
65	114	120	126	132	138	144	150	156	162	168	174	180	186
66	118	124	130	136	142	148	155	161	167	173	179	186	192
67	121	127	134	140	146	153	159	166	172	178	185	191	198
68	125	131	138	144	151	158	164	171	177	184	190	197	203
69	128	135	142	149	155	162	169	176	182	189	196	203	209
70	132	139	146	153	160	167	174	181	188	195	202	209	216
71	136	143	150	157	165	172	179	186	193	200	208	215	222
72	140	147	154	162	169	177	184	191	199	206	213	221	228
73	144	151	159	166	174	182	189	197	204	212	219	227	235
74	148	155	163	171	179	186	194	202	210	218	225	233	241
75	152	160	168	176	184	192	200	208	216	224	232	240	248
76	156	164	172	180	189	197	205	213	221	230	238	246	254

Source: National Institutes of Health; National Heart, Lung, and Blood Institute

OBESE									EXTREME OBESITY				
32	33	34	35	36	37	38	39	40	41	42	43	44	45
Body Weight (pounds)													
153	158	162	167	172	177	181	186	191	196	201	205	210	215
158	163	168	173	178	183	188	193	198	203	208	212	217	222
163	168	174	179	184	189	194	199	204	209	215	220	225	230
169	174	180	185	190	195	201	206	211	217	222	227	232	238
175	180	186	191	196	202	207	213	218	224	229	35	240	246
180	186	191	197	203	208	214	220	225	231	237	242	248	254
186	192	197	204	209	215	221	227	232	238	244	250	256	262
192	198	204	210	216	222	228	234	240	246	252	258	264	270
198	204	210	216	223	229	235	241	247	253	260	266	272	278
204	211	217	223	230	236	242	249	255	261	268	274	280	287
210	216	223	230	236	243	249	256	262	269	276	282	289	295
216	223	230	236	243	250	257	263	270	277	284	291	297	304
222	229	236	243	250	257	264	271	278	285	292	299	306	313
229	236	243	250	257	265	272	279	286	293	301	308	315	322
235	242	250	258	265	272	279	287	294	302	309	316	324	331
242	250	257	265	272	280	288	295	302	310	318	325	333	340
249	256	264	272	280	287	295	303	311	319	326	334	342	350
256	264	272	279	287	295	303	311	319	327	335	343	351	359
263	271	279	287	295	304	312	320	328	336	344	353	361	369

BODY MASS INDEX CHARTS FOR CHILDREN AND ADOLESCENTS

2 to 20 years: Boys
Body mass index-for-age percentiles

NAME ______________________

RECORD # ______________

Date	Age	Weight	Stature	BMI*	Comments

***To Calculate BMI**: Weight (kg) ÷ Stature (cm) ÷ Stature (cm) x 10,000
or Weight (lb) ÷ Stature (in) ÷ Stature (in) x 703

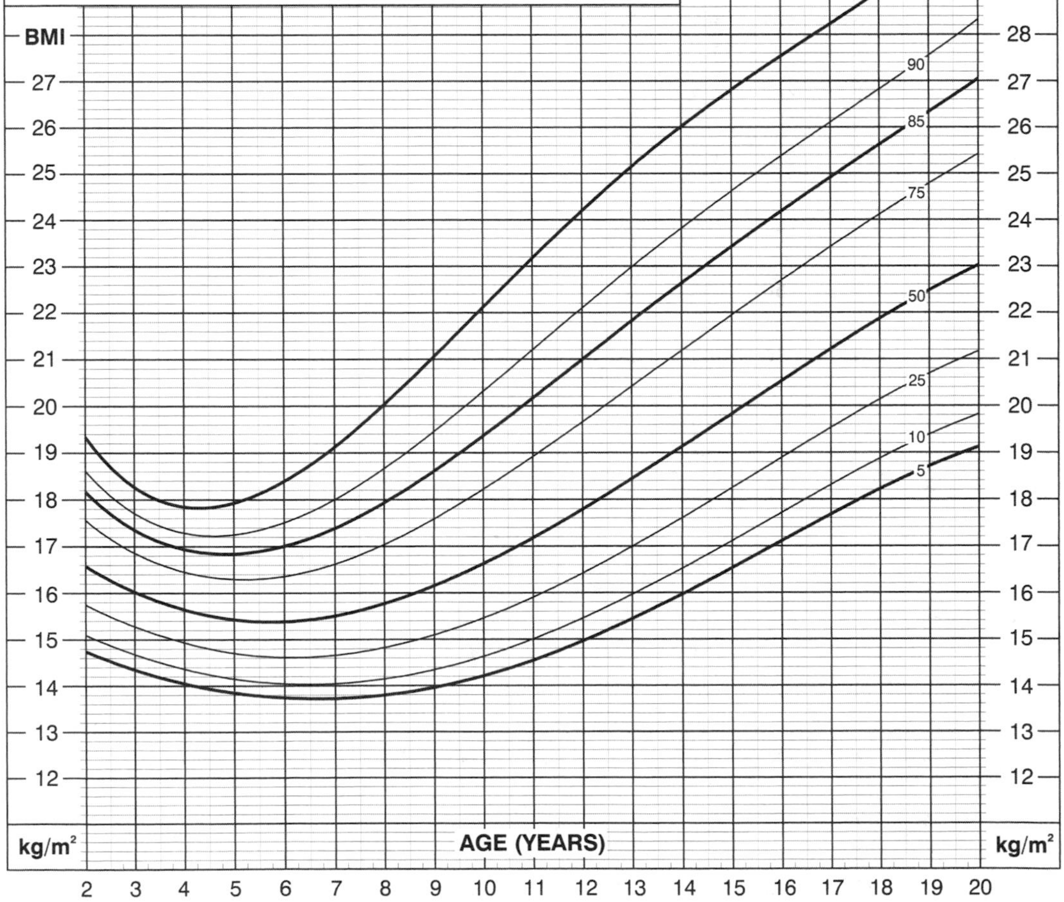

Published May 30, 2000 (modified 10/16/00).
SOURCE: Developed by the National Center for Health Statistics in collaboration with
the National Center for Chronic Disease Prevention and Health Promotion (2000).
http://www.cdc.gov/growthcharts

CDC
SAFER • HEALTHIER • PEOPLE™

2 to 20 years: Girls
Body mass index-for-age percentiles

NAME ______________________

RECORD # ______________

Date	Age	Weight	Stature	BMI*	Comments

***To Calculate BMI**: Weight (kg) ÷ Stature (cm) ÷ Stature (cm) x 10,000
or Weight (lb) ÷ Stature (in) ÷ Stature (in) x 703

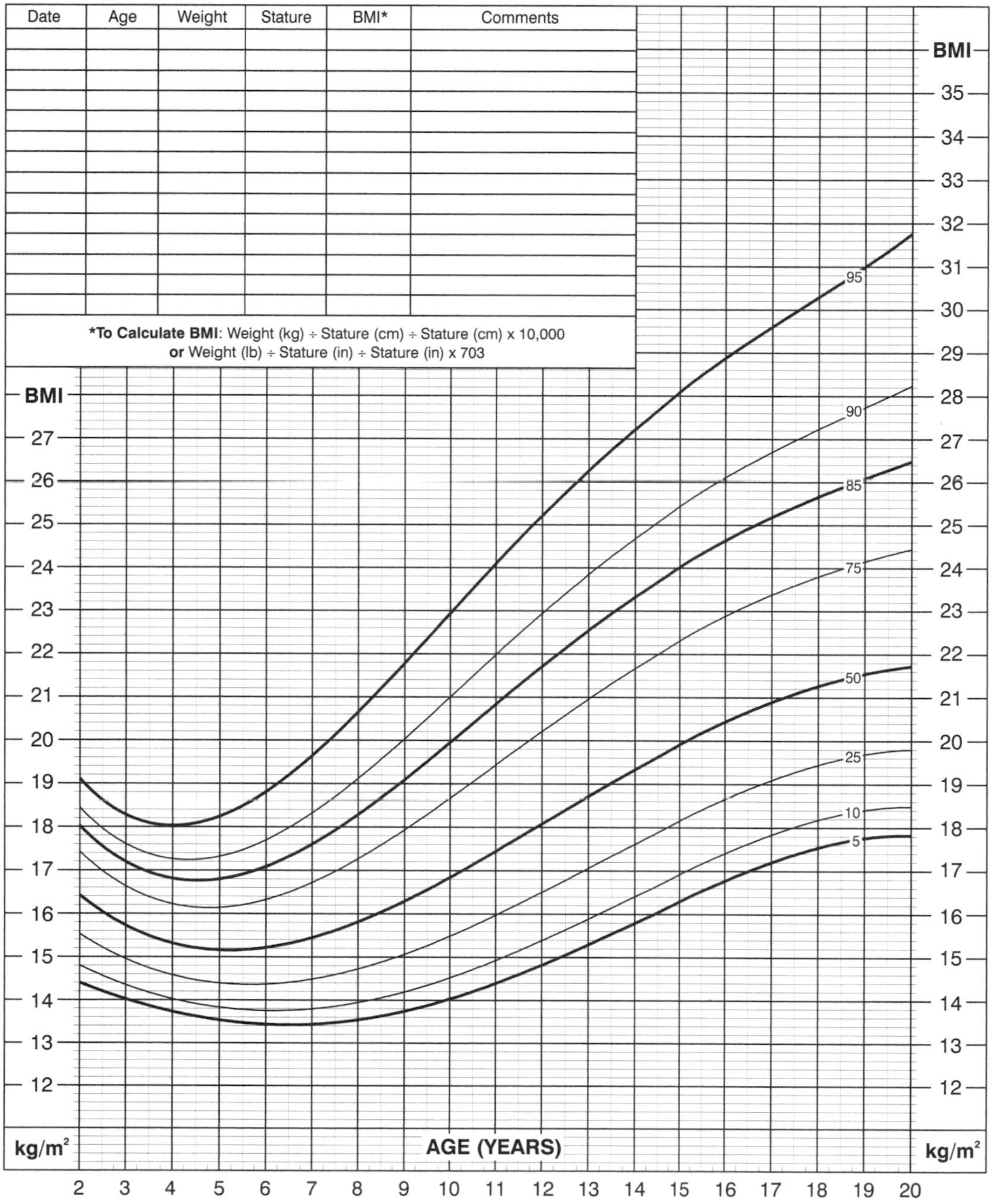

Published May 30, 2000 (modified 10/16/00).
SOURCE: Developed by the National Center for Health Statistics in collaboration with the National Center for Chronic Disease Prevention and Health Promotion (2000).
http://www.cdc.gov/growthcharts

CDC
SAFER • HEALTHIER • PEOPLE™

APPENDIX D

Strength Training and Stretching Exercises

As we described in chapter 7, strength training (also called resistance exercise) isn't just for young hunks looking to bulk up. For men and women of all ages, strength training helps maintain a healthy body weight and can be an effective component of any effort to lose excessive fat. As people approach and enter the senior years, resistance exercise helps maintain the muscles needed to perform ordinary tasks that require a modest degree of physical strength. It also maintains or increases bone density and physical coordination, thus reducing the risk for common strains, sprains, and falls—or the fractures that might result from them.

Resistance training doesn't require fancy equipment or the weight machines found in gyms (although there's nothing wrong with using these if you have access to them and know how to use them properly). Elastic exercise bands or tubes and free weights such as dumbbells or barbells are relatively inexpensive and can be a great investment in your health. However, almost anything around your house that can be grasped easily and lifted can provide resistance. For example, a beginner who wants to start strengthening muscles can lift soup cans or milk jugs. Other resistance exercises (such as push-ups) require only the weight of your body.

Do I Need a Personal Trainer?

Before you begin a resistance training program, you may wish to consider hiring a personal trainer, either to help you get started or for the long term. Even those who are relatively experienced with resistance exercises may find it helpful to work with a trainer, at least for a while. Not long ago, personal trainers were an option only for the wealthy. Today, not only are the rates charged by trainers more affordable, but hiring a personal trainer is also easier. In addition to assisting you at health clubs and gyms, many trainers will come to your home.

Why consider a personal trainer? A personal trainer can help you define your goals and understand the amount of time it may take you to reach them. He or she can then work with you to design a personalized exercise program to achieve your goals and provide ongoing encouragement to stick with it. A trainer will also help you become familiar with the various resistance exercises and show you how to do them properly. This is important, because there are right and wrong ways to do even the simplest exercises. Improper form not only will cause your exercise routine to be less effective but will also greatly increase your risk of injury.

You can find the names of personal trainers in the telephone book, but how will you know if he or she is the right one for you? Here are some points to consider when choosing a trainer.

- Your trainer should have an educational background in physiology, kinesiology, athletics, or a similar field and be certified by an agency such as the American College of Sports Medicine, the National Strength and Conditioning Association, the American Council on Exercise, or another reputable certifying body. A good trainer should also keep up with current research and new techniques to provide the safest and most effective instruction for his or her clients.

- A qualified trainer should be able to explain clearly his or her policies concerning services offered, fees, and cancellations. To get an idea of what sounds reasonable (and what doesn't), call some local gyms or friends who have used trainers to get a range of typical charges in your area.

- A trainer should be certified in first aid and CPR, and should also carry liability insurance.

- A reputable personal trainer will provide references. You should call two or three of the trainer's clients and ask for candid and specific feedback regarding their level of satisfaction.

- You should avoid hiring a trainer of the opposite sex, since some physical contact, however limited, is virtually inevitable during the training process. This is especially important if you are planning to have a trainer come to your home. Needless to say, if he or she seems interested in pursuing anything beyond a professional relationship, you should find a new trainer.

- Finally and most important, you should feel comfortable with your trainer, as well as his or her communication style and approach to fitness. The trainer should be willing to work with you at your current level of fitness and should answer your questions clearly, using vocabulary you understand. If you don't know your "lats" from your "quads," the trainer should be willing and able to explain unfamiliar terminology.

Important: If you don't understand what a trainer is telling you to do for a certain exercise, do not proceed until you do understand. (He or she may need to demonstrate and walk you through the exercise.) Also, it is likely that you may not remember all of the fine points (or even some of the simple ones) of a new exercise from one session to the next. Be sure to review your exercises with the trainer until you are consistently doing them correctly. If you feel that a trainer is becoming bored or impatient with your questions or need for review, consider making a change.

Resistance Training Done Right

To get the most benefit out of resistance training, let's recap some advice given in chapter 7.

- **How often should I exercise?** To gain the most benefit from resistance training, you should perform your strength training routine two or three times each week, allowing a day or two between sessions. Muscles recover, and consequently grow stronger, during periods of rest following exercise.
- **How many muscle groups should I exercise?** For most people, exercising eight to ten of the major muscles or muscle groups will provide a good all-around benefit. During your workouts, it is important to exercise opposing muscle groups. For example, if you exercise the muscles in your abdomen, you should also exercise those in your lower back. By increasing the strength of both sets of muscles, you reduce the risk of injury in weaker muscles when stronger ones are used.
- **How many repetitions (or reps) of a given exercise should I perform?** For each muscle/muscle group, eight to twelve reps are appropriate for those younger than fifty to sixty years of age. Ten to fifteen reps, using a lower resistance, are appropriate for people over fifty or for those with heart disease (with the approval of their physician). Seniors who exercise are less likely to be injured if they do a greater number of repetitions with less resistance.
- **How many sets should I do?** One set of reps per workout is appropriate for those starting a new exercise regimen, for those who are starting up again after not exercising for an extended length of time,

or for those just looking to perform some basic health maintenance. Those looking to increase their strength should consider increasing to two sets per workout after several weeks of exercising.

- **How much resistance is appropriate?** If you are just starting out, it's wise to go easy. If lifting, use a light weight that will allow you to perform ten to twelve reps. Once this becomes somewhat easy, increase the weight by about 5 percent. Do not increase weights beyond your ability to perform at least eight reps. However, very light resistance that allows you to perform dozens of reps will not result in increased strength.

Getting Started

Safety is a priority for anyone undertaking a new resistance-training regimen. As a first step, anyone with one or more of the following medical problems should consult a physician before undertaking an exercise program:

- A history of heart disease, including coronary artery disease, congestive heart failure, an irregular rhythm, an abnormal valve, or a congenital (present from birth) abnormality.
- Symptoms that suggest something may be wrong with the heart, including episodes of chest pain or pressure, pounding, or fluttering sensations in the chest (known as palpitations), or shortness of breath from mild exertion such as climbing a flight of stairs or walking a short distance. Remember that chest discomfort arising from an area of heart muscle that is short on oxygen may not even be felt in the chest. It may instead be noticed in the left arm, jaw, or upper abdomen.

In addition, men over forty and women over fifty who plan to begin exercising vigorously or to advance from moderate to more intense exercise should be cleared by their physician, even if they feel perfectly well.

Even if you have none of the problems listed above, or if you have one or more medical issues but your health-care provider has cleared you to exercise, use common sense when working out. If you've suffered an injury, take extra care not to aggravate it. Try to avoid exercises that use muscles in the injured or affected area unless otherwise directed by your health-care provider. If you experience pain during any exercise, stop immediately.

Once you are ready to start exercising, make sure you warm up properly. Plunging into a heavy resistance routine without properly warming up and lightly stretching muscles can lead to painful strains. Most trainers recommend doing some brief low-intensity aerobic exercise (such as brisk walking) to warm up muscles before doing more vigorous exercise. This increases blood flow and prepares your muscles and your heart for increased activity. Gently stretching the muscles will also help prevent injury. Remember to stretch slowly and gently rather than "bouncing" or jerking the muscles. For more information on helpful stretches, see pages 940–943.

Most trainers also recommend cooling down after a workout to allow the heart to return to its resting rate gradually. A low-intensity aerobic exercise, such as brisk walking, is a great way to cool down. Likewise, resistance exercises should be followed by some brief stretching exercises. These will not only help reduce tightness but can help the muscles recover more quickly after a workout.

While exercising, be sure to stand on a nonskid surface, with feet wide enough apart to allow you to keep your balance comfortably. Some exercises such as crunches or push-ups from the knees can be uncomfortable if done on a hard floor. A cushioned exercise mat is a good investment if you plan to do these types of exercise. A weight bench—although not necessary for many common resistance exercises (including most of those listed on the next few pages)—can also be helpful, especially if you wish to increase your repertoire of weight-lifting exercises.

During the lift phase of an exercise, take about two seconds to lift the weight, and lower the weight over a span of about four seconds. The object is not to move the weight to its final destination as fast as possible, but to exercise the lifting muscle efficiently. While lifting and lowering, breathe evenly and steadily, exhaling on the lift and inhaling on the lowering. Try to avoid grunting or holding your breath during lifts.

Keep a log, recording which exercises you do, how many reps and sets of each are done, and how much weight you lift during each exercise. This will allow you to track your progress and will help you pace yourself as you work to maintain or increase your strength.

Which Muscles Should I Exercise?

There are literally hundreds of different resistance exercises, some involving a large number of muscles and others focused on only one or a few. The person who wants to achieve wide-ranging benefits from strength training should adopt a basic routine that engages a broad spectrum of muscles of the arms, legs, chest, abdomen, and back. (This should be modified, of course, if you have had an injury or are dealing with other limitations in one of these areas. In such cases you should check with your physician or a physical therapist before exercising that area.) On the following six pages, you'll find examples of some basic exercises for the major muscle groups of the body.

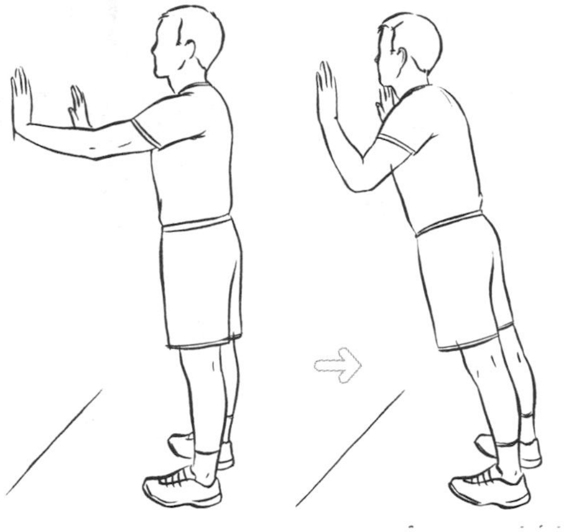

Chest

Exercises that target the muscles of the chest also provide a good workout for the upper arms. These chest exercises are listed in order of increasing difficulty and intensity.

Wall push-ups

1. Stand facing a wall, with your feet about one or two feet from the wall and a comfortable distance apart.
2. Place your hands against the wall and lean toward it.
3. Push away from the wall, then slowly lean forward again.

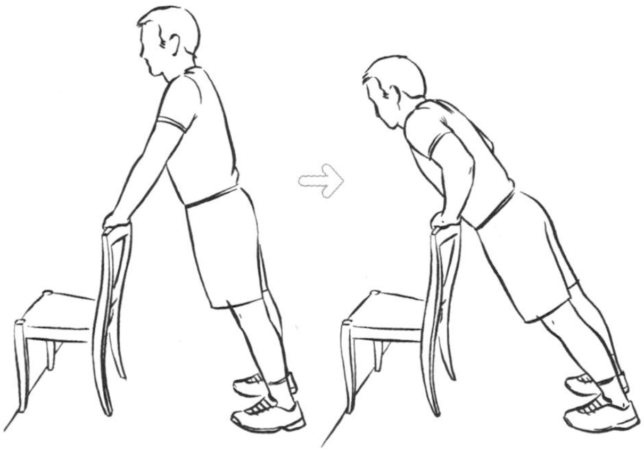

Chair push-ups

1. Position a stable chair against a wall so that it will not shift or tilt when your weight is pressed against it.
2. Standing two to three feet away from the chair, place your hands on the back of the chair and slowly lower your body forward, with your back kept straight.
3. Extend your arms to push away from the chair.

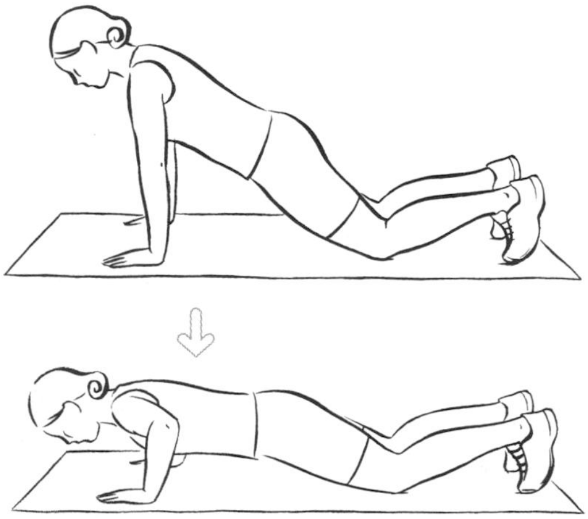

Push-ups from knees

1. Lying facedown on a cushioned exercise mat, place your hands directly under your shoulders and push your body up, pivoting the lower body from the knees. Keep your back straight.
2. Slowly bend your elbows and return to the facedown position.

Push-ups from toes
1. Lying facedown on a cushioned exercise mat, place your hands under your shoulders and push your body up, pivoting the lower body from the toes. Keep your back straight.
2. Slowly bend your elbows and return to the facedown position.

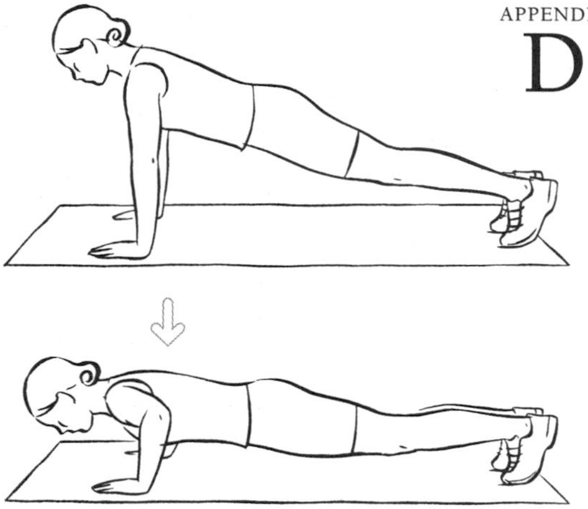

Upper back
One-arm row
This exercise also works the upper arms.
1. Hold a dumbbell with one hand and rest the opposite knee on a bench.
2. Bend forward, keeping your free hand on the bench to support your upper body. Keep your back straight, bending from the hips.
3. Slowly lift the weight by drawing your elbow upward until your upper arm is close to your body and parallel to the floor, and your elbow is bent at a ninety-degree angle.

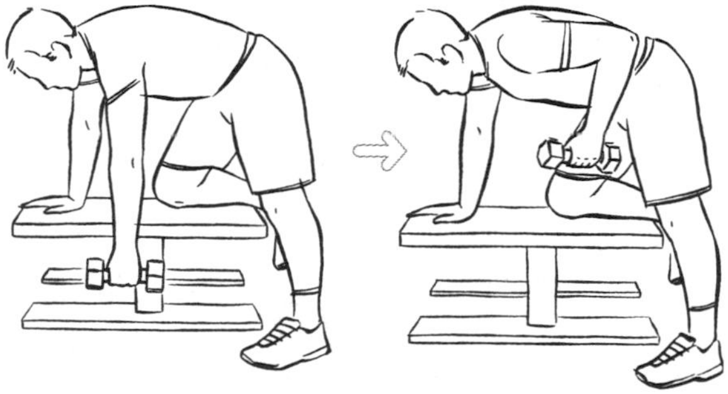

Upright row
This exercise also works the shoulders and forearms.
1. With feet spaced comfortably apart, hold a barbell with both hands, palms inward, near the middle of the bar. Your hands should be six to eight inches apart.
2. Draw the bar upward toward your chin, keeping your elbows higher than your wrists.

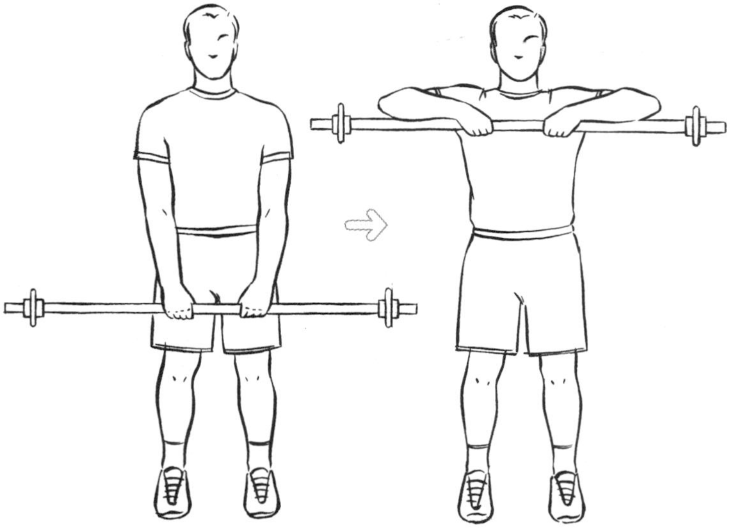

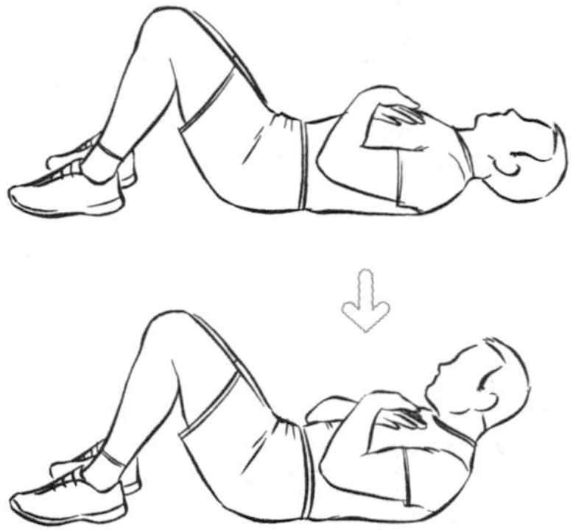

Abdomen

Crunches

1. Lie faceup on a cushioned exercise mat, with your knees bent at a ninety-degree angle.
2. You can cross your arms in front of your chest or place your hands behind or on the sides of your head to support it. Do not use your hands to pull your head forward.
3. Keeping the neck aligned straight with the spine, use your abdominal muscles to lift your upper body slowly so that your shoulder blades are off the mat.
4. Slowly relax the crunch so that your back is flat on the mat.

Lower back

These exercises are listed in order of increasing difficulty and intensity.

Prone neck lifts

1. Lie facedown on an exercise mat with your arms at your sides.
2. Using the muscles of the lower back, lift your head and torso off the mat. Try to keep your neck straight with your back.

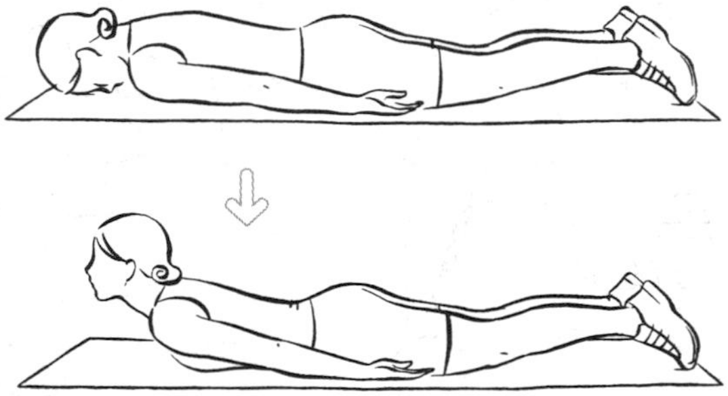

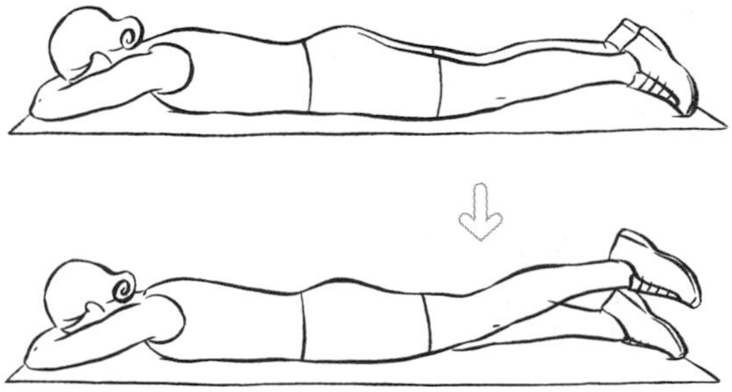

Prone leg lifts

1. Lie facedown on an exercise mat with arms at your sides or under your forehead for comfort.
2. Lift one leg off the mat six to twelve inches, keeping the knee straight.
3. Slowly lower your leg and repeat with the other leg.

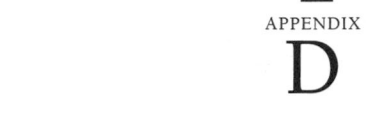

Prone leg and neck lifts

1. Lie facedown on an exercise mat with your hands palm-down on the mat, above the shoulders.
2. Using the muscles of the lower back, lift your head and torso off the mat while lifting one leg off the mat six to twelve inches.
3. Keep the knee of the lifted leg straight, and use your hands only for maintaining stability, not for lifting.
4. Try to keep your neck straight with your back, and keep your hips in contact with the floor.

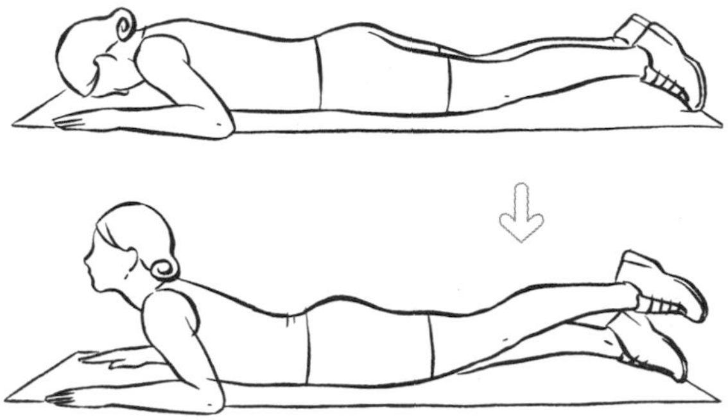

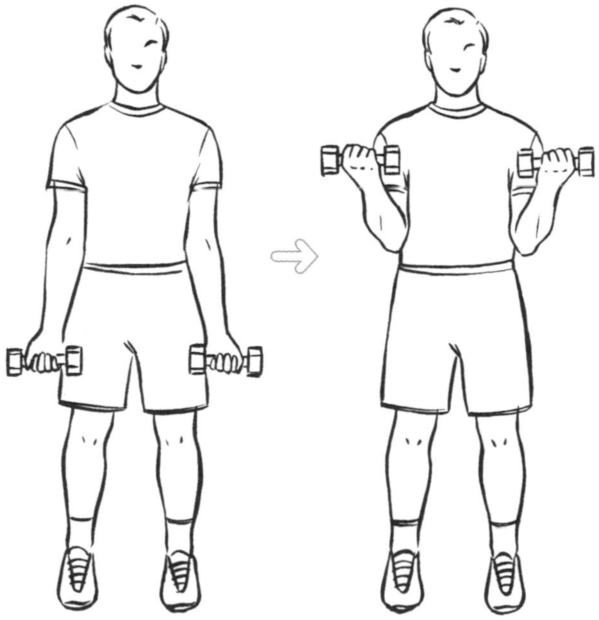

Upper arms (biceps)

Dumbbell curls

1. With arms at your sides, hold weights in each hand so that palms are facing upward.
2. Bending your arms at the elbow, lift the weights toward your shoulders.

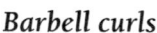

Barbell curls

1. With arms at your sides, hold the barbell so that your palms are facing outward.
2. Bending your arms at the elbow, lift the barbell toward the shoulders.

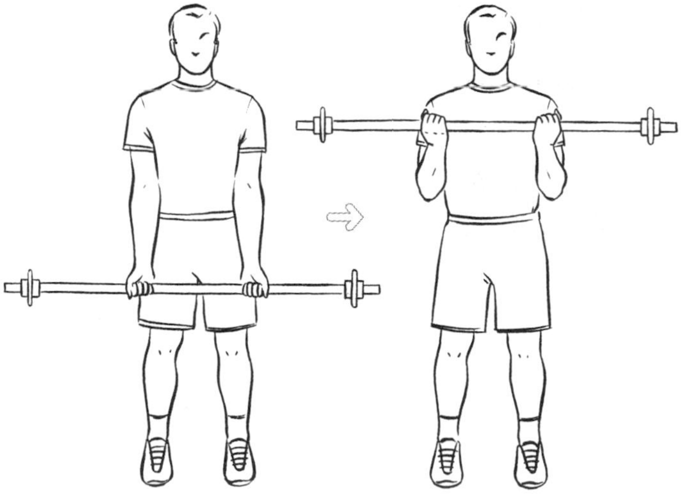

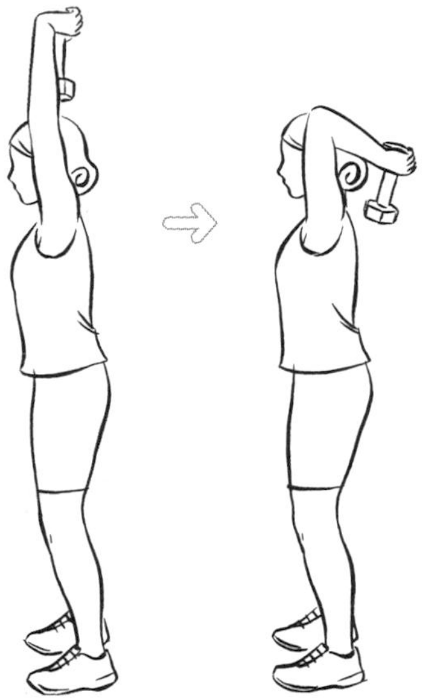

Upper arms (triceps)

Triceps extension

1. Use both hands to grasp one end of a dumbbell, allowing the other end to hang downward.
2. Position the dumbbell overhead, keeping the elbows straight.
3. Slowly lower the dumbbell behind your head by bending your elbows, keeping your upper arms close to your head.
4. Slowly lift the dumbbell above your head.

Triceps kickback

1. Hold a dumbbell with one hand and rest the opposite knee on a bench.
2. Lean forward, keeping your free hand on the bench to support your upper body.
3. Position the arm holding the weight so that the upper arm is close to the body and parallel to the floor, with the elbow bent at a ninety-degree angle.
4. Slowly move the weight by extending your forearm backward until your entire arm is parallel to the floor.

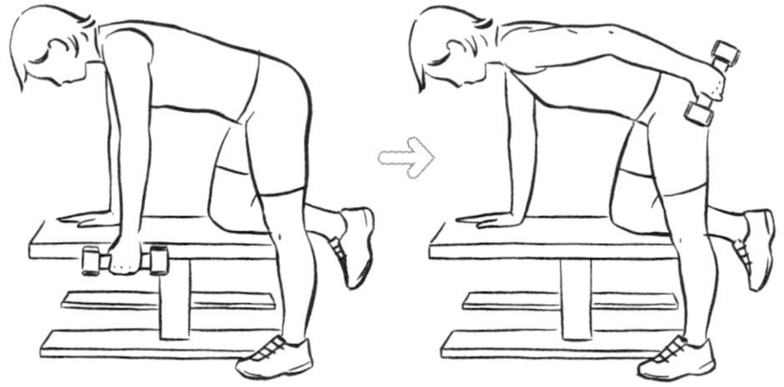

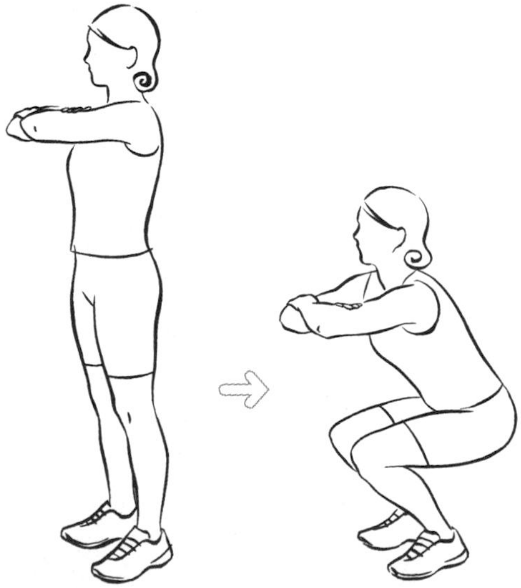

Legs

Squats

This exercise strengthens the quadriceps but also works the buttocks and hamstrings.

1. Cross your arms at your chest and stand with your feet slightly apart.
2. Flex your knees until your thighs are parallel to the floor.
3. Extend your knees and hips until you are standing upright again.
4. For increased intensity, hold dumbbells at your sides while doing this exercise.

Lunges

This exercise works the quadriceps (front of thighs) as well as the hamstrings (back of thighs) and the buttocks.

1. Stand with both feet flat on the floor.
2. With your left foot, take one large step forward, leaving the right foot in its starting position.
3. Slowly flex the left hip and knee and lower the right knee until it almost touches the ground. Your weight should be evenly distributed between your left foot (planted flat on the floor) and the ball of your right foot, while your back remains straight and perpendicular to the ground.
4. Return to the upright position by extending your left hip and knee.
5. Bring the left foot back to the starting position. Repeat the exercise with the right foot forward. The intensity of this exercise can be increased by holding dumbbells or other weights in each hand.

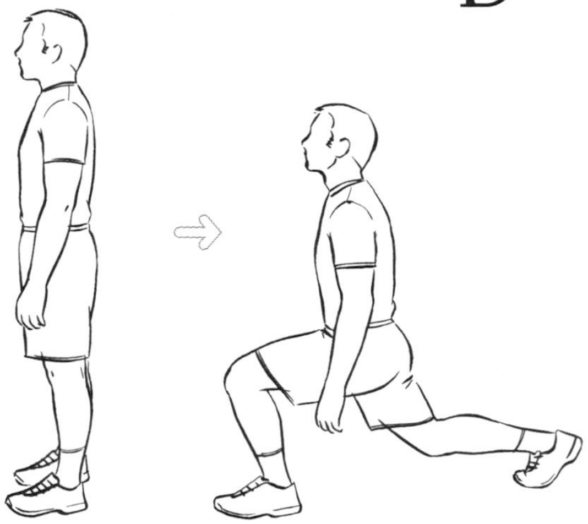

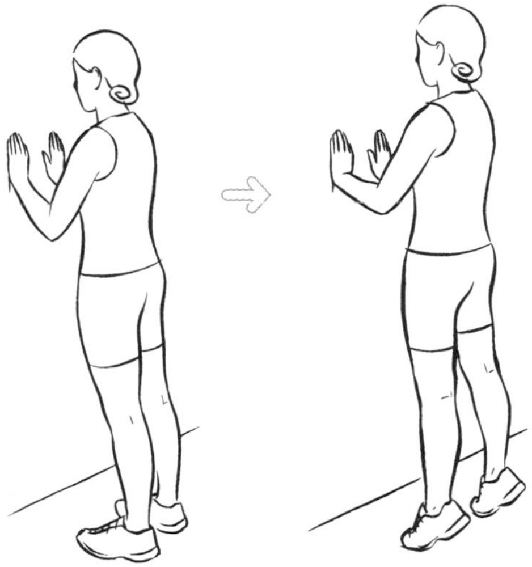

Calf raises

1. Starting with your feet flat on the floor and holding on to a secure surface for support, push upward on your toes as high as you can.
2. For a more intense workout, stand with the balls of the feet on a secure raised surface, such as a two-by-four, and start with the heels below the level of the raised surface.
3. Holding dumbbells while performing this exercise will also increase its intensity.

STRETCHING

When encouraged to do stretching exercises, some people protest, "I'm not flexible enough to do that." They may have the misconception that stretching is for gymnasts or contortionists. They also may have noticed enough stiffness, creaks, and groans from their joints and muscles to decide that stretching is literally out of their reach. Yet the point of stretching is not to become a human pretzel or to learn how to bend over backward to tie one's shoes. The major goal of stretching for most of us is to maintain whatever flexibility and range of motion we already have. As we grow older, stretching becomes more and more important to preserve our ability to move our joints and muscles freely. A second major goal, as discussed in chapter 7, is to fend off exercise-induced pains and strains. Failing to stretch properly before a brisk workout or burst of activity can lead to muscle or joint injury. In addition, stretching can be a great way to relax and reduce muscle tension.

Getting Started

Your health and safety are of primary importance. Be sure to consult your health-care provider before you start a stretching program if any of the following apply to you:

- You have been sedentary for a significant length of time.
- You have any type of musculoskeletal disorder.
- You have been injured recently.
- You have undergone surgery recently.

As with all types of exercise, it is unwise to begin a stretching routine without first warming up. "Cold" muscles do not like to be stretched and are apt to quickly and painfully indicate their displeasure when rapidly or intensely stretched. A low-intensity aerobic exercise, such as brisk walking, is a good way to warm up muscles before starting your stretching routine. As you do these exercises, stretch slowly until you feel mild tension but not pain. Increase tension steadily, maintain it for the prescribed time, then release tension slowly. Do not overstretch, and do not bounce or jerk the muscles. Breathe normally during the stretch to relax as much as possible.

What to Stretch

Just about every muscle in the body can be stretched, from facial muscles to those in the feet. If you are preparing to exercise a particular part of your body, it is important to warm up and stretch the muscles in that area. For example, if you are planning to lift weights, it is important to prepare and stretch the muscles of the upper body, including the arms, chest, and back. If you are planning on walking or running, you should stretch the muscles of the calves and thighs.

Listed below are just a few of the many stretches that can help you maintain flexibility, feel less tense, and prepare your muscles for exercising. An excellent resource with more information is *Stretching* by Bob Anderson (Bolinas, Calf.: Shelter Publications, 1980, 2000). This comprehensive and well-illustrated book walks readers through a wide variety of stretches for various parts of the body.

Neck

1. Tilt your head toward your left shoulder, using your left hand, with the palm on top of your head, to hold your head gently in this position. Hold for ten seconds.
2. Release the stretch slowly and repeat, tilting the head to the right.
3. Perform this stretch twice for each side.

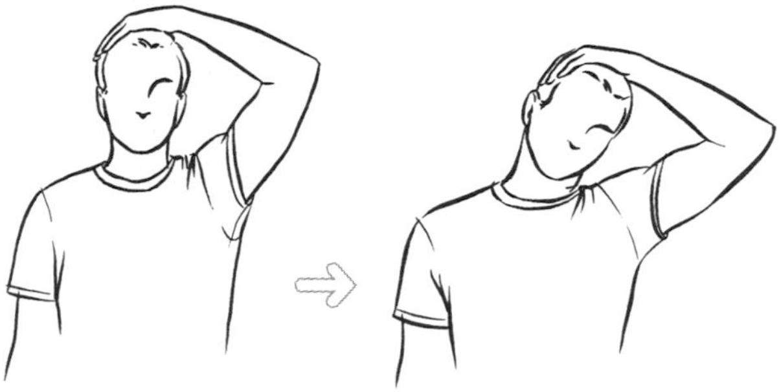

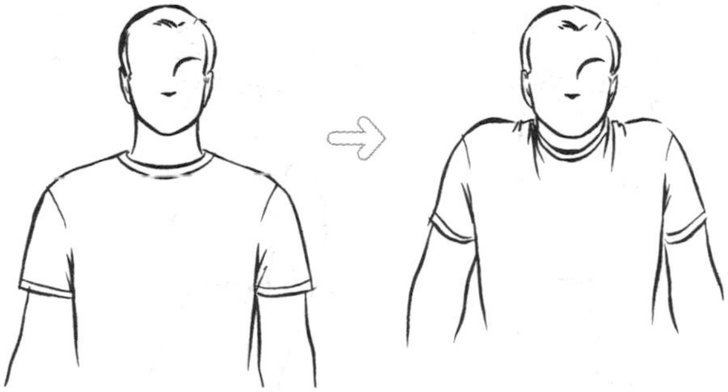

Shoulders

1. Raise both shoulders up toward your ears, as if you're shrugging. Hold for five seconds.
2. Slowly relax and completely release the shoulders downward and toward the back, so that you feel your shoulder blades come closer together. (This will help improve your posture.) Perform two to four times.

Upper arms and shoulders

1. Bring your right hand across your chest and place it on your left shoulder.
2. Place your left hand on your right arm just above the elbow, and gently pull toward your left shoulder. Hold this stretch for ten seconds.
3. Repeat with the other side, stretching the left upper arm and shoulder.

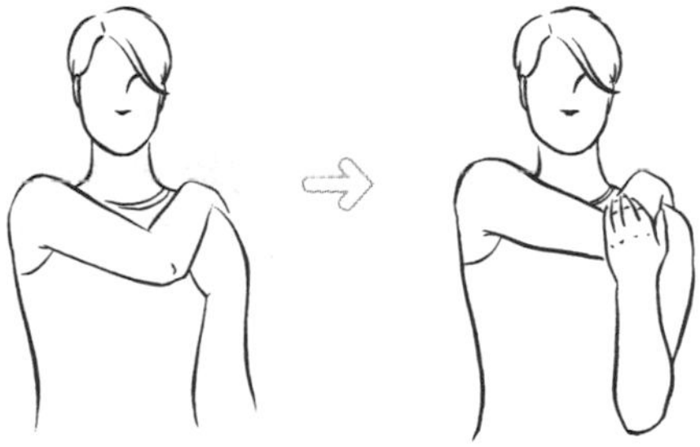

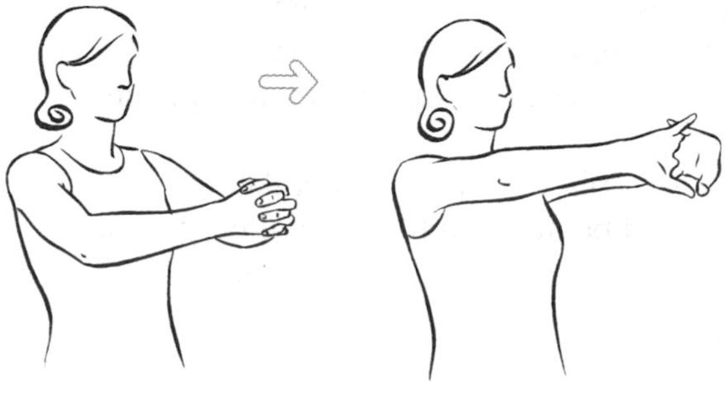

Upper and lower arms

1. Interlace fingers of both hands and turn palms outward in front of you at shoulder height.
2. Gently extend arms in front of you. Hold stretch for fifteen to twenty seconds.

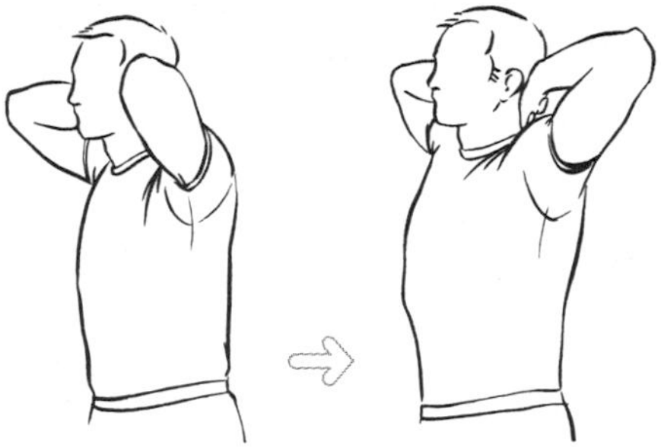

Upper back

1. Interlace fingers of both hands behind your head.
2. Without pushing forward on your head with your hands, gently draw elbows backward and pull shoulder blades together until mild tension is felt.
3. Hold the stretch for ten seconds, then gently relax.

Lower back

1. Stand with feet placed comfortably apart and knees slightly bent.
2. Place your hands on your lower back above the hips, and push your palms forward to gently arch the lower back. Hold the stretch for ten seconds.

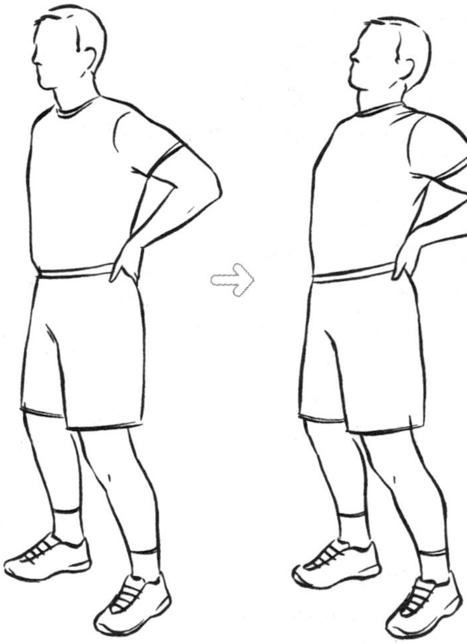

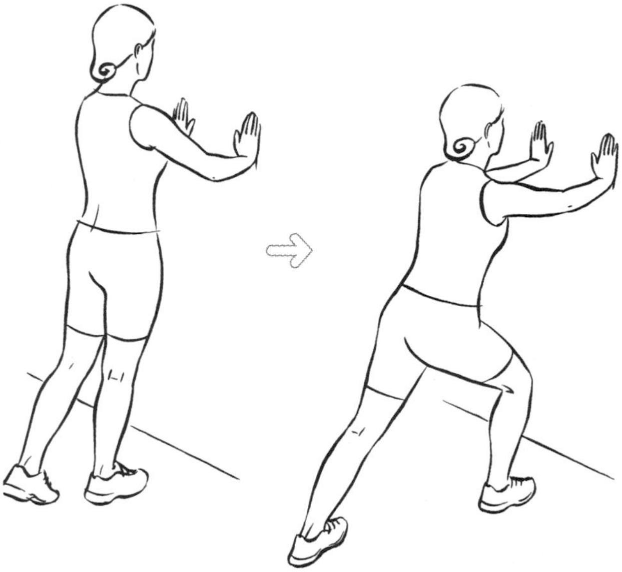

Calves

1. Lean forward against a wall, bend your right leg, and place your right foot flat on the ground in front of you.
2. Place your left foot flat on the ground behind you, with the left knee straight.
3. Slowly move your hips forward to stretch the left calf. Hold the stretch for ten to fifteen seconds.
4. Repeat, placing the right foot flat on the ground behind you to stretch the right calf.

Quadriceps (front of thighs)

You can stretch this large muscle group while lying down or standing up. If you have any problems with balance, do this exercise lying down.

Lying position:

1. Lie on your left side, supporting your head with your left hand.
2. Bend your right knee and reach back with your right hand to grasp the top of your right foot, pulling it gently toward your right buttock. Hold the stretch for ten to twenty seconds.
3. Repeat to stretch the left quadriceps, lying on your right side.

Standing position:

1. Stand on your left foot, steadying yourself with your left hand by leaning against an immovable object.
2. Bend your right knee and reach back with your right hand to grasp the top of your right foot, pulling it gently toward your right buttock. Hold the stretch for ten to twenty seconds.
3. Repeat to stretch the left quadriceps, standing on your right foot.

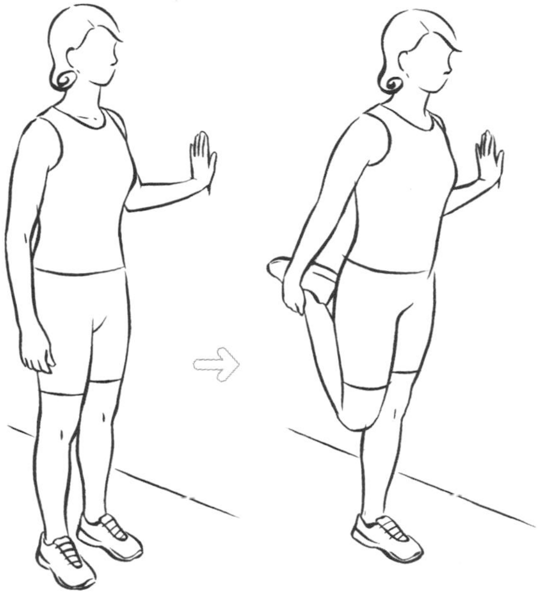

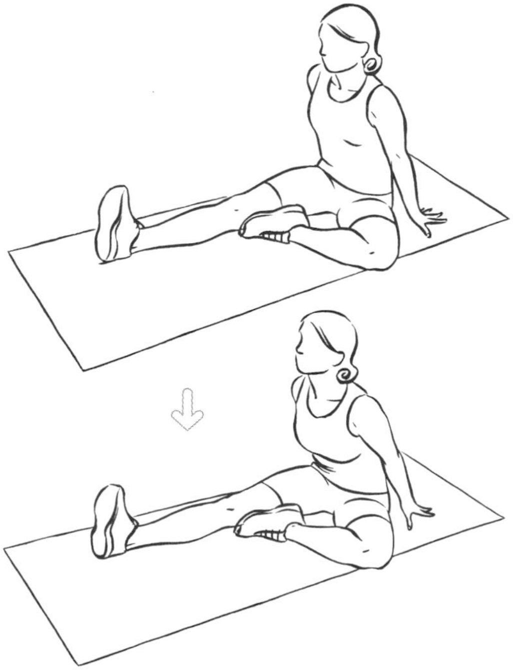

Hamstrings (back of thighs)

1. Sit on the floor with your left knee bent and the sole of your left foot touching your right inner thigh. Extend your right leg.
2. Gently bend forward from your hips to create mild tension in the back of the right leg.
3. Repeat to stretch the left hamstring, bending the right leg and keeping the left leg straight.

APPENDIX E

Common Sexual Dysfunctions

As we mentioned in chapter 12, both men and women can experience sexual dysfunction. This can arise from medical, physiological, psychological, or relational causes, or a combination of factors. Our intention here is to provide a basic overview of the more common sexual dysfunctions and to help an individual or couple begin a conversation with a counselor, physician, or both to find help and healing.

Sexual Dysfunction in Men

Sexual dysfunction is estimated to affect nearly one in three men between the ages of eighteen and fifty-nine.[1] The three most common types of problems are decreased sexual desire, erectile dysfunction, and ejaculatory disorders.

About one in seven men will admit to feeling **decreased desire** for sex, a problem that becomes more common with age.[2] Poor general health, fatigue, emotional stress, lack of sleep, and overuse of alcohol can have a negative impact on a man's sexual desire. Disturbances in levels of various hormones—especially low **testosterone** or thyroid levels, or increased secretions of a pituitary hormone called **prolactin**—can cause decreased libido. (More on low testosterone levels in a moment.)

In addition, many types of medications can cause not only decreased libido but other sexual problems as well, especially erectile dysfunction. (See sidebar on the next page, "Medications That May Cause Sexual Dsyfunction.") Childhood molestation or sexual activity with another male (past or present) may have an impact on marital sex later in life. Finally, a decrease in sexual desire is a hallmark of depression for both men and women. Unfortunately, while antidepressants often help improve mood, with one notable exception (bupropion, or Wellbutrin) they often have a negative impact on both erectile function in men and libido in both sexes.

A low level of testosterone affects approximately 2 to 4 million men in the United States and becomes more common with advanced age. When associated with specific symptoms, this condition is called **hypogonadism**, and when it occurs in an older man it is often called **andropause**. Strictly speaking, this is not the equivalent of menopause, because while menopause occurs universally in women, hypogonadism does not affect all men. It does, however, become more common with advancing age.

Not surprisingly, low testosterone may be associated with sexual problems such as decreased libido, erectile dysfunction, and difficulty achieving an orgasm. But more generalized symptoms may occur as well, including decreased energy or overt fatigue, depression, decreased muscle mass and strength, and anemia (low red blood cell count). When appropriately treated with supplemental testosterone, men with hypogonadism may experience improvements in many of these symptoms. Until relatively recently, testosterone could only be given by injection every few weeks, but now it can be obtained through the daily application of a testosterone patch or gel that is absorbed through the skin. While testosterone replacement can be helpful when true hypogonadism is present—very often a man who believes he has a low testosterone level in fact does not—safe and appropriate use of this medication requires ongoing medical supervision.

Many men have sporadic or chronic **erectile dysfunction (ED)**. In one study of the prevalence of sexual dysfunctions, 7 percent of men in their twenties complained of difficulty obtaining or maintaining an erection adequate for

MEDICATIONS THAT MAY CAUSE SEXUAL DYSFUNCTION

A number of drugs can cause erectile problems in men or loss of libido in both men and women. Some of the more common offenders include:

- Certain types of antihypertensive (blood pressure–lowering) medications, especially beta-blockers (such as propranolol and metoprolol), alpha-blockers (such as prazosin and terazosin). Diuretics such as hydrochlorothiazide and spironolactone, may also cause sexual dysfunction, though less frequently than beta- and alpha-blockers. Two older antihypertensives that are rarely used today, methyldopa and reserpine, also commonly caused sexual dysfunction.
- Antidepressant medications, many of which are associated with both loss of libido and erectile dysfunction. This can create a dilemma when a drug significantly improves mood but interferes with sexual function. The widely used selective serotonin reuptake inhibitors (SSRIs) as well as the older tricyclic antidepressants commonly cause this problem. A number of medications used to treat psychosis and bipolar disorder may have sexual side effects as well. (We review these types of drugs in more detail in chapter 8, beginning on page 342.)
- Some nonprescription antihistamines and decongestants (used to relieve symptoms of colds and allergies), which may cause both erection and ejaculation problems. ■

initiating or completing intercourse.[3] The Massachusetts Male Aging Study reported that more than 50 percent of men between ages forty and seventy have some degree of erectile dysfunction, and that 5 percent of men at forty have complete absence of erectile function. By age seventy, this number rises to 15 percent.[4] A variety of factors can contribute to ED, and more than one may be present in the same individual. Up to 80 percent of cases are **organic** in origin, involving vascular, neurological, hormonal, or medication-induced mechanisms. A smaller percentage are **psychogenic** in origin (including cases where sexual performance is affected by circumstances and surroundings), and a number of cases involve both organic and psychogenic factors. Often a failure to obtain a satisfactory erection, for whatever reason, will in turn provoke psychogenic ED, and even a reluctance to have sex, as a result of anxiety about future sexual performance. Sorting out the specific cause(s) of ED is important, because a shortage of testosterone, as we just noted, can also lead to a combination of erectile dysfunction and loss of interest in sex.

Of all of the reasons for erectile dysfunction, the most common involves a malfunction of **vascular endothelium**, the cells that form the inner lining of blood vessels. There is often an important link between ED and underlying atherosclerosis, the diffuse disease of blood vessels that can lead to heart attack and stroke. The common risk factors for atherosclerosis, including hypertension (high blood pressure), elevated cholesterol levels, diabetes, and cigarette smoking, are also associated with erection problems, and ED may be the first indication that a man has this common condition. (For a detailed review of atherosclerosis, see chapter 3, beginning on page 45.)

Erectile dysfunction, previously referred to as **impotence**, has caused a great deal of distress to men from time immemorial, and the concoctions and devices that have been deployed over the centuries in an attempt to treat it occupy a colorful corner of medical history. Prior to the introduction of the drug **sildenafil (Viagra)** in 1998, the treatments utilized for ED were not terribly effective and often uncomfortable. This drug and its cousins **vardenafil (Levitra)** and **tadalafil (Cialis)** drastically improved the outlook for men with this problem and, not surprisingly, have been best sellers ever since. All are quite effective at improving erectile function, whether of organic or psychogenic origin, over a narrow time frame (a few to several hours after a dose of Viagra and Levitra, and about thirty-six hours after Cialis is taken). None of these drugs provoke a nonstop erection for several hours—indeed, if this occurs one should seek immediate medical attention—but rather the erection occurs in response to sexual stimulation. Also, while they may help restore a man's sexual confidence, these medications are not aphrodisiacs—that is, they don't increase libido.

Aggressive marketing of ED drugs to the general public, including invitations for men to ask for free samples from their physician, has had the positive response of starting much-needed discussions about this subject in the doctor's office, but often these begin just as a visit for some other problem is wrapping up.

(Medical professionals refer to this as the "doorknob sign" that indicates a problem with erectile dysfunction—the doctor is about to leave the exam room at the end of a visit when the patient suddenly asks, "By the way, Doc, could I get a sample of Viagra?") Here's an important tip: Primary-care physicians and urologists are usually more than willing to discuss this subject, but it involves more than simply handing out a sample. The doctor will need to gather some basic information about your experience with this problem, including its history, other medical issues (especially cardiovascular risk factors), and current medications. In particular, ED drugs and nitroglycerin (whether used in a tablet, spray, or topical form to relieve or prevent angina, the chest pain related to inadequate blood flow to the heart) do not mix well. Their combined action can cause a dramatic and hazardous fall in blood pressure. Nitroglycerin should be avoided for twelve hours after a dose of Viagra or Levitra (or for forty-eight hours after a dose of Cialis). In an emergency situation involving chest pain or pressure, medical personnel should be informed if and when one of these drugs has been taken so that blood pressure can be appropriately monitored if nitroglycerin must be given.

The most common of the **ejaculatory disorders** is **premature ejaculation**. One-third of men ejaculate sooner than they would like. Unlike erectile dysfunction, this problem occurs with similar frequency across a broad age spectrum. A climax occurring before or at the time of penetration can be particularly disturbing for both husband and wife who would prefer intercourse to last longer. Premature ejaculation can be managed using behavioral techniques, marital therapy that helps a couple verbalize feelings and expand their sexual repertoire, and even a low dose of one of the SSRI antidepressants, which often causes delayed ejaculation. (While this side effect can be helpful for men with premature ejaculation, for those without this problem the use of an SSRI may lead to delayed or inhibited ejaculation, which can be quite troublesome. More detailed information about SSRIs may be found in chapter 8 beginning on page 342.) **Retrograde ejaculation** occurs when, at orgasm, seminal fluid literally flows in the wrong direction: into the bladder rather than through the urethra and the end of the penis. This may occur after surgery involving the bladder or prostate, or more commonly may result from **diabetic neuropathy**—a complication of diabetes affecting nerve function in various parts of the body. Any new onset of delayed, absent, or retrograde ejaculation should be evaluated medically.

F.Y.I.

A detailed discussion of premature ejaculation, and some basic techniques to deal with it, may be found in *The Gift of Sex: A Guide to Sexual Fulfillment* by Dr. Clifford and Joyce Penner (Nashville: W Publishing Group, revised edition 2003).

Sexual Dysfunction in Women

An estimated 43 percent (about 40 million) of American women experience some form of sexual dysfunction, compared with 31 percent of men.[5] Interestingly, one research study involving a review of primary care physicians' office charts revealed that a sexual problem was noted in only 2 percent of adult female patients.[6] This may well reflect not only physicians' lack of awareness or inclination to broach this subject, but also female patients' reluctance to ask their physicians (especially male doctors) about sexual problems. Nevertheless, because sexual dysfunctions are often related to gynecological or other medical conditions, a candid discussion with a primary care physician or gynecologist is usually the first step toward resolving a sexual dysfunction.

There are four kinds of sexual problems in women:

- **Decreased desire** means just that—a lack of interest in having sex, or a loss of desire compared to some previous time in life.
- In an **arousal disorder**, a woman doesn't feel a physical sexual response even though she has the desire for sex, or she begins to feel a response but cannot sustain it.
- A woman with an **orgasmic disorder** has difficulty achieving an orgasm or experiences pain during orgasm.
- A **sex pain disorder** involves discomfort during or after sex. The medical term for pain associated with sex is **dyspareunia**, and three basic types have been identified. **Superficial dyspareunia** is pain when penetration is attempted and is usually caused by an anatomic condition or vaginismus. **Vaginal dyspareunia** is discomfort that occurs because of inadequate lubrication, which results in painful friction during intercourse. **Deep dyspareunia** arises from the pelvis and is associated with the thrusting of intercourse.

The female sexual experience involves a complex interaction between anatomy, physiology, hormonal status, medical conditions, emotions, relational context, stage of life, prior sexual experiences, and her moral and spiritual values. Similarly, the causes of sexual dysfunction in women are often complex and interrelated. For example, recurring episodes of pain with intercourse are likely to have a serious dampening effect on a woman's desire for sex, and this will be even more profound if her relationship with her husband is turbulent. Several important factors need to be considered when dealing with female sexual problems:

Age and seasons of life very often are associated with predictable changes in a woman's interest in sex. For example, a woman's sexual appetite is likely to increase when she desires to become pregnant and decrease during the weeks after she delivers a baby. Physical and hormonal changes related to menopause may reduce a woman's sex drive and cause increased physical discomfort during intercourse because of thinning and drying of the vaginal lining, as well as other changes in the pelvis. These are but a few of the many scenarios in which consultation with a trusted primary care physician or gynecologist is important to determine whether specific interventions—for example, estrogen therapy to improve the lining and lubrication of the vagina after menopause—are appropriate.

Medical conditions such as the following can profoundly influence a woman's sexual experience:

- Physical abnormalities of the genitalia or pelvis that are congenital or develop later in life, including those that result from injury or medical procedures such as surgery or radiation therapy
- A mastectomy, which can cause a woman to feel less desirable and thus affect her sexual interest and response
- Infections such as genital herpes, human papillomavirus (HPV), or *Candida* vaginitis
- Involuntary contractions of the vaginal muscles, known as vaginismus
- Any ongoing or recurrent medical problem that affects her sense of well-being—chronic pain, cancer and its treatment, obesity, arthritis, recurrent headaches, intestinal problems such as irritable bowel syndrome or colitis, and so on
- Medications for a variety of conditions that dampen sexual interest and response, including those noted in the sidebar: "Medications That May Cause Sexual Dysfunction" on page 946.

Relational, psychological, and emotional issues often have a profound impact on a woman's sexual desire and response. These can include marital conflict, stress and fatigue related to the everyday demands of parenting or career, depression and self-image concerns (including negative perceptions of her physical appearance and overall worthiness, especially in comparison with impossibly sleek and stylish models and movie stars). Remember also that a number of medications effective in treating depression frequently diminish both libido and physical response to sex.

Negative or conflicted attitudes about sexuality may seriously dampen a woman's interest in sex. These might arise from a family, cultural, or religious background that views sexuality as shameful. Sexual abuse or rape as a child, teen, or adult can have lifelong repercussions, not only on a woman's attitude and response to sex but her life as a whole. Of particular importance is her first experience with sex—her **sexual debut**, as it is called in the medical literature. As we discussed in chapter 12, a woman's overall perspective on sex is likely to be strongly affected by the setting and quality of this experience.

A thorough exploration of the diagnosis and treatment of female sexual dysfunctions cannot be covered here. However, a few observations about some specific problems might be helpful:

Arousal disorders become more common as a woman ages, for two primary reasons. First, older women need more stimulation to reach levels of arousal that were more easily attained at a younger age. Solutions often involve nonmedical approaches such as adequate foreplay, a warm bath before intercourse, and strategies to reduce anxiety. Second, postmenopausal changes in the vagina and pelvis can cause discomfort during intercourse. This can often be alleviated with estrogen supplementation (including vaginal preparations for women who do not want to use oral or patch forms that increase levels throughout the body) or nonprescription lubricants. (See "When the Cycles End—Menopause and Its Aftermath" in chapter 13, beginning on page 653, for more information on hormone therapy.)

An **orgasmic disorder** may have several causes, including sexual inexperience, lack of stimulation, the side effects of a medication, or chronic disease. One of many reasons for confining sex to a loving, permanent relationship is the fact that nonmarital intercourse, especially at a young age, may contribute to difficulty achieving orgasms later in life. The female orgasm is often related to the length of time spent during lovemaking, as well as a woman's feelings of emotional connectedness with her partner. Women who begin their sexual experiences as unmarried teenagers are likely to be involved with men who do not selflessly dedicate themselves to their partner. For most women, an orgasm is not automatic; it is a work of art that may take years under the right circumstances to perfect.

Women with orgasmic disorder usually feel a tremendous amount of shame about their "defect." Many adult women who are well-informed about other areas of life may be unsure what an orgasm even *is*. They usually have heard a lot about this phenomenon (and have seen a male partner routinely enjoying his sexual climax) but are not sure they have ever experienced one. Women who have their first orgasm after years of having sex without it are usually surprised, because they assumed that any rising excitement they felt during sex was, by itself, the orgasm. They didn't understand that an orgasm is an unmistakable event. However, they may have an idea what it looks and sounds like (especially if they have seen films with sexual content) and may make enough of the "right sounds" to convince their partner that they have, indeed, arrived at sexual ecstasy. Why do many women fake having an orgasm? Because the popular media has convinced them that *every* normal woman has an orgasm *every* time, and they are too ashamed to admit that they don't, let alone seek help for it. So they keep on pretending, and they grow increasingly miserable over the years because they feel like such a failure in this area.

The good news is that of all the female sexual dysfunctions, this one is the most responsive to therapy, beginning with a trip to the doctor's office to rule out any medical issues (especially medications that interfere with sexual response). After that, a woman and her partner generally need some education about how the body works. Because most women report that orgasm is directly related to clitoral stimulation, she may need to get a book and a mirror and find out what and where the clitoris is. She and her partner need to explore it; the proper amount and timing of clitoral stimulation is often the key to overcoming orgasmic difficulties.

Because orgasmic disorders may be emotional in origin, counseling may be very important in dealing with issues such as marital dissatisfaction, childhood sexual abuse, poor self-concept, negative messages about sex from the family while growing up, and religious inhibitions. Other techniques for both husband and wife may be helpful, including:

- Learning how to talk openly about their sexual relationship to decrease anxiety surrounding sex
- **Sensate focus**, which involves exploring each other's bodies in an ordered way, beginning with nonsexual touch and then progressing to sexual intercourse after many sessions
- **Systematic desensitization**, which allows a woman to practice deep relaxation exercises as she deliberately imagines scenarios of sexual situations that she finds threatening

Evaluation of sex pain disorders should begin with a medical consultation, ideally with someone who has experience in this area. This will usually be a gynecologist, who in some cases may refer a woman to a local or regional specialist who has expertise in addressing this problem The physical exam will typically include an effort to pinpoint the exact location of the pain in order to better understand its origin. **Vaginismus** (the involuntary contraction of the muscles of the outer third of the vagina) is often associated with sexual phobias or past sexual trauma. It may occur only during attempts at intercourse and thus may be difficult to reproduce in the physician's examination room. Treatment for vaginismus includes progressive muscle relaxation and vaginal dilation, which may involve inserting commercial dilators or tampons of increasing diameter into the vagina twice daily for fifteen minutes. Working with a counselor who specializes in the healing of sexual trauma is also recommended.

A final thought on sexual dysfunctions: It is critical that problems with sex in marriage not be swept under the bed, so to speak, but addressed honestly, carefully, and patiently. God designed sex for our enjoyment and fulfillment, and this area of life deserves to be properly nurtured and maintained as much as any other aspect of health. Even if you feel hesitant to do so, don't neglect seeking help from a qualified physician or counselor if your sexual experience is unsatisfying, uncomfortable, or a source of turbulence in your marriage.

APPENDIX F

Hormone Therapy Controversies: A Closer Look at the HERS and WHI Studies

Until the 1990s, most of the conclusions about hormone therapy (HT) and its effects on women were drawn from **observational studies**. These gather information about people's lives and habits in order to determine how various factors impact health or disease, without attempting to influence what happens. They can provide illuminating information about health matters—for example, they have established the link between tobacco use and many forms of cancer and heart disease—but they are not considered the gold standard in research. That title is reserved for what is called a **randomized placebo-controlled double-blind study,** which theoretically can control more variables than an observational one. (For a more detailed look at this important aspect of medical research, see the section in chapter 17, "A Primer on Research and Evidence: How Do We Know What Causes What?") As it turns out, two studies of the latter type have had a profound effect on attitudes regarding HT among women and their physicians over the past few years. Because of their impact on the use—or non-use—of hormones after menopause in the United States (and elsewhere), we are going to examine these studies in some detail.

In 1998 the *Journal of the American Medical Association* published the **Heart and Estrogen/Progestin Replacement Study (HERS)**, a randomized, placebo-controlled, double-blind study that was intended to address the effects of hormone therapy on women with known coronary heart disease (CHD). More than 2,700 women with CHD were recruited, with an average age of sixty-seven at the beginning of the study. Half of these received a combination estrogen/progestin pill and the other half a placebo. (Remember that progestin is a synthetic form of the hormone progesterone.) They were followed for an average of about four years, and while several outcomes were evaluated, the primary focus was on nonfatal heart attack and death due to CHD.

As we just mentioned, previous observational studies suggested that taking HT from the onset of menopause would cut a woman's risk of a future heart attack in half. However, the HERS study found that overall there were no significant differences between the estrogen/progestin group and the placebo group in the number of women who would have a heart attack or die from CHD. Additional analysis of the data showed that women who took the hormones had *more* CHD events in the first year of the study but experienced *fewer* in the fourth and fifth years, compared to the placebo group. Moreover, women who received the hormones developed blood clots in the deep veins of the leg or pelvis (called **deep vein thrombosis** or **DVT**) two to three times as frequently as women who took the placebo. These require treatment with anticoagulant medications to reduce the likelihood that they will increase in size or break loose and float into one of the arteries supplying the lung, a potentially dangerous event called a **pulmonary embolus**.

Because the women who received estrogen and progestin appeared to experience a reduction in CHD events during the fourth and fifth years of the study, researchers began a second phase (designated HERS II) to determine whether this apparent protection would continue over a longer period of time. It didn't. After less than three additional years of follow-up, the HERS women who continued taking hormone supplements did not fare any better from a coronary heart disease standpoint than those who did not. Furthermore, HERS II looked at a number of other outcomes, including blood clots, cancer, fractures, and total mortality (that is, death from all causes). The news was not particularly good: Throughout a period of roughly seven years encompassed by HERS and HERS II, older women with existing cardiovascular disease who took estrogen and progestin were more likely to have venous blood clots and biliary tract surgery than those who did not take hormones.

The biliary tract includes the gallbladder and the bile ducts, the tubes that transport bile from the liver to the intestine. The most common type of surgery in this area is removal of the gallbladder, usually to relieve pain and other problems arising from gallstones.

The rates of cancer, fracture, and total mortality were not significantly different between the HT and placebo groups.

Needless to say, the announcement of the results of these studies seriously undermined the widespread confidence in HT as a defender of a woman's cardiovascular health. In fact, based on HERS and HERS II data, professional organizations such as the American Heart Association recommended that menopausal women *not* utilize HT solely for the specific purpose of protecting the heart against CHD. Some experts questioned whether HT offered any significant health benefits at all.

While the HERS and HERS II data were disconcerting to a lot of women and their doctors, many looked forward to the results of another ongoing study that was supposed to be more definitive—the **Women's Health Initiative (WHI)**.

The component of WHI that looked specifically at hormone therapy (which we will refer to as the WHI hormone study) included many more participants (16,608 to be exact) and was designed to examine the effects not only of estrogen plus progestin but also of estrogen alone in menopausal women.[1] (Recall that progestin is used to counteract the stimulating effects of estrogen on the endometrium. Women who have had their uterus removed have no need of progestin and can take estrogen alone for treatment of menopausal symptoms.)

F.Y.I.

The Women's Health Initiative (WHI) was a massive, fifteen-year study sponsored by the National Institutes of Health (NIH) and the National Heart, Lung and Blood Institute (NHLBI). The project was launched in an effort to identify strategies to prevent heart disease, cancer of the breast and colon, and osteoporosis in postmenopausal women, with a particular emphasis on hormone therapy, dietary habits, and the use of calcium and vitamin D supplements. Altogether more than 160,000 women between the ages of fifty and seventy-nine were enrolled in various components of the study.

This was important because physicians wanted to know if the effects seen with HT (good or bad) were due solely to estrogen or if any of them could be attributed to progestin (or progestin's effects when combined with estrogen). The WHI hormone study was designed to look at a wide range of advantages and disadvantages of HT, including possible effects on cardiovascular disease, bone loss, stroke, and blood clots, as well as cognitive decline and dementia. In short, many hoped that WHI would shed a great deal of light on these subjects, if not provide the "final word"—but ultimately it raised almost as many questions as it answered.

In one component of the study (known in research lingo as an *arm*), WHI researchers assigned women with an intact uterus to receive either estrogen plus progestin or placebo. (The hormone preparation used was Prempro, a popular and widely used combination of Premarin and medroxyprogesterone.) It was scheduled to run for eight and a half years, but in July 2002 the study's directors sent shock waves through the medical community by discontinuing it after only a little more than five years. The safety monitoring board overseeing the study recommended that it be stopped ahead of schedule because women receiving HT were found to have a 26 percent higher **relative risk** for invasive breast cancer than women in the placebo group. (The term relative risk is an important one, and we will come back to it shortly.)

Researchers also calculated that HT recipients had a 29 percent higher risk of coronary heart disease, a 41 percent higher risk of stroke, and a twofold risk of pulmonary embolism. On the positive side, the study found that women on HT had about a 34 percent lower risk of hip and vertebral fracture and a 37 percent lower risk of colorectal cancer. Nevertheless, the study's researchers considered the risks to be greater than the benefits. When the news media announced the shutdown of this arm of the WHI study, many women called their doctors looking for alternatives to HT, and many doctors began steering their patients away from combined estrogen/progestin therapy.

Because the aborted first arm of the WHI study was designed to examine the effects of estrogen combined with progestin, many hoped that estrogen alone would be found to be beneficial for menopausal women without a uterus. In the second arm of the WHI hormone study, women who had previously undergone hysterectomy were assigned to receive either estrogen (Premarin) alone or a placebo. This was carried out concurrently with the first arm (comparing estrogen/progestin vs. placebo), and when that part of the study was ended prematurely, the estrogen-only arm continued . . . for a while. Yet it too was brought to a halt prematurely in February 2004, when the safety monitoring board determined that women receiving estrogen had a 39 percent higher risk of stroke. Again, some benefits of estrogen therapy were identified, including a 39 percent risk reduction of hip fracture and even a slight reduction in the risk of developing breast cancer, but these advantages were seen to be outweighed by potential dangers.

The medical community was stunned once more by this announcement, and women lost even more confidence in HT. Further analyses of the WHI data suggested that estrogen and estrogen plus progestin do not protect against mild cognitive impairment in women sixty-five and older, as had previously been hypothesized. Estrogen alone appeared not to offer any protection against dementia, while estrogen plus progestin slightly *increased* the risk of dementia in older women.

In the span of a few years, hormone therapy underwent a transformation from a highly regarded and popular treatment to a suspect program that should be used for a short time, if at all. Media reports on the HERS and WHI studies seemed to trumpet a single message: "The risks of hormone therapy outweigh the benefits," and millions of women began asking their doctors for alternatives or simply quit taking the hormones on their own. Yet an important question remains: Did this research warrant a mass exodus from hormone therapy?

Now that experts have had more time to sift through the data and consider what these numbers really mean, one emerging observation is that these results might not be applicable to all menopausal women. For example, the average age of the participants in HERS and HERS II was about sixty-seven at the beginning of the study and seventy-four at its completion. Yet the average age at which women enter menopause is just over fifty-one. Researchers are uncertain (and many physicians doubt) whether the data and conclusions from HERS/HERS II apply to younger women—the ones who would be far more likely to begin taking hormones for vasomotor symptoms such as hot flashes. Additionally, the women in HERS/HERS II had coronary artery disease at the beginning of the study. It cannot be known whether the HERS conclusion that HT did not offer protection against this disease would apply to women with healthy hearts.

Similarly, the WHI study was designed in a way that didn't actually answer the question faced by menopausal women who are having flashes and flushes but wondering whether HT would be safe for them. Why? Because in order to be a participant in this study, a woman had to be free of these symptoms. And why was that? Because women having symptoms would almost certainly be able to tell whether the drug they received was hormone or placebo, thus defeating one of the key controls of the study. As a result, most of the women in the WHI hormone study were several years beyond the typical onset of menopause: More than two-thirds of the participants were over sixty years of age.

Furthermore, the media pronouncements concerning HERS and WHI were interpreted by many in a way that greatly overestimated the risks of HT. Let's consider the risk of breast cancer as a prime example of this problem. Remember that the oversight board for WHI halted that study because it saw a 26 percent increase in relative risk for invasive breast cancer in women taking estrogen plus progestin, compared to women taking only a placebo. But some misunderstood that to mean that their overall chance of getting breast cancer (that is, their absolute risk) would be about one in four if they used HT. Obviously, a medication that caused a one in four chance of developing cancer would represent a serious threat to health, a cure far worse than whatever disease it might treat.

The confusion between relative and absolute risk demonstrates how misunderstandings about statistics can lead to alarming conclusions. They also underscore the importance of knowing a little basic statistical terminology.

Relative risk can be defined as the incidence of an effect in women who received hormones divided by the incidence of the effect in women who did not receive hormones. Absolute risk can be defined as the incidence of an effect throughout the entire population. If this sounds confusing, bear with us.

Here's an actual example from the WHI: Among the women in that study who did not take hormones, in one year the risk of being diagnosed with breast cancer was about 30 out of 10,000, or an absolute risk of about 0.30 percent. Among the women who took estrogen plus progestin, the one-year incidence of breast cancer rose to about 38 in 10,000, or an absolute risk of about 0.38 percent. The difference between the groups—thirty-eight cases in one group, thirty in the other—represents a 26 percent increase in relative risk. But the increase in absolute risk was 8 in 10,000, or .08 percent in one year—a relatively small number. Extrapolated over ten years, this would suggest that a woman taking estrogen and progestin for a decade would have an absolute risk of developing breast cancer less than one percent higher than that of a woman of the same age who didn't take hormones. This is not to say that the question of breast cancer should be ignored—on an individual level, every case is of immense significance. But it serves as a reminder that a decision to take or abstain from hormone supplements, or for that matter any drug (including those sold without prescription), should be considered with an accurate understanding of the benefits and risks.

APPENDIX G

Chronic Fatigue Syndrome

In 1984, internists Paul Cheney and Daniel Peterson, who practiced in the resort community of Incline Village, Nevada, noted an unusual influx of patients complaining of profound fatigue, often accompanied by low-grade fever, sore throat, swollen lymph nodes, and a variety of psychological disturbances. Their physical examinations were not particularly striking, laboratory studies were usually normal, and various attempts at straightforward treatment were unsuccessful. Most significantly, the patients had previously been in excellent health and did not seem to be candidates for depression or other psychological disorders that might present as fatigue.

The apparent epidemic of severe fatigue at Incline Village became a national news item, and by 1985 the medical literature began reporting this and other instances of similar cases. Because in some ways the illness reminded clinicians of infectious mononucleosis, and because some of the patients had unusually high blood levels of antibodies against the **Epstein-Barr virus (EBV)**, which is the most common cause of mononucleosis, a cause and effect relationship was assumed prematurely. Word spread through the lay and professional press that the Incline Village outbreak and others like it represented "chronic Epstein-Barr virus syndrome." In a way this sounded plausible, since EBV is a member of the herpesvirus family, whose members are notorious for living permanently (although usually dormant) in the people they infect. If the lowly chickenpox virus (varicella) can reactivate and cause shingles, could the equally common EBV come to life in some people and wreak havoc in its own way?

Before long, tired patients all over the country were asking for blood tests for EBV antibodies, and many of them were given the diagnosis of chronic Epstein-Barr virus syndrome.

Because no cure appeared to be at hand, some practitioners became self-appointed EBV "specialists" offering unproven, unorthodox, and often expensive treatments. Meanwhile, rank-and-file physicians began to notice that virtually every adult they screened had antibodies against EBV. Furthermore, more careful analysis revealed that the antibody patterns of people diagnosed as having chronic EBV syndrome were also present in many people who felt perfectly well.[1] Eventually the entire diagnosis became suspect. Since many cases involved professional young adults, the syndrome received less respectful titles such as "yuppie flu" and "affluenza." But even though the notion of a chronic EBV syndrome was eventually discarded, a number of patients had case histories so striking as to warrant clarification and further research. Finally in 1988 the Centers for Disease Control and Prevention (CDC) published a "working case definition" of what is now called **chronic fatigue syndrome**, or **CFS.**

Chronic fatigue syndrome is, fortunately, *not* the diagnosis for the vast majority of people who feel tired on an ongoing basis. According to the new case definition (revised in 1994) from the CDC:

> Chronic fatigue syndrome, or CFS, is a debilitating and complex disorder characterized by profound fatigue that is not improved by bed rest and that may be worsened by physical or mental activity. Persons with CFS most often function at a substantially lower level of activity than they were capable of before the onset of illness. In addition to these key defining characteristics, patients report various nonspecific symptoms, including weakness, muscle pain, impaired memory and/or mental concentration, insomnia, and post-exertional fatigue lasting more than 24 hours. In some cases, CFS can persist for years.[2]

Chronic fatigue syndrome has also been called chronic fatigue and immune dysfunction syndrome (CFIDS) since patients with CFS may have problems with immune function. These issues have not been clearly defined, and this term is now used less often. Throughout our discussion we will use the term *chronic fatigue syndrome* (and the initials *CFS*).

CFS is not your run-of-the-mill case of the blahs. Furthermore, as we will see in a moment, it is not a problem like diabetes or pneumonia for which a diagnosis is made or confirmed by a straightforward lab test or X ray. Rather, it is defined by a number of key symptoms and an *absence* of specific physical, laboratory, or other diagnostic findings that would point toward a different diagnosis. According to the CDC, a case of CFS is defined as persistent or relapsing chronic fatigue with the following features:

- The feeling of exhaustion is either new or had a definite onset sometime in the past (as opposed to being lifelong). The person who says "I've been tired ever since I can remember" does not have CFS.
- It is not the result of ongoing exertion and is not substantially relieved by rest.
- It results in a significant reduction in activity that may impact job, home, school, or social life, or all of these areas.
- It is not explained by some other medical or psychiatric diagnosis after an appropriate and thorough clinical evaluation. Note that one cannot self-diagnose CFS because the diagnosis requires that an appropriate medical evaluation to rule out other causes of fatigue has been carried out.

The diagnosis of CFS requires that fatigue as described above has been present for six or more consecutive months and that at least four of the following (known as primary symptoms) have also been present during the same time frame:

- Impairment in short-term memory or concentration that is significant enough to cause a substantial reduction in activities affecting home, work, school, and social life
- Sore throat
- Tender lymph nodes
- Muscle pain
- Pain in multiple joints, but without swelling or redness
- Headache of a new type, pattern, or severity
- Unrefreshing sleep
- Malaise lasting more than twenty-four hours after exertion[3]

In addition to having at least four of these eight primary symptoms, 20 to 50 percent of people with CFS have one—or several—of the following symptoms: abdominal pain, alcohol intolerance, bloating, chest pain, chronic cough, diarrhea, dizziness, dry eyes or mouth, earaches, irregular heartbeat, jaw pain, morning stiffness, nausea, night sweats, psychological problems (such as depression, irritability, anxiety, or panic attacks), shortness of breath, skin sensations, tingling sensations, and weight loss.

A case of **idiopathic chronic fatigue** is defined by the CDC as one that is clinically evaluated but is otherwise unexplained by the presence of other illness, and also fails to meet the criteria for CFS. Idiopathic is a medical adjective that means "we don't know what the cause is, but this big word makes it sound like we do."

A typical early presentation of CFS might be debilitating fatigue that lasts weeks or months and is not relieved by a few restful days and nights of good sleep. The onset of CFS may appear to follow an otherwise innocuous infection or illness such as a cold, bronchitis, or a stomach virus. For some it may follow a bout of infectious mononucleosis (the familiar "mono" most often seen among teenagers and young adults), or it may begin after a period of unusual stress or high workload. For many people with CFS, symptoms develop gradually, with no obvious illness or precipitating event.

It is important—and often challenging—to distinguish chronic fatigue syndrome from neuropsychiatric diagnoses, for which both treatment and prognosis can be very different. As we have already noted, anxiety and depression are commonly accompanied by fatigue. In addition, some individuals (who nearly always have underlying anxiety and depression) have what are called **somatoform disorders**, characterized by a host of physical symptoms for which no underlying general medical condition can be identified as an explanation. Common symptoms include headaches, back pain, abdominal cramping, and pelvic pain, and often a number of these are present at the same time. As you might guess from the definition of CFS, it may be difficult to decide where mood and somatoform disturbances end and CFS begins.

Who Gets Chronic Fatigue Syndrome, and What Causes It?

The CDC estimates that 500,000 people in the United States currently have either chronic fatigue syndrome or a CFS-like condition. CFS is diagnosed two to four times more often in women than in men, with an average age of onset estimated to be thirty years. Some adolescents meet the symptom criteria for CFS, but very few studies have examined this subgroup of patients. Overall CFS appears to be much less common in adolescents than in adults, and there is some disagreement as to whether it occurs in children under the age of twelve.

At this point there is no clearly established cause for CFS, which is one of many reasons why this disorder is so frustrating and why definitive treatment remains so elusive. A host of mechanisms have been proposed as the cause of CFS over the past two decades, including anemia, chronic Epstein-Barr virus infection, various environmental allergies, low blood sugar, and infection with the yeast *Candida albicans*. None of these have held up as likely explanations in the face of ongoing research. There is also no scientific evidence that CFS is caused by a nutritional deficiency, although people with this disorder commonly report intolerance to certain substances such as aspartame or alcohol.

There is no credible scientific evidence that CFS is contagious or transmissible (that is, one that can be spread from person to person). As we noted at the beginning of this appendix, what appeared to be a mini-epidemic of severe fatigue at Incline Village, Nevada, brought this disorder to public attention in 1984. Nevertheless, subsequent research has indicated that CFS does not seem to occur in clusters of cases (more commonly referred to as **outbreaks**) that would suggest it is caught from others or transmitted in some other way (for example, through insect or tick bites). Also, CFS is not typically associated with behaviors—high-risk sexual activity, intravenous drug abuse, exposure to animals, or travel to areas of the world where dangerous infections are more common, for example—that would lead one to suspect that a contagious disease is involved. However, it is still possible that infectious agents or a reactivation of illness can play a role in the development of the disease. Indeed, CFS may prove to be an end point of disease arising from multiple precipitating causes.

Much of the current interest and research in CFS is focused on the possibility of an abnormal interaction between the immune system and the central nervous system. Many researchers suspect that CFS involves a malfunction of the immune system, such as an inappropriate level of proteins called **cytokines** or changes in the functions of cells that play a necessary role in normal immune function, including natural killer cells or T-cells.

Cytokines are proteins secreted by cells of the lymphatic system. They affect inflammation, a complex response of the body to injury or infection.

Investigators have observed measurable defects in the number and function of these cells in some—but not all—people with CFS, and the relationship between the illness and these defects is not clear. Furthermore, one might expect an increased risk of cancer or infectious diseases as a result of these dysfunctions, but none is observed in people with CFS. Some investigators have found evidence of autoimmune or "anti-self" antibodies, as is seen in autoimmune diseases (such as rheumatoid arthritis, systemic lupus erythematosus, and scleroderma, among others), but demonstrable tissue damage, which might be expected in their presence, is lacking.

Diagnosing and Managing CFS

A person who is suffering from severe ongoing fatigue should undergo a thorough medical evaluation, as described in chapter 16. This should include a comprehensive history and physical examination, including a review of all prescription and nonprescription medications, as well as supplements, in past and current use. A basic mental status examination should be done to identify any abnormalities in mood, intellectual function, memory, and personality, with particular attention to indications of any psychiatric or neurological disorder. In addition, a battery of basic laboratory screening tests should be done. Typically this includes a complete blood count, a panel of metabolic blood chemistries (including electrolytes and liver and kidney functions), thyroid functions, urinalysis, and a marker for inflammation known as the erythrocyte sedimentation rate ("sed rate" for short).

Any abnormal result revealed by this evaluation must be pursued, and other tests may be indicated as well, depending on the individual clinical situation and presentation. These might include elaborate imaging studies such as MRIs, CT scans, radionuclide scans and PET scans, tests of immunologic function, serologic tests for various viruses, and many others. It is important to note that at present no tests can *prove* someone has chronic fatigue syndrome. (As of this book's publication, any practitioner's claim to have "the test" for CFS involves the use of an unproven and probably unreliable method.) The diagnosis of CFS is made when a person has a fatigue problem that fits the CDC case definition described earlier, and a thorough evaluation has not identified another definitive medical or psychiatric cause.

Since the cause of CFS is unknown at this time, it should come as no surprise that a reliable and effective treatment for this disorder has yet to be found. (Unproven treatment options, on the other hand, are abundant.) CFS is a problem that is thus *managed* rather than *cured,* though for many people there is a gradual resolution of symptoms over a few years. A number of possible measures may be helpful:

Physical activity and exercise. People with CFS have two strikes against them when it comes to physical activity. They are so exhausted that they may have difficulty completing the most basic and necessary activities for living, so exercising may seem out of the question. In addition, sustained exertion (especially on a day when they feel somewhat better) may provoke a "crash," in which symptoms worsen for one or more days afterward. CFS patients may need to adjust their basic activity level at home and work, a prospect that may be both worrisome and frustrating for family members and employers alike. Their physicians may need to educate concerned parties in this regard. Nevertheless, ongoing lack of activity will only lead to deconditioning, making recovery of normal stamina even more difficult.

In addition, a physical therapist or rehabilitation specialist, if available, can be a valuable resource for planning and supervising a graduated exercise program—one that allows for slow but steady progress without aggravating fatigue after a given session. People with chronic fatigue syndrome need to do as much exercise as they can tolerate every day, but not so much as to provoke a postexercise crash the next day. Walking is one of the best forms of exercise for increasing stamina.

Medications that may benefit those with CFS usually target specific symptoms. They must be used with care, however, because individuals with CFS tend to be sensitive to drugs, especially those that impact the central nervous system. Medications are best started at a very low dose and gradually increased as needed and tolerated. Some of the most common are:

- Pain relievers such as acetaminophen (Tylenol), and nonsteroidal anti-inflammatories (NSAIDs)—both nonprescription (such as ibuprofen, naproxen, or ketoprofen) and prescription—may help with muscle aches, headache, and tender joints.
- Antidepressants may serve a twofold purpose for those with CFS. The older tricyclic antidepressants (such as amitriptyline, doxepin, desipramine, and nortriptyline) are often prescribed for CFS patients at very low doses, with a goal of improving sleep and reducing generalized pain rather than treating depression. Side effects of these drugs—especially dry mouth, weight gain, and drowsiness—are milder and less common (or for many, nonexistent) at the lower doses. The newer antidepressant medications known as selective serotonin reuptake inhibitors (SSRIs) have also been shown to be helpful for some persons with CFS, especially those who have depression in addition to their CFS symptoms. (Two-thirds of CFS patients have signs of major depression, and half of all patients with CFS previously experienced at least one episode of major depression.[4]) Examples of SSRIs include fluoxetine (Prozac), sertraline (Zoloft), paroxetine (Paxil), and venlafaxine (Effexor). Other antidepressants, including trazodone (Desyrel) and bupropion (Wellbutrin), have also been used, with variable results. (These medications are discussed in more detail in chapter 8, beginning on page 342.)
- Antibiotics (including antiviral agents) are *not* used as a primary treatment for CFS, since no organism has been identified as the cause

of this problem. (Specific infections—for example, sinusitis or a bladder infection—should of course be treated if and when they occur.)

- Antihistamines likewise are *not* recommended as an "anti-allergy" treatment for CFS. If specific allergic symptoms such as sneezing or a runny nose occur, the newer *nonsedating* antihistamines should be favored over the older drugs (such as diphenhydramine or chlorpheniramine) that tend to be sedating. Examples of the non-sedating antihistamines are loratadine (Claritin), fexofenadine (Allegra), cetirizine (Zyrtec), and desloratadine (Clarinex).
- Other types of medications, including stimulants, corticosteroids, gamma globulin injections, DHEA, and drugs that increase blood pressure (since some CFS patients have been found to have low pressure), are among many that have been tried or are undergoing research as potential treatments for CFS or accompanying symptoms. Their use should be considered experimental at best, and none should be considered (even on a trial basis) without a careful review of potential benefits and risks with a physician who is knowledgeable of CFS and its management.

Counseling (ideally with a professional who has some familiarity with CFS) can help with a number of issues, including adjusting to the limitations of this problem, dealing with emotional responses (anxiety, anger, and guilt, among others), developing strategies to manage home and work responsibilities, and responding to possible negative feedback from family, friends, coworkers, and even health-care professionals. Because CFS can have a significant impact on one's activities and interactions with spouse, children, and other relatives, family counseling and education may be an important focus for these conversations.[5]

A sleep evaluation may be appropriate because so many with CFS suffer from insomnia or nonrestorative sleep. The evaluation can help identify and treat any concurrent sleep disorders that could aggravate CFS symptoms and guide decisions regarding any medications that might be considered to assist sleep. For example, if the evaluation uncovers obstructive sleep apnea, treatment (specifically the use of continuous positive airway pressure, or CPAP) occasionally brings about a dramatic and immediate improvement in energy. (For more information about sleep and the disorders that can disrupt it, including sleep apnea, see chapter 15.)

Alternative therapies are often promoted as helpful for managing CFS, as might be expected when confronting a distressing problem for which causes and effective treatments have eluded conventional medicine. Supplement packages, herbal remedies, colonic irrigation, yoga, acupuncture/acupressure, and scores of other alternative approaches have been touted as beneficial for both chronic fatigue in general and CFS in particular. Supporting evidence for these is usually anecdotal—in other words, based on the response of one or a few individuals—and often involves theories (such as manipulating flows of invisible energy) that are at odds with well-established understandings of biology. They may also have spiritual underpinnings that are incompatible with biblical teachings on the nature of God and human beings. We look at the realm of alternative therapy in more detail in chapter 17 (see page 819), but we advise caution when considering an investment of time and money in unconventional treatments for CFS (and other problems as well).

More information on chronic fatigue syndrome is available from the CFIDS Association of America (http://www.cfids.org), which both promotes research and disseminates educational material regarding this syndrome for patients, their families, and health-care providers. While most of the content of this organization's Web site is both informative and reasonable, note that some of its material and links dealing with alternative therapies steer patients toward approaches that are scientifically unsound or that have metaphysical underpinnings that neither Focus on the Family nor its Physicians Resource Council can endorse. (See chapter 17 beginning on page 819 for a more detailed discussion of the issues raised by a number of alternative therapies.) It is important that individuals and families dealing with chronic fatigue syndrome discuss any treatment suggestions with their physician(s) and carefully consider the potential benefits and risks.

Do People Recover from CFS?

This is a difficult question to answer, because the long-term course of chronic fatigue syndrome can vary considerably from person to person. Symptoms often escalate early in the illness and then plateau, after which they may then wax and wane for months or even years. Some individuals recover completely from CFS, although the exact percentage is unknown. Part of this uncertainty arises from variable definitions of recovery, which could range from being able to resume activities at home and work (even if not feeling entirely well) to a complete restoration of previous health.

Estimates of the number of people who improve enough to consider themselves recovered range from as low as 10 to 20 percent to as high as about 60 percent, occurring within five years after the onset of symptoms.[6] Some long-term research has suggested that most of those with CFS remain functionally impaired for at least several years.[7] No distinguishing characteristics predict who will recover, or who may worsen over time. Generally, a person with CFS should be reevaluated each year, or sooner if there are changes in symptoms.

Endnotes

Note: All information from Web sites was originally accessed between January 2002 and September 2005. Links have been updated whenever possible.

Chapter 1: In Pursuit of Health

1. United Nations, Food and Agricultural Organization, *The State of Food Insecurity in the World 2002*, http://www.fao.org/docrep/005/y7352e/y7352e00.htm.
2. World Health Organization, "What Is Malaria? Roll Back Malaria Information Sheet," http://rbm.who.int/cmc_upload/0/000/015/372/RBMInfosheet_1.htm.
3. William R. Jarvis, "Infection Control and Changing Health-Care Delivery Systems," *Emerging Infectious Diseases* 7, no. 2 (March/April 2001), http://www.cdc.gov/ncidod/eid/vol7no2/jarvis.htm#1.
4. Jennifer Ragland and William Lobdell, "Party Drug Takes Toll on Teen and Her Family," *Los Angeles Times*, December 3, 2001, B1.

Chapter 3: Three Common Health Problems You Want to Avoid

1. American Heart Association, *Heart Disease and Stroke Statistics—2005 Update* (Dallas: American Heart Association, 2005).
2. Ibid.
3. American Heart Association, "Risk Factors and Coronary Heart Disease," http://www.americanheart.org/presenter.jhtml?identifier=4726.
4. "What Are the Odds?" is a simple exercise that will give you a rough idea of the likelihood that you will develop coronary artery disease during the next decade. It is derived from statistics generated by the Framingham Heart Study, one of the most important and influential research projects in the history of American medicine. Launched in 1948, the study enrolled more than five thousand residents of Framingham, Mass., in an effort to understand the causes of the rising tide of cardiovascular disease in the United States. For more than fifty years, data obtained from Framingham have generated more than one thousand research papers and identified the major risk factors associated with heart attack, stroke, and other diseases. "What Are the Odds?" does not include all of the known risk factors for coronary disease, but it is based on those factors for which some of the most abundant Framingham data are available.
5. National Institutes of Health, National Heart, Lung, and Blood Institute, *The Sixth Report of the Joint National Committee on Prevention, Detection, Evaluation and Treatment of High Blood Pressure,* NIH Publication No. 98-4080 (November 1997): 20.
6. Ibid., 22.
7. Ibid., 23.
8. Harold G. Koenig et al., "The Relationship between Religious Activities and Blood Pressure in Older Adults," *International Journal of Psychology in Medicine* 28, no. 2 (1998): 189–213, http://www.nihr.org/programs/researchreports/bloodpressure.cfm.
9. Guidelines from the U.S. Preventive Services Task Force, the American Academy of Family Physicians and the American College of Physicians.
10. American Diabetes Association, "National Diabetes Fact Sheet," http://www.diabetes.org/diabetes-

statistics/national-diabetes-fact-sheet.jsp. See also Centers for Disease Control and Prevention, "National Diabetes Fact Sheet," http://www.cdc.gov/diabetes/pubs/general.htm#top.
11. Carol Lewis, "Diabetes: A Growing Public Health Concern," *FDA Consumer* magazine 36, no. 1 (January/February 2002), http://www.fda.gov/fdac/features/2002/102_diab.html.

Chapter 4: Health Screening in Adults

1. This recommendation was made in the *Third Report of the National Cholesterol Education Program (NCEP) Expert Panel on Detection, Evaluation and Treatment of High Blood Cholesterol in Adults,* NIH Publication No. 01-3670 (May 2001).
2. American College of Physicians, "Clinical Guideline, Part I: Guidelines for Using Serum Cholesterol, High-Density Lipoprotein Cholesterol, and Triglyceride Levels as Screening Tests for Preventing Coronary Heart Disease in Adults," *Annals of Internal Medicine* 124 (1996): 515–517.
3. American Diabetes Association, "Position Statement: Screening for Diabetes," *Diabetes Care* 25, 2002.
4. American Heart Association, "Homocysteine, Folic Acid and Cardiovascular Disease," http://www.americanheart.org/presenter.jhtml?identifier=4677. See also C. Starr, "Emerging Cardiac Risk Factors," *Patient Care* (May 30, 2001): 38–50.
5. National Cancer Institute, "Genetic Testing for BRCA1 and BRCA2: It's Your Choice" (February 2002), http://cis.nci.nih.giv/fact/3_62.htm.
6. American Cancer Society, "Do Breast Self-Exams Make a Difference?" (October 2, 2002), www.cancer.org/eprise/main/docroot/NWS/content/NWS_1_1x_Do_Breast_Self-Exams_Make_A_Difference. Original study written by David Thomas et al., appeared in *Journal of the National Cancer Institute* 94, no. 19 (2002): 1420–1421, 1445–1457.
7. American Cancer Society, "Smoking Linked to Colorectal Cancer," http://www.cancer.org/docroot/nws/content/nws_1_1x_smoking_linked_to_colorectal_cancer.asp. See also American Cancer Society, "Latest Study Confirms Folate Lowers Colorectal Cancer Rate," http://www.cancer.org/docroot/nws/content/nws_2_1x_latest_study_confirms_folate_lowers_colorectal_cancer_risk.asp.
8. J. V. Lacey et al., "Menopausal Hormone Replacement Therapy and Risk of Ovarian Cancer," *Journal of the American Medical Association* 288 (2002): 334–341. Cited in the National Cancer Institute, "Increased Risk of Ovarian Cancer Is Linked to Estrogen Replacement Therapy" (July 16, 2002), http://www.cancer.gov/newscenter/Laceyovarian.
9. Mayo Foundation for Education and Research, "Ovarian Cancer," http://www.mayoclinic.com/invoke.cfm?id=DS00293.
10. To read the American College of Radiology's statement on total body CT screening, go to their Web site: http://www.acr.org/s_acr/doc.asp?TrackID=&SID=1&DID=16014&CID=2192&VID=2&RTID=0&CIDQS=&Taxonomy=False&specialSearch=False.
11. U.S. Food and Drug Administration, Center for Devices and Radiological Health, "Whole-Body CT Screening—Should I or Shouldn't I Get One?" http://www.fda.gov/cdrh/ct/screening.html.
12. Ibid.

Chapter 5: Some Food for Thought on Food

1. Blake Sperry Bowden and Jennie M. Zeisz, "Supper's On! Adolescent Adjustment and Frequency of Family Mealtimes" (paper presented at American Psychological Association meeting, Chicago, August 16, 1997), http://www.scienceblog.com/community/older/1997/A/199700122.html.
2. Economic Research Service, "Sugar and Sweeteners," (Washington, D.C.: U.S. Department of Agriculture, June 20, 2003), http://www.ers.usda.gov/briefing/sugar/.
3. Center for Science in the Public Interest, "Sugar Intake Hit All-Time High in 1999," news release, May 18, 2000, http://www.cspinet.org/new/sugar_limit.html.
4. Sally Squires, "Sweet but Not So Innocent? High-Fructose Corn Syrup, Ubiquitous in the American Diet, May Act More like Fat than Sugar in the Body" *Washington Post,* March 11, 2003.
5. See http://www.foodreference.com/html/fcerealgrains.html.
6. C. S. Fuchs et al., "Dietary Fiber and the Risk of Colorectal Cancer and Adenoma in Women," *New England Journal of Medicine* 340 (1999): 169–176.
7. Institute of Medicine, *Dietary Reference Intakes for Energy, Carbohydrate, Fiber, Fat, Fatty Acids, Cholesterol, Protein, and Amino Acids (Macronutrients),* http://www.iom.edu/report.asp?id=4340.
8. Harvard School of Public Health, "Fiber: Start Roughing It!" http://www.hsph.harvard.edu/nutritionsource/fiber.html.
9. Mayo Foundation for Medical Education and Research, "Flaxseed and Flaxseed Oil" (January 1, 2004). See also P. L. Horn-Ross et al., "Phytoestrogen Intake and Endometrial Cancer Risk," *Journal of the National Cancer Institute* 95, no. 15 (August 6, 2003): 1158–1164.
10. Findings from the ongoing Nurses' Health Study and the Health Professionals Follow-up Study, summarized in Walter Willett, *Eat, Drink and Be Healthy: The Harvard Medical School Guide to Healthy Eating* (New York: Fireside, 2001).

11. Ancel Keys, *Seven Countries: A Multivariate Analysis of Death and Coronary Heart Disease* (London: Harvard University Press, 1980).
12. M. de Lorgeril et al., "Mediterranean Alpha-Linolenic Acid-Rich Diet in Secondary Prevention of Coronary Heart Disease," *Lancet* 343 (1994): 1454–1459. [Erratum, *Lancet* 345 (1995): 738.]
13. Antonia Trichopoulou et al., "Adherence to a Mediterranean Diet and Survival in a Greek Population," *New England Journal of Medicine* 348, no. 26 (June 26, 2003): 2599–2608.
14. M. F. K. Fisher, *The Art of Eating* (New York: Macmillan, 1954). See http://www.foodreference.com/html/qbread.html.
15. American Cancer Society, "Common Questions about Diet and Cancer," http://www.cancer.org/docroot/ped/content/ped_3_2x_common_questions_about_diet_and_cancer.asp.
16. Harvard School of Public Health, "Fruits and Vegetables May Reduce Risk of Stroke: Findings Support Recommended 5 Servings a Day," news release, October 5, 1999, http://www.hsph.harvard.edu/press/releases/press10051999.html.
17. Harvard School of Public Health, "Fruits and Vegetables," http://www.hsph.harvard.edu/nutritionsource/fruits.html.

Chapter 6: Dealing with Excess Weight

1. Robert Kuczmarski and K. M. Flegal, "Criteria for Definition of Overweight in Transition: Background and Recommendations for the United States," *American Journal of Clinical Nutrition* 72, no. 5 (November 2000): 1074–1081.
2. National Institutes of Health, *Clinical Guidelines on the Identification, Evaluation, and Treatment of Overweight and Obesity in Adults—The Evidence Report,* NIH Publication No. 98-4083 (September 1998): 56–58.
3. Allison A. Hedley et al., "Prevalence of Overweight and Obesity among US Children, Adolescents, and Adults, 1999-2002," *Journal of the American Medical Association* 291, no. 23 (June 16, 2004): 2847–2850. See also http://win.niddk.nih.gov/statistics/index.htm#what.
4. Ibid.
5. World Health Organization, "Obesity and Overweight: Fact Sheet" (2003), http://www.who.int/nut/index.htm#obs.
6. E. E. Calle et al., "Overweight, Obesity, and Mortality from Cancer in a Prospectively Studied Cohort of U.S. Adults," *New England Journal of Medicine* 348, no. 17 (2003): 1625–1638.
7. National Institute of Diabetes and Digestive and Kidney Diseases, "Statistics Related to Overweight and Obesity," http://win.niddk.nih.gov/statistics/index.htm#preval.
8. National Heart, Lung, and Blood Institute, "Psychological Aspects of Overweight and Obesity," in *Guidelines on Overweight and Obesity: Electronic Textbook,* http://www.nhlbi.nih.gov/guidelines/obesity/e_txtbk/index.htm.
9. National Association to Advance Fat Acceptance information index, http://www.naafa.org/documents/brochures/naafa-info.htm#whatis.
10. Eleanor Whitney and Sharon Rolfes, *Understanding Nutrition* (Belmont, Calif.: Wadsworth/Thomson Learning, 2002), 247.
11. Donald Hensrud, ed., *Mayo Clinic on Healthy Weight: Answers to Help You Achieve the Weight That's Right for You* (Rochester, Minn.: Mayo Clinic, 2000), 8.
12. Ibid.
13. Ibid.
14. M. F. Gallo, D. A. Grimes, and K. F. Schulz et al., "Combination Contraceptives: Effects on Weight" in *The Cochrane Library, Issue 2* (Oxford, UK: Update Software, 2003). Cited at http://www.fhi.org/en/AboutFHI/News+Releases/pr2003/april222003researchfindsno.htm.
15. Susan Gilbert, *Weigh Less, Live Longer* (Boston: Harvard Health Publications, 2001), 38.
16. See, for example, Dr. Ornish's answer to a question regarding yoga on WebMD at http://my.webmd.com/content/pages/2/3079_1705.htm.
17. Willow Lawson, "The Need to Feed: How the Stomach Talks to the Brain," *Psychology Today* (September 2, 2003), http://cms.psychologytoday.com/articles/index.php?term=PTO-20030902-000009.
18. Bonnie Liebman, "Fat—More than Just a Lump of Lard," *Nutrition Action Health Letter* (October 2004).
19. Jessica Schulman, "Nutrition Education in Medical Schools: Trends and Implications for Health Educators," *Medical Education Online* 4, no. 4 (1999), http://www.msu.edu/dsolomon/f0000015.pdf.
20. See, for example, the Nutritional Academic Award program funded by the National Heart, Lung, and Blood Institute since 1998, http://www.nhlbi.nih.gov/funding/training/naa/about.htm.
21. Institute of Medicine of the National Academies, "Childhood Obesity in the United States: Facts and Figures" fact sheet (September 2004), http://www.iom.edu/report.asp?id=22596. The IOM fact sheets are derived from: Jeffrey P. Koplan, Catharyn T. Liverman, and Vivica A. Kraak, eds.,

Preventing Childhood Obesity—Health in the Balance (Washington, D.C.: The National Academies Press, 2005).
22. Ibid.
23. R. Sinha et al., "Prevalence of Impaired Glucose Tolerance among Children and Adolescents with Marked Obesity," *New England Journal of Medicine* 346 (2002): 802–810. Cited in Alison Hoppin, "Assessment and Management of Childhood and Adolescent Obesity," *Medscape CME,* June 25, 2004.
24. Institute of Medicine of the National Academies, "Childhood Obesity in the United States."
25. M. H. Fishbein et al., "The Spectrum of Fatty Liver in Obese Children and the Relationship of Serum Aminotransferases to Severity of Steatosis," *Journal of Pediatric Gastroenterology and Nutrition* 36, no. 1 (January 2003): 54–61. Cited in Hoppin article mentioned in note 23.
26. A. Fowler-Brown and L. Kahwati, "Prevention and Treatment of Overweight in Children and Adolescents," *American Family Physician* 69 (2004): 2592–2598.
27. If you would like more details on this diet, check your local library for a copy of *The Stoplight Diet* by Leonard Epstein and Sally Squires (New York: Little, Brown and Company, 1988).

Chapter 7: Born to Move: Exercise and Physical Fitness

1. U.S. Department of Health and Human Services, "National Institutes of Health Consensus Development Conference Statement: Physical Activity and Cardiovascular Health" (December 18–20, 1995) in *Physical Activity and Health: A Report of the Surgeon General* (Atlanta: U.S. Department of Health and Human Services, Centers for Disease Control and Prevention, National Center for Chronic Disease Prevention and Health Promotion, 1996), 42–43.
2. Ibid, 43.
3. U.S. Department of Health and Human Services, *Physical Activity and Health*, 177.
4. American Heart Association, "Risk Factors: Statistics on Physical Inactivity and Obesity," http://www.justmove.org/fitnessnews/healthf.cfm?Target=/riskfacts.html.
5. S. N. Blair et al., "Changes in Physical Fitness and All-Cause Mortality: A Prospective Study of Healthy and Unhealthy Men," *Journal of the American Medical Association* 273, no. 14 (April 1995): 1093–1098.
6. J. Myers et al., "Exercise Capacity and Mortality among Men Referred for Exercise Testing," *New England Journal of Medicine* 346, no. 11 (March 2002): 793–801.
7. American Heart Association, "Physical Activity and Cardiovascular Health Fact Sheet," http://www.americanheart.org/presenter.jhtml?identifier=820.
8. Ibid.
9. U.S. Department of Health and Human Services, *Physical Activity and Health,* 125–129.
10. Diabetes Prevention Program Research Group, "Reduction in the Incidence of Type 2 Diabetes with Lifestyle Intervention or Metformin," *New England Journal of Medicine* 346, no. 6 (February 2002): 393–403.
11. Harold Elrick, "Commentary: Exercise Is Medicine," *The Physician and Sportsmedicine* 24, no. 2 (February 1996).
12. U.S. Department of Health and Human Services, *Physical Activity and Health,* 112–124.
13. William J. Cromie, "Exercise Reduces Cancer Risk," *Harvard Gazette,* May 11, 2000, http://www.news.harvard.edu/gazette/2000/05.11/exercise.html.
14. B. Rockhill et al., "A Prospective Study of Recreational Physical Activity and Breast Cancer Risk," *Archives of Internal Medicine* 159, no. 19 (October 1999): 2290–2296.
15. U.S. Department of Health and Human Services, *Physical Activity and Health,* 141–142.
16. Ibid., 135–141.
17. Michael L. Pollock et al., "ACSM Position Stand: The Recommended Quantity and Quality of Exercise for Developing and Maintaining Cardiorespiratory and Muscular Fitness, and Flexibility in Adults," *Medicine & Science in Sports & Exercise* 30, no. 6 (June 1998): 975–991.

Chapter 8: The Emotional Weather

1. Unless otherwise specified, statistics in this segment regarding anxiety disorders come from National Institute of Mental Health, "Anxiety Disorders," NIH Publication 02-3879 (Bethesda, Md.: National Institute of Mental Health, National Institutes of Health, U.S. Department of Health and Human Services), http://www.nimh.nih.gov/publicat/NIMHanxiety.pdf.
2. R. C. Kessler et al., "The Epidemiology of Major Depressive Disorder: Results from the National Comorbidity Survey Replication (NCS-R)," *Journal of the American Medical Association* 289, no. 23 (June 18, 2003): 3095–3105.
3. *DSM-IV,* quoted in Bowes et al., "Diagnosis and Management of Mood Disorders," *American Family Physician Monograph* (2004).

4. This section is adapted from Paul Reisser, *Parents' Guide to Teen Health* (Colorado Springs: Focus on the Family, 1997), 238–242.
5. Mayo Clinic, "St. John's Wort (Hypericum Perforatum L.)," http://www.mayoclinic.com/invoke.cfm?objectid=17D60310-508B-D3DD-17558C382919DC5B.
6. C. S. Lewis, *The Screwtape Letters* (San Francisco: HarperSanFrancisco, 2001), 71–72.
7. Richard A. Swenson, *Margin: Restoring Emotional, Physical, Financial, and Time Reserves to Overloaded Lives*, rev. ed. (Colorado Springs: NavPress, 2004), 69.
8. Attributed to Charles Thomas Studd (1860–1931), English missionary to China, India, and Africa.
9. This section has been adapted and updated from the *Parents' Guide to Teen Health*, 79–85.

Chapter 9: More Than Molecules: Spiritual Health

1. Richard Morin, "Do Americans Believe in God?" *On Politics: Online Extras/What Americans Think*, WashingtonPost.com, April 24, 2000, http://www.washingtonpost.com/wp-srv/politics/polls/wat/archive/wat042400.htm.
2. Gowri Anandarajah and Ellen Hight, "Spirituality and Medical Practice: Using the HOPE Questions as a Practical Tool for Spiritual Assessment," *American Family Physician* 63, no. 1 (January 1, 2001): 81–88, http://www.aafp.org/afp/20010101/81.html. See also Claudia Kalb, "Faith and Healing," *Newsweek*, November 10, 2003, 44–46.
3. Dale A. Matthews with Connie Clark, *The Faith Factor: Proof of the Healing Power of Prayer* (New York: Viking, 1998).
4. References for these conclusions include Harold G. Koenig et al., *Handbook of Religion and Health* (New York: Oxford University Press, 2001), note especially page 99; Anandarajah and Hight, "Spirituality and Medical Practice"; and studies referenced in Walter Larimore with Traci Mullins, *10 Essentials of Highly Healthy People* (Grand Rapids: Zondervan, 2003), especially pages 164–166 and footnotes.
5. Dale A. Matthews et al., "Religious Commitment and Health Status," *Archives of Family Medicine* 7, no. 2 (March 1998): 118–124.
6. K. I. Pargament et al., "Religious Struggle as a Predictor of Mortality among Medically Ill Elderly Patients: A Two-Year Longitudinal Study," *Archives of Internal Medicine* 161 (2001): 1881–1885, http://www.dukespiritualityandhealth.org/research/abstracts.
7. Anandarajah and Hight, "Spirituality and Medical Practice."
8. Herbert Benson, *Timeless Healing: The Power and Biology of Belief* (New York: Scribner, 1996); referenced in Anandarajah and Hight, "Spirituality and Medical Practice."
9. Benedict Carey, "Can Prayers Heal? Critics Say Studies Go Past Science's Reach," *New York Times*, October 10, 2004, http://www.nytimes.com/2004/10/10/health/10prayer.html.
10. W. S. Harris et al., "A Randomized, Controlled Trial of the Effects of Remote, Intercessory Prayer on Outcomes in Patients Admitted to the Coronary Care Unit," *Archives of Internal Medicine* 159 (1999): 2273–2278.
11. Claudia Kalb, "Faith and Healing," *Newsweek*, November 10, 2003, 49, reporting on a presentation by Mitchell Krucoff, at the October 14, 2003, Second Conference on the Integration of Complementary Medicine into Cardiology, sponsored by the American College of Cardiology. Dr. Krucoff presented preliminary data (yet unpublished as of March 2005) on phase two of the MANTRA Project. (MANTRA stands for "Monitoring and Actualization of Noetic Training.") The pilot for this study was published as Mitchell Krucoff et al., "Integrative Noetic Therapies as Adjuncts to Percutaneous Intervention during Unstable Coronary Syndromes: Monitoring and Actualization of Noetic Training (MANTRA) Feasibility Pilot," *American Heart Journal* 142, no. 5 (2001): 760–767.
12. See, for example, *Prayer Is Good Medicine* (San Francisco: HarperSanFrancisco, 1996).
13. Paul Reisser et al., *Examining Alternative Medicine* (Downers Grove, Ill.: InterVarsity Press, 2001). See also Larry Dossey and Harold Koenig, "Health-Prayer Studies," *Science and Spirit* (March–April 2002), http://www.science-spirit.org/article_detail.php?article_id=295.
14. See, for example, L. Roberts, I. Ahmed, and S. Hall, "Intercessory Prayer for the Alleviation of Ill Health," *The Cochrane Database of Systematic Reviews* 2000, issue 2, article no. CD000368. See also John Astin, Elaine Harkness, and Edzard Ernst, "The Efficacy of 'Distant Healing': A Systematic Review of Randomized Trials," *Annals of Internal Medicine* 132, no. 11 (June 6, 2000): 903–910.
15. C. S. Lewis, "The Efficacy of Prayer," in *The World's Last Night: And Other Essays* (New York: Harcourt Brace Jovanovich, 1960), 4–5, 8.
16. C. S. Lewis, *Mere Christianity: A Revised and Amplified Edition, with a New Introduction, of the Three Books, "Broadcast Talks," "Christian Behaviour," and "Beyond Personality"* (San Francisco: HarperSanFrancisco, 2001), 52.
17. Philip Yancey, *The Jesus I Never Knew* (Grand Rapids: Zondervan, 1995), 179–180.
18. John Ortberg, *The Life You've Always Wanted: Spiritual Disciplines for Ordinary People* (Grand Rapids: Zondervan, 2002), 51.

19. Matthias Claudius, "We Plow the Fields," trans. Jane Montgomery Campbell, www.musicanet.org/robokopp/hymn/weplowth.htm.
20. Ortberg, *The Life You've Always Wanted,* 170.
21. C. S. Lewis, *The Screwtape Letters* (San Francisco: HarperSanFrancisco, 2001), 44.
22. Ibid., 53–54.

Chapter 10: Bad Habits: Tobacco, Alcohol, and Drugs

1. Glen R. Hanson and Ting-Kai Li, "Public Health Implications of Excessive Alcohol Consumption," *Journal of American Medical Association* 289, no. 8 (February 26, 2003): 1031–1032.
2. *I Love Lucy* trivia at http://www.imdb.com/title/tt0043208/trivia.
3. Gene Borio, *The History of Tobacco: Part III,* http://www.historian.org/bysubject/tobacco3.htm. See also http://www.cdc.gov/tobacco/research_data/economics/consump1.htm.
4. American Cancer Society, "Cancer Facts & Figures 2005."
5. World Health Organization, "The Tobacco Atlas," http://www.who.int/tobacco/resources/publications/tobacco_atlas/en/. See also United States Department of Agriculture, Economic Research Service, *Tobacco Outlook* TBS–258 (April 22, 2005): 4.
6. Federal Trade Commission, "Report to Congress for the Years 1998 and 1999" (issued 2001), http://ftc.gov/reports/tobacco/smokeless98_99.htm.
7. American Lung Association, "Trends in Tobacco Use," http://lungusa.org/atf/cf%7B7A8D42C2-FCCA-4604-8ADE-7F5DE762256%7D//TRENDS_IN_TOBACCO-USE_2003.PDF.
8. Centers for Disease Control and Prevention, "Cigarette Smoking among Adults—United States, 2003," *Morbidity and Mortality Weekly Report* 54, no. 20 (May 27, 2005), http://www.cdc.gov/mmwr/preview/mmwrhtml/mm5420a3.htm.
9. Centers for Disease Control and Prevention, "Smoking during Pregnancy—United States, 1990–2002," *Morbidity and Mortality Weekly Report* 53, no. 39 (October 8, 2004): 911–915, http://www.cdc.gov/mmwr/preview/mmwrhtml/mm5339a1.htm.
10. Centers for Disease Control and Prevention, "Tobacco Use, Access, and Exposure to Tobacco in Media among Middle & High School Students—United States, 2004," *Morbidity and Mortality Weekly Report* 54, no. 12 (April 1, 2005): 297–301, http://www.cdc.gov/mmwr/PDF/wk/mm5412.pdf.
11. American Lung Association, "Trends in Tobacco Use."
12. Centers for Disease Control and Prevention, "Tobacco Use, Access, and Exposure," table 2.
13. Centers for Disease Control and Prevention, "Adult Tobacco Use in the United States," see http://www.cdc.gov/tobacco/statehi/htmltext/Us_sh.htm.
14. Federal Trade Commission, "Federal Trade Commission Cigarette Report for 2002," (2004), http://www.ftc.gov/reports/cigarette/041022cigaretterpt.pdf.
15. Centers for Disease Control and Prevention, "Annual Smoking-Attributable Mortality, Years of Potential Life Lost, and Economic Costs—United States, 1997–2001," *Morbidity and Mortality Weekly Report* 54, no. 25 (July 1, 2005), http://www.cdc.gov/mmwr/PDF/wk/mm5425.pdf.
16. Highlights from the 1999 National Household Survey on Drug Abuse, a project of the Substance Abuse and Mental Health Services Administration, http://www.health.org/govstudy/bkd376/.
17. U.S. Department of Health and Human Services, "Preliminary Estimates from the 1995 National Household Survey on Drug Abuse: Advance Report 18," http://www.health.org/govstudy/ar018.default.aspx.
18. Centers for Disease Control and Prevention, "Annual Smoking-Attributable Mortality—1997–2001."
19. Ibid.
20. Ibid.
21. American Cancer Society, "Tobacco-Related Diseases Kill Half of All Smokers," http://www.cancer.org/docroot/PED/content/PED_10_2X_Smoking_and_Cancer_Mortality_Table.asp.
22. American Cancer Society, "Smoking and Cancer Mortality Table," http://www.cancer.org/docroot/PED/content/PED_10_2X_Smoking_and_Cancer_Mortality_Table.asp.
23. American Cancer Society, "Tobacco-Related Diseases."
24. American Heart Association, "Cigarette Smoking and Cardiovascular Diseases," http://www.americanheart.org/presenter.jhtml?identifier=4545.
25. National Digestive Diseases Information Clearinghouse, "Smoking and Your Digestive System," NIH Publication No. 02-949 (March 2002), http://digestive.niddk.nih.gov/ddiseases/pubs/smoking/index.htm.
26. Mayo Foundation for Medical Education and Research, "Nicotine Dependence," http://mayoclinic.com/invoke.cfm?objectid_E730A942-E51B-4419-950BE71044E9F4AF.
27. The American Academy of Periodontology, "Tobacco Use and Periodontal Disease," http://perio.org/consumer/smoking.htm.
28. See http://www.lungusa.org for more information on smoking during pregnancy.
29. National Center for Tobacco-Free Kids, "Philip Morris' New Virginia Slims Advertising Campaign

Insults and Degrades Women," news release, February 1, 2001, http://tobaccofreekids/org/Script/DisplayPressRelease.php3?Display=334.
30. American Cancer Society, "Guide for Quitting Smoking," http://www.cancer.org/docroot/ped/content/ped_10_13x_quitting_smoking.asp?sitearea=ped&viewmode=print.
31. American Lung Association, "Smoking Fact Sheet," http://www.lungusa.org/site/apps/s/content.asp?c=dvLUK9O0E&b=34706&ct=66713.
32. Ibid.
33. The American Academy of Periodontology, "Cigar and Pipe Smoking Are as Dangerous as Cigarettes to Periodontal Health," http://www.perio.org/consumer/cigars.htm.
34. American Cancer Society, "Cigar Smoking," http://www.cancer.org/docroot/PED/content/PED_10_2X_Cigar_Smoking_and_Cancer.asp?sitearea=PED&viewmode=print&.
35. See, for example, "Smokeless Tobacco: Addictive and Harmful" at http://www.mayoclinic.com/invoke.cfm?id=CA00019.
36. Ibid.
37. American Cancer Society, "What Are the Risk Factors for Oral Cavity and Oropharyngeal Cancer?" http://www.cancer.org/docroot/CRI/content/CRI_2_4_2X_What_are_the_risk_factors_for_oral_cavity_and_oropharyngeal_cancer_60.asp?sitearea=CRI.
38. Gene Borio, *The History of Tobacco: Part IV,* http://www.historian.org/bysubject/tobacco4.htm.
39. Centers for Disease Control and Prevention, "Tobacco Products: Fact Sheet," http://www.cdc.gov/tobacco/sgr/sgr_2000/factsheets/factsheets_tobacco.htm.
40. Ibid.
41. National Cancer Institute, "Cigarette Smoking and Cancer: Questions & Answers," http://cis.nih.gov/fact/10_14.htm. See also National Cancer Institute, "Smokeless Tobacco and Cancer: Questions and Answers," http://cis.nci.nih.gov/fact/10_15.htm.
42. John R. Hall Jr., "The Smoking-Material Related Problem: Executive Summary" (report prepared for the National Fire Protection Association, November 2004).
43. American Cancer Society, "Child and Teen Tobacco Use: Facts about Kids and Tobacco," http://www.cancer.org/docroot/PED/content/PED_10_2X_Child_and_Teen_Tobacco_Use.asp?sitearea=PED.
44. Michael C. Fiore et al., *Treating Tobacco Use and Dependence: A Public Health Service* (Rockville, Md.: Department of Health and Human Services, Public Health Service, June 2000), 1.
45. Ibid., 9.
46. American Cancer Society, "Guide for Quitting Smoking."
47. National Institute on Alcohol Abuse and Alcoholism, *Helping Patients with Alcohol Problems: A Health Practitioner's Guide,* NIH Publication No. 03-3769 (January 2003). Derived from unpublished data from the 1992 Longitudinal Alcohol Epidemiologic Survey, a nationwide household survey of 42,863 U.S. adults eighteen and older.
48. National Institute on Alcohol Abuse and Alcoholism, *What You Don't Know Can Harm You,* NIH Publication No. 99-4323, http://www.niaaa.nih.gov/publications/WhatUDon'tKnow_HTML/Don'tKnow.pdf.
49. J. G. Wiese et al., "The Alcohol Hangover," *Annals of Internal Medicine* 132, no. 11 (June 6, 2000): 897–902.
50. National Institute on Alcohol Abuse and Alcoholism, "Fetal Alcohol Exposure and the Brain," *Alcohol Alert* 50 (December 2000), http://www.niaaa.nih.gov/publications/aa50.htm.
51. Task Force of the National Advisory Council on Alcohol Abuse and Alcoholism, *A Call to Action: Changing the Culture of Drinking at U.S. Colleges* (April 2002), 4.
52. American Medical Association, "Fact Sheet: Effects of Alcohol on Brains of Adolescents," http://www.ama-assn.org/ama/pub/category/9416.html. For more information on the risks to young people who drink, see the National Institute on Alcohol Abuse and Alcoholism's online booklet, "Make a Difference," http://www.alcoholfreechildren.org/pubs/html/makeadifference.htm.
53. Michele G. Cyr and Kelly A. McGarry, "Alcohol Use Disorders in Women: Screening Methods and Approaches to Treatment," *Postgraduate Medicine* 112, no. 6 (December 2002): 31–47, http://www.postgradmed.com/issues/2002/12_02/cyr2.htm.
54. S. A. Smith-Warner et al., "Alcohol and Breast Cancer in Women: A Pooled Analysis of Cohort Studies," *Journal of the American Medical Association* 279, no. 7 (February 18, 1998): 535–540.
55. National Institute on Alcohol Abuse and Alcoholism, "Helping Patients with Alcohol Problems." The four CAGE questions were introduced by J. A. Ewing in "Detecting Alcoholism: The CAGE Questionnaire," *Journal of the American Medical Association* 252, 1905–1907. Used with the permission of the Bowles Center for Alcohol Studies, the University of North Carolina at Chapel Hill, where Ewing was the founding director.
56. National Institute on Drug Abuse, "Marijuana: Facts Parents Need to Know," http://www.nida.nih.gov/MarijBroch/Marijparentstxt.html.

57. Lloyd D. Johnston et al., *Monitoring the Future National Results on Adolescent Drug Use: Overview of Key Findings, 2004,* NIH Publication No. 05-5726 (Bethesda, Md.: National Institute on Drug Abuse, 2005).
58. National Institute on Drug Abuse, "Marijuana," http://drugabuse.gov/Infofax/marijuana.html.
59. Lloyd D. Johnston et al., *Monitoring the Future Overview of Key Findings, 2004.*
60. Substance Abuse and Mental Health Services Administration, *Overview of Findings from the 2004 National Survey on Drug Use & Health* NSDUH Series H-27, DHHS Publication No. SMA 05-4061 (Rockville, Md.: Office of Applied Studies, 2005).
61. National Institute on Drug Abuse, "Hallucinogens and Dissociative Drugs," NIH Publication No. 01-4209 (March 2001).
62. Substance Abuse and Mental Health Services Administration, *Overview of Findings from the 2004 National Survey on Drug Use & Health.* See also Centers for Disease Control and Prevention, "Youth Risk Behavior Surveillance—United States, 2003," *Morbidity and Mortality Weekly Report* 53, no. SS-2.
63. SAMHSA, *2004 National Survey on Drug Use & Health.* See also Johnston et al., *Monitoring the Future: Overview of Key Findings,* 2004.
64. SAMHSA, *2004 National Survey on Drug Use & Health.*
65. The Twelve Steps are reprinted with permission of Alcoholics Anonymous World Services, Inc. (A.A.W.S.). Permission to reprint the Twelve Steps does not mean that A.A.W.S. has reviewed or approved the contents of this publication, or that A.A.W.S. necessarily agrees with the views expressed herein. A.A. is a program of recovery from alcoholism only—use of Twelve Steps in connection with programs and activities which are patterned after A.A., but which address other problems, or in any other non-A.A. context, does not imply otherwise. Additionally, while A.A. is a spiritual program, A.A. is not a religious program. Thus, A.A. is not affiliated or allied with any sect, denomination, or specific religious belief.
66. LifeRing Secular Recovery, "Frequently Asked Questions," http://www.unhooked.com/lsr/faq.htm.
67. See http://www.rational.org/html_public_area/dpi.html.
68. International Association of Christian Twelve Step Ministries, "Statement of Shared Principles," http://www.iactsm.com/dox/shared.htm.
69. Ibid.

Chapter 11: Safety First (and Last)

1. Centers for Disease Control and Prevention, "Deaths: Final Data for 2002," *National Vital Statistics Reports* 53, no. 5 (October 12, 2004), http://www.cdc.gov/nchs/data/nvsr/nvsr53/nvsr53_05acc.pdf.
2. National Safety Council, "Report on Injuries in America, 2003," http://www.nsc.org/library/report_injury_usa.htm. See also Centers for Disease Control and Prevention, "National Hospital Ambulatory Medical Care Survey: 2003 Emergency Department Summary," *Advance Data from Vital and Health Statistics* no. 358 (May 26, 2005), table 9, http://www.cdc.gov/nchs/data/ad/ad358.pdf.
3. Department of Health and Human Services, Centers for Disease Control and Prevention, and National Center for Injury Prevention and Control, *CDC Injury Research Agenda* (Atlanta, Ga.: June 2002), http://www.cdc.gov/ncipc/pub-res/research_agenda/Research%20Agenda.pdf.
4. National Highway Traffic Safety Administration, "Attitudes Concerning the Utility of Seat Belts, Risk Perception, and Fatalism," in *1998 Motor Vehicle Occupant Safety Survey: Volume 2: Seat Belt Report* (March 2000), http://www.nhtsa.dot.gov/people/injury/research/SafetySurvey/Chapter3.html.
5. Rana Balci, Alicia Vertz, and Wenqi Shen, "Comfort and Usability of the Seat Belts," *Human Factors in Automotive Design,* SAE Technical Paper Series, table 2 (Detroit: SAE 2001 World Congress, March 5–8, 2001), http://www.delphi.com/pdf/techpapers/2001-01-0051.pdf.
6. NHTSA, "Attitudes Concerning the Utility of Seat Belts."
7. Balci, Vertz, and Shen, "Comfort and Usability of the Seat Belts."
8. National Safety Council, "Report on Injuries in America, 2002."
9. Michael J. Karter, *Fire Loss in the United States during 2004* (Quincy, Mass.: National Fire Protection Association, Fire Analysis and Research Division, September 2005), http://www.nfpa.org/assets/files/pdf/os.fireloss.pdf.
10. The statistics in this section on the causes of residential fires come from the National Fire Protection Association. To access any of their fact sheets on the various causes of fires in the home, see http://www.nfpa.org/categoryList.asp?categoryID=246&URL=Research%20&%20Reports/Fact%20sheets/Home%20safety.
11. National Fire Protection Association, "Smoke Alarms: Make Them Work for Your Safety," http://www.nfpa.org/categoryList.asp?categoryID=278&URL=Research%20&%20Reports/Safety%20fact%20sheets/Fire%20protection%20equipment/Smoke%20alarms.
12. National Library of Medicine and National Institutes of Health, "Hemoglobin Derivatives," in *Medical Encyclopedia,* MedlinePlus, http://www.nlm.nih.gov/medlineplus/ency/article/003371.htm.

13. National Safety Council, "Carbon Monoxide Fact Sheet," April 5, 2004, http://www.nsc.org/library/facts/carbmono.htm. See also Jean C. Mah, *Non-Fire Carbon Monoxide Deaths and Injuries Associated with the Use of Consumer Products: Annual Estimates* (Bethesda, Md.: Consumer Product Safety Commission, October 2000), http://www.cpsc.gov/LIBRARY/co00.pdf. This report lists the average number of deaths due to accidental carbon monoxide poisoning between 1993 and 1997 as 534, with about 61 percent of these due to motor-vehicle exhaust.
14. William A. Watson, Toby L. Litovitz, Wendy Klein-Schwartz et al., "2004 Annual Report of the American Association of Poison Control Centers Toxic Exposure Surveillance System," *American Journal of Emergency Medicine* 23, no. 5 (September 2005): 589–666.
15. Office of Statistics and Programming, National Center for Injury Prevention and Control, Centers for Disease Control and Prevention, "10 Leading Causes of Nonfatal Unintentional Injury, United States 2001, All Races, Both Sexes, Disposition: All Cases," http://www.cdc.gov/ncipc/wisqars/nonfatal/quickpicks/quickpicks_2001/unintall.htm.
16. Watson, Litovitz, Klein-Schwartz et al., "2004 Annual Report of Poison Control Centers."
17. Information on the symptoms and treatment of poisoning is excerpted from *Focus on the Family Complete Book of Baby and Child Care* (Colorado Springs, Colo.: Focus on the Family, 1997), 800–802.
18. Watson, Litovitz, Klein-Schwartz et al., "2004 Annual Report of Poison Control Centers."
19. American Academy of Pediatrics Committee on Injury, Violence, and Poison Prevention, "Policy Statement: Poison Treatment in the Home," *Pediatrics* 112, no. 5 (November 2003): 1182–1185.
20. Ibid.
21. Material in this section has been excerpted from *Focus on the Family Complete Book of Baby and Child Care.*
22. National Rifle Association, "Firearm Facts 2004," http://www.nraila.org.
23. Kenneth D. Kochanek, Sherry L. Murphy, Robert N. Anderson, and Chester Scott, "Deaths: Final Data for 2002," *National Vital Statistics Report* 53, no. 5 (October 12, 2004): 32. In 2002, 31,655 Americans took their own lives, and of these, 17,108 suicides were accomplished by firearms.
24. American Academy of Orthopaedic Surgeons, "Low Back Pain," http://orthoinfo.aaos.org/brochure/thr_report.cfm?Thread_ID=10&topcategory=Spine.
25. J. T. Wassell, L. I. Gardner, D. P. Landsittel et al., "A Prospective Study of Back Belts for Prevention of Back Pain and Injury," *Journal of the American Medical Association* 284, no. 21 (December 6, 2000): 2727–2732.
26. National Highway Traffic Safety Administration, "Motor Vehicle Traffic Crash Fatality Counts and Injury Estimates for 2004," DOT HS 809 923, http://www-nrd.nhtsa.dot.gov/pdf/nrd-30/NCSA/PPT/809923/809923.htm.
27. Insurance Institute for Highway Safety and Highway Loss Data Institute, "Q&A: Daytime Running Lights," March 2004, http://www.iihs.org/safety_facts/qanda/drl.htm.
28. Donna Glassbrenner, *Estimating the Lives Saved by Safety Belts and Air Bags* (Washington, D.C.: National Center for Statistics and Analysis, National Highway Traffic Safety Administration, paper no. 500), http://www-nrd.nhtsa.dot.gov/pdf/nrd-01/esv/esv18/CD/Files/18ESV-000500.pdf.
29. Donna Glassbrenner, *The New Methodology for Calculating the Lives Saved by Safety Belts and Air Bags* (presentation given to the Federal Committee on Statistical Methodology), http://www-nrd.nhtsa.dot.gov/pdf/nrd-30/NCSA/PPT/PresLivesSaved.pdf.
30. Ann Carter, "Automobile Safety," iMcKesson Clinical Reference Products, http://www.apria.com/resources/0,2725,48-49-A-3409,00.html.
31. Ibid.
32. National Highway Traffic Safety Administration, "Pregnancy: Protecting Your Unborn Child in a Car," *NHTSA Facts* (Washington, D.C.: U.S. Department of Transportation, Summer 1996), http://ntl.bts.gov/lib/6000/6700/6783/preg.pdf.
33. National Highway Traffic Safety Administration, "Motor Vehicle Occupant Protection Facts," http://www.nhtsa.dot.gov/people/injury/airbags/OccupantProtectionFacts/children_youth.htm.
34. The information on child restraints in this paragraph comes from NHTSA's Web page, "Child Passenger Safety." See http://www.nhtsa.dot.gov. See also http://www.nhtsa.dot.gov/CPS/safetycheck/TypeSeats/ for illustrations of these types of seats.
35. B. E. Cody, A. D. Mickalide, H. P. Paul, J. M. Colella, *Child Passengers at Risk in America: A National Study of Restraint Use* (Washington, D.C.: Safe Kids Worldwide, February 2002). See http://www.safekids.org/content_documents/ACFD68.pdf.
36. Donna Glassbrenner, *Child Restraint Use in 2002: Results from the 2002 NOPUS Controlled Intersection Study* (NTSA and National Center for Statistics and Analysis, February 5, 2003), http://www.nhtsa.dot.gov/CPS/ChildRestraints/ChildRestraintPPT.pdf.
37. National Highway Traffic Safety Administration, "Counts for Air Bag Related Fatalities and Seriously

Injured Persons," http://www-nrd.nhtsa.dot.gov/pdf/nrd-30/NCSA/SCI/4Q_2002/HTML/QtrRpt/ABFSISR.htm.
38. National Highway Traffic Safety Administration, "What You Need to Know about Air Bags," November 2002, http://www.nhtsa.dot.gov/people/injury/airbags/airbags03/index.html.
39. NHTSA, "Counts for Air Bag Related Fatalities."
40. These guidelines come from the National Highway Traffic Safety Administration, "Air Bag Safety: Buckle Everyone! Children in Back!" http:/www.nhtsa.dot.gov/people/injury/airbags/AirBagFlr/Abgaflr.htm.
41. National Highway Traffic Safety Administration, *Traffic Safety Facts 2003 Data: Overview,* http://www-nrd.nhtsa.dot.gov/pdf/nrd-30/NCSA/TSF2003/809767.pdf.
42. National Safety Council, "Speeding," May 24, 2004, http://www.nsc.org/nsm/speeding.htm.
43. National Highway Traffic Safety Administration, *Traffic Safety Facts 2002: Alcohol,* http://www-nrd.nhtsa.dot.gov/pdf/nrd-30/NCSA/TSF2002/2002alcfacts.pdf.
44. National Highway Traffic Safety Administration, "0.08 BAC Illegal Per Se Level," *State Legislative Fact Sheets,* http://www.nhtsa.dot.gov/people/outreach/safesobr/19qp/factsheets/bac.html.
45. National Highway Traffic Safety Administration, "National Survey of Drinking and Driving Attitudes and Behaviors: 2001," *Traffic Tech,* June 2003, http://www.nhtsa.dot.gov/people/injury/alcohol/traffic-tech2003/TT280.pdf. See also National Institute on Alcohol Abuse and Alcoholism, "Epidemiology and Consequences of Drinking and Driving" by Ralph Hingson and Michael Winter (December 2003), http://pubs.niaaa.nih.gov/publications/arh27-1/63-78.htm.
46. DrowsyDriving.org, "Facts and Stats," http://www.sleepfoundation.org/hottopics/index.php?secid=10&id=226.
47. Ibid.
48. Most of the recommendations in this paragraph are taken from the National Sleep Foundation, "Millions Drive Drowsy and Fall Asleep at the Wheel, Says New Poll," DrowsyDriving.org, November 20, 2002, http://www.drowsydriving.org/press_room/news_stories/millionsdrowsy.cfm.
49. The Gallup Organization, "National Survey of Distracted and Drowsy Driving Attitudes and Behaviors: 2002" (Volume 1 Findings Report submitted to the National Highway Traffic Safety Administration, March 2003).
50. D. A. Redelmeier and R. J. Tibshirani, "Association between Cellular-Telephone Calls and Motor Vehicle Collisions," *New England Journal of Medicine* 336, no. 7 (February 13, 1997): 453–458.
51. D. L. Strayer and W. A. Johnston, "Driven to Distraction: Dual-Task Studies of Simulated Driving and Conversing on a Cellular Telephone," *Psychological Science* 12, no. 6 (November 2001): 462–466.
52. This sidebar is adapted from *Focus on the Family Parents' Guide to Teen Health*, 248–251. A few minor updates were made with regard to endnoted data.
53. National Highway Traffic Safety Administration, "Motor Vehicle Traffic Crash Fatality Counts, 2004."
54. National Highway Traffic Safety Administration, *Saving Teenage Lives: A Case for Graduated Driver Licensing,* http://www.nhtsa.dot.gov/people/injury/newdriver/SaveTeens/.
55. National Highway Traffic Safety Administration, "Motor Vehicle Traffic Crash Fatality Counts, 2004."
56. National Highway Traffic Safety Administration, *Traffic Safety Facts 2002,* table 81, http://www-nrd.nhtsa.dot.gov/pdf/nrd-30/NCSA/TSFAnn/TSF2002Final.pdf.
57. Centers for Disease Control and Prevention, "Youth Risk Behavior Surveillance—United States, 2003," *Morbidity and Mortality Weekly Report* 53, no. SS-2.
58. Anita Smith, "Putting Science into Practice: Tips for Parents on Teen Driving," *The Youth Connection* (a bimonthly publication of the Institute for Youth Development) 3, no. 2 (March–April 2000), http://www.youthdevelopment.org/download/news0300.pdf.
59. Centers for Disease Control and Prevention, "Youth Risk Behavior Surveillance—2003."
60. Skateboardermag.com, "Fox Sports Net Launches 54321," *Skateboarder* magazine, February 1, 2003, http://skateboardermag.com/news/54321launch/index1.html
61. National Highway Traffic Safety Administration, Bureau of Transportation Statistics, *2002 National Survey of Pedestrian and Bicyclist Attitudes and Behaviors* (2003), http://www.bicyclinginfo.org/pdf/bikesurvey.pdf.
62. National Highway Traffic Safety Administration, "Motor Vehicle Traffic Crash Fatality Counts, 2004," 142.
63. Centers for Disease Control and Prevention, "National Hospital Ambulatory Medical Care Survey: 2003 Emergency Department Summary." See http://www.cdc.gov/nchs/data/ad/ad358.pdf.
64. Safe Kids Worldwide, "Injury Facts: Bike Injury," http://www.usa.safekids.org/tier3_cd.cfm?content_item_id=1010&folder_id=540.
65. Safe Kids Worldwide, "Facts about Childhood Recreational Injuries," http://www.usa.safekids.org/content_documents/Rec_facts.pdf.
66. Ibid.

67. American Academy of Pediatrics Committee on Injury and Poison Prevention, "Policy Statement: Skateboard and Scooter Injuries," *Pediatrics* 109, no. 3 (March 2002): 542–543.
68. Safe Kids Worldwide, "Childhood Recreational Injuries."
69. American Academy of Pediatrics, Committee on Injury and Poison Prevention, "All-Terrain Vehicle Injury Prevention: Two-, Three- and Four-Wheeled Unlicensed Motor Vehicles," *Pediatrics* 105, no. 6 (June 2000): 1352–1354, http://aappolicy.aappublications.org/cgi/content/full/pediatrics;105/6/1352.
70. National Children's Center for Rural and Agricultural Health and Safety, *Snowmobile Injury: Fact Sheet,* November 2000, http://research.marshfieldclinic.org/children/Resources/Snowmobile/FactSheet.html.
71. American Academy of Pediatrics, Committee on Injury and Poison Prevention, "Personal Watercraft Use by Children and Adolescents," *Pediatrics* 105, no. 2 (February 2000): 452–453, http://aappolicy.aappublications.org/cgi/content/full/pediatrics;105/2/452.
72. Centers for Disease Control and Prevention, *Water-Related Injuries: Fact Sheet,* http://www.cdc.gov/ncipc/factsheets/drown.htm.
73. Centers for Disease Control and Prevention, National Center for Injury Prevention and Control, *Injury Fact Book 2001–2002* (November 2001): 117, http://www.cdc.gov/ncipc/fact_book/ptp-z919.pdf.
74. Ibid.
75. National Center for Injury Prevention and Control, Centers for Disease Control and Prevention, *Boating Safety,* http://www.cdc.gov/ncipc/duip/safeboatingweek.htm.
76. U.S. Coast Guard, *Federal Requirements and Safety Tips for Recreational Boats,* http://www.uscgboating.org/safety/fedreqs/intro.htm.
77. National Safe Boating Council, *Four Principles of Boating Safety* and *Boating Fatality Facts,* http://www.safeboatingcouncil.org/principles.htm.
78. National Center for Injury Prevention and Control, *Boating Safety.*
79. Centers for Disease Control and Prevention, *Polio: The Disease*, http://www.cdc.gov/nip/publications/Parents-Guide/pg-polio.pdf.
80. Statistics on the incidence of common childhood diseases before the introduction of vaccines to prevent them are found at the Web site of the National Immunization Program of the Centers for Disease Control and Prevention, *What Would Happen If We Stopped Vaccinations?* http://www.cdc.gov/nip/publications/fs/gen/WhatIfStop.htm.
81. Centers for Disease Control and Prevention and National Center for Health Statistics, *Health, United States, 2004—With Chartbook on Trends in the Health of Americans,* table 51, http://www.cdc.gov/nchs/data/hus/hus04trend.pdf#051. See also World Health Organization, "Measles," *Initiative for Vaccine Research*, http://www.who.int/vaccine_research/diseases/measles/en/.
82. E. J. Gangarosa, A. M. Galazka, and C. R. Wolfe et al., "Impact of Anti-Vaccine Movements on Pertussis Control: The Untold Story," *Lancet* 351 (1998): 356–361.
83. National Immunization Program, Centers for Disease Control and Prevention, *What Would Happen If We Stopped Vaccinations?*
84. A. J. Wakefield et al., "Ileal-Lymphoid-Nodular Hyperplasia, Non-Specific Colitis, and Pervasive Developmental Disorder in Children," *Lancet* 351 (1998): 637–641.
85. Paul A. Offit et al., "Addressing Parents' Concerns: Do Multiple Vaccines Overwhelm or Weaken the Infant's Immune System?" *Pediatrics* 109, no. 1 (January 2002): 124–129.
86. National Immunization Program, Centers for Disease Control and Prevention, *The Safety of Multiple Vaccines: Multiple Vaccines and the Immune System*, http://www.cdc.gov/nip/vacsafe/concerns/gen/multiplevac.htm.

Chapter 12: Healthy Sexuality

1. For statistics on teenage pregnancy, see the Alan Guttmacher Institute, "U.S. Teenage Pregnancy Statistics with Comparative Statistics for Women Aged 20–24" (February 19, 2004), http://www.agi-usa.org/pubs/teen_stats.html. See also Joyce Martin et al., "Births: Final Data for 2002," *National Vital Statistics Report* 52, no. 10 (Hyattsville, Md.: National Center for Health Statistics, 2003) and the National Campaign to Prevent Teen Pregnancy, "Fact Sheet: How Is the 34% Statistic Calculated?" (February 2004), http://www.teenpregnancy.org/resources/reading/pdf/35percent.pdf. The last two resources are cited in Patricia Sulak and Sarah Herbelin, "Teenagers and Sex: Delaying Sexual Debut," *The Female Patient* 30, no. 4: (April 2005) 29–35.
2. Rebecca Maynard ed., *Kids Having Kids: A Robin Hood Foundation Special Report on the Costs of Adolescent Childbearing* (New York: Robin Hood Foundation, 1996): 1, 12, http://www.robinhood.org/approach/KHK.pdf.
3. National Institute of Child Health and Human Development, "Sexually Transmitted Diseases and Infections (STDs and STIs) and HIV/AIDS Research," http://www.nichd.nih.gov/womenshealth/STDHIV.cfm#stdsgen.

4. Centers for Disease Control and Prevention, "Summary of Notifiable Diseases—United States 2003," *Morbidity and Mortality Weekly Report* 52, no. 54 (April 22, 2005): 16–17, http://www.cdc.gov/mmwr/PDF/wk/mm5254.pdf. See also Hillard Weinstock, Start Berman, and Willard Cates, "Sexually Transmitted Diseases among American Youth: Incidence and Prevalence Estimates, 2000," *Perspectives on Sexual and Reproductive Health* 36, no. 1 (January/February 2001): 6–10. See also Centers for Disease Control and Prevention, "U.S. Disease Burden Data, 1980–2003 (2002), http://www.cdc.gov/ncidod/diseases/hepatitis/resource/dz_burden02.htm. See also Centers for Disease Control and Prevention, "Genital HPV Infection—CDC Fact Sheet," see http://www.cdc.gov/std/HPV/STDFact-HPV.htm.
5. Centers for Disease Control and Prevention, "Genital Herpes—CDC Fact Sheet," http://www.cdc.gov/std/Herpes/STDFact-Herpes.htm.
6. Philip Disaia and William Creasman, *Clinical Gynecologic Oncology*, 5th ed. (St. Louis: Mosby, 1997); cited in Patricia Sulak and Sarah Herbelin, "Teenagers and Sex: Delaying Sexual Debut," *The Female Patient* 30, no. 4 (April 2005): 29–35.
7. Centers for Disease Control and Prevention, *HIV/AIDS Surveillance Report* 15, http://www.cdc.gov/hiv/stats/2003surveillancereport.pdf.
8. Weinstock, Berman, and Cates, "Sexually Transmitted Diseases among American Youth."
9. Denise L. Jacobson, "Concordance of Human Papillomavirus in the Cervix and Urine among Inner City Adolescents," *Pediatric Infectious Disease Journal* 19, no. 8 (August 2000): 722–728.
10. Gloria Y. Ho et al., "Natural History of Cervicovaginal Papillomavirus Infection in Young Women," *New England Journal of Medicine* 338, no. 7 (February 12, 1998): 423–428.
11. Sulak and Herbelin, "Teenagers and Sex: Delaying Sexual Debut."
12. Bradley Boekeloo and D. E. Howard, "Oral Sexual Experience among Young Adolescents Receiving General Health Examinations," *American Journal of Health Behavior* 26, no. 4 (July/August 2002): 306–314.
13. M. A. Schuster, R. M. Bell, and D. E. Kanouse, "The Sexual Practices of Adolescent Virgins: Genital Sexual Activities of High School Students Who Have Never Had Vaginal Intercourse," *American Journal of Public Health* 86, no. 11 (November 1, 1996): 1570–1576.
14. P. F. Horan, J. Phillips, and N. E. Hagen, "The Meaning of Abstinence for College Students," *Journal of HIV/Aids Prevention & Education for Adolescents and Children* 2, no. 2 (1998): 51–66.
15. Medical Institute for Sexual Health, "The Facts about Oral Sex & STDs," http://www.medicalinstitute/includes/downloads/2_oralsexstd.pdf.
16. Lee Warner, Robert A. Hatcher, and Markus J. Steiner, "Male Condoms," in *Contraceptive Technology*, 18th edition, ed. Robert A. Hatcher et al. (New York: Ardent Media, 2004), see table 9–2.
17. M. J. Steiner et al., "Contraceptive Effectiveness of a Polyurethane Condom and a Latex Condom: A Randomized Controlled Trial," *Obstetrics and Gynecology* 101, no. 3 (March 2003): 539–547. See also "Workshop Summary: Scientific Evidence on Condom Effectiveness for Sexually Transmitted Disease (STD) Prevention," National Institute of Allergy and Infectious Diseases, National Institute of Health, Department of Health and Human Services, http://www.niaid.nih.gov/dmid/stds/condomreport.pdf. See also Ron G. Frezieres et al., "Evaluation of the Efficacy of a Polyurethane Condom: Results from a Randomized, Controlled, Clinical Trial," *Family Planning Perspectives* 31, no. 2 (March/April 1999): 81–87. See also M. Macaluso et al., "Mechanical Failure of the Latex Condom in a Cohort of Women at High STD Risk," *Sexually Transmitted Diseases* 26, no. 8 (September 1999): 450–458. See also J. Thomas Fitch et al., "Condom Effectiveness: Factors That Influence Risk Reduction," *Sexually Transmitted Diseases* 29, no. 12 (December 2002): 811–817.
18. Karen R. Davis and Susan C. Weller, "The Effectiveness of Condoms in Reducing Heterosexual Transmission of HIV," *Family Planning Perspectives* 31, no. 6 (November/December 1999): 272–279.
19. Saifuddin Ahmed et al., "HIV Incidence and Sexually Transmitted Disease Prevalence Associated with Condom Use: A Population Study in Rakai, Uganda," *AIDS* 15, no. 16 (November 9, 2001): 2171–2179. See also Jared M. Baeten et al., "Hormonal Contraception and Risk of Sexually Transmitted Acquisition: Results from a Prospective Study," *American Journal of Obsetrics and Gynecology* 183 (August 2001): 380–385. See also Lee Warner et al., "Condom Effectiveness for Reducing Transmission of Gonorrhea and Chlamydia: The Importance of Assessing Partner Infection Status," *American Journal of Epidemiology* 159 no. 3 (February 1, 2004): 242–251. See also Judith Shlay et al., "Comparison of Sexually Transmitted Disease Prevalence by Reported Level of Condom Use among Patients Attending an Urban Sexually Transmitted Disease Clinic," *Sexually Transmitted Diseases* 31, no. 3 (March 2004): 154–160. See also King K. Holmes, Ruth Levine, and Marcia Weaver, "Effectiveness of Condoms in Preventing Sexually Transmitted Infections," *Bulletin of the World Health Organization* 82, no. 6 (June 2004): 454–461.
20. Julie Gerberding, *Report to Congress: Prevention of Genital Human Papillomavirus Infection* (Atlanta: Centers for Disease Control and Prevention, January 2004). On pages 15–16 of this report, Dr. Gerberding says, "The cumulative body of available scientific evidence suggests that condoms may

provide some protection in preventing transmission of HPV infection but that protection is partial at best. The available scientific evidence is not sufficient to recommend condoms as a primary prevention strategy for the prevention of genital HPV infection." See also Lisa Manhart and Laura Koutsky, "Do Condoms Prevent Genital HPV Infection, or Cervical Neoplasia? A Meta-Analysis," *Sexually Transmitted Diseases* 29, no. 11 (November 2002): 725–735.

21. Robert T. Michael et al., *Sex in America: A Definitive Survey* (Boston: Little, Brown and Company, 1994), 124.
22. Richard Foster, *The Challenge of the Disciplined Life: Christian Reflections on Money, Sex and Power* (San Francisco: HarperSanFrancisco, 1985), 92.
23. Ibid., 117–118.
24. Pornography statistics come from TopTenREVIEWS, "Internet Pornography Statistics," http://internet-filter-review.toptenreviews.com/internet-pornography-statistics.html; Mike Genung, "Statistics and Information on Pornography in the USA" (Colorado Springs: Blazing Grace Ministries, 2005), http://www.blazinggrace.org/pornstatistics.htm; and Donna Rice Hughes, "Recent Statistics on Internet Dangers," http://www.protectkids.com/dangers/stats.htm.
25. Senate Committee on Commerce, Science and Transportation, "Hearing on the Science behind Pornography Addiction and the Effects of Addiction on Families and Communities" (testimony of Dr. James Weaver given on November 18, 2004), http://commerce.senate.gov/hearings/testimony.cfm?id=1343&wit_id=3911.
26. Senate Committee on Commerce, Science and Transportation, "Hearing on the Science behind Pornography Addiction and the Effects of Addiction on Families and Communities" (testimony of Dr. Mary Anne Layden given on November 18, 2004), http://commerce.senate.gov/hearings/testimony.cfm?id=1343&wit_id=3912.
27. Adapted from Paul C. Reisser, *Focus on the Family Parents' Guide to Teen Health* (Colorado Springs, Colo.: 1997), 164–165.
28. Rape, Abuse & Incest National Network, "The Facts about Rape," http://www.rainn.org/statistics.html.
29. Burt Bacharach and Hal David, "Wives and Lovers," copyright © 1963.
30. Bacharach and David, "Wives and Lovers."
31. Michael et al., *Sex in America*, 116.

Chapter 13: Selected Topics in Women's Health

1. Material in this section has been adapted from *Focus on the Family Parents' Guide to Teen Health* (Colorado Springs, Colo.: 1997), 29–54.
2. Material in this section has been adapted from *Focus on the Family Complete Book of Baby and Child Care* (Colorado Springs, Colo.: 1997), 4–24.
3. H. S. Klonoff-Cohen et al., "The Effect of Passive Smoking and Tobacco Exposure through Breast Milk on Sudden Infant Death Syndrome," *Journal of the American Medical Association* 273, no. 10 (March 8, 1995): 795–798.
4. J. Trussell and L. Grummer-Strawn, "Contraceptive Failure of the Ovulation Method of Periodic Abstinence," *Family Planning Perspectives* 22, no. 2 (March–April 1990): 65–75.
5. U.S. Public Health Service, *Bone Health and Osteoporosis: A Report of the Surgeon General* (2004), http://www.hhs.gov/news/press/2004pres/20041014.html.

Chapter 14: Senior Maintenance

1. Centers for Disease Control and Prevention, *The State of Aging and Health in America 2004,* http://www.cdc.gov/aging/pdf/State_of_Aging_and_Health_in_America_2004.pdf.
2. K. Tomaselli, "Senior Moments: A Simple Change Could Have a Big Impact on Your Patient's Health," *American Medical News* 38, no. 1 (January 3–10, 2005).
3. Laurie A. Kamimoto, Alyssa N. Easton, Emmanuel Maurice, Corinne G. Husten, and Carol A. Macera, "Surveillance for Five Health Risks among Older Adults—United States, 1993–1997, *MMWR* 48, no. SS08 (December 17, 1999): 89–130. See http://www.cdc.gov/mmwr/preview/mmwrhtml/ss4808a5.htm.
4. See E. W. Gregg, J. A. Cauley, K. Stone et al., "Relationship of Changes in Physical Activity and Mortality among Older Women," *Journal of the American Medical Association* 289, no. 18 (May 14, 2003): 2379–2386; and A. A. Hakim, J. D. Curb, H. Petrovich et al., "Effects of Walking on Coronary Heart Disease in Elderly Men," *Circulation* 100, no. 1 (July 6, 1999): 9–13.
5. Monika Guttman, "The Aging Brain," *USC Health* (Spring 2001), http://www.usc.edu/hsc/info/pr/hmm/01spring/brain.html.
6. National Institute on Aging, Alzheimer's Disease Education and Referral Center, *2003 Progress Report on Alzheimer's Disease: Research Advances at NIH,* October 2004, http://www.alzheimers.org/pr03/2003_Progress_Report_on_AD.pdf.
7. R. Brookmeyer, S. Gray, and C. Kawas, "Projections of Alzheimer's Disease in the United States and

the Public Health Impact of Delaying Disease Onset," *American Journal of Public Health* 88, no. 9 (1998): 1337–1342, quoted in F. Pilot, "Caring for the Elderly: A Case-Based Approach," *American Family Physician* monograph, August 2004.

8. National Institute on Aging, *2003 Progress Report on Alzheimer's Disease.*
9. Richard Goldberg, "Alzheimer's Disease: Your Role in Identifying and Managing It," *Patient Care* (December 2004): 34, http://www.patientcareonline.com/patcare/article/articleDetail.jsp?id=138156.
10. Peter P. Zandi et al., "Reduced Risk of Alzheimer Disease in Users of Antioxidant Vitamin Supplements," *Archives of Neurology* 61, no. 1 (January 2004): 82–88, http://archneur.ama-assn.org/cgi/content/abstract/61/1/82.
11. National Institute on Aging, *2003 Progress Report on Alzheimer's Disease.*
12. Federal Interagency Forum on Aging-Related Statistics, *Older Americans 2004: Key Indicators of Well-Being,* November 2004, http://www.agingstats.gov/chartbook2004/default.htm.
13. Ibid.
14. Ibid., table 25.
15. American Geriatrics Society, AGS Ethics Committee, *Health Screening Decisions for Older Adults,* AGS Position Paper, 2002, http://www.americangeriatrics.org/staging/products/positionpapers/stopscreeningPF.shtml.
16. Centers for Disease Control and Prevention, *The State of Aging and Health in America 2004.*
17. Ibid.
18. American Dental Association, *Oral Health Topics A–Z,* "Oral Changes with Age: Frequently Asked Questions," http://www.ada.org/public/topics/oral_changes_faq.asp#6.
19. Centers for Disease Control and Prevention, *The State of Aging and Health in America 2004.*
20. Melanie Johns Cupp, "Herbal Remedies: Adverse Effects and Drug Interactions," *American Family Physician* 59, no. 5 (March 1, 1999): 1239–1245, http://www.aafp.org/afp/990301ap/1239.html.
21. National Institutes of Health, "Underusing Medications Because of Cost May Lead to Adverse Health Outcomes," news release, June 25, 2004, http://www.nih.gov/news/pr/jun2004/nia-25.htm.
22. Centers for Disease Control and Prevention, National Center for Injury Prevention and Control, *Older Adult Drivers: Fact Sheet,* http://www.cdc.gov/ncipc/factsheets/older.htm.
23. National Institute for Highway Safety, *Fatality Facts: Older People 2003,* http://www.highwaysafety.org/safety_facts/fatality_facts/olderpeople.htm.
24. Centers for Disease Control and Prevention, *Older Adult Drivers.* See also National Institute for Highway Safety, *Fatality Facts.*
25. Linda F. McCaig and Catharine W. Burt, "National Hospital Ambulatory Medical Care Survey: 2003 Emergency Department Summary," *Advance Data from Vital and Health Statistics* no. 358 (May 26, 2005), http://www.cdc.gov/nchs/data/ad/ad358.pdf. See also Centers for Disease Control and Prevention Injury Center, "The Effects of Unintentional Injury," http://www.cdc.gov/ncipc/pub-res/unintentional_activity/02_effects.htm.
26. Centers for Disease Control and Prevention, National Center for Injury Prevention and Control, "Falls and Hip Fractures among Older Adults," http://www.cdc.gov/ncipc/factsheets/falls.htm.
27. National Osteoporosis Foundation, "Osteoporosis and Its Most Serious Consequence," news release, January 17, 2001, http://www.nof.org/news/pressreleases/background_hipfracture.html. See also National Osteoporosis Foundation, *Putting Osteoporosis on the Map: Annual Report 2002,* http://www.nof.org/aboutnof/2002_nof_annual_report.pdf.
28. This list is adapted from the Center of Disease Control and Prevention's "What *You* Can Do to Prevent Falls"; see http://www.cdc.gov/ncipc/pub-res/toolkit/Falls%20BrochB_W%20panels.pdf.
29. American Geriatrics Society, *Prevention and Treatment of Influenza in the Elderly*, AGS Position Statement, February 2003, http://www.americangeriatrics.org/products/positionpapers/influe96.shtml.
30. Federal Interagency Forum on Aging-Related Statistics, *Older Americans 2004: Key Indicators of Well-Being.*
31. Ibid.
32. American Geriatrics Society, *Clinical Guidelines for Alcohol Use Disorders in Older Adults,* November 2003, http://www.americangeriatrics.org/products/positionpapers/alcohol.shtml.
33. "Substance Abuse among Older Adults," *The NHSDA (National Household Survey on Drug Abuse) Report*, November 23, 2001, figure 1, http://www.oas.samhsa.gov/2k1/olderadults/olderadults.htm.
34. P. Ciechanowski, E. Wagner, K. Schmaling et al., "Community-Integrated Home-Based Depression Treatment in Older Adults," *Journal of the American Medical Association* 291, no. 13 (April 7, 2004): 1569–1577.
35. See N. Frasure-Smith, F. Lesperance, and M. Talajic, "Depression Following Myocardial Infarction: Impact on 6-Month Survival," *Journal of the American Medical Association* 270, no. 15 (October 20, 1993): 1819–1825. See also B. W. Rovner, P. S. German, and L. J. Brant et al., "Depression and

Mortality in Nursing Homes," *Journal of the American Medical Association* 265, no. 8 (February 27, 1991): 993–996.
36. National Institute of Mental Health, *Older Adults: Depression and Suicide Facts*, 2003, http://www.nimh.nih.gov/publicat/elderlydepsuicide.cfm#1.
37. Anxiety Disorders Association of America, "Anxiety in the Elderly," *Anxiety Disorders Information,* http://www.adaa.org/AnxietyDisorderInfor/AnxietyElderly.cfm.
38. P. B. Thapa, P. Gideon, and T. W. Cost et al., "Antidepressants and the Risk of Falls among Nursing Home Residents," *New England Journal of Medicine* 339, no. 13 (September 24, 1998): 875–882.

Chapter 15: To Sleep . . .

1. National Sleep Foundation, "Let Sleep Work for You" and "ABCs of ZZZs." See http://www.sleepfoundation.org/sleeplibrary.
2. National Sleep Foundation, "Summary of Findings: 2005 Sleep in America Poll," http://www.sleepfoundation.org/_content/hottopics/2005_summary_of_findings.pdf
3. William Shakespeare, *Henry IV*, part 2, act 3, scene 1.
4. A complete summary of "Sleep in America: 1995 Gallup Poll" can be found at http://www.stanford.edu/~dement/95poll.html.
5. National Institute of Child Health and Human Development, "A Frequently Asked Question about Bed Sharing," May 2003, http://www.nichd.nih.gov/sids/FQ_bed_sharing.htm#aap.
6. Consumer Product Safety Commission, "CPSC Cautions Caregivers about Hidden Hazards for Babies on Adult Beds," CPSC Document #5091, http://cpsc.gov/CPSCPUB/PUBS/5091.html.
7. National Sleep Foundation, "Dozing Off in Class?" http://www.sleepfoundation.org/hottopics/index.php?secid=18&id=202.
8. A. R. Wolfson and M. A. Carskadon, "Sleep Schedules and Daytime Functioning in Adolescents," *Child Development* 69, no. 4 (August 1998): 875–887; cited in National Sleep Foundation, *Adolescent Sleep Needs and Patterns,* http://www.sleepfoundation.org/_content/hottopics/sleep_and_teens_report1.pdf.
9. National Highway Traffic Safety Administration, "Crashes and Fatalities Related to Driver Drowsiness/Fatigue," *Research Notes* 1994; cited in National Sleep Foundation, *Adolescent Sleep Needs and Patterns.*
10. M. A. Carskadon et al., "Pubertal Changes in Daytime Sleepiness," *Sleep* 2 (1980): 453–460; cited in National Sleep Foundation, *Adolescent Sleep Needs and Patterns.*
11. Wolfson and Carskadon, "Sleep Schedules"; cited in National Sleep Foundation, *Adolescent Sleep Needs and Patterns.*
12. Franklin Brown, Barlow Soper, and Walter C. Buboltz Jr., "Prevalence of Delayed Sleep Phase Syndrome in University Students," *College Student Journal* (September 2001), http://www.findarticles.com/p/articles/mi_m0FCR/is_3_35/ai_80744660.

Chapter 16: "Why Am I So Tired All the Time?" The Problem of Fatigue

1. K. Kroenke et al., "Chronic Fatigue in Primary Care: Prevalence, Patient Characteristics, and Outcome," *Journal of the American Medical Association* 260, no. 7 (August 19, 1988): 929–934. Abstract available at http://jama.ama-assn.org/cgi/content/abstract/260/7/929.
2. William G. Crook, *The Yeast Connection: A Medical Breakthrough* (Jackson, Tenn.: Professional Books, 1983).
3. The following suggestions have been adapted from the *Focus on the Family Complete Book of Baby and Child Care* (Colorado Springs, Colo.: Focus on the Family, 1997), 461–463.

Chapter 17: Health-Care Discernment: How to Be a Wise Consumer

1. David L. Sackett et al., "Evidence Based Medicine: What It Is and What It Isn't," *British Medical Journal,* 312 (January 13, 1996): 71–72.
2. These categories are more extensively explained in Paul C. Reisser, Dale Mabe, and Robert Velarde, *Examining Alternative Medicine: An Inside Look at the Benefits and Risks* (Downers Grove, Ill.: InterVarsity Press, 2001).
3. U.S. Department of Health and Human Services, Health Resource and Services Administration, *U.S. Health Workforce Personnel Factbook 2002*, table 507. See also Eisenberg et al., "Trends in Alternative Medicine Use in the United States, 1990–1997: Results of a Follow-up National Survey," *Journal of the American Medical Association* 280 (1998): 1569–1575. See also T. J. Kaptchuk and D. Eisenberg, "Chiropractic: Origins, Controversies and Contributions," *Archives of Internal Medicine* 158 (1998): 2215–2224.
4. See, for example, "What Is Causing the Asthma Epidemic?" at the American Chiropractic Association Web site, http://www.amerchiro.org/media/tips/asthma.shtml.
5. See Gary D. Foster et al., "A Randomized Trial of a Low-Carbohydrate Diet for Obesity," *New England*

Journal of Medicine 348, no. 21 (May 22, 2003): 2082–2090; see also Michael L. Dansinger et al., "Comparison of the Atkins, Ornish, Weight Watchers, and Zone Diets for Weight Loss and Heart Disease Risk Reduction," *Journal of the American Medical Association* 293, no. 1 (January 5, 2005): 43–53.

6. Linda Rosa et al., "A Close Look at Therapeutic Touch," *Journal of the American Medical Association* 279, no. 13 (April 1, 1998): 1005–1010. This experiment, which was actually designed and carried out by a nine-year-old as a fourth-grade science project, is a model for the basic type of reality check to which many alternative therapies should be subjected.
7. See *ACNielsen Consumer Trends and Market Report, 2004,* http://us.acnielsen.com/pubs/documents/2004_q3_ci.pdf. See also "Cholesterol Agents Lead All Therapeutic Classes in Prescription Drug Sales," *Drug Benefit Trends* 16, no. 5 (June 17, 2004): 232–233, http://www.medscape.com/viewarticle/479951.
8. Consumer Healthcare Products Association, "OTC Facts and Figures," http://www.chpa-info.org/web/press_room/statistics/otc_facts_figures.aspx.
9. Consumer Healthcare Products Association, "Dietary Supplement Facts and Figures," http://www.chpa-info.org/web/press_room/statistics/supplement_facts_figures.aspx.
10. "More Americans Take Prescription Medication," *Drug Benefit Trends* 7, no. 2 (February 2005): 55, http://www.medscape.com/viewarticle/500164.
11. Consumer Healthcare Products Association, "OTC Facts and Figures."
12. J. Lazarou, B. H. Pomeranz, and P. N. Corey, "Incidence of Adverse Drug Reactions in Hospitalized Patients: A Meta-Analysis of Prospective Studies," *Journal of the American Medical Association* 279, no. 15 (April 15, 1998): 1200–1205.
13. U.S. Food and Drug Administration, Center for Food Safety and Applied Nutrition, "Dietary Supplement Health and Education Act of 1994," http://www.cfsan.fda.gov/~dms/dietsupp.html.
14. Shari Roan, "Alternative Medicine: The 18 Billion Dollar Experiment," *Los Angeles Times*, September 1, 1998; cited in Paul Reisser, D. Mabe, and R. Velarde, *Examining Alternative Medicine: An Inside Look at the Benefits and Risks* (Downers Grove, Ill.: InterVarsity Press, 2001).
15. R. J. Ko, "Adulterants in Asian Patent Medicine," *New England Journal of Medicine* 339, no. 12 (September 17, 1998): 847. See also R. B. Saper et al., "Heavy Metal Content of Ayurvedic Herbal Medicine Products," *Journal of the American Medical Association* 292, no. 23 (December 15, 2004): 2868–2873.
16. See Varro Tyler, *Tyler's Honest Herbal* (Birmingham, N.Y.: Haworth Press/Pharmaceutical Products Press, 1993) and *Tyler's Herbs of Choice: The Therapeutic Use of Phytomedicinals* (Birmingham, N.Y.: Haworth Press/Pharmaceutical Products Press, 1994).
17. See, for example, the June 16, 2004, release from the Federal Trade Commission: "FTC Testifies on the Marketing of Dietary Supplements to Children," http://www.ftc.gov/opa/2004/06/kidsupp.htm.
18. Melissa Thomasson, "Health Insurance in the United States," *EH.Net Encyclopedia,* edited by Robert Whaples, April 18, 2003, http://www.eh.net/encyclopedia/article/thomasson.insurance.health.us.
19. National Health Care Anti-Fraud Association, "Health Care Fraud: A Serious and Costly Reality for All Americans," April 2005.
20. Mark Jewell, "Harvard Study: Illness, Medical Bills Account for Half of All Bankruptcies," Associated Press (February 1, 2005).

Appendix A: Abortion: A Risk Factor for Breast Cancer?

1. M. Segi, I. Fukushima et al., "An Epidemiological Study on Cancer in Japan," *GANN* 48 (1957): 1–63.
2. American Cancer Society, "Overview: Breast Cancer," http://www.cancer.org/docroot/CRI/content/CRI_2_2_2X_What_causes_breast_cancer_5.asp?sitearea=.
3. J. Brind et al., "Induced Abortion as an Independent Risk Factor for Breast Cancer: A Comprehensive Review and Meta-Analysis," *Journal of Epidemiology and Community Health* 50 (1996): 441–496.
4. National Cancer Institute, "Summary Report: Early Reproductive Events and Breast Cancer Workshop" (meetings held February 24–26, 2003), http://www.cancer.gov/cancerinfo/ere-workshop-report.
5. Angela Lanfranchi, "The Abortion–Breast Cancer Link Revisited," *Ethics and Medics* 29, no. 11 (November 2004).
6. Collaborative Group on Hormonal Factors in Breast Cancer, "Breast Cancer and Abortion: Collaborative Reanalysis of Data from 53 Epidemiological Studies, Including 83,000 Women with Breast Cancer from 16 Countries," *Lancet* 363 (March 27, 2004): 1007–1016.
7. NCI, "Early Reproductive Events."

Appendix B: Vitamins and Minerals: What Each One Does and How Much We Need

1. Janet Hunt and Johanna Dwyer, "Position of the American Dietetic Association: Food Fortification and

Dietary Supplements," *Journal of the American Dietetic Association* 101, no. 1 (January 2001), 115–125. See also "Panel Urges U.S. Standards for Dietary Supplements," *USA Today*, January 12, 2005.
2. Lina Balluz et al., "Vitamin and Mineral Supplement Use in the United States: Results from the Third National Health and Nutrition Examination Survey," *Archives of Family Medicine* 9 no. 3 (March 2000): 258–262.
3. Peter R. Martin, Charles K. Singleton, and Susanne Hiller-Sturmhöfel, "The Role of Thiamine Deficiency in Alcoholic Brain Disease," prepared July 2004 for the National Institute on Alcohol Abuse and Alcoholism, http://pubs.niaaa.nih.gov/publications/arh27-2/134-142.htm.
4. Walter C. Willett, *Eat, Drink, and Be Healthy* (New York, Fireside Books: 2001), 155.
5. Roy Porter, *The Greatest Benefit to Mankind: A Medical History of Humanity* (New York: W. W. Norton and Company, 1997), 295.
6. Willett, *Eat, Drink, and Be Healthy,* 160.
7. Emma Hitt, "Vitamin C May Fight Colds After All," *WebMDHealth* (March 12, 2003), http://my.webmd.com/content/article/62/71548.htm?z=1728_00000_1000_ln_01.
8. Porter, *The Greatest Benefit to Mankind*, 296.
9. World Health Organization, "Combating Vitamin A Deficiency," http://www.who.int/nut/vad.htm.
10. World Health Organization, "Measles," http://www.who.int/vaccine_research/diseases/measles/en/.
11. Edgar Miller et al., "Meta-Analysis: High Dosage Vitamin E Supplementation May Increase All-Cause Mortality," *Annals of Internal Medicine* 142, no. 1 (January 4, 2005), http://www.annals.org/cgi/content/full/0000605-200501040-00110v1.
12. World Health Organization, "Battling Iron-Deficiency Anemia," http://www.who.int/nut/ida.htm.
13. World Health Organization, "Micronutrient Deficiencies: Eliminating Iodine Deficiency Disorders," http://www.who.int/nut/idd.htm.
14. Peter P. Zandi et al., "Reduced Risk of Alzheimer Disease in Users of Antioxidant Vitamin Supplements: The Cache County Study," *Archives of Neurology* 61, no. 1 (January 2004): 82–88, http://archneur.ama-assn.org/cgi/content/abstract/61/1/82.

Appendix E: Common Sexual Dysfunctions

1. Edward O. Laumann, Anthony Paik, and Raymond C. Rosen, "Sexual Dysfunction in the United States: Prevalence and Predictors," *Journal of the American Medical Association* 281 (February 10, 1999): 537–544.
2. Ibid.
3. Ibid.
4. H. A. Feldman et al., "Impotence and Its Medical and Psychosocial Correlates: Results of the Massachusetts Male Aging Study," *Journal of Urology* 151, no. 1 (1994): 54–61.
5. Laumann, "Sexual Dysfunction in the United States."
6. S. Read, M. King, and J. Watson, "Sexual Dysfunction in Primary Medical Care: Prevalence, Characteristics and Detection by the General Practitioner," *Journal of Public Health Medicine* 19 (1997): 387–391.

Appendix F: Hormone Therapy Controversies: A Closer Look at the HERS and WHI Studies

1. American College of Obstetricians and Gynecologists, "Statement on the Estrogen Plus Progestin Trial of the Women's Health Initiative by the American College of Obstetricians and Gynecologists," news release, July 9, 2002, http://www.acog.org/from_home/publications/press_releases/nr07-09-02.cfm.

Appendix G: Chronic Fatigue Syndrome

1. W. C. Hellinger et al., "Chronic Fatigue Syndrome and the Diagnostic Utility of Antibody to Epstein-Barr Virus Early Antigen," *Journal of the American Medical Association* 260, no. 7 (August 19, 1988): 971–973, http://jama.ama-assn.org/cgi/content/abstract/260/7/971.
2. Centers for Disease Control and Prevention, "Chronic Fatigue Syndrome: What Is CFS?" http://www.cdc.gov/ncidod/diseases/cfs/about/what.htm.
3. Centers for Disease Control and Prevention, "Chronic Fatigue Syndrome: The Revised Case Definition" (abridged version), http://www.cdc.gov/ncidod/diseases/cfs/about/definition/case_def_abridged.htm.
4. Timothy Craig and Sujani Kakumanu, "Chronic Fatigue Syndrome: Evaluation and Treatment," *American Family Physician* 65, no. 6 (March 15, 2002): 1083–1090.
5. Penny Whiting et al., "Interventions for the Treatment and Management of Chronic Fatigue Syndrome," *Journal of the American Medical Association* 286, no. 11 (September 19, 2001): 1360–1368, http://jama.ama-assn.org/cgi/content/abstract/286/11/1360.

6. Alfred M. Pheley et al., "Can We Predict Recovery in Chronic Fatigue Syndrome?" *Minnesota Medicine* 82 (November 1999): 62–66, http://www.mmaonline.net/publications/MnMed1999/November/Pheley.cfm.
7. A. Wilson et al., "Longitudinal Study of Outcome of Chronic Fatigue Syndrome," *British Medical Journal* 308 (March 19, 1994): 756–759.

Index

Note: Page numbers in italics refer to charts and tables.

G

H

I

J

K

L

M

N

O

P

T

U

V

W

X

Y

Z

FOCUS ON THE FAMILY®

Welcome to the Family!

Whether you received this book as a gift, borrowed it from a friend, or purchased it yourself, we're glad you read it! It's just one of the many helpful, insightful, and encouraging resources produced by Focus on the Family.

In fact, that's what Focus on the Family is all about—providing inspiration, information, and biblically based advice to people in all stages of life.

It began in 1977 with the vision of one man, Dr. James Dobson, a licensed psychologist and author of 18 best-selling books on marriage, parenting, and family. Alarmed by the societal, political, and economic pressures that were threatening the existence of the American family, Dr. Dobson founded Focus on the Family with one employee—an assistant—and a once-a-week radio broadcast, aired on only 36 stations.

Now an international organization, Focus on the Family is dedicated to preserving Judeo-Christian values and strengthening the family through more than 70 different ministries, including eight separate daily radio broadcasts; television public-service announcements; 10 publications; and a steady series of books and award-winning films and videos for people of all ages and interests.

Recognizing the needs of, as well as the sacrifices and important contributions made by, such diverse groups as educators, physicians, attorneys, crisis pregnancy center staff members, and single parents, Focus on the Family offers specific outreaches to uphold and minister to these individuals too. And it's all done for one purpose, and one purpose only: to encourage and strengthen individuals and families through the life-changing message of Jesus Christ.

For more information about the ministry, or if we can be of help to your family, simply write to Focus on the Family, Colorado Springs, CO 80995 or call 1-800-A-FAMILY (1-800-232-6459). Friends in Canada may write to Focus on the Family, P.O. Box 9800 Stn. Terminal, Vancouver, BC V6B 4G3 or call 1-800-661-9800. Visit our Web site at www.family.org to learn more about Focus on the Family or to find out if there is an associate office in your country.

We'd love to hear from you!

Other Faith and Family Strengtheners from Focus on the Family®

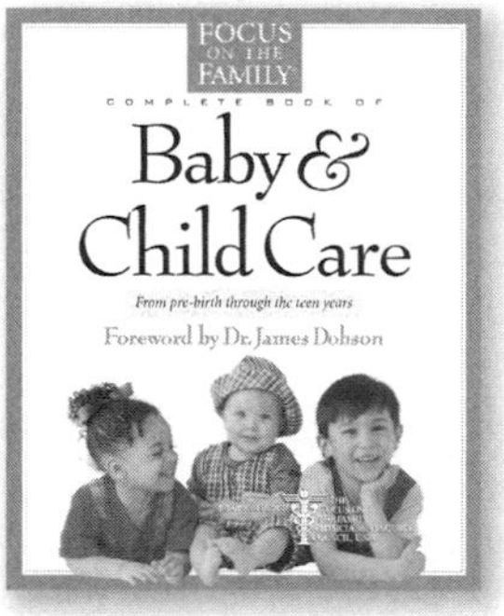

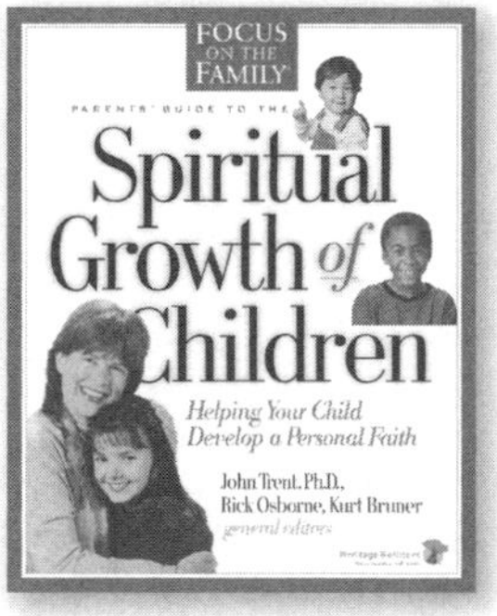

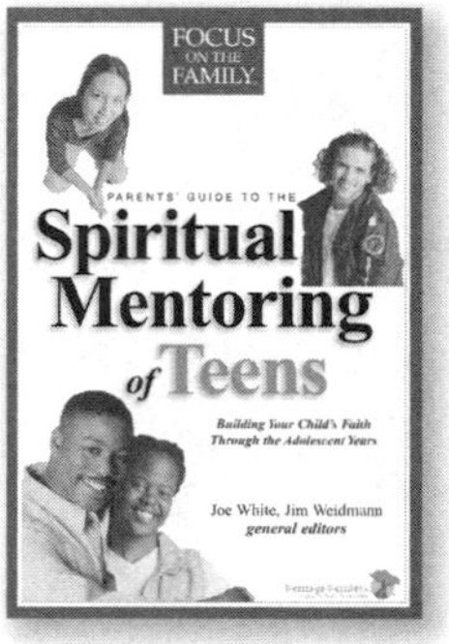

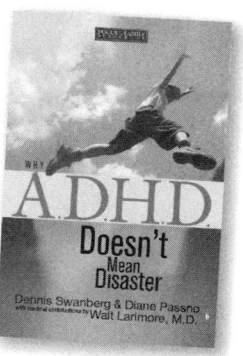

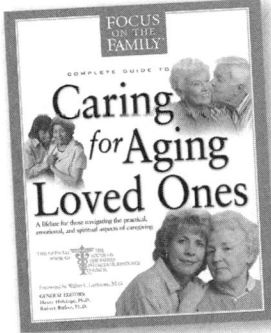

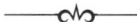

Complete Guide to Caring for Aging Loved Ones

Whether you're preparing for the responsibility or are in the midst of caring for an elderly loved one, this complete guide from Focus on the Family provides the practical information you need—and a spiritual and emotional lifeline. Topics covered include: burnout; physical, emotional, and mental changes in aging; medical, financial, and legal help; elder abuse; choosing a care facility; and end-of-life decisions. True stories throughout the guide illustrate common concerns and offer a sense of support from "those who have been there."

Why ADHD Doesn't Mean Disaster

Discovering your child has attention deficit hyperactivity disorder (ADHD) can be a traumatic moment. Until recently, little was known beyond the label. Along with the latest information about the disorder and expert medical advice, *Why ADHD Doesn't Mean Disaster* offers a biblical perspective, devotional thoughts, reflective questions, and encouraging insights from those who have lived with the disorder.

Look for these special books in your Christian bookstore or request a copy by calling 1-800-A-FAMILY (1-800-232-6459) or writing to Focus on the Family, Colorado Springs, CO 80995. Friends in Canada may write Focus on the Family, P.O. Box 9800 Stn. Terminal, Vancouver, BC V6B 4G3 or call 1-800-661-9800. Visit our Web site at www.family.org to learn more about Focus on the Family or to find out if there is an associate office in your country.